618 GOO

Management of Common Problems in Obstetrics and Gynecology

EDITED BY

T. Murphy Goodwin MD

Professor, Department of Obstetrics and Gynecology, Keck School of Medicine, University of Southern California, Los Angeles, CA, USA

Martin N. Montoro MD

Professor of Clinical Medicine and Obstetrics & Gynecology, Keck School of Medicine, University of Southern California, Los Angeles, CA, USA

Laila I. Muderspach MD

Chairman, Department of Obstetrics and Gynecology, Keck School of Medicine, University of Southern California, Los Angeles, CA, USA

Richard J. Paulson MD

Professor, Department of Obstetrics and Gynecology, Keck School of Medicine, University of Southern California, Los Angeles, CA, USA

Subir Roy MD

Professor, Department of Obstetrics and Gynecology, Keck School of Medicine, University of Southern California, Los Angeles, CA, USA

FIFTH EDITION

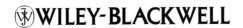

A John Wiley & Sons, Ltd., Publication

This edition first published 2010, © 2002, 2010 by Blackwell Publishing Ltd

Blackwell Publishing was acquired by John Wiley & Sons in February 2007. Blackwell's publishing program has been merged with Wiley's global Scientific, Technical and Medical business to form Wiley-Blackwell.

Registered office: John Wiley & Sons Ltd, The Atrium, Southern Gate, Chichester, West Sussex, PO19 8SQ, UK

Editorial offices: 9600 Garsington Road, Oxford, OX4 2DQ, UK
111 River Street, Hoboken, NJ 07030-5774, USA
The Atrium, Southern Gate, Chichester, West Sussex, PO19 8SQ, UK

For details of our global editorial offices, for customer services and for information about how to apply for permission to reuse the copyright material in this book please see our website at www.wiley.com/wiley-blackwell

The right of the author to be identified as the author of this work has been asserted in accordance with the Copyright, Designs and Patents Act 1988.

Wiley also publishes its books in a variety of electronic formats. Some content that appears in print may not be available in electronic books.

Designations used by companies to distinguish their products are often claimed as trademarks. All brand names and product names used in this book are trade names, service marks, trademarks or registered trademarks of their respective owners. The publisher is not associated with any product or vendor mentioned in this book. This publication is designed to provide accurate and authoritative information in regard to the subject matter covered. It is sold on the understanding that the publisher is not engaged in rendering professional services. If professional advice or other expert assistance is required, the services of a competent professional should be sought.

The contents of this work are intended to further general scientific research, understanding, and discussion only and are not intended and should not be relied upon as recommending or promoting a specific method, diagnosis, or treatment by physicians for any particular patient. The publisher and the author make no representations or warranties with respect to the accuracy or completeness of the contents of this work and specifically disclaim all warranties, including without limitation any implied warranties of fitness for a particular purpose. In view of ongoing research, equipment modifications, changes in governmental regulations, and the constant flow of information relating to the use of medicines, equipment, and devices, the reader is urged to review and evaluate the information provided in the package insert or instructions for each medicine, equipment, or device for, among other things, any changes in the instructions or indication of usage and for added warnings and precautions. Readers should consult with a specialist where appropriate. The fact that an organization or Website is referred to in this work as a citation and/or a potential source of further information does not mean that the author or the publisher endorses the information the organization or Website may provide or recommendations it may make. Further, readers should be aware that Internet Websites listed in this work may have changed or disappeared between when this work was written and when it is read. No warranty may be created or extended by any promotional statements for this work. Neither the publisher nor the author shall be liable for any damages arising herefrom.

Library of Congress Cataloging-in-Publication Data
Management of common problems in obstetrics and gynecology / edited by T. Murphy Goodwin . . . [et al.].—5th ed.
    p. ; cm.
  Includes bibliographical references and index.
  ISBN 978-1-4051-6916-5
  1. Pregnancy—Complications. 2. Generative organs, Female—Diseases. I. Goodwin, T. Murphy.
  [DNLM: 1. Genital Diseases, Female—therapy. 2. Pregnancy Complications—therapy.
WP 140 M266 2010]
  RG571.M23 2010
  618—dc22

                                                                                            20010012059

ISBN: 978-1-4051-6916-5

A catalogue record for this book is available from the British Library.

Set in 9.25/12pt Palatino by MPS Limited, A Macmillan Company
Printed in Singapore
1 2010

Contents

Preface

For over 25 years, and through four prior editions, this book has espoused the "USC way" of managing clinical problems in obstetrics and gynecology. This fifth edition, again exclusively organized and written by the department faculty, fellows and residents, continues the tradition. Major milestones in our specialty, electronic fetal monitoring, ultrasound, colposcopy, and laparoscopy, formed an impressive panoply of techniques that were refined and firmly established in the last part of the previous century. Since the fourth edition was published 8 years ago, other advances have occurred, which will be addressed in this edition.

Maternal fetal medicine (obstetrics) has improved enormously in its ability to diagnose maternal and fetal changes during pregnancy. Fetal heart rate monitoring terminology has undergone refinement and standardization. As evidenced by the burgeoning use of three- and four-dimensional ultrasound, obstetric ultrasonography continues to advance its clarity and efficiency. The diagnosis and prevention of preterm birth are improving dramatically through the evolution of ultrasound cervical length, fetal fibronectin testing, and prophylactic progesterone therapy. A new chapter on fetal interventions emphasizes another exciting area of advancement in maternal fetal medicine. The difficulties and dangers presented by the mature gravida, who has delayed childbearing or conceived via assisted reproductive technologies, comprise another new chapter. Obesity has become a significant entity in today's society, and another new chapter looks at its impact on the pregnant woman and her passenger.

Gynecologic oncology has made major strides in introducing minimally invasive surgical techniques, especially with the advent and ongoing evolution of robotic surgery. In addition, new biologic therapies are being developed and will improve and increase before the next edition of this book. Cancer prevention strategies, as evidenced by the HPV vaccine, should lead to the future promise of a reduction in invasive malignancies. To the practicing physician, understanding the nuts and bolts of gynecologic oncology is important for recognizing the signs and symptoms of cancer, especially in its neophyte stages, and for knowing when to refer patients to gynecologic oncology. To assess all the above, the gynecologic oncology chapters in this edition have been updated.

Gynecology has been specialized by the addition of female pelvic medicine and reconstructive surgery (urogynecology). Advances in the areas of endometriosis, uterine myomas, and pelvic infection have not been as dramatic as those in urogynecology. Laparoscopic and robotic surgical approaches to endometriosis and uterine myomata have reduced hospital stays and made for shorter recovery times, while medical therapies for these conditions have remained stable with limited effectiveness. Preventive techniques have reduced the severity of pelvic infection and more specific antibiotic therapies have improved treatment. These chapters have been updated, but the largest revision of the gynecology section is the increased number and coverage of the urogynecology chapters, e.g. fistulae, voiding dysfunction, and urethral disorders. Since the fourth edition, interstitial cystitis (painful bladder syndrome) has become a major gynecologic entity and a new chapter looks at its diagnosis and treatment.

Differentiation of the various urinary incontinence diagnoses has become an important part of gynecologic testing and the practitioner will benefit from an updated look at these procedures. Additionally, the development of newer techniques for sling placement is reviewed, including the transobturator route where the needle does not pass retropubically, thus minimalizing complications. As with many other fading traditional surgical approaches in our specialty, single-incision sling procedures are evolving, which may allow this surgery to become an outpatient clinic operation.

With sexuality becoming more public in our society, a new chapter looks at female sexual dysfunction. Family planning remains important and the traditional methods are reviewed along with indepth analysis of new hormonal contraceptive techniques. The medically complicated patient deserves contraception and these patients are discussed as well.

Reproductive endocrinology and infertility (REI) is always newsworthy, and keeping up with its philosophy and changes must be important to the practicing clinician.

The biggest advance in REI is that assisted reproductive technologies, because of their increasing reliability and success in treating all infertility presentations, are replacing virtually all traditional fertility therapies. Intracytoplasmic sperm injection (ICSI) has made fertility possible for thousands of men who have limited sperm production, but who previously had to rely solely on donor insemination for successful fertilization. ICSI is discussed in the *in vitro* fertilization chapter, and a separate, new chapter has been added on egg donation.

With the increasingly successful treatment of malignancies, a fertility need has been created for those women who survive their cancers but, as a result of gonadotoxic treatments, lose ovarian function. A new chapter on fertility preservation and oocyte cryopreservation addresses this major issue. Polycystic ovarian syndrome is a common entity in an office-based practice. The previous chapter has been updated and now includes therapy with insulin-sensitizing agents, such as metformin. Unexplained infertility is well explained in another new chapter.

As has always been the case, *Management of common problems in obstetrics and gynecology* is written for all healthcare providers who diagnose and treat women.

While this group includes practicing obstetricians/ gynecologists and residents in training, it also pertains to family and internal medicine physicians as well as nurse practitioners and physician assistants working in the field of obstetrics and gynecology. Although not designed as an all-inclusive, indepth text for medical students, it could assist them as they rotate through our specialty.

The editors would like to thank all the residents, fellows, and faculty in the department for the time and effort they expended in organizing, writing, and completing the fifth edition of this ongoing effort. Contributing chapters to a textbook may be tedious and time-consuming, but the contribution to individuals treating women, and their patients, is enormous. Additionally, the editors are grateful for the patience, advice, and co-operation of the publisher, who stayed the course on a long journey.

T. Murphy Goodwin
Martin N. Montoro
Laila I. Muderspach
Richard J. Paulson
Subir Roy
Los Angeles

Abbreviations

AC	abdominal circumference	CDC	Centers for Disease Control and Prevention
ACE	angiotensin-converting enzyme		
ACOG	American College of Obstetricians and Gynecologists	CDH	congenital diaphragmatic hernia
		CF	cystic fibrosis
ACTH	adrenocorticotropic hormone	cfu	colony-forming units
ADA	American Dietetic Association	CHD	coronary heart disease
AED	antiepileptic drug	CI	cervical insufficiency; confidence interval
AFI	Amniotic Fluid Index		
AΦΠ	α-fetoprotein	CIC	clean intermittent catheterization
AGC	atypical glandular cells	CIN	cervical intraepithelial neoplasia
AI	anal incontinence	CMV	cytomegalovirus
AIUM	American Institute of Ultrasound in Medicine	CNS	central nervous system
		COC	combination oral contraceptive
AMA	advanced maternal age	COX	cyclo-oxygenase
AMH	antimullerian hormone	CPK	creatine phosphokinase
ANA	antinuclear antibodies	CPP	central precocious puberty; chronic pelvic pain
aPTT	activated partial thromboplastin time		
APS	antiphospholipid syndrome	CPR	cardiopulmonary resuscitation
ARDS	acute respiratory distress syndrome	CRL	crown–rump length
ART	assisted reproductive technology	CST	contraction stress test
ASA	acetylsalicylic acid	CT	computed tomography; *Chlamydia trachomatis*
ASC	abdominal sacral colpopexy; typical squamous cells		
		CVS	chorionic villus sampling
ATFP	arcus tendineus fascia pelvis		
ATP	adenosine triphosphate	D&C	dilation and curettage
AVM	arteriovenous malformation	DCIS	ductal carcinoma *in situ*
		D&E	dilation and evacuation
BE	barium enema	DES	diethylstilbestrol
BMD	bone mineral density	DESD	detrusor–external sphincter dyssynergia
BMI	Body Mass Index		
BPD	biparietal diameter; bipolar disorder	DEXA	dual-energy x-ray absorptiometry
BPP	biophysical profile	DHEAS	dehydroepiandrosterone sulfate
BSO	bilateral salpingo-oopherectomy	DHT	dihydrotestosterone
BUN	blood, urea, nitrogen	DIC	disseminated intravascular coagulation
BV	bacterial vaginosis		
		DMPA	depot medroxyprogesterone acetate
CAH	congenital adrenal hyperplasia		
CBC	complete blood count	DMSO	dimethyl sulfoxide
CBE	clinical breast exam	DO	detrusor overactivity
CC	clomiphene citrate	DTR	deep tendon reflexes
CCAM	congenital cystic adenomatoid malformation	DUB	dysfunctional uterine bleeding
		DVT	deep vein thrombosis

EAS	external anal sphincter	HRT	hormone replacement therapy
EASI	extra-amniotic saline infusion	HSDD	hypoactive sexual desire disorder
EC	emergency contraception	HSG	hysterosalpingogram/graphy
ECG	electrocardiogram	HSIL	high-grade intraepithelial lesion
EDC	estimated date of confinement	HSV	herpes simplex virus
EEG	electroencephalogram	HTLV	human T-lymphotropic virus
EGA	estimated gestational age		
EMG	electromyography	IAS	internal anal sphincter
ENT	ear, nose and throat	IBC	inflammatory breast cancer
ERCP	endoscopic retrograde	IBD	inflammatory bowel disease
	cholangiopancreatography	IC	interstitial cystitis
ET	embryo transfer	ICI	intracervical insemination
		ICP	intrahepatic cholestasis of pregnancy
FAS	fetal alcohol syndrome	ICS	International Continence Society
FDA	Food and Drug Administration	ICSI	intracytoplasmic sperm injection
fFN	fetal fibronectin	IDDM	insulin-dependent diabetes mellitus
FFP	fresh-frozen plasma	IM	intramuscular
FGR	fetal growth restriction	INR	international normalized ratio
FHA	functional hypothalamic amenorrhea	ITP	immune thrombocytopenia
FHR	fetal heart rate	IUA	intrauterine adhesions
FI	fecal incontinence	IUD	intrauterine device
FL	femur length	IUGR	intrauterine growth restriction
FLM	fetal lung maturity	IUI	intrauterine insemination
FMH	fetomaternal hemorrhage	IUT	intrauterine transfusion
FNA	fine needle aspiration	IV	intravenous
FSH	follicle-stimulating hormone	IVF	*in vitro* fertilization
FVL	factor V Leiden	IVF-ET	*in vitro* fertilization-embryo transfer
GABA	γ-aminobutyric acid	IVH	intraventricular hemorrhage
GAG	glycosaminoglycan	IVM	*in vitro* maturation
GBS	group B streptococcus	IVP	intravenous pyelogram
GCT	glucose challenge test		
GDM	gestational diabetes mellitus	LABA	long-acting β2-agonists
GH	growth hormone	LAC	lupus anticoagulant
GIFT	gamete intrafallopian tube transfer	LAVH	laparoscopically assisted vaginal hysterectomy
GnRH	gonadotropin-releasing hormone	LDH	lactic dehydrogenase
GTN	gestational trophoblastic neoplasia	LDL	low-density lipoprotein
		LH	luteinizing hormone
HAART	highly active combination antiretroviral therapy	LHR	lung-to-head ratio
		LLD	lupus-like disease
HC	head circumference	LMP	last menstrual period
hCG	human chorionic gonadotropin	LMWH	low molecular weight heparin
HDL	high-density lipoprotein	LPP	leak point pressure
HELLP	hemolysis, elevated liver enzymes, low platelets	L/S ratio	lecithin/sphingomyelin ratio
		LSIL	low-grade intraepithelial lesion
HG	hyperemesis gravidarum	LUTO	lower urinary tract obstruction
HIT	heparin-induced thrombocytopenia	LUTS	lower urinary tract symptoms
HIV	human immunodeficiency virus	LVSI	lymph-vascular space invasion
HLA	human leukocyte antigen		
HLHS	hypoplastic left heart syndrome	MAS	meconium aspiration syndrome
hMG	human menopausal gonadotropin	MBL	menstrual blood loss
hpf	high-power field	MBPP	modified biophysical profile
HPO	hypothalamic-pituitary-ovarian	MCA	middle cerebral artery
HPT	hypothalamic-pituitary-testicular	MCV	mean corpuscular volume
HPV	human papilloma virus		

MI	Morphology Index; myocardial infarction		POF	premature ovarian failure
MIS	mullerian inhibiting substance		POP	pelvic organ prolapse
MMI	methimazole		PPHN	persistent pulmonary hypertension of the newborn
MODY	maturity-onset diabetes of the young		PPP	peripheral precocious puberty
MPA	medroxyprogesterone acetate		PPROM	preterm premature rupture of membranes
MPV	mean platelet volume		PPTD	postpartum thyroid dysfunction syndrome
MRA	magnetic resonance angiography			
MRI	magnetic resonance imaging		PPUG	positive pressure urethrography
MRKH	Mayer Rokitansky Kuster Hauser syndrome		PPV	positive predictive value
			PRBC	packed red blood cells
MRSA	methicillin-resistant *Staph. aureus*		PS	pulmonary sequestration
MSAFP	maternal serum α-fetoprotein		PST	potassium sensitivity test
			psv	peak systolic velocity
NEC	necrotizing enterocolitis		PTL	preterm labor
NICU	neonatal intensive care unit		PTT	partial thromboplastin time
NIDDM	noninsulin-dependent diabetes mellitus		PTU	propylthiouracil
NPV	negative predictive value		PUBS	percutaneous umbilical blood sampling
NS	normal saline		PVR	postvoid residual
NSAID	nonsteroidal anti-inflammatory agent			
NST	nonstress test		RBC	red blood cell
NSV	nonspecific vaginitis		RCT	randomized controlled trial
NT	nuchal translucency		RDS	respiratory distress syndrome
NV	nausea and vomiting		RI	Resistive Index
NVP	nausea and vomiting of pregnancy		RPL	recurrent pregnancy loss
			RPR	rapid plasma reagent
OA	occiput anterior		RR	relative risk
OAB	overactive bladder			
OCD	obsessive-compulsive disorder		SBE	self breast exam
OCP	oral contraceptive pill		SBO	small bowel obstruction
OCT	oxytocin challenge test		SCCA	squamous cell carcinoma
OGTT	oral glucose tolerance test		SD	standard deviations
OHSS	ovarian hyperstimulation syndrome		SERM	selective estrogen receptor modulator
OP	occiput posterior		SGA	small for gestational age
OR	odds ratio		SHBG	sex hormone-binding globulin
			SIUGR	selective intrauterine growth restriction
PAT	pregnancy-associated thrombocytopenia		SK	streptokinase
			SLE	systemic lupus erythematosus
PBS	painful bladder syndrome		SLL	second-look laparoscopy
PCOS	polycystic ovarian syndrome		SLPCV	selective laser photocoagulation of communicating vessels
PCR	polymerase chain reaction			
PDA	patent ductus arteriosus		SLS	sacrospinous ligament suspension
PE	pulmonary embolism		SNRI	selective norepinephrine reuptake inhibitor
PEFR	peak expiratory flow rate			
PET	positron emission tomography		SSRI	selective serotonin reuptake inhibitor
PG	phosphatidylglycerol; prostaglandin		STI	sexually transmitted infection
PGSI	prostaglandin synthetase inhibitor		SUI	stress urinary incontinence
PI	Pulsatility Index			
PICC	peripherally inserted central catheter		TAH	total abdominal hysterectomy
PID	pelvic inflammatory disease		TBG	thyroxine-binding globulin
PMD	premenstrual disease		TCA	trichloroacetic acid
PMDD	premenstrual dysphoric disorder		TENS	transcutaneous electrical nerve stimulation
PMS	premenstrual syndrome			
PNTML	pudendal nerve terminal motor latency		TET	tubal embryo transfer
POC	products of conception			

TLH	total laparoscopic hysterectomy	USLS	uterosacral ligament suspension
TMP-SMX	trimethoprim/sulfamethoxazole	UTI	urinary tract infection
TOL	trial of labor	UUI	urge urinary incontinence
TPA	tissue plasminogen activator	UVJ	urethrovesical junction
TRAP	twin reversed arterial perfusion		
TRH	thyrotropin-releasing hormone	VAIN	vaginal intraepithelial neoplasia
TSH	thyroid-stimulating hormone	VAS	vibroacoustic stimulation
TSI	thyroid-stimulating immunoglobulin	VBAC	vaginal birth after cesarean
TTTS	twin–twin transfusion syndrome	VDRL	Venereal Disease Reseach Laboratory test
TVH	total vaginal hysterectomy		
TVS	transvaginal ultrasonography	VEGF	vascular endothelial growth factor
TVT	tension-free vaginal tape	VIN	vulvar intraepithelial neoplasia
TVUS	transvaginal ultrasound	VTE	venous thromboembolism
		VZV	varicella zoster virus
UAE	uterine artery embolization		
UGTI	upper genital tract infection	WBC	white blood cell
UH	unfractionated heparin	WHO	World Health Organization
UK	urokinase		
USI	urodynamic stress incontinence	ZIFT	zygote intrafallopian tube transfer

Chapter 1
Cervical Insufficiency and Cerclage

Bhuvan Pathak, James A. McGregor and T. Murphy Goodwin
Department of Medicine and Obstetrics and Gynecology, Keck School of Medicine, University of Southern California, CA, USA

Introduction

Primary cervical insufficiency (CI) is the preferred term for the clinical findings of cervical shortening (≤ 25 mm), funneling and/or cervical dilation during the second trimester in the absence of cervical trauma or other abnormality. Secondary CI includes cervical change in the setting of prior trauma, frequently with a history of prior preterm births in the absence of clear clinical preterm labor. CI is a complication which affects up to 1% of all pregnancies and up to 8% of pregnancies with a history of recurrent second-trimester loss. Given a lack of consensus on its diagnostic criteria, its etiology, and its treatment, there is much variation in its reported incidence. CI is a potentially preventable cause of second-trimester loss and extreme prematurity, with associated low birthweight and other sequelae. Preterm birth, regardless of its etiology, remains the leading cause of neonatal morbidity and mortality.

Diagnosis

Unfortunately, there is no clear consensus for the diagnosis of CI despite its relatively common occurrence. Recurrent, relatively painless, second-trimester fetal losses or preterm births in the absence of contractions or vaginal bleeding remains the gold standard for diagnosis. Therefore, it is crucial that a careful and thorough obstetric and gynecologic history is taken at the onset of prenatal care. Although this presentation is classic, it is clearly recognized that cervical competence is a continuous variable and cannot simply be categorized as "competent" or "incompetent." For example, contractions may be present as a late sign of CI after prolonged exposure of the membranes to the vaginal flora. Furthermore, with the increasing use of transvaginal ultrasound, cervical shortening and dilation of the internal os can be recognized prior to the onset of symptoms and even without digital examination of the cervix.

Transvaginal sonography of the cervix can be easily performed as early as 14–16 weeks of gestation, when the lower segment of the uterus is developed well enough to allow reproducible measurements of cervical length and architecture of the internal os. Ultrasound cervical length screening at 18–22 weeks' gestation has been proposed. A length of less than 25 mm is generally considered shortened and suggestive of CI, although the probability of preterm delivery at a given cervical length varies according to gestational age. Also important is any dynamic change noted after Valsalva or mild fundal pressure, as well as differences in cervical appearance or length between consecutive measurements. Other changes which have been described include dilation and funneling of the internal os.

In nonpregnant patients, several tests including physical examination and ultrasound or radiographic studies are available to facilitate the diagnosis of CI. On physical examination, the easy passage of a number 8 Hagar dilator or a number 15 Pratt dilator is essentially diagnostic of CI. Hysterosalpingography showing dilation of the internal os to greater than 6 mm is also diagnostic of CI. These tests are both inconvenient and of limited diagnostic utility as they often yield equivocal results in patients with an unclear history.

Etiology

Although there are several postulated causes of CI, it is believed that ascending intrauterine infection with inflammation and cervical trauma are the most common causes. Cervical trauma most commonly results from surgical interventions including conization, loop electrosurgical excision procedures, repetitive or second-trimester therapeutic terminations, and obstetric injuries. More than one first-trimester termination or a single second-trimester

Management of Common Problems in Obstetrics and Gynecology, 5th edition. Edited by T.M. Goodwin, M.N. Montoro, L. Muderspach, R. Paulson and S. Roy. © 2010 Blackwell Publishing Ltd.

termination increases the incidence of CI. Obstetric injuries include compression necrosis of the cervix due to a prolonged second stage of labor, and spontaneous as well as iatrogenic lacerations of the cervix such as Duhrssen's incisions performed during vaginal delivery. Further obstetric injury may include extension of the uterine incision into the cervix at the time of cesarean section.

Congenital defects including mullerian anomalies, exposure to diethylstilbestrol, maternal deficiencies in elastin or collagen polymorphisms are less common causes of CI. Rarely, acquired anatomic defects such as large polyps or cervical myomata may be associated with CI. Premature signaling of "cervical ripening," molecular signals from fetal, trophoblast or maternal sources, is increasingly studied and may explain inconsistent CI in consecutive pregnancies in the same mother.

Management

Once a diagnosis of CI has been established or the need for intervention is identified, treatment has traditionally been by surgical correction using an encircling or cerclage suture. The most commonly used technique is the McDonald cerclage, which was described in 1957. With this, a purse-string suture of four or five bites is placed around the cervix. The material most commonly used is 5 mm Mersilene tape. Mersilene provides better tensile strength and is less likely to pull through the cervix in later gestation. Prolene and nylon are both more easily passed through the cervical tissue but are also more likely to pull through the tissues, given their smaller calibers. The suture is placed below the level of the internal os and must be placed deep into the substance of the cervix to prevent lacerations. The lateral blood supply should be left outside the purse-string suture. The knot is then placed anteriorly and one end left long enough to facilitate removal at 36–37 weeks' gestation. The McDonald technique differs from the modified Shirodkar cerclage described below in that more suture is left exposed within the vagina.

The Shirodkar cerclage was described 2 years earlier in 1955, using maternal fascia lata as the suture material. Today, a 5 mm Mersilene tape is again the suture material most commonly used. The modified Shirodkar has now replaced the original version due to it simplicity. Transverse incisions are made in the cervix anteriorly and posteriorly, and the suture is passed between the fibromuscular substance of the cervix and the lateral blood supply. The knot is again tied anteriorly and some surgeons anchor the tape anteriorly and/or posteriorly to the cervical tissue using a second suture to avoid slippage of the tape. While the originally described Shirodkar cerclage requires increased dissection of both the bladder and rectum superiorly, as well as entailing increased operative time, bleeding, cervical scarring, and cesarean delivery rates, the modified Shirodkar avoids these complications. The Shirodkar is less commonly employed but may still be indicated in cases where a previous McDonald cerclage has failed or when the cervix is significantly shortened due to congenital abnormalities or surgical intervention.

In cases where vaginal cerclage has failed or when there is marked scarring, shortening or deformation of the cervix, precluding vaginal placement, transabdominal cerclage may be employed. Given the inherently more invasive nature of the abdominal route, maternal and fetal risks are significantly increased. An abdominal incision is made and the lower uterine segment exposed. The uterine vessels are located and withdrawn laterally, and a Mersilene tape is placed in the avascular space between the retracted vessels and the uterine isthmus. The suture is passed anteriorly and tied anteriorly and overlies the uterosacral ligaments without penetrating the myometrium. Delivery in these cases must be by cesarean section and the cerclage is usually kept in place for subsequent pregnancies. Fetal salvage is reported to be up to 90%. Several cases of abdominal laparoscopic cerclage placement have been described.

Cerclage placement may be performed on an elective or prophylactic basis, as a therapeutic measure or on an emergency basis, often referred to as a "rescue" cerclage. When the obstetric history is diagnostic for CI, as in the patient with classic repetitive, painless dilation described above, a prophylactic cerclage may be placed in the late first trimester, usually after 10 weeks' gestation. This usually allows for placement after the gestational age at which most inevitable miscarriages would occur. This timing also allows for documentation of fetal viability and exclusion of major malformations and certain lethal anomalies such as anencephaly, which are usually visible in the late first trimester. In cases where the history is suggestive of CI but not clearly diagnostic, there remains controversy as to the ideal management. Examples of patients at a possibly elevated risk of CI are listed in Box 1.1.

There are differing views as to the specific situations in which elective cerclages should be placed. One view is that of the American College of Obstetricians and Gynecologists which recommends that elective cerclage placement based only on historical factors should be confined to patients with three or more otherwise unexplained second-trimester losses or preterm births. It should be noted that even in women with a history of three or more unexplained second-trimester deliveries, there is still an approximately 50% chance of delivering at term without cerclage placement. Other experts suggest confirmation

---

Box 1.1 Patients at risk of cervical incompetence without a history of incompetence

- Procedures with no intervening normal pregnancy
- Cone biopsy or loop excision
- More than one first-trimester abortion
- A single second-trimester abortion
- Spontaneous preterm premature rupture of membranes or preterm birth less than 28 weeks' gestation
- Preterm birth at any time in gestation with progress in labor out of proportion to uterine activity
- Congenital uterine anomaly without prior loss
- Multiple gestation

---

of cervical change using ultrasound surveillance. Severe restriction of activities or bedrest is less effective but is frequently employed after 24 weeks' gestation.

Therapeutic or urgent cerclage is often placed in women with a shortened cervix or evidence of funneling on ultrasound. These women are often being assessed by ultrasound due to a history placing them at risk for CI, or symptoms or findings on physical examination placing them at risk. The randomized studies examining cerclage placement in these situations contain small numbers of subjects and have yielded conflicting results. It appears, however, that cerclage may prolong pregnancy in a woman with a shortened cervix who is at high risk for CI based on history as well. In otherwise low-risk patients with a shortened cervix, cerclage placement has not been shown to significantly prevent preterm birth. Bedrest or a modified version of it is commonly employed for women with a shortened cervix who do not undergo cervical cerclage.

Finally, emergency or "rescue" cerclage is sometimes placed in women with advanced cervical dilation although the supporting data are rather limited. These women must be thoroughly evaluated prior to surgical intervention. Most importantly, chorio-amnionitis must be ruled out. There should also be no vaginal bleeding, no rupture of membranes, and a viable fetus with no major anatomic abnormalities visible. There should be no uterine activity or an excellent response to short-term tocolytics. Evaluation includes but is not necessarily limited to physical examination, cultures of the urine, cervix, and vagina, and a complete blood count. If the patient is deemed to be an appropriate candidate for an emergency cerclage, she should be placed on bedrest and broad-spectrum antibiotics for 12–24 hours prior to the procedure. Adequate uterine relaxation, anesthesia, and visualization of the anatomy are key to

the successful placement of an emergency cerclage. This is usually attained by the use of spinal anesthesia as well as with uterine relaxants including terbutaline or nitroglycerine. Other techniques to assist in the reduction of possibly protuberant membranes include placing the patient in the Trendelenburg position, and gentle pressure using a 30 cc Foley catheter balloon and/or moistened gauzes on sponge sticks. Some authors even advocate the use of transabdominal amnioreduction to further reduce the bulging membranes. Postsurgical treatment with up to a 3 week course of broad-spectrum antibiotics and short-term prostaglandin synthase inhibitors for 24–48 hours is also recommended.

Prior to or concurrent to any cerclage, the mother should be screened and treated for common genitourinary tract infections including urinary tract infection, bacteriuria, vaginitis, cervicitis, bacterial vaginosis, and prevalent sexually transmitted infections. Optimal results are obtained with perioperative antibiotic use, tocolytics such as calcium channel blockers, prostaglandin synthase inhibitors, and nitroglycerine, and with serial treatments of progesterone.

Overall success rates with cervical cerclage placement vary widely given the wide variation in studies and controls used. Some authors report no differences with or without cerclage placement, while others report infant viability rates of up to 90% following surgical intervention. For emergency cerclage placement, success rates and neonatal survival vary by both gestational age and cervical dilation, with rates ranging from 33% to 83%.

Finally, the use of rigid pessaries, although not common in the United States, is popular in some European countries. These studies are small with poorly described selection criteria.

Complications

Although not an extremely invasive procedure, the risks with cerclage placement include those related to the operative procedure itself, as well as those related to the prevention of possible subsequent preterm birth. The most commonly encountered complications are chorio-amnionitis and rupture of membranes, both of which have increased rates with advancing gestational age. Rupture of membranes is also greater with emergency cerclage than with elective cerclage and occurs up to 45% of the time in the former situation. In cases where there is subsequent rupture of membranes, we feel that cerclages should generally be removed promptly to avoid chorio-amnionitis and its associated maternal and neonatal morbidity. In the well-counseled patient with rupture of membranes at previable or extremely premature gestational ages, the cerclage may be left in place and the patient closely monitored for any signs of chorio-amnionitis. Other complications include intraoperative bleeding which requires transfusion in 6% of transabdominal procedures. An increased risk of hospitalization for pre-term labor, as well as an increased use of tocolytics, has been shown with cerclage use. Cervical lacerations at the time of delivery have been noted in 10% of cases, and chronic fistula formation with long-term cerclage place-ment has also been reported. Finally, cerclage placement in the setting of twins has been associated with a sig-nificantly higher incidence of preterm birth and should therefore be avoided.

Once a cerclage has been placed, a baseline ultrasound should be obtained for cervical length. This allows for accu-rate assessment of any further changes that may present.

Conclusion

As mentioned above, CI is a complication of pregnancy that is not uncommonly encountered. Despite this, there is not always clear consensus as to its diagnostic criteria and management regimens. A thorough obstetric history is therefore of the utmost importance in these situations. Cerclage placement is commonly employed in patients with a classic history of CI on an elective basis, in the patient with a shortened cervix as a therapeutic measure, or in the patient with advanced dilation on an emergency basis. The most common complications of cerclage placement include rupture of membranes and chorio-amnionitis, both of which should be monitored for, with removal of the suture if necessary.

Suggested reading

Althuisius SM, Dekker GA, Hummel P, Bekedam DJ, van Geijn HP. Final results of the cervical incompetence prevention randomized cerclage trial (CIPRACT): therapeutic cerclage with bed rest ver-sus bed rest alone. *Am J Obstet Gynecol* 2001; 185(5): 1106–1112.

Berghella V, Odibo AO, To MS, Rust OA, Althuisius SM. Cerclage for short cervix on ultrasononography; meta-analysis of trials using individual patient level data. *Obstet and Gynecol* 2005; 106(1): 181–189.

Berghella V, Roman A, Daskalakis C, Ness A, Baxter J. Gestational age at cervical length measurement and incidence of preterm birth. *Obstet Gynecol* 2007; 110(2): 311–317.

Cervical insufficiency. *ACOG Pract Bull* 2003; 48.

Drakeley AJ, Roberts D, Alfirevic Z. Cervical stitch (cerclage) for preventing pregnancy loss in women. *Cochrane Database Syst Rev* 2003; 1: CD003253.

Fox NS, Chervenak FA. Cervical cerclage: a review of the evi-dence. *Obstet Gynecol Surv* 2008; 63(1): 58–65.

Jorgensen AL, Alfirec Z, Smith CT, Williamson PR. Cervical stitch (cerclage) for preventing pregnancy loss: individual patient data meta-analysis. *BJOG* 2007; 114(12): 1460–1476.

Medical Research Council/Royal College of Obstetricians and Gynecologists Working Party on Cervical Cerclage. Final report of the Medical Research Council/Royal College of Obstetricians and Gynecologists multicenter randomised trial of cervical cer-clage. *BJOG* 1993; 100(6): 516–523.

Rust OA, Roberts WE. Does cerclage prevent preterm birth? *Obstet Gynecol Clin* 2005; 32: 441–456.

Rust OA, Atlas RO, Jones KJ, Benham BN, Balducci J. A randomized trial of cerclage versus no cerclage among patients with ultra-sonographically detected second-trimester preterm dilatation of the internal os. *Am J Obstet Gynecol* 2000; 183(4): 830–835.

Simcox R, Shennan A. Cervical cerclage in the prevention of pre-term birth. *Best Pract Res Clin Obstet Gynecol* 2007; 21(5): 831–842.

Chapter 2
Preterm Premature Rupture of the Membranes

Paola Aghajanian

Department of Medicine and Obstetrics and Gynecology, Keck School of Medicine, University of Southern California, CA, USA

Introduction

Preterm premature rupture of the membranes (PPROM) is defined as rupture of membranes occurring prior to the onset of contractions and prior to 37 weeks' gestation. It complicates 3% of pregnancies and precedes approximately one-third of preterm births. PPROM is associated with oligohydramnios, placental abruption, cord prolapse, and intrauterine infection and hence places the fetus at risk before delivery. When PPROM occurs remote from term, there are significant risks of neonatal morbidity and mortality. To date, there are no reliable means of predicting and preventing PPROM. The physician caring for the woman with PPROM is therefore in a unique position to intervene in an attempt to improve perinatal outcome.

Etiology

At term, rupture of fetal membranes occurs as a normal part of labor due to a combination of cellular apoptosis and increased collagenase activity. Shearing forces accompanying uterine contractions aid this process. The etiology of PPROM is multifactorial, involving mechanical, infectious and inflammatory processes. Mechanical forces encountered in preterm labor, cervical incompetence or polyhydramnios can all induce the production of prostaglandins. This increases uterine irritability, decreases synthesis of fetal membrane collagen and increases collagenase activity. The subsequent exposure of the membranes to vaginal flora increases the likelihood of attack by bacterial proteases, endotoxins and enzymes such as phospholipase. The role of infection in the causation of PPROM is supported by the identification of pathologic micro-organisms in human vaginal flora soon after membrane rupture. An association between colonization of the genital tract by group B streptococci (GBS), *Ureaplasma urealyticum, Chlamydia trachomatis,* and *Neisseria gonorrhoeae* has been established. Although earlier smaller studies showed an association between bacterial vaginosis (BV) and PPROM, prospective studies have found that BV is not a risk factor for PPROM at less than 35 weeks. In general, intrauterine infection may predispose women to PPROM through the secretion of bacterial proteases that induce the degradation of collagen and the extracellular matrix. Additionally, the host inflammatory response to bacterial infection mediated by cytokines and prostaglandins produced by neutrophils and macrophages may predispose the patient to PPROM. In the majority of cases, however, the exact etiology of PPROM is not known. The risk of recurrence of preterm birth from PPROM in a future pregnancy approaches 14%.

Prevention

The population at risk for PPROM is similar to the population at risk for preterm birth. Risk factors associated with PPROM include a history of preterm birth or PPROM in a previous pregnancy, preterm labor in the current pregnancy, cervical insufficiency, cervical conization, cerclage, maternal smoking, low socio-economic status, low maternal Body Mass Index, second-trimester vaginal bleeding, and amniocentesis. Additionally, a substantial portion of PPROM cases are related to urinary tract infections and sexually transmitted infections (STI). Patients with a history of PPROM or spontaneous preterm birth should therefore be screened for the presence of genitourinary infections and STI in early pregnancy and treated accordingly. Of note, evaluation for asymptomatic BV and its treatment have not proven effective in preventing PPROM.

Diagnosis

The first step in the management of PPROM is confirmation of the diagnosis. In most cases, the history and physical examinations will provide ample evidence for a diagnosis

Management of Common Problems in Obstetrics and Gynecology, 5th edition. Edited by T.M. Goodwin, M.N. Montoro, L. Muderspach, R. Paulson and S. Roy. © 2010 Blackwell Publishing Ltd.

of PPROM, with patient history having an accuracy of 90%. If the clinical history is equivocal, a sterile speculum examination is undertaken. Visualization of amniotic fluid passing from the cervix or the presence of pooling in the posterior fornix of the vagina is diagnostic. Amniotic fluid is more alkaline (pH > 6) than vaginal secretions and will stain pH-sensitive indicators such as nitrazine paper blue. False-positive results on nitrazine testing may be seen with blood or semen contamination, antiseptic solutions or bacterial vaginosis. Microscopic evaluation of amniotic fluid allowed to dry on a clean slide will reveal the characteristic pattern of ferning. This is due to the interaction of amniotic fluid, proteins and salts. A false-positive but atypical ferning pattern may be seen when contamination with cervical mucus is present. On the other hand, false-negative ferning or nitrazine testing can occur with prolonged leakage.

If the diagnosis of PPROM is strongly suspected but cannot be confirmed by the tests above, an ultrasound examination showing diminished amniotic fluid volume (AFI) is supportive of the diagnosis. If the diagnosis remains in doubt, dilute indigo carmine may be injected into the uterine cavity and its egress detected on a vaginal tampon or perineal pad.

At the time of the initial speculum examination, the cervix should be inspected for evidence of cervicitis or umbilical cord prolapse. Cervical effacement and dilation can be evaluated visually (correlation coefficient with digital examination = 0.74) in order to reduce infectious morbidity, as digital examinations have been associated in multiple studies with a significantly shortened latency.

Maternal and fetal risks associated with preterm premature rupture of the membranes

After PPROM, the latency period from membrane rupture to delivery decreases inversely with advancing gestational age. For example, at 20–26 weeks' gestation, the mean latency period is close to 12 days; at 32–34 weeks' gestation, it is only 4 days. The natural history of PPROM therefore allows significant prolongation of pregnancy in some cases of PPROM. A central tenet of care of the patient with PPROM is that pregnancy prolongation should be considered only when significant fetal benefit could be expected, in the absence of significant fetal and maternal risk.

The principal maternal risk with PPROM and prolonged membrane rupture is chorio-amnionitis, which may result from ascending bacterial infection before or after membrane rupture. Notably, at the time of presentation with PPROM in the absence of labor, the rate of subclinical chorio-amnionitis (defined as positive amniotic fluid cultures obtained by transabdominal amniocentesis) has been reported to be as high as 40%. Clinical chorio-amnionitis, on the other hand, is present in 1–2% of women who present with PPROM. Subsequently, chorio-amnionitis develops clinically in 3–8% of these women. Placental abruption also occurs in a significant number of cases, as does a retained placenta or postpartum hemorrhage requiring dilation and curettage. Maternal sepsis and death occur rarely, at 0.8% and 0.14% respectively.

The principal fetal risks after PPROM result from maternal intrauterine infection, umbilical cord prolapse, umbilical cord compression and placental abruption. Following rupture of fetal membranes before fetal viability (less than 24 weeks' gestation), pulmonary hypoplasia and skeletal deformities may be seen due to the presence of persistent oligohydramnios. Either of the latter two complications is found to some degree in about 30% of early rupture cases. However, the primary determinant of infant morbidity and mortality is gestational age at delivery. In general, infant morbidity in PPROM is similar to that of infants born at the same gestational age without PPROM (assuming absence of pulmonary hypoplasia). Patients with PPROM, especially if it occurs before 24 weeks, should be extensively counseled about the associated maternal and neonatal risks and outcomes. In certain instances of PPROM prior to viability, where the patient chooses to continue the pregnancy, outpatient management may be considered.

Management

In certain cases, delivery is indicated after PPROM regardless of the gestational age. If overt chorio-amnionitis, nonreassuring fetal status, significant bleeding from placental abruption and/or advanced labor are present, expeditious delivery is required. Otherwise, if the mother and fetus are clinically stable, gestational age will be the primary factor determining management. The benefits of expectant management mainly involve decreasing the gestational age-related morbidity from prematurity.

Preterm premature rupture of the membranes diagnosed before 32 weeks' gestation is associated with significant neonatal morbidity and mortality. In the absence of indications for immediate delivery, women with PPROM at 23–32 weeks should be expectantly managed in the hope of prolonging the latency period and reducing neonatal morbidity due to prematurity.

When PPROM is diagnosed between 32 and 33 weeks, neonatal survival is likely although the risk of respiratory distress syndrome remains if fetal pulmonary testing shows immaturity. Conservative management in this gestational age only briefly prolongs pregnancy without significantly reducing neonatal morbidity. Therefore, if fetal pulmonary maturity can be demonstrated via vaginal pool fluid or transabdominal amniocentesis, delivery should be considered. Vigilance for evidence of infection must be heightened, as there is little long-term benefit in prolonging pregnancy after 32 weeks' gestation.

At 34–36 weeks' gestation, the occurrence of severe neonatal complications due to immaturity is low.

Expectant management in this group of women leads to a significant increase in the risk of chorio-amnionitis and a lower umbilical cord pH without any benefit to the fetus. Therefore, if PPROM occurs between 34 and 36 weeks, delivery should proceed expeditiously.

Exceptions to expectant management at any gestational age include maternal HIV, primary maternal herpes simplex virus infection and fetal malpresentation in cases of advanced cervical dilation. In cases of conservative management, antenatal fetal surveillance is recommended in order to assess for signs of fetal compromise due mainly to umbilical cord compression and/or chorio-amnionitis. Initially, continuous electronic fetal heart rate (FHR) and contraction monitoring should be conducted for 48 hours. If testing reveals reassuring fetal status with adequate AFI, then the patient can be observed on the antepartum ward with daily nonstress testing and twice-weekly AFI evaluation. Twice-weekly biophysical profiles for those patients with an AFI greater than 5 are also acceptable. At this time, there is no evidence to guide the frequency of fetal surveillance in this population. During hospitalization, modified bedrest with deep venous thrombosis prophylaxis should be employed. Digital pelvic examinations should be avoided unless labor ensues or delivery is indicated.

A number of tests have been studied for their ability to identify fetal infection during the period of expectant management for PPROM. Tests of maternal blood such as the white blood cell (WBC) count and C-reactive protein are not routinely used in clinical practice. However, if clinical findings are suspicious, gram stain, culture, WBC count, and glucose levels of the amniotic fluid may prove beneficial in diagnosing intra-amniotic infection. Interleukin-6 appears to be the best biomarker for intra-amniotic infection but is unavailable in most hospitals. Clinical chorio-amnionitis is diagnosed by the presence of uterine tenderness, maternal fever greater than or equal to 100.4°F, and maternal or fetal tachycardia in the absence of other sources of infection. As chorio-amnionitis is associated with "fetal inflammatory syndrome" (elevated amniotic fluid cytokines and fetal systemic inflammation), which may lead to subsequent adverse neurologic sequela (cerebral palsy, cystic periventricular leukomalacia), a diagnosis of intra-amniotic infection, clinical or subclinical, necessitates expeditious delivery of the pregnancy complicated by PPROM.

Antibiotics, steroids, and tocolysis

A number of broad-spectrum antibiotic regimens have been shown to prolong the latent phase in PPROM. Multiple prospective randomized trials have been published regarding this issue. The NICHD-MFMU study found that antibiotic treatment of expectantly managed women with PPROM between 24 and 32 weeks' gestation prolongs pregnancy and reduces the risk of delivery at 1, 2, and 3 weeks by 50%. Furthermore, treatment with antibiotics has been proven to reduce amnionitis, neonatal sepsis, and intraventricular hemorrhage. The most widely used antibiotic regimen is intravenous ampicillin and erythromycin for 2 days followed by 5 days of oral amoxicillin and erythromycin. Any woman with PPROM in whom vaginal delivery is imminent also needs appropriate antibiotic therapy to prevent the vertical transmission of group B streptococcus (GBS), unless an already prescribed antibiotic regimen provides appropriate coverage or a recent anovaginal culture is negative for GBS.

The benefit of antenatal steroids in the presence of ruptured membranes has been thoroughly investigated. In a recent meta-analysis, corticosteroids were shown to significantly reduce the risks of respiratory distress syndrome (RR 0.56), intraventricular hemorrhage (RR 0.47) and necrotizing enterocolitis (RR 0.21). The risk of neonatal death may also be reduced (RR 0.68). Antenatal corticosteroids do not appear to increase the risk of infection in the mother or infant. The 2000 NIH Consensus Panel recommended that antenatal corticosteroids be administered to all pregnant women at risk of delivery between 24 and 34 weeks' gestation, although it is acceptable to administer corticosteroids between 32 and 34 weeks' gestation only in the case of documented immaturity or if fluid for testing cannot be obtained. Antenatal steroid therapy should not be routinely repeated in patients with PPROM.

The benefit of tocolytic therapy is less firmly established in the presence of PPROM as compared to patients with intact membranes. Studies suggest that tocolysis after PPROM may increase short-term latency to allow more time for antenatal corticosteroid and antibiotic administration. Therefore, tocolysis can be used to achieve 48 hours of corticosteroid administration in the absence of any evidence of infection or other contraindications to labor inhibition. The current literature does not support the use of maintenance tocolysis beyond the initial 48-hour steroid window. The fetal benefits of tocolysis in this setting are unclear.

Special circumstances related to PPROM

When PPROM occurs before 23 weeks' gestation, the prognosis is guarded. Many patients will choose termination of pregnancy because of the poor prognosis for the fetus and in order to reduce the risk of ascending infection in the mother. Nevertheless, intact survival of the newborn has been described even with PPROM before 20 weeks' gestation. The risks and benefits of expectant management with antibiotic therapy compared to termination of pregnancy should be thoroughly reviewed with the patient in such cases. If previable PPROM has occurred after amniocentesis, the prognosis is more favorable and expectant management with broad-spectrum antibiotic therapy may be employed. In 2.6–13% of cases, cessation of fluid leakage will occur.

Cervical cerclage, especially when placed as an emergency, is a common risk factor for PPROM. There are no prospective trials dictating the optimal management of PPROM in the setting of a cervical cerclage. When the cerclage is removed at the time of presentation with PPROM, the risk of adverse perinatal outcome appears not to be increased. No controlled studies have demonstrated a significant reduction in infant morbidity with retention of the cerclage. Given the potential risks associated with a retained cerclage without evident neonatal benefit, it is recommended that the cerclage be removed on presentation with PPROM. In selected patients without evidence of infection but with a history of cervical insufficiency, the cerclage may be left in place until the patient has received antenatal corticosteroids and antibiotic therapy. The patient should undergo thorough counseling on the benefits and risks of each option and be an active participant in the decision-making process throughout the management of PPROM.

Suggested reading

American College of Obstetricians and Gynecologists. Premature rupture of membranes. ACOG Practice Bulletin No. 80. *Obstet Gynecol* 2007; 109: 1007–1019.

Canavan TP, Simhan HN, Caritis S. An evidence-based approach to the evaluation and treatment of premature rupture of membranes. *Obstet Gynecol Surv* 2004; 59: 669–689.

Epstein FH. Premature rupture of the fetal membranes. *NEJM* 1998; 338: 663–670.

Greig PC. The diagnosis of intrauterine infection in women with preterm premature rupture of the membranes (PPROM). *Clin Obstet Gynecol* 1998; 41: 849–863.

Harding JE, Pang J, Knight DV, Liggins GC. Do antenatal corticosteroids help in the setting of preterm rupture of membranes? *Am J Obstet Gynecol* 2001; 184: 131–139.

Kenyon SL, Taylor DJ, Tarnow-Mordi W, for the ORACLE Collaborative Group. Broad-spectrum antibiotics for preterm, prelabour rupture of fetal membranes: the ORACLE I randomised trial. *Lancet* 2001; 357(9261): 979–988.

Kominiarek MA, Kemp A. Perinatal outcome in preterm premature rupture of membranes at < or = 32 weeks with retained cerclage. *J Reprod Med* 2006; 51: 533–538.

Lee MJ, Davies J, Guinn D, *et al.* Single versus weekly courses of antenatal corticosteroids in preterm premature rupture of membranes. *Obstet Gynecol* 2004; 103: 274–281.

Mercer BM. Preterm premature rupture of the membranes: current approaches to evaluation and management. *Obstet Gynecol Clin North Am* 2005; 32: 411–428.

Mercer BM. Is there a role for tocolytic therapy during conservative management of preterm premature rupture of the membranes? *Clin Obstet Gynecol* 2007; 50: 487–496.

Mercer BM, Miodovnik M, Thurnau GR, *et al.* Antibiotic therapy for reduction of infant morbidity after preterm premature rupture of the membranes: a randomized controlled trial. *JAMA* 1998; 278: 989–995.

O'Connor S, Kuller JA, McMahon MJ. Management of cervical cerclage after preterm premature rupture of membranes. *Obstet Gynecol Surv* 1999; 54: 391–394.

Steer P, Flint C. ABC of labor care: preterm labor and premature rupture of membranes. *BMJ* 1999; 318: 1059–1062.

Chapter 3
Preterm Labor: Diagnosis and Management

Joseph G. Ouzounian and T. Murphy Goodwin
Department of Medicine and Obstetrics and Gynecology, Keck School of Medicine, University of Southern California, CA, USA

Incidence and complications

Preterm birth is defined as delivery occurring at less than 37 completed weeks' gestation, and is a major cause of neonatal morbidity and mortality in developed countries. In the United States, preterm birth is the second leading cause of infant mortality (after congenital malformations). Moreover, the incidence of preterm birth has increased, from 9.4% in 1981 to 10.9% in 2005. This is due, at least in part, to rising rates of multiple gestations. In 1989, there were 2529 triplet gestations delivered in the United States, but 6800 cases in the year 2000. Infants born prematurely are at risk for respiratory distress syndrome (RDS), patent ductus arteriosus (PDA), intraventricular hemorrhage (IVH), necrotizing enterocolitis (NEC), and sepsis. They are also at risk for poor school performance, mental retardation, and growth delay. Cerebral palsy is a nonprogressive motor dysfunction disorder, which can have an onset near the time of delivery. Its incidence is 2:1000 births in the general population, but as high as 10% in infants born before 28 weeks' gestation.

Risk factors for preterm birth

Risk factors for preterm birth include: preterm labor; prior preterm birth; multifetal gestation; second-trimester vaginal bleeding; low socio-economic status; familial history; chronic stress; poor nutrition; and chronic stress. However, more than 50% of preterm births occur in women with no identifiable risk factors. Furthermore, approximately one-third of preterm births are due to maternal or fetal complications (hypertensive disorders, placental abruption, placenta previa, multiple fetal pregnancy, congenital malformations), one-third is due to preterm premature rupture of membranes (PPROM), and one-third is idiopathic (with intact membranes).

Maternal infections outside the uterus (e.g. pneumonia, pyelonephritis, viral syndromes) are associated with an increased risk for preterm labor (PTL). Asymptomatic urinary tract infection with PTL is also associated with PTL.

Anatomic abnormalities of the uterus may account for up to 15% of PTL cases, with or without relative cervical insufficiency. Important congenital anomalies include septate and/or bicornuate uteri. Cervical insufficiency itself is recognized as a continuum and is responsible for at least some cases of preterm birth. Premature shortening and dilation of the cervix may result in exposure of the fetal membranes to bacteria. The anatomic and inflammatory components of preterm birth are thus often intermingled.

Congenital anomalies of the fetus, especially those associated with fetal hydrops or severe oligohydramnios, can also result in PTL. Uterine overdistension with severe polyhydramnios or multiple gestation is also associated with PTL. The high frequency of growth-restricted infants among those delivered preterm supports the association of placental insufficiency with PTL. Trauma is an uncommon but well-documented cause of PTL.

Subclinical genital tract infection leading to intra-amniotic infections by the ascending route has been shown to cause as much as 30% of spontaneous preterm birth and even a greater percentage of PPROM. Bacterial vaginosis and colonization with gonorrhea and chlamydia are associated with PTL and PPROM as well.

Diagnosis and treatment of preterm labor

The strict definition of PTL requires evidence of cervical change in response to regular uterine contractions. Nevertheless, in clinical practice therapy is commonly initiated on the basis of persistent contractions alone out of concern for difficulty in stopping advanced labor, which can lead to preterm birth. Interestingly, if the diagnosis is based solely on the presence of uterine contractions, studies have shown that up to 60% of patients are falsely

Management of Common Problems in Obstetrics and Gynecology, 5th edition. Edited by T.M. Goodwin, M.N. Montoro, L. Muderspach, R. Paulson and S. Roy. © 2010 Blackwell Publishing Ltd.

diagnosed. In a patient without documented cervical change, a period of several hours of bedrest with monitoring may clarify the situation. The decision whether or not to initiate therapy can be guided with the addition of cervical length measurement via transvaginal ultrasonography (TVS) and/or assessment of fetal fibronectin (fFN) status. A patient with a cervical length ≥ 3.0 cm is very unlikely to deliver early. Similarly, a patient with a negative fFN has only a 3% or less chance of delivering within 2 weeks of the negative test.

Utilization of TVS or fFN testing (the choice of approach may depend on availability, cost, and local turnaround time) provides improved triaging of patients who are at low risk for active PTL and thus limits needless therapy. During this observation period, the mother and fetus should be evaluated for conditions that may play a role in the onset of labor (e.g. PPROM, polyhydramnios, multifetal gestation, trauma) and for conditions that would preclude inhibition of labor (e.g. fetal demise, fetal anomaly incompatible with life, severe intrauterine growth restriction, maternal hemorrhage, severe hypertensive disease, chorio-amnionitis or evidence of fetal maturity, etc.). A history and physical examination, urinalysis, complete blood count, and cervical culture for GBS should be performed, along with a complete ultrasound. If intrauterine infection is suspected but not clinically obvious, amniocentesis for gram stain, culture, and cell count may be useful.

All patients with progressive PTL should receive antibiotics to prevent transmission of GBS from mother to infant at the time of birth. The most common regimens are intravenous penicillin or ampicillin. Our preferred regimen is intravenous penicillin G 5 million units initially then 2.5 million units every 4 hours until delivery. Penicillin-allergic patients may be treated with clindamycin or erythromycin. If the GBS culture returns negative, then the antibiotics may be discontinued.

Maternal steroid therapy

The two main objectives of tocolytic therapy for symptomatic PTL are to delay delivery to facilitate maternal transport to a hospital with an appropriate neonatal intensive care unit, and to allow for administration of corticosteroids to enhance fetal lung maturity. Both of these interventions reduce perinatal mortality and morbidity. Tocolytic therapy is restricted typically to gestations between 24 and 34 weeks. Prior to 24 weeks and between 34 and 37 weeks, therapy may be individualized. In the latter gestational age group, amniocentesis to document fetal lung maturity should be considered prior to instituting tocolytic therapy or proceeding with elective delivery.

Commonly used regimens of corticosteroids for fetal lung maturity include two doses of betametasone, 12 mg

intramuscularly 24 hours apart, or dexamethasone, 6 mg given twice daily for a total of four doses. The beneficial effect appears to extend from 24 hours of initiation of the regimen up to 7 days. While current evidence does not support serial dosing of corticosteroids for women at high risk for early delivery, this is an area of active research and recommendations continue to evolve.

Tocolysis with magnesium sulfate

While ritodrine is the only FDA-approved drug for the indication of PTL, magnesium sulfate has gained in popularity due to its similar efficacy to ritodrine with fewer side effects. An absolute contraindication to magnesium sulfate use is maternal myasthenia gravis. Renal insufficiency is a relative contraindication. The most common side effects (chest pain, severe nausea, flushing, drowsiness or weakness) are seen in less than 5% of patients. Magnesium toxicity, which can result in respiratory arrest, is counteracted immediately by the administration of 1 ampoule (10 mL) of 10% calcium gluconate. This should be kept readily available. Fluid intake and output should be monitored closely to ensure adequate renal excretion of magnesium and to prevent pulmonary edema. A magnesium serum concentration of 5–8 mg/dL is desirable. The protocol used for magnesium sulfate tocolysis at our institution is shown in Box 3.1.

Box 3.1 Tocolysis with magnesium sulfate

- Hydrate patient with 500 mL isotonic crystalloid over 20 min
- Maintain strict intake and output
- Solution: 10 g magnesium sulfate in 100 mL saline
- Loading dose: 4 g bolus/20 min
- Start constant infusion 2 g/h
- Increase infusion rate 0.5 g/h every 20 min until tocolysis achieved
- Continue infusion at lowest effective dose for 12 h once tocolysis achieved
- Vital signs every 15 min during loading and hourly while on maintenance
- Check deep tendon reflexes (DTR) hourly while on maintenance
- Discontinue infusion and call doctor if:
  - no DTR
  - respirations less than 12/min
  - chest pain or tightness
  - urine output less than 30 mL/h
- Doses of magnesium sulfate above 3 g/h require continuous ECG monitoring and serum magnesium levels every 6 h

β-Mimetics and other tocolytics

The use of intravenous β-mimetics for tocolysis has been associated with a variety of maternal complications, including death due to pulmonary edema. Many centers, including our own, no longer employ these agents by the intravenous route. However, subcutaneous terbutaline 0.25 mg every 3 hours may be employed during the initial evaluation of a patient with preterm contractions to help distinguish inconsequential preterm contractions from true PTL. During this time, patient assessment and consideration for definitive therapy can continue. Some have advocated the subcutaneous terbutaline pump based on the theory that downregulation of β-receptors can be diminished with continuous low-dose administration of the drug combined with intermittent demand boluses. Unfortunately, there have been no controlled trials documenting the efficacy of this expensive regimen.

Prostaglandin synthetase inhibitors, such as indometacin, can be given orally or rectally and appear to have efficacy comparable to intravenous agents. Questions of their safety for the fetus have been raised but most complications appear to be associated with long-term usage. We generally use indometacin (25–50 mg orally or by rectum every 6 h) as a second-line tocolytic agent between 24 and 32 weeks for not more than 48 hours. Calcium channel blockers, such as nifedipine, appear to have equal efficacy to other tocolytics and have been a promising alternative to intravenous therapy. Many centers now advocate nifedipine as a first-line agent.

There are no data to indicate that oral maintenance therapy prolongs pregnancy after successful intravenous treatment.

Prevention of preterm birth

While numerous risk assessment strategies for PTL have been devised and assessed, collectively they have yielded a positive predictive value of 25% or less.

Patient education regarding the warning signs and symptoms of PTL is an important part of PTL prevention. Such symptoms include rhythmic backache, a sensation of pelvic pressure, a change in vaginal discharge (heavier), vaginal spotting and abdominal cramping. All patients should be encouraged to report these symptoms, since earlier recognition of PTL allows more efficacious treatment. Unfortunately, studies of home uterine activity monitoring have not demonstrated a consistent benefit and so we do not use this tool at our institution.

Treatment of women with bacterial vaginosis who are at high risk for spontaneous preterm birth can reduce the preterm birth rate significantly. We screen such high-risk patients for the presence of bacterial vaginosis between 14 and 20 weeks and treat them with oral metronidazole.

Assessment of cervical length with TVS can also be helpful in managing high-risk patients. Our approach is to use TVS in patients at high risk for preterm birth, in particular those with a history of preterm birth less than 32 weeks' gestation or patients with multifetal gestation. These patients are instructed at length regarding the warning signs and symptoms of PTL. TVS of the cervix is performed between 18 and 20 weeks' gestation. If the cervical length is suspicious (2.0–2.9 cm), the TVS is repeated in 1–2 weeks; the work routine is modified or the patient may be placed on bedrest, depending on the exact length. If the cervical length is less than 2.0 cm, bedrest and/or cerclage are considered.

Patients at high risk for preterm birth can also benefit from progesterone therapy. Studies have demonstrated that treatment of high-risk patients with weekly 17-OH progesterone caproate significantly reduces the recurrence of preterm birth. The treatment regimen is weekly 250 mg intramuscular injections from 18 to 34 weeks' gestation. Treatment with micronized progesterone vaginal suppositories 200 mg twice daily has also been shown to delay delivery in patients with asymptomatic cervical shortening noted on TVS. Progesterone therapy is not effective for patients diagnosed with active PTL. Since fFN cannot be used before 24 weeks of gestation, its principal role is in the assessment of patients who present with preterm contractions, and it is generally not effective as a screening tool.

Suggested reading

Colombo DF, Iams JD. Cervical length and preterm labor. *Clin Obstet Gynecol* 2000; 43(4): 735–745.

Fanaroff AA, Stoll BJ, Wright LL, *et al.*, for the NICHD Neonatal Research Network. Trends in neonatal morbidity and mortality for very low birthweight infants. *Am J Obstet Gynecol* 2007; 196: 147.

Gomez R, Romero R, Medina L, *et al.* Cervicovaginal fibronectin improves the prediction of preterm delivery based on sonographic cervical length in patients with preterm uterine contractions and intact membranes. *Am J Obstet Gynecol* 2005; 192: 350–359.

Guinn DA, Goepfert AR, Owen J, *et al.* Management options in women with preterm uterine contractions: a randomized clinical trial. *Am J Obstet Gynecol* 1997; 177: 814–818.

Matijevic R, Grgic O, Vasili O. Is sonographic assessment of cervical length better than digital examination in screening for preterm delivery in a low-risk population? *Acta Obstet Gynecol Scand* 2006; 85: 1342–1347.

McIntire DD, Leveno KJ. Neonatal mortality and morbidity rates in late preterm births compared with births at term. *Obstet Gynecol* 2008; 111: 35–41.

Chapter 4
Post-Term Pregnancy

Patrick M. Mullin and David A. Miller

Department of Medicine and Obstetrics and Gynecology, Keck School of Medicine, University of Southern California, CA, USA

Introduction

Post-term pregnancy is defined as a gestation that has progressed to 42 completed weeks (294 days) from the first day of the last menstrual period (LMP). Historically, post-term pregnancy has been associated with increased perinatal morbidity and mortality. In 1963, McClure-Browne reported that, compared to term, perinatal mortality doubled after 42 completed weeks, tripled after 43 weeks, and quadrupled after 44 weeks [1]. Reports continue to demonstrate increased perinatal morbidity compared to term, but not a significantly higher rate of perinatal death. This difference probably reflects improvements in prenatal care, assessment of fetal status, and neonatal management. Recent trials indicate that delivery at 41 completed weeks compared with post-term is associated with lower rates of perinatal morbidity and cesarean delivery. Perinatal morbidity in post-term pregnancies is attributable, primarily, to fetal macrosomia, birth trauma, placental insufficiency, oligohydramnios, intrapartum fetal distress, meconium aspiration, and postmaturity syndrome. The rate of labor induction for post-term pregnancy has more than doubled since 1991, making it the most common indication for labor induction [2].

Incidence

The reported incidence of post-term pregnancy is 3–15%, with an average of approximately 10%. This relatively wide range reflects, in part, the difficulty inherent in accurately defining pregnancy dates. The most common criterion used to establish gestational age is the menstrual history. However, numerous reports suggest that menstrual history alone is unreliable. Warsof reported

uncertain menstrual histories in 45% of 4000 pregnancies in a 5-year study [3]. Using the LMP as the sole dating criterion, 11% of pregnancies were considered post term, compared to 6% when pregnancy dates were established by early ultrasound. Among 15,241 pregnancies, Tunon reported a post-term incidence of 10% using menstrual dating criteria compared to 4% using sonographic criteria [4]. Mongelli *et al.* studied 34,249 computer files of singleton pregnancies with "certain" menstrual dates and sonographic biometry [5]. Compared to menstrual history alone, sonographic estimation of dates yielded a 70% reduction in post-term pregnancies. A systematic review of nine trials by Neilson reported similar findings. Routine ultrasound resulted in reduced rates of labor induction for post-term pregnancy [6]. These reports are consistent with the experience of most obstetricians that the menstrual history is unreliable as the sole criterion for pregnancy dating.

Sonographic assessment of gestational age is most precise when performed early in pregnancy. A crown–rump length between 5 and 12 weeks is accurate to within ±5 days (±2 SD). The fetal biparietal diameter is accurate to ±8 days at 12–20 weeks, ±14 days at 20–30 weeks, and ±21 days beyond 30 weeks. The femur length is accurate to ±7 days at 12–20 weeks, ±11 days at 20–30 weeks, and ±16 days beyond 30 weeks. During the late second trimester, the best estimate is obtained from the average of the biparietal diameter, head circumference, abdominal circumference, and femur length. If the estimated gestational age (EGA) by these measurements differs from that derived by the LMP by more than 2 weeks in the second trimester, consideration should be given to recalculating the dates. During the third trimester, sonographic gestational age assessment is of limited use in dating a pregnancy.

Complications

Macrosomia

Macrosomia, defined as a birthweight in excess of 4500 g, has been reported in 2.8–5.4% of post-term infants compared

Management of Common Problems in Obstetrics and Gynecology,
5th edition. Edited by T.M. Goodwin, M.N. Montoro,
L. Muderspach, R. Paulson and S. Roy. © 2010 Blackwell
Publishing Ltd.

to 0.8% of term infants. At any gestational age, fetal macrosomia is associated with increased risks of shoulder dystocia (14% vs 0.3%), birth trauma (11% vs 2%), and cesarean delivery (35% vs 17%).

Oligohydramnios

Oligohydramnios is observed with increased frequency in the post-term gestation. Phelan reported that the amniotic fluid volume, as estimated by the Amniotic Fluid Index, increased steadily in the first half of pregnancy, reaching a plateau of approximately 12 cm during the third trimester [7]. Between 40 and 42 weeks, it declined by as much as 30%. Using dye dilution, Beischer *et al.* demonstrated that the amniotic fluid volume declined by 30% after 42 weeks and by 50% after 43 weeks. The increased morbidity associated with oligohydramnios is well documented. Crowley *et al.* [9] and Leveno *et al.* [10] observed increased incidences of meconium-stained amniotic fluid and cesarean section for fetal distress in association with diminished amniotic fluid volume. Other associations include lower Apgar scores and umbilical artery pH values, and increased rates of fetal distress, cesarean delivery, meconium aspiration syndrome, and umbilical cord compression leading to variable FHR decelerations.

Meconium

Numerous reports have described an increased frequency of meconium passage in post-term pregnancies. The incidence of 25–30% represents a twofold increase over that observed at term. In the presence of diminished amniotic fluid volume, the incidence may be as high as 71%. However, meconium passage alone is not a reliable indicator of intrauterine fetal compromise. In many cases, meconium passage may simply reflect a maturing fetal vagal system. Alternatively, it may reflect stimulation of the vagal system by relatively mild degrees of fetal stress. Even when meconium passage is not secondary to fetal stress or distress, it poses the risk of meconium aspiration syndrome (MAS). The risk is compounded by diminished amniotic fluid volume, resulting in thick, undiluted meconium that is more likely to obstruct the airways. The incidence of MAS in the presence of meconium-stained amniotic fluid is approximately 2–4.5%. Reduction in MAS has been reported following adequate suctioning of the oropharynx prior to the first breath. MAS is encountered most often in high-risk gestations exhibiting abnormal FHR findings, but has been described in the absence of observed fetal distress.

Postmaturity

Approximately 10–20% of post-term fetuses exhibit clinical signs of the "postmaturity" or "dysmaturity" syndrome, including reduced subcutaneous tissue, dry, wrinkled, peeling skin, and meconium staining. Other observations include hypothermia, hypoglycemia, polycythemia, and hyperviscosity. These findings, present in 3% of term infants, are thought to reflect subacute placental insufficiency leading to nutritional deprivation, fetal wasting, decreased fat and glycogen stores, and chronic hypoxemia with compensatory hematopoiesis. Although the late consequences of this disorder are incompletely understood, infants have been reported to regain weight rapidly and exhibit few long-term neurologic sequelae.

Management

In an accurately dated pregnancy, the evidence suggests that a fetus stands to gain nothing by remaining *in utero* beyond 41 weeks. On the contrary, continuing the pregnancy beyond this time exposes the fetus to many potential complications. Therefore, expectant management may be considered a reasonable option only if there is some anticipated benefit to offset the fetal risks. Historically, the major purported benefit of expectant management over induction has been a lower rate of cesarean delivery.

The largest randomized trial evaluating routine induction versus expectant management in post-term pregnancies was reported in 1992 by the Canadian Multicenter Post-term Pregnancy Trial Group [11]. A total of 3418 women were randomized at 41 weeks or later to induction or expectant management. The expectantly managed group had higher rates of intrapartum fetal distress (12.8% vs 10.3%, $p = 0.023$) and meconium staining (28.7% vs 25%, $p = 0.015$); however, there were no significant differences between the groups with respect to 26 other measures of neonatal morbidity. There were two stillbirths in the expectant group and none in the induction group. The cesarean section rate in the expectantly managed group (24.5%) was significantly higher than that in the induction group (21.2%). This difference was attributable primarily to a higher rate of cesarean section for fetal distress in the expectant group (8.3% vs 5.7%, $p = 0.003$). The authors concluded that inducing labor in women with post-term pregnancies resulted in a lower rate of cesarean section and no difference in perinatal outcome.

In 1994, the Network of Maternal–Fetal Medicine Units reported a multicenter trial of labor induction versus expectant management in post-term pregnancy [12]. Four hundred and forty women with uncomplicated pregnancies at 41 weeks' gestation were randomized to expectant management ($n = 175$), induction with intracervical prostaglandin gel, amniotomy and oxytocin ($n = 174$) or induction with intracervical placebo, amniotomy and oxytocin ($n = 91$). Primary outcome variables included perinatal death, maternal death, and perinatal morbidity (neonatal seizures, intracranial hemorrhage, need for mechanical ventilation, brachial plexus or facial nerve injury). Cesarean section rates were similar among the three groups; however, the study was halted due to the low incidence of the primary outcome measures.

More recently, Gülmezoglu *et al.* completed a systematic review of labor induction at or beyond term [13]. The analysis, which included 19 trials and a total of 7984 women, found that a policy of labor induction at 41 weeks or beyond resulted in fewer perinatal deaths (1/2986 versus 9/2953). Rates of cesarean delivery did not differ (RR 0.92, 95% confidence interval (CI) 0.76–1.12; RR 0.97, 95% CI 0.72–1.31) for women induced at 41 and 42 weeks respectively. Limiting the analysis to include women with unfavorable cervical examinations, expectant management yielded three perinatal deaths in 386 pregnancies versus no perinatal deaths in 695 pregnancies induced at or beyond term (RR 0.32, 95% CI 0.05–2.02). Expectant management in women with unfavorable cervical examinations resulted in significantly higher rates of MAS (RR 0.27, 95% CI 0.11–0.68). To date, the literature does not provide convincing evidence that expectant management beyond 41 weeks results in a lower cesarean section rate, even in the setting of an unfavorable cervical examination. Therefore, in an accurately dated pregnancy at or beyond 41 weeks, the increased fetal risks of expectant management and the lack of evidence confirming a benefit favor induction of labor.

Given the limitations of the available data, this approach must be tempered with clinical judgment. For example, the effect of parity has not been evaluated separately in prospective trials. Present data, derived from women of varying parity and cervical status, might not be applicable to a nullipara with a very unfavorable cervix. Such cases require individualized management based upon analysis of the pertinent risks and benefits. Early pregnancy dating is essential to optimal management of the pregnancy. Antepartum surveillance should begin by 40 weeks and cervical status should be assessed frequently. The protocol for the management of pregnancy at or beyond 41 weeks at the University of Southern California is summarized in Box 4.1.

Antepartum surveillance

Antepartum testing at the University of Southern California employs the modified biophysical profile (MBPP) as the primary test and the complete biophysical profile (BPP) as the back-up test. The MBPP utilizes the nonstress test (NST) as a short-term marker of fetal status and the Amniotic Fluid Index (AFI) as a marker of longer-term placental function. Testing is initiated at 40 weeks and is performed twice weekly. In the post-term population, the incidence of fetal death within 1 week of a normal test is approximately 0.9 per 1000 women tested. In a pregnancy

---

Box 4.1 Antepartum management of pregnancy at or beyond 41 weeks

- Establish EDC with best available criteria
- Initiate antepartum fetal surveillance by 40 weeks
- Examine the cervix frequently
- *Reliable dates*: deliver by 41 weeks with few exceptions
- *Unreliable dates*: deliver by 41 weeks if the cervix is favorable
- If expectant management is continued beyond 41 weeks:
  - examine the cervix frequently and deliver if favorable
  - daily fetal movement counts
  - deliver no later than 43 weeks, regardless of cervical status

---

at or beyond 41 weeks, an abnormal antepartum test is an indication for delivery, regardless of cervical status.

Intrapartum management

Intrapartum management should include sonographic estimation of fetal weight and amniotic fluid volume. An estimated fetal weight greater than 4500 g should prompt a frank discussion with the patient regarding the risks associated with macrosomia, including shoulder dystocia and attendant birth trauma. Elective cesarean delivery may be considered. At estimated weights between 4000 and 4500 g, the decision to attempt a vaginal delivery should take into account such factors as obstetric history, clinical pelvimetry, maternal obesity, and diabetes.

In the intrapartum period, there is increased risk for the sequelae of uteroplacental insufficiency, including meconium passage, oligohydramnios, and umbilical cord compression. Therefore, continuous FHR monitoring is recommended. In the presence of oligohydramnios and fetal heart rate abnormalities, intrapartum saline amnioinfusion has been shown to reduce the incidence and severity of variable decelerations as well as the rates of fetal distress, fetal acidemia, and cesarean section for fetal distress. In the absence of fetal heart rate abnormalities, there does not appear to be a benefit of prophylactic amnio-infusion [14]. When meconium staining of the amniotic fluid is observed, amnio-infusion has not been shown to significantly reduce the incidence of meconium aspiration and MAS [15]. Infusion via intrauterine catheter of 250 mL of normal saline should increase the AFI by 4 cm. An AFI of greater than or equal to 10 cm is desirable. Management at delivery should include suctioning of the fetal oropharynx prior to the first breath. In the presence of thick meconium, intubation and suctioning of the airways are often performed immediately after delivery.

Conclusion

The first priority in the management of post-term pregnancy is to confirm the reliability of the dates. The estimated date of confinement (EDC) should be established by the best available criteria.

In women with well-established dates, antepartum testing and weekly cervical examinations should be initiated by 40 weeks. When the MBPP is used, antepartum testing should be performed twice weekly. If fetal surveillance is abnormal or if medical or obstetric complications arise, delivery should be accomplished. With few exceptions, induction should be undertaken if spontaneous labor has not occurred by 42 weeks.

Women with unreliable dating criteria should begin antepartum testing and weekly cervical examinations by 40 weeks, calculated from the best EDC. If the cervix becomes favorable, induction should be undertaken at 41 weeks. If the cervix remains unfavorable beyond 41 weeks, a finite period of expectant management is reasonable.

Regardless of the reliability of the dating criteria, all women not delivered by 41 weeks must be followed closely with antepartum testing and frequent examinations. Daily fetal movement counts are recommended. Delivery should be accomplished if the cervix becomes favorable, antepartum testing is abnormal or suspicious, medical or obstetric indications for delivery arise, or the pregnancy progresses to 42–43 weeks. Beyond 42–43 weeks, the safety of expectant management has not been established.

References

1. McClure-Brown JC. Postmaturity. *Am J Obstet Gynecol* 1963; 85: 573–582.
2. Yawn BP, Wollan P, McKeon K, Field CS. Temporal changes in rates and reasons for medical induction of term labor, 1980–1996. *Am J Obstet Gynecol* 2001; 184(4):611–619.
3. Warsof SL, Pearce JM, Campbell S. The present place of routine ultrasound screening. *Clin Obstet Gynecol* 1983; 10: 445–557.
4. Tunon K, Eik Nes SH, Grottum P. A comparison between ultrasound and a reliable LMP as predictors of the day of delivery in 15,000 examinations. *Ultrasound Obstet Gynecol* 1996; 8: 178–185.
5. Mongelli M, Wilcox M, Gardosi J. Estimating the date of confinement: ultrasonographic biometry versus certain menstrual dates. *Am J Obstet Gynecol* 1996; 174: 278–281.
6. Neilson JP. Ultrasound for fetal assessment in early pregnancy. *Cochrane Database Syst Rev* 2000; 2: CD000182.
7. Phelan JP, Smith CV, Broussard P, Small M. Amniotic fluid volume assessment with four-quadrant technique at 36–42 weeks' gestation. *J Reprod Med* 1987; 32: 540–542.
8. Beischer NA, Brown JB, Townsend L. Studies in prolonged pregnancy. 3. Amniocentesis in prolonged pregnancy. *Am J Obstet Gynecol* 1969; 103(4):496–503.
9. Crowley P, O'Herlihy C, Boylan P. The value of ultrasound measurement of amniotic fluid volume in the management of prolonged pregnancies. *BJOG* 1984; 91: 444–448.
10. Leveno KJ, Quirk JG, Cunningham G, *et al.* Prolonged pregnancy. I. Observations concerning the causes of fetal distress. *Am J Obstet Gynecol* 1984; 150: 465–473.
11. Hannah ME, Hannah WJ, Hellmann J, *et al.*, for the Canadian Multicenter Post-term Pregnancy Trial Group. Induction of labor as compared with serial antenatal monitoring in post-term pregnancy. A randomized controlled trial. *NEJM* 1992; 326: 1587–1592.
12. National Institute of Child Health and Human Development Network of Maternal–Fetal Medicine Units. A clinical trial of induction of labor versus expectant management in post term pregnancy. *Am J Obstet Gynecol* 1994; 170: 716–723.
13. Gülmezoglu AM, Crowther CA, Middleton P. Induction of labour for improving birth outcomes for women at or beyond term. *Cochrane Database Syst Rev* 2006; 4: CD004945.
14. Hofmeyr GJ. Prophylactic versus therapeutic amnioinfusion for oligohydramnios in labour. *Cochrane Database Syst Rev* 2000; 2:CD000176.
15. Xu H, Hofmeyr J, Roy C, Fraser W. Intrapartum amnioinfusion for meconium-stained amniotic fluid: a systematic review of randomised controlled trials. *BJOG* 2007;114(4):383–390.

Suggested reading

American College of Obstetricians and Gynecologists. *Diagnosis and management of post term pregnancy.* ACOG Technical Bulletin no. 130. Washington, DC: American College of Obstetricians and Gynecologists, 1989.

American College of Obstetricians and Gynecologists. *Ultrasonography in pregnancy.* ACOG Technical Bulletin no. 187. Washington, DC: American College of Obstetricians and Gynecologists, 1993.

Hofmeyr GJ. Prophylactic versus therapeutic amnioinfusion for oligohydramnios in labor. *Cochrane Database Syst Rev* 2000; 2: CD000176.

Iams JD, Gabbe SG. Intrauterine growth retardation. In: Iams, JD, Zuspan, FP, Quilligan, EJ (eds) *Manual of obstetrics and gynecology*, 2nd edn. St Louis: Mosby, 1990: 165–172.

Miller DA, Rabello YA, Paul RH. The modified biophysical profile: antepartum testing in the 1990s. *Am J Obstet Gynecol* 1996; 174: 812–817.

Miller FC, Sachs DA, Yeh SY, *et al.* Significance of meconium during labor. *Am J Obstet Gynecol* 1975; 122: 573–580.

Miyazaki FS, Taylor NA. Saline amnioinfusion for relief of variable or prolonged decelerations. A preliminary report. *Am J Obstet Gynecol* 1983; 146: 670–678.

Product information. *Cervidil brand of dinoprostone vaginal insert.* St Louis, MO: Forest Pharmaceuticals, 1995.

Shime J. Influence of prolonged pregnancy on infant development. *J Reprod Med* 1983; 33: 277–284.

Strong TH Jr, Hetzler G, Sarno AP, Paul RH. Prophylactic intrapartum amnioinfusion: a randomized clinical trial. *Am J Obstet Gynecol* 1990; 162: 1374–1375.

Xu H, Hofmeyr J, Roy C, *et al.* Intrapartum amnioinfusion for meconium-stained amniotic fluid: a systematic review of randomized controlled trials. *BJOG* 2007; 114(4): 383–390.

Yawn BP, Wollan, P, McKeon K, *et al.* Temporal changes in rates and reasons for medical induction of term labor, 1980–1996. *Am J Obstet Gynecol* 2001; 184: 611–619.

Chapter 5
Multiple Gestations

Ramen H. Chmait

Department of Medicine and Obstetrics and Gynecology, Keck School of Medicine, University of Southern California, CA, USA

Introduction

The rate of multiple gestations in the United States is rising dramatically. This is of concern because multiple gestations contribute disproportionately to the incidence of perinatal morbidity and mortality. Fortunately, recent advances in perinatal medicine have resulted in improved overall outcomes in pregnancies complicated by multiple gestations.

Chorionicity

The fetus develops within the amniotic sac, which consists of two fetal membranes called the chorion and the amnion. The outer layer, which is in closer proximity to the mother, is the chorion. A segment of the chorion contains the chorionic villi, which invade the uterine decidua to eventually form the placenta. The villi in the remaining chorion undergo atrophy, thus forming the smooth opaque outer layer of the fetal membranes. The inner layer of the fetal membranes is the translucent amnion. In the case of twins, dichorionic twins have entirely separate placentas and fetal membranes, while monochorionic twins share the same placenta.

Multiple gestations should be classified based on chorionicity (Figure 5.1). Chorionicity can be diagnosed in the first or early second trimester with over 95% accuracy by ultrasound evaluation of the dividing membranes' insertion site. Dividing membranes are defined as the portion of the fetal membranes in which the two separate twin gestational sacs are in contact. All twins, except monochorionic monoamniotic twins, have dividing membranes. In the case of dichorionicity, the dividing membranes have intervening chorion, thereby forming a "twin peak" or "lambda" sign at the junction between the two placentas. In the case of

monochorionic diamniotic twins, the dividing membrane is composed of only two abutting amnions. Thus, the dividing membranes of a monochorionic placenta are thin and insert perpendicularly into the placenta in the so-called "T" sign.

It is important that chorionicity be established as early in pregnancy as possible. Aside from gender discordance, which would confirm dichorionicity, all ultrasound markers of chorionicity become less accurate as the pregnancy progresses. Ultrasound views of the dividing membranes' insertion site are hampered in the latter half of pregnancy. Also, the placentas in a dichorionic twin gestation often adjoin one another, appearing as one placental mass, in the late second and third trimester.

Clinical significance of monochorionicity

Monochorionic twins are associated with significant increased perinatal morbidity and mortality as compared to dichorionic twins and singletons. One factor associated with this increased risk is the presence of vascular communications in the shared placenta. The vascular communications are important in the development of twin–twin transfusion syndrome and twin reverse arterial perfusion sequence, both of which have high perinatal mortality rates. Also, because the circulatory systems of the twins are linked together by the vascular anastomoses, the death of one twin may lead to an immediate hypotensive episode in the live twin due to exsanguination into the dead twin. The acute hemodynamic instability may result in death or injury to the co-twin. Another placental factor that contributes to the disproportionate rate of perinatal complications in monochorionic twins is unequal partitioning of the single placental mass, which may manifest clinically as selective intrauterine growth restriction. Finally, the risk of structural or chromosomal anomalies is increased in monochorionic twins. Anomalies of the central nervous system, heart, gastrointestinal tract and anterior abdominal wall occur at a higher rate in monochorionic twins as compared to dichorionic twins and

Management of Common Problems in Obstetrics and Gynecology, 5th edition. Edited by T.M. Goodwin, M.N. Montoro, L. Muderspach, R. Paulson and S. Roy. © 2010 Blackwell Publishing Ltd.

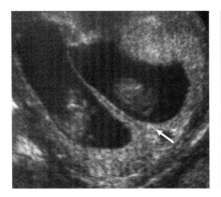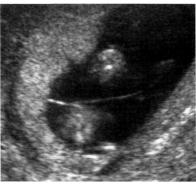

Figure 5.1 First trimester ultrasound of dichorionic twins (left) and monochorionic twins (right). The image on the left shows the "twin peak" sign (arrow), which is indicative of dichorionic twins. The image on the right shows a thin dividing membrane inserting into the common placenta, called a "T sign", which is an ultrasound marker for monochorionic twins.

singletons. Despite being monozygotic, the rate of discordance in anomalies between monochorionic twins may reach 80%, meaning that only one "identical" twin may have a structural abnormality.

Zygosity

A zygote is a cell that results from fertilization of an ovum and a sperm. Dizygotic twins result from fertilization of two separate ova by two separate sperm. The twins are genetically distinct, with as much commonality as ordinary siblings. The two zygotes each develop their own placentas and surrounding membranes, resulting in dichorionic diamniotic twins.

Monozygotic twinning results from a "split" of a single zygote into two or more embryos. The etiology of this division is unknown, although some view it as an anomalous embryonic event. The timing of the division determines both the chorionicity and amnionicity. Division within 3 days of fertilization results in the development of a dichorionic diamniotic twin gestation because the division occurred prior to the differentiation of the chorion. Approximately 30% of monozygotic twins are dichorionic diamniotic. If the division occurs between days 4 and 8 after fertilization, monochorionic diamniotic twin gestation develops. In this case, the twinning happens after differentiation of the chorion but before differentiation of the amnion. Monochorionic diamniotic twins make up almost 70% of monozygotic twins. A monochorionic monoamniotic twin gestation results from division after day 9 from fertilization, after the differentiation of the amnion; this occurs in about 1% of monozygotic twins. Incomplete embryonic division occurs after day 13, resulting in the rare condition of conjoined twins. Although monozygotic twins typically have an identical genetic make-up, genetic and/or phenotypic discordance can arise due to postzygotic perturbations.

Zygosity testing is feasible during pregnancy. One method is via DNA testing of amniocytes (fetal cells suspended in amniotic fluid) using PCR to identify discordance between variable number tandem repeats and other polymorphisms. However, aside from rare uses in prenatal diagnosis of genetic diseases, zygosity testing is not often utilized during pregnancy. As already mentioned, it is primarily the chorionicity, not zygosity, which determines the risks of the pregnancy.

Epidemiology

The incidence of twins and higher order multiples has been increasing significantly in the past few decades. Twinning occurs naturally in approximately 1.3% of all pregnancies in the US. However, in the past decade the rate of twins has increased to 3–4% of all pregnancies. The rate of triplets and high-order multiples has increased by over 400%. The increase in multiples is attributed mostly to infertility therapy, although other factors such as advanced maternal age may also independently contribute to the current multiple gestation epidemic. The vast majority of these additional multiple gestations are dizygotic, thus dichorionic. The rate of monochorionic twins is relatively constant at approximately 0.4% of all pregnancies. There has been a small but measurable increase in the rate of monochorionic twins attributed to assisted reproductive technology.

Diagnosis

The ubiquitous use of ultrasound during pregnancy has resulted in a nearly 100% rate of identification of multiples prior to birth. However, caution is advised when multiple gestations are detected very early in gestation because of the possibility of spontaneous loss of one twin, the so-called "vanishing twin" syndrome. Based on early sonographic examinations, there appears to be an attrition rate of about 36% in twin conceptions prior to 7 weeks' gestation. Ultrasound is also critical to determine chorionicity, which is then used to triage the pregnancy to differing levels of surveillance. Factors that would prompt an ultrasound to identify multiples include increased levels of analytes in the maternal serum biochemical tests, such as chorionic gonadotropin and α-fetoprotein, more than one fetal heart rate identified on Doppler auscultation, and increased fundal height on physical examination.

Perinatal complications

Multiple gestation is a risk factor for several pregnancy-related complications. Compared to singletons, the risk of pre-eclampsia is increased approximately twofold in twins and three- to fourfold in triplets. An interesting observation is that the spontaneous demise of one fetus in a multiple gestation has resulted in resolution or amelioration of the pre-eclampsia. The diagnosis and management of pre-eclampsia in multiple gestations are akin to those of singletons. Multiple gestations also increase the risk of acute fatty liver, thromboembolism, maternal anemia, gestational diabetes, and urinary tract infections.

Preterm birth represents the single most important factor in the increased perinatal morbidity and mortality risk of multiple gestations. The risk of prematurity increases with the number of fetuses. The mean gestational age at delivery is approximately 35.5 weeks in twins and 32.0 weeks in triplets, with approximately 10% of twins and 25% of triplets delivering before 32 weeks' gestation. In appropriately grown multiples, the perinatal morbidity and mortality rates are akin to gestational age-matched singletons. Unfortunately, there is no efficacious treatment to prevent preterm labor in multiple gestations. Oral or subcutaneous prophylactic tocolysis, continuous or periodic home uterine activity monitoring, prophylactic cervical cerclage, and progesterone therapy have not been shown to be of benefit and are not recommended at this time.

Monochorionic twins are associated with unique complications. One condition with a high perinatal mortality rate is twin–twin transfusion syndrome (TTTS), which develops in 10–15% of monochorionic twins due to unbalanced sharing of blood through vascular communications in the shared placenta. Blood from one twin, referred to as the "donor," is preferentially shunted through the vascular anastomoses to the second twin, referred to as the "recipient." The donor twin develops anuria and oligohydramnios, while the recipient twin has polyuria and polyhydramnios. TTTS is diagnosed by noting on ultrasound a single maximum vertical pocket of amniotic fluid of 2 cm or less on one side of the dividing membranes and greater than or equal to 8 cm on the other side. Significant improvement in perinatal outcomes has been reported using various fetal interventions. Recent studies have shown favorable outcomes after operative fetoscopic-guided laser ablation of the vascular communications. The treatment options for TTTS are reviewed in detail in Chapter 49.

Monochorionic twins are associated with an increased risk of anomalies, most of which are discordant, i.e.

occurring in only one of the twins. A discordant anomaly unique to monochorionic twins is twin reversed arterial perfusion (TRAP) sequence. In this condition, one fetus (often called the "acardiac" twin) is supplied with blood in a reversed fashion. This leads to severe maldevelopment of cephalic, thoracic, and upper extremity structures, and results in a condition that is not compatible with life outside the womb for that fetus. Because the heart of the other fetus (often called the "pump" twin) must pump blood for both fetuses, there is a 50–75% risk of heart failure and demise in the pump twin, particularly if the acardiac mass is relatively large. In the presence of pump twin heart failure or a large acardiac twin, fetoscopic umbilical cord occlusion of the acardiac fetus has been shown to improve perinatal outcomes in the pump twin.

Although growth abnormalities are relatively common in all types of twins, poor fetal growth is more prevalent in one of a monochorionic twin pair and poses a significant clinical dilemma. In this condition of selective intrauterine growth restriction (SIUGR), one twin measures less than the 10th percentile for the given gestational age. SIUGR appears to be a distinct condition from TTTS, although there may be overlap in some cases. The SIUGR fetus is at relatively high risk of spontaneous intrauterine demise, which may result in concomitant demise or severe neurologic handicap to the co-twin. Treatment of this condition is clinically challenging, as standard treatment requires attempting to time delivery prior to the demise of the SIUGR fetus.

Monochorionic monoamniotic twins occur in approximately 1% of monozygotic gestations. In this condition, the twins share the same placenta and amniotic sac. This can lead to umbilical cord entanglement in approximately two-thirds of cases. The perinatal mortality rate has historically been very high due to cord strangulation, but that risk has decreased substantially with intensive fetal heart rate monitoring in the third trimester and elective cesarean section at approximately 34 weeks' gestation.

Conjoined twinning is a rare condition that occurs when the embryonic disk fails to divide completely. The twins may be joined at various sites, and it is the shared anatomy that is used to classify conjoined twins. Management usually entails elective cesarean section, with subsequent surgical separation by a co-ordinated multidisciplinary surgical team.

Antepartum management

The antenatal course of multiple gestations is more likely to be encumbered by complications than are singleton gestations. Thus, one of the primary goals in antenatal management is the prevention and early identification of complications. The first step in management of a pregnancy complicated by multiple gestations is to establish the chorionicity. First- and early second-trimester ultrasound is highly accurate in determining chorionicity, and should be performed to allow for appropriate triage and management of the pregnancy.

There are no standardized recommendations for the ultrasound surveillance required in multiple gestations. In monochorionic twins, we suggest ultrasound be performed at least once every 2 weeks in the second and early third trimester to monitor amniotic fluid volumes and cervical length. Fetal growth should be assessed every 3 or 5 weeks thereafter. Special attention is given to the evaluation for ultrasound evidence of TTTS, TRAP sequence, and SIUGR. If the pregnancy is dichorionic, then a single scan in the mid-trimester to assess fetal anatomy and cervical length, followed by growth scans every 6 weeks, is recommended. If one of the perinatal complications described previously is suspected, then the frequency of ultrasound should be adjusted accordingly.

Important considerations should be borne in mind regarding prenatal diagnosis and genetic counseling in pregnancies with multiple gestations. First, maternal serum biochemical testing for aneuploidy and neural tube defects is not as accurate in multiple gestations compared to singletons. Second, the risk of aneuploidy is increased in dizygotic twins because each fetus has an independent risk for chromosomal abnormality. This is not the case in monozygotic twins which theoretically are genetically identical, although there are rare cases of discordant genetic make-up due to postzygotic nondisjunction. Third, invasive genetic testing poses unique challenges. Genetic amniocentesis is complicated by the need to sample both amniotic sacs. The amniocentesis is performed under direct ultrasound guidance, aspirating 15–20 mL from one sac, followed by instillation of 2 mL of 0.1% indigo carmine dye. A second amniocentesis is then performed on the second sac and its success is verified by the absence of a blue color in the fluid. Chorionic villus sampling can also be performed in twins, although as many as 4% of specimens may contain tissue from the co-twin.

Ongoing fetal evaluation is an integral part of antenatal care. The frequency of routine prenatal visits is increased to every 3 weeks until 28 weeks, then every 2 weeks until 34 weeks, followed by weekly visits until delivery. Increased prenatal visits are instituted in the case of multiple gestations with the goal that maternal complications such as pre-eclampsia, gestational diabetes, and urinary tract infections will be diagnosed and managed in a timely fashion. The NST combined with ultrasonographic evaluation of the fetal status (amniotic fluid volume or full biophysical profile) are the best indicators of fetal status. The same criteria for assessing fetal well-being by NST apply to twin gestations as to singletons. In general, the NST is initiated at 34 weeks' gestation.

The increased metabolic burden of multiples on the mother requires that she increase caloric intake by at least 300 kcal per day. Because of the increased risk of maternal anemia, at least 60 mg of elemental iron and 1 mg of folic acid supplementation are provided.

Intrapartum management

Spontaneous labor occurs earlier on average in multiple gestations than in singleton pregnancies and its onset is inversely proportional to the number of fetuses present. Multiple gestations should not continue past 40 completed weeks of gestation and it is our practice to recommend delivery by 38 weeks. Patients presenting in labor or for induction of labor should have an ultrasonographic examination to document the fetal positions. Pharmacologic labor induction and augmentation in twin gestation is not contraindicated and follows the same guidelines as in singleton gestations.

Intrapartum electronic fetal heart rate monitoring is essential in the management of labor of multiple gestations. Both fetuses should be simultaneously monitored and the same criteria applied to interpretation of the FHR pattern as with singletons. Difficulty arises in situations where only the second fetus demonstrates an abnormal pattern and cannot be further evaluated. If no assurance of fetal well-being can be obtained, prompt delivery is advised.

The route of delivery depends on the presentation, estimation of birthweights, experience of the obstetrician, and compliance of the patient. In the majority of situations the first twin will present by the vertex and a trial of vaginal delivery may be attempted in some cases. When both twins present vertex, a trial of vaginal delivery may be attempted regardless of the estimated fetal weights. In situations where presentation of the second twin is not vertex and its estimated fetal weight is greater than 2000 g, a trial of vaginal delivery may be undertaken with either external or internal version of the second twin after delivery of the first. Hazards of this routine involve relative inexperience of the obstetrician, lack of patient acceptance, and lack of immediate surgical back-up. In cases of a nonvertex second twin with estimated fetal weight less than 2000 g, cesarean section has been advocated to prevent increased morbidity and mortality of vaginally delivered breech fetuses in this weight range. There is little information on the safety of external cephalic version in this setting.

Cesarean section is advised in the circumstance of first twins presenting other than vertex regardless of second twin presentation and in cases of monoamniotic and conjoined twin gestations. It should be noted that cesarean section may, on occasion, be required for delivery of second twins only, most commonly as a result of fetal distress. The same criteria of cesarean section for documented fetal distress or failure to progress in labor are applied to remaining second twins as would be applied to singleton gestations. Exceptions can be made when there is an ability to perform a prompt, atraumatic delivery through the fully dilated cervix. Judicious augmentation of labor for second twins is often useful, since a period of relative uterine dysfunction sometimes occurs after delivery of the first twin. Decisions on cesarean sections in twin gestations should be tempered with reasonable estimates of fetal survivability.

Suggested reading

Benirschke K, Masliah E. The placenta in multiple pregnancy: outstanding issues. *Reprod Fertil Dev* 2001; 13(7–8): 615–622.

Dube J, Dodds L, Armson BA. Does chorionicity or zygosity predict adverse perinatal outcomes in twins? *Am J Obstet Gynecol* 2002; 186(3): 579–583.

Heyborne KD, Porreco RP, Garite TJ, Phair K, Abril D. Improved perinatal survival of monoamniotic twins with intensive inpatient monitoring. *Am J Obstet Gynecol* 2005; 192(1): 96–101.

Ong SS, Zamora J, Khan KS, Kilby MD. Prognosis for the co-twin following single-twin death: a systematic review. *BJOG* 2006; 113(9): 992–998.

Quintero R, Morales W, Allen M, Bornick P, Johnson P, Krueger M. Staging of twin–twin transfusion syndrome. *J Perinatol* 1999; 19: 550–555.

Quintero RA, Chmait RH, Murakoshi T, *et al.* Surgical management of twin reversed arterial perfusion sequence. *Am J Obstet Gynecol* 2006; 194(4): 982–991.

Russell RB, Petrini JR, Damus K, Mattison DR, Schwarz RH. The changing epidemiology of multiple births in the United States. *Obstet Gynecol* 2003; 101(1): 129–135.

Shetty A, Smith AP. The sonographic diagnosis of chorionicity. *Prenat Diagn* 2005; 25(9): 735–739.

Chapter 6
Fetal Growth Restriction

Patrick M. Mullin and Marc H. Incerpi
Department of Medicine and Obstetrics and Gynecology, Keck School of Medicine, University of Southern California, CA, USA

Introduction

Abnormalities of fetal growth represent a significant complication of pregnancy. Perinatal mortality for growth-restricted infants is 6–10 times greater than for normally grown infants, and fetal growth restriction (FGR) is the second leading contributor to the perinatal mortality rate. Intrapartum asphyxia in the presence of FGR has been reported to be as high as 50%. Moreover, up to 30% of stillbirths are growth restricted. Recent data suggest long-term morbidity with reduction in both physical and mental development in children affected by FGR when compared with normal controls. In addition, underlying placental dysfunction predisposes these infants to the sequelae of asphyxia, including hypoxic encephalopathy, congestive heart failure, necrotizing enterocolitis, intracranial hemorrhage, and persistent fetal circulation. Metabolic derangements such as hypoglycemia, hypocalcemia, and polycythemia are also common in newborns with FGR.

Definition

The term FGR was created for fetuses with predicted weight below the 10th percentile for a given gestational age. The original standards for fetal growth were based on work carried out by Lubchenco *et al.* in Denver [1]. Subsequent studies undertaken in differing populations have produced newer adjusted growth curves. In contrast to FGR, which refers to abnormal growth, small for gestational age (SGA) is a quantitative description of infants with birthweights below the 10th percentile, including those who are constitutionally small. Since fetuses that are SGA are not necessarily growth restricted,

Management of Common Problems in Obstetrics and Gynecology, 5th edition. Edited by T.M. Goodwin, M.N. Montoro, L. Muderspach, R. Paulson and S. Roy. © 2010 Blackwell Publishing Ltd.

a more exact definition of FGR is a fetus that fails to reach its growth potential, and is therefore at risk for adverse perinatal morbidity and/or mortality.

Etiology

Fetal growth restriction is a syndrome with various etiologies. The risk factors for FGR can be separated into fetal, placental, and maternal origins. Growth restriction is classified as symmetric or asymmetric ("head sparing"). Early fetal insult or intrinsic abnormalities resulting in a reduction in fetal cell number produce symmetric growth restriction. Asymmetric growth restriction is thought to result from an inadequate transfer of nutrients and oxygen to the fetus, which evolves over the course of the pregnancy. Therefore, asymmetric FGR manifests later in gestation. "Head sparing" develops when the fetus responds to a limited nutritional source by selectively supporting the brain and vital organs as well as minimizing growth and activity to reduce metabolic demands.

Fetal

Intrauterine infection has long been associated with FGR. Although it probably accounts for less than 10% of all cases, infectious agents can produce disruption of cell growth, potentially resulting in significant residual deficits. The children have a higher incidence of mental deficiencies and are less likely to have normal growth in childhood. Herpes, cytomegalovirus, rubella, and toxoplasmosis have all been demonstrated to produce growth restriction. Similarly, many chromosomal abnormalities such as trisomies 13, 18 and 21 and malformation syndromes result in a reduced cell number which leads to early onset of growth impairment.

A more common cause of FGR is multifetal gestation. Approximately 20% of these pregnancies are complicated by impaired growth of one or more fetuses. The most common reasons for FGR in these cases are the relative decrease in placental mass, abnormal placentation, and placental vascular anastomoses. In twin pregnancies, fetal growth begins to decrease, relative to singletons, at approximately 32 weeks, and FGR is the second most likely cause of morbidity after prematurity.

Placental

Decreases in the functional mass of the placenta can compromise fetal growth by limiting the transfer of necessary nutrients. Growth restriction has also been described in pregnancies in which there is placental mosaicism, meaning the placenta is made up of both normal and aneuploid cell lines. Abnormal placentations such as circumvallate placenta, partial placental abruption or infarction, placenta previa or placenta accreta can result in FGR. Hemangiomas or other placental tumors can also shunt substrate away from the fetus and restrict growth. Other umbilical–vascular abnormalities associated with FGR include single umbilical artery and velamentous cord insertion. Studies have found that women with an unexplained elevation in maternal serum α-fetoprotein or human chorionic gonadotropin in the second trimester have an increased risk of having a fetus with FGR. This may be explained by abnormal placentation.

Maternal

Poor nutrition and poor weight gain have both been associated with FGR. While the severity of nutritional restriction necessary to produce reduction in fetal size is unclear, pregnant women living in famine conditions produce smaller infants. However, women with limited gastrointestinal absorption secondary to diseases such as ulcerative colitis or Crohn's disease have not been reported to have a significantly greater risk of FGR. Even patients who have undergone ileojejunal bypass for weight control produce infants which, although smaller than average, do not fall below the 10th percentile.

Maternal ingestion of teratogenic medications can also adversely affect fetal growth. Both therapeutic medication (anticonvulsants, coumarin) and illicit drugs (narcotics, cocaine) have been associated with poor fetal weight gain.

Alcohol has a linear dose-related association with impaired fetal growth, and up to 30% of fetuses of heavy drinkers (five or more drinks per day) will display features of fetal alcohol syndrome. Tobacco has long been documented to impair fetal growth. This may be due to chronic fetal hypoxia, since the decrement in fetal size is directly proportional to the number of cigarettes smoked. Nicotine alone is not associated with FGR.

Maternal vascular diseases, such as those found with chronic hypertension, diabetes or collagen vascular disorders (systemic lupus erythematosus, antiphospholipid antibody syndrome), all predispose to FGR. Vascular disease reduces uteroplacental blood flow and transfer of nutrients to the fetus. Pre-eclampsia is associated with abnormal trophoblastic invasion of maternal spiral arterioles, which ultimately results in luminal narrowing and diminished placental blood flow. Sickle cell disease is also associated with FGR, because of local hypoxia secondary to poor uterine perfusion rather than maternal hypoxemia.

Finally, conditions in which there is chronic maternal hypoxia (cyanotic heart disease, pulmonary disease, and high altitude) or maternal anemia reducing oxygen transfer to the fetus are risk factors for compromised fetal growth.

Diagnosis

Identification of patients at high risk of developing IUGR begins with a thorough history. Social history, dietary habits, use of medication, as well as history of infectious symptomatology during the pregnancy, are important. Elucidation of the previous obstetric history, with particular reference to birthweights, gestational ages, and neonatal development, is also essential as the history of a previous infant with FGR is the strongest predictor for delivery of an affected infant.

An accurate determination of the gestational age of the pregnancy is an important initial step in the diagnosis of growth restriction. Sonographic assessment of gestational age is most precise when performed early in pregnancy. A crown–rump length between 5 and 12 weeks is accurate to within ±5 days (±2 SD). During the second trimester, the best estimate is obtained from the average of the biparietal diameter, head circumference, abdominal circumference, and femur length. If the estimated gestational age (EGA) by these measurements differs from that derived by the LMP by more than 2 weeks, consideration should be given to recalculating the dates. During the third trimester, sonographic gestational age assessment is of limited use in dating a pregnancy. Serial ultrasounds at 3-week intervals can be used in an attempt to establish an estimated due date.

The physical examination is also vital in any investigation of FGR. However, studies have produced conflicting results on the effectiveness in detecting growth restriction. Belizan *et al.* were able to identify 86% of SGA fetuses in gestations with a 4 cm or greater lag in expected fundal height [2]. Other authors have found fundal height to be a poor predictor of IUGR, with sensitivities in the range of 30–40%. Therefore, when there is clinical suspicion of FGR, ultrasound is the best modality to evaluate fetal size.

Ultrasound estimation of fetal weight is calculated from measured fetal head, abdomen and femur dimensions. The cumulative error present can be significant. Furthermore, these measurements are compared to cross-sectional birthweight data that have limited accuracy secondary to the prevalence of FGR in prematurely delivered fetuses. Therefore, the best approach is to plot each measured fetal value on a standard growth curve. Sequential ultrasound evaluations should be similarly plotted so that growth trends can be assessed.

Abdominal circumference (AC) is the single most important measurement to use in serial evaluation. Eighty percent of the explained variance in fetal weight prediction models is due to the AC measurement and studies have shown that estimated fetal weight based on AC alone is almost always within 10% of actual birthweight. The liver composes the largest portion of the cross-sectional area that is used to calculate the AC, and reduced glycogen stores in a nutritionally deprived fetus result in a smaller abdominal size. Most importantly, the AC should also be examined in proportion to other fetal measurements to control for questionable pregnancy dating criteria.

Comparison of the AC to head circumference (HC) or femur length (FL) can also be used to decrease false-negative results, as these measurements should be relatively spared in asymmetric FGR. The HC/AC ratio should exceed 1.0 prior to 32 weeks of gestation, reach 1.0 at 32–34 weeks, and fall below 1.0 from 34 weeks onward. When a fetus has asymmetric FGR, the disproportionate decrease in AC will result in an increased HC/AC ratio for gestational age. Similarly, FL is unaffected in asymmetric FGR and a ratio greater than 23.5 after the 21st week of gestation is suggestive of FGR. Importantly, serial measurements taken at least 2 weeks apart are necessary to determine interval growth. This is critical because growth restriction should be considered if the growth curve of the fetus does not maintain an upward slope, even if the measurements are still within the normal percentile range. If the interval growth continues at a constant rate the fetus is probably growing normally.

Ultrasound also provides an assessment of amniotic fluid. Oligohydramnios can precede and can be an indicator of early changes in pregnancies complicated by poor fetal growth. Studies have indicated that the smaller the fluid pocket, the greater the risk of FGR and perinatal morbidity. A normal amniotic fluid volume, on the other hand, does not eliminate the possibility of FGR.

Doppler evaluation of the uterine artery has been investigated as a screening tool for pregnancies at risk of developing FGR. Blood flow at the end of diastole typically increases as the gestational age of the pregnancy increases. Failure of normal trophoblastic invasion can result in increased placental vascular resistance, leading to an increased risk of growth restriction. The associated uterine artery Doppler findings have been reported as decreased end-diastolic flow and/or a "notch" noted at the end of systole.

Management

Management of symmetric FGR should begin with a detailed ultrasound evaluation for fetal malformations.

Consideration should also be given to amniocentesis or percutaneous fetal blood sampling to detect chromosomal abnormalities and/or infectious etiologies. This is most important in very early-onset FGR where a genetic abnormality or infection is more likely.

Management of asymmetric FGR is contingent on the gestational age at diagnosis. If the patient is at or near term, then delivery is probably indicated. If oligohydramnios is present at 34 weeks of gestation or greater, delivery is warranted. However, if the amniotic fluid volume is normal, antepartum testing is reassuring, and if the fetus is still showing interval growth then delivery may be delayed to 37 weeks or until fetal lung maturity is documented by amniocentesis. With either type of FGR, some authors recommend screening for toxoplasmosis, rubella, syphilis, cytomegalovirus, herpes, and other viral illnesses, but these studies have a low yield and probably add little to the management.

If the diagnosis is made prior to 34 weeks and oligohydramnios is not present, antepartum surveillance should be initiated. Ultrasound should be repeated every 2–3 weeks to assess interval growth and AFI. Poor or absent interval growth should suggest the need for delivery. Antepartum FHR testing with AFI assessment ("modified biophysical profile") should begin either at the time of diagnosis or at viability and continue for the duration of the pregnancy every 3–4 days. Spontaneous variable decelerations during testing suggest oligohydramnios with cord compression. This finding is associated with a higher perinatal mortality rate. A nonreactive NST has a high false-positive rate and should be further evaluated with a BPP. This is especially important in immature fetuses where morbidity secondary to premature delivery can result. Additionally, maternal assessment of fetal activity can aid in optimizing pregnancy outcome.

Doppler ultrasonography has been used as an adjunct in the diagnosis and management of FGR. The assessment of umbilical cord blood flow is based on the premise that in cases of increased placental vascular resistance, low-pressure flow during fetal cardiac diastole decreases, producing an increased systolic to diastolic blood flow ratio (S/D ratio) and an increased Pulsatility Index (PI). The low sensitivity (15–30%) seen with the use of Doppler velocimetry as a predictor of FGR in a normal population precludes its use as a screening test. Although there is no consensus on the management of pregnancies with slightly abnormal S/D ratios, if absent or reversed flow is present intervention is often necessary. Reversed end-diastolic flow is indicative of severe fetal compromise and is associated with a perinatal mortality rate of 50–64%. This finding is an indication for immediate delivery. Absent end-diastolic flow, although also associated with both acute and chronic hypoxia, has been reported to improve with bedrest and may not progress to reversal for days to weeks. Depending on the gestational age, these pregnancies may be managed with either delivery or intensive fetal monitoring with delivery for worsening fetal status.

More recent studies have investigated the Doppler assessment of fetal cerebral blood flow. In a growth-restricted fetus, blood flow is redistributed to more essential areas such as the heart, adrenal glands, and brain. While the fetal cerebral vessels are normally an area of low impedance, additional lowering of vascular resistance permits the redirection of blood flow in pregnancies complicated by FGR. Doppler evaluation of the middle cerebral arteries detects this lowered impedance as a decrease in the PI.

Doppler assessment of the fetal venous circulation has also been described. Absent or reversed ductus venosus blood flow during atrial systole of the fetal cardiac cycle has been identified as an ominous finding and provides additional evidence for delivery. The temporal relationship of the Doppler flow findings associated with FGR has been reported as a progression of abnormal flow noted initially in the umbilical artery, followed by the middle cerebral artery, and ultimately in the ductus venosus.

Several therapies have been investigated. Since FGR and its associated placental dysfunction have vascular disease as the underlying cause, vasodilators and antiplatelet medications have been proposed as possible treatments. Wallenberg & Rotmans in 1987 produced significant reductions in FGR with the use of aspirin and dipyridamole [3]. In 1991, the Essai Pre-eclampsia Dipyridamole Aspirin (EPREDA) trial also found lower rates of FGR, stillbirth, and abruption with the use of aspirin [4]. However, the Collaborative Low-dose Aspirin Study in Pregnancy (CLASP) trial in 1994 [5], as well as the Italian Study of Aspirin in Pregnancy in 1991 [6], did not find any improvement in these factors with the administration of low-dose aspirin. These more recent studies do not support the use of therapeutic aspirin in the treatment of FGR.

Maternal hyperoxygenation has also been attempted as a means to improve outcome. Nicolaides has shown that administration of O_2 via a facemask prolonged pregnancy and improved neonatal blood gases, but other neonatal indices were unimproved or worsened [7]. Since several other studies have confirmed that maternal hyperoxygenation allowed for safe short-term prolongation of these pregnancies, it may be a viable option for pregnancies extremely remote from term or to allow time for the administration of corticosteroids.

Delivery

Growth-restricted fetuses are at high risk of intrapartum asphyxia and should have continuous FHR monitoring. Pre-existing compromise in placental function can worsen during labor, and oligohydramnios can precipitate

cord compression and heart rate decelerations. *In utero* meconium passage is likely secondary to hypoxia and may necessitate amnio-infusion if associated with FHR abnormalities. Cesarean delivery is also more common in this group because of abnormal fetal heart tracings, increased rate of breech presentation, and unfavorable cervices in preterm gestations. Because of the increased risk for these complications, a neonatal resuscitation team should be present at the time of delivery.

Neonatal outcome

The immediate neonatal period is a time of great risk for the FGR infant. Because of intrauterine malnutrition, stores of glycogen and fat are low, leading to hypoglycemia and poor neonatal temperature control. Hypocalcemia, probably due to relative hypoparathyroidism, is also common and may present as a jittery infant or as neonatal convulsions. Polycythemia and increased blood viscosity may cause sludging in capillaries, predisposing to thrombosis and pulmonary hypertension, cerebral infarction, and necrotizing enterocolitis. Red cell destruction results in a high incidence of hyperbilirubinemia as well. Long-term prognosis for these infants is still unknown, but FGR has been linked to various long-term complications such as developmental delay, lagging growth, and neurologic sequelae. In addition, it may predispose to diseases of adulthood including cardiovascular disease, obesity, non-insulin-dependent diabetes mellitus, and hyperlipidemia.

Conclusion

Growth restriction remains a major complication of pregnancy. Once the diagnosis is made, antepartum testing consisting of an NST with an AFI or a BPP, maternal fetal activity charting, and serial ultrasounds to assess fetal growth and Doppler velocimetry should be instituted to minimize perinatal morbidity and mortality. Delivery should be undertaken for worsening fetal status or fetal maturity. Even with optimal antepartum care, these infants are susceptible to complications in the nursery as well as long-term sequelae.

References

1. Lubchenco LO, Hansman C, Boyd E. Intrauterine growth in length and head circumference as estimated from live births at gestational ages from 26 to 42 weeks. *Pediatrics* 1966; 37: 403–408.
2. Belizan JM, Villar J, Nardin JC, *et al.* Diagnosis of intrauterine growth retardation by a simple clinical method: measurement of uterine height. *Am J Obstet Gynecol* 1978; 131: 643–646.
3. Wallenberg HC, Rotmans N. Prevention of recurrent idiopathic growth retardation by low-dose aspirin and dipyridamole. *Am J Obstet Gynecol* 1987; 157: 1230–1235.

4. Uzan S, Beaufils M, Breart G, *et al.* Prevention of fetal growth retardation with low-dose aspirin: findings of the EPREDA trial. *Lancet* 1991; 337: 1427–1431.

5. Collaborative Low-dose Aspirin Study in Pregnancy. A randomized trial of low-dose aspirin for the prevention and treatment of preeclampsia among 9364 pregnant women. *Lancet* 1994; 343: 619–629.

6. Italian Study of Aspirin in Pregnancy. Low-dose aspirin in prevention and treatment of intrauterine growth retardation and pregnancy-induced hypertension. *Lancet* 1993; 341: 396–400.

7. Nicolaides KH, Bradley RJ, Soothill PW, *et al.* Maternal oxygen therapy for intrauterine growth retardation. *Lancet* 1987; 1: 942–945.

Suggested reading

Alexander GR, Himes JH, Kaufman RB, *et al.* A United States national reference for fetal growth. *Obstet Gynecol* 1996; 87: 163–168.

Baschat AA, Gembruch U, Weiner CP, *et al.* Qualitative venous Doppler waveform analysis improves prediction of critical perinatal outcomes in premature growth-restricted fetuses. *Ultrasound Obstet Gynecol* 2003; 22: 240–245.

Brar HS, Platt LD. Reverse end-diastolic flow velocity on umbilical artery velocimetry in high-risk pregnancies: an ominous finding with adverse pregnancy outcome. *Am J Obstet Gynecol* 1988; 159: 559–561.

Chien PF, Arnott N, Gordon A, *et al.* How useful is uterine artery Doppler flow velocimetry in the prediction of pre-eclampsia, intrauterine growth retardation and perinatal death? An overview. *BJOG* 2000; 107(2): 196–208.

Fong KW, Ohlsson A, Hannah MR, *et al.* Prediction of perinatal outcome in fetuses suspected to have intrauterine growth restriction: Doppler US study of fetal cerebral, renal, and umbilical arteries. *Radiology* 1999; 213: 681–689.

Gonen R, Perez R, David M, *et al.* The association between unexplained second trimester maternal serum hCG elevation and pregnancy outcome. *Obstet Gynecol* 1992; 80: 83–86.

Manning FA, Hohler C. Intrauterine growth retardation. Diagnosis, prognostication, and management based on ultrasound methods. In: Fleisher AC, Romero R, Manning FA, *et al.* (eds) *The principles and practice of ultrasonography in obstetrics and gynecology,* 5th edn. Norwalk, CT: Appleton and Lange, 1996: 517.

Neerhof MG. Causes of intrauterine growth restriction. *Clin Perinatol* 1995; 22: 375–385.

Robinson L, Grau P, Crandall BF. Pregnancy outcomes after increasing maternal serum alpha-fetoprotein levels. *Obstet Gynecol* 1989; 74: 17–20.

Williams RL. Intrauterine growth curves. Intra- and international comparisons with different ethnic groups in California. *Prevent Med* 1975; 4: 163–172.

Chapter 7
Rhesus Disease and Isoimmunization

Ramen H. Chmait

Department of Medicine and Obstetrics and Gynecology, Keck School of Medicine, University of Southern California, CA, USA

Introduction

Isoimmunization is an immune-mediated process that is caused by maternal antibodies directed toward fetal red cell antigens, and results in extravascular hemolysis in the fetus. This condition, also referred to as hemolytic disease of the fetus and newborn, ranges from mild to severe disease. In mild cases the fetus has slight anemia with reticulocytosis. In cases of severe isoimmunization, the fetus develops profound anemia, hydrops fetalis, and eventual demise. Prevention and treatment strategies for this condition have significantly improved fetal and neonatal outcomes. This chapter will review the pathogenesis, management, and prevention of red blood cell isoimmunization.

Pathogenesis

Red blood cell (RBC) isoimmunization develops after an initial exposure of foreign erythrocyte surface antigens to the maternal immune system, referred to as the sensitization event. The most common sensitization event is a prior pregnancy in which the fetal erythrocytes contained paternally inherited antigens that were not present on the maternal erythrocytes. The highest risk of sensitization is at time of delivery, whether at term or at time of miscarriage or abortion, although fetal-maternal transfusion may occur at any time during pregnancy. Nonpregnancy-related causes of sensitization include blood transfusions and shared needles. Once erythrocytes containing nonnative surface antigens enter into the maternal circulation, maternal B-lymphocyte clones recognize the erythrocyte antigens as foreign and antibodies directed

Management of Common Problems in Obstetrics and Gynecology,
5th edition. Edited by T.M. Goodwin, M.N. Montoro,
L. Muderspach, R. Paulson and S. Roy. © 2010 Blackwell
Publishing Ltd.

to those antigens are produced. The initial maternal antibody response results in IgM production, which does not cross the placenta. A gradual rise in maternal IgG production, which can cross the placenta and enter the fetal circulation, occurs 6–16 weeks after the initial sensitization event.

Subsequent antigenic exposure during a succeeding pregnancy in an isoimmunized mother can result in significant increase in maternal antibody titer. Maternal memory B-lymphocytes differentiate into plasma cells and IgG antibodies are produced. The maternal IgG antibodies cross the placenta and target the fetal erythrocytes. The "sensitized" fetal RBC are destroyed by hemolysis via macrophages in the fetal spleen, resulting in fetal anemia. The most common cause of RBC isoimmunization used to be the Rhesus (D) (Rh(D)) antigen but the practice of Rh(D) immune prophylaxis has reduced the frequency of isoimmunization from Rh disease, resulting in relatively increased rate of sensitization to non-Rh(D) antigens (irregular antigens). A second mechanism of fetal anemia, unique to the Kell antigen system, results from erythropoietic suppression due to direct destruction of Kell antigen containing fetal erthroid progenitor cells.

The hypoxemia that ensues due to severe fetal anemia stimulates increased fetal erythropoiesis. Whereas the bone marrow is the primary site of blood cell formation in the normal fetus by mid-pregnancy, additional erythropoietic sites, primarily the fetal liver, are stimulated under this hypoxemic stress to produce red cells. The name of this condition, erythroblastosis, arises from the appearance of red cell precursors, erythroblasts, in the peripheral circulation of the fetus. As hematopoietic tissue supplants liver parenchyma, liver functions, including protein synthesis, are impaired. High cardiac output, a compensatory response to anemia and hypoxemia, leads to cardiac failure. Hypoproteinemia and impaired cardiac function combine to produce fetal body cavity effusions and generalized edema, the clinical picture referred to as hydrops fetalis. Untreated, hydrops fetalis results in perinatal death.

Rhesus blood group system

Several dozen red cell antigens have been associated with isoimmunization. However, the Rh blood group system has historically had the greatest clinical impact with regard to the number of affected cases and severity of disease. Typically, when healthcare providers are discussing a patient's Rh status, they are referring exclusively to the Rh(D) status. In fact, the Rh blood group system can produce five potential antigens: D, C, c, E, and e. The Rh(D) antigen is the most immunogenic of the five main Rh antigens. Two genes on chromosome 1, the RhD gene and the RhCE gene, encode the various antigens. The single RhCE gene produces two different gene products due to alternative mRNA splicing. Slight variation in amino acid composition results in the antigenically distinct C versus c and E versus e.

Understanding the genetics of the RhD gene locus is important for appropriate interpretation of tests that ascertain serologic versus genotypic status. Patients who are referred to as serologically negative for Rh(D) antigen either are missing the RhD gene from both alleles or have an RhD pseudogene. The RhD pseudogene, which occurs in about one-quarter of African Americans, contains a stop codon within the gene that does not allow translation of the mRNA product. Because there is no gene product, patients who have the RhD pseudogene exclusively are serologically Rh(D) negative but genotypically RhD positive. Thus, these patients are at risk for isoimmunization. Patients who are serologically Rh(D) antigen positive have either one or two RhD alleles. A subgroup of patients, particularly African Americans and Asians, may have a modified version of the gene, called RhDu, which produces an abridged gene product. Laboratories often will report that these patients are serologically weakly positive or are Rh(Du) positive. These patients are not at risk of Rh(D) isoimmunization.

In summary, it is the patient's serologic status that confers risk for isoimmunization. This has important implications with regard to prenatal diagnosis.

Irregular antibodies

Antibodies to erythrocyte antigens other than the Rh blood group system are referred to as irregular antibodies. The most common irregular antibodies are to the Kell, Duffy, MNS, and Kidd blood group systems. These antibodies are more often produced in response to maternal blood transfusion, and have a higher likelihood of being absent in specimens from the father and fetus. It is important to note that the assessment and management of isoimmunization are dependent on the type of antibody. Unless otherwise specified, this chapter will focus on the management of Rh(D) isoimmunization.

Identifying the at-risk fetus

All gravid patients undergo blood typing and antibody screening at their first prenatal visit. A positive antibody screen means that the fetus is at risk for hemolytic disease. If the antibody screen is positive, the laboratory performs antibody identification and titer on the maternal specimen. Not all types of maternal antibodies to erythrocyte antigens cause hemolytic disease of the fetus and newborn. A reference table should be used to ascertain fetal risk if an irregular antibody is identified. The antibody titers can then be followed during the pregnancy on a monthly basis until 24 weeks' gestation and every 2 weeks thereafter. If the maternal titer rises above a critical level, further testing is indicated. A titer of 1:8 to 1:32 is considered critical, depending on the laboratory and the type of isoimmunization. Monitoring of maternal antibody titers is useful in the evaluation of the index pregnancy, but has limited utility in monitoring patients with a prior affected pregnancy.

Once a maternal antibody has been identified, it is important to determine if the fetal erythrocytes express the target antigen. There are three methods currently employed to identify the at-risk fetus. The first is to obtain paternal blood testing for antigen status. If the father is antigen positive, then the fetus is at 100% risk if the father is homozygous and 50% risk if he is heterozygous. In the case of Rh(D), paternal zygosity can be estimated based on serology, ethnicity, and history of prior affected offspring. If the father of the baby is serologically negative, then the fetus is theoretically not at risk, although it should be noted that the rate of erroneous paternity in the United States has been estimated at 10%.

The second method of identifying the at-risk fetus is to directly determine fetal blood type by DNA testing of amniocytes obtained by amniocentesis. Amniocytes are fetal cells that are shed into and suspended in the amniotic fluid. Because this tests fetal genotype, not serologic status, rare false positives and negatives may occur. Potential errors are reduced with the addition of parental blood DNA testing. The risk of this approach is that it requires an amniocentesis, a procedure in which a 22 gauge spinal needle is inserted through the maternal abdomen into the amniotic fluid. This invasive test has been shown to occasionally worsen the isoimmunization by causing increased maternal antibody titers due to procedure related fetal-to-maternal transfusion.

A third recently developed technique for identifying the at-risk fetus takes advantage of the presence of cell-free fetal DNA circulating in the plasma of pregnant women. The detection of fetal DNA sequences of RhD has been shown to be highly accurate, although there remains the risk of false positives and negatives akin to the above-mentioned tests that assess fetal genotype rather than serology. The advantage of this method is that it avoids amniocentesis, thereby reducing the theoretical risk of exacerbation of the isoimmunization. This test is widely used in Europe, but has not yet been adopted into clinical practice in the United States.

Prenatal diagnosis of fetal anemia

The next clinical step in the evaluation of the isoimmunized patient is determination of the severity of disease. Three methods are currently used to ascertain if the at-risk fetus is actually anemic. The first utilizes spectrophotometry to quantify the bilirubin level in the amniotic fluid acquired via amniocentesis. The bilirubin level in the amniotic fluid correlates with the degree of hemolysis. The result is expressed as the change in absorbance at 450 nm, or δ OD450, and is plotted on a normative curve based on gestational age. This semi-logarithmic graph, called the Liley curve, is separated into three zones. Patients who fall into zone I are at low risk of fetal anemia, although there remains the risk that a neonatal exchange transfusion may be required. Patients in zone II are at mild to moderate risk of fetal anemia. Zone III patients have severe fetal anemia with high probability of fetal death in 7–10 days. Serial amnioceuteses are performed to establish a trend of the bilirubin measurement. Measurements that are trending up to upper zone II or zone III require intervention.

The Liley curve is predictive of fetal anemia from 27 weeks onwards. Modification of the curve to allow assessment of amniotic fluid bilirubin at earlier gestational ages has been advocated, but is used with less confidence. This approach often requires multiple amniocenteses, so there is a risk of worsening isoimmunization or other amniocentesis-related complications such as rupture of membranes. Because the mechanism of fetal anemia in the case of Kell isoimmunization involves erythropoietic suppression as well as RBC hemolysis, amniotic fluid bilirubin determination does not accurately reflect disease severity in this condition.

The second method utilizes ultrasound to assess for fetal anemia. Overt evidence of fetal hydrops on ultrasound is an end-stage sign of severe fetal anemia. Obviously, the goal of fetal surveillance is to identify the anemic fetus prior to the onset of hydrops. The ultrasound-acquired Doppler measurement of the middle cerebral artery (MCA) peak systolic velocity (psv) has been shown to accurately identify moderate to severe fetal anemia even in nonhydropic fetuses. Using a cut-off of greater than 1.5 multiples of the median, at-risk fetuses with elevated MCA psv were noted to have a high risk

for moderate to severe anemia. The increased cerebral blood flow has been attributed to the low viscosity of the blood, although cerebral autoregulatory mechanisms to preserve delivery of oxygen to the brain may play a role as well. Because this technique is noninvasive and has been shown to be more accurate than the Liley curve, the MCA Doppler has largely replaced serial amniocenteses in current clinical practice.

The third method for fetal anemia assessment, and the gold standard to which all are compared, is fetal blood sampling. This procedure is the most invasive and thus carries the highest risk. A needle is placed through the maternal abdomen into a fetal vessel via direct ultrasound guidance, and 1–2 mL of fetal blood is obtained. Preparations for intrauterine transfusion should be in place at the time of fetal blood sampling to proceed with transfusion if necessary.

Fetal treatment

Severe fetal anemia is treated in the prenatal period via intrauterine transfusion (IUT). IUT is performed under direct ultrasound guidance using a 20–22 gauge needle. The procedure was first carried out using an intraperitoneal route. Red blood cells are placed into the fetal peritoneal cavity where they are subsequently absorbed through the diaphragmatic lymphatics. This approach is advantageous when fetal vascular access is difficult. However, intraperitoneal IUT is not the preferred approach because of the 7–10 days' delay in absorption of the cells in nonhydropic fetuses and significantly impaired absorption in hydropic fetuses. In cases of fetal hydrops, intraperitoneal IUT has been shown to result in almost half the perinatal survival rate compared to intravenous IUT.

Intravenous IUT is performed by accessing the umbilical vein either in the umbilical cord at the placental cord insertion site (umbilical cord IUT) or in the fetus where the umbilical vein traverses the liver (intrahepatic IUT). Both methods have similar procedure loss rates of approximately 1% in nonhydropic fetuses and 7% in hydropic fetuses. Umbilical cord IUT is the most common method used in the US today. Risks of IUT include fetal bradycardia, hemorrhage, infection, and rupture of membranes. The overall fetal survival rates in pregnancies complicated by severe fetal anemia and treated by IUT are approximately 92% for nonhydropic fetuses and 70% in hydropic fetuses. Normal neurologic outcome can be expected in over 90% of surviving infants even if hydrops was noted at the time of the first IUT.

The frequency of transfusions over the course of the pregnancy can be guided by MCA psv Doppler. The threshold value used to trigger another transfusion is somewhat higher, at 1.69 multiples of the median, after the first IUT. This may be the case because adult RBC have different flow characteristics within the cerebral vessels compared to fetal RBC. In general, the second IUT is usually necessary in 10–14 days, while subsequent IUT are usually required every 3–4 weeks. A general rule is that the fetal hematocrit declines approximately 1% per day after the first transfusion. Most centers perform IUT up to 35 weeks' gestation, after which delivery and neonatal transfusion are recommended.

Other treatment options have been developed for the management of isoimmunization. Combined maternal plasmapheresis and intravenous immunoglobulin has been successfully utilized in the treatment of isoimmunization in which fetal access for transfusion is technically prohibitive. For example, this approach has been used to treat the rare patient who had a prior intrauterine fetal demise before 20 weeks' gestation due to isoimmunization. This regimen is instituted from 12 weeks' to 20 weeks' gestation, at which time the fetal blood sampling and IUT may be performed if necessary.

Summary of contemporary management of isoimmunization

Paternal and, if necessary, fetal antigen status is determined to identify the at-risk fetus. Surveillance for severe fetal anemia is performed via Doppler assessment of the MCA psv. In pregnancies with a previously affected fetus or infant, MCA Doppler measurements are initiated at 18 weeks' gestation and repeated every 1–2 weeks. In the first affected pregnancy, maternal antibody titers can be used to guide surveillance. Antibody titers are obtained monthly until 24 weeks and then every 2 weeks thereafter. MCA Doppler studies are initiated once a critical titer has been reached. Many centers are relying less on maternal antibody titers and more on MCA Doppler studies regardless of patient history. If severe anemia is suspected, then fetal blood sampling is performed and transfusion is given if the hematocrit measures less than 30%. Antenatal testing should be initiated at approximately 32 weeks' gestation. Delivery should occur between 35 and 38 weeks' gestation, depending on the timing of the prior transfusion and the suspicion of recurrent severe fetal anemia.

Prevention of Rhesus (D) disease

The frequency of Rh(D) isoimmunization has decreased precipitously since the introduction of Rh-immune globulin. The exact mechanism by which Rh-immune globulin suppresses the immune response has not yet been defined. A dose of Rh-immune globulin is given to an Rh(D)-negative mother within 72 hours of delivery if the infant is found to be Rh(D) positive. Because there is approximately a 2% risk of maternal sensitization during the course of the pregnancy, it is standard in the US to administer Rh-immune globulin at 28 weeks' gestation as well. Other indications for Rh-immune prophylaxis include any procedures that may result in fetal-to-maternal hemorrhage, such as amniocentesis and external cephalic version.

Approximately 0.1% of deliveries are associated with excessive fetal-to-maternal hemorrhage, of which 50% are without risk factors. The Kleihauer–Betke test approximates the volume of fetal blood transfused into the maternal circulation, and can be used to determine the required Rh-immune globulin dose. One ampoule of Rh-immune globulin is sufficient to prevent sensitization to less than 30 mL of fetal whole blood. For example, if the Kleihauer–Betke test estimated 45 mL of whole fetal blood in the maternal circulation, then two ampoules of Rh-immune globulin are required to prevent maternal sensitization.

Conclusion

The perinatal mortality rate from isoimmunization has fallen sharply over the past half century due to the preventive and treatment strategies described in this chapter. It is instructive to review historical accounts of this disease to fully appreciate the magnitude of this achievement. The remarkable diminution in the frequency of isoimmunization has resulted in a significant decrease in the number of patients needing treatment. For this reason, patients who require intrauterine transfusion are often referred to centers that specialize in fetal therapy.

Suggested reading

American College of Obstetricians and Gynecologists. Practice Bulletin No. 75: management of alloimmunization. *Obstet Gynecol* 2006; 108(2): 457–464.

Geifman-Holtzman O, Grotegut CA, Gaughan JP. Diagnostic accuracy of noninvasive fetal Rh genotyping from maternal blood – a meta-analysis. *Am J Obstet Gynecol* 2006; 195(4): 1163–1173.

Kumpel BM. On the immunologic basis of Rh immune globulin (anti-D) prophylaxis. *Transfusion* 2006; 46(9): 1652–1656.

Oepkes D, Seaward PG, Vandenbussche FP, *et al.* Doppler ultrasonography versus amniocentesis to predict fetal anemia. *NEJM* 2006; 355(2): 156–164.

Ruma MS, Moise KJ Jr, Kim E, *et al.* Combined plasmapheresis and intravenous immune globulin for the treatment of severe maternal red cell alloimmunization. *Am J Obstet Gynecol* 2007; 196(2): 138.

Scheier M, Hernandez-Andrade E, Fonseca EB, Nicolaides KH. Prediction of severe fetal anemia in red blood cell alloimmunization after previous intrauterine transfusions. *Am J Obstet Gynecol* 2006; 195(6): 1550–1556.

Chapter 8
Diagnosis and Management of Macrosomia

Joseph G. Ouzounian and T. Murphy Goodwin

Department of Medicine and Obstetrics and Gynecology, Keck School of Medicine, University of Southern California, CA, USA

Introduction

Suspected fetal macrosomia is encountered commonly in the practice of obstetrics. The delivery of large fetuses remains clinically important because of the increased potential for maternal and neonatal complications. Data from the National Center for Health Statistics shows that 10% of liveborn infants in the Unites States weigh more than 4000 gm at birth, and about 1.5% weigh more than 4500 gm. Potential maternal risks of macrosomia include abnormal labor, uterine rupture, postpartum hemorrhage, lacerations, and infection. Potential risks to the fetus include shoulder dystocia (see also Chapter 12, "Shoulder Dystocia"), brachial plexus injury, bone fractures, and in rare cases asphyxial injury. Some studies have also suggested that fetal macrosomia can lead to childhood obesity, glucose intolerance, and development of metabolic syndrome.

Definition of macrosomia

The terms *macrosomia* and *large for gestational age* (*LGA*) both refer to excessive fetal growth. Even though there is no universal agreement regarding the absolute threshold for macrosomia, historically it has been defined as a birth weight exceeding 4000 gm independent of gestational age. The term "large for gestational age" refers to infants whose birth weight exceeds the 90th percentile for growth at a specific gestational age. Birth weight data from the National Center for Health Statistics is listed in Table 8.1. The American College of Obstetricians and Gynecologists acknowledges that there is increased morbidity in infants with a birth weight > 4000 gm, but they recommend that macrosomia be defined as any infant with an estimated fetal weight above 4500 gm. This recommendation is

most likely based on data regarding birth injury and the difficulty in assessing fetal weight accurately prior to delivery. It should also be noted that male infants, on average, have higher birth weights than female infants, and that racial and ethnic differences can also influence birth weight.

Risk factors for macrosomia

There are several historic risk factors described in association with macrosomia. These include: maternal diabetes, multiparity, male fetus, advanced maternal age, maternal obesity (or high body mass index), prior history of macrosomia, postterm pregnancy, maternal birth weight over 4000 gm, Hispanic or African-American ethnicity, and excessive weight gain in pregnancy. Approximately one-third of all neonates over 4000 gm at birth are born to diabetic mothers. Even though the risk of accelerated

Table 8.1 Percentiles of birth weight (grams) by gestational age: U.S. singleton births, 1991

Gestational age, weeks	5th percentile	10th percentile	50th percentile	90th percentile
26	529	625	899	1362
27	591	702	1035	1635
28	670	798	1196	1977
29	772	925	1394	2361
30	910	1085	1637	2710
31	1088	1278	1918	2986
32	1294	1495	2203	3200
33	1513	1725	2458	3370
34	1735	1950	2667	3502
35	1950	2159	2831	3596
36	2156	2354	2974	3668
37	2357	2541	3117	3755
38	2543	2714	3263	3867
39	2685	2852	3400	3980
40	2761	2929	3495	4060
41	2777	2948	3527	4094
42	2764	2935	3522	4098

Source: Alexander *et al.* (1996).

Management of Common Problems in Obstetrics and Gynecology, 5th edition. Edited by T.M. Goodwin, M.N. Montoro, L. Muderspach, R. Paulson and S. Roy. © 2010 Blackwell Publishing Ltd.

fetal growth in infants of diabetic mothers increases with increasing hyperglycemia, there is no universal threshold value of hyperglycemia that predisposes the fetus to becoming macrosomic. Conversely, in diabetic women with good glycemic control, the rate of macrosomia approaches that of the general population (10–13%). There are also rare causes of genetic macrosomia, such as in fetuses with Beckwith-Wiedemann or Weaver syndromes.

Poorly understood factors which relate to increased fetal growth include genetic predisposition, fetal intrauterine metabolism and placental nutrient transport. Some or all of these factors likely contribute to the intrauterine environment and influence fetal growth. Fetal hyperinsulinism, a finding integral to the pathophysiology of diabetic fetopathy, is an example of altered fetal metabolism that can lead to excessive intrauterine growth and increase the risk for type 2 diabetes in later life for these infants. However, fetal hyperinsulinism appears to affect only a minority of pregnancies complicated by diabetes and does not correlate well with maternal glycemic control. This lack of association between fetal hyperinsulinism and maternal glucose levels may explain why good glycemic control does not eliminate the risk of macrosomia in some diabetic pregnancies.

Finally, note that many of the risk factors for macrosomia (male gender, parity, prior history of macrosomia, and maternal prepregnancy weight) are not modifiable and are already determined at the time of conception. Overall, less than 40% of macrosomic infants are born to women with identifiable risk factors.

Diagnosis of macrosomia

The available methods for diagnosis of macrosomia are ultrasound measurements, clinical assessment via Leopold's maneuvers or fundal height measurement, and maternal estimation. Unfortunately, accurate detection of macrosomia prior to birth remains a clinical conundrum. Accelerated growth of the fundal height as estimated by measurement and palpation of the uterine fundus may provide an early clinical clue for suspected macrosomia, but fundal height measurements are not reliable with birth weight > 4000 gm. With birth weights between 2500 and 4000 gm, there is good evidence that demonstrates the superiority of ultrasound-derived fetal weight estimates over clinical estimation. However, all techniques lose accuracy as birth weight rises. The American Institute of Ultrasound in Medicine reports that even the best fetal weight detection methods yield error rates of $+/- 15\%$. Other reports show error rates as high as 20% in infants weighing over 4500 gm.

There are over 30 different formulas for ultrasound estimates of fetal weight, but most use the fetal biparietal diameter, head circumference, abdominal circumference, or femur length alone or in combination to predict the fetal weight. Ultrasound estimates of fetal weight have a low sensitivity, but a high specificity and negative predictive value for detecting macrosomia. A recent review showed a sensitivity of 12–75% and a specificity of 68–99% for ultrasonographic prediction of macrosomia.

Clinical estimates of fetal weight can be accomplished by abdominal palpation (Leopold's maneuvers) and/or fundal height measurements. Some studies have shown that in experienced hands, clinical estimates approach the accuracy of ultrasound estimates for fetal weight. Other studies have shown that a mother's estimate of her own baby's weight can be as accurate as clinical or ultrasound estimates.

In clinical practice, it is reasonable to use maternal and clinical estimates to estimate fetal weight, but in cases where macrosomia is suspected, ultrasound examination could be helpful. Despite the inherent limitations of ultrasound, a combination of clinical estimates, ultrasound assessment, and clinical history can help craft an appropriate management plan when macrosomia is suspected. In pregnancies complicated by diabetes, the ratio of head circumference (HC) to abdominal circumference (AC) may indicate disproportionate fetal growth. An HC/AC ratio of less than 0.80 suggests disproportionate central body growth and raises the risk for shoulder dystocia and potential birth trauma.

Management of suspected macrosomia

Macrosomia technically is a statistical definition and not a true "disease." Nevertheless, because of the potential for serious maternal, fetal, and neonatal morbidity, cases with suspected macrosomia require thoughtful management plans.

In nondiabetic patients, once macrosomia is suspected in the antepartum period, clinical interventions aimed at impeding fetal growth are very limited. Even though maternal obesity and excessive weight gain are known risk factors for macrosomia, there are no randomized clinical trials evaluating the clinical effectiveness of caloric restriction on reducing fetal growth. Existing clinical studies have shown conflicting results. In diabetic patients, it has been shown that improved glycemic control (with the addition of insulin therapy) in patients with suspected macrosomia in the second trimester can have a small but measurable reduction of birth weight at term.

The clinical dilemma encountered most often by clinicians managing a patient with suspected macrosomia at term is whether or not to allow labor or proceed with elective Cesarean section. Unfortunately, the effectiveness of prophylactic Cesarean delivery in reducing fetal and neonatal morbidity in these cases has not been evaluated in randomized clinical trials. In addition, as outlined earlier in this chapter, available techniques to estimate fetal weight are not very accurate. Finally, Cesarean section reduces, but does not eliminate, the risk for birth trauma and brachial plexus injury associated with vaginal birth. Thus, while clinically it may be tempting to select a route of delivery based solely on estimated fetal weight, such a decision should take into account all pertinent risk factors as well as the patient's desires after detailed informed consent. Current guidelines from the American College of Obstetricians and Gynecologists do not support a planned Cesarean delivery unless estimated fetal weight exceeds 5000 gm (4500 gm in diabetics). Equally important, current evidence does not support early induction of labor in patients with suspected macrosomia. In these patients, careful monitoring is required during labor, and operative vaginal delivery, especially midpelvic procedures, should be avoided. Finally, suspected macrosomia is not an absolute contraindication for vaginal birth after Cesarean section.

Suggested readings

Alexander GR, Himes JH, Kaufman RB, *et al*. United States national reference for fetal growth. *Obstet Gynecol* 1996; 87: 163–168.

Alsulyman OA, Ouzounian JG, Kjos SL. The accuracy of sonographic fetal weight estimation in diabetic pregnancies. *Am J Obstet Gynecol* 1997; 177: 503–506.

American College of Obstetricians and Gynecologists. *Fetal macrosomia*. Practice Bulletin no. 22. Washington, DC: ACOG, 2000.

American College of Obstetricians and Gynecologists. *Gestational Diabetes*. Practice Bulletin no. 30. Washington, DC: ACOG, 2001.

American Institute of Ultrasound in Medicine, *Practice Guideline for the Performance of Obstetric Ultrasound Examinations*, October, 2007.

Chauhan SP, Grobman WA, Gherman RA, *et al*. Suspicion and treatment of the macrosomic fetus: A review. *Am J Obstet Gynecol* 2005; 193: 332–340.

Combs CA, Singh NB, Khoury JC. Elective induction versus spontaneous labor after sonographic diagnosis of fetal macrosomia. *Obstet Gynecol* 1993; 81: 492–496.

Lipscomb KR, Gregory K, Shaw K. The outcome of macrosomic infants weighing at least 4500 grams: Los Angeles County. University of Southern California experience. *Obstet Gynecol* 1995; 85: 558–564.

Naylor CD, Sermer M, Chen E, Sykora K. Cesarean delivery in relation to birthweight and gestational glucose tolerance: pathophysiology or practice style. *JAMA* 1996; 265: 1165–1170.

Ouzounian JG. Effective management of shoulder dystocia. *OBG Management* 1997; 28–32.

Ouzounian JG, Gherman RB. Shoulder dystocia: Are historic risk factors reliable predictors? *Am J Obstet Gynecol* 2005; 192: 1933–1938.

Ouzounian JG, Korst LM, Phelan JP. Permanent Erb's palsy: A lack of a relationship with obstetrical risk factors. *Am J Perinatol* 1998; 15(4): 221–223.

Rouse DJ, Owen J, Goldenberg RL, Oliver SP. The effectiveness and costs of elective cesarean delivery for fetal macrosomia diagnosed by ultrasound. *JAMA* 1996; 276: 1480–1486.

Sacks DA, Chen MS. Estimating fetal weight in the management of macrosomia. *Obstet Gynecol Surv* 2000; 55: 229–239.

Zhang X, Decker A, Platt RW, Kramer MS. How big is too big? The perinatal consequences of fetal macrosomia. *Am J Obstet Gynecol* 2008; 198: 517–521.

Chapter 9
Labor Induction

Patrick M. Mullin

Department of Medicine and Obstetrics and Gynecology, Keck School of Medicine, University of Southern California, CA, USA

Introduction

Labor induction is the process of achieving vaginal delivery by initiating uterine activity before the onset of spontaneous labor. Labor induction in the United States is at an all-time high; its use is reported in up to 25% of pregnancies. A similar trend is described in both Canada and Europe. The decision to initiate an induction of labor must take into account the risks to mother and fetus from the induction process versus the risks to continuing the pregnancy. The availability of methods to stimulate uterine activity has expanded as labor induction rates have increased.

Indications and contraindications

Post-term pregnancy is the most commonly cited indication for labor induction. Data from several large multicenter randomized studies have reported favorable outcomes with routine induction as early as 41 weeks. One of the largest studies included 3407 low-risk women randomized at 41 weeks to expectant management versus labor induction. A significantly lower cesarean rate was noted in the electively induced group, 21.2% versus 24.5%, a difference thought to be due to fewer cesareans performed for nonreassuring fetal heart rate tracings [1]. While a review of 19 studies investigating routine labor induction after 41 weeks found no difference in the cesarean delivery rate, a lower rate of perinatal mortality was noted. Additionally, no effect was seen in the instrumental delivery rate, use of analgesia or incidence of fetal heart rate abnormalities [2]. In a report describing the changing patterns in labor induction, the average gestational age at induction for the indication of post-term pregnancy was noted to have declined from 41.9 weeks to 41 weeks [3].

Other indications for proceeding with labor induction include pre-eclampsia, eclampsia, abruptio placentae, chorio-amnionitis, fetal demise, premature rupture of membranes, isoimmunization, fetal growth restriction, and maternal medical conditions such as diabetes and chronic hypertension.

Additionally, elective inductions for logistic or psychosocial reasons have become more common. There has been at least a 15-fold rise in the number of elective inductions since 1990. While benefits cited for initiating an elective induction include avoiding a rapid delivery away from the hospital and minimizing any disruption to the patient's and provider's work and nonwork responsibilities, risks include increased iatrogenic prematurity, increased healthcare costs, and increased rates of operative delivery [4]. The greatest risk appears to involve elective induction of nulliparous patients, particularly those with an unfavorable cervix. In an investigation comparing 7683 nulliparous women who were electively induced to a matched cohort of 7683 nulliparous women who had spontaneous labors, the electively induced group had higher rates of cesarean delivery (10% vs 7%), instrumental delivery (32% vs 29%), and use of epidural anesthesia (80% vs 58%). Similar findings were reported in other studies with all showing an approximate twofold increased risk of cesarean delivery.

Prior to initiating a labor induction for logistic or psychosocial indications, the American College of Obstetricians and Gynecologists suggests that fetal lung maturity be established or one of the following criteria met: fetal heart tones have been documented for 20 weeks by nonelectronic fetoscopy or for 30 weeks by Doppler; it has been 36 weeks since a positive serum or urine human chorionic gonadotropin pregnancy test was performed by a reliable lab; an ultrasound measurement of the crown–rump length, obtained at 6–12 weeks, supports a gestational age of at least 39 weeks; or an ultrasound obtained at 13–20 weeks confirms the gestational age of at least 39 weeks determined by clinical history and physical examination [5].

Management of Common Problems in Obstetrics and Gynecology, 5th edition. Edited by T.M. Goodwin, M.N. Montoro, L. Muderspach, R. Paulson and S. Roy. © 2010 Blackwell Publishing Ltd.

Contraindications to labor induction include: prior classic uterine incision, active genital herpes infection, placenta or vasa previa, and transverse fetal lie. There are other conditions which are not necessarily contraindications, but caution and judgment should be exercised when managing them. These include: multiple gestation, maternal cardiac disease, grand multiparity, breech presentation, abnormal fetal heart rate patterns that do not require immediate delivery, and severe hypertension.

Requirements for induction

Before beginning a labor induction, the risks, alternatives, and potential need for cesarean delivery should be thoroughly discussed with the patient. Additionally, the following should be completed: a review of the gestational age; estimation of the fetal size and position; and assessment of the patient's pelvis and cervical status. The Bishop score is the method most commonly used to assess the cervix. It was originally developed to describe the state of multiparous cervices prior to the onset of spontaneous labor. Four characteristics of the cervical exam are used to tabulate a Bishop score: effacement, dilation, consistency, and position. In 1966, Friedman studied the Bishop score of 408 multiparous patients before labor, many of which were elective inductions. Labor induction was successful in all patients with a Bishop score of 9 or greater while 20% of inductions failed in patients with a Bishop score of 4 or less. A score between 5 and 8 resulted in a 4.8% failure rate. Investigators have demonstrated that cervical dilation is the most important component of the Bishop score in predicting success of a labor induction. Effacement, station and consistency were found to have about half of the influence while position had little effect as compared with cervical dilation.

Additional methods investigated for predicting success of labor induction have included cervical length and fetal fibronectin. A meta-analysis of seven studies compared the usefulness of a cervical length to the Bishop score. Both measures were found to be equally predictive of successful induction and of vaginal delivery. Similarly, increased levels of fetal fibronectin have been associated with successful labor induction. In comparison to the Bishop score, neither measure was found to be superior [6].

Cervical ripening

The goal of cervical ripening is to create a more favorable cervix prior to beginning a labor induction. Cervical effacement and dilation result from chemical changes within the cervix through breakdown of collagen fibrils and increased water content within the cervix. The benefits include a more rapid labor and a greater potential for vaginal delivery. Current methods include membrane stripping, prostaglandin compounds, and mechanical dilation.

Membrane stripping, which involves separating the fetal membranes from their attachment to the lower uterine segment, is a common office procedure used to begin cervical ripening. Membrane stripping results in local release of prostaglandins and mechanical dilation of the cervix. A meta-analysis of 22 investigations studying the efficacy of membrane stripping found the procedure was associated with fewer pregnancies continuing beyond 41 and 42 weeks of gestation and reduced need for formal induction. The cesarean delivery rate did not differ between the comparison groups and there was no difference in maternal or neonatal outcome [7].

There are two approved prostaglandin E2 preparations available in the US – Prepidil and Cervidil. Cervidil is the more commonly used preparation and consists of 10 mg of dinoprostone in a vaginal insert, which releases 0.3 mg of dinoprostone per hour. The vaginal insert is left in place until active labor begins or for up to 12 hours. An oxytocin infusion can then be initiated 30–60 minutes later. The efficacy of prostaglandin E2 was reported in a review of 52 studies. Compared to placebo, the prostaglandin preparations were noted to provide improved cervical ripening, a lower oxytocin requirement, and a higher delivery rate within 24 hours. There was no difference in the cesarean delivery rates [8].

Misoprostol is a prostaglandin E1 preparation used to treat gastric ulcer disease. It has also been used off-label in labor induction. A meta-analysis indicated that misoprostol compared favorably with prostaglandin E2 preparations and was found to be more effective in achieving vaginal delivery within 24 hours while requiring less oxytocin administration. Again, cesarean rates were not different. Misoprostol, however, was found to be associated with a higher rate of hyperstimulation [9]. Most commonly, misoprostol is administered at a dose of 25 μg every 3–6 hours until active labor is achieved or up to 24 hours total. Oxytocin augmentation is usually initiated 4 hours later.

Mechanical dilation works, at least in part, by causing the release of prostaglandin F2-α from the decidua and adjacent membranes or prostaglandin E1 from the cervix. Today, the most common method used is the balloon catheter. A Foley catheter is inserted through the cervix and the balloon is distended with 30–60 cc of saline. Once the balloon is distended, it is retracted to allow placement against the internal cervical os. Gentle traction can be applied when taping the balloon to the inner thigh. Attaching the balloon to a weighted object such as an IV bag has not been shown to enhance cervical ripening. In most cases, the balloon is extruded within 12 hours. Otherwise, it can be left in place for up to 24 hours. Randomized trials have demonstrated balloon catheters to be as effective as prostaglandins. There does not appear to be any benefit of adding a prostaglandin while the balloon catheter is in place.

Extra-amniotic saline infusion (EASI) involves infusion of normal saline through the central port of a Foley balloon placed above the internal cervical os. A continuous infusion rate of 30 cc per hour is typically used. Randomized trials have not shown a benefit in using the EASI protocol over the Foley catheter alone. Furthermore, a meta-analysis failed to show a benefit of EASI over induction with prostaglandins [10]. The efficacy of the EASI protocol, however, appears enhanced with the addition of concomitant oxytocin administration.

Hygroscopic dilators have been utilized primarily in pregnancy termination, but have also been shown to be safe and effective in term pregnancies. Laminaria tents are made from natural seaweed. Among the commercially available options is Lamicel. The synthetic tents are designed to expand within the cervical canal. These devices probably function by disrupting the chorio-amniotic decidual interface, causing lysosomal destruction and prostaglandin synthesis. These events also lead to active stretching of the cervix beyond the passive mechanical stretching by the tent itself. Clinical trials comparing hygroscopic dilators to prostaglandin E2 gel demonstrate that both methods are similar in terms of cervical change; however, PGE2 is associated with a higher success rate of induction and the dilators have a higher incidence of postpartum maternal and fetal infections.

Labor induction

Intravenous oxytocin infusion is the standard method for labor induction. Oxytocin stimulates contractions in myometrial smooth muscle by increasing intracellular calcium levels through the activation of the phospholipase C-inositol pathway. Oxytocin is the most potent uterotonic agent known; its plasma half-life is 3–6 minutes. As pregnancy progresses, the number of oxytocin receptors increases 300-fold. Complications of oxytocin use include uterine hyperstimulation and, with excessive doses, hypotension, water intoxication, and neonatal hyperbilirubinemia. Numerous intravenous oxytocin regimens have been studied and the optimal protocol remains uncertain. Low-dose regimens commonly begin with a 1 mU per minute initial dose, increased by 1 mU per minute at 40–60-minute intervals. This regimen attempts to mimic the physiologic release of oxytocin. High-dose regimens begin with an initial dose of 6 mU per minute, increased by 6 mU per minute every 15 minutes. Labor and delivery protocols typically include a maximum infusion rate of 40 mU per minute. Various intermediate regimens have also been studied. A literature review by Patka *et al.* in 2005 included all investigations of oxytocin induction published from 1966 to 2003. The high-dose protocol, while associated with a more rapid

initiation of induction to delivery time, was also found to have a higher rate of hyperstimulation. Cesarean delivery rates did not differ between the various protocols [11].

At the Los Angeles County – University of Southern California Women's and Children's Hospital, a continuous infusion of oxytocin is started at a dose of 1 mU per minute, and increased linearly by 1 mU/min every 30 minutes to a maximum of 22 mU per minute. In addition, when no contraindications exist, early amniotomy is used to shorten the duration of labor and increase the chances of a successful induction. The use of amniotomy in combination with oxytocin administration was found to be more effective than oxytocin alone in achieving delivery within 24 hours. The risks of amniotomy include infection, bleeding, and cord prolapse.

Conclusion

The rate of labor induction continues to increase, with post-term pregnancy being the most common indication reported. While the ideal method of labor induction has yet to be identified, oxytocin remains the method of choice in women with favorable cervical examinations. Cervical ripening can be used to create a more favorable cervix prior to beginning a labor induction. Patients with an unfavorable cervix may benefit from membrane stripping, prostaglandin compounds or mechanical dilation.

References

1. Hannah ME, Hannah WJ, Hellmann J, *et al*. Induction of labor as compared with serial antenatal monitoring in post-term pregnancy. A randomized controlled trial. The Canadian Multicenter Post-term Pregnancy Trial Group. *NEJM* 1992; 326: 1587–1592.
2. Gülmezoglu AM, Crowther CA, Middleton P. Induction of labour for improving birth outcomes for women at or beyond term. *Cochrane Database Syst Rev* 2006; 4: CD004945.
3. Yawn BP, Wollan, P, McKeon K, *et al*. Temporal changes in rates and reasons for medical induction of term labor, 1980–1996. *Am J Obstet Gynecol* 2001; 184: 611–619.
4. Wing DA. Elective induction of labor in the USA. *Curr Opinion Obstet Gynecol* 2000; 12: 457–462.
5. American Congress of Obstetricians and Gynecologists Practice Bulletin Number 107, *Induction of Labor*, August 2009, Washington, DC: American Congress of Obstetricians and Gynecologists.
6. Crane JMG. Factors predicting labor induction success: a critical analysis. *Clin Obstet Gynecol* 2006; 49(3): 573–584.
7. Boulvain M, Stan C, Irion O. Membrane sweeping for induction of labour. *Cochrane Database Syst Rev* 2005; 1: CD000451.
8. Kelly AJ, Kavanagh J, Thomas J. Vaginal prostaglandin (PGE2 and PGF2a) for induction of labour at term. *Cochrane Database Syst Rev* 2003; 2: CD003101.
9. Hofmeyer GJ, Gülmezoglu AM. Vaginal misoprostol for cervical ripening and induction of labour. *Cochrane Database Syst Rev* 2003; 1: CD000941.

10. Boulvain M, Kelly A, Lohse C, *et al*. Mechanical methods for induction of labour. *Cochrane Database Syst Rev* 2001; 4: CD 001233.
11. Patka JH, Lodolce AE, Johnston AK. High- versus low-dose oxytocin for augmentation or induction of labor. *Ann Pharmacother* 2005; 39: 95.

Suggested reading

Brindley BA, Sokol RJ. Induction and augmentation of labor: basis and methods for current practice. *Obstet Gynecol Surv* 1988; 43: 730–743.

Hannah ME, Ohlsson A, Farine D, *et al*. Induction of labor compared with expectant management for prelabor rupture of the membranes at term. *NEJM* 1996; 334: 1005–1010.

Hauth JC, Hankins GDV, Gilstrap LC, *et al*. Uterine contraction pressures with oxytocin induction/augmentation. *Obstet Gynecol* 1986; 68: 305–309.

Keirse MJNC. Prostaglandins in preinduction cervical ripening. Meta-analysis of worldwide clinical experience. *J Reprod Med* 1993; 38: 89–100.

Lyndrup J, Nickelson C, Weber T, *et al*. Induction of labor by balloon catheter with extra-amniotic saline infusion (BCEAS): a randomised comparison with PGE2 vaginal pessaries. *Eur J Obstet Gynecol* 1994; 53: 189–197.

St Onge RD, Connors GT. Preinduction cervical ripening. A comparison of intracervical prostaglandin E2 gel versus the Foley catheter. *Am J Obstet Gynecol* 1995; 172: 687–690.

Wing DA, Rahall A, Jones MM, *et al*. Misoprostol: an effective agent for cervical ripening and labor induction. *Am J Obstet Gynecol* 1995; 172: 1811–1816.

Chapter 10
Abnormal Labor

Emiliano Chavira and T. Murphy Goodwin
Department of Medicine and Obstetrics and Gynecology, Keck School of Medicine, University of Southern California, CA, USA

Introduction

Labor is defined as "uterine contractions of sufficient intensity, frequency, and duration to bring about demonstrable effacement and dilation of the cervix." Abnormal prolongation of labor, or labor dystocia (derived from the Greek *dys + tokos*, difficult birth), is important to recognize because it has been associated with adverse consequences for the fetus and mother. Morbidities that have been attributed to prolonged labor include fetal and maternal infections, uterine rupture, postpartum hemorrhage, obstetric fistulae, and perineal injuries. This chapter will detail the factors which distinguish normal from abnormal labor, discuss underlying etiologies, and finally address management options in the setting of labor dystocia.

Normal and abnormal labor patterns

Normal labor occurs in four stages. The first stage is cervical dilation, the second is delivery of the fetus, the third is placental expulsion, and the fourth is recovery. The first stage is subdivided into latent and active phases. The latent phase, the earlier of the two, is characterized by regular contractions perceived by the mother and relatively slow cervical dilation. According to Friedman, who began analyzing normal labor progress as early as 1954, the mean duration of the latent phase in nulliparous women is 8.6 hours, and 5.3 hours in multiparous women. Using two standard deviations as the outer limit of normal, the latent phase should be less than 20 hours in nulliparae and less than 14 hours in multiparae. Friedman's work has been one of the foundations of labor and delivery management for decades, although some authors have questioned the definition and even the existence of the latent phase.

Active labor, the second phase of the first stage, is characterized by an accelerated rate of cervical dilation. Technically speaking, the precise onset of active labor can only be determined retrospectively after graphically plotting the labor curve for any given patient. Clinically, most women transition from the latent to the active phase when the cervix is between 3 and 4 cm dilated, although in one series 30% of women reached 5 cm of cervical dilation prior to entering active labor. Thus, the combination of regular uterine contractions and cervical dilation between 3 and 5 cm is a useful clinical marker for active labor. In Friedman's graphical analysis of labor, the mean duration of the active phase among nulliparous women was 4.9 hours but a wide range was observed. Thus, the rate of cervical dilation in active labor varies, but should proceed at a minimum of 1.2 cm/h for nulliparae and 1.5 cm/h for multiparae. Gravid women who have entered into active labor and who dilate at a slower rate are said to have protracted labor or labor dystocia, whereas those whose cervix is unchanged over a period of 2 hours are said to have an arrest of dilation.

The second stage of labor begins when cervical dilation is complete and ends with the expulsion of the fetus. Although the cardinal fetal movements in labor occur primarily in the second stage, descent of the fetal head is usually noted beginning around 7–8 cm of dilation. Thus, fetal descent bridges the first two stages of labor. The rate of this descent was also quantified in Friedman's work and proceeds at least 1 cm/h in nulliparae and 2 cm/h in multiparae. Arrest of descent is diagnosed if the fetus does not advance in station over a period of 1 hour. The total duration of the second stage of labor should be less than 2 hours in nulliparae and less than an hour in multiparae. These limits are extended by an hour if regional anesthesia is used.

The origin of these guidelines is difficult to determine, but they were already established by the time the first edition of *Williams' Obstetrics* was published in 1903 and currently remain widely accepted. In fact, the American College of Obstetricians and Gynecologists (ACOG) uses these same parameters to define both prolonged second

Management of Common Problems in Obstetrics and Gynecology, 5th edition. Edited by T.M. Goodwin, M.N. Montoro, L. Muderspach, R. Paulson and S. Roy. © 2010 Blackwell Publishing Ltd.

stage as well as second-stage arrest. Strict adherence to these limits may lead to unnecessary cesarean or forceps deliveries. More recent data suggest that prolonged second stages in closely monitored patients, even in cases where the second stage exceeds 6 hours, are not associated with adverse outcomes such as low Apgar scores, NICU admissions, neonatal seizures or neonatal death. Being mindful of the usual limits for the second stage of labor, the provider nevertheless has some leeway to exercise judgment regarding operative delivery versus continued observation, depending on the specific clinical situation, in particular continued progress in descent. In any event, if one does decide to allow the second stage to continue beyond the usual parameters, thorough documentation of the rationale behind this decision is critical.

Etiologic factors underlying labor dystocia

In labors which are progressing slowly, a combination of several variables may be involved. These are commonly summarized as "the passage, the passenger, and the powers." Although these factors are considered separately in the ensuing discussion, they are probably not always independent. For example, inadequate uterine activity may result from an excessively large or malpositioned fetus attempting to pass through a narrow pelvis.

Abnormalities of the birth canal, or "passage," may predispose to labor dystocia. Adequacy of the pelvis is assessed clinically, although the ability of clinical pelvimetry to accurately predict whether labor dystocia will be encountered is poor. Abnormally small diameters of the pelvic inlet, mid-pelvis, and outlet can be identified using x-ray or CT imaging techniques. Indeed, pelvic contractures so identified have been associated with increased incidence of labor dystocias. However, many women with increased risk of dystocia identified radiographically deliver vaginally. Thus, the positive predictive values of these instruments for obstructed labor are poor. Combinations of imaging technologies such as ultrasound and MRI have also been investigated and show some promise, but at this point such techniques are investigational. In general, in the absence of a deforming bony disease, a pelvic fracture or a soft tissue abnormality such as a cervical myoma, a narrow pelvis is unlikely to be the sole cause of abnormal labor. In any event, it is a variable that cannot be altered and at most may alert the clinician to a risk factor for prolonged or arrested labor.

The development, size, and position of the fetus, or "passenger," may also contribute to abnormal labor. Certain fetal anomalies such as macrocephaly, arthrogryposis or conjoined twins will obstruct labor. Given the widespread use of antenatal ultrasound, such anomalies are most often identified before labor. Still, in women who present in labor without having had prenatal care, the possibility of an undiagnosed fetal anomaly should be considered. On the other hand, fetal macrosomia is a condition that will be encountered more frequently. Increasing fetal weight is associated with slow progress in labor as well as with birth trauma. Despite this, fetuses over 4000 g represent a small minority of term births, and most macrosomic fetuses who deliver vaginally do so without trauma. Fetal size alone, therefore, is usually not sufficient to prevent vaginal delivery. Fetal malpresentation, however, is a common explanation for labor abnormalities. There are many variants of malpresentation, and asynclitism, persistent occiput posterior and compound presentations are the most commonly encountered examples. Although there are some exceptions, in most instances these cannot easily be remedied by the obstetrician during labor.

One common cause of protracted or arrested labor is persistent occiput posterior (OP) position. Somewhere between 15% and 25% of term fetuses begin labor in this position, but around 85% of these eventually rotate into the occiput anterior (OA) position. Fetuses that persist in OP position often undergo operative delivery. Ultimately, only about a quarter of fetuses with persistent OP position in nulliparae deliver vaginally, whereas more than half deliver vaginally if the mother is parous. Forceps delivery, forceps rotation, and manual rotation have all been utilized for persistent OP position. Vacuum delivery is attractive in this setting because it can facilitate flexion of the head and rotation of the fetus into OA position. In this sense, OP position (and similarly, asynclitism) can sometimes be corrected with a vacuum device, although the vacuum itself is not rotated. Obviously, adequate training, selection of appropriate candidates, and correct technique are required to minimize complications associated with vacuum delivery.

The third variable to be considered in labor disorders is the frequency and intensity of uterine contractions, or "the powers." In contrast to the other variables, uterine activity can be readily influenced during labor. If assessment of a patient who is not progressing reveals insufficient uterine activity, the diagnosis of active phase arrest should not be made until adequate contractions have been present for a period of at least 2 hours. Adequate uterine activity in a patient with an external tocodynamometer is defined as at least three contractions in a 10-minute period, with adequate intensity assessed via manual palpation (inability to indent the fundus of the uterus at the peak of a contraction). In patients who are monitored with an intrauterine pressure catheter, adequacy of contractions is assessed by summing the pressures generated during each contraction over a 10-minute period. The value for each individual contraction is the difference between the baseline and peak pressures, in mmHg. The number of Montevideo units thus calculated should be at least 200 to be considered adequate.

Management options in abnormal labor

In the 3–4% of patients who present with a protracted latent phase, Friedman advocated therapeutic rest via administration of parenteral sedation. Of women thus treated, 85% awoke in active labor, 10% ceased contracting (false labor), and 5% persisted in abnormal latent labor. These 5% Friedman augmented with oxytocin. Term patients who are not in active labor and who have no indication for delivery can also be sent home in expectation of active labor. This is an acceptable option if the patient has ready access to the hospital within a reasonable time frame, if pain is not excessive, and if there is no history of precipitate delivery (defined as delivery within 3 hours of the onset of contractions).

In the active phase, protracted labor should trigger a reassessment of the maternal pelvis, fetal size and position, and uterine activity. If inadequacy of contractions is a contributing factor, then amniotomy or administration of oxytocin can be employed to increase uterine activity. Both measures have been shown to independently shorten the course of labor. So-called active management of labor, a strict labor management protocol involving high-dose oxytocin augmentation and applied principally to nulliparous women in active labor with cephalic presentation, was associated with low rates of cesarean delivery when first described in Ireland. Application of this management scheme in two trials in the US resulted in shortened time to delivery, but effects on the cesarean delivery rate were mixed. Whether active management of labor should be universally applied is open to debate.

Augmentation of labor with oxytocin is widely practiced, yet dosing regimens vary considerably. Variables include starting dose, incremental dosage increase, and time interval between dose changes. High-dose protocols are characterized by any combination of higher starting doses, shorter intervals between dose increases, and larger increments at each dose change. Although low-dose regimens have been associated with a lower incidence of uterine hyperstimulation, high-dose regimens have been found in several randomized trials to result in shorter times to delivery with either no change or a decrease in cesarean delivery rates. In our center, oxytocin is begun at 1 mU/min and is titrated upward every 30 minutes until adequate uterine activity results. The following dosage levels (in mU/min) are used: 1, 2, 3, 4, 6, 8, 10. If the oxytocin has reached 10 mU/min and uterine activity is still inadequate, an order is written for maximum pitocin. The maximum pitocin protocol also increases every 30 minutes to the following dosages (again, in mU/min): 12, 16, 22. Thus, the maximum dose of oxytocin administered in our center is 22 mU/min. The dose is reduced if uterine activity is excessive, defined as six or more contractions per 10 minutes.

If labor arrests altogether prior to complete cervical dilation, then abdominal delivery is indicated. The only question left for the clinician is when labor has truly arrested. According to traditional criteria, if adequate uterine activity is present for 2 hours with no progress, then labor is arrested and the fetus should be delivered by cesarean. This 2-hour limit was challenged in a study protocol that required 4 hours of no cervical change prior to diagnosing active phase arrest. In almost 550 subjects, there was a 92% vaginal delivery rate without an increase in adverse maternal or fetal outcomes. Ultimately, the optimal time to intervene in a patient who appears to have an arrest disorder depends on the maternal and fetal status, the circumstances and capabilities of the facility, the values and wishes of the patient herself, and the experience and skill of the physician. Documentation of the management rationale is essential, in case of any untoward outcome.

In active labor, especially among nulligravidae, epidural analgesia is commonly used. It is recognized that parturients with an epidural in place have a longer second stage, as described above. In these patients, there is often a clinical window during which cervical dilation is complete and yet the patient does not feel the urge to push. The fetal station may be above + 2, and attempts at pushing may be ineffectual. This has led to the common practice of "laboring down" during which maternal pushing is deferred for some time to allow fetal descent to occur. Although "laboring down" is a colloquialism without a formal definition, the practice of delaying maternal pushing has been studied in several trials. In a large trial in Canada, nulliparous patients with an epidural who reached complete cervical dilation were randomized to either commence pushing or to wait for at least 2 hours prior to pushing. Although the mean time to delivery was about an hour longer for the delayed pushing group compared to the immediate pushing group, the pushing time was much shorter, the spontaneous vaginal delivery rate was slightly higher, and the difficult delivery rate was lower when maternal pushing efforts were delayed. In this trial, the "passive time" during which the patient was completely dilated but not yet pushing was not included in the 3-hour time limit for the second stage. If a patient is to be allowed to "labor down," the time from complete dilation as well as the time from active pushing should be noted along with a careful description of the rationale for exceeding the usual limits of the second stage.

Abnormally slow progress in the second stage of labor requires the application of clinical judgment. If the fetus is beyond the safe reach of either forceps or a vacuum device, then the options include expectant management, continuation of maternal pushing efforts, augmentation of uterine contractions with oxytocin, and cesarean delivery. Which of these options is most appropriate for any given patient depends on the specific mix of the variables described above. Resorting immediately to cesarean delivery in all cases is not ideal. In the 2003 ACOG practice bulletin on labor dystocia, it is emphasized that "contemporary practice patterns may be associated with more variation in duration of the second stage of labor. If progress is being made, the duration of the second stage alone does not mandate intervention by operative delivery."

When fetal descent slows or arrests at a sufficiently low station where operative vaginal delivery is an additional option, the decision algorithm becomes somewhat more complex. First, it must be decided whether continuation of labor is safe for the mother and fetus or whether it is more prudent to proceed with expeditious delivery. If delivery is decided upon, the clinician must make a judgment as to which route of delivery can be most safely achieved.

Conclusion

Labor occurs in four stages: cervical dilation, delivery of the fetus, expulsion of the placenta, and recovery. The latent phase of the first stage should last less than 20 hours in the nullipara, less than 14 in the multipara. Active labor is diagnosed when regular uterine contractions are present in association with cervical dilation between 3 and 5 cm. Active labor proceeds at a minimum rate of 1.2 cm/h in nulliparous women and 1.5 cm/h in women who have borne children. Protraction of active phase labor should prompt reassessment of the maternal pelvis, fetal size and position, and the quantity of uterine activity. If deemed appropriate, protracted labor can be augmented with amniotomy or intravenous oxytocin. Arrested labor is traditionally defined as no cervical change over 2 hours during active labor in the presence of adequate uterine contractions. When labor is arrested, delivery is effected via cesarean section, unless fetal station and clinical circumstances permit operative vaginal delivery.

While these specific timeframes and guidelines must play some role in decision making, the precise timing and mode of delivery for a given patient must be individualized, and sound clinical judgment is paramount.

Suggested reading

American College of Obstetricians and Gynecologists. Dystocia and augmentation of labor. ACOG Practice Bulletin No. 49. *Obstet Gynecol* 2003; 102: 1445–1454.

Cheng YW, Hopkins LM, Caughey AB. How long is too long: does a prolonged second stage of labor in nulliparous women affect maternal and neonatal outcomes? *Am J Obstet Gynecol* 2004; 191: 933–938.

Cunningham FG, Gant NF, Leveno KJ, Gilstrap LC, Hauth JC, Wenstrom KD. *Williams' obstetrics*, 21st edn. New York; McGraw Hill, 2001.

Ness A, Goldberg J, Berghella V. Abnormalities of the first and second stages of labor. *Obstet Gynecol Clin North Am* 2005; 32: 201–220.

Patka JH, Lodolce AE, Johnston AK. High- versus low-dose oxytocin for augmentation or induction of labor. *Ann Pharmacother* 2005; 39: 95–101.

Plunkett BA, Lin A, Wong CA, *et al.* Management of the second stage of labor in nulliparas with continuous epidural analgesia. *Obstet Gynecol* 2003; 102: 109–114.

Chapter 11
Operative Vaginal Delivery

Marc H. Incerpi

Department of Medicine and Obstetrics and Gynecology, Keck School of Medicine, University of Southern California, CA, USA

Introduction

One of the areas of obstetrics that has dramatically changed in the past several years is operative vaginal delivery. In 1970 the operative vaginal delivery rate in the United States was approximately 30%. By 1997 this rate had decreased to less than 10%. The most current statistics show the operative vaginal delivery rate to be approximately 6%. At the same time the number of forceps-assisted vaginal deliveries has decreased, while vaginal deliveries using the vacuum extractor have increased as a proportion of operative deliveries. The reasons that are often cited as contributing to the decline in the use of forceps are: fear of litigation, reliance on cesarean section as a remedy for abnormal labor and suspected fetal jeopardy, perception that the vacuum is easier to use and less risky to the fetus and mother, and decreased number of programs that are actively training residents in the use of forceps. These factors have resulted in a cycle, in which less teaching has led to a decline in technical skills. This decline in technical skills may increase adverse outcomes and fear of litigation, resulting in a further decrease in the use of forceps.

Indications and prerequisites for operative vaginal delivery

The indications for operative vaginal delivery are the following: nonreassuring fetal heart rate pattern, impairment of maternal health due to pushing during the second stage, and poor maternal expulsive efforts in the second stage of labor. This latter indication most commonly applies when the second stage of labor is prolonged. According to the American College of Obstetricians and Gynecologists

(ACOG), the second stage of labor is considered prolonged in a nulliparous patient if it lasts greater than 3 hours for a woman with a regional anesthetic or more than 2 hours for a woman without a regional anesthetic. In a multiparous patient, greater than 2 hours with a regional anesthetic or more than 1 hour without a regional anesthetic constitute a prolonged second stage of labor.

In order for a patient to be considered a candidate for an operative vaginal delivery, the following prerequisites must be met:
- complete cervical dilation
- ruptured membranes
- vertex presentation (unless forceps application during vaginal breech delivery)
- fetal head engaged with fetal head position known
- empty bladder
- absence of evidence of cephalopelvic disproportion
- adequate analgesia
- cesarean section capability
- experienced operator

In 1988 the classification of forceps deliveries was redefined by the ACOG (see Box 11.1). The same classification should be applied to vacuum delivery. Only very rarely should an attempt be made at operative vaginal

---

Box 11.1 ACOG forceps classification

Outlet forceps
Fetal scalp visible at introitus without separating the labia
    Fetal skull has reached the pelvic floor
    Sagittal suture is in the anterior-posterior diameter or in the right or left occiput anterior or posterior position
    Fetal head at or on the perineum
    Rotation ≤45°

Low forceps
Leading point of fetal skull at ≥ station 2:
  – with rotation ≤45°
  – or rotation ≥45°

Midforceps
Above +2 station with head engaged

Management of Common Problems in Obstetrics and Gynecology, 5th edition. Edited by T.M. Goodwin, M.N. Montoro, L. Muderspach, R. Paulson and S. Roy. © 2010 Blackwell Publishing Ltd.

delivery above station +2. Because of safety concerns, the prior classification of high forceps application was eliminated. Under no circumstances should forceps or vacuum be applied to an unengaged head.

Forceps delivery

Types of forceps

While it is beyond the scope of this chapter to discuss all the different varieties of forceps and their indications, it is appropriate to briefly comment on the more common types. Simpson or Elliot forceps are most often used for outlet vaginal deliveries. Kielland or Tucker–McLane forceps are used for rotational deliveries. Lastly, Piper forceps are used to assist in delivery of the aftercoming head for breech deliveries. The pelvic and cephalic curves, shanks, blades, and locks are different for each type of forceps. These features determine the types of forceps that are best suited for the given indication. The Piper forceps, for example, have a reverse pelvic curve suitable for delivery of the aftercoming head. The Simpson forceps have blades that are best suited for application to the molded fetal head, while those of the Kielland forceps are more appropriate for application to the fetal head with little or no molding.

Forceps application

What follows is a brief description of how forceps should be applied. For a more thorough discussion on the application of forceps, the reader is referred to additional references cited at the end of the chapter.

The concept underlying the correct application of forceps is finesse rather than force. Before actually applying the forceps to the fetal head, a "phantom application" should be performed first. The forceps are inspected to make sure that there is a complete and matched set, and that the forceps articulate (lock) easily. Forceps should be applied in a delicate fashion in order to avoid potential injury to the vagina and perineum. The goal is for the blades to fit the fetal head as evenly and symmetrically as possible. The blades should lie evenly against the side of the head, covering the space between the orbits and ears. After the forceps have been applied, they should articulate easily. If this does not occur, the forceps should be removed and a second attempt should be made. The forceps should never be forced or "jammed" into the vagina!

After the forceps have been comfortably applied to the fetal head and have been locked into place, the following safety checks should be performed for delivery of an occiput anterior position before any traction is applied to the fetal head.
• The sagittal suture should be perpendicular to the plane of the shanks.
• The posterior fontanelle should be one finger breadth away from the plane of the shanks, equidistant from the sides of the blades, and directly in front of the locked forceps.
• If fenestrated (open) blades are used, the amount of fenestration in front of the fetal head should admit no more than the tip of one finger.
Only after these checks have been performed, and the operator is confident of a correct application, can traction can be applied to the fetal head.

Traction forces should be applied in the plane of least resistance, and follow the pelvic curve. This can best be accomplished by applying downward pressure on the shanks with outward pressure exerted upon the handle of the forceps. Once the fetal head begins to emerge out of the vagina, the forceps are usually disarticulated and the head is delivered via a modified Ritgen maneuver. After delivery, it is important to identify any vaginal or perineal lacerations, paying particular attention to deep lateral vaginal sidewall (sulcal) lacerations. If lacerations are present they should be repaired in the usual fashion. A detailed delivery note should be written and preferably dictated after a forceps delivery.

Relative safety of forceps

Despite the fact that forceps have fallen into disfavor over the last several years, there have been few studies to prospectively evaluate the safety of forceps. Both maternal and fetal injuries have been reported in association with forceps deliveries. Maternal complications include lacerations of the vagina and cervix, episiotomy extensions involving the anal sphincter and rectal mucosa, pelvic hematomas, urethral and bladder injuries, and uterine rupture. In addition, the estimated blood loss and need for blood transfusions are increased in forceps deliveries. Fetal complications include minor facial lacerations, forceps marks, facial and brachial plexus palsies, cephalohematomas, skull fractures, intracranial hemorrhage, antenatal depression, and seizures. Most reports demonstrate that maternal and/or fetal complications are more common with mid forceps than low or outlet forceps deliveries. Nonetheless, it is the concern for fetal and maternal injury that has contributed to the widespread decline in the use of forceps and the increasing popularity of vacuum deliveries.

Vacuum delivery – general principles

The vacuum extractor currently employed in the United States is either a disposable, pliable, plastic cup with tubing that attaches to a separate nondisposable hand-held pump with a gauge or a disposable self-contained unit that includes the cup and the pumping mechanism and gauge all in one single device. Whichever device is being used, the basic principles are the same. The pump mechanism delivers a certain amount of suction pressure that is delivered to the fetal head in order to effect delivery. The vacuum extractor works by allowing the external traction forces applied to the scalp to be transmitted to the fetal head. In order for delivery to be accomplished, both traction on the fetal scalp and compression of the fetal head occur. The prerequisites for vacuum delivery are the same as those listed above for forceps delivery.

Vacuum application

The application of the vacuum is perceived by many to be much simpler than that of forceps, but careful attention is required. The vacuum system should be assembled to ensure that no leaks are present. The cup should then be inserted into the vagina by directing pressure toward the posterior aspect of the vagina, away from the urethra. The objective is to place the center of cup on the fetal scalp over the sagittal suture toward the occiput in order to maintain flexion of the fetal head. This area is called the median flexion point, and is located 3 cm in front of the posterior fontanelle. There should be no maternal tissue included under the cup margin.

While holding the cup firmly against the fetal head with the nondominant hands or fingers, the pressure is increased to approximately 600 mmHg at the beginning of a uterine contraction. As the mother pushes, traction is applied along the pelvic axis. If more than one contraction is necessary before the fetal head delivers, it is our practice to lower the vacuum pressure between contractions. While the fetal head is delivering, the cup should then assume a 90° orientation to the horizontal as the head is extended. Once the head has completely delivered through the vagina, the suction is withdrawn and the cup is removed.

Effectiveness and safety of vacuum delivery

Most reports demonstrate that the vacuum is quite effective, with a failure rate less than 10%. There are few data comparing different vacuum devices and cups to one another to determine if one is more effective than another.

Concern over the safety of the vacuum has significantly increased in recent years. There have been multiple reports in the literature of fetal injuries associated with vacuum delivery. These have ranged from benign superficial scalp abrasions to serious incidents of intracranial hemorrhage. The most common neonatal complication is retinal hemorrhage, which may occur as often as 50% of the time. Fortunately, this rarely has any clinical significance. Cephalohematoma occurs when bleeding is present below the periosteum, and complicates approximately 6% of all vacuum deliveries. Because the bleeding is underneath the periosteum, this very rarely results in significant blood loss due to the inability of the blood to cross the suture lines. Subgaleal hematoma is a rare but serious complication, occurring in approximately 50 out of every 10,000 vacuum deliveries. The subgaleal space extends from the nape of the neck posteriorly to the orbits anteriorly. When a subgaleal hematoma occurs, the bleeding is located above the periosteum within the loose subaponeurotic tissues of the scalp. Since there are no suture lines to contain the amount of blood, there is the potential for life-threatening hemorrhage. Lastly, the incidence of intracranial hemorrhages with vacuum delivery is approximately 0.35%, and includes subdural, subarachnoid, intraventricular, and/or intraparenchymal hemorrhage.

The issues surrounding potential neonatal complications from vacuum-assisted vaginal delivery were addressed by the FDA in a statement issued in 1998 requiring that all such complications be reported.

An awareness of the potential complications of the vacuum has led us to adopt the following safety guidelines at our institution.
• The vacuum should only be used when a specific obstetric indication is present.
• Traction is applied only when the patient is actively pushing.
• Applying torsion or twisting the cup in order to attempt to rotate the head is prohibited.
• The time from the first application of the cup to delivery of the infant should not exceed 20 minutes.
• The procedure should be abandoned after the cup has dislodged from the fetal head ("popped off") two times.
• The procedure should be abandoned if there is no fetal descent after a single pull.
• The vacuum should not be used if the estimated fetal weight is less than 2500 g or greater than 4000 g. It should not be used prior to 34 weeks of gestation.
• The operator should not switch from vacuum to forceps or vice versa.
• Neonatal staff who are knowledgeable about the complications of vacuum delivery should be present in the delivery room, and all those caring for the infant should be made aware that vacuum was used.
A detailed written and dictated delivery note should accompany each vacuum delivery. The medical record should document the indication for the procedure, the fetal station and head position at the time of the vacuum application, the type of vacuum device, the total vacuum application time, the number of applications, pulls and "pop-offs," and subsequent mode of delivery if vacuum was not successful.

While it is unrealistic to expect the patient to sign an informed consent prior to the application of the vacuum, to the extent possible, the risks of the procedure should be explained to the patient and documented in the hospital chart.

Vacuum versus forceps

Somewhat surprisingly, there have been relatively few randomized, prospective studies comparing vacuum with forceps. After surveying the medical literature, the following conclusions can be drawn in determining the success, fetal outcome, and maternal outcome of the two types of instrumental vaginal delivery.

On the whole, the vacuum extractor is significantly less likely to achieve a successful vaginal delivery than the forceps. The vacuum is significantly less likely to cause serious maternal injury than is the forceps. Although the vacuum extractor is associated with more cephalohematomas, other facial/cranial injuries are more common with forceps. In comparing Apgar scores, there is a trend toward lower Apgar scores at 5 minutes in the vacuum extractor group. Thus, it appears that the overall reduction in severe maternal injuries is the most important immediate benefit associated with the use of the vacuum extractor. However, it remains to be shown which instrument results in fewer adverse neonatal effects.

Before an operative vaginal delivery is attempted, the operator should conduct a realistic appraisal regarding likelihood for success. When an operative vaginal delivery using either forceps or vacuum fails, and the patient is delivered via cesarean section, there is a greater tendency for neonatal injury. This was illustrated by a study that examined the neonatal complications that occurred after operative vaginal delivery was attempted. The investigators reported increased rates of subdural or cerebral hemorrhage, facial nerve injury, convulsions, central nervous system depression, and mechanical ventilation in infants delivered by cesarean section after a failed attempt at operative vaginal delivery.

A discussion on operative vaginal delivery would not be complete without mentioning shoulder dystocia and its inherent complications. It has been demonstrated that the incidence of shoulder dystocia is increased with instrumental delivery. Moreover, it has been shown that shoulder dystocia is more likely to occur with vacuum rather than forceps, and more likely when the birthweight is greater than 4000 g or the total time to complete delivery is greater than 6 minutes.

Conclusion

While both forceps and vacuum have been proven to be useful in assisting with vaginal delivery, the vacuum is quickly becoming the preferred instrument of choice.

Both devices have the potential to cause fetal and maternal injury. However, the incidence of maternal injury is less with the vacuum than the forceps. In order to minimize both maternal and fetal risks, operators must be familiar with the indications, contraindications, application, and use of the particular instrument. Safe and effective guidelines similar to those outlined in this chapter should facilitate safe and effective deliveries.

Suggested reading

American College of Obstetricians and Gynecologists. *Delivery by vacuum extraction.* Committee Opinion No. 208. Washington, DC: American College of Obstetricians and Gynecologists, 1998.

American College of Obstetricians and Gynecologists. *Operative vaginal delivery.* Practice Bulletin No. 17. Washington, DC: American College of Obstetricians and Gynecologists, 2000.

Bofill JA, Rust OA, Schorr SJ, *et al.* A randomized prospective trial of the obstetric forceps versus the M-cup vacuum extractor. *Am J Obstet Gynecol* 1996; 175: 1325–1330.

Bofill JA, Rust OA, Devidas M, *et al.* Shoulder dystocia and operative vaginal delivery. *J Matern Fetal Med* 1997; 6: 220–224.

Center for Devices and Radiological Health. FDA Public Health Advisory: need for caution when using vacuum assisted delivery devices. May 21, 1998. Available at http://www.fda.gov/cdrh/fetal598.html

Clark SL, Belfort MA, Hankins GDV, *et al.* Variation in the rates of operative delivery in the United States. *Am J Obstet Gynecol* 2007; 196(6): 526.

Fitzpatrick M, Behan M, O'Connell R, *et al.* Randomized clinical trial to assess anal sphincter function following forceps or vacuum assisted vaginal delivery. *BJOG* 2003; 110: 424–429.

Hagadorn-Freathy AS, Yeomans ER, Hankins GDV. Validation of the 1988 ACOG forceps classification system. *Obstet Gynecol* 1991; 77: 35–60.

Hankins GDV, Rowe TF. Operative vaginal delivery – year 2000. *Am J Obstet Gynecol* 1996; 175: 275–282.

McQuivey RW. Vacuum-assisted delivery: a review. *J Matern Fetal Neonatal Med* 2004; 16: 171–179.

Towner DR, Ciotti MC. Operative vaginal delivery: a cause of birth injury or is it? *Clin Obstet Gynecol* 2007; 50: 563–581.

Vacca A. Operative vaginal delivery: clinical appraisal of a new vacuum extraction device. *Aust NZ J Obstet Gynecol* 2001; 41: 156–160.

Vacca A, Grant AM, Wyatt G, *et al.* Portsmouth operative delivery trial. A comparison of vacuum extraction and forceps delivery. *BJOG* 1983; 90: 1107–1112.

Williams MC. Vacuum assisted delivery. *Clin Perinatol* 1995; 22: 933–952.

Chapter 12
Shoulder Dystocia

Joseph G. Ouzounian and T. Murphy Goodwin
Department of Medicine and Obstetrics and Gynecology, Keck School of Medicine, University of Southern California, CA, USA

Definition and incidence

Shoulder dystocia occurs when further delivery of the fetal head and body is prevented by impaction of the shoulders anteriorly behind the maternal symphysis pubis, or in some cases posteriorly behind the maternal sacral promontory. Most commonly, shoulder dystocia is defined as the need for additional maneuvers after gentle downward traction is insufficient to effect delivery of the fetal head. Shoulder dystocia is an obstetric emergency, with an incidence of 0.2 to 3% of all births.

Pathophysiology

Shoulder dystocia results from a persistent anterior-posterior position of the fetal shoulders during fetal descent in labor. Normally, the fetal bisacromial diameter (the distance between the outermost points of the fetal shoulders) enters the pelvis at an oblique angle. The shoulders rotate to an anterior-posterior position with external rotation of the fetal head, which allows the anterior shoulder to slide under the symphysis pubis. With shoulder dystocia, the shoulders remain in an anterior-posterior position during descent, or descend simultaneously (rather than sequentially), leading to impaction. Either anterior impaction under the symphysis pubis or posterior impaction behind the sacral promontory can occur. Increased resistance between the fetal skin and vaginal walls (as in cases of macrosomia), or cases where truncal rotation does not occur (as in precipitous labor), can lead to shoulder dystocia. In some cases, stretching of the nerves in the brachial plexus during labor and/or fetal descent can result in nerve injury.

Management of Common Problems in Obstetrics and Gynecology, 5th edition. Edited by T.M. Goodwin, M.N. Montoro, L. Muderspach, R. Paulson and S. Roy. © 2010 Blackwell Publishing Ltd.

Risk factors

Numerous risk factors have been described for the occurrence of shoulder dystocia. Even though about 50% of cases occur in infants weighing less than 4000 gm, the incidence of shoulder dystocia increases progressively as birth weight rises. An infant weighing between 4000 and 4500 gm has an 8–10% chance of shoulder dystocia, as compared to a 20–30% chance if the infant weighs more than 4500 gm. The most commonly used threshold for macrosomia is a birthweight over 4000 gm. Of note, fetal body configuration may be more important than birthweight per se, as macrosomic infants have a trunk or chest circumference larger than the head circumference in addition to an increased bisacromial diameter. These factors impede normal shoulder rotation and can lead to the shoulder impaction.

Diabetes mellitus is another risk factor reported in association with shoulder dystocia. Many macrosomic infants are delivered from women with diabetes. As such, the incidence of shoulder dystocia in diabetic mothers is higher than that in the general population (9–33%). Moreover, infants of diabetic mothers experience a significantly higher shoulder dystocia rate than infants of nondiabetics of a similar birthweight. ACOG advises against a trial of labor in patients with maternal diabetes and an estimated fetal weight > 4500 gm.

Other historically reported antepartum risk factors for shoulder dystocia include postdates gestation, advanced maternal age, multiparity, excessive maternal weight or weight gain, oxytocin use, epidural use, and prior shoulder dystocia. Intrapartum risk factors include a protracted first stage, prolonged deceleration phase (between 8 and 10 cm), and epidural anesthesia.

Prediction

Attempts at predicting the occurrence of shoulder dystocia have been disappointing. Even though it is evident that shoulder dystocia rates increase with increasing birthweight, efforts to predict birthweight accurately

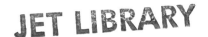

with antepartum or intrapartum assessments remain very poor. Ultrasound estimates of fetal weight are often no better than clinical estimates in predicting macrosomia, and have an inherent error rate of $+/-15\%$ in estimating the actual birthweight. Furthermore, weight estimates become increasingly inaccurate as birthweight increases. As such, numerous studies have demonstrated that while many of the risk factors noted above are indeed associated with a higher incidence of shoulder dystocia (macrosomia in particular), their positive predictive value remains very low (1–3%). Studies have demonstrated that induction of labor for suspected macrosomia (as compared to expectant management) does not decrease the incidence of shoulder dystocia or brachial plexus injury and only results in an increased rate of cesarean delivery. Thus, in practical terms, the presence of one or more risk factors should lead to a heightened awareness of the chance for shoulder dystocia, but elective cesarean section for suspected fetal macrosomia should be reserved for cases with an estimated fetal weight > 5000 gm (4500 gm in diabetics).

Management

Shoulder dystocia is a true obstetric emergency, and its occurrence requires a rapid and well-coordinated stepwise plan. Because shoulder dystocia is so difficult to predict, the presence of one or more risk factors may trigger an informed consent discussion with the patient regarding the risks and benefits of prophylactic cesarean section, and careful monitoring during labor and delivery. Operative vaginal delivery should be avoided in patients with prolonged labor and concomitant fetal macrosomia.

Shoulder dystocia is often heralded by the classic "turtle sign." After the fetal head delivers, it retracts back onto the maternal perineum. As maternal efforts to expel the fetal body continue, the shoulders become further impacted behind the symphysis pubis. Once shoulder dystocia is diagnosed additional support should be called for. Anesthesia personnel, additional nursing support, and pediatrics should be summoned. Time spent suctioning the nares or relieving a tight nuchal cord should be minimized, and the mother should be instructed to stop pushing. All attendants should refrain from applying fundal pressure, as this has been shown to worsen the impaction and increase the chance of brachial plexus injury.

While no sequence or combination of maneuvers has been shown to be superior in the management of shoulder dystocia, it is reasonable to implement the McRoberts maneuver as the initial technique for disimpaction of the anterior shoulder. Studies have shown that the McRoberts maneuver alone alleviates the dystocia in approximately 40% of cases. Objective testing has also shown that this maneuver may reduce fetal shoulder extraction forces and brachial plexus stretching.

The McRoberts maneuver involves exaggerated hyperflexion of the patient's legs, resulting in a straightening of the maternal sacrum relative to the lumbar spine with consequent cephalic rotation of the symphysis pubis. The effects of this position enhance passage of the posterior fetal shoulder over the sacrum and through the pelvic inlet, positioning the plane of the pelvic inlet to its maximal dimension perpendicular to the maximum maternal expulsive force. Limitations to the technique include the need for two assistants and the extra time required to elevate and flex the patient's legs. Potential difficulty can also be encountered in moving the very obese patient or the patient with a dense epidural motor blockade.

The need for additional maneuvers after McRoberts has been associated with larger fetal birth weights, longer active phases, and longer second stages of labor. Simultaneous suprapubic pressure, applied either posteriorly or laterally, can displace the impacted shoulder into the oblique diameter and effect delivery. The need for a proctoepisiotomy is best left to the clinical judgment of the physician or midwife in attendance at the delivery. In some cases it can help in implementation of various maneuvers, and in other cases it is unnecessary.

By applying pressure on the anterior surface of the posterior shoulder, the Woods' (corkscrew) maneuver attempts to push the posterior shoulder through a clockwise 180° arc. In the reverse of Woods', the Rubin's maneuver, pressure is applied to the posterior surface of the anterior shoulder in order to effect counterclockwise rotation of the posterior shoulder.

Should the above maneuvers fail, the physician's hand can be passed into the vagina following the posterior arm to the elbow. After pressure is applied at the antecubital fossa in order to flex the fetal forearm, the arm is swept out over the infant's chest and delivered over the perineum. Rotation of the fetal trunk to bring the posterior arm anteriorly may be required.

If all of the above maneuvers fail, they should be re-attempted with the patient under adequate anesthesia. If delivery is still unsuccessful, then heroic next steps (Zavanelli maneuver and symphysiotomy) may be in order.

In the Zavanelli maneuver, the head is rotated back to a direct occiput anterior position and then flexed. Constant firm pressure is used to push the head back into the vagina; a cesarean section subsequently is performed. To perform a symphysiotomy, the patient should be placed in an exaggerated lithotomy position and have a Foley catheter placed to identify the urethra. With the physician's index and middle finger displacing the urethra laterally, the cephalad portion of the symphysis is incised with a scalpel blade. Fracture of the clavicle may be attempted by applying direct pressure away from the fetal lung. In reality, however, this is difficult to accomplish in the setting of shoulder dystocia.

It is important to document the sequence and types of maneuvers used in the management of shoulder dystocia, and maintain a consistent plan. Shoulder dystocia drills, like medical simulations used for other types of emergencies, can be helpful in ensuring that the entire healthcare team is prepared for this unpredictable event.

Complications

Maternal complications of shoulder dystocia include postpartum hemorrhage, cervical and/or vaginal lacerations, bladder atony, and in rare cases uterine rupture. Symphyseal separation and transient maternal femoral neuropathy have been reported with use of the McRoberts maneuver. Studies have reported fetal injury rates as high as 25% with shoulder dystocia. Brachial plexus injury can occur in up to 17% of shoulder dystocia cases. Approximately 80% of these involve the upper nerve roots at C5–C7 (Erb–Duchenne palsy), with lower C8–T1 nerve root involvement (Klumpke's palsy) occurring less often. Over 90% of brachial plexus palsies resolve by one year of life. Those that persist beyond that time are usually considered permanent injuries. It is important to note that while these injuries frequently do occur in cases of shoulder dystocia, they are also known to occur in the posterior shoulder of infants with anterior shoulder dystocia, in spontaneous vaginal deliveries, and with cesarean section. Equally important, their occurrence has no relation to the number or type of maneuvers used to disimpact the shoulder. Clavicular and humeral fractures may also occur in up to 10% of shoulder dystocia cases, although most of these usually resolve without any long-term sequelae. Permanent neurologic injury can also occur. One study demonstrated a mean head-shoulder interval of 7 minutes in cases of neonatal brain injury after severe shoulder dystocia. While the fetal pH has been shown to decline at a rate of approximately 0.04 units/min between delivery of the head and trunk (due to cord occlusion), fetal death due to shoulder dystocia is quite rare.

Suggested readings

Gherman RB, Ouzounian JG, Goodwin TM. Obstetric maneuvers for shoulder dystocia and associated fetal morbidity. *Am J Obstet Gynecol* 1998; 178(6): 1126–1130.

Gherman RB, Ouzounian JG, Incerpi MH, Goodwin TM. Symphyseal separation and transient femoral neuropathy associated with the McRoberts maneuver. *Am J Obstet Gynecol* 1998; 178(3): 609–610.

Gherman RB, Goodwin TM, Souter I, Ouzounian JG, Paul RH. The McRoberts maneuver for the alleviation of shoulder dystocia: how successful is it? *Am J Obstet Gynecol* 1997; 176: 656–661.

Gherman RB, Ouzounian JG, Satin AG, Goodwin TM, Phelan JP. A comparison of shoulder dystocia-associated transient and permanent brachial plexus palsies. *Obstet Gynecol* 2003; 102(3): 544–548.

Gherman RB, Ouzounian JG, Miller DA, *et al*. Spontaneous vaginal delivery: a risk factor for Erb's palsy? *Am J Obstet Gynecol* 1998; 178(3): 423–427.

Goodwin TM, Banks E, Millar LK, Phelan JP. Catastrophic shoulder dystocia and emergency symphysiotomy. *Am J Obstet Gynecol* 1997; 177: 463–464.

Gross SJ, Shime J, Farine D. Shoulder dystocia. Predictors and outcome. *Am J Obstet Gynecol* 1987; 156: 334–336.

Gross TL, Sokol RJ, Williams T, Thompson K. Shoulder dystocia: a fetal–physician risk. *Am J Obstet Gynecol* 1987; 156: 1408–1418.

Lipscomb KR, Gregory K, Shaw K. The outcome of macrosomic infants weighing at least 4500 grams: Los Angeles County University of Southern California experience. *Obstet Gynecol* 1995; 85: 558–564.

McFarland MB, Langer O, Piper JM, Berkus MD. Perinatal outcome and the type and number of maneuvers in shoulder dystocia. *Int J Gynecol Obstet* 1996; 55: 219–224.

Ouzounian JG. Effective management of shoulder dystocia. *OBG Management* 1997; 28–32.

Ouzounian JG, Gherman RB. Shoulder dystocia: Are historic risk factors reliable predictors? *Am J Obstet Gynecol*, 2005; 192: 1933–1938.

Ouzounian JG, Korst LM, Phelan JP. Permanent Erb's palsy: A lack of a relationship with obstetrical risk factors. *Am J Perinatol* 1998; 15(4): 221–223.

Ouzounian JG, Phelan JP, Korst LM. Permanent Erb palsy: A traction-related injury? *Obstet Gynecol* 1997; 89: 139–141.

Ouzounian JG, Korst LM, Ahn MO, *et al*. Shoulder dystocia and neonatal brain injury: Significance of the head-shoulder interval. *Am J Obstet Gynecol* 1998; 178: S76.

Ouzounian JG, Naylor CS, Gherman RB, *et al*. Recurrent shoulder dystocia: How high is the risk? *Am J Obstet Gynecol* 2001; 185: S108.

Phelan JP, Ouzounian JG, Gherman RB, *et al*. Shoulder dystocia and permanent Erb's palsy: the role of fundal pressure. *Am J Obstet Gynecol* 1997; 176: S138.

Rouse DJ, Owen J, Goldenberg RL, Cliver SP. The effectiveness and costs of elective cesarean delivery for fetal macrosomia diagnosed by ultrasound. *JAMA* 1996; 276: 1480–1486.

Chapter 13
Chorio-Amnionitis and Postpartum Endometritis

Marc H. Incerpi

Department of Medicine and Obstetrics and Gynecology, Keck School of Medicine, University of Southern California, CA, USA

Chorio-amnionitis

Strictly defined, chorio-amnionitis is an infection of the amniotic cavity, fetal membranes, placenta, and/or decidua. Other terms used to describe this condition are intra-amniotic infection, amnionitis, and amniotic fluid infection. This is usually a polymicrobial infection involving organisms commonly found in the vagina. Research studies indicate that chorio-amnionitis complicates 0.5–10% of all pregnancies. A distinction between histologic chorio-amnionitis and clinical amnionitis is often made. The former is defined by infiltration of the fetal membranes with polymorphonuclear leukocytes. It occurs more often than clinical chorio-amnionitis, and usually is discovered in cases in which there are no clinical signs or symptoms of infection as discussed below. Up to 20% of term deliveries and nearly half of preterm deliveries are associated with histologic chorio-amnionitis. Clinical chorio-amnionitis is seen in 1–2% of term and 5–10% of preterm births. Despite continued advances in antibiotic therapy, intra-amniotic infection is associated with increased maternal and neonatal morbidity and mortality.

Etiology

While the majority of cases of chorio-amnionitis are due to an ascending infection from the vagina and cervix, intra-amniotic infection may also occur via the hematogenous route or after invasive procedures such as amniocentesis, chorionic villous sampling or cerclage. Any factor that increases the risk of prolonged exposure of the fetal membranes and/or uterine cavity to ascending bacteria from the vagina will increase the risk of chorio-amnionitis. Such factors include prolonged rupture of membranes, frequent vaginal examinations, prolonged labor, premature labor, nulliparity, internal fetal monitoring, and meconium-stained amniotic fluid.

Clinical features

The diagnosis of chorio-amnionitis is based on observation of the following reactions of the patient and her fetus to an intra-amniotic infection.
• Maternal temperature greater than 100.4°F or 38°C in the absence of any obvious causes of fever
• Maternal tachycardia
• Uterine tenderness
• Malodorous or purulent amniotic fluid
• Elevated white blood cell count (>15,000 mL)
• Fetal tachycardia
• Fetal heart rate pattern with decreased variability and/or decelerations

In situations in which the diagnosis is unclear, the gold standard is a positive amniotic fluid culture and gram stain obtained via amniocentesis. It is not essential for an amniocentesis to be performed in all cases in which chorio-amnionitis is suspected. Most often, the diagnosis is made on the basis of the clinical observations noted above. Amniocentesis should be considered in those patients in preterm labor without obvious signs of intra-amniotic infection who fail to respond to tocolysis with a single agent or in those patients who have recurrent preterm labor. The presence of low amniotic fluid glucose levels (<15 mg/dL) or elevated cytokines (interleukin-1, interleukin-6, and tumor necrosis factor) has been associated with the histologic diagnosis of chorio-amnionitis. Unfortunately, testing amniotic fluid for the presence of cytokines is not routinely available. Testing maternal blood for elevated C-reactive protein provides little if any diagnostic information.

Perinatal complications

The risk of fetal infection associated with chorio-amnionitis is 10–20%. Potential infectious morbidities include pneumonia, meningitis, and sepsis. In addition, greater evidence is accumulating to implicate the role of intra-amniotic infection in neurodevelopmental delay

Management of Common Problems in Obstetrics and Gynecology,
5th edition. Edited by T.M. Goodwin, M.N. Montoro,
L. Muderspach, R. Paulson and S. Roy. © 2010 Blackwell
Publishing Ltd.

and cerebral palsy. These complications are more severe in premature infants. While the exact etiology of neurodevelopmental delay and cerebral palsy in infants born to mothers with chorio-amnionitis is not known with certainty, the leading theory suggests that it is due to an elevation in fetal cytokine levels as part of the fetal inflammatory response syndrome. The elevation in cytokines has been associated with destruction of the white matter within the brain (cystic periventricular leukomalacia) and the development of neurologic delay or cerebral palsy. Lastly, chorio-amnionitis can lead to fetal or neonatal death.

Maternal complications

While not as common as fetal and neonatal complications, chorio-amnionitis may result in significant maternal morbidity ranging from pelvic infection to septic shock. With continuing advances in medical care, maternal mortality due to chorio-amnionitis is exceedingly rare. In fact, in four relatively recent studies involving more than 700 women with chorio-amnionitis, no maternal deaths were reported.

Management

After a diagnosis of chorio-amnionitis is made, parenteral antibiotics should be started followed by delivery regardless of gestational age. Antipyretic therapy with acetaminophen and/or cooling blankets help to decrease febrile morbidity. Since many different organisms have been associated with intra-amniotic infection (Box 13.1), most

---

Box 13.1 Organisms commonly associated with chorio-amnionitis

Aerobic
Gram negative
Escherichia coli
Other gram-negative bacilli
Gram positive
Streptococcus agalactiae
Enterococcus faecalis
Staphylococcus aureus
Streptococcus species

Anaerobic
Gram negative
Bacteroides fragilis
Fusobacterium species
Gardnerella vaginalis
Gram positive
Peptostreptococcus species
Peptococcus species
Clostridium species

Other
Mycoplasma hominis
Ureaplasma urealyticum

---

authorities recommend combination antibiotics or single-agent broad-spectrum antibiotics. Many different regimens have been proposed but ampicillin given along with an aminoglycoside such as gentamicin has proven to be safe and effective. In cases in which anaerobic organisms are suspected or recovered, an antimicrobial with anaerobic coverage such as clindamycin or metronidazole is recommended. Similarly, either clindamycin or metronidazole should be added if cesarean section is performed.

Cesarean section should be reserved for usual obstetric indications. There is no evidence to suggest that cesarean delivery offers any advantage over vaginal birth in the setting of chorio-amnionitis. Intra-amniotic infection is often associated with poor uterine contractility and dysfunctional labor. Not only is oxytocin augmentation often necessary, but also uterine atony is much more common after delivery, because of the diminished ability of the uterus to contract after delivery. Consequently, the incidence of postpartum hemorrhage is increased in patients with chorio-amnionitis.

Summary

The diagnosis of chorio-amnionitis is made primarily on clinical criteria based on maternal and fetal manifestations including fever, uterine tenderness, and both maternal and fetal tachycardia. Early diagnosis and prompt treatment remain the cornerstones of management so that a favorable outcome for both mother and baby can be achieved.

Postpartum endometritis

Endometritis refers to infection of the endometrium or decidua, often with extension into the myometrium or parametrial tissues. Although endometritis can theoretically occur at any time, the following discussion will center on infection occurring in the postpartum period. The incidence varies depending on population studied and route of delivery. After vaginal delivery, the incidence is only 3%, while after cesarean delivery it ranges from 15% to 85%, with most studies reporting a range of 30–40%. With the routine use of prophylactic antibiotics, the incidence can be reduced dramatically. As is the case with chorio-amnionitis, postpartum endometritis is most commonly a polymicrobial infection.

Etiology

The majority of cases of postpartum endometritis arise from an ascending infection from organisms that are part of the normal vaginal flora. The following risk factors are associated with the development of endometritis: prolonged labor, prolonged rupture of membranes, number of vaginal examinations, internal monitoring, lower socioeconomic status, and route of delivery. While all of these may play a role in the patient developing endometritis, the most important is route of delivery. As stated previously, the incidence after vaginal delivery approximates 2–3% and after cesarean delivery, 10–85%. Reports in the literature have demonstrated that the major reason for such a wide range is primarily the population of patients studied, and whether they fall into high-risk versus low-risk groups. The former would include women who have prolonged rupture of membranes, prolonged labor, multiple vaginal examinations, and those who have been diagnosed with chorio-amnionitis. The latter includes women who undergo repeat cesarean section with intact membranes and no labor.

Clinical features

Patients with postpartum endometritis will commonly present with fever ($\geq$100.4°F or 38°C) without obvious source of infection (e.g. urinary tract infection, mastitis). The majority of cases develop within the first week after delivery. Additional findings on physical examination include uterine tenderness, abdominal tenderness, and foul-smelling lochia. Patients will commonly have an elevated white blood cell count. The diagnosis is based on clinical findings. There is little if any role for obtaining cultures from the cervix or endometrium in patients suspected of having postpartum endometritis.

Management

After the clinical diagnosis of postpartum endometritis is made, treatment with parenteral antibiotics should be initiated immediately. Since a variety of microbes have been associated with postpartum endometritis (Box 13.2), most authorities recommend combination therapy. Unlike the organisms associated with chorio-amnionitis, anaerobic organisms predominate in patients with endometritis. The gold standard has been clindamycin and gentamicin. Reports in the literature demonstrate that this regimen will result in a cure rate greater than 90%. Some investigators have reported very good success with single-agent treatment using either a broad-spectrum second- or third-generation cephalosporin (e.g. cefoxitin, cefoperazone) or a β-lactamase inhibitor with an extended-spectrum penicillin (e.g. ampicillin/sulbactam). Cure rates in the range of 80–90% have been reported using single-agent therapy.

Antibiotics should be continued for a period of 48–72 hours. If the patient has an adequate clinical response, she can then be discharged home without further antibiotics. However, if there has been no clinical improvement after 48–72 hours of antibiotics, the patient should be re-examined for possible complications such as cellulitis, pelvic abscess, abdominal wound infection or septic pelvic thrombophlebitis. The addition of ampicillin may also prove beneficial in order to treat an infection due to *Enterococcus* or other gram-positive aerobic bacteria. A CT scan or MRI of the abdomen and pelvis is indicated in such cases where pelvic abscess or septic

---

Box 13.2 Organisms commonly associated with postpartum endometritis

Aerobic
Gram positive
Streptococcus agalactiae
Streptococcus viridans
Streptococcus faecalis
Streptococcus species
Staphylococcus aureus
Staphylococcus epidermidis
Enterococcus species

Gram negative
Escherichia coli
Klebsiella pneumoniae
Enterobacter aerogenes
Gardnerella vaginalis
Morganella morganii

Anaerobic
Gram positive
Peptococcus species
Peptostreptococcus species
Clostridium species
Gram negative
Bacteroides bivius
Bacteroides fragilis
Bacteroides species
Fusobacterium necrophorum
Fusobacterium nucleatum

---

pelvic thrombophlebitis is suspected. The former may potentially be drained surgically or via CT or ultrasound guidance, while the latter may respond with the addition of heparin. Pelvic ultrasound can sometimes identify retained products of conception within the uterus. If retained tissue is seen then uterine curettage should be performed after the patient has received at least a single course of antibiotics.

Prevention

It appears that the best way to prevent patients from developing postpartum endometritis is to decrease the incidence of chorio-amnionitis by limiting vaginal examinations, especially in patients who have ruptured membranes. The judicious use of internal monitors may also help to decrease this complication. Lastly, if cesarean section is to be done, patients should receive prophylactic antibiotics. It has been a long-standing belief that in order to optimize neonatal outcome, antibiotics should be administered after the umbilical cord has been clamped. However, a recent study indicated that the incidence of postpartum infection was significantly decreased, while neonatal outcome was unchanged, when prophylactic antibiotics were given prior to the skin incision. Studies have also demonstrated decreased incidence of postpartum infection when the placenta was spontaneously delivered as opposed to being manually removed at the time of cesarean section.

Summary

The diagnosis of postpartum endometritis is made on clinical criteria, keeping in mind that the route of delivery is the most significant risk factor. The patient must be examined to rule out other causes of postpartum fever such as atelectasis, urinary tract infection, wound infection, drug reaction, and thromboembolic events. In addition, other conditions unique to the postpartum period should be considered including vaginal or pelvic hematoma, vaginal or pelvic abscess, mastitis, septic pelvic thrombophlebitis, and ovarian vein thrombosis. Taking a detailed history and performing a thorough physical examination can distinguish most of these conditions. Prompt antibiotic management is the mainstay of therapy. A favorable response is the rule rather than the exception. Appropriate antibiotic therapy should be continued until the patient has been asymptomatic and afebrile for 48 hours. There is no proven benefit to continuing oral antibiotics after the patient has been discharged from the hospital.

Suggested reading

Bracci R, Buonocore G. Chorio–amnionitis: a risk factor for fetal and neonatal morbidity. *Biol Neonate* 2003: 83: 85–96.

Burrows LJ, Meyn LA, Weber AM. Maternal morbidity associated with vaginal versus cesarean delivery. *Obstet Gynecol* 2004; 103: 907–912.

Casey BM, Cox SM. Chorio-amnionitis and endometritis. *Infect Dis Clin North Am* 1997; 11: 203–222.

di Zerega G, Yonekura L, Roy S, *et al*. A comparison of clindamycin-gentamicin and penicillin-gentamicin in the treatment of post-cesarean section endomyometritis. *Am J Obstet Gynecol* 1979; 134: 238–242.

Edwards RK. Chorio-amnionitis and labor. *Obstet Gynecol Clin North Am* 2005; 32: 287–296.

Gaudet LM, Smith GN. Cerebral palsy and chorio-amnionitis: the inflammatory-cytokine link. *Obstet Gynecol Surv* 2001; 56: 433–436.

Hauth JC, Gilstrap LC, Hankins GDV, *et al*. Term maternal and neonatal complications of acute chorio-amnionitis. *Obstet Gynecol* 1985; 66: 59–62.

Lasley DS, Eblen A, Yancey MK, *et al*. The effect of placental removal method on the incidence of post-cesarean infections. *Am J Obstet Gynecol* 1997; 176: 1250–1254.

Ledger WJ. Post-partum endomyometritis diagnosis and treatment: a review. *J Obstet Gynaecol Res* 2003; 29: 364–373.

Mittendorf R, Montag AG, MacMillan W, *et al*. Components of the systemic fetal inflammatory response syndrome as predictors of impaired neurologic outcomes in children. *Am J Obstet Gynecol* 2003; 188: 1438–1446.

Newton ER, Prihoda TJ, Gibbs RS. A clinical and microbiologic analysis of risk factors for puerperal endometritis. *Obstet Gynecol* 1990; 75: 402–406.

Soper DE, Mayhall CG, Dalton HP. Risk factors for intra-amniotic infection: a prospective epidemiologic study. *Am J Obstet Gynecol* 1989; 161: 562–566.

Sullivan SA, Smith T, Chang E, *et al*. Administration of cefazolin prior to skin incision is superior to cefazolin at cord clamping in preventing post cesarean infectious morbidity: a randomized, controlled trial. *Am J Obstet Gynecol* 2007; 196: 455.

Trochez-Martinez RD, Smith P, Lamont RF. Use of C-reactive protein as a predictor of chorio-amnionitis in preterm prelabour rupture of membranes: a systemic review. *BJOG* 2007; 114: 796–801.

Wu JW, Escobar GJ, Gretther JK, *et al*. Chorio-amnionitis and cerebral palsy in term and near-term infants. *JAMA* 2003; 290: 2677–2684.

Chapter 14
Vaginal Birth After Cesarean

David A. Miller

Department of Medicine and Obstetrics and Gynecology, Keck School of Medicine, University of Southern California, CA, USA

Introduction

Between 1965 and 1988, the cesarean rate in the United States increased from 4.5% to 24.7%, prompting efforts to minimize unnecessary operative deliveries [1]. Obstetric practice at that time was heavily influenced by the dictum of "once a cesarean, always a cesarean"[2]. Vaginal birth after cesarean (VBAC) was uncommon, and repeat cesarean sections accounted for approximately one-third of all abdominal deliveries. In 1980, the National Institute of Health convened a Consensus Development Conference on Cesarean Childbirth, recommending that a trial of labor (TOL) be considered an option for women with a previous cesarean delivery [1]. With growing support from the American College of Obstetricians and Gynecologists (ACOG), the national VBAC rate increased from approximately 1% in 1970 to a high of 28.3% in 1996, contributing to a fall in the overall cesarean section rate to 20.7% [3]. However, enthusiasm for VBAC was dampened by a number of reports of adverse outcomes related to uterine rupture. Since 1996, the VBAC rate in the United States has been on the decline, reaching a low of 9.2% in 2004 [4]. Due in part to the falling rate of VBAC, the overall cesarean section rate in the United States reached a new high of 31.1% in 2006 [5].

During the 20th century, the classic uterine incision gave way to the low-transverse incision. Early experience suggested that the low-transverse uterine incision conferred a much lower risk of subsequent uterine rupture than did its predecessor. Lavin reviewed the English language literature between 1950 and 1980 and reported the outcomes of 3214 trials of labor in women with previous cesarean sections [6]. The vaginal delivery rate was 66.7%, and 21 women (0.7%) experienced uterine rupture.

Since 1980, more than 24,000 trials of labor have been reported in the literature, with a mean success rate of approximately 80%, and uterine rupture rates as low as 0.2–0.8%. In 2004, Guise published a review of the literature from 1980 to 2002 and reported a rate of rupture of 0.38% [7].

Benefits and risks

The principal anticipated benefits of VBAC include avoidance of the morbidity, mortality and cost of a major abdominal operation. The major risks of VBAC are those associated with intrapartum separation of the uterine scar. With respect to severity, scar separation may be classified as dehiscence or rupture. Uterine scar dehiscence is asymptomatic and is encountered incidentally during uterine exploration following vaginal delivery or at the time of cesarean section for an unrelated indication. Uterine rupture is defined as a defect that: (1) involves the entire thickness of the uterine wall, and (2) is associated with at least one of the following:
• laparotomy for control of hemorrhage from the uterine defect
• hysterectomy due to hemorrhage from the uterine defect
• repair of damage to the uterus or surrounding organs caused by uterine scar separation
• extrusion of any part of the fetus, placenta or umbilical cord through the uterine defect
• cesarean section for acute fetal compromise
Overall, more than 80% of women who attempt VBAC are successful. However, several factors can influence the likelihood of success and the risk of uterine rupture [8].

Type of previous incision
Prospective data are limited but estimated risks of uterine rupture range from less than 1% with a single previous low-transverse uterine incision to approximately 4–9% with a classic or T-shaped incision [8]. With a previous low-vertical incision, reported rates range from 1% to 7% [9].

Management of Common Problems in Obstetrics and Gynecology, 5th edition. Edited by T.M. Goodwin, M.N. Montoro, L. Muderspach, R. Paulson and S. Roy. © 2010 Blackwell Publishing Ltd.

Number of previous cesareans

With two previous low-transverse cesarean deliveries, reported rates of uterine rupture range from 1% to almost 4%. In one study, the success rate of VBAC was 75% among women undertaking a TOL with two previous cesareans [10]. One or more previous successful vaginal deliveries may reduce the rupture rate and increase the success rate significantly [11].

Indication for previous cesarean

The indication for the previous cesarean section can influence the likelihood of a successful VBAC. In women with previous cesarean sections for "dystocia" or "failure to progress," reported success rates range from 54% to 77%, with an average of approximately 65%. The risk of uterine rupture does not appear to be increased.

Fetal macrosomia

Although fetal macrosomia may lower the likelihood of successful VBAC, the impact on the rate of uterine rupture may be limited to those women who have not had a previous vaginal delivery.

Maternal age

While some studies demonstrate a lower VBAC success rate in women aged 35 and older, there is no established consensus regarding the impact of maternal age on the risk of uterine rupture [12].

Cervical status

Cervical status prior to induction has been reported to influence the likelihood of successful VBAC as well as the risk of uterine rupture. Among women with modified Bishop scores of 0–2, Bujold reported a successful VBAC rate of 57.8% and a rupture rate of 0.21%, compared to a success rate of 97% and a rupture rate of 0% among those with a Bishop score 9 or greater [13].

Layers of uterine closure

In women with a previous single-layer uterine closure, one study reported a sixfold higher rate of uterine rupture (3.1%) than in women with a previous double-layer closure (0.5%). After correcting for other factors such as prior vaginal delivery, birthweight and interdelivery interval, the risk was still four times higher with a previous single-layer uterine closure [14].

Interdelivery interval

An interdelivery interval of less than 18 months has been reported to increase the risk of uterine rupture threefold. Interdelivery intervals of at least 2 years are associated with uterine rupture rates less than 1%, while rupture rates of more than 4% have been reported when the interdelivery interval is 1 year or less [15]. The impact on TOL success rates has not been established.

Thickness of the lower uterine segment

Although data are limited, one study reported a higher rate of uterine scar separation among women with a sonographically measured lower uterine segment thickness of 2.5 mm or less. A measurement less than 3.5 mm had a positive predictive value for uterine scar separation of 11.8% and a negative predictive value of 99.3% [16]. Lower uterine segment thickness has an unknown effect on the likelihood of successful VBAC.

Dystocia in the current labor

Dystocia is a recognized risk factor for failed VBAC. In at least one case–control study, dysfunctional labor was significantly more common among women with uterine rupture than among controls without scar separation [17]. Arrest of dilation was 10 times more likely in cases than controls.

Oxytocin and prostaglandin

Labor induction and augmentation have been reported to increase the risk of uterine rupture. In one study of 2214 women with one prior cesarean section who entered labor spontaneously, the rate of uterine rupture was 0.7% compared to a rate of 2.3% in 560 women who had labor induction or augmentation [18]. Among 20,095 women with one previous cesarean, Lydon-Rochelle reported a uterine rupture rate of 1.6 per 1000 with no labor, 5.2 per 1000 with spontaneous labor, 7.7 per 1000 if labor was induced without prostaglandin and 24.5 per 1000 if labor was induced with prostaglandin [19]. Higher reported uterine rupture rates associated with prostaglandins have led the ACOG to discourage the use of prostaglandins for induction of labor in most women with a previous cesarean delivery [8].

Consequences of uterine rupture

Maternal and perinatal morbidity rates in 99 cases of uterine rupture reported by Leung are summarized in Table 14.1 [20]. These risks must be weighed against the risks associated with elective repeat cesarean section. Flamm reported a significantly higher rate of low 5-minute Apgar scores with a trial of labor, but longer

Table 14.1 Uterine rupture-related maternal and perinatal morbidity

Event	% of ruptures	Per 1000 trials of labor
Hysterectomy	21	1.5
Bladder rupture	10	0.7
Transfusion	30	2.1
Fetal extrusion	31	2.2
Perinatal asphyxia	5.1	0.4

hospital stays, more blood transfusions, and more febrile morbidity among women undergoing routine, elective repeat cesarean sections than among those attempting VBAC [21]. McMahon reported more major complications (hysterectomy, uterine rupture, operative injury) among women undertaking a TOL than in those undergoing elective repeat cesarean section [22]. Mozurkewich and Hutton conducted a meta-analysis of the literature between 1989 and 1999 and reported significantly higher rates of uterine rupture, fetal mortality and low 5-minute Apgar scores and significantly lower rates of maternal fever, transfusion and hysterectomy in association with a TOL compared to elective repeat cesarean delivery [23]. Available evidence suggests that maternal risks are slightly higher with elective repeat cesarean and fetal risks slightly higher with TOL.

Recommendations for vaginal birth after cesarean

Recommendations published in ACOG Practice Bulletin Number 54 are summarized below.
• Most women with one previous cesarean delivery with a low-transverse incision are candidates for VBAC and should be counseled about VBAC and offered a trial of labor.
• Epidural anesthesia may be used for VBAC.
• Women with a vertical incision within the lower uterine segment that does not extend into the fundus are candidates for VBAC.
• The use of prostaglandins for cervical ripening or induction of labor in most women with a previous cesarean delivery should be discouraged.
• Because uterine rupture may be catastrophic, VBAC should only be attempted in institutions equipped to respond to emergencies with physicians immediately available to provide emergency care.
• After thorough counseling that weighs the individual benefits and risks of VBAC, the ultimate decision to attempt this procedure or undergo a repeat cesarean delivery should be made by the patient and her physician. This discussion should be documented in the medical record.
• Vaginal birth after a previous cesarean delivery is contraindicated in women with a previous classic uterine incision or extensive transfundal uterine surgery.
• A trial of labor is not recommended in patients at high risk for uterine rupture, including:
  – previous classic or T-shaped incision or extensive transfundal uterine surgery
  – previous uterine rupture
  – medical or obstetric complication that precludes vaginal delivery

  – inability to perform emergency cesarean delivery because of unavailable surgeon, anesthesia, sufficient staff or facility
  – two prior uterine scars and no vaginal deliveries.
Women who are candidates for VBAC should be counseled regarding the risks and benefits of a trial of labor. Counseling should take place during the prenatal period, well in advance of delivery, and the patient's decision should be documented in the medical record. At the University of Southern California, women with previous cesarean sections account for approximately 14% of all deliveries. Among these, approximately 80% have had one previous cesarean and 20% have had two or more. Women with one previous low-transverse cesarean who are determined to be candidates are offered the option of VBAC. After thorough counseling regarding a lower likelihood of successful VBAC and a higher risk of uterine rupture, women with two previous cesarean sections who wish to attempt VBAC are not discouraged from doing so. Women who do not desire a trial of labor are scheduled for elective repeat cesarean section.

Controversies

Many issues pertaining to VBAC remain unresolved. Although a classic uterine incision is a contraindication to labor, there is limited information to generate recommendations regarding previous low-vertical or undocumented incisions. At our institution, lack of documentation of the previous incision type does not preclude a trial of labor, provided that the history is not suggestive of a classic incision. The management of previous low-vertical incisions is individualized. The risks related to VBAC in women with twins are not well established. One study, including 92 trials of labor in women with twins, reported no uterine ruptures [24]. However, the number of patients encompassed by published reports is insufficient to support a recommendation on the issue. Similarly, there is insufficient evidence to support recommendations regarding breech presentation or external cephalic version.

Regional anesthesia is not associated with adverse maternal or perinatal outcomes and is not contraindicated. While the pain associated with uterine rupture may be diminished somewhat by regional anesthesia, it is not masked entirely. Moreover, an abnormal fetal heart rate pattern, not abdominal pain, is the most common clinical finding in uterine rupture.

Manual exploration of the uterus following vaginal delivery is performed routinely at our institution. However, the discovery of an incisional defect is not necessarily an indication for surgical repair. A dehiscence that is hemostatic and does not extend into the peritoneal cavity rarely requires treatment. Labor is discouraged, however, in subsequent pregnancies.

Management of uterine rupture

When uterine rupture is diagnosed or strongly suspected, prompt surgical intervention is critical. Fetal distress appears to be the earliest and most sensitive indicator of uterine rupture. Among 99 cases reported by Leung, 92% were associated with fetal heart rate abnormalities, including fetal tachycardia, recurrent variable decelerations, late decelerations or prolonged decelerations [20]. Other clinical findings include maternal tachycardia, hypotension, hematuria or the acute onset of lower abdominal pain. In cases of fetal extrusion into the maternal abdomen, fetal parts may be palpated through the abdominal wall. Intrapartum hemorrhage, loss of intrauterine pressure recorded by an intrauterine pressure catheter, and loss of station of the fetal presenting part are infrequent observations.

In earlier reports of uterine rupture, 58–87% were managed with hysterectomy. In contrast, nearly 80% of the cases reported by Leung were managed by repair of the defect [20]. This approach raises the possibility of rupture recurrence in a subsequent pregnancy, an event with a reported incidence of 4.3–19%. Women with previously repaired uterine ruptures or unrepaired dehiscences are advised not to attempt labor in subsequent pregnancies. Ideally, a repeat cesarean section should be performed prior to the onset of uterine contractions.

Approximately 10% of uterine ruptures involve the urinary bladder. Uncomplicated defects involving the dome of the bladder usually are amenable to layered closure. Intraoperative urologic consultation should be considered if the defect involves the trigone or the ureters. If hysterectomy is required, the decision to proceed with total versus supracervical hysterectomy must be made by the responsible surgeon.

Conclusion

A trial of labor is an acceptable alternative to repeat abdominal birth in many women with previous cesarean sections. In women with one previous low-transverse cesarean section, a trial of labor should be offered. The overall likelihood of success is approximately 80%, and the risk of uterine rupture is low (less than 1%). Although a trial of labor is reasonable in women with two or more previous low-transverse cesarean sections, the likelihood of success is significantly lower (75%) and the risk of uterine rupture is nearly threefold higher.

In all candidates for VBAC, the risks associated with a trial of labor must be weighed against the risks of elective repeat cesarean section.

References

1. National Institutes of Health. Consensus Development Conference on Cesarean Childbirth, September 1980, sponsored by NICHD. NIH Pub. No. 82-2067. Bethesda, MD: National Institutes of Health, 1981.
2. Craigin EB. Conservatism in obstetrics. *NY Med J* 1916; 104: 1–3.
3. Centers for Disease Control and Prevention. Vaginal birth after cesarean birth – California, 1996–2000. *MMWR* 2002; 51: 996–998.
4. Martin JA, Hamilton BE, Sutton PD, *et al. Births: final data for 2004.* National Vital Statistics Reports. Vol 55, no. 1. Hyattsville, MD: National Center for Health Statistics, 2004.
5. Hamilton BD, Martin JA, Ventura SJ. *Births: preliminary data for 2006.* National Vital Statistics Reports. Vol 57, no. 7. Hyattsville, MD: National Center for Health Statistics, 2006.
6. Lavin JP, Stephens RJ, Miodovnik M, Barden TP. Vaginal delivery in patients with a prior cesarean section. *Obstet Gynecol* 1982; 59(2): 135–148.
7. Guise JM, McDonagh MS, Osterweil P, Nygren P, Chan BKS, Helfand M. Systematic review of the incidence and consequences of uterine rupture in women with previous cesarean section. *BMJ* 2004; 329(7456): 19–25.
8. American College of Obstetricians and Gynecologists. Vaginal birth after previous cesarean delivery. ACOG Practice Bulletin No. 54. *Obstet Gynecol* 2004; 104: 203–212.
9. American College of Obstetricians and Gynecologists. *Vaginal birth after previous cesarean delivery.* ACOG Practice Bulletin No. 5. Washington, DC: American College of Obstetricians and Gynecologists, 1999.
10. Miller DA, Diaz FG, Paul RH. Vaginal birth after cesarean: a 10-year experience. *Obstet Gynecol* 1994; 84: 255–258.
11. Caughey AB, Shipp TD, Repke JT, Zelop CM, Cohen A, Lieberman E. Rate of uterine rupture in women with one or two prior cesarean deliveries. *Am J Obstet Gynecol* 1999; 181: 872–876.
12. Bujold E, Hammoud AO, Hendler I, *et al.* Trial of labor in patients with a previous cesarean section: does maternal age influence the outcome? *Am J Obstet Gynecol* 2004; 190: 1113–1118.
13. Bujold E, Blackwell SC, Hendler I, Berman S, Sorokin Y, Gauthier RJ. Modified Bishop's score and induction of labor in patients with a previous cesarean delivery. *Am J Obstet Gynecol* 2004; 191: 1644–1648.
14. Bujold E, Bujold C, Hamilton EF, Harel F, Gauthier RJ. The impact of a single-layer or double-layer closure on uterine rupture. *Am J Obstet Gynecol* 2002; 186: 1326–1330.
15. Bujold E, Mehta SH, Bujold C, Gauthier RJ. Interdelivery interval and uterine rupture. *Am J Obstet Gynecol* 2002; 187: 1199–1202.
16. Rozenberg P, Goffinet F, Phillippe HJ, Nisand I. Ultrasonographic measurement of lower uterine segment to assess risk of defects of scarred uterus. *Lancet* 1996; 347: 281–284.
17. Leung AS, Farmer RM, Leung EK, *et al.* Risk factors associated with uterine rupture during trial of labor after cesarean delivery: a case control study. *Am J Obstet Gynecol* 1993; 168: 1358–1363.

18. Zelop CM, Shipp TD, Repke JT, Cohen A, Caughey AB, Lieberman E. Uterine rupture during induced or augmented labor in gravid women with one prior cesarean delivery. *Am J Obstet Gynecol* 1999; 181: 882–886.

19. Lydon-Rochelle M, Holt VL, Easterling TR, Martin DP. Risk of uterine rupture during labor among women with a prior cesarean delivery. *NEJM* 2001; 345(1): 3–8.

20. Leung AS, Leung EK, Paul RH. Uterine rupture after previous cesarean delivery. Maternal and fetal consequences. *Am J Obstet Gynecol* 1993; 169: 945–950.

21. Flamm BL, Newman LA, Thomas SJ, *et al.* Vaginal birth after cesarean delivery: results of a 5-year multicenter collaborative study. *Obstet Gynecol* 1990; 76: 750–754.

22. McMahon MJ, Luther ER, Bowes WA Jr, Olshan AF. Comparison of a trial of labor with an elective second cesarean section. *NEJM* 1996; 335: 689–695.

23. Mozurkewich EL, Hutton EK. Elective repeat cesarean delivery versus trial of labor: a meta-analysis of the literature from 1989 to 1999. *Am J Obstet Gynecol* 2000; 183(5): 1187–1197.

24. Miller DA, Mullin P, Hou D, Paul RH. Vaginal birth after cesarean in twin gestation. *Am J Obstet Gynecol* 1996; 175: 194–198.

25. Committee on Obstetrics. Maternal and fetal medicine. Guidelines for vaginal delivery after a previous cesarean birth. Committee Opinion No. 64. Washington, DC: American College of Obstetricians and Gynecologists, 1988.

Chapter 15
Placenta Previa and Abruptio Placentae

David A. Miller

Department of Medicine and Obstetrics and Gynecology, Keck School of Medicine, University of Southern California, CA, USA

Placenta previa

Placenta previa is a condition in which the placenta implants in the lower portion of the uterus and covers all or part of the internal cervical os. The incidence at term is approximately 1 in 200 births. Although the etiology remains unclear, the risk factors listed in Box 15.1 implicate previous decidual damage and/or large placental surface area. Three categories are defined below. An additional form of abnormal placentation is the low-lying placenta, in which the placental edge extends to within 2 cm of the internal cervical os.

- *Complete placenta previa*: placenta completely covers internal cervical os
- *Partial placenta previa*: placenta partially covers internal cervical os
- *Marginal placenta previa*: placenta extends to the margin of the internal cervical os

During routine second-trimester ultrasound, the placenta is observed to cover the cervical os in 5–20% of pregnancies. However, differential growth of the uterus and placenta throughout gestation results in realignment of the placenta with respect to the internal cervical os. By term, more than 90% of early placenta previas convert to a normal location. Conversion to normal location is less common in centrally located complete placenta previa.

Clinical presentation

Placenta previa is characterized by painless vaginal bleeding in the late second or third trimester. However, uterine pain and/or contractions do not preclude the diagnosis in a woman who presents with vaginal bleeding. In many cases, placenta previa remains asymptomatic throughout pregnancy.

Historically, placenta previa has been associated with increased maternal and perinatal morbidity and mortality. Preterm delivery and complications of prematurity are the most common sources of perinatal morbidity, occurring in nearly two-thirds of cases. Among 590 women with placenta previa, Miller and colleagues reported an average gestational age at delivery of 34.9 weeks. Delivery occurred before 37 weeks in 63% and before 34 weeks in 32%. Increased maternal morbidity and mortality are attributable primarily to hemorrhage and complications of cesarean delivery. Blood product replacement is necessary is one-third to one-half of cases. Approximately 10% of cases of placenta previa are associated with placenta accreta, an abnormally firm adherence of the placenta to the uterine wall. Placenta accreta is discussed in detail in Chapter 16.

Diagnosis

Placenta previa is most often diagnosed by routine sonography. In other cases, the initial diagnosis is made at the time of presentation for vaginal bleeding during the second half of pregnancy. In such cases, sonographic confirmation of placental location is recommended prior to digital cervical examination. Transabdominal ultrasound may confirm the suspicion of placenta previa. When adequate visualization of the relationship between the placenta and the internal cervical os is not possible with transabdominal ultrasound, the transperineal or transvaginal approach may be beneficial. Careful transvaginal sonography does not appear to increase the risk of hemorrhage in placenta previa.

Box 15.1 Risk factors for placenta previa

Previous cesarean section
Multiparity
Advanced maternal age
Multiple gestation
Erythroblastosis fetalis

Management of Common Problems in Obstetrics and Gynecology,
5th edition. Edited by T.M. Goodwin, M.N. Montoro,
L. Muderspach, R. Paulson and S. Roy. © 2010 Blackwell
Publishing Ltd.

Management of placenta previa without hemorrhage

Placenta previa diagnosed by routine second-trimester sonography is managed expectantly. The patient can be reassured that the likelihood of spontaneous resolution is greater than 90%. It is reasonable to recommend avoidance of strenuous activity, but further limitations probably are not necessary early in pregnancy. Placental location should be re-evaluated at 28–30 weeks. If placenta previa persists, the patient should be cautioned that rigorous activity and/or intercourse might provoke bleeding. If complete placenta previa persists beyond 32–34 weeks, resolution by term is unlikely. Cesarean delivery should be scheduled at a gestational age that will maximize the likelihood of fetal maturity and minimize the risk of hemorrhage that may result from the normal onset of uterine contractions. In the asymptomatic patient, amniocentesis should be considered at 34–36 weeks to assess fetal pulmonary maturity. If the test result is consistent with pulmonary maturity, delivery is indicated. If the test suggests pulmonary immaturity, decisions regarding corticosteroid administration and delivery timing must be individualized, taking into account such factors as obstetric history, gestational age, L/S ratio, phosphatidylglycerol level, fetal status, amniotic fluid volume and uterine activity. Beyond 37 weeks, expectant management should not be expected to yield a substantial benefit for the fetus or mother.

Management of placenta previa with hemorrhage

The management of placenta previa complicated by acute hemorrhage is directed at optimizing the outcomes of the mother and the fetus. In many cases, bleeding resolves spontaneously and the patient may be managed expectantly. In other cases, severe hemorrhage may require intervention. Detailed management of hemorrhage is discussed below.

Expectant management: inpatient versus outpatient

If the initial episode of bleeding resolves, the mother and fetus remain stable, and the fetus is premature, a period of expectant management may be appropriate. Bedrest usually is prescribed, antenatal corticosteroids are administered to accelerate fetal maturation, Rh immune globulin is given if indicated, and blood product availability is confirmed. In women who remain stable for a period of days after an initial episode of bleeding, the benefit of continued hospitalization is controversial. Wing and colleagues randomized 53 such women to receive either inpatient or outpatient expectant management after ≥72 hours of observation. There were no differences between the groups with respect to gestational age at delivery, birthweight, transfusion requirements, neonatal morbidity

or mortality. Although outcomes were similar with inpatient and outpatient management, 62.3% of patients had recurrent episodes of bleeding. Among these, more than three-quarters required expeditious delivery. The authors concluded that outpatient management of placenta previa following an initial episode of bleeding appears to be an acceptable approach in stable, carefully selected patients.

Delivery

Cesarean delivery is recommended in nearly all cases of placenta previa. Preparations should be made prior to delivery to ensure adequate venous access and ready availability of blood products and uterotonic agents. Informed consent should include the possibility of hysterectomy and blood transfusion. The management of placenta accreta encountered at cesarean section is discussed elsewhere in detail.

Abruptio placentae

Abruptio placentae is defined as the premature detachment of a normally implanted placenta after the 20th week of gestation. The reported incidence ranges from 1 in 75 to 1 in 225 births, with an average of approximately 1 in 120. Placental abruption accounts for 10–15% of all third-trimester fetal deaths. Reported perinatal mortality rates range from 21% to 35%, and 1 in 8 survivors may exhibit long-term neurodevelopmental impairment. Maternal mortality rates of 0.5–5% have been reported.

Etiology

The etiology of abruptio placentae is not known but several associated factors are recognized. Hypertensive disorders are present in 25–50% of cases. Among women with eclampsia, the incidence approaches 25%. Abruption rates as high as 17.3% have been reported among women using cocaine, possibly due to disruption of spiral arteries caused by vasoconstriction and subsequent dilation. Trauma (motor vehicle accidents, falls, assaults) accounts for 1–5% of abruptions. Women who experienced abruptio placentae in a previous pregnancy face a 4.0–16.7% risk of recurrence. With two previous abruptions, the recurrence risk is 25%. Cigarette smoking, high parity and advanced maternal age have been implicated as risk factors in some studies. Other reported associations include preterm, premature rupture of membranes, chorio-amnionitis, male fetus, short umbilical cord, uterine leiomyoma and sudden uterine decompression during the delivery of twins or rupture of membranes in cases of polyhydramnios.

Pathophysiology

The initiating event in placental abruption is hemorrhage into the decidua basalis, leading to the formation of a retroplacental hematoma. Expansion of the hematoma separates the decidua from the basal plate, disrupting adjacent vessels and causing further hemorrhage. When this process progresses to the placental margin, blood may dissect along the plane between the membranes and the uterine wall and escape via the cervix, resulting in clinically evident vaginal bleeding. In approximately 20% of cases, the expanding hematoma is retained behind the placenta or the membranes and the hemorrhage remains concealed. Blood may rupture through the membranes into the amniotic cavity, or hemoglobin breakdown products may diffuse across the membranes, imparting a dark red ("port wine") color to the amniotic fluid. Extravasation of blood into the uterine musculature and beneath the serosa may result in a bruised appearance characteristic of the Couvelaire uterus. In nontraumatic abruptio placentae, placental separation rarely disrupts the intervillous spaces, and fetomaternal hemorrhage is uncommon.

Diagnosis
Placental abruption classically presents with vaginal bleeding and a tender, rigid uterus. Contractions are frequent, intense and often prolonged. Baseline uterine tone is elevated. In 20% of cases, bleeding is not evident externally. Severe hypertension, pre-eclampsia or eclampsia may be present. Alternatively, maternal hypotension, tachycardia and oliguria may signal hemorrhagic shock. Fetal death complicates 15% of cases. If the fetus is alive, electronic FHR monitoring may reveal fetal tachycardia, loss of variability, loss of accelerations and recurrent or prolonged decelerations. Dark red amniotic fluid or blood may be observed at amniotomy. Occasionally, ultrasound examination will demonstrate a retroplacental hematoma but normal sonographic findings do not exclude the diagnosis of abruptio placentae.

Laboratory evaluation may reveal severe anemia, thrombocytopenia, low serum fibrinogen, elevated lactate dehydrogenase and prolonged prothrombin and activated partial thromboplastin times. Significant proteinuria and elevated serum transaminases may indicate severe pre-eclampsia or HELLP syndrome.

Clinical and laboratory findings are used to grade the severity of placental abruption as follows.
• *Grade 1*: minimal vaginal bleeding and uterine activity. Normal maternal blood pressure and fibrinogen level. Normal FHR pattern.
• *Grade 2*: moderate vaginal bleeding and uterine activity. Tetanic contractions may be present. Normal maternal blood pressure. Elevated pulse rate and postural changes may be present. Fibrinogen level 150–250 mg%. FHR monitoring reveals evidence of fetal distress.
• *Grade 3*: severe vaginal bleeding or concealed hemorrhage. Tetanic contractions and uterine pain present. Maternal hypotension. Fibrinogen level <150 mg%. Fetal death. Evidence of disseminated intravascular coagulation.

Management of severe hemorrhage

Placenta previa, accreta or abruption may be accompanied by significant bleeding and evidence of hemorrhagic shock. In the case of placental abruption, shock may be out of proportion to the observed blood loss. Hemorrhage in excess of 2 L may remain concealed behind the placenta or membranes. In the early stage of hemorrhagic or hypovolemic shock, compensatory tachycardia, peripheral vasoconstriction and renal fluid conservation are sufficient to maintain cardiac output and blood pressure. However, if blood loss is not corrected, shock may become progressive. Decreasing functional circulatory volume can lead to inadequate tissue perfusion and cellular hypoxia. Lactic acidosis results from the accumulation of organic acid byproducts of anaerobic cellular metabolism. Finally, shock may advance to the irreversible stage in which severe acidosis disables vasomotor reflexes, and the resultant arteriolar dilation causes blood to pool in the peripheral microvasculature. Diminished venous return further compromises cardiac output, and widespread tissue hypoxia may lead to multiple organ failure and death.

Disseminated intravascular coagulation
Disseminated intravascular coagulation (DIC) is a thrombo-hemorrhagic disorder characterized by activation of the coagulation cascade, generation of microthrombi throughout the microcirculation, and consumption of clotting factors and platelets. The most common obstetric cause of DIC is abruptio placentae. Hemorrhage is the dominant clinical feature. The inciting event is the release of decidual thromboplastins into the maternal circulation, activating the extrinsic pathway of the coagulation cascade. Resultant widespread microthrombosis consumes clotting factors and platelets. Fibrin monomers, produced by the clotting cascade, are deposited in the microvasculature, causing vascular occlusion, tissue ischemia and microangiopathic hemolysis. Secondary activation of plasminogen leads to fibrinolysis and degradation of coagulation factors V and VIII. Fibrin degradation products, formed by the cleavage of fibrin by plasmin, possess antithrombin activity and act as inhibitors of platelet aggregation and fibrin polymerization. When abruptio placentae is complicated by severe shock, DIC may be exacerbated by an additional triggering mechanism. Hypoxia and acidosis may cause widespread endothelial damage, increasing endothelial surface expression of tissue factor and activating the intrinsic pathway of the coagulation cascade. The combined effect of these processes is a severe hemorrhagic diathesis.

Management
When the diagnosis of severe obstetric hemorrhage is made, rapid assessment of maternal and fetal status is critical. Clinical evidence of severe maternal hypovolemia

may include pale, cool skin and mucous membranes, tachycardia, hypotension, delayed capillary refill in the nail beds, and a diminished volume of dark, concentrated urine. Simultaneous assessment of the fetus includes rapid estimation of the gestational age and fetal weight. If the fetus is alive, continuous electronic FHR monitoring should be instituted. The FHR tracing may reveal evidence of disrupted fetal oxygenation (late, variable or prolonged decelerations) and/or metabolic acidemia (fetal tachycardia, loss of variability, loss of accelerations). Occasionally, sonography may confirm the presence of a retroplacental hematoma but the absence of such a finding does not preclude abruptio placentae. Laboratory evaluation includes a blood type and cross-match (at least two units of packed red cells), complete blood count, prothrombin time, activated partial thromboplastin time and fibrinogen level.

The initial therapeutic objectives are to ensure adequate maternal oxygenation and to stabilize the maternal hemo-dynamic status. Continuous pulse oximetry is applied if necessary, and supplemental oxygen is administered by tight-fitting nonrebreather facemask at a rate of 10 L/min. The patient is placed in the Trendelenburg position. At least two large-bore intravenous lines are placed, and fluid resuscitation initiated immediately with isotonic crystalloid solutions. Central venous access and pulmonary artery catheterization may be necessary. In acute, severe hypotension, temporizing measures include administration of ephedrine (5–10 mg), placement of military antishock trousers and/or aortic compression. Blood product replacement is initiated as rapidly as possible.

In the setting of active hemorrhage (clinically evident or concealed), imminent surgery or shock with a hematocrit less than 25%, rapid transfusion of packed red blood cells (PRBC) and aggressive fluid replacement are indicated. One unit of PRBCs will raise the hematocrit by 3–4%. Ideally, a hematocrit of at least 30% should be maintained. If hemorrhage is complicated by evidence of coagulopathy, fresh-frozen plasma (FFP) is indicated. FFP contains all coagulation factors, including fibrinogen, and one unit will raise the serum fibrinogen level by 10 mg/dL. When possible, a fibrinogen level of at least 100 mg/dL should be maintained. Platelet transfusion is indicated in the setting of hemorrhage or imminent surgery when the platelet count is less than 50,000/mm³. One unit of random donor platelets contains 5.5 [mult] 10^{10} platelets and will increase the platelet count by 5000–8000/mm³.

In some cases, immediate delivery may not be necessary. For example, if the fetus is premature and the fetus and mother are stable, perinatal outcome may be improved by delaying delivery for 24–48 hours to allow administration of corticosteroids. Close observation is essential during this period. If tocolysis is necessary, magnesium sulfate is the agent of choice. β-Mimetics may cause maternal and fetal tachycardia, masking the clinical signs of hypovolemia and anemia.

Tocolysis is contraindicated in the following settings:
- deteriorating maternal hemodynamic status despite appropriate therapy
- uncontrolled hemorrhage
- gestational age ≥36 weeks
- estimated fetal weight ≥2500 g
- fetal death or deteriorating fetal status despite appropriate therapy.

If expeditious delivery is indicated, the route is determined by the status of the mother and the fetus as well as the rate of progress of labor. If the maternal hemodynamic status is stable, FHR monitoring reveals no evidence of acute deterioration and labor is progressing rapidly, vaginal delivery may be possible. On the other hand, if the maternal status is unstable and vaginal delivery cannot be accomplished within an acceptable period of time, cesarean may be necessary.

Conclusion

Placenta previa complicates approximately 1 in 200 pregnancies and is associated with a high incidence of preterm birth. When placenta previa is identified in the setting of a previous cesarean section, the possibility of placenta accreta should be anticipated. Placental abruption is an obstetric emergency that is associated with high rates of maternal and perinatal morbidity and mortality. Rapid assessment and initiation of therapeutic measures are critical. In selected, mild cases of abruption, immediate delivery may not be necessary. In most cases, however, rapid delivery is indicated. Delivery route is determined by maternal and fetal condition as well as rate of progress of labor.

Suggested reading

American College of Obstetricians and Gynecologists. *Blood component therapy*. ACOG Technical Bulletin No. 199. Washington, DC: American College of Obstetricians and Gynecologists, 1994.

Ananth CV, Wilcox AJ. Placental abruption and perinatal mortality in the United States. *Am J Epidemiol* 2001; 153: 332–337.

Baglin T. Disseminated intravascular coagulation: diagnosis and treatment. *BMJ* 1996; 312: 683.

Clark SL, Koonings P, Phelan JP. Placenta previa/accreta and prior cesarean section. *Obstet Gynecol* 1985; 66: 89–92.

Development Task Force of the College of American Pathologists. Practice parameters for the use of fresh-frozen plasma, cryoprecipitate and platelets: fresh-frozen plasma, cryoprecipitate and platelets administration practice guidelines. *JAMA* 1994; 271: 777–781.

Miller DA, Chollet JA, Goodwin TM. Clinical risk factors for placenta previa – placenta accreta. *Am J Obstet Gynecol* 1997; 177: 210–214.

Oyelese Y, Ananth CV. Placental abruption. *Obstet Gynecol* 2006; 108: 1005–1016.

Oyelese Y, Smulian JC. Placenta previa, placenta accreta, and vasa previa. *Obstet Gynecol* 2006; 107: 927–941.

Pritchard J. The genesis of severe placental abruption. *Am J Obstet Gynecol* 1970; 208: 22.

Royal College of Obstetricians and Gynaecologists. *Placenta praevia and placenta praevia accreta: diagnosis and management.* London: Royal College of Obstetricians and Gynaecologists, 2005.

Wing DA, Paul RH, Millar LK. Management of the symptomatic placenta previa: a randomized controlled trial of inpatient versus outpatient expectant management. *Am J Obstet Gynecol* 1996; 175: 806–811.

Chapter 16
Placenta Accreta

Richard H. Lee and David A. Miller

Department of Medicine and Obstetrics and Gynecology, Keck School of Medicine, University of Southern California, CA, USA

Introduction

Placenta accreta is defined as an abnormally firm attachment of placental villi to the uterine wall with the absence of the normal intervening decidua basalis and fibrinoid layer of Nitabuch. Collectively termed "placenta accreta," three variants of the condition are recognized. In the most common form, accreta, the placenta is attached directly to the myometrium. This variant accounts for approximately 75–78% of all cases. In approximately 17% of cases, the placenta extends into the myometrium and is termed placenta increta. In the remaining 5–7%, the placenta extends through the entire myometrial layer and is termed placenta percreta.

Over the past two decades, the reported incidence of placenta accreta has ranged from 1 in 533 to 1 in 2510 deliveries [1,2]. The latter incidence reflects the observed number of histologically confirmed placenta accreta cases from 1985 to 1994 at the University of Southern California. These numbers are considerably higher than what has been reported in the past. A major contributor to this rise appears to be the increasing incidence of previous cesarean delivery.

A characteristic feature of placenta accreta is the absence or attenuation of the decidua basalis. This abnormality permits the trophoblasts to come into direct contact with, and invade into, the underlying myometrium. The resultant abnormally firm placental attachment prevents the placenta from separating normally after delivery and interferes with uterine contraction that is essential to postpartum hemostasis. In the majority of cases placenta accreta remains asymptomatic until delivery. Although antepartum hemorrhage is not uncommon, it is more likely attributable to placenta previa which often accompanies it than to placenta accreta itself.

Intractable hemorrhage and the operative procedures performed in an attempt to control the bleeding are the major sources of maternal morbidity and mortality in cases of placenta accreta. Subsequently, additional complications can occur such as hysterectomy, ureteral/bladder injury, visceral injury, disseminated intravascular coagulopathy, ARDS, renal failure, and death. In a review of 109 cases of placenta percreta, O'Brien *et al.* reported 44 cases (40%) requiring greater than 10 units of blood transfusion, five cases (5%) with ureteral ligation or fistula formation, 31 cases (28%) of infection, 10 cases (9%) of perinatal death, and eight cases (7%) of maternal death. Of particular interest were the three cases of uterine rupture [3]. The blood loss from such cases is considerable. At the University of Southern California, among 62 cases of placenta accreta the estimated blood loss exceeded 2000 mL in 41 cases (66%), 5000 mL in nine (15%), 10,000 mL in four (6.5%), and 20,000 mL in two (3%). Thirty-two women (55%) required blood transfusions. Blood product replacement exceeded 5 units in 13 (21%), 20 units in five (8%), and 70 units in three (5.5%). Three cases required ureteral transaction and reimplantation or reanastomosis. Additional morbidity included disseminated intravascular coagulation (five), hypotensive shock (two), reoperation from control of hemorrhage (two), and enterotomy (one) [4]. There were no maternal deaths [1].

The principal perinatal complication of placenta accreta is prematurity. O'Brien *et al.* reported that among 109 cases of placenta percreta, there were 10 perinatal deaths. Six of the 10 cases were due to extreme prematurity with a median gestational age of 22 weeks and two were associated with concomitant maternal death [3]. Alternatively, among 62 cases of placenta accreta at the University of Southern California, there were no perinatal deaths. This may be attributed to the mean gestational age at delivery which was 34.6 weeks.

Risk factors

Several risk factors for placenta accreta have been identified (Box 16.1). Among these, the two most important

Management of Common Problems in Obstetrics and Gynecology, 5th edition. Edited by T.M. Goodwin, M.N. Montoro, L. Muderspach, R. Paulson and S. Roy. © 2010 Blackwell Publishing Ltd.

Box 16.1 Risk factors for placenta accreta

- Placenta previa
- Previous cesarean section
- Advanced maternal age
- Placental location with respect to uterine scar
- Multiparity
- Previous uterine curettage
- Previous myomectomy

Box 16.2 Sonographic findings in placenta accreta

- Loss of the normal retroplacental hypoechoic zone
- Thinning or disruption of the hyperechoic interface between the uterine serosa and the bladder
- Intraplacental vascular lacunae
- Loss of the normal venous flow pattern of the peripheral placental margin
- Myometrial thickness of <1 mm under the placenta

Table 16.1 Estimated risk of placenta accreta among women with placenta previa

Previous cesareans	Placenta *not* overlying uterine scar		Placenta overlying uterine scar	
	Age <35	Age ≥35	Age <35	Age ≥35
None	2.1% (6/288)	6.3% (9/144)	N/A –	N/A –
One	3.7% (1/27)	9.1% (1/11)	15.9% (7/44)	30% (6/20)
Two or more	5.2% (1/19)	20% (1/5)	38.5% (15/39)	38.1% (8/21)

N/A, not applicable.

appear to be prior cesarean delivery and placenta previa. Placenta accreta complicated 9.3% of 590 cases of placenta previa at the University of Southern California from 1985 to 1994. Among 155,080 women without placenta previa, the incidence of placenta accreta was 1 in 22,154. In women with placenta previa, the incidence of placenta accreta appears to correlate with the number of previous cesarean sections. Clark *et al.* reported a 5% incidence of placenta accreta among women with placenta previa and no previous cesarean sections [5]. The incidence increased to 24% with one previous cesarean section and to 45% with two or more. Among 723 women with cesarean delivery and previa, Silver *et al.* reported the risk for accreta to be 3%, 11%, 40%, 61%, and 67% for one, two, three, four, and five or more cesarean deliveries. Among 29,409 women with cesarean delivery and no previa, the risk for accreta was 0.03%, 0.2%, 0.1%, 0.8%, 0.8%, 4.7% for one, two, three, four, five, and six or more cesarean deliveries [6].

Advanced maternal age and placental location with respect to the previous uterine scar also have been reported to be independent risk factors for placenta accreta among women with placenta previa. Miller reported a 2.1% incidence of accreta in women with placenta previa who were less than 35 years of age and had no previous cesareans. The incidence increased to 38.1% in women who were 35 years of age or older with two or more previous cesarean sections and a placenta previa overlying the uterine scar (Table 16.1) [1]. Information is limited

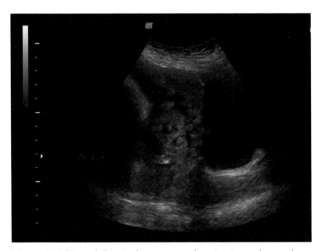

Figure 16.1 Transabdominal sonogram showing intraplacental vascular lacunae.

regarding the risks associated with previous uterine curettage or myomectomy.

Diagnosis

Placenta accreta should be suspected in all women with placenta previa. The risk factors listed in Box 16.2 may be helpful in quantifying the risk, selecting candidates for detailed sonographic evaluation, and planning for delivery. A definitive diagnosis of accreta is often not possible prior to delivery but ultrasonographic diagnosis has yielded encouraging results. The use of sonographic criteria listed in Box 16.2 has yielded sensitivities of approximately 80% and specificities of approximately 95% for the detection of accreta [7,8] Figures 16.1 and 16.2. Using ultrasound color flow mapping, Twickler found that if the myometrial thickness under the placenta was less than 1 mm, this was predictive of myometrial invasion with a sensitivity of 100%, specificity 72%, PPV 72% and NPV 100% [4]. Warshak *et al.* evaluated the accuracy of sonography and MRI in the antenatal diagnosis of placenta accreta. Of 39 cases of confirmed placenta accreta, sonography had a sensitivity of 77% and specificity of 96% whereas

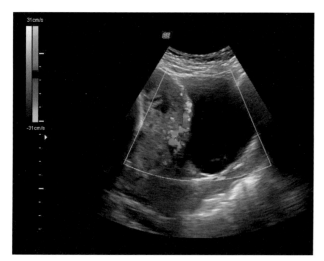

Figure 16.2 Transabdominal color Doppler sonogram demonstrating increased vascular flow at the utero–vesical interface.

gadolinium-enhanced MRI had a sensitivity of 88% and specificity of 100% and was able to exclude placenta accreta in 14/14 cases [9]. The use of MRI must take into account cost, accessibility and, if gadolinium is used, the risks and benefits of fetal exposure to contrast agents. We currently use sonography as our primary means of diagnosing accreta.

Management

In women with placenta previa who are considered to be at high risk for placenta accreta, cesarean delivery should be timed to allow the assembly of resources in anticipation of massive hemorrhage. The patient should be counseled preoperatively regarding the risks of hemorrhage, transfusion, and hysterectomy. The operating room should be staffed by experienced personnel, and equipped with hysterectomy instruments and blood salvage equipment. The placement of prophylactic intravascular balloon catheters for placenta accreta has failed to produce any substantial decrease in maternal morbidity [10].

Hysterectomy remains the procedure of choice (Figures 16.3, 16.4, 16.5). When placenta accreta is suspected at cesarean section, we advise proceeding with a vertical midline skin incision in order to provide optimal exposure to the surgical field. If possible, we begin by carefully creating a bladder flap in order to facilitate the hysterectomy if needed. Occasionally, in the setting of increta, the placenta can be visualized underneath the uterine serosa. A hysterotomy is made away from the placenta, which often requires a classic incision near the uterine fundus. The fetus is delivered, spontaneous delivery of the placenta is awaited or gentle traction is applied on the cord to await delivery of placenta.

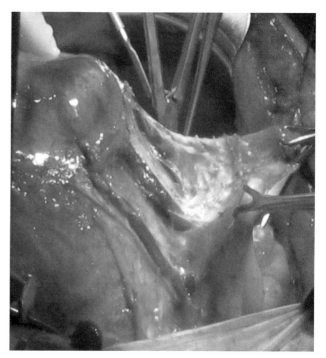

Figure 16.3 Intraoperative findings demonstrating the placenta underneath the uterine serosa.

We do not attempt to manually deliver the placenta as this can cause massive hemorrhage if there is indeed a placenta accreta. If placental delivery is unsuccessful or if uncontrollable hemorrhage ensues, the surgeon should leave the placenta in place, close the uterus rapidly, and proceed with hysterectomy. Although more expedient than total hysterectomy, supracervical hysterectomy may not always be possible in cases of placenta accreta attached near the cervix. Selection of the appropriate procedure must be made by the surgeon. Care is taken to locate the ureters as the lower uterine segment can be bulbous, which can distort the normal anatomic relationship between the ureters and the cervix. The vaginal cuff and pedicles are carefully inspected for hemostasis. If integrity of the bladder is in question, we fill the bladder in retrograde fashion with methylene blue diluted in normal saline and observe for any leakage.

Control of potentially life-threatening hemorrhage is the first priority; however, the patient's desire for future fertility must be taken into consideration. If the patient is hemodynamically stable and strongly desires future fertility, conservative management may be cautiously considered, bearing in mind that the literature regarding conservative management is based on case series or reports. The risks of conservative management include delayed hemorrhage (requiring reoperation) and infection. *If the patient is unstable, conservative management is not an option.* Techniques that have been described include curettage, oversewing the placental bed or wedge resection of the area of accreta with subsequent repair of the

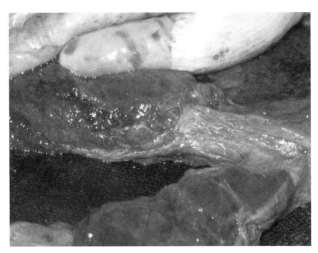

Figure 16.5 Gross section demonstrating nearly full-thickness invasion of the placenta into the myometrium.

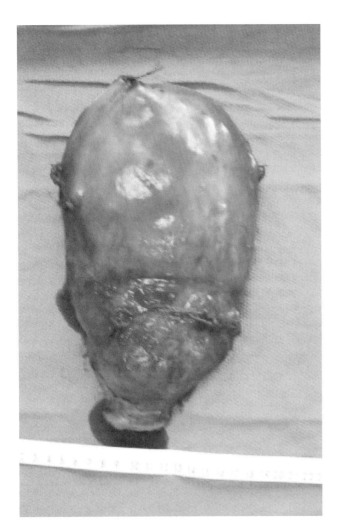

Figure 16.4 Cesarean hysterectomy specimen of a placenta increta.

myometrium. In the vast majority of cases, these techniques have been applied in the setting where a focal accreta is encountered after attempted removal of the placenta. Planned conservative management has been described in case reports when a placenta accreta is diagnosed before delivery and the patient strongly desires future fertility; this involves leaving the placenta *in situ* and thereafter adjunctive therapy is administered with uterine artery embolization, methotrexate or delayed removal.

These methods of management have not been well studied and should be considered investigational. They should only be considered in patients who strongly desire future fertility and who understand and accept the risks of delayed hemorrhage, infection, and death. The patient should be counseled that conservative management cannot be used if she has profuse bleeding or is hemodynamically unstable. Timmermans *et al.* reviewed 60 pregnancies managed conservatively. The most common complication consisted of vaginal bleeding (21/60). The timing of blood loss ranged from immediately post partum up to 3 months after delivery. Treatment failure due to vaginal bleeding occurred in 15% of cases (9/60). Fever occurred in 21/60 cases, 11/60 had endomyometritis, and 2/60 required hysterectomy for definitive treatment. Importantly, the authors caution that the number of complications may be falsely lowered due to publication bias of reported successful cases [11].

Conclusion

Placenta accreta is characterized by an absent or attenuated decidua basalis that permits trophoblastic invasion into the myometrium. Incomplete placental detachment following delivery results in profuse hemorrhage that often necessitates hysterectomy. Important clinical risk factors include placenta previa, previous cesarean section, placental implantation over the uterine scar, and advanced maternal age. Other potential risk factors include multiparity, previous uterine curettage, and previous myomectomy. Accreta complicates 9–10% of all cases of placenta previa. In the absence of placenta previa, however, accreta is rare (1 in 22,000). Prospective diagnosis may be possible with ultrasonography, color Doppler, and MRI. When placenta accreta is suspected, thorough preparation is the key to successful management. Although conservative management may be an option in a select few patients, hysterectomy remains the treatment of choice.

References

1. Miller D, Chollet J, Goodwin T. Clinical risk factors for placenta previa-placenta accreta. *Am J Obstet Gynecol* 1997; 177: 210–214.
2. Wu S, Kocherginsky M, Hibbard J. Abnormal placentation: twenty-year analysis. *Am J Obstet Gynecol* 2005; 192: 1458–1461.

3. O'Brien J, Barton J, Donaldson E. The management of placenta percreta: conservative and operative strategies. *Am J Obstet Gynecol* 1996; 175: 1632–1638.

4. Twickler D, Lucas M, Balis A, *et al*. Color flow mapping for myometrial invasion in women with a prior cesarean delivery. *J Matern Fetal Med* 2000; 9: 330–335.

5. Clark S, Koonings P, Phelan J. Placenta previa/accreta and prior cesarean section. *Obstet Gynecol* 1985; 66: 89–92.

6. Silver R, Landon M, Rouse D, *et al*. Maternal morbidity associated with multiple repeat cesarean deliveries. *Obstet Gynecol* 2006; 107: 1226–1232.

7. Chou M, Ho E, Lee Y. Prenatal diagnosis of placenta previa accreta by transabdominal color Doppler ultrasound. *Ultrasound Obstet Gynecol* 2000; 15: 28–35.

8. Comstock C, Love J Jr, Bronsteen R, *et al*. Sonographic detection of placenta accreta in the second and third trimesters of pregnancy. *Am J Obstet Gynecol* 2004; 190: 1135–1140.

9. Warshak C, Eskander R, Hull A, *et al*. Accuracy of ultrasonography and magnetic resonance imaging in the diagnosis of placenta accreta. *Obstet Gynecol* 2006; 108: 573–581.

10. Shrivastava V, Nageotte M, Major C, Haydon M, Wing D. Case–control comparison of cesarean hysterectomy with and without prophylactic placement of intravascular balloon catheters for placenta accreta. *Am J Obstet Gynecol* 2007; 197: 402.

11. Timmermans S, van Hof A, Duvekot J. Conservative management of abnormally invasive placentation. *Obstet Gynecol Surv* 2007; 62: 529–539.

Suggested Reading

Oyelese Y, Smulian J. Placenta previa, placenta accreta, and vasa previa. *Obstet Gynecol* 2006; 107: 927–941.

Faranesh R, Shabtai R, Eliezer S, Raed S. Suggested approach for management of placenta percreta invading the urinary bladder. *Obstet Gynecol* 2007; 110: 512–515.

Oppenheimer L. Diagnosis and management of placenta previa. *J Obstet Gynaecol Can* 2007; 29: 261–273.

Bhide A, Thilaganathan B. Recent advances in the management of placenta previa. *Curr Opin Obstet Gynecol* 2004; 16: 447–451.

American College of Obstetricians and Gynecologists. Clinical management guidelines for obstetrician-gynecologists: postpartum hemorrhage. Practice Bulletin No. 76. *Obstet Gynecol* 2006; 108: 1039–1047.

Gilstrap LC, Cunningham FG, van Dorsten P (eds). *Operative obstetrics*, 2nd edn. New York: McGraw-Hill, 2002.

Chapter 17
Postpartum Hemorrhage

Richard H. Lee

Department of Medicine and Obstetrics and Gynecology, Keck School of Medicine, University of Southern California, CA, USA

Introduction

Postpartum hemorrhage is a leading cause of maternal morbidity and mortality. Classically defined as blood loss greater than 500 mL after a vaginal delivery and 1000 mL after cesarean delivery, these definitions of postpartum hemorrhage are antiquated. Although this system is easy to remember, visual estimations of blood loss are inaccurate. Clinically useful information is better conveyed if postpartum hemorrhage is classified based on a combination of estimated blood loss, patient symptoms and volume status.

The differential diagnosis of postpartum hemorrhage includes genital lacerations, uterine atony, retained placenta (including accreta), uterine inversion, uterine rupture, scar dehiscence, disseminated intravascular coagulation, consumptive coagulopathy, hematoma, thrombocytopenia, and, rarely, coagulation disorders. There are several risk factors associated with postpartum hemorrhage listed in Box 17.1.

Diagnosis and management

A rapid sequence of interventions is necessary to prevent further blood loss and maintain patient hemodynamic stability. In patients with known risk factors, a high index of suspicion should be maintained. General precautions implemented before delivery for patients at risk include establishing at least one large-bore intravenous line, ensuring the availability of uterotonics (oxytocin, methylergonovine, prostaglandins), and confirming that appropriate nursing, operating room, and anesthesia personnel are available and aware of the possibility of postpartum hemorrhage. In selected high-risk patients,

> **Box 17.1 Factors associated with uterine atony**
>
> - Prolonged labor
> - Oxytocin
> - General anesthetics (halothane)
> - Multiple gestation
> - Polyhydramnios
> - Fetal macrosomia
> - Grand multiparity
> - Couvelaire uterus
> - Dystocia
> - Infection (chorio-amnionitis)

crossmatching 2–4 units of packed red blood cells may be appropriate.

In the setting when there is excessive bleeding, a second large-bore intravenous line should be placed as well as a transurethral catheter to monitor the patient's fluid status. Crystalloid should be infused at a 3/1 ratio to the amount of blood lost. Colloid (albumin, dextran, hespan) has little added benefit compared to crystalloid in restoring intravascular volume. Furthermore, certain colloids can promote coagulopathy. The blood bank should be notified that an obstetric patient is hemorrhaging and packed red blood cells should be obtained. In the absence of cross-matched blood, O negative blood should be obtained followed by type-specific blood until cross-matched blood is available. It is also important to anticipate the need for fresh-frozen plasma and cryoprecipitate as it may take approximately 30 minutes to an hour to thaw. Replacement of blood products is addressed at the end of this chapter. Oxytocin (20–80 units diluted in 1000 mL of normal saline) should be administered intravenously and run continuously. Directly bolusing oxytocin intravenously is not recommended as this may precipitate

Management of Common Problems in Obstetrics and Gynecology, 5th edition. Edited by T.M. Goodwin, M.N. Montoro, L. Muderspach, R. Paulson and S. Roy. © 2010 Blackwell Publishing Ltd.

significant hypotension. Alternatively, if there is no intravenous access, 10 units of oxytocin can be administered intramuscularly. Concomitantly, attempts should be made to determine the cause of bleeding and proceed with treatment.

Often the clinician must multitask and assess the perineum for lacerations, palpate the uterine fundus for atony, and inspect the placenta to ensure it has delivered intact. Having an assistant push the uterus towards the vagina can facilitate evaluation for cervical lacerations. This also allows evaluation for uterine atony and visualization for any trailing membranes or placental fragments. If the uterus is firm and the bleeding is determined to be from a laceration, appropriate steps should be taken to repair the laceration. In the setting of a cervical laceration, a traction suture can be placed at the external os and the laceration can be repaired, making sure that the suture goes beyond the apex of the laceration. Often the cervix appears as if there are multiple lacerations but only those that are actively bleeding should be repaired.

The diagnosis of uterine atony is established by the combination of postpartum hemorrhage in the presence of a large, relaxed uterine fundus. Bimanual uterine massage should be applied while oxytocin and other uterotonics are administered. Bimanual uterine massage consists of elevating the uterus with one hand in the vagina and a separate hand massaging the fundus abdominally. If massage is not adequately causing the uterus to contract, bimanual compression should be applied where a fist is placed in the anterior vaginal fornix and the opposite hand firmly presses the uterine fundus to tamponade the vascular sinuses in the uterus. Additional uterotonics are given. Methylergonovine 0.2 mg can be administered intramuscularly. The dosage may be repeated every 2–4 hours. This agent is contraindicated in hypertension. An alternative uterotonic agent is 15-methyl prostaglandin F2-α. An initial dose of 0.25 mg may be administered IM following vaginal delivery or directly into the myometrium at cesarean delivery. Dosages may be repeated at intervals of 15–90 minutes as necessary. The total dosage should not exceed eight doses (2 g). This prostaglandin preparation is contraindicated in patients with asthma or glaucoma. Dinoprostone 20 mg vaginally or rectally may also be administered, but caution is advised in patients who are hypotensive. We advise starting with 10 mg and observing for any changes in blood pressure. As a third-line agent, we use misoprostol 800–1000 μg per rectum. Based on available data, the use of misoprostol as a nonsurgical intervention to treat uterine atony seems reasonable as long as the physician is aware of the potential side effects. This medication may be useful in preventing surgical interventions that would require laparotomy or hysterectomy, although further studies are needed to determine optimal route of delivery and dosage.

If the uterus remains atonic despite bimanual massage and the administration of uterotonics, the physician should undertake manual exploration of the uterine cavity. Ideally, this should be performed in the operating room and the patient should have adequate anesthesia prior to performing manual exploration, but often the very fact that the patient needs rapid evaluation makes it necessary to perform this task under suboptimal conditions. A gauntlet glove is donned and the hand is inserted into the uterus to palpate for any retained placental fragments. A second hand is placed on the fundus to control the exploration. If placental fragments are detected, a plane is created to carefully attempt to remove the fragments by inserting the finger between the placenta–decidual interface. Bedside ultrasound may assist in visualizing retained placental products. Occasionally it may be necessary to perform a gentle curettage under ultrasound guidance using a blunt curette or ring forceps. This procedure should ideally be performed in an operating room. If excessive hemorrhage occurs after such attempts or if it is difficult to find a cleavage plane, the possibility of placenta accreta should be considered (refer to Chapter 16). In women with risk factors for accreta, we do not advise manual removal of retained placental fragments as such attempts can further provoke hemorrhage. Finally, manual exploration allows the physician to assess for uterine rupture, especially in the case of a patient with prior cesarean delivery or uterine surgery. If a myometrial defect is palpated with hemorrhage, the physician should proceed to immediate laparotomy.

If bleeding persists despite these maneuvers, nursing and anesthesia personnel should be instructed to prepare for operative intervention. Blood product replacement should be instituted or continued as necessary. Bimanual uterine compression should be continued. If successful in mitigating bleeding due to atony, compression should be continued with consideration of the placement of an intrauterine balloon catheter to maintain uterine tamponade. However, if bimanual compression is unsuccessful and hemorrhage persists, transabdominal aortic compression should be performed at the level of the umbilicus while preparations are made for laparotomy.

The objective of laparotomy is to control hemorrhage as rapidly as possible. It is important to have an assistant place the patient in the "frog-leg" or dorsal lithotomy position and clear the vagina of any clots in order to achieve adequate assessment of continued blood loss. If bimanual compression was thought to be suboptimal prior to laparotomy for various reasons (i.e. maternal obesity), a second attempt at bimanual compression can be considered when the uterus is exposed. If bimanual compression is effective at tamponading bleeding at the time of laparotomy, consideration should be given to placing a uterine compression suture. Several brace sutures have been described in the literature. At the University of Southern California we have had success using the brace suture described by B-Lynch. Alternatively, a balloon catheter (Bakri) can be placed vaginally and observed to see if further hemorrhage occurs. Other methods of tamponading bleeding from atony include the use of gauze packing, placement of one or more Foley balloons or a Sengstaken–Blakemore tube.

If bimanual compression was optimally applied prior to laparotomy without success in controlling hemorrhage from uterine atony, the physician should bypass attempts at uterine packing, balloon tamponade or using a brace suture. Instead, the practitioner should proceed directly towards ligating the blood supply to the uterus. The first step involves bilateral ligation of the uterine arteries. Absorbable sutures may be passed through the lower uterine segment on each side and passed around the uterine vessels. Caution must be exercised to avoid the bladder and the ureters. If uterine artery ligation is unsuccessful, the next series of sutures can be placed around the utero-ovarian arteries in the cornual regions. Successful pregnancies have been reported following ligation of all major uterine vessels. Occlusion of the hypogastric arteries has fallen out of favor as a procedure as this requires familiarity with the retroperitoneum and carries a risk of serious complications, including lace-ration of the hypogastric, external iliac or common iliac veins, and inadvertent ligation of the ureter, external iliac artery or hypogastric trunk. Unless there is someone skilled with retroperitoneal dissections, such as a gynecologic oncologist, we generally avoid this step. In some settings, interventional radiology may provide an additional alternative in the form of angiographic embolization of pelvic arteries with gelatin sponge particles or spring coils. Although successful control of hemorrhage has been reported in small series, this option may not be available in emergency situations and in all practical senses is not suitable for an unstable patient.

If conservative measures fail to achieve hemostasis, hysterectomy may be necessary. Supracervical hysterectomy is the fastest and safest approach in a hemodynamically unstable patient. Moreover, cervical dilation and effacement often obscure the boundary between the cervix and vagina, resulting in the removal of more upper vaginal tissue than intended. The decision to proceed with total versus subtotal hysterectomy must be made by the responsible surgeon. General anesthetic agents that diminish uterine tone (halothane, isoflurane) should be avoided, if possible.

Uterine inversion

Another cause for postpartum hemorrhage is uterine inversion. This can be diagnosed when a bulbous mass protrudes through the cervix and may be visible or feel similar to an aborting myoma. The primary setting in which this occurs is when excessive cord traction is applied to remove a fundal placenta. Massive hemorrhage and shock can ensue. The principal method of management is to attempt to replace the uterus as rapidly as possible without removing the placenta. If oxytocin is being administered, it should be discontinued. The palm of the hand should be placed on the fundus with the fingers extended circumferentially outward. The uterus should be replaced with the "last out, first in" principle, meaning the lower segment is replaced first, then the upper segment, and lastly the fundus, which is replaced with the palm of the hand. Occasionally, the cervix or uterus may have contracted, making replacement difficult; in this setting an uterorelaxant should be given (magnesium sulfate, terbutaline, nitroglycerine, halothane) and attempts to replace the uterus should resume. Once the uterus is replaced, the uterorelaxants are discontinued and an uterotonic is given and the hand removed once the uterus is contracted, at which point gentle manual removal of the placenta is attempted. However, occasionally the uterus cannot be returned vaginally, at which time laparotomy may need to be performed. An assistant should attempt to return the uterus from below while the surgeon places traction on the round ligaments. Alternatively, if there is a thick constriction band preventing the uterus returning, a midline incision is made on the posterior wall of the uterus, which should relieve tension from the band. The uterus is replaced and the incision repaired.

Hematomas

Hematomas can be vulvar, vulvovaginal, paravaginal or retroperitoneal. Hematomas can cause considerable pain and discomfort. Importantly, the clinical diagnosis based on appearance and palpation must not overlook the fact that bleeding may extend into the retroperitoneum, causing a significant amount of blood loss. Small vulvar hematomas are managed expectantly but large hematomas should be evaluated surgically, with any bleeding vessels ligated. If no bleeding is noted, the vagina should be packed (after the placement of a transurethral catheter) for 24 hours. Serial hemoglobin levels should be assessed. If there is a significant decrease in hemoglobin levels, the hematoma may be extending into the retroperitoneum. Occasionally laparotomy may be necessary. If the patient is hemodynamically stable, embolization can be considered.

Blood product replacement

Careful attention must be given to the replacement of blood products. Hemoglobin, platelets, fibrinogen, electrolytes (including calcium), and coagulation studies should be obtained at baseline, as clinically necessary, and for every

5–7 units of packed red blood cells transfused. Packed red blood cells (PRBC) are prepared in a volume of 200–250 cc per unit. Transfusion of PRBC is indicated in the setting of massive hemorrhage or shock or hemoglobin less than 7 g/dL. Each unit of PRBC has a hematocrit of 60–70% and should raise the maternal hemoglobin by 1 g/dL, in the absence of continued bleeding. The target hemoglobin is between 7–10 g/dL depending on the patient's age, condition, and risk for future hemorrhage.

Massive hemorrhage may deplete platelets and clotting factors, leading to disseminated intravascular coagulation, and compounding the problem of hemostasis. Clotting factors are replaced with FFP prepared in volumes of 200–250 mL per unit. Transfusion of FFP is indicated when active bleeding is accompanied by evidence of coagulopathy, including a serum fibrinogen level less than 100 mg/dL and/or prolongation of the prothrombin or activated partial thromboplastin times (greater than 1.5 times normal). FFP contains all coagulation factors and fibrinogen. If a patient is in DIC, we start by administering 4 units of FFP (one unit per 15–20 kg). One unit of FFP contains approximately 500 mg of fibrinogen and will increase clotting protein levels by 8%. Hemostasis is usually maintained when coagulation proteins are 25% of normal. Each unit of FFP will raise the serum fibrinogen level by 10–15 mg/dL, and a fibrinogen level of at least 100 mg/dL should be maintained.

Transfusion of platelets is indicated in the setting of active bleeding or imminent surgery when the platelet count is less than 50,000/mm^3. Platelets can be administered either as random donor units or as pheresis units. One unit of random donor platelets will raise the platelet count by 5000 mm^3 and is suspended in approximately 50 mL of plasma. Random donor units are typically administered as six units ("six pack"). One pheresis unit of platelets is approximately equivalent to 6–10 random donor units and contains a volume of approximately 300 mL. A pheresis unit has the advantage of being collected from a single donor, thus potentially avoiding exposure to multiple donors as is the case when more than one random donor unit is administered. Platelets, ideally, should be matched to the patient's blood type and Rh status. The practitioner is advised to consult their blood bank and inquire how platelets are collected and supplied at their institution.

Cryoprecipitate is indicated when volume status is of concern and there is a need to replace fibrinogen. Cryoprecipitate contains fibrinogen, von Willebrand factor, factor XIII, and factor VIII. It is prepared in a volume of 10–15 mL per unit. Usually 10 units of cryoprecipitate are administered, which contains approximately 2 g of fibrinogen and will raise the fibrinogen level by 70 mg/dL. The use of recombinant factor VIIa (90–100 μg/kg) has been described

in the setting of massive obstetric hemorrhage when traditional treatment of DIC has failed with donated blood products. The mechanism of action is thought to be stimulation of thrombin generation at the site of vessel injury and stimulating the extrinsic coagulation pathway. We have had success using this product in several cases.

Conclusion

Prompt recognition and appropriate intervention are the cornerstones of successful management in cases of postpartum hemorrhage. Fluids, blood, platelets and clotting factors must be replaced as needed. Conservative measures for control of hemorrhage due to uterine atony include uterine massage, uterine compression, and administration of uterotonic agents. An intrauterine balloon catheter or uterine artery brace suture should only be placed in patients who respond to bimanual uterine compression. The next step should incorporate sequential ligation of the uterine blood supply; however, if these measures are unsuccessful or if the patient is hemodynamically unstable, hysterectomy should be considered. Other causes of postpartum hemorrhage include lacerations, retained placental fragments, uterine inversion, and hematomas.

Suggested reading

Alfirevic Z, Elbourne D, Pavord S, *et al.* Use of recombinant activated factor VII in primary postpartum hemorrhage: the Northern European Registry 2000–2004. *Obstet Gynecol* 2007; 110: 1270–1278.

American College of Obstetricians and Gynecologists. Clinical management guidelines for obstetrician-gynecologists: postpartum hemorrhage. Practice Bulletin No. 76. *Obstet Gynecol* 2006; 108(4): 1039–1047.

Bakri YN, Amri A, Abdul Jabbar F. Tamponade balloon for obstetrical bleeding. *Int J Obstet Gynecol* 2001; 74: 139–142.

B-Lynch C, Coker A, Lawal AH, Abu J, Cowen MJ.The B-Lynch surgical technique for the control of massive postpartum haemorrhage: an alternative to hysterectomy? Five cases reported. *BJOG* 1997: 104: 372–375.

Gilstrap LC, Cunningham FG, van Dorsten P (eds). *Operative obstetrics*, 2nd edn. New York: McGraw-Hill, 2002.

Loudoun B, Smith MP. Recombinant factor VIIa as an adjunctive therapy for patients requiring large volume transfusion: a pharmaco-economic evaluation. *Int Med J* 2005; 35: 463–467.

O'Brien P, El-Refaey H, Gordon A, Geary M, Rodeck CH. Rectally administered misoprostol for the treatment of postpartum hemorrhage unresponsive to oxytocin and ergometrine: a descriptive study. *Obstet Gynecol* 1998; 92: 212–214.

Segal S, Shemesh IY, Blumental R, *et al.* The use of recombinant factor VIIa in severe postpartum hemorrhage. *Acta Obstet Gynecol Scand* 2004; 83: 771–772.

Chapter 18
Fetal Death

Marc H. Incerpi and Ronna Jurow
Department of Medicine and Obstetrics and Gynecology, Keck School of Medicine, University of Southern California, CA, USA

Introduction

The expectation of every pregnancy is that a healthy patient and baby will be the outcome. Unfortunately, we know all too well that this is not always the case. One of the most devastating situations is when fetal death occurs. Fortunately, the occurrence of fetal death is rare in the United States. The most recent statistics demonstrate a fetal death rate of 7/1000 total births. While there is still no standard that is applied universally, the definition most commonly used for fetal death or stillbirth, including the American College of Obstetricians and Gynecologists, is when a fetus that weighs 500 g or more or has attained a gestational age of 20 weeks or greater is delivered without any signs of life (Apgar scores 0,0).

Fetal mortality rates over the last several decades have decreased significantly in the United States. In 1950, the fetal death rate was approximately 18/1000 total births. Since then, we have seen a steady decline in the rate of stillbirths. Many factors have contributed to this decrease. Probably, the most obvious is the improvement in obstetric care. The implementation of antenatal testing for high-risk patients has also resulted in fewer stillbirths. The almost universal application of ultrasound and increased ability to diagnose fetal chromosomal and congenital anomalies have resulted in elective termination of fetuses that would likely result in stillbirth. Lastly, as neonatal care has improved, many fetuses that would have potentially expired *in utero* are delivered at earlier gestations. Thus, an increase in iatrogenic early preterm deliveries has evolved.

Benefits of fetal death evaluation

As stated earlier, when a stillbirth occurs it is often devastating to the parents, family, and caregivers. While it is clear that nothing can be done to prevent a stillbirth after it has occurred, there is a great deal of benefit that can be obtained by performing a thorough evaluation in hopes of identifying reasons why the fetal death happened. While it is very difficult to state definitively that a specific circumstance or condition caused the fetal death, a comprehensive stillbirth evaluation will at least allow one to identify potential associations.

Probably the most practical and important benefit of performing a complete evaluation is to help with parental grieving and the parental right to know. Almost invariably there is a sense of guilt that is felt by the mother. What did I do wrong? How could I have prevented this from happening? The parents have a strong desire, and deserve, to obtain information that will help them understand why this happened, and whether it may happen again. The answers will often assist and influence their reproductive decision-making.

A thorough stillbirth evaluation will also assist the physician with prenatal assessment, intervention, and management in future pregnancies. For example, if a patient had a prior stillbirth associated with anencephaly, she would best be served by undergoing genetic counseling and ultrasound evaluation. On the other hand, if a patient had a prior stillbirth that was associated with poorly controlled diabetes mellitus, she would best benefit from preconception counseling and obtaining good glycemic control before becoming pregnant.

Stillbirth evaluation is also important and beneficial to the physician in helping to decrease inappropriate litigation. When fetal death occurs it is not uncommon for the physician to be blamed. Sentiments such as "The doctor should have known something was wrong" or "The doctor must have missed something" are common after fetal death. Very often a comprehensive evaluation will demonstrate that the physician was not at fault, and that the fetal death could not have been prevented.

Lastly, studying fetal death has increased scientific understanding of the causes of stillbirth. This has allowed us to identify patients who might be at risk for

Management of Common Problems in Obstetrics and Gynecology,
5th edition. Edited by T.M. Goodwin, M.N. Montoro,
L. Muderspach, R. Paulson and S. Roy. © 2010 Blackwell
Publishing Ltd.

stillbirth, and has assisted with a variety of interventions to help minimize this risk.

Causes of fetal death

The causes of fetal death are many and varied. Early reports in the literature centered primarily on maternal medical conditions. Very little information was available regarding the association of fetal abnormalities and placental abnormalities with fetal death. Consequently, a large percentage of stillbirths were classified as unexplained. However, as we have gained a greater understanding of fetal abnormalities through ultrasound and autopsy, and have become more proficient at examining the placenta for specific abnormalities, the number of unexplained stillbirths has decreased.

In 1997 a review of causes of fetal death was published. By this time, greater emphasis was placed on the importance of autopsy and placental pathology. In addition, antepartum testing was being performed almost uniformly for maternal medical conditions such as chronic hypertension and pregestational diabetes. As a result, this review seemed to de-emphasize maternal conditions as a separate cause of fetal deaths, comprising only 5–10%. Instead, intrinsic fetal anomalies were noted as being associated with fetal death and 25–40% of stillbirths were attributed to fetal causes. These were broken down as follows: 6–13% chromosomal, 10–17% non-chromosomal, 10% non-immune hydrops, and 5–12% fetal infections. Placental abnormalities were identified as the cause 25–35% of the time. Therefore, the percentage of unexplained stillbirths had decreased to 25–35%.

A variety of demographic factors have been associated with fetal death. Advanced maternal age of 35 years or more doubles the risk. Obesity is also a known risk factor and women weighing 85 kg or more (BMI $\geqslant$30 kg/m^2) have a 2–3-fold increase in fetal death. African American women have a stillbirth risk 1.5 times that of Caucasian women, and smokers also have an increased risk of fetal death compared to nonsmokers. Thus, there are some demographic risk factors that can be potentially modified.

Several maternal medical diseases are associated with increased fetal death rates (see table 18.1). In addition, increased fetal death rates have been observed in patients with underlying thrombophilias. These can be either inherited (antithrombin deficiency, protein C deficiency, protein S deficiency, factor V Leiden mutation, prothrombin gene mutation or methylene tetrahydrofolate reductase deficiency) or acquired thrombophilias, in which lupus anticoagulant, anticardiolipin antibodies or anti-β2 glycoprotein antibodies are present.

Another potential etiology for stillbirth is fetal hemorrhage. This can be ascertained by performing a Kleihauer–Betke test, which looks at the number of fetal cells present in the maternal circulation. Based on the

Table 18.1 Maternal medical diseases

Condition	Estimated stillbirth rate
All pregnancies	6–7/1000
Chronic hypertension	5–25/1000
Severe preeclampsia	21/1000
HELLP syndrome	51/1000
Gestational diabetes	5–10/1000
Type 1 diabetes	6–10/1000
Type 2 diabetes	6–20/1000
SLE	40–150/1000
Intrahepatic cholestasis	12–30/1000

Simpson LL. Semin Perinatol 2002; 26: 42–50

number of fetal cells present, one can then calculate if a significant fetal hemorrhage has occurred that may have been responsible for the fetal death. While the Kleihauer–Betke test is commonly performed in cases of maternal trauma, it has proven to be useful in cases of otherwise unexplained fetal death.

Infections are another broad category that can cause fetal death via a variety of mechanisms. Some of the most common bacterial agents are *E. coli, Mycoplasma,* and *Listeria. Treponema pallidum,* a spirochete that causes syphilis, is a potentially lethal congenital infection. *Toxoplasma* is a protozoan that can lead to fetal death by causing severe hydrops. Lastly, multiple viral infections such as parvovirus B19 and cytomegalovirus are associated with stillbirth. Commonly the patient herself is entirely asymptomatic.

There are also a variety of genetic causes that may lead to fetal death by causing congenital abnormalities. The most common genetic factors are sporadic conditions, which make up approximately 33% of genetic causes. Cytogenetic abnormalities such as trisomy 18 or trisomy 21 comprise approximately 25%. Multifactorial processes such as complex congenital heart defects account for about 12%. Mendelian disorders are responsible for 5% of the genetic causes. Environmental exposures are thought to contribute to 5% as well. Lastly, 20% of genetic causes are nonspecific.

Umbilical cord accidents are often cited as causing stillbirths. Since approximately one-third of all deliveries of normal infants are associated with a nuchal cord, one must be very careful to state that a nuchal cord was the cause of the stillbirth without ruling out other potential etiologies. There are, however, a variety of umbilical cord conditions that are seen in fetal death. True knots in the umbilical cord are uncommon, comprising only 1% of all deliveries. However, when they are seen, there is a four-fold increase in fetal death. Cord insertion abnormalities, such as marginal and velamentous cord insertions, are associated with fetal death. Cord prolapse can also lead to stillbirth. Lastly constriction of the umbilical cord via a wide array of mechanisms can lead to anoxia and fetal death. These are very uncommon but include stenosis, torsion, intravascular cord thrombosis, and obliteration of the cord vessels. In order to prove that an umbilical cord accident is the true cause of fetal death, one must be able not only to document cord occlusion and fetal hypoxia, but also to exclude other causes.

Lastly, a variety of placental abnormalities, both intrinsic and others associated with maternal medical conditions such as antiphospholipid syndrome, have been associated with fetal death. Placental abruption is the most frequent cause of stillbirth. Other placental abnormalities include acute chorio-amnionitis, placental infarcts, occlusive vasculopathy, and villitis.

Components of the stillbirth evaluation

Since there are several potential etiologies for fetal death, it is clear that the stillbirth evaluation should be comprehensive. Unless the cause is immediately recognized, such as in the case of anencephaly, the stillbirth evaluation should include a complete clinical examination incorporating a thorough review of the prenatal records, as well as genetic evaluation. Appropriate laboratory tests should be conducted as indicated. Placental pathology should be obtained and autopsy should also be performed. Since the identification of an underlying thrombophilia can have profound and potentially lifelong implications, a thrombophilia work-up should be undertaken as well.

There are very good data that demonstrate the value of a comprehensive stillbirth evaluation. One of the best studies examined the results of a statewide stillbirth evaluation project in Wisconsin. When a comprehensive stillbirth assessment was performed significant information was obtained to guide practitioners with future pregnancies. The most profound of these was a 40% change in recurrence risk. For instance, a fetal condition that was initially thought to be multifactorial was later determined to be sporadic. A thorough stillbirth evaluation was noted to change the prenatal diagnosis 21% of the time. Other areas that were influenced as a result of a comprehensive evaluation included pre-conceptual treatment as well as prenatal, perinatal and neonatal treatments.

At our own institution we discovered that when placental pathology was added to the stillbirth evaluation, significant placental pathology was observed 30% of the time. Multiple studies have documented the value of autopsy. We have determined that in otherwise unexplained stillbirths, autopsy determined a cause 30% of the time. Other investigators have noted that 35% of stillborn infants have congenital structural anomalies. In evaluating recurrence risk, autopsy findings significantly altered recurrence risk factors 26% of the time.

In the case of fetal death, the autopsy should be complete and include the following components: complete medical record review to obtain clinical history, birthweight and external measurements, photographs and x-rays, gross external examination of the stillborn, placenta, and cord, gross examination and weight of major fetal organs, microscopic examination of fetal organs, placenta, and cord, bacterial cultures of fetal blood and lung, and cytogenetic studies when appropriate. Therefore, when all components are performed as listed above, autopsy can identify malformations, metabolic abnormalities, hypoxia, and infection. While the value of autopsy cannot be overestimated, autopsy is only obtained in half the cases. A variety of reasons are responsible for this low number.

Since there are several factors that may be responsible for fetal death, and since performing a comprehensive evaluation can be expensive, evaluations that are universally recommended are the following: perinatal autopsy, placental pathology, karyotype, Kleihauer–Betke test, urine toxicology, and parvovirus serology. Depending on the clinical picture, tests to evaluate for underlying thrombophilias can be added. At our institution, we have created the following algorithm. At the initial evaluation, all prenatal records are thoroughly reviewed, including past obstetric history and genetic history. Initial tests include routine labs (type, Rh, antibody screen, CBC, serum glucose). Additional lab tests include a Kleihauer–Betke test, urine toxicology, and glycosylated hemoglobin if the patient has an elevated serum glucose or known history of diabetes. After the fetus is delivered, a detailed physical examination of the stillborn is performed, and a detailed fetal death/stillborn evaluation form is completed. The placenta is sent to pathology in all cases, and in all cases we attempt to obtain parental consent for autopsy. In cases in which there are obvious fetal anomalies, tissue is sent for karyotype. In otherwise unexplained cases, a thrombophilia work-up is performed. This consists of testing for the presence of lupus anticoagulant, anticardiolipin antibodies, anti-β2 glycoprotein antibodies, and factor V Leiden. In addition, serum homocysteine levels are evaluated. If there is a high suspicion for underlying thrombophilia (e.g. placental pathology demonstrates the presence of multiple infarcts, fetus with severe intrauterine growth restriction) additional tests are performed for the presence of prothrombin gene mutation, protein C or protein S deficiency, or antithrombin deficiency. Lastly, the patient is given a postpartum evaluation in 1 week to assess her condition and to review the above studies.

Timing of delivery and delivery method

Once the patient has been told that her baby is no longer living, a tremendous surge of emotions is common. While many patients report that they had a premonition that something was wrong, the vast majority of individuals are understandably confused, angry and sad. They report an unreal or numbing feeling, feelings that they have never experienced before.

While most women desire delivery soon after the diagnosis is made, some will prefer to wait for a period of time. Most authorities recommend that a period of time be allowed to elapse between diagnosis and induction, if possible. This will allow the patient to gain motivation for a vaginal delivery, achieve some physical and mental rest before the birth of the baby, and prepare psychologically to meet and hold the baby. Some patients will elect to wait and let labor occur spontaneously. While this may be an option, the patient must be made aware of the potential risks, including intrauterine infection and maternal coagulopathy. If the stillborn has not delivered within 4 weeks of diagnosis, there is a 25% risk of disseminated intravascular coagulation (DIC). In these rare cases, it would be reasonable to determine CBC and fibrinogen on a weekly basis. The patient needs to understand that the risks of infection and/or DIC can lead to significant morbidity and, in some cases, maternal death.

The delivery method may be surgical via a cervical dilation and evacuation (D&E) or via cesarean delivery (hysterotomy). Conversely, the patient may elect to proceed with labor induction. The agent most commonly used for labor induction is misoprostol. At less than 28 weeks of gestation, the dose commonly given is $400\mu g$ every 4 hours. In patients beyond 28 weeks, misoprostol can be given as a $25\mu g$ initial dose, followed by $25–50\mu g$ every 4 hours. It is important to realize that in patients with a history of prior uterine surgery or cesarean section, misoprostol has been associated with uterine rupture. Therefore, in these cases, it should be used very judiciously or not at all. Misoprostol is an effective agent and is tolerated well with minimal side effects.

After delivery, it is important that the patient and family be given the opportunity to hold the infant and keep mementos such as pictures, footprints, and handprints. Most hospitals have grief counselors, spiritual counselors, and social work services available for patients to help them cope with such a devastating loss. In addition, a variety of support groups are available in the Internet as well.

Prenatal evaluation of the patient with a prior stillbirth

What should be done for those patients who have previously had a fetal death and then become pregnant again? It is important to understand and appreciate the level of anxiety that the patient will experience during the prenatal course. It is therefore vital that everything be done to provide the patient with as much reassurance as possible that the outcome will be different this time.

A comprehensive evaluation regarding the prior stillbirth should be attempted. Every effort should be made to determine the potential etiology of the previous stillbirth. This should include prior prenatal care and hospital records. Placental pathology and autopsy reports should be obtained if possible. Lab tests should also be reviewed. If a thorough evaluation was not performed initially, and if no cause could be determined, then it is reasonable to obtain lab tests for an underlying thrombophilia as discussed previously.

The goal with a subsequent pregnancy is to assess the likelihood of recurrence and help to minimize the risk. Sometimes it will involve genetic counseling and amniocentesis or it could involve treating the patient medically (e.g. with heparin if a thrombophilia was diagnosed). The course of the pregnancy is often managed similarly to other pregnancies. However, in a pregnancy complicated by a prior fetal death, increased fetal surveillance via either non-stress testing or by biophysical profile is recommended. At our institution, we commonly begin twice-weekly antepartum testing with amniotic fluid volume assessment (modified biophysical profile) at 32 weeks of gestation. Delivery is anticipated to occur at term with labor induction or cesarean section for usual obstetric indications.

Future goals and directions

It is clear that our understanding of stillbirth is still incomplete. There are many limitations to assessment of stillbirth. Throughout the United States stillbirths are under-reported. The completeness of fetal death certificates varies. There is no standardized classification system that exists currently. There is no existing standardized protocol for postmortem investigation of stillbirths. Fetal autopsy rates are low. Lastly, there are few geographic population-based detailed investigations.

The National Institute for Child and Human Development (NICHD) has recognized the above limitations and the need for a standardized protocol. The NICHD has established the Stillbirth Collaborative Research Network (SCRN) to study stillbirths in the United States. This will be a 5-year study examining approximately 500 fetal deaths. The major goals of this study will be to (1) determine causes of stillbirth using a standardized stillbirth postmortem protocol to identify genetic, maternal, and environmental influences, (2) obtain a geographic and population-based determination of the incidence of stillbirth, and (3) elucidate risk factors for stillbirth.

Conclusion

It is clear that there are a variety of potential etiologies for stillbirth. The stillbirth evaluation should be systematic and comprehensive, incorporating placental pathology and autopsy. The value of autopsy should not be underestimated given that studies have consistently demonstrated that up to 30% of stillbirths may be due to congenital anomalies. Lastly, we are optimistic that data from the SCRN and other such studies will provide valuable information to help us better understand and potentially prevent this devastating entity.

Suggested reading

Cunningham FG, Holier LM: Fetal death. In Williams Obstetrics, 20th ed (Suppl 4). Norwalk, Conn, Appleton & Lange. Aug-Sept 1997.

Faye-Peterson O, Guinn DA, Wenstron KA. Value of perinatal autopsy. *Obstet Gynecol* 1999; 94: 915–920.

Fretts RC. Etiology and prevention of stillbirth. *Am J Obstet Gynecol* 2005; 193: 1923–1935.

Incerpi MH, Miller DA, Samadi R, *et al.* Stillbirth evaluation: what tests are needed? *Am J Obstet Gynecol* 1998; 178: 1121–1125.

Michalski ST, Porter J, Pauli RM. Costs and consequences of comprehensive stillbirth assessment. *Am J Obstet Gynecol* 2002; 186: 1027–1034.

Mueller RF, Sybert VP, Johnson J, *et al.* Evaluation of a protocol for post-mortem examination of stillbirths. *New Engl J Med* 1983; 309: 586–590.

National Center for Health Statistics. *Infant mortality rates, fetal mortality rates, and perinatal mortality rates according to race. United States, selected years 1950–2002.* Atlanta, GA: National Center for Health Statistics, 2001.

Pitkin RM. Fetal death: diagnosis and management. *Am J Obstet Gynecol* 1987; 157: 583–589.

Preston FE, Rosendaal FR, Walker ID, *et al.* Increased fetal loss in women with heritable thrombophilia. *Lancet* 1996; 348: 913–916.

Rayburn W, Sander C, Barr M, *et al.* The stillborn fetus: placental histologic examination in determining a cause. *Obstet Gynecol* 1985; 65: 637–640.

Reddy UM, Ko CW, Willinger M. Maternal age and risk of stillbirth throughout pregnancy in the United States. *Am J Obstet Gynecol* 2006; 195: 764–770.

Robertson L, Wu O, Langhorne P, *et al.* Thrombophilia in pregnancy: a systemic review. *Br J Haematol* 2005; 132: 171–196.

Silver RM. Fetal death. *Obstet Gynecol* 2007; 109: 153–167.

Simpson LL. Maternal medical disease: risk of antepartum fetal death. *Semin Perinatol* 2002; 26: 42–50.

Smith GC, Fretts RC. Stillbirth. *Lancet* 2007; 370: 1715–1725.

Smulian JC, Ananth CV, Vintzileos AM, *et al.* Fetal deaths in the United States: influence of high-risk conditions and implications for management. *Obstet Gynecol* 2002; 100: 1183–1189.

Tolfvenstam T, Papadogiannakis N, Norbeck O, *et al.* Frequency of human parvovirus B19 infection in intrauterine fetal death. *Lancet* 2001; 357: 1494–1497.

Trulsson O, Radestad I. The silent child – mothers' experiences before, during, and after stillbirth. *Birth* 2004; 31: 189–195.

Weeks JW, Asrat T, Morgan MA, *et al.* Antepartum surveillance for a history of stillbirth: when to begin? *Am J Obstet Gynecol* 1995; 172: 486–492.

Chapter 19
Assessing the Obstetric Role in the Brain-Damaged Newborn

David A. Miller

Department of Medicine and Obstetrics and Gynecology, Keck School of Medicine, University of Southern California, CA, USA

Introduction

The objective of intrapartum fetal heart rate (FHR) monitoring is to prevent fetal injury that might result from interruption of normal fetal oxygenation during labor. The underlying assumption is that interruption of fetal oxygenation leads to characteristic physiologic changes that can be detected by changes in the FHR. Understanding the physiologic basis for electronic FHR monitoring requires a realistic appraisal of this basic assumption. This chapter will review the physiology underlying fetal oxygenation, including transfer of oxygen from the environment to the fetus and the subsequent fetal response.

Transfer of oxygen from the environment to the fetus

Oxygen is carried from the environment to the fetus by maternal and fetal blood along a pathway that invariably includes the maternal lungs, heart, vasculature, uterus, placenta and umbilical cord. Interruption of oxygen transfer can occur at any or all the points along the oxygen pathway.

External environment

In inspired air, the partial pressure exerted by oxygen gas is approximately 150 mmHg. As oxygen is transferred from the environment to the fetus, the partial pressure steadily declines. By the time oxygen reaches fetal umbilical venous blood, the partial pressure is as low as 30–35 mmHg. After oxygen is delivered to fetal tissues, the PO_2 of deoxygenated blood in the umbilical arteries returning to the placenta is in the range of 15–25 mmHg [1-4].

The sequential transfer of oxygen from the environment to the fetus and potential causes of interruption at each step are described below.

Maternal lungs

Inspiration carries oxygenated air from the external environment to the distal air sacs of the lung – the alveoli. Normal alveolar PO_2 is in the region of 105 mmHg. Interruption of normal oxygen transfer from the environment to the alveoli can result from upper airway obstruction or from interruption of breathing caused by depression of central respiratory control (narcotics, magnesium, seizure). From the alveoli, oxygen diffuses into maternal pulmonary capillary blood across a thin "blood–gas" barrier consisting of a single-cell layer of alveolar epithelium, an interstitial collagen layer and a single-cell layer of pulmonary capillary endothelium. Interruption of normal oxygen transfer from the alveoli to the pulmonary capillary blood can be caused by a number of factors including ventilation-perfusion mismatch and diffusion defects. Pulmonary causes of interrupted oxygenation may include respiratory depression due to medication or seizure, pulmonary embolus, pulmonary edema, pneumonia, asthma, atelectasis or adult respiratory distress syndrome.

Maternal blood

In maternal arterial blood, more than 98% of oxygen combines with hemoglobin in maternal red blood cells. Approximately 1–2% remains dissolved in the blood and is measured by the partial pressure of dissolved oxygen (PaO_2). A normal adult PaO_2 value of 95–100 mmHg results in hemoglobin saturation of approximately 95–98%. A number of factors affect the affinity of hemoglobin for oxygen. In general, the tendency for hemoglobin to release oxygen is increased by factors that signal an increased requirement for oxygen such as anaerobic glycolysis (reflected by increased 2,3-DPG concentration), production of hydrogen ions (reflected by decreased pH) and heat. Interruption of oxygen transfer from the environment to the fetus due to abnormal maternal oxygen-carrying capacity can result from severe anemia or from

Management of Common Problems in Obstetrics and Gynecology, 5th edition. Edited by T.M. Goodwin, M.N. Montoro, L. Muderspach, R. Paulson and S. Roy. © 2010 Blackwell Publishing Ltd.

hereditary or acquired abnormalities affecting oxygen binding (hemoglobinopathies or methemoglobinemia). Reduced maternal oxygen-carrying capacity is an uncommon cause of reduced fetal oxygenation.

Maternal heart

From the lungs, pulmonary veins carry oxygenated maternal blood to the heart. Blood enters the left atrium with a PaO_2 of approximately 95 mmHg. Oxygenated blood passes from the left atrium, through the mitral valve into the left ventricle and out the aorta for systemic distribution. Interruption of oxygen transfer from the environment to the fetus at the level of the maternal heart can be caused by any condition that reduces cardiac output, including altered heart rate (arrhythmia), reduced preload (hypovolemia, compression of the inferior vena cava), impaired contractility (ischemic heart disease, diabetes, cardiomyopathy, congestive heart failure) and increased afterload (hypertension). In addition, structural abnormalities of the heart and/or great vessels may impede the normal ability to pump blood (valvular stenosis, valvular insufficiency, pulmonary hypertension, coarctation of the aorta). In a healthy obstetric patient, the most common cause of reduced cardiac output is reduced preload (hypovolemia, compression of the inferior vena cava).

Maternal vasculature

Oxygenated blood leaving the heart is carried by the systemic vasculature to the uterus. The path includes the aorta, common iliac artery, internal iliac artery, anterior division of the internal iliac artery and the uterine artery. From the uterine artery, oxygenated blood travels through the arcuate arteries, the radial arteries and finally the spiral arteries before exiting the maternal vasculature and entering the intervillous space of the placenta. Interruption of normal oxygen transfer from the environment to the fetus at the level of the maternal vasculature commonly results from hypotension (for example, regional anesthesia, hypovolemia, impaired venous return, impaired cardiac output, medications). Alternatively, it may result from vasoconstriction of distal arterioles in response to endogenous vasoconstrictors or medications. Conditions associated with chronic vasculopathy, such as chronic hypertension, long-standing diabetes, collagen vascular disease, thyroid disease and renal disease, may result in chronic suboptimal transfer of oxygen and nutrients to the fetus. Pre-eclampsia is associated with abnormal vascular remodeling at the level of the spiral arteries and can impede normal perfusion of the intervillous space. Catastrophic vascular injury (trauma, aortic dissection) is rare.

Uterus

Between the maternal uterine arteries and the intervillous space of the placenta, the arcuate, radial and spiral arteries traverse the muscular wall of the uterus. Interruption of normal oxygen transfer from the environment to the fetus at the level of the uterus commonly results from uterine contractions that compress intramural blood vessels and impede the flow of blood. Excessive uterine activity and uterine injury (rupture, trauma) are the most common causes of acute interruption of fetal oxygenation at this level.

Placenta

The placenta is the maternal–fetal interface that facilitates the exchange of gases, nutrients, wastes and other molecules (for example, antibodies, hormones, medications) between maternal blood in the intervillous space and fetal blood in the villous capillaries. On the maternal side of the placenta, oxygenated blood exits the spiral arteries and enters the intervillous space to surround and bathe the chorionic villi. On the fetal side of the placenta, paired umbilical arteries carry blood from the fetus through the umbilical cord to the placenta. At term, the umbilical arteries receive 40% of fetal cardiac output.

Upon reaching the placental cord insertion site, the umbilical arteries divide into multiple branches and fan out across the surface of the placenta. At each cotyledon, placental arteries dive beneath the surface *en route* to the chorionic villi. The chorionic villi are thousands of tiny branches of trophoblast that protrude into the intervillous space. Each branch of trophoblast is perfused by a fetal capillary bed that represents the terminal distribution of an umbilical artery. At term, fetal villous capillary blood is separated from maternal blood in the intervillous space by a thin "blood–blood" barrier similar to the "blood–gas" barrier in the maternal lung. The placental "blood–blood" barrier consists of a layer of placental trophoblast and a layer of fetal capillary endothelium with intervening basement membranes and villous stroma. Oxygen is transferred from the intervillous space to the fetal blood by a complex process that depends upon the PaO_2 of maternal blood perfusing the intervillous space, maternal blood flow within the intervillous space, chorionic villous surface area and diffusion across the placental "blood–blood" barrier.

Although many conditions can interfere with the normal transfer of oxygen across the placenta, most involve the microvasculature and can be confirmed only by histopathology [5–7]. Clinically, the most common cause of interrupted oxygen transfer at the level of the placenta is abruption or premature separation of placenta previa. Fetal–maternal hemorrhage and vasa previa should be considered in the appropriate clinical setting.

Fetal blood

After oxygen has diffused from the intervillous space across the placental "blood–blood" barrier and into fetal blood, the PaO_2 is in the region of 30 mmHg and fetal hemoglobin saturation is between 50% and 70%. Although fetal PaO_2 and hemoglobin saturation are low in comparison to adult values, adequate delivery of oxygen to the fetal tissues is maintained by a number of compensatory mechanisms. For example, fetal cardiac output per unit weight is 3–4 times greater than that of the adult. Hemoglobin concentration and affinity for oxygen are greater in the fetus as well, resulting in increased oxygen-carrying capacity. Finally, oxygenated blood is directed preferentially toward vital organs by way of anatomic shunts at the level of the ductus venosus, foramen ovale and ductus arteriosus. Conditions that can interrupt the normal transfer of oxygen from the environment to the fetus at the level of the fetal blood are uncommon, but may include fetal anemia (alloimmunization, viral infections, fetomaternal hemorrhage, vasa previa) and conditions that reduce oxygen-carrying capacity (Bart's hemoglobinopathy, methemoglobinemia).

Umbilical cord

After oxygen combines with fetal hemoglogin in the villous capillaries, oxygenated blood returns to the fetus by way of villous veins that coalesce to form placental veins on the surface of the placenta. Placental surface veins unite to form a single umbilical vein within the umbilical cord. Interruption of the normal transfer of oxygen from the environment to the fetus at the level of the umbilical cord most often results from simple mechanical compression. Other uncommon causes may include vasospasm, thrombosis, atherosis, hypertrophy, hemorrhage, inflammation or a "true knot."

Oxygen transfer from the environment to the fetus represents the first basic component of fetal oxygenation. The second basic component of fetal oxygenation involves the fetal physiologic response to interrupted oxygen transfer.

Fetal response to interrupted oxygen transfer

Depending upon frequency and duration, interruption of oxygen transfer at any point along the oxygen pathway may result in progressive deterioration of fetal oxygenation. The cascade begins with hypoxemia, defined as decreased oxygen content in the blood. At term, hypoxemia is characterized by an umbilical artery PaO_2 below the normal range of 15–25 mmHg. Recurrent or sustained hypoxemia can lead to decreased delivery of oxygen to the tissues and reduced tissue oxygen content, or hypoxia. Normal homeostasis requires an adequate supply of oxygen and fuel in order to generate the energy required by basic cellular activities. When oxygen is readily available, aerobic metabolism efficiently generates energy in the form of ATP. Byproducts of aerobic metabolism include

carbon dioxide and water. When oxygen is in short supply, tissues may be forced to convert from aerobic to anaerobic metabolism, generating energy less efficiently and resulting in the production of lactic acid.

Accumulation of lactic acid in the tissues results in metabolic acidosis. Lactic acid accumulation can lead to utilization of buffer bases (primarily bicarbonate) to help stabilize tissue pH. If the buffering capacity is exceeded, the blood pH may begin to fall, leading to metabolic acidemia. Eventually, recurrent or sustained tissue hypoxia and acidosis can lead to loss of peripheral vascular smooth muscle contraction, reduced peripheral vascular resistance and hypotension.

Acidemia is defined as increased hydrogen ion content (decreased pH) in the blood. With respect to fetal physiology, it is critical to distinguish between respiratory acidemia, caused by accumulation of CO_2, and metabolic acidemia, caused by accumulation of fixed (lactic) acid. These distinct categories of acidemia have entirely different clinical implications and will be discussed later in this chapter.

Mechanisms of injury

If interrupted oxygen transfer progresses to the stage of metabolic acidemia and hypotension, as described above, multiple organs and systems (including the brain and heart) can suffer hypoperfusion, reduced oxygenation, lowered pH and reduced delivery of fuel for metabolism. These changes can trigger a cascade of cellular events including altered enzyme function, protease activation, ion shifts, altered water regulation, interrupted neurotransmitter metabolism, free radical production and phospholipid degradation. Interruption of normal cellular metabolism can lead to cellular dysfunction, tissue dysfunction and even death.

Injury threshold

The relationship between interrupted fetal oxygenation and neurologic injury is complex. Electronic FHR monitoring was introduced with the expectation that it would significantly reduce the incidence of neurologic injury (specifically cerebral palsy) caused by intrapartum interruption of fetal oxygenation. In recent years, it has become apparent that most cases of cerebral palsy are unrelated to intrapartum events and therefore cannot be prevented by intrapartum FHR monitoring. Nevertheless, a significant minority of such cases may be related to intrapartum events and continue to generate controversy.

In January, 2003, the ACOG and the American Academy of Pediatrics jointly published a monograph entitled *"Neonatal encephalopathy and cerebral palsy: defining the pathogenesis and pathophysiology"* summarizing the world literature regarding the relationship between intrapartum events and neurologic injury [8]. Agencies and professional organizations that reviewed and endorsed the report include the Centers for Disease Control, the Child Neurology Society, the March of Dimes Birth Defects Foundation, the National Institute of Child Health and Human Development, the Royal Australian and New Zealand College of Obstetricians and Gynecologists, the Society for Maternal-Fetal Medicine and the Society of Obstetricians and Gynaecologists of Canada. The consensus report established four essential criteria defining an acute intrapartum event sufficient to cause cerebral palsy (Box 19.1).

The first criterion provides crucial information regarding the threshold of fetal injury in the setting of intrapartum interruption of oxygenation. Specifically, it indicates that intrapartum interruption of fetal oxygenation does not result in injury unless it progresses at least to the stage of significant metabolic acidemia (umbilical artery $pH < 7$ and base deficit ≥ 12 mmol/L). It is important to note that fetal injury is uncommon even when metabolic acidemia is present. It is also important to understand that respiratory acidemia is not a recognized risk factor for fetal injury. This information has significant implications for the interpretation and management of intrapartum FHR patterns.

The second criterion highlights an equally important point. Specifically, intrapartum interruption of fetal oxygenation does not result in cerebral palsy unless it first causes moderate-to-severe neonatal encephalopathy. The report further clarified that neonatal encephalopathy has many possible causes. "Hypoxic-ischemic" encephalopathy resulting from intrapartum interruption of fetal oxygenation represents only a small subset of the larger category of neonatal encephalopathy.

The third criterion emphasizes that different subtypes of cerebral palsy have different clinical origins. Spastic quadriplegia is associated with injury to the parasagittal cerebral cortex and involves abnormal motor control of all four extremities. The dyskinetic subtype of cerebral palsy is associated with injury to the basal ganglia and involves disorganized, choreo-athetoid movements. The report concluded that these are the only two subtypes of cerebral palsy that are associated with term "hypoxic-ischemic" injury. Specifically, spastic diplegia, hemiplegia, ataxia and hemiparetic cerebral palsy are "unlikely to result from acute intrapartum hypoxia." The report further concluded that other conditions, including epilepsy, mental retardation and attention deficit hyperactivity disorder, do not result from "birth asphyxia" in the absence of cerebral palsy.

The fourth criterion underscores the fact that intrapartum "hypoxic-ischemic" injury is a potential factor in only a small subset of all cases of cerebral palsy. Most cases of cerebral palsy are unrelated to intrapartum events.

Conclusion

The physiology of fetal oxygenation involves the sequential transfer of oxygen from the environment to the fetus and the subsequent fetal response. Interruption of normal oxygen transfer can occur at any point along the oxygen pathway. Recurrent or sustained interruption of normal oxygen transfer can lead to progressive deterioration of fetal oxygenation and eventually to potential fetal injury. However, the joint ACOG-AAP consensus report defined significant metabolic acidemia (umbilical artery $pH < 7.0$ and base deficit ≥ 12 mmol/L) as an essential precondition to intrapartum hypoxic injury. With respect to the relationship between fetal oxygenation and potential injury, there is consensus in the literature that interrupted oxygenation does not result in fetal injury unless it progresses at least to the stage of significant metabolic acidemia.

References

1. Richardson, B, Nodwell A, Webster K, Alshimmiri M, Gagnon R, Natale R. Fetal oxygen saturation and fractional extraction at birth and the relationship to measures of acidosis. *Am J Obstet Gynecol* 1998; 178: 572–579.
2. Nodwell A, Carmichael L, Ross M, Richardson B. Placental compared with umbilical cord blood to assess fetal blood gas and acid-base status. *Obstet Gynecol* 2005; 105: 129–138.
3. Helwig JT, Parer JT, Kilpatrick SJ, Laros RK. Umbilical cord blood acid-base state: what is normal? *Am J Obstet Gynecol* 1996; 174: 1807–1812.
4. Victory R, Penava D, Da Silva O, Natale R, Richardson B.Umbilical cord pH and base excess values in relation to adverse outcome events for infants delivering at term. *Am J Obstet Gynecol* 2004; 191(6): 2021–2028.
5. Giles WB, Trudinger BJ, Baird PJ. Fetal umbilical artery flow velocity waveforms and placental resistance: pathological correlation. *BJOG* 1985; 92: 31–38.

> **Box 19.1 Essential criteria that define an acute intrapartum hypoxic event sufficient to cause cerebral palsy (must meet all four)**
>
> - Umbilical cord arterial blood $pH < 7$ and base deficit ≥ 12 mmol/L
> - Early onset of severe or moderate neonatal encephalopathy in infants born at 34 or more weeks of gestation
> - Cerebral palsy of the spastic quadriplegic or dyskinetic type
> - Exclusion of other identifiable etiologies such as trauma, coagulation disorders, infectious conditions or genetic disorders

6. Fetus and Neonate: Physiology and Clinical Applications, Volume 1, The Circulation. Mark A. Hanson, John A.S. Spencer, Charles H. Rodeck editors Cambridge, United Kingdom: Cambridge University Press, 1993:323–38.

7. Arabin B, Jimenez E, Vogel M, Weitzel HK. Relationship of utero- and fetoplacental blood flow velocity wave forms with pathomorphological placental findings. *Fetal Diagn Ther* 1992; 7(3-4): 173–179.

8. American College of Obstetricians and Gynecologists' Task Force on Neonatal Encephalopathy and Cerebral Palsy, American College of Obstetricians and Gynecologists, American Academy of Pediatrics. *Neonatal encephalopathy and cerebral palsy: defining the pathogenesis and pathophysiology*. Washington, DC: American College of Obstetricians and Gynecologists, 2003.

Chapter 20
Lactation Management

Brendan Grubbs

Department of Medicine and Obstetrics and Gynecology, Keck School of Medicine, University of Southern California, CA, USA

Benefits of breastfeeding

The American Academy of Pediatrics recognizes multiple benefits of breastfeeding to both the term and premature newborn, particularly with regard to protection from infectious agents. Studies have demonstrated decreased rates of bacteremia, meningitis, respiratory and urinary tract infections, necrotizing enterocolitis, and otitis media among breastfed infants. There are multiple advantages to the new mother who chooses to breastfeed, both immediate and long term. Right after birth, breastfeeding initiates bonding between the mother and the child. Lactational amenorrhea allows for decreased menstrual blood loss and increased pregnancy spacing. Women who breastfeed also experience a more rapid return to their pre-pregnancy weight, and reduce their future risks of breast and ovarian cancer. These health advantages of breastfeeding also translate to lower costs to both the individual (cost of formula, increased doctor visits, medications) and to society (WIC, missed work due to doctor visits, insurance costs, contraception).

Physiology

The breast is both factory and depot for milk. Milk is produced and stored in glands, which attach radially to a central nipple with 15–20 ejection ducts. An infant initiates the milk ejection reflex by grasping and deforming the nipple and areola. This not only causes milk release, but also sends a feedback signal to the pituitary gland causing a rise in serum prolactin and oxytocin levels. Serum oxytocin augments milk ejection by stimulating myoepithelial cells surrounding the milk glands to contract, forcing the milk into ducts within the nipples.

Prolactin stimulates an increase in new milk production. The infant begins sucking as a series of rapid compressions, which enhance milk ejection, then slows to a sucking/swallowing rhythm. In the absence of active sucking, the nipple regains its compact shape and thus will not drip continuously. It is during this phase that the infant will be able to swallow effortlessly. This is in contrast to the manufactured rubber nipple, which maintains a continuous flow throughout the feeding cycle. An infant feeding from a bottle must compress his/her lips or perform a tongue thrust to interrupt this flow and allow unimpeded swallowing. The differences in milk delivery between bottle and breast nipples form the basis for "nipple confusion" in which the infant cannot distinguish which type of activity will result in comfortable swallowing.

Technique

While milk letdown may be a reflex, the act of breastfeeding is complex and all women can benefit from instruction in the proper technique. Breastfeeding is best initiated in a quiet, stress-free environment. Special consideration should be given to positioning, latch-on, and nipple care. Adequate nutrition, rest and fluid intake are needed to maintain milk supply. A lactating woman needs approximately 300 kCal/day above her maintenance caloric requirement. She should also drink adequate amounts of fluid; however, increased intake will not solve problems of milk production. If weight loss in excess of 1 lb (0.45 kg) per week occurs, caloric intake should be increased.

When initiating breastfeeding, one must first assure the baby is alert and ready to feed. Infants who have been given formula in the nursery while the mother is recovering may not readily initiate suckling. Acceptable strategies to awaken a baby include cheek strokes, back rubs, tickling the feet, and undressing an infant to improve skin-to-skin contact. Several positioning holds have been described, with the most common being the cuddle hold and the football hold. The cuddle hold supports the infant

Management of Common Problems in Obstetrics and Gynecology,
5th edition. Edited by T.M. Goodwin, M.N. Montoro,
L. Muderspach, R. Paulson and S. Roy. © 2010 Blackwell
Publishing Ltd.

along the length of the forearm, crossing the maternal abdomen while using the contralateral hand to position the breast near the infant's mouth. The football hold presents the ipsilateral breast to the infant while supporting the infant along the side. The football hold has advantages when the breasts are especially pendulous or during feeding of twins. In all cases, the use of a nursing pillow helps the mother decrease strain along the upper back and neck.

Proper latch-on occurs when the baby grasps the nipple and areola, pressing its nose directly up to the breast. Painful latch-on is tantamount to recognition of improper latch-on or sucking. Once latch-on has occurred, the infant initiates a series of quick suckling motions that stimulate a "pins and needles" sensation of milk letdown. A baby should be encouraged to nurse for at least 10–15 minutes at each breast during a feeding. Once satiated, the infant will cease suckling, but may hold the nipple lightly to maintain contact. Breastfeeding can occur "on demand" or on schedule, but most infants respond best to an on-demand system. As many delivery units have adopted policies encouraging the baby to room in with the mother, the popularity of "on-schedule" nursing has declined.

After nursing, women should be encouraged to express some residual breast milk onto the nipple and areola and allow the area to air-dry for a few minutes. The immunoglobins in the milk protect against cracking and dryness, and air-drying prevents yeast infections. Women should be cautioned against using creams or lotions. Often, these preparations clog milk ducts and carry a perfume or taste which is unappealing to the infant.

Once an infant masters sucking and latch-on, the prognosis for success over the next 2–4 weeks is good. Unfortunately, minor problems during this time period can evolve as barriers to continued breastfeeding if the mother does not receive advice to overcome them. In addition to the physician, there are several resources available. Most delivery units have trained lactation specialists who will assist with telephone advice or home visits. Most metropolitan areas boast several commercial businesses as well as free support groups to assist with questions about breastfeeding.

Challenges to continued breastfeeding

Problems of supply and demand
Most commonly, imbalances in supply and demand occur during the initiation period of breastfeeding, during infant growth spurts and after 6 months of lactation. During the first 1–3 days post partum, most women do not experience breast fullness or sensation of letdown when nursing. This leads to the understandable concern that the baby is not receiving nourishment and needs

supplementation with bottle feeding. Bottle feeding at this time interferes with establishment of breastfeeding by inducing nipple confusion and by decreasing suckling time at the breast. Women should be reassured that as long as the baby is nursing every 2–3 hours and five or six wet diapers are noted each day, supplementation with bottle feeding is not necessary. If supplementation is indicated, it should occur after at least 10–15 minutes of suckling efforts at the breast.

After about 3 days, normal breast fullness occurs which can progress to engorgement. Proper therapy for engorgement includes frequent nursing, gentle breast massage during nursing, and attention to proper latch-on technique. Acetaminophen or ibuprofen may be used if desired. An overabundant milk supply may be noted in the first 2 months, before the breasts soften and enlarge to contain milk production.

The first growth spurt usually occurs at about 2–3 weeks of age, and during this time milk production lags behind the infant's demand for a few days. During this time, babies will want to nurse more frequently and are generally more irritable. More frequent nursing is indicated during times of growth spurts. Another growth spurt usually occurs at about 6 weeks of age. Knowing when these normal appetite spurts occur can reassure the mother that there is nothing wrong with her milk supply and that supplementary feedings are not indicated. At about 6 months, several things occur in association with a growth spurt that may impact the continuation of breastfeeding. Babies become very distractible when nursing and may not suckle well. Their gums may be sore due to impending eruption of the first teeth. There is increased interest in solid foods and a developing infant independence. At the same time, menstruation cycles usually re-establish themselves at about 6 months. All these factors decrease milk supply at a time when demand increases. Some mothers maintain breastfeeding in the face of these challenges while others decide to use this time to transition to weaning.

Refusal to nurse
Occasionally, babies who have initiated breastfeeding will develop a refusal to nurse. Physical discomfort and maternal dietary intake are frequently found to be the cause of a sudden refusal to continue feeding. Ear infections and thrush often cause pain during feeding and may lead to the baby pulling away. A pediatrician should evaluate ear infections. Oral candida infections (thrush), however, are easily identified. The infant will have a thick whitish coating of the tongue and may also have a bright red diaper rash. Burning pain and redness of the nipples is also common in thrush infections.

Babies who are colicky may be reacting either to changes in the mother's diet or to substances applied to the breast.

Creams, lotions and perfumes should not be applied to the areola or the breast. If it is suspected that the infant is responding to maternal dietary changes, the mother should keep a dietary log. The culprit spice or food is usually ingested 3–6 hours before the breastfeeding event that initiates the infant's discomfort. Common culprits include the theobromides found in chocolate, citrus, green vegetables, and onions. Garlic, on the other hand, has been reported to please most infants' taste buds. If an infant is getting supplemental bottle feedings based on cow's milk, consider switching to a soy-based formula or eliminating maternal dairy intake.

Engorgement and mastitis

Engorgement may affect both breasts globally or may be limited to one area of milk stasis. Overall engorgement is most common during the first few weeks of breastfeeding and usually dissipates as the breast enlarges to more efficiently store the milk produced. Engorgement may progress to milk stasis or "plugged ducts." Milk stasis is the result of incomplete emptying of one part of the breast. Treatment of milk stasis includes frequent breastfeeding with initiation of each breastfeeding event on the affected side, application of moist heat, and gentle massage of the area during breastfeeding to relieve the obstruction and allow complete drainage. If these treatment measures do not result in significant improvement in 24 hours, or if the mother develops a fever, she should be seen by her physician and evaluated for the presence of mastitis.

Mastitis may be of epidemic or nonepidemic type. The epidemic type, associated with *Staphylococcus aureus* infections in hospital nurseries, has declined as the average length of postpartum stay has declined. The nonepidemic type represents a progression of disease from milk stasis to painful inflammation, erythema, and edema. Approximately 10% of nursing women will develop mastitis. When the physician is evaluating a patient for mastitis, a breastfeeding history should be obtained. Frequently, there will be a history of missed or irregular feedings, cracked nipples on the affected side, or one-sided breastfeeding. Physical examination typically reveals a firm, tender mass and a unilateral V-shaped area of erythema. Milk stasis can be differentiated from mastitis by culture and leukocyte count in expressed milk.

If a woman has already unsuccessfully applied the measures listed above to relieve engorgement, then antibiotics and antipyretics should be added. Optimal oral antibiotic therapy is best provided using penicillin, amoxicillin or a synthetic penicillin such as dicloxacillin. Abscesses should be drained when identified and intravenous antibiotics administered. Women with mastitis should not be advised to stop breastfeeding, as this will increase the engorgement and risk for abscess formation. Women taking these antibiotics do not need to withhold their milk from their infants.

Returning to work

Few mothers returning to work are aware of the supports available to them to continue breastfeeding while working. Others are hesitant to ask their employer about flexitime, use of childcare facilities at work or part-time employment. Fortunately, many national companies have recognized that it is to their ultimate benefit to retain a trained employee by offering such arrangements. If bringing the baby to the workplace is not possible, the use of a breast pump will ensure continued feeding. Portable breast pumps may be purchased or rented. Choices include manual pumps, hand-operated battery pumps, and fully electric models. Electric pumps are more expensive to buy or rent but are also more efficient in the extraction of breast milk. Women using electric pumps require less pumping time, are better able to maintain an adequate milk supply, and have fewer problems with nipple soreness. Women who wish to continue breastfeeding after returning to work should be informed that many rental services also offer information and advice about the process of storing milk and pumping in the workplace.

Use of medications during breastfeeding

The American Academy of Pediatrics has published a list of drugs considered compatible with breastfeeding. Drugs that are absolutely contraindicated during breastfeeding are bromocriptine, ergotamine, lithium, methotrexate, cyclophosphamide, ciclosporin, doxorubicin, and phenindione, as well as "street drugs." All radiopharmaceuticals require temporary cessation of breastfeeding until cleared from breast milk. Mothers undergoing diagnostic studies using radiopharmaceuticals should be encouraged to pump a supply of breast milk prior to the study. After the study, pumping should continue to maintain milk supply but the milk should be discarded until radioactivity excretion times have passed. Drugs that should be used with extreme caution include aspirin and phenobarbital. The drugs classified as anxiolytics, antidepressants, and antipsychotics are in general considered to be of some concern. Anti-infectives are generally considered compatible with breastfeeding, although mothers taking chloramphenicol or metronidazole should temporarily cease breastfeeding.

The use of angiotensin-converting enzyme inhibitors or warfarin is contraindicated during pregnancy. However, they are not considered to be contraindicated for use during breastfeeding. There may be an increased risk of development of jaundice in the newborn, so it is prudent to check with the pediatrician in individual cases. If, for example, a premature infant is receiving treatment for hyperbilirubinemia, a mother taking these drugs should discard her milk until the neonate has recovered.

Medical contraindications to breastfeeding

Few medical conditions preclude breastfeeding. An absolute contraindication is the presence of congenital galactosemia in the newborn. Preterm delivery, multiple births or the birth of a baby with cleft palate do not preclude breastfeeding. Women with diabetes should be encouraged to breastfeed, as it may prolong the "honeymoon" period during which insulin requirements are low. Special care should be taken to prevent sore nipples, and surveillance for yeast infections or mastitis should be vigilant. The nursing mother with diabetes should plan to see her doctor frequently when weaning her infant. Thyroid disease should not prevent breastfeeding, nor should hypertension. Women with seizure disorders, unless being treated with phenobarbital, can breastfeed. All women taking medications should be advised to breastfeed prior to ingesting their medication, as this will limit the baby's exposure to peak drug levels.

Special concern exists for transmission of maternal diseases to the neonate, whose immune system remains immature at birth. Women with herpes infections may develop active lesions following delivery. The lesion should be covered when the baby is in contact with the mother, and strict handwashing guidelines adhered to. Unless the lesion is on the nipple or areola, breastfeeding does not need to be interrupted. Hepatitis B is not a contraindication to breastfeeding, as long as the infant receives vaccination and an immunoglobins preparation. Hepatitis A and C infections are currently considered compatible with breastfeeding by both the ACOG and the Centers for Disease Control. In the United States, women with HIV should be advised not to breastfeed due to the risk of transmission. This contraindication should be considered relative in the setting of developing countries where access to adequate nutrition and clean water is limited. HTLV types I and II should also be considered contraindications to breastfeeding. Lastly, women with active tuberculosis should not breastfeed or even room in with their infant until they have received at least 2–3 weeks of adequate treatment.

Prior breast surgery

Women with a history of breast surgery can usually breastfeed. When examining a patient and evaluating her ability to breastfeed, the most important factor is whether or not the milk ducts have been severed. A scar along the circumference of the areola usually indicates that the milk ducts have been surgically cut in the past. Simple breast biopsies rarely involve the milk ducts, nor do breast augmentation procedures commonly disturb the areola. Women who have undergone breast reduction surgery can safely attempt to breastfeed. If an adequate breast milk supply cannot be provided, supplementation with formula can allow breastfeeding to continue.

Women with flat or inverted nipples can also attempt to breastfeed. An examination of the breast in the third trimester will identify the presence of inverted nipples. The use of breast shells placed in the nursing bra will assist in maintaining the nipple in an everted position. The application of ice to the nipple just before breastfeeding will also cause the nipple to become erect and assist in easy latch-on. Women with inverted nipples should not try to make the nipple stand out by pinching, as this just causes further inversion. Instead, the areola should be grasped between thumb and forefingers and pressure applied to the chest wall.

Weaning

Often, the choice to wean an infant is influenced by factors other than maternal or infant readiness. The need to return to work, cultural traditions and difficulties in maintaining an adequate milk supply may be paramount. Assuming that a woman has sufficient resources to nurse for as long as she wishes, it should be noted that infants infrequently choose to wean themselves before 1 and 2 years of age. However, there are developmental events occurring at 7–12 months that distract the infant from breastfeeding. The period of increasing independence is associated with less interest in breastfeeding, and many women choose this time to wean. Weaning should be gradual, substituting a supplemental feeding and extra attention for a session of breastfeeding. Slowly, breastfeeding can decrease in frequency until milk production ceases. If weaning occurs suddenly, there is an increased incidence of milk stasis and mastitis. Once a woman has decided to wean her infant, she should be encouraged not to reverse the decision, as this will make later weaning more difficult and also increase the risk for mastitis. When weaning occurs suddenly, breast binders, ice and analgesics usually provide relief from engorgement within 3–5 days.

Medical suppression of lactation is rarely indicated. Estrogenic (diethylstilbestrol) and estrogenic/androgenic (Deladumone) preparations have been used in the past. Their use raises concerns of possible increased risk for thrombotic complications, although these data come mainly from retrospective studies. Uterine subinvolution may occur more frequently with the use of estrogenic-only regimens. When compared to breast binding alone, hormonal preparations provide more relief in the early postpartum period, but about half of patients experience rebound engorgement after discharge. Estrogenic compounds must be given prior to the initiation of breastfeeding in order to be effective. Bromocriptine has also been used to suppress lactation and is effective if given after breastfeeding has begun. However, about half of patients experience rebound lactation requiring an additional course of therapy. Side effects, including hypotension, headache, gastrointestinal disorders and rash, occur in at least 25% of women. The frequency and potential severity of the side-effects led the Food and Drug Administration to remove lactation suppression from the list of diagnoses for which bromocriptine may be administered.

Suggested reading

American Academy of Pediatrics. Policy statement. *Pediatrics* 2005; 115: 496–506.

Auerbach KG. Breastfeeding fallacies: their relationship to understanding lactation. *Birth* 1990; 17: 44–49.

Ball TM, Bennett DM. The economic impact of breast feeding. *Pediatr Clin North Am* 2001; 48(1): 253–262.

Briggs GG, Freeman RK, Yaffe SJ. *Drugs in pregnancy and lactation: a reference guide to fetal and neonatal risk,* 5th edn. Baltimore, MD: Lippincott, Williams and Wilkins, 1998.

Hager WD. Puerperal mastitis. *Contemp Obstet Gynecol* 1998; 43: 27–33.

Hale RW. Breastfeeding: maternal and infant aspects. *ACOG Clin Rev* 2008; 12(1): 1S–16S.

Huggins K. The reward period: from two to six months. In: *The nursing mother's companion,* 3rd edn. Boston, MA: Harvard Common Press, 1995.

Schwartz DJ, Evans PC, Garcia LR, *et al.* A clinical study of lactation suppression. *Obstet Gynecol* 1973; 42: 599–606.

Chapter 21
Heart Disease in Pregnancy

Uri Elkayam and T. Murphy Goodwin
Department of Medicine and Obstetrics and Gynecology, Keck School of Medicine, University of Southern California, CA, USA

Introduction

Maternal heart disease complicates the management of about 1% of pregnancies. While few obstetrician-gynecologists will be called upon to manage heart disease during pregnancy, the diagnostic work-up is often initiated because of findings elicited by the obstetrician. This chapter will describe an approach to the common complaints of pregnancy that may be indicative of cardiac disease. The initial investigations as well as issues related to counseling to assess the risks of pregnancy will be discussed.

Cardiovascular changes in pregnancy

The maternal heart rate increases by 10–15 beats per minute, from 70 to 85 beats per minute. In addition to the increase in heart rate, there is an increase in the occurrence of arrhythmias, which are usually benign. Total blood volume increases by 40–50% above pre-pregnancy values. The plasma volume expands proportionately more than the increase in red blood cell mass, accounting for the physiologically lower hematocrit during pregnancy. The maximum increase in plasma volume occurs between 20 and 30 weeks' gestation, a time of increased risk for mothers with heart disease sensitive to volume overload. By 30 weeks' gestation, the cardiac output will be 30–50% higher than before pregnancy. Seventeen percent of the cardiac output goes to the uterus.

Maternal body position, labor and anesthesia can affect the cardiovascular status. Prolonged standing causes venous pooling and decreases venous return to the heart, which in turn decreases cardiac output and may provoke syncope. Supine hypotension may occur when the gravid uterus compresses the vena cava and impairs venous return to the heart, causing a fall in cardiac output and blood pressure.

Pain from uterine contractions causes maternal tachycardia, which may have unfavorable hemodynamic effects because it reduces the diastolic filling time. Effective analgesia will blunt this effect. For nearly all types of cardiac disease, epidural anesthesia is preferred for either vaginal or cesarean deliveries. However, it must be administered with care to avoid hypotension. The narcotic epidural or combined narcotic epidural and spinal may be used in patients who are very sensitive to changes in systemic resistance.

During the second stage of labor, the maternal Valsalva maneuver from bearing-down efforts decreases venous blood return to the heart because it increases intrathoracic pressure. There is a simultaneous increase in peripheral resistance as well but because of the decreased cardiac output, the blood pressure does not increase. When the straining is stopped, there is a rapid increase in cardiac output and blood pressure. The consequences of the Valsalva maneuver may affect cardiac conditions that are sensitive to decreased filling pressure or increased systemic resistance.

In the immediate postpartum period there is an abrupt increase in cardiac output by 60%. This is due to re-entry of blood, which was previously diverted to the uterus or pooled in the partially obstructed venous circulation of the lower extremities, into the central circulation. Stroke volume is increased, and there is a reflexive fall of heart rate.

The normal physiologic changes associated with pregnancy are well tolerated by women with normal hearts. Patients with cardiac disease who are unable to tolerate these changes may decompensate and develop congestive heart failure.

Approach to common complaints possibly representing cardiac disease

Normal pregnant women frequently have symptoms and signs that could be interpreted as indicative of heart

Management of Common Problems in Obstetrics and Gynecology, 5th edition. Edited by T.M. Goodwin, M.N. Montoro, L. Muderspach, R. Paulson and S. Roy. © 2010 Blackwell Publishing Ltd.

disease in the nonpregnant state. Dyspnea occurs in up to 60% of pregnant women. It is usually described as "a sense of not being able to breathe quite deeply enough to get all the air one needs." Increased fatigue is a common complaint, especially during the first and last trimesters. Lower-extremity edema is commonly seen in the third trimester.

Apart from a history of known cardiac disease, the most common reasons for cardiac evaluation in our experience are heart murmur, palpitations, syncope, and chest pain. Most women with these complaints are healthy. Certain findings, however, deserve indepth evaluation and are listed in Box 21.1.

When heart disease is suspected, an ECG is done and, in almost all cases, an echocardiogram as well. Echocardiography is the mainstay of diagnosing anatomic abnormalities, intra- and extracardiac shunts, and can also estimate valve orifice size. A chest radiograph (shielding the uterus from the radiation) and at times a baseline arterial oxygen saturation determination are appropriate. The evaluation of arrhythmias may be done with a 24-hour Holter monitor or with an event monitor.

The New York Heart Association classification continues to be useful for management and prognosis.
- Class I   Asymptomatic
- Class II   Symptoms with greater than normal activity
- Class III Symptoms with normal activity
- Class IV   Symptoms at rest

Because this functional classification system relies heavily on subjective findings, it is important to use additional diagnostic tools to obtain objective information about the anatomic and physiologic abnormalities. Box 21.2 combines structural and anatomic factors.

Preconception counseling and antepartum screening

Congenital heart disease occurs in approximately 8 per 1000 livebirths. As many as 16% of women with a major heart defect will also have a fetus with a heart defect. Thus, all women with a congenital heart defect should undergo fetal echocardiography at 18–20 weeks' gestation.

Women with cyanotic congenital heart disease have increased rates of spontaneous abortion, preterm delivery, and small for gestational age infants. The risk of worsening cardiac status or congestive heart failure during pregnancy is 2–3 times greater for women with cyanosis compared to acyanotic patients. Surgical correction, if possible prior to pregnancy, will improve obstetric outcome. Fifteen percent of patients with cardiac disease may develop pregnancy-induced or associated hypertension, compared to 5% in the general obstetric population.

Certain patients have a very high (10–50%) risk of death if pregnancy is attempted. This group includes patients with severe pulmonary hypertension due to

---

Box 21.1 Clinical cardiovascular findings that merit further evaluation

Symptoms
Dyspnea that limits activity
Progressive orthopnea or paroxysmal nocturnal dyspnea
Syncope with exertion
Palpitations
Chest pain
Hemoptysis

Signs
Pulse >100 or <60 beats/min
Arrhythmia
Cyanosis or clubbing
Diastolic murmur
Systolic murmur:
- grade III/VI
- grade II, with radiation to axilla or carotid
- associated with abnormal S2
- maximum intensity at other than the 2nd left intercostal space

---

Box 21.2 Maternal risk of pregnancy according to anatomic findings and symptoms

Group 1: Slightly increased risk
Mild valvular stenosis
    Moderate valvular regurgitation with normal chamber size and normal blood pressure
    NYHA class I–II

Group 2: Moderately increased risk
Moderate valvular stenosis
    Valve regurgitation with enlarged chamber size
    Prosthetic heart valve with normal hemodynamic function
    NYHA class II

Group 3: Considerably increased risk
Severe valvular stenosis or regurgitation
    Atrial fibrillation
    Prosthetic heart valve with compensated heart failure
    NYHA class II

Group 4: Extremely high risk
Congestive heart failure unresponsive to treatment
    Pulmonary arterial hypertension
    Eisenmenger's syndrome
    Marfan's syndrome with incompetent valve or aortic root dilation
    Symptoms with less than usual activity or at rest (NYHA class III or IV) with treatment

increased pulmonary vascular resistance (Eisenmenger's syndrome, idiopathic pulmonary arterial hypertension, collagen vascular disease, etc.), Marfan's syndrome with evidence of valvular incompetence or a dilated aortic root, and peripartum cardiomyopathy with persistent cardiac dysfunction.

Antepartum management

A team including an obstetrician and cardiologist should carry out antepartum care of the pregnant cardiac patient. Consultation with a geneticist if the disease is inheritable, a fetal echocardiographer, and a nutritionist is often appropriate. Patients with few symptoms and a low-risk lesion (group 1 or 2, Box 21.2) may be seen every 2–4 weeks until 24 weeks, then 1–2 weeks thereafter. Patients with significant symptoms or a moderate-risk lesion (group 3) should be seen every 1–2 weeks. Patients with symptoms at rest (group 4) may require hospitalization for most of the pregnancy. Antepartum fetal testing is generally reserved for group 3 or 4 patients.

Knowledge of the normal changes of pregnancy and labor described above allows the physician to anticipate when and how such changes will affect a given lesion or condition. At each visit, weight gain, heart rate, blood pressure, and pulse pressure are carefully noted. A pulse rate greater than 100 beats per minute or rapid weight gain are often signs of impending heart failure. Pregnant patients with decompensated congestive failure should be hospitalized. Bedrest will reduce the demand for increased cardiac output by limiting oxygen consumption. In patients whose status is tenuous, fetal growth and well-being may be monitored by serial ultrasound examinations and antepartum surveillance.

Rheumatic heart disease

Patients with rheumatic heart disease should receive prophylaxis against recurrent group A β-hemolytic streptococcal infection which causes initial and recurrent attacks of rheumatic fever. The regimen is benzathine penicillin G 1.2 million units intramuscularly given monthly. Alternative regimens include potassium penicillin V 125–250 mg orally twice daily or, for the penicillin-allergic patient, sulfadiazine 1 g daily. The American Heart Association recommends that this regimen be continued until age 40 or until regular contact with children ceases.

Anticoagulation and drug therapy

It is our practice to treat pregnant patients who require anticoagulation for mechanical valves or chronic atrial fibrillation with subcutaneous unfractionated or low molecular weight heparin at 12-hour intervals, rather than with warfarin. The degree of anticoagulation required in these women is intense (activated partial thromboplastin time (aPTT) 2.5 times normal or anti-factor Xa level in the upper therapeutic range). Rarely, warfarin may have to be considered, after the first trimester, and continued until about 35–36 weeks when it should be stopped and heparin resumed. These patients are advised to withhold heparin when labor begins to avoid being anticoagulated during labor (see Chapter 27). Digoxin or β-adrenergic blockers such as metoprolol may be used to control the rapid ventricular response to atrial fibrillation. Digoxin is also used for its positive inotropic effect in chronic congestive heart failure. The preferred agent for afterload reduction is hydralazine, as angiotensin-converting enzyme (ACE) inhibitors are contraindicated during pregnancy.

Management of labor

Patients in functional class I, II or compensated III may await the onset of spontaneous labor at term. Common maternal reasons for preterm delivery include pre-eclampsia or cardiac decompensation. Fetal indications for early delivery include growth retardation or abnormal fetal testing.

Intrapartum management of the cardiac patient is challenging. A team including an obstetrician, an anesthesiologist, and a critical care nurse should be available. The patient should labor in the lateral recumbent position if the cardiac output seems to be compromised. Pain relief is best obtained with epidural anesthesia. Delivery should be planned at a hospital where an anesthetist skilled in this technique is available. If the patient has been recently anticoagulated, aPTT or anti-factor Xa levels should be determined before inserting an epidural catheter.

Endocarditis prophylaxis is given, as needed, according to prescribed regimens (Boxes 21.3, 21.4). It is our practice *not* to assume that a delivery will be "uncomplicated" and that endocarditis prophylaxis be given to all at-risk patients. This opinion is due to the frequent need for instrumental delivery in cardiac patients, and to a not negligible incidence of endometritis with bacteremia after cesarean and vaginal deliveries.

If the mother has a condition sensitive to the changes of the Valsalva maneuver, the second stage of labor should be shortened, when possible, by an instrument-assisted delivery. The Sims position is desirable for spontaneous vaginal delivery. The lithotomy position is usually required for an instrument-assisted delivery, although the uterus should be displaced to the left side. Cesarean delivery is reserved for obstetric indications or cardiac decompensation.

Box 21.3 Cardiac conditions and endocarditis prophylaxis

Endocarditis prophylaxis recommended
High risk – prosthetic cardiac valves, previous bacterial endocarditis, complex cyanotic congenital heart disease
   Moderate risk – most other congenital cardiac malformations, rheumatic and other acquired valvular dysfunction (even after valvular surgery), hypertrophic cardiomyopathy, mitral valve prolapse with valvular regurgitation or thickened leaflets

Endocarditis prophylaxis not recommended
Isolated secundum atrial septal defect
   Surgical repair without residual beyond 6 months of secundum atrial septal defect, ventricular septal defect or patent ductus arteriosus
      Previous coronary artery bypass graft surgery
      Mitral valve prolapse without valvular regurgitation
      Physiologic, functional or innocent heart murmurs
      Previous Kawasaki's disease without valvular dysfunction
      Previous rheumatic fever without valvular dysfunction
      Cardiac pacemakers and implanted defibrillators

Box 21.4 Regimens for genitourinary/ gastrointestinal procedures

Although the American Heart Association recommendations apply only to high-risk patients for vaginal delivery or uninfected cesarean, it has been our practice to apply them to all patients at risk since chorio-amnionitis is common and unpredictable.

High and moderate risk
Ampicillin 2.0 g IV 30 min before procedure

Ampicillin/amoxicillin/penicillin-allergic patient regimen
Vancomycin 1.0 g IV over 1–2h, to be completed within 30 min of starting the procedure

Immediately post partum, cardiac output increases. Patients with volume-sensitive conditions such as mitral stenosis may develop pulmonary edema at this time. This can be avoided with careful monitoring of the patient's fluid status by means of a pulmonary artery (Swan–Ganz) catheter during labor.

Contraception in heart disease

Patients desiring sterilization and who are well compensated can be considered for postpartum tubal ligation. In the poorly compensated patient, it is best to delay sterilization until the cardiovascular system has returned to a normal status, at least until 6 weeks post partum. Many cardiac patients will not tolerate the pneumoperitoneum

needed for laparoscopic tubal ligation and will require a laparotomy under epidural anesthesia.

Women with valvular heart disease or congestive heart failure are at increased risk for thromboembolic events and they should not be prescribed estrogen-containing contraceptives unless they are already anti-coagulated. Injectable or implanted progestins are alternatives for these patients. An intrauterine device can be considered for patients who are not at risk of bacterial endocarditis.

Suggested reading

Elkayam U, Bitar F. Valvular heart disease and pregnancy: part I: native valves. *J Am Coll Cardiol* 2005; 46: 223–230.

Elkayam U, Bitar F. Valvular heart disease and pregnancy: part II: prosthetic valves. *J Am Coll Cardiol* 2005; 46: 403–410.

Elkayam U, Gleicher N. *Cardiac problems in pregnancy: diagnosis and management of maternal and fetal disease,* 3rd edn. New York: Alan R. Liss, 1998.

Goland S, Elkayam U. Cardiovascular problems in pregnant women with Marfan's syndrome. *Circulation* 2009; 119: 619–623.

Hameed A, Karaalp IS, Padmini PP, *et al.* The effect of valvular heart disease on maternal and fetal outcome of pregnancy. *J Am Coll Cardiol* 2001; 37: 893–899.

Chapter 22
Asthma during Pregnancy

Martin N. Montoro
Department of Medicine and Obstetrics and Gynecology, Keck School of Medicine, University of Southern California, CA, USA

Introduction

Asthma is the most common and potentially serious respiratory illness encountered during pregnancy. Inflammation of the bronchial mucosa is currently thought to play a dominant role in the pathogenesis of increased bronchial airway obstruction and hyper-responsiveness. In the definition of asthma provided by the National Asthma Education Program, the three key components are: reversible airway obstruction, airway inflammation, and increased airway responsiveness to a variety of stimuli.

Frequency

Asthma is not only the most common respiratory illness seen in pregnant women but also one of the most common medical illnesses encountered during pregnancy. The most recent estimates from national health surveys give an asthma prevalence of 3.7–8.4% in pregnant women and women of childbearing age in the United States. During the last decade a 29% higher worldwide prevalence has been seen, as well as a threefold increase in emergency room visits and hospital admissions. Also, a 31% higher mortality has been reported which, unfortunately, includes many young people. The increased prevalence involves urban more commonly than rural populations, with industrial pollution being quoted as a major factor. However, there are unexplained marked geographic variations possibly related to differences in genetic susceptibility.

Genetic predisposition plays a role as well, although no clear genetic pattern has yet been described. There is great interest in the population of the small island of Tristan da Cunha in the southern Atlantic Ocean. These people are thousands of miles from the stress and pollution of urban life but half of the population suffers from asthma. Two of the original settlers had asthma, and the gene or genes responsible for asthma susceptibility were passed down through the inbred generations. Scientists working on the human genome have collected samples from most of the island's residents for clues to the genetic basis of asthma.

Effect of asthma on reproduction and pregnancy

Fertility
There is no evidence that fertility rates of women with asthma, eczema or hay fever are lower than those of women in the general population.

Menstrual cycle
The severity of asthma may show variations during the menstrual cycle, with premenstrual worsening being more common. It is speculated that estrogen and progesterone may modulate the smooth muscle adrenergic response to catecholamines.

Pregnancy
Pregnancy has not been observed to have a consistent effect on asthma, either worsening or improvement. This has led to the belief that the variability of its course during gestation may be related to the natural history of the disease rather than to the influence of pregnancy. Subsequent responses, however, tend to be similar to what happened during the first pregnancy. No particular trimester has been associated with worsening or improvement.

Nevertheless, some of the changes, either worsening or improvement, may actually be related to what some women do with their medications, without necessarily informing their doctors, when they realize they are pregnant. Some believe that the medications may be harmful to the fetus and stop taking them and therefore their asthma will get worse. These patients will be included in the group

Management of Common Problems in Obstetrics and Gynecology,
5th edition. Edited by T.M. Goodwin, M.N. Montoro,
L. Muderspach, R. Paulson and S. Roy. © 2010 Blackwell
Publishing Ltd.

that "gets worse during pregnancy." Others become more compliant when they realize that most medications are safe and that well-controlled asthma will provide better oxygen delivery to the fetus. These patients will be included in the group that "experienced improvement" during pregnancy.

Potential maternal complications include hyperemesis gravidarum, pre-eclampsia, vaginal hemorrhage, placental abruption, more complicated labors, higher rate of cesarean deliveries and depression. In addition, women with asthma account for up to 60% of pneumonia cases reported during pregnancy.

Possible fetal complications may include increased perinatal mortality, intrauterine growth retardation, preterm birth, low birthweight, and neonatal hypoxia. Studies show that women with severe asthma are at the highest risk, but when asthma is properly controlled there is little or no increased risk to mother or fetus. Patients should be made aware that most women with asthma can be managed effectively.

Diagnosis and classification

The diagnosis of asthma during pregnancy is usually not difficult provided that an adequate history and physical examination are performed. Most patients will have been diagnosed prior to pregnancy and will already be on some form of therapy. In a few, the diagnosis may not be obvious and a more detailed evaluation is needed. Pulmonary function studies are valuable and important to confirm the diagnosis. Occasionally, bronchospasm may be caused by a disease process other than asthma, such as acute left ventricular heart failure ("cardiac asthma"), pulmonary embolism, chronic bronchitis, carcinoid tumors, upper airway obstruction (e.g. laryngeal edema) or foreign bodies.

Common triggers of asthma include upper respiratory infections (more frequently viral), β-blockers, aspirin and nonsteroidal anti-inflammatory agents, sulfites and other food preservatives, allergens (pollen, animal dander, etc.), smoking, gastric reflux, certain environmental factors (e.g. occupational asthma), and exercise or hyperventilation from other causes. Asthma is classified as mild, moderate or severe for diagnostic and therapeutic considerations (Tables 22.1, 22.2).

Treatment

The goals of therapy are directed toward the maintenance of normal or near normal pulmonary function, control of symptoms, maintenance of normal levels of activity, prevention of exacerbations and avoidance of medication side effects in order to give birth to a healthy baby. This can only be achieved if adequate oxygenation of the fetus is maintained.

Table 22.1 Types of asthma

Allergic (one-third of patients)	Idiosyncratic (two-thirds of patients)
Positive family history of asthma	Negative family history
Past history of allergies[a]	No history of allergies[a]
Elevated serum IgE	Normal serum IgE
Positive provocative tests	Negative provocative tests

[a] Rhinitis, urticaria, eczema.
Note: inhalation of an allergen leads to bronchospasm; intradermal injection of an allergen causes a wheal.

Table 22.2 Severity of asthma

	Mild	Moderate	Severe
Wheezing	Exp	Insp+Exp	Insp only
Dyspnea	+	++	Profound
Breath sounds	Nl	Nl	Decreased
Accessory muscle use	–	–	+
Costal Retraction	–	–	+
Fatigue	–	–	+
Insp/Exp ratio*	<1/3	>1/3	>1/3
Tachycardia	–	+	>120 beats/min
Pulsus paradoxus	–	–	>18 mmHg
FEV1	>70%	<70% but >50%	<50%

* Normals 1/2.
Abbreviations: Exp: Expiratory breath. Insp: Inspiratory breath.
Nl: Normal. FEV1: Forced expiratory volume in 1 second.

Patient education is an extremely important aspect of the treatment of patients with asthma. Pregnant women are usually very receptive, thus providing an excellent opportunity for education in asthma management skills that they can continue to use after delivery.

However, there is a perception among a large segment of the lay population that all medications taken during pregnancy are harmful. Nevertheless, the risk of uncontrolled asthma is far greater, with potential maternal morbidity and hypoxemia in the fetus. Moreover, some women may have minimal clinical symptoms but their pulmonary function is abnormal enough to compromise fetal oxygenation. During an acute asthma attack, maternal oxygenation must be carefully monitored. A decrease in maternal PO_2, particularly to below 60 mmHg, may result in marked fetal hypoxia. In addition, maternal hyperventilation and hypocarbia may result in decreased uterine blood flow. Fetal distress may occur even in the absence of maternal hypotension or hypoxia because compensatory mechanisms tend to maintain systemic arterial pressure and oxygenation in vital maternal organs at the expense of uterine blood flow. Fetal monitoring is essential during episodes of acute asthma exacerbation.

Objective measurements of lung function are preferable because the patient's perception and the clinical signs of asthma severity are frequently inaccurate. Some patients may have minimal symptoms but their pulmonary function can be impaired enough to cause fetal hypoxia. Measuring the peak expiratory flow rate (PEFR) correlates well with the forced air expired in 1 second after a maximal inspiration (FEV1) and can be done with inexpensive, portable peak flow meters. They can be used at home to assess the course of asthma throughout the day, detect signs of early deterioration even before symptoms appear, and evaluate the response to therapy. In the hospital or at the office, a spirometer can be used for diagnosis or to more fully evaluate the severity of asthma.

Diet

Evidence is accumulating about the importance of some dietary factors in pregnant women with asthma and other allergic disorders. In 1998 the United Kingdom government recommended that women with a history of asthma, hay fever or eczema should avoid peanuts or products containing peanuts during pregnancy and breastfeeding because of the belief that allergy to peanuts may develop *in utero*. However, whether this advice has been beneficial is still uncertain. Adequate maternal intakes of fish (probably due to omega-3 content), apples, vitamin E, zinc and vitamin D have all been reported to be protective against the development of asthma and atopy in the offspring.

Exercise

Pregnant women with asthma should be able to continue their regular activities. Those on adequate treatment should be controlled well enough so that an attack is not provoked by exercise. For other women, exercise-induced asthma may be prevented by the inhalation of a β2-agonist or cromolyn sodium within an hour of beginning exercise. The beneficial effect lasts several hours.

Other factors

Avoidance of asthma triggers (allergens and irritants) is an important component of therapy. It may be necessary to remove pets, encase mattresses and pillows in airtight covers, wash bedding carefully, keep humidity below 50%, avoid vacuuming (or at least wear a mask), use air conditioning and air filters, and avoid outdoor activities when allergen concentration and air pollution are high. Other irritants should be avoided as well, particularly tobacco smoke. Other potential triggers to be avoided include strong odors, air pollutants, food additives, aspirin, and β-blockers.

Immunotherapy has been shown to prevent allergic inflammation and reduce symptoms provoked by allergen exposure. The concern is that if anaphylaxis occurs, it may induce uterine contractions with potential fetal morbidity and mortality. The current advice is that immunotherapy should not be started *de novo* during pregnancy and that ongoing immunotherapy may be continued but without further increasing the dose. However, there are no specific studies in pregnant women on this topic.

Influenza vaccine is strongly recommended for patients with asthma every year and there is no risk to mother or fetus because it is based on a killed virus. Patients with moderate and severe asthma should also receive the pneumococcal vaccine but preferably prior to becoming pregnant.

Treating associated conditions such as rhinitis and sinusitis is an important aspect of therapy because both are capable of exacerbating co-existing asthma. For rhinitis, environmental control to reduce antigen exposure is important. If not sufficient, intranasal cromolyn may be used followed by antihistamines (tripelennamine or chlorpheniramine) if necessary. Intranasal corticosteroids are preferred by others. For sinusitis, after an accurate diagnosis, amoxicillin is the initial antibiotic of choice and erythromycin for those allergic to penicillin. Other antibiotics may be needed depending on the infective micro-organism. Oxymethazoline (nose spray or drops) and pseudoephedrine may be helpful adjunctive, symptomatic therapy. For the vasomotor rhinitis of pregnancy, a buffered saline nose spray may be helpful. Exercise, within the limitations of pregnancy, may help because it induces physiologic nasal vasoconstriction. If additional treatment is needed, pseudoephedrine is recommended.

Avoiding exposure to infections *in utero* and therefore the need to use antibiotics (more than two courses) also decreases the incidence of asthma and other allergic diseases in the offspring.

Pharmacologic therapy

Inhaled β2-agonists

Patients with mild asthma may be controlled with inhaled β2-agonist bronchodilators alone. These are patients who experience symptoms (wheezing, coughing, difficulty breathing) less than twice a week, and nocturnal wheezing and cough less than twice a month; they are free of symptoms in between episodes. The usual dosage is two puffs every 6 hours as needed. A long-acting oral β2-agonist may be given, once daily in the evening, to patients who have symptoms primarily at night. However, patients must be made aware that a need for medication on a daily basis, or even more often than three times per week, indicates more severe asthma and the need for additional treatment. Experience in humans is extensive and there is no evidence of harm to the fetus from either systemic or inhaled use of short-acting β2-agonists. Albuterol has the most data available on safety during pregnancy.

However, the data for long-acting β2-agonists (LABA) are limited although they are thought to be safe for the fetus when used by inhalation. In addition, their general safety has been questioned following reports of increased asthma mortality with LABA use, and strong warnings recommended if used alone. They are believed to be safer when used in combination with an inhaled corticosteroid. Nevertheless, more recent reviews with large patient populations have not been conclusive. In these reports there is no specific mention of risks in pregnant women. LABA should not be used intravenously because of adverse effects observed in animal studies. The two most commonly used are salmeterol and formoterol.

Anti-inflammatory medication

Daily anti-inflammatory medication is recommended for patients with moderate asthma in order to suppress and/or prevent airway inflammation. These medications help to decrease airway responsiveness as well. Inhaled corticosteroids decrease the need for systemic steroids. They have become a very important part of the treatment because airway inflammation plays a critical role in the pathogenesis of asthma. Their use is now recommended at a much earlier stage in treatment. They provide effective control with minimal side effects if the recommended guidelines are followed. Full therapeutic benefits may not be seen for 2–4 weeks after the initiation of therapy. The dosage is 2–4 puffs 2–4 times daily when inhaled or two sprays in each nostril, twice daily, when used intranasally for allergic rhinitis. The use of a spacer, when inhaled, is strongly recommended in order to reduce side effects, which may include oropharyngeal candidiasis, dysphonia, and hoarseness. The spacer will also improve respiratory tract penetration and reduce the possibility of systemic steroid effects. Inhaled corticosteroids, particularly budesonide and beclometasone, have not been associated with fetal anomalies in human studies.

Cromolyn sodium has an anti-inflammatory effect as well but its efficacy is less predictable than that of the inhaled steroids and, in addition, the beneficial effect may take 4–6 weeks to be seen. However, it is essentially free of side effects for both mother and fetus.

Bronchodilators

Sustained-release theophylline has a long duration of action and administration once a day, in the evening, may be helpful for patients who experience symptoms primarily at night. The dose should be titrated to reach a serum level of 8–12 μg/mL. Infants born to mothers receiving theophylline may develop jitteriness, tachycardia and vomiting but only when their serum levels are higher than 12 μg/mL and this is the reason not to exceed that

level in the mother. Extensive human experience has not shown other complications in the fetus or newborn up to this time.

Systemic corticosteroids

A short, tapering course of oral corticosteroids (usually prednisone, 40 mg/day for 1 week and then tapering for another week) should be considered when asthma is not controlled by bronchodilators, cromolyn sodium, and inhaled corticosteroids. However, if this short course fails to control symptoms or if it is effective for less than 2 or 3 weeks, the patient is considered to have severe asthma and additional therapy is needed. Oral corticosteroids on a long-term basis may be required in some patients with severe asthma, and in this case the lowest single daily dose possible or alternate-day therapy should be used. With prolonged use of these medications there is an increased risk of developing diabetes mellitus, preeclampsia, intrauterine growth retardation, and premature delivery. First-trimester use should be avoided if possible, as recent data support an association with facial clefts in the fetus.

In an effort to reduce the amount of systemic steroids, a high dose of inhaled steroids (800 μg/day or more) may be given. When considering stopping systemic steroids after a period of prolonged use, adrenal insufficiency may occur and these patients need to be monitored closely. Stress steroid coverage during labor may be needed as well.

Pregnant women with severe asthma are best managed in conjunction with an asthma expert as well as an obstetrician specializing in high-risk pregnancies.

Other asthma medications

Nonselective β-agonists such as epinephrine and isoproterenol are sometimes given subcutaneously during acute asthma attacks. However, during pregnancy epinephrine may cause vasoconstriction and therefore reduced fetal oxygenation. There are reports of teratogenesis in animals and humans. Isoproterenol has been associated with anomalies in animal embryos but not in humans. Since there are safe and effective alternatives to both, epinephrine and isoproterenol are best avoided during pregnancy.

A number of drugs that modify the leukotriene pathway have been recently introduced for the treatment of asthma. Clinical trials have shown benefit in exercise-induced, cold air hyperventilation-induced, allergen-induced and aspirin-induced asthma. Zileuton is teratogenic in animals and its use is not recommended in pregnancy. Zafirlukast and montelukast have been shown to be safe for the fetus in animal studies but there is little information about their use in pregnant women at this time and their use is limited to recalcitrant asthma, which responded to this type of medication prior to pregnancy.

Nedocromil sodium is similar in action to cromolyn; there are no reports of its use in human pregnancies but studies in animals have not shown significant complications. Anticholinergics such as atropine, ipatropium, and glycopyrrolate block bronchoconstriction caused by inhaled irritants. Atropine may alter heart rate and inhibit breathing in the fetus but no developmental anomalies have been described in humans or animals. There are no human studies on ipratropium but reports in animals have not shown teratogenic effects. Glycopyrrolate use in pregnant women near term is safe and no increase in birth defects has been reported in animals.

Acute asthmatic attack

Symptoms of worsening asthma include increasing dyspnea, cough, wheezing, chest tightness, and a decrease in expiratory air flow. Patients who are well educated may recognize early symptoms of an exacerbation and be able to manage at home while in close communication with the healthcare team. However, serious exacerbations are better managed in hospital or at least in the emergency room, where repetitive measurements of lung function, intensified treatment, and fetal monitoring can be performed. Maternal PO_2 must be kept ≥ 70 mmHg and the oxygen saturation 95% or greater to ensure adequate fetal oxygenation.

If admission to the hospital becomes necessary, it is better to reassure the patient rather than to use sedatives, which may depress respiration. It is also advisable to avoid iodine-containing mucolytics and expectorants because fetuses exposed to iodine may develop large goiters, with the potential for mechanical asphyxia in the newborn. Hydration is best accomplished with intravenous fluids in the form of 0.45 or 0.9 normal saline (NS). A chest x-ray, with abdominal shielding, should be taken in any patient sick enough to require hospitalization. The routine use of antibiotics is not recommended and evidence of a bacterial infection should be required for the use of antibiotics. To ensure adequate fetal oxygen supply at all times, maternal oxymetry must be monitored closely and the PO_2 maintained at greater than 70 mmHg (>95% saturation).

Some pregnant patients receiving large amounts of intravenous fluids, β2-agonists and corticosteroids have developed pulmonary edema and therefore close monitoring is mandatory. A few patients may continue to deteriorate and require endotracheal intubation and mechanical ventilation.

In the hospital, a nebulized, short-acting β2-agonist is administered every 3–6 hours. Intravenous methylprednisolone, 0.5–1 mg/kg, is given twice daily. Theophylline is rarely needed with early use of steroids. When the patient improves, an attempt to switch to oral therapy should be made. The β2-agonist aerosol is continued as before and inhaled corticosteroids are resumed. Prednisone is given by mouth, 0.5 mg/kg/day, and tapered gradually.

Management during labor and delivery

The medications that the patient has been using should be continued as scheduled. Peak flow measurements should be taken on admission and at regular intervals thereafter. Adequate hydration and pain relief are necessary in order to decrease the risk of bronchospasm. Patients on chronic steroid therapy must be given stress doses for adequate coverage (hydrocortisone 100 mg every 8 h) until 24 hours after delivery. Thereafter, rapid tapering can proceed if there were no complications.

Medications to avoid include prostaglandin F2-α because it may trigger bronchospasm. Prostaglandin E2, either suppositories or gel, may be used because it does not cause bronchospasm.

Oxytocin is safe for patients with asthma and the agent of choice for induction of labor. For analgesia, avoid analgesics and narcotics that cause histamine release because they may precipitate bronchospasm as well as respiratory depression. Epidural analgesia is beneficial for asthma patients because it helps to reduce oxygen consumption and minute ventilation. General anesthesia may trigger an asthma attack and, when necessary, pretreatment with atropine and glycopyrrolate offers a bronchodilatory effect. In addition, low concentrations of halogenated anesthetics may provide bronchodilation as well. Ketamine is the recommended agent of choice for induction of anesthesia. Post partum, ergot derivative compounds are best avoided because they may precipitate bronchospasm. In cases of postpartum hemorrhage, oxytocin is the medication of choice. If a prostaglandin is being considered, the E2 or E (misoprostol) appears to be safe.

The use of indometacin is relatively contraindicated because 3–8% of patients with asthma will develop profound, sometimes even life-threatening bronchoconstriction (as well as naso-ocular, dermal, and gastrointestinal responses).

For asthmatic pregnant women requiring treatment for premature labor, magnesium sulfate is the recommended medication but caution should be exercised to avoid overdosing and respiratory depression.

Enlisting the aid of an anesthesiologist who is knowledgeable about asthma management will be invaluable during labor and delivery, particularly if a cesarean section becomes necessary. There is no evidence that the form of delivery (use of forceps, breech delivery or cesarean section) has any effect on the development or course of allergic diseases.

Box 22.1 Asthma management – summary

Before pregnancy

Reassure that most patients do well if the asthma is controlled. The best for the fetus is well-controlled maternal asthma.

Inform about effects of pregnancy on asthma and possible medication effect (or lack of) on the fetus.

Provide education regarding the proper use of inhalers, peak flow meters and a stepwise approach to adjusting medication.

Have a clear plan of action including specific guidelines as to when to contact the healthcare team.

Prepare the house, work environment, etc. to minimize allergen exposure and asthma triggers.

Smoking cessation in smokers should be a strong priority.

Consider pneumococcal vaccine if not already done.

During pregnancy

Diet: avoid peanuts? Eat fish that is safe for pregnancy or consider omega-3 supplements, eat fresh fruits, take prenatal multivitamins daily.

Consider a higher dose than the 400 IU of vitamin D in the prenatal vitamins (800–1000 IU/day).

Exercise: maintain normal activity, walk 30 min/day if possible.

Influenza vaccine.

Medications: adjust as needed to stay free of symptoms and be able to maintain regular daily activities and moderate exercise.

Continue regular (twice-daily) use of peak flow meter (keep records and bring them to the doctor's visits).

Have supplemental O_2 available in case of exacerbations to insure adequate oxygenation.

Continue to adhere to the Specific Guidelines About Asthma action plan.

Labor and delivery

Continue all medications. If unable to use by mouth or inhaler, use parenterally.

Monitor oxygenation (maintain O_2 saturation > 95% at all times).

Control pain.

If cesarean section anticipated, obtain anesthesiology consult.

If on chronic steroids, provide stress coverage.

After delivery

Consult respiratory therapy to prevent atelectasis (particularly after a cesarean)

Continue asthma medications

Encourage breastfeeding if at all possible

Fetal monitoring

An early ultrasound (12–20 weeks) will help to date the pregnancy and to provide a baseline for serial fetal growth assessments at later dates. Serial evaluations are recommended for women with moderate and severe asthma or in any other patient if growth retardation is suspected. No specific guidelines for antepartum fetal surveillance have been issued except "when needed in the third trimester to assure fetal well-being." It seems reasonable to recommend fetal surveillance once or twice a week after 32–34 weeks for those women with moderate and severe disease and at any other time during the third trimester if there is exacerbation of asthma. Daily recordings of fetal activity with reporting of any changes are encouraged as well. Fetal monitoring during labor is essential, particularly in patients with moderate and severe asthma.

Breastfeeding

Inhaled corticosteroids, β2-agonists, cromolyn sodium, theophylline, and ipratropium have been considered safe while breastfeeding. Oral or parenteral corticosteroids may enter into breast milk but in small amounts and are unlikely to cause significant clinical effects at doses below 40 mg per day of prednisone or equivalent dose of other corticosteroids. Breast milk levels of zafirlukast are 20% of the maternal serum level and the manufacturers of all leukotriene synthesis inhibitors recommend against the use of these compounds while breastfeeding.

Suggested reading

Alati R, Al Mamun A, O'Callaghan M, *et al.* In utero and post-natal maternal smoking and asthma in adolescence. *Epidemiology* 2006; 17: 138–144.

Carmichael SL, Shaw GM, Chen MA, *et al.* Maternal corticosteroid use and orofacial clefts. *Am J Obstet Gynecol* 2007; 197 (6): 585–592.

Cates CJ, Lasserson TJ, Jaeschke R. Reegular treatment with salmeterol and inhaled steroids for chronic asthma: serious adverse effects. *Cochrane Database Syst Rev* 2009; 3: CD006922.

Chatenoud L, Malvezzi M, Pitrelli A, *et al.* Asthma mortality and long-acting beta2-agonists in five major European countries,1994–2004. *J Asthma* 2009; 46(6): 546–551.

Hourihane JO, Aiken R, Briggs R, *et al.* The impact of government advice to pregnant mothers regarding peanut avoidance on the prevalence of peanut allergy in United Kingdom children at school entry. *J Allergy Immunol* 2007; 119(5): 1197–1202.

Källén B, Rydhstroem H, Åberg A, *et al.* Asthma during pregnancy – a population study. *Eur J Epidemiol* 2000; 16(2): 167–171.

Kattan M, Stearns SC, Crain EF, *et al.* Cost-effectiveness of home-based environmental observation for inner city children with asthma. *J Allergy Clin Immunol* 2005; 116(5): 1058–1063.

Kwon HL, Belanger K, Bracken MB, *et al.* Asthma prevalence among pregnant and childbearing-aged women in the United States: estimates from national health surveys. *Ann Epidemiol* 2003; 13(5): 317–324.

Namazy JA, Schatz M. Treatment of asthma during pregnancy and perinatal outcomes. *Curr Opin Allergy Clin Immunol* 2005; 5: 229–233.

National Institutes of Health. *Managing asthma during pregnancy. Recommendations for pharmacologic treatment.* NIH Publication No. 05-3279. Bethesda, MD: National Institutes of Health, 2004.

National Institutes of Health. *Guidelines for the diagnosis and management of asthma.* Expert Panel Report 3. NIH Publication No. 08-4051. Bethesda, MD: National Institutes of Health, 2007.

Salam MT, Milstein J, Li YF, *et al*. Birth outcomes and prenatal exposure to ozone, carbon monoxide and particulate matter: results from the Children Health Study. *Environ Health Perspect* 2005; 113: 1638–1644.

Tata LJ, Hubbard RB, McKeever TM, *et al*. Fertility rates in women with asthma, eczema, and hay fever: a general population-based cohort study. *Am J Epidemiol* 2007; 165(9): 1023–1030.

Willers SM, Devereux G, Craig LC, *et al*. Maternal food consumption during pregnancy and asthma, respiratory and atopic symptoms in 5-year old children. *Thorax* 2007; 62(9): 772–778.

Chapter 23
Thyroid Disease in Pregnancy: Hyperthyroidism

Martin N. Montoro and T. Murphy Goodwin
Department of Medicine and Obstetrics and Gynecology, Keck School of Medicine, University of Southern California, CA, USA

Thyroid function tests

The following tests are useful in selected situations.

Total thyroxine (T$_4$)

The upper normal range is higher during pregnancy because of the increase in the levels of thyroxine-binding globulin (TBG). To ascertain the normal pregnancy range, the normal nonpregnant T$_4$ level (5–12 μg/dL by most laboratories) should be multiplied by 1.5 to calculate the normal range for pregnancy (e.g. 7.5–18 μg/dL). This calculation will be more dependable until the problems associated with the free T$_4$ immunoassays during pregnancy are resolved.

Free Thyroxine Index (FT$_4$I)

Many commercial laboratories have discontinued offering the FT$_4$I in favor of direct free T$_4$ determinations by immunoassay which are more convenient in general practice outside pregnancy. If available, it will remain a useful test until the limitations of the freeT$_4$ immunoassays during pregnancy are overcome.

Free thyroxine (FT$_4$)

The levels of free T$_4$ when measured by immunoassay have been shown to steadily decrease as pregnancy advances. These immunoassays are influenced by the changes in TBG and albumin levels that occur during pregnancy and are considered to be less reliable under conditions of altered protein binding. In addition, the normal reference ranges provided have been determined using nonpregnant individuals and are therefore not valid during pregnancy. At this time there is no consensus as to what the normal pregnancy levels should be for each trimester, which makes the usefulness of the current free T$_4$ immunoassays limited. Trimester-specific reference intervals have been published using tandem mass spectrometry, a method that has been found to be accurate and reliable during pregnancy (first trimester: 1.13 ± 0.23 ng/dL, second trimester: 0.92 ± 0.30 ng/dL, third trimester: 0.86 ± 0.21 ng/dL [mean ± standard error]).

Total tri-iodothironine (T$_3$)

The level of T$_3$ is higher during pregnancy also due to increased levels of the thyroid hormone carrier proteins, mainly TBG and albumin. To calculate the normal pregnancy values, the nonpregnant reference levels are multiplied by 1.5 in the same manner described above to determine T$_4$. Measuring T$_3$ may be helpful when the serum thyroid-stimulating hormone (TSH) is suppressed but the total and/or free T$_4$ levels are normal. An elevation in T$_3$ is consistent with the diagnosis of T$_3$ thyrotoxicosis, seen mainly in patients with hyperthyroidism caused by autonomous thyroid nodules and in the early phase of Graves' disease. T$_3$ is usually not elevated in the transient hyperthyroidism of hyperemesis gravidarum, and if elevated, usually not as high as in Graves' disease or in toxic nodules.

Serum TSH

Serum TSH (ultrasensitive, at least third or fourth generation assays) is the best screening test for thyroid disease. However, during pregnancy TSH levels are influenced by the elevated concentration of human chorionic gonadotropin (hCG) and therefore, using the normal nonpregnant TSH levels will often lead to misdiagnosis. Several recent publications recommend the following trimester-specific reference values obtained from populations of normal pregnant women without thyroid antibodies: first trimester 0.10–2.5 μIU/L, second trimester 0.10–3 μIU/L, third trimester 0.13–3 μIU/L, although the first trimester normal lower limit has been reported to be as low as 0.03 μIU/L. An elevated value is diagnostic of hypothyroidism due to intrinsic thyroid disease. A suppressed or undetectable value is normally consistent with the

Management of Common Problems in Obstetrics and Gynecology, 5th edition. Edited by T.M. Goodwin, M.N. Montoro, L. Muderspach, R. Paulson and S. Roy. © 2010 Blackwell Publishing Ltd.

diagnosis of hyperthyroidism. However, many women will be misdiagnosed, particularly during the first and second trimesters, if the general TSH reference values specified by the majority of laboratories (0.4–4.0 µIU/L) are used as the normal range for pregnancy.

Thyroid antibodies (thyroid peroxidase antibodies (TPO-Ab)) and antithyroglobulin antibodies (TG-Ab)

The presence of these antibodies in the serum is diagnostic of autoimmune thyroid disease and affected women are at risk of developing thyroid insufficiency as pregnancy progresses and for postpartum thyroiditis as well. They are most useful in the evaluation of goiter or hypothyroidism.

Serum thyroglobulin (Tg)

This test is used to monitor patients after treatment for thyroid carcinoma. It is an early marker for recurrence of the disease.

TSH receptor-binding antibodies (TSHR-Ab)

These antibodies are markers for Graves' disease and include a group of immunoglobulins that compete with TSH for binding to its receptor. The currently commercially available tests report the percentage of inhibition of TSH binding to its receptor but do not specifically measure the antibodies' ability to stimulate or inhibit the TSH receptor. To measure the specific stimulating receptor antibodies, it should be indicated that a thyroid-stimulating immunoglobulin (TSI) is the test desired. TSH receptor antibodies are present in up to 80% of women with present or past history of Graves' disease. A significant elevation in maternal titer (>50%) may identify infants at risk for neonatal hyperthyroidism.

Transient hyperthyroidism of hyperemesis gravidarum

The symptoms of hyperemesis gravidarum include nausea and vomiting, greater than 5% weight loss, and large ketonuria. It is our experience that as many as 65% of patients with hyperemesis gravidarum also have at least one thyroid test in the hyperthyroid range (i.e. suppressed TSH, elevated T_4 or, in 12% of cases, elevated T_3). This is a self-limited abnormality and no specific antithyroid therapy is indicated although some authors have recommended treatment with antithyroid medication if there are clinical symptoms of overt hyperthyroidism and very high T_4 and T_3 concentrations, greater than 50% above the pregnancy-adjusted normal values. However, unnecessary treatment with antithyroid medications should be avoided unless there is evidence of Graves' or a toxic nodule.

It may not be easy to differentiate the chemical hyperthyroidism of hyperemesis gravidarum from the hyperthyroidism of other causes. The following points may be helpful in the differential diagnosis: no history or symptoms of thyroid disease preceding pregnancy, negative family history, absence of goiter, negative thyroid antibodies, and symptom resolution and normalization of thyroid tests by 20 weeks in most cases.

Goiter

Goiter is defined as an enlargement of the thyroid gland, which normally weighs between 15 and 25 g and in general is not palpable. In areas of normal dietary iodine ingestion, the thyroid gland enlarges during pregnancy, as shown by studies using serial sonography, but usually not enough to be detected clinically. Therefore, any enlargement noted by physical examination should be considered abnormal and deserving of careful evaluation, including a thyroid ultrasound. The physician should be able to describe the size, consistency, symmetry, and tenderness, along with the presence of nodularity or adenopathy. The determination of T_4 and TSH levels will define the functional status of the goiter. The presence of thyroid antibodies is suggestive of autoimmune thyroid disease as the etiology of the goiter.

A fine needle aspiration biopsy should be considered in the presence of a single or any dominant nodule larger than 1 cm, to rule out thyroid cancer. Interruption of pregnancy is not justified when thyroid malignancy is found, since there is no evidence that pregnancy worsens the prognosis of well-differentiated thyroid cancer. However, there are insufficient data to also recommend this approach for those patients with advanced disease or more aggressive tumors such as medullary, undifferentiated or anaplastic carcinomas.

It is generally recommended to avoid surgery in the first and third trimesters but it should be offered in the second trimester, preferably before 22 weeks. Nevertheless, surgery may be postponed until after delivery in patients reluctant to undergo this procedure while pregnant. When the decision is made to postpone surgery until after delivery, thyroid suppression with exogenous levothyroxine is recommended for TSH suppression but making sure that the freeT_4 and/or total T_4 levels do not rise above the upper normal range for pregnancy.

Hyperthyroidism

Frequency

Hyperthyroidism complicates 0.1–0.4% of pregnancies in the USA. In most cases the symptoms precede pregnancy, although they may appear for the first time during pregnancy or recur in a patient previously in remission. Hyperthyroidism due to autoimmune thyroid disease may spontaneously recur or worsen during pregnancy. The exacerbations tend to occur more often during the first trimester or in the postpartum period, and the improvements in the second half of pregnancy.

Etiology

Hyperthyroidism due to Graves' disease accounts for over 85% of cases, excluding the transient hyperthyroidism of hyperemesis gravidarum. Other causes include toxic nodular goiter (single nodule or multinodular), chronic thyroiditis and, less commonly, thyrotoxicosis from excess exogenous thyroid intake or hydatidiform molar disease. Hyperemesis gravidarum as a cause of biochemical hyperthyroidism was discussed previously. It is the most common cause of elevated thyroid function tests, in the hyperthyroid range, during pregnancy.

Diagnosis

Clinical diagnosis during pregnancy could be difficult at times because many women show hyperdynamic signs similar to those of mild hyperthyroidism such as heat intolerance, warm, moist skin and a rapid pulse rate. Classic symptoms are considered to be weight loss, palpitations, nervousness, personality changes, irritability, heat intolerance, muscle weakness, insomnia, and hyperdefecation. The two more reliable signs are weight loss, or failure to gain, and a resting pulse over 100 beats/minute. On physical examination, a diffuse painless goiter is found in over 90% of cases; warm and moist skin, eye changes, tachycardia, wide pulse pressure, hyper-reflexia, and proximal muscle weakness are other common findings. A suppressed serum TSH and an elevated free T_4, total T_4, free T_4I and T_3 levels confirm the diagnosis. Most patients with Graves' disease will also have detectable TSHR-Ab.

Complications

The TSHR-Ab crosses the placenta and may cause fetal and/or neonatal hyperthyroidism. Fortunately, this occurs rarely, in 1–5%, and mostly when the maternal TSHR-Ab titer is high, > 50%. The diagnosis is suspected when the fetus develops tachycardia, growth restriction, a goiter, heart failure or hydrops.

Other adverse pregnancy outcomes include miscarriage, pre-eclampsia, preterm delivery, IUGR, stillbirth, maternal cardiac arrhythmias (atrial fibrillation is the most common), congestive heart failure and thyroid storm. These complications are much more likely to occur in women with poorly controlled hyperthyroidism.

Treatment

Once the diagnosis is confirmed, medical therapy is the treatment of choice during pregnancy. Propylthiouracil (PTU) and methimazole (MMI) are the two antithyroid medications available in the USA. MMI has been associated with aplasia cutis as well as choanal and esophageal atresia when used during embryogenesis. There is no unanimous agreement that the data linking MMI exposure to congenital anomalies are strong enough to prevent its use but since PTU has not been associated with congenital malformations, it has been generally preferred as the initial therapy during pregnancy. Until now, PTU was preferred for the reasons given above and also later in the pregnancy because of the belief that it crossed the placenta less readily than MMI even though more recent studies have not confirmed that result. Recently, there has been great concern about severe liver failure associated with PTU and it has been recommended that its use be restricted. In view of this information, we have modified our treatment approach and now use PTU only during the first trimester and then switch to methimazole once embryogenesis has been completed. It is recommended that the minimum amount of antithyroid medication be used to keep the mother clinically and biochemically euthyroid since these medications cross the placenta and could affect fetal thyroid function. To minimize the risk of causing fetal hypothyroidism, the maternal levels of total free T_4 index and free T_4 should be kept in the upper third of the of the normal reference range. Clinic visits should be scheduled every 2–4 weeks. The two clinical signs that correlate best with the thyroid function tests are maternal weight gain and pulse rate.

The initial PTU dose is 200–400 mg and for methimazole is 20–40 mg daily, given in divided doses. MMI has a longer half-life which allows more widely spaced doses, even once a day, and therefore it is preferable for less compliant patients since PTU requires taking more tablets more often. The thyroid tests will improve in 2–3 weeks and normalize in 3–6 weeks. The dose should be reduced as soon as the tests improve; adjustments are made every 2–3 weeks to the minimum effective medication dose that keeps the mother stable. Maternal hypothyroidism must be avoided and care should be taken to keep the T_4 and T_3 levels in the upper normal range to minimize the risk of fetal hypothyroidism. There is no need to recheck the serum TSH since in the majority of cases it will remain suppressed for weeks or months even after normalization of the T_4 and T_3 levels.

Antithyroid medication may be discontinued in the last 4–6 weeks of gestation in patients who have maintained prolonged euthyroidism on minimum amounts, especially in patients with small goiters and short duration of disease. The purpose is to allow the fetus to clear the medication before delivery. The mother would be unlikely to relapse during that short period of time without medication.

A serious side effect of both PTU and MMI is agranulocytosis, reported in 0.03% of patients. The patient should be advised to discontinue the use of antithyroid drugs in the presence of a sore throat, fever or gingivitis and to consult her physician at once. Severe liver damage has been associated with the use of PTU, not predictable by periodic determinations of liver function, and this is the reason for restricting its use as mentioned above.

Hospitalization should be reserved for patients with uncontrolled disease, poorly compliant patients, those seen for the first time in the third trimester with severe disease, and those with fetal growth retardation or superimposed toxemia. If the mother is kept euthyroid during pregnancy, fetal morbidity and mortality are similar to the general population. Long-term follow-up of infants exposed to antithyroid medications *in utero* has not shown significant sequelae.

β-Blockers (usually propanolol) may be used temporarily at the time of diagnosis in very symptomatic patients but they are discontinued when the symptoms improve. They could also be used in preparation for thyroidectomy. There are no reports of teratogenic effects in animals or humans. If long-term use of β-blockers is considered, monitoring of fetal growth is advised because of case reports of IUGR. When used in late pregnancy, the neonate may experience hypoglycemia, apnea, and bradycardia.

Thyroid surgery during pregnancy is considered only when there are no medical options left and, if at all possible, it should be performed in the second trimester. A brief course of iodides could be given in preparation for thyroidectomy but only if strictly necessary and if β-blockers are not sufficient or cannot be used. Long-term iodide use in pregnancy has been associated with hypothyroidism and goiter in the newborn; the goiters sometimes have been large enough to cause tracheal obstruction and asphyxiation. It goes without saying that any radio-active iodine diagnostic or therapeutic procedures are contraindicated during pregnancy. All reproductive-age women contemplating radio-active iodine administration should have a prior pregnancy test to avoid inadvertent use in a pregnant woman.

Fetal surveillance

There are no specific published guidelines. We recommend serial assessments of fetal growth in an effort to detect potential complications such as fetal growth restriction, advanced bone age, goiter, tachycardia, heart failure and hydrops. Antepartum testing twice weekly is initiated at 34 weeks. This type of surveillance will be of benefit mainly to those patients with uncontrolled hyperthyroidism and those with very high titers of TSHR-Ab regardless of their thyroid function status. Well-controlled patients will rarely show any of the complications mentioned above.

Lactation and postpartum follow-up

Patients need to be followed in the postpartum period because recurrences of hyperthyroidism may occur. Infants of hyperthyroid mothers should also be evaluated and followed by a pediatrician, since transient abnormalities in thyroid function may be present in 2–10% of these infants.

Breastfeeding may be allowed when the total amount of medication is less than 300 mg/day of PTU or less than 20 mg/day of methimazole. Recent studies have reported no alterations in thyroid function in infants of mothers taking antithyroid medications up to these doses. The drug should be administered just after infant suckling. The pediatrician should be informed and the infant followed with the appropriate thyroid function tests.

Postpartum thyroid dysfunction syndrome

Women with autoimmune thyroid disease frequently develop thyroid abnormalities within 1 year of delivery. The incidence of these abnormalities in the USA has been reported to be between 3% and 8% of all pregnancies. Women with type 1 diabetes mellitus have a very high prevalence of TPO antibodies and their incidence of PPTD is higher than in the general population and reported to occur in 18–25% of these women. There can be considerable variability in the clinical course. Some patients may go directly into a hypothyroid stage without a preceding hyperthyroid phase. In an occasional patient, the hyperthyroid phase is followed by complete recovery without a subsequent hypothyroid stage. Only those patients with PPTD who develop a thyrotoxic phase as part of their postpartum thyroid dysfunction will be discussed in this section.

Patients with a history of Graves' disease may present with an exacerbation of hyperthyroid symptoms 1–3 months after delivery, occasionally later. The hyperthyroid symptoms tend to be more severe than those occurring during the thyrotoxic phase of chronic thyroiditis and will persist indefinitely if the patient is not treated. The presence of extrathyroidal signs of Graves' disease (ophthalmopathy, pretibial myxedema) will corroborate the diagnosis. Also, nearly 95% of patients with Graves' disease relapsing post partum will test positive for TSHR-Ab. The[131]I thyroid uptake, if performed, will be elevated and consistent with Graves' disease.

In contrast, patients with chronic thyroiditis who develop an initial hyperthyroid phase will do so 1–6 months post partum, usually 3 months, and will not last longer than 1–2 months even if not treated. Within 3 months of delivery these women may complain of enlargement of the thyroid gland and mild, nonspecific symptoms such as tiredness, fatigue, nervousness, heat intolerance, and personality changes. These symptoms are often attributed to postpartum depression. Thyroid tests are in the hyperthyroid range and thyroid antibodies (TPO) are positive, with titers even higher than during pregnancy. The presence of positive TPO antibodies in the first trimester of pregnancy in a euthyroid woman is predictive of the development of PPTD. If a ^{131}I thyroid uptake is obtained, it will be low (near 0%), and will help to differentiate this condition from Graves' disease. Without specific therapy, hypothyroidism ensues within a few months, frequently with few symptoms. Spontaneous recovery occurs within 4–6 months with normalization of thyroid function, but the thyroid antibodies remain elevated. The goiter may decrease somewhat in size.

Therapy with β-blockers, usually propranolol (20 mg twice to four times a day), is indicated for the occasional patient with significant hyperthyroid symptoms; conversely, thyroid hormone therapy may be necessary for some patients during the hypothyroid phase if there are significant symptoms present, if they are planning to get pregnant or if the TSH level is higher than 10 μIU/L. It should be emphasized that those women who experienced PPTD and who plan to become pregnant again should be treated, particularly during the hypothyroid stage, to ensure that they will not be hypothyroid during a subsequent pregnancy.

Long-term follow-up of these patients indicates a significant incidence of permanent hypothyroidism and therefore periodic evaluations are recommended. Prediction of progression to overt hypothyroidism can be estimated using a recently published scoring system.

Suggested reading

Abalovich M, Amino N, Barbour LA, *et al*. Management of thyroid dysfunction during pregnancy and postpartum: an Endocrine Society clinical practice guideline. *J Clin Endocrinol Metab* 2007; 92: S1-S47.

Cooper DS, Rivkees SA. Putting propylthiouracil in perspective. *J Clin Endocrinol Metab* 2009: 94(6): 1881–1882.

Goodwin TM, Hershman JM. Hyperthyroidism due to inappropriate production of human chorionic gonadotropin. *Clin Obstet Gynecol* 1997; 40: 32–44.

Goodwin TM, Montoro M, Mestman JH. Transient hyperthyroidism and hyperemesis gravidarum: clinical aspects. *Am J Obstet Gynecol* 1992; 167: 648–652.

Goodwin TM, Montoro MN, Mestman JH, Pekary AE, Hershman JM. The role of chorionic gonadotropin in transient hyperthyroidism of hyperemesis gravidarum. *J Clin Endocrinol Metab* 1992; 75: 1333–1337.

Kahric-Janicic N, Soldin SJ, Soldin OP, West T, Gu J, Jonklaas J. Tandem mass spectrometry improves the accuracy of free thyroxine measurements during pregnancy. *Thyroid* 2007; 17: 303–311.

Lee RH, Spencer CA, Mestman JH, *et al*. Free T4 immunoassays are flawed during pregnancy. *Am J Obstet Gynecol* 2009; 200: 260.

Mestman JH. Hyperthyroidism in pregnancy. *Best Pract Res Clin Endocrinol* 2004; 18: 267–288.

Mestman JH, Goodwin TM, Montoro MN. Thyroid disorders in pregnancy. *Endocrinol Metab Clin North Am* 1995; 24: 41–71.

Millar LK, Wing DA, Leung AS, Koonings PP, Montoro MN, Mestman JH. Low birth weight and preeclampsia in pregnancies complicated by hyperthyroidism. *Obstet Gynecol* 1994; 84: 946–949.

Strieder TGA, Tijssen JGP, Wenzel BE, *et al*. Prediction of progression to overt hypothyroidism or hyperthyroidism in female relatives of patients with autoimmune thyroid disease using the thyroid events Amsterdam (THEA) score. *Arch Intern Med* 2008; 168(15): 1657–1663.

Wing DA, Millar LK, Koonings PP, Montoro MN, Mestman JH. A comparison of propylthiouracil and methimazole in the treatment of hyperthyroidism in pregnancy. *Am J Obstet Gynecol* 1994; 170: 90–95.

Chapter 24
Thyroid Disease in Pregnancy: Hypothyroidism

Martin N. Montoro

Department of Medicine and Obstetrics and Gynecology, Keck School of Medicine, University of Southern California, CA, USA

Frequency

Most reports do not provide enough information to ascertain the incidence of overt hypothyroidism during pregnancy. In our institution during the 10-year period from 1981 to 1990, there were 101 cases and 164,611 deliveries for an incidence of 1 in 1629 (0.06%). In Australia and during a similar period of time (1980–89), there were 26 cases in 51,407 deliveries for an incidence of 1 in 1977 (0.05%). More recent reports give a frequency of 0.3–0.5% for overt hypothyroidism (low free thyroxine (FT_4) and elevated thyroid-stimulating hormone (TSH)), 2–3% for subclinical hypothyroidism (normal FT_4 and elevated TSH concentrations) and a fairly high frequency, 5–15%, of positive thyroid antibodies without thyroid dysfunction. Whether or not the incidence of hypothyroidism during pregnancy is higher than in women of similar age who are not pregnant remains to be elucidated.

Etiology of hypothyroidism during pregnancy

When first diagnosed during pregnancy, most women will have autoimmune thyroid disease. Lymphocytic infiltration is the cause of the thyroid enlargement (goitrous form), although in some cases, usually late in the disease course, the thyroid may become atrophic and nonpalpable. The majority of the cases not caused by autoimmune thyroiditis are secondary to destruction or removal of the thyroid gland (radio-active iodine ablation or surgery) as part of the treatment for hyperthyroidism, thyroid cancer, suspicious nodules or toxic nodular goiter. Rare causes include the transient hypothyroidism that may be seen in silent (painless) and subacute thyroiditis, drug-induced hypothyroidism, high-dose external neck radiation (e.g. for Hodgkin's lymphoma), congenital hypothyroidism, inherited metabolic disorders of the thyroid, and thyroid hormone resistance syndromes. Secondary hypothyroidism may be seen in pituitary or hypothalamic diseases. Several drugs may cause hypothyroidism if taken during pregnancy. Iodine, lithium, propylthiouracil, and methimazole interfere with thyroid hormone synthesis and/or its release. Carbamazepine, phenytoin, and rifampin increase thyroxine (T_4) clearance. Amiodarone decreases the conversion from T_4 to triiodothyronine (T_3) and also inhibits T_3 action. Aluminum oxide, cholestyramine, sucralfate, and particularly ferrous sulfate interfere with the intestinal absorption of T_4. Therefore, it is important to make sure that women on levothyroxine replacement take these medications at least 2 hours apart, and perhaps 4 hours might be even better (especially when taking ferrous sulfate which is very commonly given to pregnant women).

Diagnosis

The diagnosis of hypothyroidism is difficult to make on clinical grounds alone and therefore it will remain unsuspected and undiagnosed until it is profound and the symptoms very obvious. In addition, only one-third of hypothyroid pregnant women show the classic symptoms, another third will have moderate symptomatology, and the rest will have few or no symptoms despite very abnormal thyroid function tests. Symptoms may include fatigue, sleepiness, lethargy, mental slowing, depression, cold intolerance (which is very unusual in normal pregnancy), decreased perspiration, hair loss, dry skin, deeper voice or hoarseness, weight gain despite poor appetite, constipation, arthralgias, muscle aching, and stiffness and paresthesias. There might be history of menstrual irregularities before pregnancy. On physical examination, signs that may be present include general slowing of speech and movements, dry and pale (or at times yellowish) skin, sparse thin hair, deep or hoarse voice, bradycardia (also unusual in pregnancy),

Management of Common Problems in Obstetrics and Gynecology, 5th edition. Edited by T.M. Goodwin, M.N. Montoro, L. Muderspach, R. Paulson and S. Roy. © 2010 Blackwell Publishing Ltd.

myxedema (nonpitting edema), hyporeflexia, prolonged relaxation phase of the deep tendon reflexes, carpal tunnel syndrome, and a diffuse or a nodular goiter.

The best laboratory test to diagnose hypothyroidism is the TSH except in the rare cases of hypothalamic or pituitary disease. Current sensitive TSH assays make it possible to diagnose hypothyroidism very early and allow monitoring thyroxine replacement therapy very accurately. Other tests include the total T_4 (TT_4) and free T_4 index (FT_4I), FT_4, thyroid peroxidase antibodies (TPO-Ab), and antithyroglobulin antibodies (ATG-Ab). The levels of total T_4 are higher during pregnancy due to an increase in thyroxine-binding globulin (TBG). The pregnancy range is calculated by multiplying the normal nonpregnant TT_4 value (5–12 μg/dL for most laboratories) by 1.5 (e.g. 7.5–18 μg/dL). Caution is needed to interpret the current FT_4 levels during pregnancy because the normal ranges have been determined using nonpregnant individuals. In addition, the FT_4 assays currently in use are influenced by the changes in TBG and albumin that occur during pregnancy. Therefore, until normal FT_4 values that are specific for pregnancy are determined, the utility of present FT_4 assays will be limited (see Chapter 23). TT_4 and FT_4I may provide a more reliable estimate for the time being since they retain an appropriate inverse relationship with TSH throughout pregnancy.

Anemia may be found in 30–40% of patients, usually secondary to decreased erythropoiesis, but at times it may also be due to vitamin B12, folic acid or iron deficiencies. Serum lipids and creatine phosphokinase (CPK – of muscle origin) may be elevated. Mild, reversible abnormalities of liver function have also been described.

Maternal and fetal complications of hypothyroidism during pregnancy

Increased risk of spontaneous abortion to twice the normal rate has been reported in at least six studies in women with elevated titers of thyroid antibodies (TPO-Ab, ATG-Ab) but some studies have not reported an increased risk. The women in those studies were euthyroid and it was unclear if the antibodies themselves were the cause or, more likely, just markers for other immune abnormalities responsible for the miscarriages. Whether or not hypothyroidism alone is a risk for miscarriage remains unclear. Nevertheless, elevated maternal thyroid antibodies may have additional deleterious effects on the fetus and newborn. Thyroid antibodies cross the placenta and may cause hypothyroidism in the newborn. This hypothyroidism is usually transient but since it occurs at a critical period of brain development, it may lead to serious cognitive deficiencies if not treated in a timely manner. It has also been reported that children born to euthyroid women but with elevated titers of TPO-Ab had lower IQs than children born to antibody-negative women. It is not known by what mechanism the antibodies may harm the fetus but it is speculated that they might have caused hypothyroidism at some critical stage of fetal brain development. One recent study did report that women with positive TPO antibodies and normal FT_4 and TSH levels had fewer miscarriages and preterm deliveries if treated with levothyroxine even though they were not hypothyroid.

Women with positive thyroid antibody titers are also at risk for developing postpartum thyroiditis and this condition is reported in about 7% of women in the postpartum period. Although this condition is considered to be transient, it increases the risk of permanent hypothyroidism later in life.

The role of the maternal thyroid status on fetal development is still incompletely understood. However, it is now accepted that during the first trimester and probably until mid-gestation, the fetus is not able to provide enough thyroid hormone and it is therefore dependent on the mother for thyroid hormone supply. Afterwards, the contribution of mother and fetus to the total fetal thyroid hormone pool is not well known. Much of the information currently available comes from animal studies (mostly in the rat) and how much can be applied to humans remains to be seen. None of the more recent publications has reported an increased frequency of congenital anomalies in infants born to hypothyroid mothers.

Other publications have suggested that mild maternal hypothyroidism, subclinical hypothyroidism and even low normal maternal thyroid hormone levels (below the 10th percentile) may be a cause of deficient neuropsychologic development of the child. It is not known at what gestational age the developing fetus may be most susceptible but presumably early in gestation. It is unknown if these deficits could be prevented by maternal thyroid therapy or iodine supplementation even in iodine-replete areas. Further research is needed to confirm these findings and to clarify if the thyroid level is the only cause or if other factors could also responsible.

Some authors now advocate universal screening of pregnant women for hypothyroidism while others state that there are insufficient data at this time. Until this point is clarified we strongly recommend routine screening for hypothyroidism during pregnancy in certain high-risk groups. Those at highest risk include women previously treated for hyperthyroidism, previous neck irradiation, previous postpartum thyroiditis, a palpable goiter, family history of thyroid disease, women with type 1 diabetes mellitus, and treatment with amiodarone or any of the other medications listed above (see "Etiology of hypothyroidism during pregnancy"). At less risk but still deserving screening are patients with any other endocrinopathy, any autoimmune disorder, particularly systemic lupus erythematosus, exposure to certain industrial or chemical substances, and hyperlipidemia. Nevertheless, a recent publication indicates that limiting screening to only those considered to be high risk will miss 30% of cases of overt or subclinical hypothyroidism during pregnancy. These data would support the recommendation for universal thyroid screening during pregnancy.

The main maternal complication reported in almost all the papers published in the past 20 years is a high risk of pre-eclampsia. Frequently, this complication leads to premature delivery with its related morbidity, mortality, and the very high cost for care of these newborns. Those women who are euthyroid at the time of conception and remain euthyroid during pregnancy are at low risk. No special monitoring is needed except for periodic measurements of thyroid function to ensure that it remains in the normal range for pregnancy. The women who are hypothyroid at conception but who become euthyroid with treatment still have a 15–30% risk of pre-eclampsia but the hypertension tends to be milder and to develop later in gestation than in those women who remain hypothyroid. One study reported fetal distress during labor in women who were hypothyroid in early gestation even if they improved with treatment, but no other papers have confirmed this finding. Patients who are still hypothyroid by the end of the second trimester have an even higher risk of pre-eclampsia and premature delivery (22–44%) and of placental abruption and postpartum hemorrhage as well. Why hypertension occurs more frequently in thyroid disorders is not yet fully understood. In hypothyroidism, cardiac output is reduced and the arterial peripheral resistance is higher, probably secondary to an increased sympathetic nervous tone and also to an increased α-adrenergic response. High levels of endothelin, a potent vasoconstrictor peptide produced after a vascular injury, have been associated with decreased T_4 and elevated TSH levels.

Antepartum fetal surveillance is not routinely recommended for hypothyroid women except when indicated for other reasons such as concurrent diabetes mellitus or chronic hypertension. However, it is difficult to make firm recommendations at this time because the total number of hypothyroid pregnant women published to date remains relatively small and from different institutions. At ours, we initiate antepartum fetal surveillance twice a week starting at 34 weeks of gestation. The overall outcome of pregnancy in hypothyroid women has been much improved in the last 15–20 years than in reports prior to that time. Hypothyroidism is nowadays diagnosed and treated earlier, which is probably a major contributing factor to the improved outcome. Other factors have undoubtedly contributed to improved outcomes, such

as more effective fetal monitoring techniques, earlier diagnosis of fetal distress, timely delivery if indicated, and more effective neonatal care.

Treatment

Hypothyroid pregnant women should be made euthyroid as soon as possible and the euthyroid state maintained throughout pregnancy. Ideally, hypothyroid women should be made euthyroid before pregnancy (normal FT4 and a TSH below 2.5 μIU/mL) and the treatment readjusted whenever needed, because up to 60–70% of patients may require higher replacement doses during pregnancy. The treatment of hypothyroidism is simple and inexpensive, particularly if we consider the very high cost of managing the complications in untreated patients.

Levothyroxine is considered the drug of choice. The hormonal content of the synthetic drugs is more reliably standardized, and they have replaced the desiccated thyroid compounds as the mainstay of therapy. The administration of T_4 alone is generally recommended; T_4 is de-iodinated to T_3 in the extrathyroidal tissues and it is considered that this most closely resembles the normal physiologic process. In one study, therapy with a combination of T_4 and T_3, approximating the ratio normally secreted by the thyroid gland, resulted in improvement in mood and neuropsychologic function in some patients as compared with administering T_4 alone and also may cause maternal hypothyroxinemia and less T_4 reaching the fetus. However, subsequent studies have failed to show that the T_4/T_3 combination is more effective than T_4 alone. The best time to take levothyroxine is early in the morning, on an empty stomach, but women experiencing nausea and vomiting should be allowed to take it later in the day until they improve. If ferrous sulfate is also being given, the ingestion of these two medications should be separated by at least 2 hours and preferably 4 hours.

There are numerous reports indicating increased thyroxine requirements during pregnancy. The initial dose should be 100–150 μg per day or, perhaps even better, titrated by bodyweight at 2μg per kilogram (of actual bodyweight). Further adjustments are made according to the TSH level and the goal of treatment is to keep it within the normal range (< 2.5 μIU/mL in the first and second trimesters and < 3 μIU/mL in the third. The lower normal TSH limits are 0.10 μIU/mL for the first and second trimesters and 0.13 μIU/mL for the third trimester). If the TSH is elevated but it is less than 10 μIU/mL, the replacement dosage should be increased by 25–50 μg per day. It the TSH is over 10 and below 20 μIU/mL, add 50–75 μg per day and if above 20 μIU/mL, 75–100 μg per day should be added to the previous dose. However, dosage changes made at less than 4-week intervals may lead to overtreatment.

Women already on levothyroxine replacement before pregnancy are very likely to need higher doses during gestation and they should be monitored at regular intervals. It has even been recommended that the dose be increased by a third as soon as the pregnancy is diagnosed in those patients who, for whatever reason, cannot see a physician and have thyroid function tests done soon after the pregnancy is detected.

The following schedule is suggested to measure thyroid function studies: every 4–5 weeks until 16–20 weeks and less frequently afterwards because the increased demands occur early in gestation and much less after the first half of pregnancy. The necessary readjustments are made in the replacement dose when indicated by the thyroid function studies. After delivery, the dosage should be reduced to the pre-pregnancy amount and a TSH measured 4–8 weeks post partum to verify the adequacy of the therapy.

Breastfeeding is encouraged and patients should be reassured that it is safe while taking levothyroxine. In women with pituitary or hypothalamic disease in whom the TSH cannot be used to guide the treatment, the total and free T_4 index should be kept in the upper third of the normal range.

Women with a history of thyroid carcinoma are treated with larger doses of levothyroxine in order to inhibit TSH secretion to undetectable levels, since the growth of differentiated thyroid carcinomas may be dependent on thyrotropin. The free T_4 index levels are kept in the upper normal or slightly above the normal range. There is no need to change the goals of treatment in these women since subclinical hyperthyroidism has not been associated with adverse pregnancy outcomes. Pregnancy has not been reported to adversely influence the long-term prognosis of differentiated thyroid carcinoma or the outcome of pregnancy if it is delayed for 1 year after the administration of high doses of radio-active iodine.

Pregnancy and lactation increase iodine demands and sufficient iodine intake (250 μg/day average) is necessary. It is now recommended that additional iodine intake (150 μg/day) be provided during pregnancy even to women residing in iodine-sufficient countries. Prescribing a prenatal vitamin preparation that also contains iodine is the easiest way to accomplish this advice.

Suggested reading

Alexander EK, Marqusee E, Lawrence J, Jarolim P, Fischer GA, Larsen PR. Timing and magnitude of increases in levothyroxine requirements during pregnancy in women with hypothyroidism. *NEJM* 2004; 351: 241–249.

Fisher DA. Fetal thyroid function: diagnosis and management of fetal thyroid disorders. *Clin Obstet Gynecol* 1997; 40: 16–31.

Glinoer D, Rovet J. Gestational hypothyroxinemia and the beneficial effects of early dietary iodine fortification. *Thyroid* 2009; 19: 431–434.

Haddow JE, Palomaki GE, Allan WC, *et al*. Maternal thyroid deficiency during pregnancy and subsequent neuropsychological development of the child. *NEJM* 1999; 341: 549–555.

Lee RH, Spencer CA, Mestman JH, *et al*. Free T4 immunoassays are flawed during pregnancy. *Am J Obstet Gynecol* 2009; 200: 260.

Leung AS, Millar LK, Koonings PP, Montoro MN, Mestman JH. Perinatal outcome in hypothyroid pregnancies. *Obstet Gynecol* 1993; 81: 349–353.

Mestman JH, Goodwin TM, Montoro MN. Thyroid disorders of pregnancy. *Endocrinol Metab Clin North Am* 1995; 24: 41–71.

Montoro MN. Management of hypothyroidism during pregnancy. *Clin Obstet Gynecol* 1997; 40: 65–80.

Soldin OP, Tractenberg RE, Hollowell JG, Jonklaas J, Janicic N, Soldin SJ. Trimester-specific changes in maternal thyroid hormone, thyrotropin, and thyroglobulin concentrations during gestation: trends and associations across trimesters in iodine sufficiency. *Thyroid* 2004; 14: 1084–1090.

Vaidya B, Anthony S, Bilous M, *et al*. Detection of thyroid dysfunction in early pregnancy: universal screening or targeted high-risk case finding? *J Clin Endocrinol Metab* 2007; 92: 203–207.

Chapter 25
Seizure Disorders and Headaches in Pregnancy

Laura Kalayjian

Department of Neurology, Keck School of Medicine, University of Southern California, CA, USA

Epilepsy and seizures in pregnancy

Epilepsy is a common condition occurring in approximately 1% of the population. Women with epilepsy pose a difficult dilemma for their practitioner; all the antiepileptic drugs (AEDs) are pregnancy category C or D, but without the medication many patients will suffer seizures. Seizures during pregnancy may cause injury to the patient or fetus and may cause premature labor or rupture of membranes. The seizure frequency remains the same in the majority of patients with pre-pregnancy control being maintained. Preconception counseling to discuss the need for medication or to switch to a safer medication should be considered early and initiated by the practitioner since half of the pregnancies in the US are unplanned.

Diagnosing epilepsy and seizures

Epilepsy is defined as two or more unprovoked seizures. Generalized tonic clonic seizures (grand mal) last approximately 2 minutes with the entire body stiffening during the tonic phase followed by rhythmic body jerking during the clonic phase. During complex partial seizures patients stare or have impaired awareness, with one-sided body stiffening or fidgeting. The duration of these seizures is also approximately 2 minutes. A patient may become confused (postictal) after a complex partial seizure or it may progress into a tonic clonic seizure. Absence seizures (petit mal) occur less often in adults. These seizures last only a few seconds with eye blinking or staring and have no postictal confusion. Myoclonic jerks are quick single jerks of the body and are usually part of an epilepsy syndrome, juvenile myoclonic epilepsy. Simple partial seizures involve a confined area of cerebral cortex so consciousness is not impaired. Clinical symptoms of simple partial seizures depend on the location of seizure activity. If it is contained in the motor cortex, then a Jacksonian seizure of unilateral clonic activity will ensue. Auras are actually simple partial seizures and are localized to the temporal lobe when *déjà vu* or fear is experienced, or to the olfactory cortex when smell is experienced. Auras may progress into complex partial or generalized tonic clonic seizures. A detailed history from the patient and eyewitnesses can help determine the classification. An electroencephalogram (EEG) is abnormal in greater than 50% of patients with epilepsy but can be normal. A magnetic resonance image (MRI) of the brain is preferred over computed tomography (CT) since it can detect small areas of scarring or low-grade gliomas that are the seizure nidus and that CT may not detect.

Syncope is a common occurrence in the first trimester of pregnancy and can be confused with epilepsy and seizures. A good eyewitness account is paramount. Often the patient will describe tachycardia, tunnel vision, sweating and dizziness prior to fainting. After a syncopal event there should be no postictal confusion. New-onset epilepsy during pregnancy is uncommon and requires a detailed history and physical examination, and urgent evaluation with EEG and brain MRI to exclude an intracerebral hemorrhage or tumor. A history of febrile seizures, developmental delay, head trauma, meningitis or encephalitis, or a family history of epilepsy should raise the suspicion for a diagnosis of epilepsy. Later in the pregnancy, seizures may be associated with eclampsia.

Antiepileptic drug use during pregnancy

How AEDs interfere with fetal development and cause teratogenic effects is not completely known but clearly is medication dependent. Some mechanisms for teratogenicity may include folate depletion, epoxide formation, and suppression of neuronal signaling. This may lead to major malformation (neural tube, cleft lip/palate and cardiac are most common), minor malformations (nail and facial dysmorphism) or cognitive impairment in an exposed fetus. Fetal loss is also increased in women with epilepsy taking AEDs. Exposure to two or more AEDs

Management of Common Problems in Obstetrics and Gynecology, 5th edition. Edited by T.M. Goodwin, M.N. Montoro, L. Muderspach, R. Paulson and S. Roy. © 2010 Blackwell Publishing Ltd.

during pregnancy greatly increases major malformation rates, probably by introducing multiple mechanisms of teratogenicity. The older AEDs are all FDA pregnancy category D while the new AEDs are category C at this time. Many believe all AEDs will eventually be category D once more data are collected. Folic acid supplementation may be beneficial.

Valproate appears to be more teratogenic than similar medications. Recent studies and worldwide AED prospective registry data have shown that the major malformation risk is approximately 11% (6–24%) as compared to 3–4% for most other monotherapy AED exposures. The teratogenic effects are also dose dependent with higher rates seen when taking doses over 1000 mg per day. Birth defects are varied but include neural tube defects, hypospadias, renal anomalies, cardiac and limb malformations. Switching to another AED prior to conception is advised.

Phenobarbital has recently been shown to have a higher birth defect rate compared to other AEDs: 6.5% versus 3–4%. Birth defects with phenobarbital include cleft lip and/or palate, and cardiac abnormalities. Primidone is metabolized into two byproducts, one of which is phenobarbital. Therefore, it should be considered equally teratogenic. With the advent of newer AEDs, phenobarbital's use has waned in recent years although due to its low cost it is still used extensively worldwide. If this drug is to be withdrawn prior to pregnancy, it must be tapered off slowly (months) to prevent withdrawal seizures.

Phenytoin exposure *in utero* has been associated with a fetal hydantoin syndrome (craniofacial anomalies, limb defects) and has a major malformation rate of approximately 4%, cardiac abnormalities being most prevalent. Its mechanism of toxicity may be due to the epoxide byproduct.

Carbamazepine is the AED of choice for partial-onset seizures. Although it is category D, malformation rates are approximately 2.5% with cleft lip/palate 0.5% and neural tube defect ~1% predominating. Higher malformation rates were seen in the past and rates may have decreased with the ubiquitous use of folate supplementation. Oxcarbazepine is chemically similar to carbamazepine but does not form the 10,11 epoxide when metabolized. Regardless of this fact, it does not appear to be safer than carbamazepine during pregnancy.

Lamotrigine has the most pregnancy data of the newer agents, with more than 1000 monotherapy exposures registered. Although birth defect rates are comparable to other AEDs (~3%), one registry found an increase in cleft lip and/or palate (0.89%) and another registry found a dose-dependent birth defect rate for doses greater than 200 mg a day. Lamotrigine levels in particular fall dramatically during pregnancy and require frequent level checks (monthly or more) and reduction of the dose in the first 2 weeks post partum to prevent toxicity.

Leviteracetam is a widely used newer AED. Its major malformation rate is approximately 3.5%. Premature births and low birthweights have been described with its use. Topiramate, zonisamide, gabapentin and pregabalin have limited pregnancy data available. Benzodiazepines can cause a syndrome similar to fetal alcohol syndrome.

There is much debate regarding the appropriate vitamin supplementation for pregnant women with epilepsy taking AEDs. Women taking AEDs need more than the FDA recommended 0.4 mg of folic acid to prevent neural tube birth defects but the optimal dose (1–4 mg) is not known. In addition, taking a high dose of folate, 4 mg a day, prior to conception does not guarantee protection against birth defects. Supplementing with oral vitamin K 10 mg a day in the last month of pregnancy may prevent neonatal hemorrhagic syndrome due to its deficiency from AED liver enzyme induction.

A high-risk perinatologist should follow women on these AEDs. Amniocentesis should be offered early to women with carbamazepine and valproate exposures. Triple screen testing should be offered to all others. A high-level anatomy scan in the second trimester is crucial in detecting abnormalities.

Managing seizures during pregnancy and delivery

Seizures can harm both the mother and fetus during pregnancy. Seizures have been associated with premature rupture of membranes, premature labor, abruption, fetal bradycardia and hypoxia. Generalized tonic clonic seizures pose the greatest risk to the mother and fetus although complex partial seizures can also cause similar injury and prolonged fetal bradycardia. Injury to the mother occurs during falls associated with the seizure, resulting in abdominal or head trauma, bone fractures, thermal burns, and aspiration. Therefore seizures should be prevented with appropriate therapy.

Seizure control during pregnancy often reflects seizure control prior to conception but breakthrough seizures occur for a number of reasons. The most common reason is stopping AEDs abruptly when the pregnancy is discovered. Stopping phenobarbital in particular will provoke withdrawal seizures and can provoke status epilepticus. Nausea and vomiting due to morning sickness or hyperemesis gravidarum will prohibit proper ingestion and absorption of medication, leading to seizures. In those patients who are prone to seizures after sleep deprivation, seizures may also occur as sleep deteriorates in the third trimester due to discomfort.

Another factor contributing to breakthrough seizure activity is alteration of AED levels during pregnancy. Increased metabolism, renal clearance, volume of distribution and hormones can lower AED levels. Conversely, protein binding decreases during pregnancy, thereby effectively increasing the free (active) drug. Often these opposing factors will negate each other and no medication adjustment is required, with the exception of lamotrigine and oxcarbazepine. These two AEDs have been associated with the most breakthrough seizures during pregnancy and their levels need to be checked often (monthly) and dose increased accordingly. If high doses are needed to maintain levels, changing from a bid to tid dosing schedule may improve seizure coverage. In the postpartum period, lamotrigine and oxcarbazepine doses need to be lowered to avoid toxicity. Otherwise, most practitioners check AED levels each trimester and then prior to delivery. If seizure-free patients begin having auras or myoclonic jerks then medications need to be increased to prevent an impending generalized tonic clonic seizure. Having pre-pregnancy serum AED levels can help guide dose adjustments during pregnancy.

A diagnosis of epilepsy alone is not a contraindication to a vaginal delivery. If epilepsy is due to a structural lesion causing raised intracranial pressure or a vascular lesion that may rupture during delivery, a cesarean section is advised. Patients with seizures triggered by sleep deprivation may have breakthrough seizure activity if labor is prolonged with minimal rest. In addition, if patients are not allowed to take their regular AEDs during labor, a seizure may result. If no caveats exist, then vaginal delivery can occur safely.

Status epilepticus is a medical emergency and should be treated similarly to the nonpregnant state. Technically it is defined as 30 minutes of continuous seizure activity or two seizures without return to baseline consciousness although treatment should begin if seizure activity is longer than 10 minutes. Intravenous lorazepam should be given in 2 mg increments every 2 minutes up to 0.1 mg/kg. This should be followed by intravenous fosphenytoin or phenytoin 20 mg/kg. If eclampsia is suspected, intravenous magnesium should also be given.

Breastfeeding and the postpartum period

The benefits of breastfeeding and breast milk have been well documented. Antiepileptic agents do enter breast milk at variable rates. The more highly protein bound a medication is, the less it enters the breast milk (example carbamazepine, phenytoin, valproate). Since the newer AEDs are less protein bound (e.g. lamotrigine, leviteracetam, and oxcarbazepine), they are passed more freely into breast milk. Phenobarbital, although highly protein bound, can accumulate in the neonate due to decreased liver metabolism of the drug and cause excessive sedation. Therefore breastfeeding with phenobarbital is undertaken with extreme caution. Some groups advocate breastfeeding while taking AEDs since the benefit of breast milk outweighs the risk of the medication with diligent observation of the neonate for signs of sedation, poor feeding or poor weight gain. In these situations, changing over to formula is advisable. One can also obtain serum levels of the AED in the breastfed infants for closer monitoring.

Instruction in infant safety is important for women with epilepsy. Since seizures may occur without warning, mothers should not bath infants alone in standing water and should always use a strap on a changing table. Sponge baths are acceptable. Patients with frequent seizures should avoid carrying the baby up and down stairs when possible. During breastfeeding, consider sitting on the floor to avoid injury to the baby should a seizure occur. Patients who are known to have seizures triggered by sleep deprivation should get assistance with night feeds. Obtaining less than 6 hours uninterrupted sleep could put vulnerable patients at risk for seizures.

Preconception counseling and consideration of AED withdrawal

As a group, women with epilepsy do not experience decreased fertility, although women with epilepsy are more prone to polycystic ovarian syndrome and a history of irregular menstrual cycles may warrant further investigation. The etiology may be multifactorial: weight gain from antiseizure medications, the medications themselves or ongoing epileptic discharges on EEG. Women with uncontrolled seizures may also experience premature ovarian failure. These issues should be factored into family planning decisions.

The best medication for a woman with epilepsy during pregnancy is usually the medication that works the best to control her seizures. This is not the case for women taking valproate or phenobarbital; one should strongly consider changing these to another agent prior to conception due to the high birth defect rate. Phenobarbital needs to be tapered slowly over months since rapid discontinuation will lead to withdrawal seizures. Since fetal exposure to two or more medications results in higher birth defect rates, reducing the AED regimen to one agent should be considered.

Of course, if an AED is no longer needed, eliminating fetal exposure to AEDs is best. If a patient has been seizure free for greater than 2 years it may be possible to withdraw medication if the EEG and MRI are normal. Cases in which it is inadvisable to withdraw medication would be with a genetic form of epilepsy or when epilepsy is due to a structural lesion or there is a history of meningitis, febrile seizures or head trauma. In these circumstances, there is a greater than 50% recurrence if medication is withdrawn. Neurology consultation is warranted to make a final determination. If an AED is changed or stopped, driving should be suspended until the new agent is proven to be safe and effective against the woman's seizures.

Contraception will be needed until AEDs are optimized. Barrier methods are the preferred form of birth control since OCP efficacy may be reduced by medications that interfere with the P450 liver enzyme metabolism (e.g. carbamazepine, phenytoin, phenobarbital). If OCP use is needed while taking an enzyme-inducing AED, using an OCP with 50 µg of estrogen can be tried. Valproic acid, lamotrigine, and most newer agents do not interfere (see Table 25.1). Topiramate in doses > 200 mg and oxcarbazepine in doses higher than 1200 mg interfere with OCPs. Lamotrigine dose not interfere with OCP efficacy but OCPs reduce lamotrigine levels and may cause breakthrough seizures if the dose is not adjusted. Folic acid supplementation with 1 mg should be prescribed to all women taking AEDs since the rate of unplanned pregnancies is high. Up to 4 mg a day should be given to women actively attempting to conceive.

Headaches in pregnancy

Headache is a common complaint during pregnancy, especially during the first trimester. Most often it is due to a benign etiology such as migraine or tension headache but on occasion it can herald a serious neurologic condition. Some headache syndromes actually improve during pregnancy. A detailed history and physical exam can usually exclude most worrisome causes of headache. If needed, neuroimaging with MRI or CT can be done safely with precautions. On the other hand, management of headaches during pregnancy can be challenging due to limited medication options.

New-onset headache

Fortunately, most headaches that begin during pregnancy are self-limited and improve as the pregnancy progresses.

Table 25.1 Properties of antiepileptic drugs (AEDs)

AED	Significant excretion into breast milk	Interferes with OCP	Pregnancy category
Carbamazepine	No	Yes	D
Lamotrigine	Yes	No	C
Phenytoin	No	Yes	D
Topiramate	Yes	At > 200 mg	C
Gabapentin	Yes	No	C
Pregabalin	Yes	No	C
Valproic acid, divalproate	No	No	D
Phenobarbital	No*	Yes	D
Clonazepam	Yes	No	D
Zonisamide	Yes	No	C
Oxcarbazepine	Yes	At > 1200mg	C
Levetiracetam	Yes	No	C

OCP, oral contraceptive pill.
* Metabolites can accumulate in neonate.

Associated symptoms of altered consciousness, focal weakness and numbness or papilledema indicate that a headache is of a more serious nature. Headaches that are exclusively on one side of the head may represent an underlying abnormality. Acute life-threatening headaches are most often encountered in an emergency room setting and patients complain of the "worst headache of my life." Rapid-onset headaches with altered consciousness signal possible intracerebral bleeding, subarachnoid hemorrhage or meningitis.

Cerebral aneurysms and arteriovenous malformations (AVM) may grow during pregnancy and are most likely to rupture in the third trimester or early postpartum period, causing subarachnoid hemorrhage or intracerebral hemorrhage with severe headache and depressed mental sensorium. Stroke, either ischemic or hemorrhagic, can present with headache but can be painless. Patients with stroke will have acute onset of neurologic deficits due to occlusion of the cerebral blood vessel or rupture and hemorrhage into cerebral tissue. A prior hypercoagulable state can be unmasked during pregnancy and become symptomatic this way. Meningitis presents with fever, headache, stiff neck, and photophobia.

A noncontrast head CT is the best way to detect acute blood and can be obtained quickly in most emergency rooms. Some subarachnoid hemorrhage can be missed on head CT and a lumbar puncture looking for blood or degrading blood products (xanthochromia) should be performed in patients in whom there is a high suspicion for subarachnoid hemorrhage clinically but a negative head CT. MRI of the brain is sensitive for structural abnormalities and special diffusion-weighted images can detect acute strokes. A lumbar puncture is essential in diagnosing meningitis.

Less likely causes of progressive headache are pseudotumor cerebri or brain tumor resulting in raised intracranial pressure. These headaches occur daily, but are worse in the morning and improve over the day. Pseudotumor cerebri can present for the first time during pregnancy since weight gain can be a trigger. Funduscopic exam will show papilledema. If neuroimaging is normal, a lumbar puncture should be performed to measure the opening pressure and confirm the diagnosis. Repeated lumbar punctures can acutely reduce raised intracranial pressure followed by treatment with acetazolamide. Visual field monitoring is essential since persistent elevated cerebral spinal fluid pressures will damage the optic nerves. Brain tumors rarely present during pregnancy but should be considered when patients have purely unilateral headache with focal neurologic signs or seizures. Some tumors can enlarge during pregnancy, such as meningiomas and pituitary adenomas. One way to monitor pituitary adenoma growth is with visual field testing. Patients with ventriculoperitoneal shunts for hydrocephalus may experience worsening of headaches if the output drain to their shunt is blocked in the abdomen by the expanding uterus.

Migraine with aura often presents for the first time during pregnancy. The most common migraine aura is a visual disturbance of shimmering lights surrounding an expanding blind spot. Description of the visual aura can be vague and some patients will complain of loss or blurred vision prior to the headache. The "aura" is not limited to visual symptoms and some patients will experience dizziness, numbness or tingling prior to their headache. The headache pain may not be that severe and can be overlooked if no inquiry is made. Migraine with aura should be a diagnosis of exclusion only after full neurologic evaluation and neuroimaging are completed.

Chronic headaches during pregnancy

Migraine is the most common headache syndrome in women, affecting approximately one in five. Since migraine is most prevalent during the child-bearing years, it is often encountered during pregnancy. Fortunately, most migraine sufferers (50–80%) will have significant improvement or complete remission during pregnancy. Migraine without aura and menstrual migraine are more likely to improve during pregnancy than migraine with aura. If a woman has been taking preventive medication for her migraines, such as propranolol, amitriptyline, topiramate or valproic acid, and unexpectedly becomes pregnant she should stop her medication since there is a high likelihood that her migraines will improve on their own.

Migraines are easily diagnosed with a thorough history and normal exam. Migraine headaches are usually one-sided although they can occur bilaterally. Migraine pain has a throbbing quality and there is associated light and sound sensitivity. Nausea and vomiting often but not always accompany the headache. When the pain is located in the frontal and temporal regions it is often misdiagnosed as sinus headache. When migraine pain is located in the occipital region and/or neck, it is often misdiagnosed as neck strain. Regular triggers (certain foods, lack of sleep, missing meals, stress, etc.) can also help establish the diagnosis of migraine. Migraines are usually worse in the afternoon although some women can be woken from sleep with one.

Migraine treatment consists of two arms: abortive and preventive. In the acute setting, intravenous narcotics and antiemetics can be used. Intravenous magnesium (1 g magnesium sulfate) has also been used acutely with success. Other preferred abortive medications include acetaminophen, Vicodin®, and acetaminophen with codeine. Of the triptan drugs, sumatriptan (Imitrex®) has the most pregnancy data and is felt to be safe if used sparingly. Combination pills often contain caffeine and therefore are less desirable. Analgesics that were used prior to conception such as aspirin or ibuprofen should be avoided.

Strategies to prevent migraines include trigger identification, relaxation techniques, and medication. Identification and elimination of migraine triggers can limit the need for both abortive and preventive medications. Lack of sleep and missing meals are often more significant triggers than specific foods. Other common triggers are stress, glare, and strong odors. Biofeedback, prenatal yoga and other relaxation techniques may be helpful. Patients should wear dark sunglasses when going outside to avoid glare and request family members or colleagues not to wear strong perfumes. Neck massage and cold packs to the head can all be done safely.

If conservative measures fail to provide relief and migraines are frequent enough to inhibit daily activities, preventive medications should be initiated. Oral magnesium preparations (magnesium oxide 400–800 mg daily), and riboflavin (up to 400 mg a day) are known migraine prophylactic agents and can be used safely in pregnancy. Because of their safety, consider using these as the first line for prophylaxis during pregnancy. Low-dose amitriptyline or propranolol are usually first line as daily prophylaxis medication. If needed, these medications should be started in the second trimester and risks and benefits discussed with the patient.

Other chronic headaches such as tension headaches and chronic daily headaches may occur or persist during pregnancy. Tension headaches have a band-like or helmet-like pressure pain. The preventive and abortive measures described above can be tried. Some patients will experience caffeine withdrawal headaches if they abruptly stop caffeine use when the pregnancy is discovered. Reintroduction of low-dose caffeine (e.g. green tea) may be necessary. Daily use of analgesics can produce rebound headaches and overuse of prescribed medications should be monitored.

Postpartum headache and breastfeeding

In the postpartum period the most common headache is migraine. Other headaches include tension headaches, postdural puncture headaches, and pain from venous sinus thrombosis. Unfortunately, migraines that remitted during pregnancy often return in the postpartum period. Breastfeeding may delay the return of migraines but not significantly. Certain migraine medications can be used during lactation (see Table 25.2). Postdural puncture headaches are diagnosed if the patient had epidural or spinal anesthesia and the headache is better in the supine position. Conservative treatment with non-steroidal anti-inflammatory drugs and caffeine should be tried first before a blood patch is performed. Venous sinus thrombosis can present in the postpartum period with severe headache, focal neurologic signs and seizures. Emergency neurologic evaluation and treatment are needed to prevent long-term disability.

Table 25.2 Migraine medication and lactation

Compatible	Caution
Ibuprofen	Aspirin
Naprosyn	Other triptans
Acetaminophen	Ergotamine
Codeine	Caffeine combination pills
Meperidine	Amitriptyline
Sumatriptan	Valproic acid
Magnesium	

Table 25.3 Migraine prevention in pregnancy

Compound	Class of drug	Pregnancy category	FDA approved for migraine
Propranolol	β-blocker	C	
Verapamil	Calcium channel blocker	C	
Lisinoprill, candesartan	ACE/angio II	C first trimester	
		D third trimester	
Amitriptyline, nortriptyline	Tricyclic antidepressant	D	
Venlafaxine	SNRI reuptake inhibitor	C	
Valproic acid	Anticonvulsant	D	Yes
Topiramate	Anticonvulsant	C	Yes
Gabapentin	Anticonvulsant	C	
Magnesium	Alternative	B	
Riboflavin (B2)	Alternative	B	
Feverfew	Alternative	Unknown	
Butterbur	Alternative	Unknown	

Suggested reading

Epilepsy

Harden CL, Hopp J, Ting TY, *et al.* Practice parameter update: management issues for women with epilepsy – focus on pregnancy (an evidence-based review): obstetrical complications and change in seizure frequency. Report of the Quality Standards Subcommittee and Therapeutics and Technology Assessment Subcommittee of the American Academy of Neurology and American Epilepsy Society. *Neurology* 2009; 73: 126–132.

Harden CL, Meador KJ, Pennell PB, *et al.* Practice parameter update: management issues for women with epilepsy – focus on pregnancy (an evidence-based review): teratogenesis and perinatal outcomes. Report of the Quality Standards Subcommittee and Therapeutics and Technology Assessment Subcommittee of the American Academy of Neurology and American Epilepsy Society. *Neurology* 2009; 73: 133-141.

Harden CL, Pennell PB, Koppel BS, *et al.* Practice Parameter update: management issues for women with epilepsy – focus on pregnancy (an evidence-based review): vitamin K, folic acid, blood levels, and breastfeeding. Report of the Quality Standards Subcommittee and Therapeutics and Technology Assessment Subcommittee of the American Academy of Neurology and American Epilepsy Society. *Neurology* 2009; 73: 142–149.

Headache

Loder E. Migraine in pregnancy. *Semin Neurol* 2007; 27: 425–433.

Marcus DA, Scharff L, Turk D. Longitudinal prospective study of headache during pregnancy and postpartum. *Headache* 1999; 39(9): 625–632.

Sances G, Granella F, Nappi RE, *et al.* Course of migraine during pregnancy and postpartum: a prospective study. *Cephalalgia* 2003; 23(3): 197–205.

Chapter 26
Anemia and Thrombocytopenia in Pregnancy

Patrick M. Mullin and T. Murphy Goodwin

Department of Medicine and Obstetrics and Gynecology, Keck School of Medicine, University of Southern California, CA, USA

Anemia

Anemia affects more than half of pregnant women in the United States, and is one of the most common problems encountered in pregnancy. It has long been recognized that there is a "relative anemia" in pregnancy that occurs as a result of the disproportionate increase in plasma volume in relation to the red cell volume. The mean plasma volume increases in pregnancy by approximately 40–45% over the mean nonpregnant plasma volume. The result is a fall in erythrocyte count, hemoglobin, and hematocrit. The consequence of this process is a physiologic anemia, which is not a disease but rather a symptom that can be reversed in most instances.

Guidelines have been established to aid clinicians in establishing the diagnosis of nonphysiologic anemia. In the first and third trimesters, the lower limits of normal are 11 g/dL for hemoglobin and 33% for hematocrit. In the second trimester the lower limits are 10.5 g/dL for hemoglobin and 32% for hematocrit.

Etiology of anemia in pregnancy

The first step in recognizing the etiology of any anemia is to obtain the appropriate history, physical examination, and laboratory tests. This initial step will aid in the formulation of the differential diagnosis to distinguish between an acquired and inherited anemia. While pregnant patients with anemia are often asymptomatic, in part because of the increase in blood volume, clinical findings can be identified, such as glossitis (nutritional deficiencies), jaundice (hemolytic problems), petechiae (coagulopathies) or skeletal abnormalities (hemoglobin sickle cell anemias), which suggest the presence of anemia.

Management of Common Problems in Obstetrics and Gynecology, 5th edition. Edited by T.M. Goodwin, M.N. Montoro, L. Muderspach, R. Paulson and S. Roy. © 2010 Blackwell Publishing Ltd.

The basic laboratory work-up includes a complete blood count, peripheral blood smear, iron studies, and urinalysis. Patients at risk for sickle cell anemia or thalassemia should also have a hemoglobin electrophoresis.

Nutritional deficiency anemias

Iron deficiency anemia

The most common cause of anemia in pregnancy is iron deficiency – it accounts for about 95% of anemia seen during pregnancy. The ideal body iron content in the adult woman is 3.5–4 g with approximately 60–70% contained in circulating hemoglobin and the remainder stored as ferritin and hemosiderin in the liver, spleen, and bone marrow. Absence of hemosiderin in the bone marrow indicates that iron stores are exhausted.

The World Health Organization and most experts recommend prevention of iron deficiency anemia with prophylactic iron supplementation in pregnancy. Pregnancy requires an additional 700–1200 mg of iron. Of this, 200–300 mg is transferred to the fetus. Most of the iron requirements of pregnancy are in the second half of pregnancy, and they are approximately 5–6 mg/day. An average balanced diet will supply only 1–2 mg/day. Daily supplementation with 300 mg ferrous sulfate (which contains 60 mg elemental iron) will satisfy the pregnancy requirements; it is recognized that only 10–15% of the ingested iron is being absorbed.

The consequence of iron deficiency is a microcytic, hypochromic anemia with red cells showing a mean corpuscular volume (MCV) of less than 80 femtoliters (fL). Serum iron studies typically demonstrate a decrease in serum iron, low serum ferritin, and an increase in serum total iron-binding capacity.

When iron deficiency anemia is identified, the treatment requires the administration of 900 mg of oral ferrous sulfate daily. On occasion, some women will require parenteral iron therapy given as iron dextran. Each 2 mL vial of iron dextran provides 100 mg of elemental iron. The rapidity of response of parenteral therapy is the same as for oral iron.

A rise in hemoglobin concentration of 0.2 g/dL associated with an increase in reticulocyte count indicates that the patient is responding to treatment. Blood transfusion is seldom required, and the potential risks for blood-borne infections (hepatitis, cytomegalovirus, HIV) must be weighed carefully before transfusion is recommended. At hemoglobin levels of 4–6 g/dL there is some risk for high-output cardiac failure in the mother and somewhat less of a risk for fetal hypoxia.

Vitamin deficiency megaloblastic anemias

The two most common megaloblastic conditions acquired in pregnancy are caused by folate deficiency and vitamin B12 deficiency. Both vitamin B12 and folate deficiency delay DNA synthesis and can result in megaloblastic anemias. Megaloblastic anemia is a nonspecific term utilized to describe hypoproliferative disorders that have characteristic hematocytopathic features, evidence of inadequate erythropoiesis, and/or hemolysis of red blood cells. The most prominent clinical features of severe megaloblastic anemias are roughness of the skin and glossitis. Folic acid deficiency is the most common cause for megaloblastic anemia, while vitamin B12 deficiency is extremely uncommon during pregnancy.

The diagnosis of folic acid deficiency anemia is usually made late in pregnancy or in the puerperium. Diagnostic laboratory tests show a macrocytic anemia (MCV above 100 fL) with hypersegmentation of the polymorphonuclear leukocytes, decreased reticulocyte count, and a decreased serum folate (normal folate values in pregnancy are 5–10 mg/μL). The natural history of folate deficiency is such that the sequential events usually observed are: decrease in serum folate in 3 weeks, appearance of hypersegmented neutrophils in 7 weeks, a decrease in red cell folate in 18 weeks, a megaloblastic bone marrow in 19 weeks, with clinical anemia presenting in 20 weeks. Among the late fetal effects of folate deficiency are low birthweight and fetal growth restriction. An association with placental abruption and pre-eclampsia/eclampsia has been reported but not definitively established.

A variety of factors contribute to folic acid deficiency in pregnancy: multiple pregnancy, inadequate diet, excessive hyperemesis, chronic infection, ethanol, drugs (nitrofurantoin, hydantoin), and inherited defects in folate metabolism.

The recommended daily allowance of folate during pregnancy is 800 μg/day. Dietary intake of up to 400 μg of folate can be achieved with a well-rounded diet. An additional 400 μg of synthetic folate from fortified foods or supplements is recommended. The treatment of anemia caused by folate deficiency is 4 mg of folate PO per day as soon as the condition is recognized.

Vitamin B12 deficiency (pernicious anemia) is primarily caused by deficiency in oral absorption. The most common type is that caused by autoimmune atrophic gastritis, which occurs most frequently in patients of Scandinavian and Northern European ancestry as well as those of Hispanic origins. This condition usually presents in women between 30 and 40 years of age. Rare causes of vitamin B12 deficiency, which should be considered, include infection by the fish tapeworm *Diphyllobothrium latum*, and chronic conditions such as Crohn's disease. The diagnosis is made in patients demonstrating a macrocytic anemia with an abnormally low serum vitamin B12 level.

Treatment of patients with pernicious anemia is undertaken with parenteral therapy because oral absorption of vitamin B12 is deficient. Daily injections of 200 μg are given for the first week followed by weekly injections for 3 weeks and then once a month thereafter. Importantly, therapy must continue for life to prevent recurrence of anemia. Response to therapy is usually manifested by a brisk production of reticulocytes within the first few days of therapy.

Hemoglobinopathies

Sickle cell disease

Sickle cell anemia is inherited in an autosomal recessive pattern and results in the formation of hemoglobin S through the genetic substitution of valine for glutamic acid at codon 6 of the β globin chains. Hemoglobin S causes red blood cells to become sickle shaped in the presence of decreased oxygen tension. Patients homozygous for the hemoglobin S allele have "sickle cell anemia," those heterozygous have "sickle cell trait." In the USA, about 10% of African Americans have sickle cell trait, and 1 in 500 has sickle cell anemia. A relatively common associated condition is hemoglobin S/C disease. This condition occurs in people who are heterozygous for both the S and another abnormal hemoglobin allele, C. In this condition maternal mortality rates are as high as 2–3% and it is peculiarly associated with embolization of necrotic fat and cellular bone marrow with resultant respiratory insufficiency.

Screening for sickle cell disease with the Sickledex test involves mixing 2 mL of sodium dithionite reagent with 20 μL of blood. The presence of hemoglobin S causes clouding of the solution. Hemoglobin electrophoresis can then be used to differentiate between the homozygous and heterozygous states.

Prenatal genetic counseling is of great importance. If both partners have the gene for S hemoglobin, their offspring have a one in four chance of having sickle cell anemia. Fetal DNA isolated from amniotic fluid cells or via chorionic villous sampling can be evaluated by polymerase chain reaction (PCR) to detect a hemoglobinopathy in pregnancies at risk.

Pregnancy has deleterious effects on sickle cell disease. There are increased rates of maternal mortality and morbidity from hemolytic and folic acid deficiency anemias, frequent crises, pulmonary complications, congestive heart failure, infection, and pre-eclampsia/eclampsia. In addition, there is an increased incidence of early fetal wastage, stillbirth, preterm delivery, and intrauterine growth restriction. Good prenatal care, avoidance of complications, and prompt effective treatment for complications are necessary for a good outcome of pregnancy.

Sickle cell disease is characterized by chronic hemolytic anemia and other chronic problems. The most common manifestations of sickle cell disease include increased susceptibility to bacterial infection; bacterial pneumonia, segmental bronchopneumonia, and pulmonary infarction; myocardial damage and cardiomegaly; and functional and anatomic renal abnormalities in the form of sickle cell nephropathy or papillary renal necrosis, resulting in hematuria.

Acute sickle cell crisis occurs with variable frequency and severity in different patients. Pain crises involve the bones and joints. These are usually precipitated by dehydration or infection. An aplastic crisis is characterized by rapidly developing anemia. The hemoglobin decreases to 2–3 g/dL due to cessation of red blood cell production. An acute splenic sequestration crisis is associated with severe anemia and hypovolemic shock, resulting from sudden massive trapping of red blood cells within the splenic sinusoids.

While persons with sickle cell trait are not anemic and are usually asymptomatic, they have twice as many urinary tract infections as normal women. Additionally, their red blood cells tend to sickle when oxygen tension is significantly lowered; thus, hypoventilation during general anesthesia may be fatal.

Antepartum management involves ultrasound evaluation to assess fetal growth and biophysical monitoring for fetal surveillance. Adequate intrapartum pain relief is essential and hypoxia must be prevented during general anesthesia by maintaining adequate oxygenation and ventilation. Cesarean section should be carried out at the earliest sign of fetal compromise for the best perinatal outcome.

Hemolysis of the defective red blood cells and the resulting increased hematopoiesis causes a megaloblastic anemia. While iron therapy will not correct the anemia, folic acid 1 mg/day is necessary to compensate for the shortened red blood cell life span. Monthly urine cultures are recommended to screen for asymptomatic bacteriuria. Pneumococcal polyvalent vaccine has been shown to reduce the incidence of pneumococcal infection in adults with sickle cell disease, and therefore it is highly recommended. *Haemophilus influenzae* type B vaccine should be considered in patients who have undergone autosplenectomy. In the management of crises, predisposing factors should be sought and eliminated, if possible. Symptomatic treatment for a pain crisis

consists of intravenous fluid and adequate analgesics (e.g. meperidine or codeine). Bacterial pneumonia or pyelonephritis must be treated rigorously with intravenous antibiotics. In all cases, adequate oxygenation must be maintained by facemask as necessary.

The concentration of hemoglobin S should be less than 50% of the total hemoglobin to prevent crisis. Blood transfusion should be considered in cases of a fall in hematocrit to less than 25%; repeated crisis; symptoms of tachycardia, palpitation, dyspnea, or fatigue; or evidence of fetal growth restriction.

Prophylactic hypertransfusion or exchange transfusion to prevent maternal complications, improve uteroplacental perfusion, and achieve a better perinatal outcome has been advocated by some, but these methods are not universally accepted. Transfusion always carries a risk of allergic reaction, delayed hemolytic reaction with rapid fall in hemoglobin A, and transmission of HIV or hepatitis. Isoimmunization may also occur. Hemolytic disease of the newborn or transfusion reactions due to incorrect cross-matching of blood may occur if careful blood typing is not done. The use of fresh buffy coat-poor washed packed cells for exchange transfusion will help in avoiding transfusion reactions. Oral contraceptives are avoided because of the risk of thromboembolism.

Thalassemia

The thalassemias are a group of autosomal recessive disorders affecting the synthesis of the normal hemoglobin found in adults, hemoglobin A, which contains two α globin and two β globin chains ($\alpha_2\beta_2$). The two major thalassemias, α and β, are found throughout the world but are most prevalent in persons of Mediterranean, Central African, and South-east Asian descent.

Production of α globin is controlled by a total of four copies of the α globin gene, with two copies residing on each chromosome 16. Fetal hemoglobin F ($\alpha_2\gamma_2$) and all normal hemoglobins of postnatal life contain α chains. Therefore, the severity of α thalassemia is directly related to the number of deleted α globin genes. In α (0) thalassemia, also called hemoglobin Barts, all four α globin genes are deleted which prevents formation of normal hemoglobin. This results in hydrops fetalis and, typically, fetal demise. The most severe form of α thalassemia compatible with extrauterine life is hemoglobin H (β_4) disease in which three of the four α globin genes are deleted. The remaining normal α globin gene allows for the production of normal fetal hemoglobin F and adult hemoglobin A, but the overproduction of β globin chains leads to the formation of hemoglobin H as well. The presence of hemoglobin H, a poor transporter of oxygen, can cause development of hydrops fetalis. After delivery, neonatal jaundice and anemia are seen. Women with hemoglobin H disease have anemia of variable levels that is usually worsened in pregnancy.

In α thalassemia minor, two α globin genes are deleted, causing a mild hypochromic, microcytic anemia that must be differentiated from iron deficiency anemia. α Thalassemia minima results from a single α globin gene deletion and commonly has no clinical effects. Women with these conditions tolerate pregnancy well.

β Thalassemia results from impaired β globin chain production. A single β globin gene resides on each chromosome 11. β Thalassemia major is the homozygous state, in which there is little or no production of β chains. The fetus with β thalassemia major is protected from severe disease because fetal hemoglobin F ($\alpha_2\gamma_2$) contains no β globin chain. However, this protection disappears at birth, when fetal hemoglobin production terminates. At about 1 year of age, a baby with β thalassemia major usually begins to show signs (anemia, hepatosplenomegaly) and requires frequent blood transfusions. Death in the late teens or early twenties can occur because of congestive heart failure, often related to myocardial hemosiderosis, and liver failure. However, improved treatment with transfusion and iron chelation therapy has led to overall improved survival and even successful pregnancies in women with β thalassemia major.

β Thalassemia minor, the heterozygous state, is frequently diagnosed only after the patient fails to respond to iron therapy or delivers a baby with homozygous disease. Such patients usually suffer from hypochromic microcytic anemia and show an increased red blood cell count, elevated hemoglobin A_2 ($\alpha_2\delta_2$) concentrations, increased serum iron levels, and iron saturation greater than 20%. Suspected adult cases of thalassemia are diagnosed by hemoglobin electrophoresis. Antenatal diagnosis of thalassemia is possible by molecular analysis of fetal cells obtained via amniocentesis or chorionic villous sampling. Preimplantation genetic analysis is also available and allows for the transfer of unaffected embryos.

Thrombocytopenia

The approach to thrombocytopenia in pregnancy changed with the wide availability of the automated blood counts (CBC) in the mid 1980s. It is now common for the obstetrician to be faced with a low platelet count of uncertain significance.

The first step is to confirm that thrombocytopenia exists by making sure the peripheral smear does not show platelet clumping. Next, the CBC is examined to note whether white cells or red cells are affected in addition to platelets. The size of the platelets is also noted by looking at the smear or by observing the mean platelet volume (MPV) on the CBC report. In the vast majority of cases seen during pregnancy, the thrombocytopenia is isolated and the platelets are near or above the upper limit of normal size. The cause of the thrombocytopenia in such cases is peripheral destruction. If the thrombocytopenia does not fit this pattern, it is our practice to seek consultation with the hematologist promptly.

The major differential diagnosis of thrombocytopenia due to peripheral destruction includes immune mechanisms; ITP, systemic lupus erythematosus (SLE), antiphospholipid syndrome (APS), infection (HIV, hepatitis C, sepsis), medications, disseminated intravascular coagulation (DIC), pre-eclampsia, and pregnancy-associated thrombocytopenia (PAT). Our approach to this pattern of thrombocytopenia is based on an understanding of the characteristics of PAT. It is by far the most common cause of this pattern of thrombocytopenia (occurring in 5% of all pregnancies), but is of no known pathologic significance. It rarely presents before 30 weeks' gestation and the platelets rarely fall below 60,000/mm³. Thus, the initial approach to a patient with thrombocytopenia in the last trimester consists of a history and physical examination, looking for evidence of the known causes of thrombocytopenia due to peripheral destruction. No further work-up is undertaken if the history and physical examination are negative and the platelet count is above 60,000/mm³. Platelets are rechecked every 2–4 weeks. The patient may have new-onset mild ITP, but this cannot be distinguished from PAT unless the platelets continue to drop. The management of both conditions is the same (expectant) in any case.

If the platelets are less than 60,000/mm³ or if the thrombocytopenia was noted before 28 weeks' gestation and no other cause is suspected from the history and physical examination, the following laboratory tests are checked: antinuclear antibodies (ANA), anticardiolipin antibodies, lupus anticoagulant (LAC), HIV, and hepatitis C. If the laboratory work-up is negative, the presumed diagnosis is new-onset ITP. Platelet antibodies are not checked as they are of no value in distinguishing between ITP and PAT or in the management of ITP itself.

Management of immune thrombocytopenia in pregnancy

Immune thrombocytopenia, whether diagnosed for the first time in pregnancy or if it antedates pregnancy, is managed the same. If the platelet count is consistently below 50,000/mm³, the first line of therapy is prednisone in a dose of 1 mg/kg/day. A response is usually seen within 3 weeks after which the dose should be tapered to maintain a count above 50,000/mm³. ASA and nonsteroidal anti-inflammatory agents should be avoided because they interfere with platelet function.

For patients who do not respond to steroid therapy, intravenous immune globulin (IV IgG) may be given in a dose of 400 mg/kg/day for a 5-day course. A response is usually seen within 5 days. For patients who fail IV

IgG or who relapse frequently, we have had success with a regimen of dexametasone 40 mg/day orally for 4 days repeated monthly for 3 months. This latter regimen avoids the need for cytotoxic agents, which may otherwise be required in refractory ITP.

Attempts to determine which fetuses are thrombocytopenic and therefore at presumed risk for hemorrhage either poses undue risk (percutaneous umbilical sampling) or is unreliable (fetal scalp sampling). Of more importance, although 15% of newborns of mothers with ITP may have platelet counts less than $50,000/mm^3$ at birth, there is no conclusive evidence from large series of ITP cases that bleeding (in particular, intracranial hemorrhage) has occurred in the neonate that could have been altered by changing the mode of delivery. For these reasons, we manage mothers with ITP expectantly during labor, avoiding instrumental delivery.

If the maternal platelet count is less than $50,000/mm^3$, platelets should be available at the time of cesarean or vaginal delivery, but the platelets should not be given unless abnormal bleeding is encountered – an uncommon occurrence. If a cesarean birth (or other elective surgery) is planned, it is our practice to administer IV IgG in a dose of 1 g/kg daily for 2 consecutive days in addition to the above measures.

There are no exact guidelines regarding when platelets should be transfused. It is generally agreed that there is a risk of spontaneous bleeding with counts below $20,000/mm^3$; however, patients with ITP frequently tolerate lower counts without difficulty if they are not subjected to surgical or accidental trauma. If thrombocytopenia is the only hemostatic abnormality, it is unlikely that bleeding will occur with counts of $50,000/ mm^3$ or more, even during surgery. Each unit of platelets will increase the platelet count by $8000–10,000/ mm^3$. Single donor platelet pheresis packs have 8–10 units. Transfused platelets do not persist for long in the recipient because the same immune-mediated process that is causing the thrombocytopenia destroys them.

Fetal and neonatal thrombocytopenia

The neonatal platelet count reaches a nadir 2–6 days after delivery. Platelet count should be measured, although the thrombocytopenic neonate usually has petechiae. The platelet count usually returns to normal within 2 months after birth. There is a theoretical, but unlikely, risk that breast-feeding may transfer maternal antibody to the neonate.

Suggested reading

Burrows RF. Platelet disorders in pregnancy. *Curr Opin Obstet Gynecol* 2001; 13(2): 1150–119.

Burrows RF, Kelton JG. Thrombocytopenia at delivery. A prospective survey of 6715 deliveries. *Am J Obstet Gynecol* 1990; 162: 731–734.

Cook RL, Miller RC, Katz VL, Cefalo RC. Immune thrombocytopenic purpura. A reappraisal of management. *Obstet Gynecol* 1991; 78: 578–583.

Haram K, Nilsen ST, Ulvik RJ. Iron supplementation in pregnancy. Evidence and controversies. *Acta Obstet Gynecol Scand* 2001; 80: 683–688.

Koshy M, Burd L, Wallace D, Moawad A, Baron J. Prophylactic red-cell transfusions in pregnant patients with sickle cell disease. A randomized cooperative study. *NEJM* 1988; 319: 1447–1452.

Schwartz KA. Gestational thrombocytopenia and immune thrombocytopenias in pregnancy. *Hematol-Oncol Clin North Am* 2000; 14(5): 1101–1116.

Serjeant GR, Loy LL, Crowther M, Hambleton IR, Thame M. Outcome of pregnancy in homozygous sickle cell disease. *Obstet Gynecol* 2004; 103: 1278–1285.

Sloan NL, Jordan E, Winikoff B. Effects of iron supplementation on maternal hematologic status in pregnancy. *Am J Public Health* 2002; 92: 288–293.

Xiong X, Buekens P, Alexander S, Demianczuk N, Wollast E. Anemia during pregnancy and birth outcome: a meta-analysis. *Am J Perinatol* 2000; 17: 137–146.

Chapter 27
Venous Thromboembolism and Inherited Thrombophilias

Martin N. Montoro

Department of Medicine and Obstetrics and Gynecology, Keck School of Medicine, University of Southern California, CA, USA

Introduction

The risk of venous thromboembolism (VTE) is five to ten times greater during pregnancy than in age-matched nonpregnant women. It is now one of the leading causes of maternal morbidity and mortality since other complications such as infections and hemorrhage are treated more effectively. According to the Centers for Disease Control, VTE caused 20% of pregnancy-related deaths from 1991 to 1999, surpassing the 17% deaths form hemorrhage. VTE includes both deep vein thrombosis (DVT) and pulmonary embolism (PE), which are true clinical emergencies. Many of the women at risk of thromboembolism also have inherited or acquired thrombophilias and are more likely to have poor pregnancy outcomes, including fetal loss (particularly after 20 weeks), severe pre-eclampsia, eclampsia, HELLP syndrome, abruptio placentae and intrauterine growth restriction (IUGR).

Location

In pregnancy, DVT involves more frequently the iliofemoral system (72% vs 9%) and the left side (85% vs 55%). On the left side, the iliac artery crosses over the vein, resulting in additional stasis. Upper extremity VTE is exceedingly rare and should raise the suspicion of intravenous drug use (particularly cocaine), a severe hypercoagulable state or, more commonly, a needle or a catheter left in the vein too long.

Frequency

Symptomatic VTE in pregnant women without previous episodes and no obvious risk factors is 0.5–1.8 per 1000.

Management of Common Problems in Obstetrics and Gynecology, 5th edition. Edited by T.M. Goodwin, M.N. Montoro, L. Muderspach, R. Paulson and S. Roy. © 2010 Blackwell Publishing Ltd.

Older studies reported higher frequencies because objective documentation of thrombosis was not usually required. More recent publications quote 1 in 1000 deliveries. Subclinical, asymptomatic episodes of thrombosis, particularly in the calf and during the puerperium, are probably much more common and incidences as high as 3% are quoted, but no prospective trials involving pregnant or postpartum women have been done. Moreover, these quotes are extrapolated from studies in nonpregnant patients undergoing a variety of elective surgical procedures with preoperative injection of fibrinogen-labeled iodine 131, which for obvious reasons cannot be used during pregnancy.

In our own experience, during a 19-year period there were 165 VTE complicated pregnancies and 268,036 deliveries (1 per 1627 births – 0.06%). There were 127 cases of DVT and 38 cases of PE.

The recurrence rate during pregnancy in women with a previous VTE episode depends on the specific risks associated with the previous episode. The risk was higher when it was associated with a hypercoagulable state (thrombophilia) or if it was labeled as "idiopathic" and much lower if the risk factors were transient, such as trauma or surgery.

The risk of recurrence in thrombophilias, either hereditary or acquired, depends on the specific condition. Heterozygous women who are carriers of the G1691A factor V Leiden mutation have a 3–9-fold higher risk but 49–80-fold if they are homozygous. The G2021A mutation in the prothrombin gene carries a 2–9-fold higher risk for the heterozygotes and 16-fold for the homozygous carriers. If the patient happens to be heterozygote for both the factor V Leiden and prothrombin G2021A gene mutation ("compound mutation"), the risk increases by 150-fold. Antithrombin III (AT-III) deficiency increases the risk 25–50-fold, making it the single most thrombogenic condition. Protein C deficiency causes a 3–15-fold higher risk and protein S deficiency twofold. Hyperhomocysteinemia carries a 2.5–4-fold higher risk and antiphospholipid antibodies increase the risk by 5–6-fold. Women who are relatives of persons with VTE but who themselves have only laboratory evidence of risk factors, and not previous clinical VTE episodes, were found to have a 4% risk of VTE during pregnancy.

At present, 50% or more of pregnancy-related VTE cases occur in women with a hereditary or acquired thrombophilia. Those without discernible risk factors are said to have an "idiopathic episode" but they are at a high risk of recurring VTE during subsequent pregnancies. It is possible that the VTE currently labeled as "idiopathic" are actually cases of still unknown thrombophilias.

Timing in relation to pregnancy

The risk of VTE was thought to increase with progression of pregnancy but recent studies indicate that the risk is evenly divided throughout all trimesters and that it is already well established in early pregnancy, by the end of the first trimester. The immediate postpartum remains the highest risk period for PE, with $\geq 80\%$ occurring after operative deliveries. Sixty-one percent of all PE in our series occurred post partum and 82.6% of all postpartum PE occurred after cesarean sections.

The overall risk of VTE at present is still higher after delivery than antepartum. Nevertheless, the risk of postpartum VTE has decreased to a greater extent than antepartum in comparison to older studies and most likely because of changes in obstetric practices such as shorter hospital stays, earlier postpartum ambulation and bedrest not being recommended as frequently. And when bedrest is recommended, measures are generally applied to reduce risks by using elastic stockings, intermittent pneumatic leg compressors or prophylactic anticoagulation in the high-risk groups. Furthermore, estrogens are no longer used to suppress lactation.

Risk factors for venous thromboembolism

Rudolf Virchow is credited with establishing the basic risk factors for VTE in his now classic 1845 lecture, later published in 1856, and known as the "Virchow's triad": venous stasis, "alterations of the blood," and endothelial vascular injury. These risk factors are present during gestation and are believed to be the reason for the so-called "hypercoagulable state of pregnancy."
• The velocity of the venous return may decrease by as much as 50% towards the end of pregnancy due to venous dilation caused by progesterone (already present in early pregnancy) and mechanical obstruction by the fetus, which increases with the progression of pregnancy.
• There is also a 20–200% increase in the amount of clotting factors such as fibrinogen and factors II (prothrombin),

VII, VIII, X and XII, with a secondary increase after the delivery of the placenta. There is a concomitant decrease in the natural inhibitors of coagulation, indicated by lower protein S levels, and lower activity of the fibrinolytic system evidenced by higher levels of the plasminogen activator inhibitors 1 and 2 and thrombin activator fibrinolysis inhibitor.
• Endothelial vascular injury leading to release of tissue thromboplastin may occur during vaginal delivery and placental separation, but it is more pronounced after cesarean sections and traumatic deliveries with tissue rupture. Additional tissue damage by postpartum infections may further increase the risk.
Other factors that may additionally increase the risk include older age (>35 years), obesity (pre-pregnancy BMI ≥ 30 kg/m^2), bedrest, smoking, hypertension, venous damage from previous thrombosis (postphlebitic syndrome), large varicose veins, nephrotic syndrome, dehydration (e.g. in severe hyperemesis), intravenous drug abuse and long-distance air travel.

It is widely believed that there are still unknown "thrombopreventive and vasoprotective" mechanisms that seem to over-ride the thrombogenic diathesis of pregnancy in most women. It is also likely that future research will disclose more instances of coagulation abnormalities in many of the cases now labeled as "idiopathic." The reason for the overwhelming occurrence of thrombosis in veins, rather than in arteries, during pregnancy seems to be the increased venous stasis plus the fact that pregnant women are generally young and free of arterial vascular disease (e.g. plaque) predisposing to arterial thrombosis. Nevertheless, some cases of arterial thrombosis (cerebral, cardiac, peripheral) have been reported in pregnant women although almost exclusively in those with the most severe forms of the antiphospholipid syndrome.

Special risk categories: thrombophilias

An increasing number of pregnant women with VTE are being found to have an underlying hereditary or acquired thrombophilia. A mutation in the factor V gene is associated with resistance to activated protein C (APC-R). This autosomal dominant-inherited defect causes a point mutation in the gene encoding for factor V, also known as Leiden, whereby glutamine is substituted for arginine at the amino acid site 506 which renders factor V resistant to proteolytic downregulation by activated protein C, leading to thrombin generation. The prevalence of APC-R (heterozygous state) in the general population is 2–7% with variations according to ethnicity: 3–7% in Caucasians, 2.21% in Hispanic Americans, 1.25% in Native Americans, 1.23% in African Americans, and 0.45% in Asian Americans.

These patients also have an increased risk of adverse pregnancy outcomes, as stated in the introduction.

A mutation in the prothrombin G20210A gene, which results in increased levels of prothrombin, also increases the risk of thrombosis and adverse pregnancy outcomes. It occurs in 2% of the general population. Patients with both factor V and prothrombin gene compound mutation have a markedly increased thrombotic risk.

Antithrombin III deficiency is reported in 0.02–0.17% of the general population. It is considered to be a very thrombogenic condition.

The prevalence of protein S or protein C deficiencies is found in 0.14–0.5% of the general population, and the frequency during pregnancy in women with a previous VTE episode is 0–6% for protein S deficiency and 3–10% for protein C, but higher, 7–22%, among women who develop VTE post partum.

Hyperhomocysteinemia, caused by a mutation in the methylene tetrahydrofolate reductase C677T and A1298C genes, also increases the risk VTE during pregnancy and the risk of recurrent abortion by twofold. Other risks reported include neural tube defects.

Frequently, the precipitating event in persons with an inherited coagulation defect is the addition of an acquired risk for thrombosis such as the use of oral contraceptives, pregnancy, labor and delivery, immobilization, trauma or surgery.

Boxes 27.1 and 27.2 list the inherited and acquired coagulopathies that may be encountered during pregnancy as well as the maternal and fetal risks associated with these conditions.

Box 27.1 Coagulopathies in pregnancy: inherited and acquired

Inherited
Deficiency of antithrombin III, protein C, protein S, plasminogen, fibrinogen
  Resistance to activated protein C
  Hyperhomocysteinemia
  Prothrombin G mutation (G20201A)
  Paroxysmal nocturnal hemoglobinuria
  Sickle cell disease

Acquired
Antiphospholipid syndrome:
  • associated with SLE
  • independent of SLE
  • lupus anticoagulant
  • anticardiolipin antibody
Anti-β2 glycoprotein antibody:
  • antithrombin III deficiency
  • certain malignancies (rare in pregnancy)

Box 27.2 Coagulopathies in pregnancy: maternal and fetal risks

Maternal risks
Deep vein thrombosis and pulmonary embolism
  Extensive thrombosis or at unusual sites (sagittal, mesenteric, portal veins)
  Arterial occlusions
  Hemocytopenia (thrombocytopenia more commonly)
  Pre-eclampsia (early, severe, persistent postpartum, atypical HELLP, hepatic infarction)
  Postpartum autoimmune syndrome

Fetal risks
Spontaneous abortion, recurrent abortion, stillbirth, fetal death
  Intrauterine growth retardation
  Placental abruption, placental infarction
  Unexplained elevated maternal serum α-fetoprotein (MSAFP)
  Neonatal thrombosis

Diagnosis of deep vein thrombosis during pregnancy

Clinical diagnosis

The clinical manifestations of DVT may include pain, tenderness, swelling, warmth, redness, discoloration, cyanosis, a palpable cord, superficial venous dilation and, in severe cases, massive swelling and phlegmasia caerulea dolens. The diagnosis should never be made on clinical grounds alone because many other conditions may cause similar symptoms. It has been repeatedly shown that the diagnosis of DVT by clinical signs alone is accurate in less than 50% of cases, and in pregnancy, even less than 10% of suspected DVT is confirmed by ancillary testing. A careful personal and family history with emphasis on thromboembolic events should be taken.

Laboratory testing

General laboratory tests include a complete blood count (CBC), platelet count, partial thromboplastin time (PTT), thrombin clotting time and perhaps a bleeding time. A high-sensitivity D-dimer level, if not elevated, is considered strong evidence against the presence of VTE in nonpregnant patients. In pregnancy, a normal D-dimer is considered helpful if the compression ultrasound is also normal; if elevated, even if the ultrasound is negative, this indicates the need for further testing. D-dimer levels increase with the progression of pregnancy and spike if there are complications such as pre-eclampsia and placental abruption. One particular D-dimer assay (SimpliRED) might have a higher specificity, a superior negative predictive value and a lower rate of false-positive results in the first and second trimesters but it needs further validation.

Indications for thrombophilia testing include recurrent VTE, positive family history, and previous adverse pregnancy outcomes such as recurrent miscarriage (3 or more consecutive losses) before the 10th week, one or more fetal losses at or after 10 weeks, premature delivery (before 34 weeks) because of severe pre-eclampsia, eclampsia, HELLP syndrome, placental abruption, IUGR ($\leq$ 5th percentile), or a combination of these factors (see Chapter 28). Whether or not screening for thrombophilia is warranted after the first VTE episode is still a matter of debate.

Basic thrombophilia screening tests include functional AT-III assay, functional proteins C and S assays, APC resistance factor V polymerase chain reaction and/or the more specific DNA-based testing for mutation of the factor V gene, and prothrombin G20210A polymerase chain reaction. Tests for acquired thrombophilias include the lupus anticoagulant, anticardiolipin and anti-β_2 glycoprotein antibodies (IgG and IgM). Other possible factors to look for include a homocysteine level (testing 6 hours after l-methionine loading – 0.1 g/kg bodyweight – might be more accurate than just a fasting level), thrombomodulin gene variants, protein Z levels, fibrinogen, plasminogen, plasminogen activator inhibitors and fibrinolysis inhibitors.

At present, the cost of thrombophilia screening is very high for routine use. The recommendation from the most recent consensus of the American College of Obstetricians and Gynecologists is to screen patients with a history of thrombosis, unexplained fetal loss at or after 20 weeks' gestation, severe pre-eclampsia/HELLP occurring at less than 34 weeks' gestation, severe IUGR or a family history of thrombosis. The basic screening tests should include factor V Leiden mutation, prothrombin G20210A mutation, functional protein C and S deficiencies, AT-III deficiency, lupus anticoagulant, anticardiolipin, anti-β_2 glycoprotein antibodies and a homocysteine level.

Imaging

Contrast venography was, for years, the diagnostic gold standard for DVT and the sensitivity and specificity of all others tests were measured against it. It is rarely performed at present since it cannot be repeated serially because of fetal radiation and intravenous X-ray contrast exposure. It is an invasive procedure and carries risk of DVT itself.

The venous color Doppler compression ultrasound in symptomatic patients has a 95% sensitivity and a 96% specificity for the proximal (above the knee) veins but 75% sensitivity and 90% specificity for the distal veins (below the knee). It does not reliably detect isolated iliac vein thrombosis either. Nevertheless, it is currently the most widely used initial examination. When the ultrasound cannot be technically performed (in about 3% of cases) or if the DVT suspicion remains high despite a negative ultrasound, back-up testing includes magnetic resonance venography which has a 95–96% sensitivity and a 90–92% specificity for both the proximal and distal veins. The

cost is higher but its effectiveness is also higher because it includes more vein sites such as the vena cava, pelvic, thigh and popliteal veins. Helical CT contrast venography of the pelvis and lower extremities has a 95% sensitivity and a 86% specificity but the experience in pregnancy is limited and there is concern about fetal radiation although the risk is supposed to be low. The suggested diagnostic sequence for DVT can be seen in Figure 27.1.

The most frequent form of DVT, particularly postoperatively, involves the veins of the calf. Only 20% extend proximally and pose a risk of embolization when the larger veins above the knee are reached. Most authors recommend treating only those patients in whom extension is detected and consider it safe to withhold therapy if no extension is seen by serial ultrasound over a period of 10 days. There is no uniform agreement, however; some recommend treating all patients with positive tests and others withhold therapy only if the noninvasive tests are negative. The suggested sequence for the management of distal (calf) DVT is given in Figure 27.2.

Complications of deep vein thrombosis

Postphlebitic syndrome

May appear immediately or long after, even years after, the DVT episode. It is caused by damage to veins from the clot leading to valvular incompetence and/or residual venous obstruction. The true incidence is unknown but it is estimated to be as high as 50% after proximal and 30% after calf DVT. A prompt diagnosis and effective DVT treatment will prevent lasting vein damage.

Pulmonary embolism

Pulmonary embolism is the most serious complication. The PE mortality rate of untreated symptomatic DVT in older studies was 12–37% and even in asymptomatic patients it was as high as 5%. If left untreated, DVT

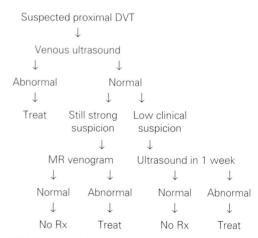

Figure 27.1 Suggested diagnostic sequence for proximal deep vein thrombosis.

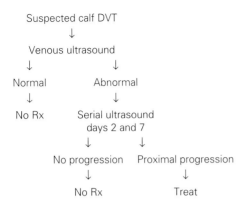

Suspected calf DVT
↓
Venous ultrasound
↓   ↓
Normal   Abnormal
↓   ↓
No Rx   Serial ultrasound
           days 2 and 7
           ↓   ↓
       No progression Proximal progression
           ↓   ↓
         No Rx   Treat

Figure 27.2 Suggested sequence for the management of distal (calf) deep vein thrombosis.

patients may have a high prevalence (50–65%) of initially silent PE. These figures underscore the importance of diagnosing and treating all cases of proximal DVT and those of distal (calf) DVT with proximal extension.

The clinical diagnosis alone is inaccurate and objective confirmation is mandatory. The clinical symptoms may be suggestive but are nonspecific. Conditions that may mimic the symptoms of submassive PE include chest wall muscle strain, rib fractures, mitral stenosis, viral or autoimmune pleuritis, pneumonia, pneumothorax or pericarditis. The differential diagnosis of massive pulmonary embolism includes aspiration of gastric contents, amniotic fluid embolism, gram-negative sepsis, mucus plug aspiration, and tension pneumothorax.

The electrocardiogram or the chest x-ray may be normal or show nonspecific changes. The blood gases usually show a decreased PO_2, which is not specific either. Other tests such as fibrin degradation products, lactic dehydrogenase (LDH), serum alanine aminotransferase (SGPT), bilirubin levels, etc. are neither sensitive nor specific. However, a high-sensitivity D-dimer may be helpful (particularly if normal) but with the limitations of its use in pregnant women (see above).

The ventilation-perfusion lung scan was for many years the first step in the diagnostic approach to suspected PE. A PE was excluded if the perfusion scan was normal and if it showed high probability, it was considered strong evidence to warrant initiation of treatment. However, performing lung scans is time consuming, the sensitivity varies widely, and in 40–70% of cases the result is indeterminate or "nondiagnostic," indicating the need for further testing. The next step in those cases was a pulmonary angiogram, considered to be the reference standard. However, a pulmonary angiogram is an invasive procedure with significant radiation to the fetus and a large dose of iodinated x-ray contrast material as well. It requires cardiac catheterization via a femoral or an internal carotid artery and carries a 0.5% risk of mortality and a 3% risk of other complications including groin hematomas, cardiac perforation, contrast-induced renal failure and respiratory failure. Therefore, an

intensive effort has been made to find an easier and safer alternative procedure. CT pulmonary angiography has emerged as more cost-effective, easier to perform, with even lower fetal radiation and able to detect other pulmonary disorders as well. It is reported to have sensitivity and specificity of 94% and 100% and a negative predictive value of 99.1%, and is considered similar to pulmonary angiography. Its usefulness and safety have also been validated in pregnancy. Because of concerns about maternal breast radiation, the use of breast shields is recommended. Magnetic resonance angiography (MRA) has a sensitivity of only 77% when compared to pulmonary angiography and in addition, there is limited experience in pregnancy. The current recommended approach to the diagnosis of PE during pregnancy is given in Figure 27.3.

Fetal radiation from various diagnostic procedures

Little radiation reaches the fetus from technetium 99 lung scans; with 1 mCi the fetal radiation is 8 mrads and 15–16 mrads if 2 mCi are used. In comparison, the old iodine 131 scans gave 130 mrads to the fetus. If the mother is post partum and breastfeeding, she should stop for 48 hours following a lung scan, after which it is safe to resume (the half-life of technetium 99 is 6 hours). The ventilation scan gives 5 mCi to the mother and variable amounts, 1–19 mrads, to the fetus; a ventilation scan is recommended only when the perfusion is abnormal and not routinely. Pulmonary angiography via the femoral route gives 221–374 mrads to the fetus but when it can be performed via the brachial route, the amount of fetal radiation is much less. CT pulmonary angiogram gives 130 μGy to the fetus, which is considered to be low, particularly considering the risk of an undiagnosed and untreated PE. However, the effect of this amount of radiation on the mother's breasts in pregnancy is not known and to reduce whatever risk exists, the use of breasts shields is recommended.

Therapy

An accurate and timely diagnosis is mandatory to prevent morbidity from venous insufficiency (postphlebitic syndrome), and mortality from pulmonary embolism. Anticoagulants are potentially dangerous and should not

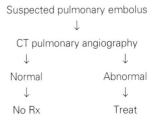

Suspected pulmonary embolus
↓
CT pulmonary angiography
↓   ↓
Normal   Abnormal
↓   ↓
No Rx   Treat

Figure 27.3 Recommended approach to the diagnosis of pulmonary embolism (PE) during pregnancy.

be used unless the diagnosis has been firmly established by *objective* ancillary testing.

Unfractionated heparin (UH) has been safe during pregnancy when properly used and monitored but low molecular weight heparin (LMWH) has become the treatment of choice in most cases. Warfarin should be avoided except in very special circumstances (e.g. older generation mechanical valves in the mitral position), and in those cases the women must be informed of the risks, which include spontaneous abortion, warfarin embryopathy, and bleeding during delivery.

Oral anticoagulants (warfarin)

The spontaneous abortion rate is reported to be 8–50%; however, in many instances the cause may be the underlying maternal disease rather than the warfarin itself because most treated patients are those with cardiac disease and prosthetic heart valves who have a higher rate of fetal loss, independent of the therapy. The risk of warfarin embryopathy is reported to be 5–10% when taken during the first trimester, but in some studies it is as high as 29–67% when geneticists examine the newborns. The risk is lower when the exposure occurs before the 6th week of gestation and highest between the 6th and 9th weeks. Fetal malformations may still occur after the first trimester, because fetal bleeding may happen at any time during gestation. Anomalies of this origin include dorsal midline dysplasia, midline cerebellar atrophy, and ventral midline dysplasia resulting in optic atrophy, microcephaly, and mental retardation.

Warfarin should be stopped and substituted with heparin no later than at 35–36 weeks of gestation. This is particularly important in women with cardiac diseases because premature delivery occurs frequently (36% in a recent study) in these women. If labor starts while on warfarin, a cesarean section is recommended to avoid the almost certain risk of fetal cerebral hemorrhage during labor. The mother should receive 2–4 units of fresh-frozen plasma and vitamin K, but since vitamin K is slow acting it should not be given as the only neutralizing agent. Breastfeeding is safe while on warfarin since it does not pass into breastmilk because it is highly bound to plasma proteins and it is not lipid soluble in its ionized form.

When used post partum, it should be given within 24 hours after the initiation of heparin, which should not be stopped until the warfarin has been therapeutic for 2–5 days. The anticoagulant effect of warfarin precedes its antithrombotic effect by 24 hours, and during that period a transient hypercoagulable state exists due to the rapid reduction of protein C levels. Warfarin-induced skin necrosis is a rare complication which may occur in patients with protein C or protein S deficiencies and it is also related to the rapid decrease in protein C levels which precede the reduction of prothrombin, factor IX and factor X levels. In these cases a loading

dose of warfarin should be avoided and warfarin not given until heparin has become therapeutic. Heparin should be continued for at least 2 days after warfarin has become therapeutic.

Monitoring warfarin therapy is necessary because of the highly individual responses; also, many drugs, especially antibiotics, interfere with its action. It is monitored by the prothrombin time expressed as the international normalized ratio (INR) and kept at two to three times the control. An INR higher than three greatly increases the risk of bleeding and it is not more effective.

Heparin

Unfractionated heparin (UH) does not cross the placenta because of its large size and it is not secreted into breast milk. It enhances antithrombin and factor Xa inhibitory activity and inhibits platelet aggregation. It does not directly destroy blood clots but stops the coagulation process, allowing the fibrinolytic system eventually to destroy the clot.

An initial intravenous bolus of 5000 IU is commonly recommended, followed by an infusion of 30,000 IU for the first 24 hours because of an increased rate of recurrence with lower initial doses. In nonpregnant individuals, the most commonly recommended doses are 80 IU/kg for the initial bolus and 18 IU/kg/h for the infusion. Frequent monitoring of the aPTT, which should be kept prolonged at 2–3 times the control, is recommended. The intravenous treatment is continued for 5–10 days, until the symptoms disappear. After this "acute phase" UH is changed to the subcutaneous route, also known as the "secondary prophylaxis" phase but at present, almost always, LMWH rather than UH is used. If for any reason UH is still desired for the subcutaneous route, the following is recommended: the total daily amount of intravenous UH needed to keep the aPTT in the therapeutic range is divided into two equal doses and given subcutaneously every 12 hours. The aPTT is checked 6 hours after the subcutaneous injection and kept at 1.5–2.0 times the control. When heparin levels by protamine titration are used to monitor UH treatment, the therapeutic range is 0.2–0.4 IU/mL and, if using antifactor Xa assays, 0.35–0.7 IU/mL. Post partum, warfarin may be used instead of heparin to complete the therapeutic cycle, depending on the specific circumstances of each case.

Because of the cumbersome dosing, need for frequent monitoring, hospitalization and potential side effects, alternative options are highly desirable. Nevertheless, there are some situations in which therapy with UH is still recommended for pregnant patients. PE should be treated in the hospital with IV UH during the acute phase, particularly if patients are not clinically stable. Women close to term who might require regional anesthesia and/or a cesarean section, and those at risk of bleeding (e.g. placental abnormalities or immediately postoperative), may benefit from the shorter half-life of UH and its ease of reversibility with protamine.

Complications

Heparin-induced thrombocytopenia (HIT)

Reported in 3–5% of patients. Type I HIT occurs soon after initiation of treatment and may be self-limiting. Type II occurs 5–14 days after starting heparin and it is defined as an absolute platelet count of less than $100,000/mm^3$ or a 50% decrease from the pretreatment count. It may have an immune basis and be IgG mediated. Platelets are monitored before treatment and on days 3, 7, 10, 14 and then monthly thereafter. If HIT occurs, heparin should be stopped and a hematology consult obtained.

Osteoporosis

The risk of fractures is 2.2% after 17 weeks of UH treatment (range 7–27 weeks). Using serial bone densitometry, there is a 30% decrease in bone density with long periods of therapy even if no fractures occur. Calcium supplementation is often recommended (1.5–2.0 g/day) but it is not known if it might be protective.

Bleeding

Major bleeding occurs in 3–5%. Risks include excessive PTT prolongation, recent surgery, liver disease, thrombocytopenia, and the concomitant use of antiplatelet agents. The treatment includes stopping heparin and using local measures against bleeding. Neutralization with protamine sulfate is rarely needed but it should be given to patients who are actively bleeding and have a prolonged PTT, and if at the time of delivery the PTT is 2.7 times the control or greater. Protamine forms a stable salt with heparin and inhibits its anticoagulant effect. One milligram of protamine neutralizes 100 IU of heparin, but giving more than 50 mg at a time is not recommended because it may cause hypotension. It must be administered slowly, over a 10-minute period.

Additional considerations about unfractionated heparin

Beginning in November 2007, there have been worldwide (at least 12 countries) reports of acute hypersensitivity reactions (hypotension, facial swelling, tachycardia, urticaria and nausea, as well as 81 deaths as of April 2008) in patients receiving unfractionated heparin manufactured in China. The cause was identified to be contamination mainly by an oversulfated form of chondroitin sulfate and some batches also by dermatan sulfate. The mechanism was activation by these contaminants of the kinin–kallikrein pathway to generate bradykinin as well as by activation of the complement system. As a consequence, there was a recall in February 2008 of unfractionated heparin (multidose, single-dose and flush vials) [1]. Hopefully, this will be a temporary problem with prompt and effective resolution.

Low molecular weight heparin

Low molecular weight heparins are fractions of standard unfractionated heparin obtained by chemical or enzymatic depolymerization, which result in fractions of heparin that are approximately one-third to one-fourth the size of UH. Their molecular weight is 4000–5000 Da. Although smaller, LMWH does not cross the placenta and is not secreted into breast milk either.

LMWH offers several advantages over UH and it has emerged as the anticoagulant of choice for the subcutaneous route. Since it does not bind to plasma proteins, its bio-availability is greater and does not change with different dosages, providing a more predictable dose response. It has a longer half-life, offering the possibility of once-daily dosing although once versus twice a day dosing is still a matter of debate. Because of its predictable response, fixed doses can be given with little or no laboratory monitoring. When monitoring is desired, however, antifactor Xa levels must be used, since the aPTT does not correlate well with the effect of LMWH. There is less risk of bleeding and a lower incidence of thrombocytopenia than with UH and no osteoporotic effect on bone. No placental abruption or neonatal bleeding has yet been reported. It may be even more effective than UH in preventing recurrences and has a good safety profile in pregnancy. However, pregnant women usually require 10–20% higher doses because of increased renal clearance. In addition, there is a slightly greater variability of binding, distribution and metabolism in pregnancy which has led some authors to propose more frequent monitoring of the factor Xa activity during pregnancy although this is still an area of debate along with once- versus twice-daily dosing and inpatient versus outpatient treatment choices.

The high cost of LMWH was an initial limiting factor. However, in selected nonpregnant patients, outpatient therapy of both DVT and even PE is safe and effective. Therefore, the possibility of outpatient treatment for many patients and the need for little or no laboratory testing greatly offset the cost and the overall treatment course is much cheaper than treatment with UH in the hospital.

Enoxaparin is the most commonly used in pregnancy followed by dalteparin. There is little or no experience with the other LMWH available in the USA at this time including nadroparin, tinzaparin, ardeparin and reviparin.

Neuroaxial anesthesia (epidural, spinal) is not recommended unless the last LMWH injection was given > 24 hours before because of danger of spinal hematoma with neurologic injury which might even include permanent paralysis. Patients are instructed to hold LMWH at the very onset of contractions and therefore 24 hours or more will have elapsed by the time of delivery in most cases. For planned labor inductions and cesarean section, LMWH is held 24 hours before.

The recommended dosages are 1 mg/kg (of actual weight) subcutaneously every 12 hours for acute-phase treatments and 0.5 mg/kg (also actual weight) subcutaneously every 12 hours for secondary prophylaxis. Lower doses are now used in some cases for primary prophylaxis (see below). Laboratory monitoring is not usually recommended. We measure antifactor Xa levels when using the higher dose, usually once, after the first 2–3 days of initiating treatment, to ensure a therapeutic effect and then monthly. The blood sample should be taken 3–4 hours after the subcutaneous injection for the peak level and the desired range is 0.6–1.0 U/mL. The sample for the trough level is taken 12 hours after the injection, just prior to the next injection, and it should be 0.2–0.4 IU/mL, but ≥ 0.5 IU/mL for the highest risk patients. For prophylaxis, the peak range is 0.2–0.4 IU/mL and through levels 0.1–0.3 IU/mL.

Management during labor and delivery

Unfractionated heparin should be stopped at the onset of contractions and, because it has a short half-life, its activity will be low or it will have completely disappeared by the time delivery occurs. The maternal risk of bleeding is low if heparin levels are less than 0.4 IU/mL during spontaneous vaginal delivery, but increased risk of hematoma formation with episiotomy has been reported. There is little information about the risk of bleeding at the time of cesarean section in these patients. Some authors allow regional anesthesia if the aPTT is normal at the time of delivery and the last dose of heparin was administered more than 4–6 hours before, but the risk of spinal hematoma is a strong deterrent to most others. Neutralization with protamine is recommended when the PTT is still 2.5 times the control or greater at the time of delivery.

In stable patients, heparin is restarted 3–8 hours post partum, but a longer waiting period (24 h or more) is recommended if there was excessive bleeding, particularly in operative delivery cases. A reloading bolus of 5000 IU is given followed by an infusion at the previous level known to be effective. If warfarin is used post partum, it should be started within 24 hours of heparin or as soon as the patient is able to resume oral intake. In patients with coagulation disorders, primarily those with protein C and protein S deficiencies, warfarin should not be given until therapeutic concentrations of heparin have been obtained and a loading dose of warfarin is avoided. Heparin should be continued until the warfarin has been therapeutic for 2–5 days (see "Oral anticoagulants (warfarin)" above). Warfarin anticoagulation should be continued until 6 weeks post partum

or until a total of 3–6 months (or longer), depending on the circumstances of each case.

However, in most cases LMWH is used post partum. It is resumed 3–6 hours after an uncomplicated vaginal delivery and 6–8 hours after an uncomplicated cesarean section. A longer waiting period is recommended if there was excessive bleeding or a traumatic or operative delivery. Most women also prefer LMWH post partum rather than warfarin or UH because they will not have to make frequent trips to the laboratory for testing at a time when they are busy with a new baby and recovering from a long pregnancy and perhaps a complicated delivery.

Inferior vena cava filters and surgical thrombectomy

The indications for inferior vena cava filters are the same as those outside pregnancy to prevent PE from clots below the inferior vena cava. They are indicated for patients with acute thromboembolism and active bleeding, recurrent PE despite adequate anticoagulation, true HIT and no therapeutic alternative, or any other contraindication to anticoagulants because of a high potential for complications. Whether or not filters are indicated for patients who are not compliant with their anticoagulants is a matter of debate.

Surgical thrombectomy may be considered in patients with pulmonary hypertension from chronic thromboembolism or in massive PE when thrombolytic therapy is contraindicated.

Thrombolytic therapy

Thrombolytic therapy is not generally recommended until 10–14 days after delivery. The complications include maternal hemorrhage, placental abruption, fetal loss, and preterm delivery. There are no controlled trials and the data available come from case reports when it was used in desperate cases of massive PE and hemodynamic instability. In the majority of those reports streptokinase (SK) was used. Urokinase (UK) and tissue plasminogen activator (TPA) have also been used in a few cases. SK and TPA do not cross the placenta in animals; UK, however, does cross the placenta although it has not been shown to be teratogenic in rats.

Outside pregnancy, the indications for thrombolytic therapy are limited to patients with extensive iliofemoral venous thrombosis and low risk of bleeding, or those with massive pulmonary embolism and hemodynamic instability. The regimens approved by the FDA are SK for extensive venous thrombosis with phlegmasia caerulea dolens, 250,000 units as a bolus dose followed by an infusion of 100,000 units per hour for up to 72 hours. For PE, 100 mg of TPA is given intravenously over a period of 2 hours. Major bleeding seems to be the major limiting factor.

Duration of anticoagulant therapy

The recurrence of thrombosis is unacceptably high (>25%) if no therapy is given after the acute phase and it is low (<4%) if secondary prophylaxis is continued for 3–6 months following acute-phase treatment. In addition, the recurrence rate remains high (12–24%) even after 3 months of anticoagulation, in cases of idiopathic or recurrent thromboembolism. However, the recurrence rate is lower (9%, none fatal) in patients treated for 6 months after an acute episode of idiopathic DVT/PE than in those treated for only 6 weeks (18% and 0.6% fatal). When the only risks are transient (e.g. surgery, including cesarean section, or trauma), treating for only 3 months may suffice since the recurrence rate is low (0–4%) in these cases.

Suggested management recommendations include the following.

• Venous thromboembolism associated with only transient risk factors: anticoagulation until 6 weeks post partum or until the risks resolve and the patient is mobile, whichever occurs later.

• Distal (calf) vein thrombosis, no previous episode and no other risk factors: anticoagulation for 3 months but if the patient is still pregnant at this point, continue until 6 weeks post partum. Withholding anticoagulants during pregnancy except when extension occurs is an accepted management by some authors.

• Proximal DVT and/or PE, no previous episode, no other risk factors: anticoagulation for 6 months and if the patient is still pregnant at that point, continue until 6 weeks post partum.

• Congenital or acquired thrombophilia with acute DVT and/or PE during pregnancy: anticoagulation for at least 6 months (as above). The treatment should be continued for 1 year or longer after two episodes and perhaps indefinitely after three episodes.

• In the unlikely case of pregnancy in a woman with cancer and venous thrombosis: long-term anticoagulation is recommended.

Prophylaxis for prevention of VTE during pregnancy and post partum

Pregnant women with a history of thromboembolism have a higher risk of recurrence until 4–6 weeks post partum. The overall quoted risk is 12–15%, but in some women it is probably higher: a previous "idiopathic" episode, an underlying hereditary or acquired thrombophilia and residual venous insufficiency (postphlebitic syndrome). If the previous episode was only related to transient risk factors (trauma or surgery), the risk of recurrence is much lower except if there was residual venous damage.

The risk of recurrence is already present in early pregnancy and prophylaxis should be initiated soon enough to be effective (at the end of the first trimester at the latest).

Pregnant women who have to be on prolonged bedrest will benefit from graded compression stockings or intermittent pneumatic leg compression even if they do not have other risks. Intermittent pneumatic leg compression should be used routinely during any operative procedure, particularly cesarean sections.

The American College of Obstetricians and Gynecologists recently issued specific recommendations for the prevention of venous thromboembolism and/or previous adverse pregnancy outcomes. The patients are grouped according to their risk category after the initial assessment.

• *Low risk*: transient risk factors, family history (but no personal history) of VTE or previous history of severe pre-eclampsia, IUGR (≤ 5th percentile) or fetal loss at ≥ 20 weeks. There are no specific recommendations other than perhaps the intrapartum use of intermittent pneumatic leg compressors.

• *Moderate risk*: history of adverse pregnancy outcome such as severe pre-eclampsia, IUGR (≤ 5th percentile), fetal loss at ≥ 20 weeks, history of VTE associated with transient risk factors (including pregnancy) and thrombophilia with family history of VTE. LMWH is recommended antepartum for prevention of adverse pregnancy outcome, either enoxaparin 40 mg subcutaneously once daily or dalteparin 5000 units subcutaneously once daily. Postpartum prophylaxis: enoxaparin 40 mg subcutaneously once daily or 30 mg twice daily or dalteparin 5000 units subcutaneously once daily.

• *High risk*: history of idiopathic VTE outside pregnancy and no other identifiable risk factors, thrombophilia with a previous VTE episode, and history of recurrent pregnancy loss. Subcutaneous LMWH antepartum, either enoxaparin 40 mg once daily or 30 mg twice daily, or dalteparin 5000 units once or twice daily. Measuring antifactor Xa levels each trimester is recommended. Anticoagulation has to be continued after delivery in women with a history of VTE or, if desired and accepted by the patient, warfarin could be used post partum to complete 4–6 weeks.

• *Highest risk*: this group includes women with active thromboembolism (venous or arterial), antiphospholipid antibody syndrome, antithrombin deficiency, homozygotes for factor V Leiden and compound heterozygotes for both factor V Leiden and prothrombin mutations. Therapeutic anticoagulation antepartum and for at least 6 weeks after delivery. Enoxaparin at 1 mg/kg of actual bodyweight, given subcutaneously every 12 hours, or dalteparin 200 units/kg once daily. It is recommended to measure antifactor Xa levels each week, keeping peak levels at 0.8–1.0 IU/mL and through levels at least 0.5 IU/mL. Post partum, warfarin could be used to keep the INR at 2–3 and not stopping heparin until the INR has been therapeutic for a minimum of 2 days (see "Oral anticoagulants (warfarin)" above).

Additional considerations

Although not specifically mentioned in the ACOG consensus, women with any condition requiring full, long-term anticoagulation should be managed as per the "highest risk" group above, and patients with residual venous insufficiency as a result of vein damage from previous DVT should be managed as outlined in the "high-risk" category. Women with antithrombin deficiency might require antithrombin III concentrate at the time of delivery to keep the AT-III level $\geq 80\%$ of normal.

All women undergoing cesarean section should have intermittent pneumatic leg compression during surgery and postoperatively, until they become ambulatory.

There might be some patients in whom antepartum anticoagulation could be safely withheld but only if they meet certain very specific conditions: a single previous VTE episode associated with transient risk factors that occurred longer than 3 months before pregnancy, a normal venous ultrasound with no evidence of residual venous damage, and the exclusion of thrombophilia or any other indication for prolonged anticoagulation. Nevertheless, after delivery they should be given prophylactic anticoagulation for 4–6 weeks as in the "moderate-risk" group above.

Factor Xa inhibitors

Factor Xa inhibitors are a new class of anticoagulants with limited experience of use during pregnancy. The first of this kind of anticoagulants to be approved for use was fondaparinux. It is a category B drug for pregnancy and animal studies have not shown an effect on fertility or harm to the fetus. However, it is secreted into breast milk. At present, treatment with fondaparinux in pregnancy is considered in patients who are unable to use any other measures and are at high risk of thrombosis.

Direct thrombin inhibitors

There is very little information about their use in pregnant women. No impairment of fertility or fetal damage has been reported from animal studies and therefore the FDA has classified them as class B drugs for pregnancy. Those approved for use in the USA include lepirudin, bivalidurin and argatroban. In animal experiments, lepirudin has been shown to cross the placenta and argatroban has been detected in breast milk but there are currently no data about their possible effects in humans.

Reference

Kishimoto TK, Viswanathan K, Ganguly T, *et al.* Contaminated heparin associated with adverse clinical events and activation of the contact system. *NEJM* 2008; 358: 2457–2467.

Suggested readings

Bates SM, Greer IA, Pabinger I, *et al.* Venous thromboembolism, thrombophilia, antithrombotic therapy and pregnancy: American College of Chest Physicians evidence-based clinical practice guidelines (8th edition). *Chest* 2008; 133(suppl): 844S–886S.

Brill-Edwards P, Ginsberg JS, Gent M, *et al.* Safety of withholding heparin in pregnant women with a history of venous thromboembolism. *NEJM* 2000; 343: 1439–1444.

Chan WS, Chunilal S, Lee A, *et al.* A red blood cell agglutination d-dimer test to exclude deep venous thrombosis in pregnancy. *Arch Intern Med* 2007; 147: 165–170.

Duhl AJ, Paidas MJ, Ural SH, *et al.* Antithrombotic therapy and pregnancy: consensus report and recommendations for prevention and treatment of venous thromboembolism and adverse pregnancy outcomes. *Am J Obstet Gynecol* 2007; 197: 457.

Gherman RB, Goodwin TM, Leung BA, *et al.* Incidence, clinical characteristics, and timing of objectively diagnosed venous thromboembolism during pregnancy. *Obstet Gynecol* 1999; 94: 730–734.

Kawamata K, Chiba Y, Tanaka R, *et al.* Experience of temporary inferior vena cava filters inserted in the perinatal period to prevent pulmonary embolism in pregnant women with deep vein thrombosis. *J Vasc Surg* 2005; 41: 652–656.

Marik PE, Plante LA. Venous thromboembolic disease and pregnancy. *NEJM* 2008; 359: 2025–2033.

Matthews S. Imaging pulmonary embolism in pregnancy: what is the most appropriate imaging protocol? *Br J Radiol* 2006; 79: 441–444.

Pillny M, Sandman W, Luther B, *et al.* Deep venous thrombosis during pregnancy and after delivery: indications for and results of thrombectomy. *J Vasc Surg* 2003; 37: 528–532.

Rosenberg VA, Lockwood CJ. Thromboembolism in pregnancy. *Obstet Gynecol Clin North Am* 2007; 34: 481–500.

Van Vlijmen EF, Brouwer JL, Veeger NJ, van der Meer J. Oral contraceptives and the absolute risk of venous thromboembolism in women with single or multiple thrombophilic defects. *Arch Intern Med* 2007; 167: 282–289.

Chapter 28
Systemic Lupus Erythematosus and The Antiphospholipid Syndrome

Martin N. Montoro and T. Murphy Goodwin
Department of Medicine and Obstetrics and Gynecology, Keck School of Medicine, University of Southern California, CA, USA

Systemic lupus erythematosus

Systemic lupus erythematosus (SLE) is a chronic autoimmune disease able to cause inflammatory damage to many different organ systems. Women are affected more often than men (10 to 1) and frequently during their reproductive years (1 in 700 women). Since fertility is generally preserved, SLE is not uncommonly encountered during pregnancy (1 in 1600 pregnancies). The diagnosis of SLE can be made with certainty when four or more of the criteria listed in Box 28.1 are fulfilled. A positive antinuclear antibody (ANA) alone, especially in low titers, does not identify patients at increased risk of pregnancy complications unless found in a suspicious clinical context. Nevertheless, even when the strict criteria for SLE are not met, women with the so-called lupus-like disease (LLD) may experience pregnancy complications.

Timing of pregnancy and disease activity

For patients seeking preconception or early pregnancy counseling, the prognosis is related to the following factors:
• current disease activity
• end organ damage (especially renal impairment)
• medications required to maintain remission
• presence or absence of the antiphospholipid antibody syndrome (APS)
• presence of autoantibodies associated with fetal damage such as anti-Ro/SS-A and anti-La/SS-B.
Knowledge of disease activity prior to pregnancy is important in estimating the risk of a SLE exacerbation and superimposed pre-eclampsia. Patients in remission for 6–12 months before pregnancy have a 35% risk of exacerbation or superimposed pre-eclampsia during pregnancy

Management of Common Problems in Obstetrics and Gynecology, 5th edition. Edited by T.M. Goodwin, M.N. Montoro, L. Muderspach, R. Paulson and S. Roy. © 2010 Blackwell Publishing Ltd.

> **Box 28.1 Criteria for the diagnosis of systemic lupus erythematosus (SLE)**
>
> A patient with any four of the following criteria, either serially or simultaneously, may be classified as having SLE.
> - **Malar rash** (fixed erythematous rash over the malar eminences, sparing the nasolabial folds)
> - **Discoid rash** (erythematous raised patch with keratotic scaling and follicular plugging; older lesions may be atrophic)
> - **Photosensitivity**
> - **Oral ulcers** (usually painless)
> - **Arthritis** (nonerosive arthritis involving two or more peripheral joints)
> - **Serositis**
>   - Pleuritis or pleural effusion or
>   - Pericarditis or pericardial effusion
> - **Renal disorder**
>   - Proteinuria of 0.5 g per day or
>   - Cellular casts
> - **Neurologic disorder**
>   - Seizures in the absence of other causes or
>   - Psychoses in the absence of other causes
> - **Hematologic disorder**
>   - Hemolytic anemia with reticulocytosis or
>   - Leukopenia $<4000/mm^3$ on at least two occasions or
>   - Lymphopenia $<1500/mm^3$ or
>   - Thrombocytopenia $<100,000/mm^3$
> - **Immunologic disorder**
>   - Positive LE cell preparation
>   - Anti-DNA antibody to native double-stranded DNA
>   - Anti-Sm antibody or
>   - False-positive serologic test for a syphilis for at least 6 months
> - **Antinuclear antibody**

and a better than 90% chance of having a viable pregnancy while the risk for patients not in remission prior to pregnancy is approximately 60% for exacerbation or superimposed pre-eclampsia and 50% for a viable pregnancy outcome. Therefore, the optimal time to plan a pregnancy should be when the SLE has been in remission for at least 6–12 months.

Lupus exacerbations have been said to occur unpredictably and at any time during pregnancy or post partum but more recent case-controlled studies have found fewer exacerbations in the third trimester. This finding has been related to lower levels of cytokines (particularly IL-6), estradiol and progesterone in SLE women than in non-SLE, normal pregnant controls. These lower levels have been attributed to a reduced placental production of these compounds and it is suggestive of placental damage in women with SLE. Other recent studies have also shown that postpartum exacerbations were not more frequent in women with SLE than in nonpregnant SLE control patients followed for a similar length of time.

Patients with active renal disease (lupus nephritis) have a poorer prognosis. Between 40% and 60% develop superimposed pre-eclampsia, which may be difficult to distinguish from an SLE exacerbation. Besides clinical symptoms, active urinary sediments, high anti-DNA antibody titers and low serum complement levels will support the diagnosis of lupus exacerbation but still it might be very difficult to differentiate superimposed pre-eclampsia from a lupus flare. Until recently, if a lupus exacerbation was felt to be present, the patient's response to specific therapy for lupus and continued observation was used to determine if a lupus flare or superimposed pre-eclampsia was the main cause of the deterioration. Lately, the Lupus Activity Index to define a lupus flare in nonpregnant patients has been validated and adapted for use in pregnancy as well. Three activity scales, specific for pregnancy, will help to better identify a lupus flare since they showed a 93% sensitivity and 98% specificity: the SLE Pregnancy Disease Activity Index (SLEPDAI), the Lupus Activity Index in Pregnancy (LAI-P), and the modified Systemic Lupus Activity Measure (m-SLAM).

Management of medications

An important goal of therapy is to reduce the number of medications to the least possible and with the safest profile for pregnancy. It is generally recommended to change nonsteroidal anti-inflammatory drugs and hydroxychloroquine to prednisone. Prednisone and other nonfluorinated steroids are preferred because lower amounts reach the fetus as opposed to the fluorinated compounds (betametasone, dexametasone), which cross the placenta in much larger amounts. Although the maternal complications of glucocorticoids could be manifold (glucose intolerance, gastric ulceration, truncal obesity, cutaneous atrophy, poor wound healing, glaucoma, cataracts, osteoporosis and,

less commonly, steroid myopathy and aseptic necrosis of the femoral head), their use during the months of pregnancy in the lowest dose possible is usually not associated with serious complications. Fetal complications such as transient fetal adrenal suppression are rare. The risk of cleft lip and cleft palate with glucocorticoid use in the first trimester is considered to be small. It has also been recently shown that preterm birth after 33 weeks may occur in as many as one-third of patients treated with 40 mg/day or more of prednisone. Breastfeeding is considered to be safe, particularly at daily doses of 40 mg or less of prednisone or equivalent steroid.

Despite the many potential complications, carefully adjusted glucocorticoid regimens are preferable to long-term use of nonsteroidal anti-inflammatory agents (NSAIDs). These compounds may not be too problematic in early pregnancy when given in moderate doses but later, they will cause constriction and/or closure of the ductus arteriosus, which could even be lethal to the fetus. After delivery, NSAIDs are considered safe during breastfeeding. Antimalarials have been generally safe although cases of fetal blindness and deafness have been reported.

The chronic use of pharmacologic doses of steroids will result in maternal adrenal suppression. These patients should be tested for evidence of adrenal insufficiency but if unable to confirm it in a timely manner, intravenous hydrocortisone 100 mg every 8 hours during periods of stress, including delivery or surgical intervention, should be given with tapering to the maintenance dose over the next few days. In addition, patients receiving glucocorticoids should be screened for evidence of tuberculosis, which may reactivate during steroid therapy, as well as for glucose intolerance.

The use of immunosuppressants is generally discouraged. Nevertheless, some of them, including azathioprine and 6-mercaptopurine, have been safer than expected although malformations have been reported with their use. Ciclosporin crosses the placenta but no malformations have been reported. Methotrexate, cyclophosphamide, mycophenolate and mofetil besides being teratogenic, may also cause miscarriage. None of these drugs should be used during lactation. Intravenous immunoglobulins are considered safe (category B) to use if needed. Tumor necrosis factor inhibitors were associated in one report with serious anomalies. If a more complex regimen (e.g. azathioprine) is required to maintain suppression of the disease, however, it should not be changed just because the patient is pregnant.

An important role of the obstetrician is to review the medications and, in most cases, allow the internist/rheumatologist to use the best regimen possible to control the disease because, in general, an active lupus is far worse than the potential medication effect for a successful pregnancy outcome.

Fetal complications of SLE

The risk of intrauterine fetal growth retardation (IUGR) is increased and there are multiple factors involved, including systemic vasculitis, renal disease, chronic hypertension, and superimposed pre-eclampsia. The presence of the antiphospholipid syndrome (see below) along with SLE may be a factor in many of these fetal and maternal complications such as maternal thromboembolic disease and placental insufficiency along with preterm labor, IUGR, pre-eclampsia and fetal death.

The fetal/neonatal lupus syndrome consists of complete congenital heart block or a typical skin rash at birth. If heart block is identified *in utero* high-dose maternal dexametasone therapy has been advocated by some authors but most studies have not shown any benefit. The presence of the maternal antibody anti-Ro/SS-A in a patient with SLE is associated with development of the transient neonatal lupus syndrome in 2–10% of the newborns.

Management guidelines

The basic management of the pregnant patient with SLE, including serologic tests, is shown in Table 28.1. Blood

Table 28.1 Management of pregnant patients with APS or active SLE

Antibody	Frequency in SLE (%)	Clinical significance associations
ANA	> 90	
Anti-ds DNA	> 80	Correlates with disease activity, specific for SLE
ACA	40	Correlates with fetal loss and thrombotic events
LAC	20	
Anti-SSA (Ro)	25	Both associated with
	20	NLE/CCHB Anti-SSB (la) and with Sjögren's syndrome
Every 2 to 3 months		
aCL[a]		Useful for following disease activity
Anti-ds DNA[a]		
Platelet count		
Timed quantification of proteinuria		

[a] If positive initially.
aCL, anticardiolipin antibodies; ANA, antinuclear antibodies; CCHB, congenital complete heart block; NLE, neonatal lupus; LA, lupus anticoagulant.
Notes:
• Visit every 2 weeks until 24 weeks; every 12 weeks thereafter.
• MSAFP at 16–20 weeks.
• Ultrasound every 4 weeks for fetal growth after 20 weeks.
• Antepartum fetal surveillance weekly between 26 and 34 weeks in patients with active disease.
• Screen for gestational diabetes at first visit; if negative, repeat at 24–26 and 32 weeks if on glucocorticoids.

pressure, proteinuria and fetal growth are monitored carefully. Delivery is often triggered by superimposed pre-eclampsia, exacerbation of the SLE or evidence of fetal compromise. However, in the patient who is stable and has a healthy fetus, labor at term can be expected. Cesarean section is done only for the usual obstetric indications.

The antiphospholipid antibody syndrome

An international panel of experts has recently updated the definition of the antiphospholipid syndrome (APS). It is present when one or more of the clinical criteria and one or more of the laboratory criteria are met (Box 28.2).

The diagnosis of APS should not be made if less than 3 months or more than 5 years separate the positive laboratory and the clinical manifestations.

The expert panel discouraged use of the terms primary or secondary APS and recommended simple documentation of the co-existence of other disease. Most patients categorized as having secondary APS usually have SLE and a few others a LLD. It is yet unknown if SLE and APS are different diseases coinciding in one individual, if SLE predisposes to the development of APS or if they are just two different elements of the same disorder.

Antiphospholipid syndrome is generally an acquired condition but an inherited form has been described in a few families. Some authors recommend testing for

---

Box 28.2 Criteria for diagnosis of APS

Clinical criteria
(1) Vascular thrombosis (venous, arterial or small vessel), which must be confirmed by unequivocal, objective testing, and/or (2) pregnancy morbidity: (a) three or more consecutive spontaneous abortions before 10th week and having excluded maternal anatomic or hormonal disturbances as well as both maternal and paternal chromosomal abnormalities, (b) one or more unexplained fetal deaths (morphologically normal fetus) at or beyond the 10th week, or (c) one or more premature deliveries (morphologically normal neonate) before 34th week because of severe pre-eclampsia/eclampsia or placental insufficiency. Accepted features of placental insufficiency include nonreactive stress testing suggestive of fetal hypoxia, abnormal Doppler waveforms, oligohydramnios (index $\leq$ 5 cm) and a birthweight below the 10th percentile for gestational age.

Laboratory criteria
Persistently positive antibody titers during a minimum of 3 months to lupus anticoagulant (LA), anticardiolipin (aCL) at medium/high titers and to β_2-glycoprotein (β_2-GPI) at medium/high titers (to IgG and/or IgM).

more extensive phospholipid antibody subgroups than those recommended by the last international consensus, arguing that almost one-third of APS patients would be missed and not otherwise diagnosed.

Category I APS includes positive tests against more than one antibody and in these cases there is a clear association with clinical events. In category II APS, the tests are positive against only one antibody and no clear association with clinical events. The significance of low-titer IgG anticardiolipin or isolated IgM and antibodies is doubtful and therapeutic decisions should not be made based on them alone. IgA anticardiolipin is not currently considered a laboratory criterion for the diagnosis of APS.

The manifestations of APS unique to pregnancy are varied and include infertility, recurrent miscarriage, IUGR, fetal death, placental abruption, unexplained high maternal serum α-fetoprotein (MSAFP), atypical pre-eclampsia (e.g. occurring very early in gestation, persisting in the postpartum period or associated with hepatic infarction) besides maternal thromboembolism.

The reported pregnancy failure rate among untreated APS women is over 90% and therefore it is unacceptable to leave them untreated. The risk is highest in women found to have an unexplained elevation of the MSAFP between 16 and 20 weeks' gestation. Early reports of improved pregnancy outcome with steroid treatment were not confirmed and besides, steroids may have considerable undesirable side effects. The addition of heparin to low-dose ASA improved the outcome considerably but it appeared that high doses of heparin were not as successful as lower ones, perhaps related to the occurrence of small placental hemorrhages. At present, the most frequently recommended approach to APS women is to start low-dose ASA (81 mg in the USA) before pregnancy if at all possible and then start heparin as soon as pregnancy is documented, either UH 5000 units every 12 hours or, more commonly, LMWH, either enoxaparin 40 mg once or twice a day or dalteparin 5000 units once a day. Obviously, patients with active thromboembolic events will require therapeutic doses of heparin. The potential side effects of both UH and LMWH are detailed in Chapter 27.

There is an accelerated form of APS that affects 1% or less of patients, called catastrophic APS, resulting in multiorgan failure, which develops in a short period of time (less than a week). There is evidence of multiple small vessel occlusion (rarely, also large vessel thrombosis) and very high titers of antiphospholipid antibodies. Usually, there is also a precipitating event, mainly an infectious process. The mortality rate is about 50% with current therapeutic efforts, probably because its rarity makes it difficult to diagnose, study and develop optimal treatment protocols. The management includes treatment of any precipitating factor including the prompt use of antibiotics for suspected infections, removal of necrotic tissues and prevention or treatment of thrombotic events. Combination therapy is reported to achieve the best results (up to 70% survival) and includes anticoagulation, corticosteroids, antibiotics, plasma exchange and intravenous gammaglobulins in addition to full support in the critical intensive care unit.

Women with APS who have had a fetal death but no thrombotic event are still at risk of developing a variety of autoimmune diseases as well as venous or arterial thromboses later in life. Guidelines for following these patients are shown in Table 28.1.

Suggested reading

Alsulyman OM, Castro MA, Zuckerman E, *et al.* Preeclampsia and liver infarction in early pregnancy associated with the antiphospholipid syndrome. *Obstet Gynecol* 1996; 88: 644–646.

Asherson RA, Cervera R, de Groot PG, *et al.* Catastrophic antiphospholipid syndrome: international consensus statement on classification criteria and treatment guidelines. *Lupus* 2003; 12: 530–534.

Bick RI. Antiphospholipid syndrome in pregnancy. *Hematol Oncol Clin North Am* 2008; 22: 107–120.

Brucato A. Prevention of congenital heart block in children of SSA-positive mothers. *Rheumatology* 2008; 47: iii35–iii37.

Doria A, Tincani A, Lockshin M. Challenges of lupus pregnancies. *Rheumatology* 2008; 47(suppl 3): iii9–iii12.

Erkan D, Patel S, Nuzzo M, *et al.* Management of the controversial aspects of the antiphospholipid syndrome pregnancies: a guide for clinicians and researchers. *Rheumatology* 2008; 47: iii23–iii27.

Hochberg MC. Updating the American College of Rheumatology revised criteria for the classification of systemic lupus erythematosus. *Arthritis Rheum* 1997; 40: 1725.

Mecacci F, Bianchi B, Pieralli A, *et al.* Pregnancy outcome in systemic lupus erythematosus complicated by anti-phospholipid antibodies. *Rheumatology* 2009; 48: 246–249.

Miyakis M, Lockshin T, Atsumi D, *et al.* International consensus statement on an update of the classification criteria for definite antiphospholipid syndrome (APS). *J Thromb Haemost* 2006; 4: 295–306.

Ruiz-Irastorza G, Khamashta MA, Gordon C, *et al.* Measuring systemic lupus erythematosus activity during pregnancy: validation of the lupus activity index activity in pregnancy scale. *Arthritis Rheum* 2004; 51: 78–82.

Chapter 29
Urinary Tract Infections in Pregnancy: from Symptomatic Bacteriuria to Pyelonephritis

Bhuvan Pathak
Department of Medicine and Obstetrics and Gynecology, Keck School of Medicine, University of Southern California, CA, USA

Introduction

Infections of the kidney and lower urinary tract are commonly encountered in pregnancy due to the marked physiologic and structural alterations in these organs that occur with advancing gestation. Caliceal dilation due to ureteral obstruction is one change that predisposes to urinary tract infection. Ureteral obstruction is more prominent on the right side and can be attributed to a number of factors including compression from uterine enlargement and relative dextrorotation, compression from the right ovarian venous plexus that crosses over the ureter, and finally from progesterone which may induce smooth muscle relaxation in the ureter. Bladder pressure and capacity are also altered due to decreased tone, all of which when combined lead to increased urinary stasis and predisposition to infection.

Asymptomatic bacteriuria

Asymptomatic bacteriuria complicates 2–10% of all pregnancies and is defined as bacterial colonization of the lower urinary tract without symptoms. The diagnosis has traditionally been established by two clean-catch urine specimens of > 100,000 colony-forming units (cfu)/mL but one midstream void of > 100,000 cfu/mL is now generally accepted as adequate for making the diagnosis. Many other screening tests for the detection of asymptomatic bacteriuria have been suggested, including urinalysis for the presence of nitrites and leukocyte esterases. This method was examined in a meta-analysis and found to have a high specificity (0.98) but a low sensitivity (0.46) in pregnant women for the detection of bacteriuria. Therefore, although the urine dipstick is effective at ruling out urinary infection, its usefulness at ruling in infection is limited and most guidelines instead recommend performing a single urine culture at the beginning of pregnancy. Some authorities recommend cultures in each trimester to improve detection rates.

As mentioned above, the incidence of asymptomatic bacteriuria is 2–10% but this varies with socio-economic status, parity, and sexual practice, as well as with certain medical conditions including sickle cell anemia and diabetes mellitus. The United States Preventative Services Task Force as well as several other international medical societies recommend screening for and treatment of asymptomatic bacteriuria. Screening and treatment of asymptomatic bacteriuria is cost-effective especially in populations where its incidence is greater than 2%. If untreated, up to 30% of cases will progress to pyelonephritis. Furthermore, asymptomatic bacteriuria has been associated with low birthweight and preterm birth. A review of randomized trials comparing antibiotic treatment versus no antibiotic treatment of asymptomatic bacteriuria revealed that the former management resulted in a greater clearance of bacteria as well as in a greater decrease in both pyelonephritis and low birthweight in babies. The rates of preterm delivery, however, were not affected by treatment. It should be noted that the overall quality of studies in this review was reported to be poor so caution in interpretation of these studies must be maintained. With proper treatment of asymptomatic bacteriuria, the number needed to treat to prevent one episode of pyelonephritis is only 7, and the rate of hospitalization for pyelonephritis is reduced to 1.4%.

As in the nonpregnant state, *E. coli* is the most common uropathogen found in asymptomatic bacteriuria, accounting for about 80% of isolates. Other pathogens include *K. pneumoniae*, *Enterococcus* species, *S. saprophyticus*, and *P. mirabilis*. Finally, group B hemolytic streptococcus (GBS) in the urine has been associated with preterm rupture of membranes and preterm delivery, as well as with early-onset neonatal sepsis and postpartum chorio-amnionitis. Antepartum treatment of GBS significantly decreases the above-mentioned complications. Further intrapartum prophylaxis for antepartum GBS

Management of Common Problems in Obstetrics and Gynecology, 5th edition. Edited by T.M. Goodwin, M.N. Montoro, L. Mudersbach, R. Paulson and S. Roy. © 2010 Blackwell Publishing Ltd.

bacteriuria is also recommended to reduce the postpartum and neonatal complications mentioned above.

A meta-analysis of 10 randomized controlled trials comparing single dose versus 4–7-day treatments of asymptomatic bacteriuria showed a nonstatistically significant higher "no cure rate" for those in the single-dose group. There were no significant differences in the rates of recurrence, preterm delivery or pyelonephritis but the studies were not sufficiently powered to detect differences in the latter two outcomes. Finally, single-dose treatments were associated with fewer adverse side effects of any kind. The study concluded that there was not enough evidence to support the use of one regimen over the other but single-dose treatment was associated with lower costs and side effects. Therefore, the recommendations for treatment of asymptomatic bacteriuria at present remain standard cystitis treatment regimens.

Patients with an initial positive urine culture are treated empirically, usually based upon local resistance patterns. A variety of antibiotics have been used to treat asymptomatic bacteriuria and appear to be equally efficacious although there has been no systematic review of the topic. The Cochrane review of treatment for symptomatic cystitis concluded that there was insufficient evidence to recommend any one regimen over another. These conclusions have been assumed to most likely be applicable to the treatment of asymptomatic bacteriuria and therefore a number of standard regimes are currently used in its treatment (Box 29.1). Single-dose regimens are also listed in Box 29.2.

When prescribing antibiotic agents, one should be familiar with the possible side effects and contraindications of various classes of drugs. For example, penicillins and cephalosporins sometimes cause allergic reactions and rarely anaphylactic reactions. Nitrofurantoin leads to hemolysis in patients with glucose-6-phosphate dehydrogenase deficiency. Sulfonamides inhibit the binding of bilirubin to albumin and are thus associated with neonatal hyperbilirubinemia and kernicterus and should be avoided in the third trimester. Regardless of the type and duration of the antibiotic course used, patients should be recultured at the culmination of treatment to ensure eradication, as well as on a monthly basis as the risk of recurrence remains elevated. Patients who have a recurrent infection with the same pathogen or who are reinfected with a different pathogen should have culture

---

Box 29.1 Seven to 21 day treatments of symptomatic or asymptomatic bacteriuria

- Amoxicillin 500 mg po tid
- Nitrofurantoin 100 mg po qid
- Cephalexin 250–500 mg po qid

Box 29.2 Single-dose treatments of symptomatic or asymptomatic bacteriuria

- Amoxicillin 3 g po
- Cephalexin 2 g po
- Nitrofurantoin 200 mg po

---

and sensitivities performed and treated accordingly. After two documented infections, consideration should be given to suppressive therapy for the remainder of the pregnancy. A commonly used suppressive regimen is nitrofurantoin 100 mg orally, nightly.

Cystitis

Acute cystitis occurs in 1–2% of pregnancies and symptoms include urinary frequency, dysuria, and urgency. Diagnosis of cystitis based on symptoms alone may be confusing as some of the above-mentioned symptoms are common in normal pregnancy, given compression of the bladder by the enlarging uterus. Factors that have been associated with cystitis in pregnancy include those associated with asymptomatic bacteriuria listed above as well as the following: anatomic abnormalities of the urinary tract, prior antenatal or pre-pregnancy urinary tract infections, history of chlamydia (in Caucasian women), less than 12 years of education, illicit drug use, unmarried status, use of nonprivate clinics, and age less than 30 years.

Given that treatment of asymptomatic bacteriuria has not been associated with a decreased incidence of cystitis, it is assumed that most cases of cystitis develop *de novo*. Treatment of cystitis is the same as that for asymptomatic bacteriuria (see Box 29.1). As mentioned above, a Cochrane review of nine studies showed that no single treatment regimen for cystitis in pregnancy was superior to another. More specifically, there were no differences with regard to cure rates, recurrent infection, preterm delivery, admission to the neonatal intensive care unit, need for change of antibiotic or prolonged pyrexia. Again, as for asymptomatic bacteriuria, cultures should be repeated at the end of therapy and on a monthly basis thereafter. Finally, in the case of persistent symptoms and negative urine cultures, consideration of other diagnoses, including cervicitis, vaginitis, and especially urethritis, should be entertained and cultures taken appropriately.

Pyelonephritis

Pyelonephritis also complicates 1–2% of pregnancies and its recurrence rate is approximately 20%. The majority of cases occur antepartum, but a significant proportion do present in the postpartum period as well. Pyelonephritis is most commonly encountered in younger, nulliparous women in their second trimester. Women with a history of pyelonephritis, renal calculi or anatomic malformations are particularly susceptible to the development of pyelonephritis and should therefore be regularly screened on a monthly basis throughout pregnancy. In a prospective study of 440 cases of antepartum pyelonephritis, there was no difference in ethnic background in women with or without pyelonephritis. In the same study, 13% had an identifiable risk factor for pyelonephritis, the most common being a previous history of pyelonephritis or asymptomatic bacteruria.

Symptoms and signs of pyelonephritis include symptoms of cystitis, chills, flank pain, nausea, vomiting, fever, and costovertebral angle tenderness. The diagnosis is made by urine culture and therefore, as for cystitis, therapy is begun on an empiric basis. One to two bacteria per high-power field (hpf) on a unspun urine sample or greater than 20 bacteria per hpf on a spun urine sample correlates with 100,000 cfu/mL. The presence of white blood cell casts on urinalysis can confirm the diagnosis as well. Other basic investigations which should be obtained include a complete blood count and a basic metabolic panel to detect the presence of thrombocytopenia, anemia due to hemolysis, hypokalemia, and a rising creatinine. These laboratory parameters, with the exception of anemia, usually normalize within several days of treatment. Blood cultures may also be obtained if the patient presents with significant fever or a septic appearance, and especially if there is a suboptimal response to antibiotics within 48 hours.

Bacteremia is present in 10–20% of patients with pyelonephritis. Standard treatment involves in-hospital administration of intravenous antibiotics for at least 48 hours afebrile. If bacteremia is present, intravenous treatment should be extended to a period of at least 5–7 days. As with cystitis, *E. coli* is the uropathogen cultured in 70–81% of cases. The most commonly used first-line regimen is a first-generation cephalosporin such as cefazolin 1–2 g every 8 hours. Other treatment options include a second- or third-generation cephalosporin, an extended-spectrum penicillin or ampicillin if local bacterial susceptibilities are high. Of note, in a trial of 179 patients with pyelonephritis prior to 24 weeks who were randomized to one of three different antibiotic regimens (IV ampicillin + gentamicin, IV cefazolin, IM ceftriaxone), there were no significant differences in clinical response or birth outcomes. Treatment with antibiotics has also been shown to decrease the frequency of uterine contractions.

A clinical response to antibiotics, as reflected by defervescence and a decrease in pain and costovertebral angle tenderness, is usually observed within 48–72 hours of treatment. If there has been no such response or only a subclinical response to treatment, then the patient must be re-evaluated and an aminoglycoside may be added if the uropathogen is susceptible to such an agent. Further evaluation involves radiologic evaluation of the kidneys and urinary tract to assess for nephrolithiasis and anatomic malformation. First-line imaging modalities include either ultrasound or a one-shot intravenous pyelogram to reduce radiation exposure to the fetus.

Following IV or IM treatment, oral antibiotics should be continued to complete a 2-week course. A urine culture should be obtained at this point to ensure eradication of bacteria. Furthermore, suppressive antibiotic therapy is recommended for the remainder of the gestation with a common choice being nitrofurantoin 100 mg orally, nightly. In noncompliant patients, monthly urine cultures should be obtained to screen for recurrent bacterial growth.

More serious complications of pyelonephritis include septic shock and pulmonary insufficiency, the latter having a reported incidence of fewer than 10%. Pregnant women are more susceptible to the effects of endotoxins and are therefore more likely to develop these complications when compared with their nonpregnant counterparts. Endotoxins can cause increased vascular and alveolar capillary permeability, decreased peripheral vascular resistance, and changes in cardiac output. A high index of suspicion for these complications must be maintained. Patients with shortness of breath, tachypnea, desaturation or decreases in blood pressure should be promptly evaluated. Evaluation should include, but not be limited to, chest radiographs and arterial blood gas determination. Care should be continued in an intensive care setting, with respiratory and vascular support promptly administered as needed. This may include intubation and vasopressive agents respectively.

Conclusion

Infections of the urinary tract are commonly encountered in pregnancy. Asymptomatic bacteriuria can lead to pyelonephritis and adverse pregnancy outcomes if left untreated and should therefore be screened for and treated promptly. There are various treatment regimens which are effective for both asymptomatic and symptomatic cystitis. Pyelonephritis is also commonly seen in pregnancy and management remains in-hospital administration of antibiotics until symptoms and fever subside. Given the uncommon but not rare progression of pyelonephritis to sepsis and pulmonary edema or adult respiratory distress syndrome, patients must be closely monitored and treated aggressively at the first sign of such conditions. Finally, patients with asymptomatic or symptomatic bacteriuria should be monitored for recurrent infection during the remainder of pregnancy, while those with pyelonephritis require daily suppressive therapy for the remainder of their gestation.

Suggested reading

Anderson BL, Simhan HN, Simons KM, Wiesenfeld HC. Untreated asymptomatic group B streptococcal bacteriuria in pregnancy and chorioamnionitis at delivery. *Am J Obstet Gynecol* 2007; 196(6): 524.

Deville WL, Yzermans JC, van Duijn NP, Bezemer PD, van der Windt DA, Bouter LM. The urine dipstick test useful to rule out infections. A meta-analysis of the accuracy. *BCM Urol* 2004; 2(4): 4.

Hill JB, Sheffield JS, McIntire DD, Wendel GD Jr. Acute pyelonephritis in pregnancy. *Obstet Gynecol* 2005; 105(1): 18–23.

Milar LK, DeBuque L, Wing DA. Uterine contraction frequency during treatment of pyelonephritis in pregnancy and subsequent risk of preterm birth. *J Perinat Med* 2003; 31(1): 41–46.

Pastore LM, Savitz DA, Thorp JM Jr. Predictors of urinary tract infection at the first prenatal visit. *Epidemiology* 1999; 10(3): 282–287.

Pastore LM, Savitz DA, Thorp JM Jr, Koch GG, Hertz-Picciotto I, Irwin DE. Predictors of symptomatic urinary tract infection after twenty weeks' gestation. *J Perinatol* 1999; 19(7): 488–493.

Sharma P, Thapa L. Acute pyelonephritis in pregnancy: a retrospective study. *Aust NZ J Obstet Gynecol* 2007; 47(4): 313–315.

Smaill F. Asymptomatic bacteriuria in pregnancy. *Best Pract Res Clinic Obstet Gynaecol* 2007; 21(3): 439–450.

Smaill F, Vazquez JC. Antibiotics for asymptomatic bacteriuria in pregnancy. *Cochrane Database Syst Rev* 2007; 2: CD000490.

Villar J, Lydon-Rochelle MT, Gulmezoglu AM, Roganti A. Duration of treatment for asymptomatic bacteriuria during pregnancy. *Cochrane Database Syst Rev* 2000; 2: CD000491.

Vazquez JC, Villar J. Treatments for symptomatic urinary tract infection during pregnancy. *Cochrane Database Syst Rev* 2003; 4: CD002256

Wing DA, Hendershott CM, Debuque L, Miller LK. A randomized trial of three antibiotics for the treatment of pyelonephritis in pregnancy. *Obstet Gynecol* 1998; 92(2) 249–253.

Chapter 30
Diabetes Mellitus in Pregnancy

Carolina Reyes

Department of Medicine and Obstetrics and Gynecology, Keck School of Medicine, University of Southern California, CA, USA

Introduction

Gestational diabetes refers to any degree of glucose intolerance with variable severity with the onset or first recognition during pregnancy. This complicates approximately 4–7% of pregnancies. The prevalence may range from 1% to 14%. About 90% of diabetes in pregnancy is gestational diabetes. This does not exclude the possibility of unrecognized pre-existing diabetes before pregnancy. Pregestational diabetes, which accounts for 5–10% of diabetes in pregnancy, refers to diabetes diagnosed before pregnancy. Diabetes mellitus is a metabolic disorder that can significantly alter the maternal and *in utero* environment, leading to complications. Optimizing maternal glucose is central to the management of diabetes in pregnancy because it has been shown that most complications in pregnancy can be prevented or controlled.

The most widely used classification of diabetes mellitus in pregnancy is the White classification. The categorization was used to indicate the duration of disease, age of onset in relation to the pregnancy, and the presence or absence of diabetic complications (Table 30.1). This classification has become less useful as the pathogenesis of diabetes and the effects of complications on the outcome of pregnancy are better understood. From a clinical management perspective, it is more useful to group patients into three functional groups.

• Gestational diabetes (patients developing diabetes for the first time during pregnancy)
• Preconceptional diabetes without diabetic sequelae (both insulin-dependent and noninsulin-dependent diabetes)
• Preconceptional diabetes with significant diabetic sequelae (nephropathy, advanced retinopathy, autonomic neuropathy or coronary artery disease)

Management of Common Problems in Obstetrics and Gynecology, 5th edition. Edited by T.M. Goodwin, M.N. Montoro, L. Muderspach, R. Paulson and S. Roy. © 2010 Blackwell Publishing Ltd.

Screening for gestational diabetes mellitus

Recommendations for screening for gestational diabetes mellitus are not universally agreed upon. The Fourth International Workshop Conference on Gestational Diabetes recommends screening for gestational diabetes based on an initial assessment of individual risk in all pregnant women (Tables 30.2, 30.3). High-risk criteria include those 25 years or older, belonging to an ethnic group with a high prevalence of type 2 diabetes, obesity, diabetes in a first-degree relative, history of glucose intolerance or prior gestational diabetes, prior history of macrosomia, unexplained stillbirth or congenital anomaly, current glycosuria. Women with high-risk factors should undergo screening at the first visit or as soon as possible, while individuals who continue to exhibit low-risk characteristics do not require screening. A 1-hour 50 g glucose challenge test performed randomly without regard

Table 30.1 Classification of diabetes during pregnancy

White's classification	Age of diagnosis or onset	Duration of diabetes	Diabetes sequelae	Physiologic classification
A	Any	Pregnancy	None	Gestational diabetes
B	> 20 years old	< 10 years	None	Pregestational diabetes
C	10–19 years old	or 10–19 years	None	Pregestational diabetes
D	< 10 years old	or > 20 years	Benign retinopathy	Pregestational diabetes
F	Any	Any	Nephropathy	Pregestational diabetes with sequelae
R	Any	Any	Proliferative retinopathy	Pregestational diabetes with sequelae
H	Any	Any	Coronary artery disease	Pregestational diabetes with sequelae

Table 30.2 Clinical screening for gestational diabetes based on clinical characteristics

	High risk (one or more)	Average risk	Low risk (all)
Clinical risk	Obesity Diabetes of first-degree relative History of GDM Prior history of macrosomia, unexplained stillbirth or anomaly Current glycosuria	Meets neither low-risk or high-risk criteria	Normal pregnancy weight and normal weight gain during pregnancy No diabetes in a first-degree relative No history of glucose intolerance No history of macrosomia, unexplained stillbirth or congenital anomaly Below age 25 Belongs to a low-risk race or ethnic group
When to screen	At initial prenatal visit or as soon as possible	Between 24 and 28 weeks of gestation	Not required
How to screen	Ingest 50 g glucose without reference to time of day or last meal Measure serum or plasma venous concentration 1 hour after Positive screen meriting oral GTT: >140 mg/dL		

* Not a high-risk race or ethnic group for type 2 diabetes, namely Hispanic, Black, Native American, South or East Asian, Pacific Islander

Table 30.3 Diagnosis of diabetes during pregnancy based on the recommendations of the Fourth International Workshop-Conference on Gestational Diabetes Mellitus

	Glucose tolerance test (mg/dL)				
	Fasting[†]	Random[‡]	1 h	2 h	3 h
Diabetes mellitus (type 1 or 2)	126	200	–	–	–
Gestational diabetes mellitus[§]					
1997 4th International Workshop-Conference on GDM	95	–	180	155	140

[†] A subsequent abnormal fasting glucose level >126 mg/dL is required to confirm the diagnosis of DM. This excludes further testing for gestational diabetes by a 3-hour GTT.

[‡] Random values are measured at any time and exclude those measured during a GCT or OGTT.

[§] The diagnosis of GDM is made by a 100 g, 3-hour oral glucose test. Two or more values must be met for the diagnosis of GDM.

to time or eating is recommended. If the initial screen is < 140 mg/dL in high-risk individuals, the screening test should be repeated or performed at 24–28 weeks' gestation. Routine screening is not required if the individual meets all low-risk criteria. Routine screening at 24–28 weeks is recommended for those not meeting low- or high-risk criteria.

The US Preventive Services Task Force states that there is insufficient evidence to assess the balance between the benefits and harm of screening for GDM either before or after 24 weeks' gestation and clinicians should discuss screening with their patients on a case-by-case basis. The American College of Obstetricians and Gynecologists recommends universal screening since there is a high prevalence of pregnant patients meeting the high-risk criteria. The Australian Carbohydrate Intolerance Study in Pregnant Women (ACHOIS), a multicenter control trial of gestational diabetes mellitus (GDM) versus routine prenatal care found a reduction in the composite of severe perinatal outcomes in the treatment group. The Hyperglycemia and Adverse Pregnancy Outcome (HAPO) study, a multi-institutional study, found strong associations between higher level of maternal glucose at 24–32 weeks, within normoglycemic levels, and adverse pregnancy outcomes. Given that hyperglycemia and pregnancy complications are strongly associated and that managing gestational diabetes reduces complications, the results support screening for GDM. Current recommendations for screening in pregnancy are being debated internationally. LAC/USC Medical Center screens every pregnant woman at the first visit and if negative, again at 24–28 weeks. This is based on the high prevalence of risk criteria in our population.

A glucose challenge test (GCT) is recommended for screening for GDM. Fifty grams of oral glucose is ingested without diet preparation, at any time of day, with a venous plasma glucose level measured 1 hour later. A positive screen is defined as greater than or equal to 140 mg/dL. Some recommend 130 mg/dL and require a follow-up oral glucose tolerance test (OGTT) to diagnose GDM. Using a cut-off of 130 mg/dL increases the sensitivity by 10% but results in almost twice as many OGTT performed. If the GCT equals or exceeds 200 mg/dL, the risk of undiagnosed diabetes is increased. We recommend measuring overnight fasting plasma glucose the next day. If the fasting plasma glucose is equal to or greater than 126 mg/dL, no further testing is necessary; the patient has undiagnosed diabetes. Otherwise an OGTT is performed after an overnight fast of 8–14 hours after 3 days of unrestricted carbohydrate intake. Venous plasma glucose levels are measured fasting and at 1, 2, and 3 hours. The diagnosis of GDM is made when two or more values meet or exceed the cut-off thresholds based on the Fourth International Conference Workshop Conference on GDM: fasting, 95 mg/dL; 1 hour, 180 mg/dL; 2 hour, 155 mg/dL; 3 hour, 140 mg/dL. Diagnosis is a vital step in the management of GDM. Once the diagnosis is made, achieving euglycemia leads to reduction of perinatal complications.

Pregestational diabetes mellitus

Women with pre-existing diabetes mellitus may have insulin-dependent (IDDM or type 1), noninsulin-dependent diabetes mellitus (NIDDM or type 2) or maturity-onset diabetes of the young (MODY). In type I diabetes, the insulin deficiency usually results from autoimmune destruction of pancreatic β cells, leading to severe or complete insulin deficiency. In type 2 diabetes, the insulin deficiency occurs due to progressive β cell dysfunction. It is recognized that both type I and type II diabetes may be heterogeneous in etiology. MODY, an autosomal dominant form of diabetes resulting from several gene-specific mutations, provides a third category of β cell dysfunction. Although the White's classification is still used for diagnosis, it is clinically more useful to categorize patients with pregestational diabetes into those with and without significant medical complications.

Pregnancy for the woman with diabetic sequelae significantly elevates the risk for maternal, fetal and neonatal morbidity and mortality and requires close and highly specialized medical care. These complications include preproliferative or proliferative retinopathy, nephropathy, autonomic neuropathy, and coronary artery disease. Many patients have multiple complications and pregnancy outcome is worse with multiple organ involvement. Women with pre-existing diabetes should undergo a baseline assessment of renal function, thyroid assessment, lipid screen. If pre-existing diabetes is greater than five years, an EKG and ophthalmology exam is also recommended.

Effects of diabetes on fetal development

Infants born to women with pregestational diabetes, type 1 or type 2 have an increased risk of major congenital anomalies. This risk increases with poor glycemic and metabolic control during embryogenesis. The overall rate of major congenital anomalies in women with type 1 and type 2 diabetes is 6–12%. With poor glycemic control, the risk increases dramatically to 22–25%. Glucose is an easily measured metabolite and provides a benchmark for assessment of metabolic regulation in diabetic pregnancies. With elevated glucose, fatty acids, ketones,

triglycerides, and amino acids may be elevated. These metabolites may also have an effect on embryonic and fetal development. This may explain why glycemic control does not completely eliminate fetal complications in pregnancy. The risk of major congenital anomalies correlates with the initial glycosolated hemoglobin level and the initial mean fasting glucose levels. The risk of spontaneous abortion is also increased with poor glycemic control. The most common major structural congenital anomalies for both type I and type 2 diabetes involve the heart (transposition of the great vessels, atrial, ventricular septal defects), the central nervous system (caudal regression, anencephaly, spina bifida, and encephalocele) and the genitourinary system (renal agenesis, cystic kidneys and duplication of the renal collecting system). Judicious use of ultrasonography provides essential information about the fetus of a woman with pre-existing diabetes. A first-trimester ultrasound should be used to date the pregnancy and to document fetal viability; a second-trimester ultrasound (18–20 weeks) involving a detailed survey of fetal anatomy and a fetal echocardiogram will rule out most major congenital anomalies.

Fetal growth is also affected, especially if the glycemia is poorly controlled. Elevated maternal glucose and abnormal levels of other nutrients cross the placenta, producing elevated fetal glucose and altered nutrient levels. The fetus in turn produces high levels of insulin – fetal hyperinsulinism. High levels of fetal insulin promote abnormal intrauterine growth or somatic and biochemical fetopathy. A newborn of a diabetic mother with poor glycemic control can exhibit abnormal adipose deposition (central obesity), visceral organ hypertrophy and hyperplasia (hypertrophic cardiomyopathy and pancreatic hyperplasia) and biochemical dysregulation (hypoglycemia, hyperbilirubinemia, hypocalcemia). Strict maternal glucose control reduces but may not completely eliminate fetal overgrowth. The goal of management is to normalize glucose levels to minimize fetal overgrowth and reduce the risks of congenital abnormalities and prevent spontaneous loss or stillbirth.

Effects of pregnancy on diabetes

Maternal metabolism alters significantly during early pregnancy to provide adequate nutritional stores for the demands later in pregnancy and during lactation. In normal pregnancy, the metabolic alterations in pregnancy lead to increased insulin resistance. This is thought to be due to several placental hormones (human placental lactogen, progesterone, cortisol, possibly placental insulinase) and cytokines elevated in the maternal circulation. The normal response to insulin resistance is to increase insulin secretion up to 3–5 times more in order to minimize the impact of insulin resistance on the circulating glucose levels. With low insulin levels, pregnant women shift to lipolysis, producing free fatty acids and ketones for energy. Women with diabetes are unable to meet the demand of increased insulin secretion. They are either unable to secrete sufficient insulin (type I DM) or they have β cell dysfunction with the inability to produce sufficient insulin (type 2I or GDM). Women with diabetes in pregnancy require increasing insulin doses as the pregnancy progresses and are at increased risk for fasting hypoglycemia, lower premeal glucose or rapid development of ketosis with low blood sugars.

Medical management of diabetes

The cornerstone of therapy, whether treating gestational or pregestational diabetes, is the maintenance of euglycemia throughout the pregnancy. This is achieved primarily through a combination of proper diet, exercise, home glucose monitoring and self-management education, insulin therapy or oral hypoglycemic agents. Medical management requires a team approach. This usually involves an obstetrician, perinatologist, endocrinologist, neonatologist, diabetes nurse specialist, a registered dietician and social work specialists. Involving the patient and her family as an equal team member in every step of her management is vital to achieving a successful outcome. Screening for psychosocial issues that may compromise compliance with treatment should be a routine part of care, such as screening for depression, domestic violence and substance use.

Medical management of diabetes in pregnancy involves a trial of dietary therapy with sufficient calories and nutrients to meet the increasing demands of pregnancy and to maintain good metabolic control. The nutritional requirements for women with diabetes are the same whether they have gestational or pregestational diabetes. For women with ideal bodyweight (BMI < 26 kg/m^2), a diet of 30 kcal per kilogram of true bodyweight is prescribed. Women who are overweight ($> 120\%$ of ideal bodyweight or a BMI of $> 26\%$), a caloric intake of 25 kcal per kg is recommended. The minimum and maximum calories prescribed are between 1800 and 2500, regardless of maternal weight. The current recommended diet for patients with diabetes includes 10–20% of calories as protein, about 50–60% as carbohydrate, less than 30% as fats and less than 10% as saturated fats. Complex carbohydrates are digested and absorbed more slowly. This results in a smaller increase in blood sugar. The ADA guidelines suggest individualizing the percentage of calories from carbohydrates. A diet that helps blunt the postprandial glucose level reduces the risk of developing macrosomia. The calories are distributed throughout the day as three meals and three snacks.

Women with gestational diabetes who maintain fasting glucose levels below 90 mg/dL and 1 hour postprandial < 135 mg/dL on diet therapy are at minimal risk for developing fetal macrosomia or other neonatal complications. As the pregnancy progresses, women who demonstrate hyperglycemia require more intense therapy.

For women with pregestational diabetes or gestational diabetes with hyperglycemia, self-monitoring of blood glucose, fasting, premeal, postmeal, and bedtime, is recommended. Over the last decade, the target glycemic levels have been reduced due to improved benefit in reducing the risk of macrosomia. The target glycemic levels are fasting, 60–90 mg/dL; before lunch, dinner and bedtime snack, 60–90 mg/dL; 1 hour postprandial, < 135 mg/dL; and 2 am–6 am, 60-90 mg/dL. Self-monitoring of glucose provides patients with immediate feedback about the effect of their meal on their glucose level. This gives patients ample opportunity to learn about the quantity and type of foods that increase postprandial glucose levels.

Daily exercise in the form of walking briskly 30 minutes/day or 15 minutes three times a day after meals is also recommended. Maternal exercise has been shown to reduce hyperglycemia in patients with gestational diabetes. Patients with long-standing diabetes should be under close observation before taking on an exercise training program.

Most patients with gestational diabetes, the most common metabolic disorder of pregnancy, are treated with diet therapy alone. Kjos *et al.* demonstrated that when glucose levels are only borderline elevated, an ultrasound to measure fetal abdominal circumference to assess excessive fetal growth is a useful modality to help identify if a fetus is at risk for macrosomia. Women with GDM and borderline hyperglycemia should have a strict regimen of diet and exercise with close monitoring to reduce the risk of unmonitored hyperglycemia.

Pharmacologic therapy

All women with pregestational diabetes and approximately 20–50% of women with gestational diabetes require pharmacologic agents for glucose control. Insulin is the mainstay of pharmacotherapy. An advantage of insulin is that it does not cross the placenta. The insulin dose should be titrated to achieve euglycemia. Patients usually require combined rapid- and /or intermediate-acting insulin given in multiple injections or an insulin pump. These patients should be managed by physicians and diabetes care teams. Significant attention is given to teaching the patient self-management skills and the understanding of diabetes in pregnancy. Patients can manage their diabetes with outpatient management and 24-hour on-call service. The insulin dose should be based on the current gestational age and bodyweight. During embryogenesis, patients with markedly elevated fasting hyperglycemia should be hospitalized for rapid glycemic control and teaching to reduce the risk of congenital anomalies.

Oral agents are used to achieve euglycemia because of their ease of administration and dosing schedule. Oral agents can cross the placenta. Glyburide is a second-generation sulfonylurea whose primary action is to suppress hepatic glucose production and improve insulin secretion after meals. Glyburide is demonstrated to be effective in patients with residual B-cell function. It was initially shown not to cross the placenta in significant amounts and was also not detectable in umbilical cord blood. A recent study reported that umbilical cord levels of glyburide averaged 70% of maternal levels when using a different modality to detect blood levels. Insulin sensitivity was five times lower in women with GDM as compared to healthy pregnant women. Current dosing recommendations may not be sufficient to achieve higher levels of insulin sensitivity. Fetal safety should be considered when administering glyburide, especially when considering higher doses.

Metformin is a biguanide that enhances insulin action by stimulating glucose uptake in the liver and by suppressing hepatic glucose output. Metformin is used for type 2 diabetes patients with residual B-cell function. It does not stimulate insulin secretion and therefore does not cause hypoglycemia. Metformin has been shown to cross the placenta and concentrate in the fetal compartment. It is classified as a class B drug but many questions remain about the fetal effects of this agent and further studies should evaluate its safety. A large randomized control trial, the Metformin in Gestational Diabetes (MiG) trial, found that 46% of women assigned to metformin required the addition of insulin to achieve glycemic goals.

Obstetric management of diabetes

Pregnancy dating is paramount in the obstetric management of diabetes patients. Unsure dating criteria or accelerated fetal growth due to uncontrolled diabetes may lead to delivery prematurely. Prenatal genetic screening includes first-trimester ultrasound and an expanded MSAFP screen at 16–20 weeks. A detailed anatomy ultrasound at 18–22 weeks to rule out major congenital abnormalities is recommended. An echocardiogragm may be warranted if the glycemic control in the first trimester was poor or if the hemoglobin A1C was above 7%.

The first prenatal visit should include a urine culture to screen for urinary infections due to increased risk of pyelonephritis. A thyroid-stimulating hormone, lipid panel and 24-hour protein and creatinine clearance are recommended. Antepartum testing is recommended in all women with pregestational diabetes or insulin-requiring GDM beginning 34 weeks or earlier if there are other medical complications. In diet-treated GDM patients, testing should begin by 40 weeks. At LAC + USC, in

the tested diabetic population, the stillbirth rate is about 1.5 per 1000 babies. Decisions regarding the timing of delivery should be individualized. Generally, elective delivery after 38.5 weeks may be considered for women with pregestational and gestational diabetes, taking into account glycemic control, estimated fetal weight, and likelihood of a successful labor induction. All diabetes patients should be delivered by 40 weeks given the increased risk of macrosomia and of stillbirth. Diabetes patients should be monitored for clinical signs of pre-eclampsia or uncontrolled hypertension.

Intrapartum maternal glycemic control

Generally, the glucose requirement in labor is less. Women with pregestational and insulin-requiring GDM need close monitoring of glucose levels during labor. Patients who are scheduled for an elective cesarean or induction of labor are instructed to enter early in the morning fasting and not take their morning insulin or oral agent. Intrapartum, patients receive continuous intravenous glucose infusion (5% dextrose NS at 125 mg/h). Insulin is administered via an intravenous pump with monitoring of glucose values every 1–2 hours. Women with insulin-requiring GDM or type 2 diabetes may not require insulin infusion. Insulin should be started if the glucose level exceeds 120 mg/dL. The insulin rate is adjusted in 0.5–1.0 unit increments for every 40 mg/dL of glucose increase. The target glucose goal is 70–119 mg/dL. For women with type I diabetes, insulin should be started at a basal rate of 0.5–1.0 units per hour.

Women requiring a long period of induction may be a candidate for oral feeding with a reduced caloric diet (1200–1400 calories) and controlled by short- and rapid-acting insulin with premeal and postmeal glucose checks. When the patient enters active labor, she can be switched to the standard intrapartum management.

Postpartum management, lactation and family planning

In the postpartum period, women with pregestational diabetes may not require insulin or only need a low dose to control their glucose levels. Short- or rapid-acting insulin should be administered on a sliding scale based on glucose levels measured every 4 hours if they are not eating or based on premeal glucose levels. In type I diabetes, insulin is generally restarted 1–5 days post partum based on 0.5–0.6 units/kg of actual bodyweight. There is very limited information about the safety of oral hypoglycemic agents if the mother is breastfeeding and they are generally not recommended for control of hyperglycemia immediately post partum. Diabetes patients should continue to monitor glucose levels and return 1–2 weeks post partum for re-evaluation. Breastfeeding can exhaust about 500 calories per day and should be encouraged. Breastfeeding reduces glucose concentration and insulin requirements.

Women with pregestational diabetes should be referred for continued management within 3–6 months. Women with gestational diabetes should be tested 4–12 weeks post partum and if negative, tested yearly thereafter. Women with gestational diabetes have a considerable risk of developing type 2 diabetes later in life. The risk is similar in all ethnic groups with GDM. There is nearly a linear increase in the cumulative incidence of diabetes during the first 10 years after pregnancy. Mestman *et al.* found in a Hispanic population that 65% of women with GDM developed diabetes during a 12–18-year period post partum. Overall, women will have more than a 50% risk of developing diabetes within 10–20 years. Factors associated with an increased risk of developing type 2 diabetes after GDM include: a previous history of GDM, high maternal age, overweight, early gestational age at diagnosis of GDM, a high fasting and 2-hour OGTT, a low fasting plasma insulin in the diagnostic OGTT, and insulin treatment during pregnancy.

All women should be encouraged to follow an ADA diet, achieve or maintain ideal bodyweight and exercise daily. Planning a future pregnancy and contraception should be addressed. Patients should be counseled about the risk of congenital anomalies with poor glucose control, and the risk of developing diabetes for both mother and child. Preconception counseling prior to a planned pregnancy is highly recommended.

Suggested reading

Crowther CA, Hiller JE, Moss JR, McPhee AJ, Jeffries WS, Robinson JS. Effect of treatment of gestational diabetes mellitus on pregnancy outcomes. *NEJM* 2005; 352: 2477–2486.

Expert Committee on the Diagnosis and Classification of Diabetes Mellitus. Diagnosis and classification of diabetes mellitus. *Diabetes Care* 2008; 31: S55–S60.

Herbert MF, Ma X, Naraharisetti SB, *et al.* Are we optimizing gestational diabetes treatment with glyburide? The pharmacologic basis for better clinical practice. *Clin Pharmacol Therapeut* 2009; 85(6): 607–614.

International Association of Diabetes and Pregnancy Study Groups Recommendations on the Diagnosis and Classification of Hyperglycemia in Pregnancy: International Association of Diabetes and Pregnancy Study Groups Consensus Panel. *Diabetes Care* 2010 March; 33(3): 676–682.

Kjos SL, Buchanan TA. Gestational diabetes mellitus. *NEJM* 1999; 341: 1749–1756.

Kjos SL, Henry OA, Montoro M, *et al.* Insulin-requiring diabetes in pregnancy: a randomized control trial of active induction of labor and expectant management. *Am J Obstet Gynecol* 1993; 169: 611–615.

Kjos SL, Leung A, Henry OA, *et al.* Antepartum surveillance in diabetic pregnancies: predictors of fetal distress. *Am J Obstet Gynecol* 1995; 173: 1532–1539.

Langer O, Conway DL, Berkus MD, Xenakis EM, Gonzales O. A comparison of glyburide and insulin in women with gestational diabetes mellitus. *NEJM* 2000; 343: 1134–1138.

Mestman JH, Anderson GV, Guadalupe V. Follow-up study of 360 subjects with abnormal carbohydrate metabolism during pregnancy. *Obstet Gynecol* 1972; 39: 41–45.

Metzger BE, Coustan DR. Summary and recommendations of the Fourth International Workshop-Conference on Gestational Diabetes Mellitus. *Diabetes Care* 1998; 21(suppl. 2): B161–167.

Paglia MJ, Coustan DR. The use of oral antidiabetic medications in gestational diabetes mellitus. *Curr Diabetes Rep* 2009: 9: 287–290.

Rowan JA, Hague WM, Wanzhen G, *et al.* Metformin versus insulin for the treatment of gestational diabetes. *NEJM* 2008; 358: 2003–2015.

US Preventive Health Services Task Force. Screening for gestational diabetes mellitus: US Preventive Health Services Task Force Recommendation Statement. *Ann Intern Med* 2008; 148: 759–764.

Chapter 31
Gastrointestinal Disorders in Pregnancy

Michael J. Fassett and Richard H. Lee
Department of Medicine and Obstetrics and Gynecology, Keck School of Medicine, University of Southern California, CA, USA

Introduction

As more patients with medical complications become pregnant, the obstetrician is placed in the unique situation of needing to combine knowledge of both internal medicine and obstetrics to effectively manage these patients. Gastrointestinal complaints, both those prior to and those arising during pregnancy, are common. This chapter will explore various gastrointestinal disorders as they affect the pregnant woman and her fetus.

Pregnancy effects on gastrointestinal physiology

The gastrointestinal tract undergoes many physiologic changes in pregnancy. With advancing gestation, increased levels of progesterone result in decreased smooth muscle activity. Esophageal motility, lower esophageal sphincter tone, as well as gastric tone and contractility are decreased during pregnancy. Small intestinal motility decreases significantly between the first and second trimesters, and remains fairly constant during the third trimester before returning to pre-pregnancy levels in the postpartum period. Biliary contractility is also similarly altered.

Gastroesophageal reflux

Heartburn occurs in nearly half of all pregnancies. It develops early in pregnancy and resolves in the postpartum period. A combination of decreased lower esophageal sphincter pressure and decreased gastric motility, with mechanical obstruction secondary to the gravid uterus, plays a contributing role. Clinical features of reflux, mainly heartburn and regurgitation, are similar to those in the

Management of Common Problems in Obstetrics and Gynecology, 5th edition. Edited by T.M. Goodwin, M.N. Montoro, L. Muderspach, R. Paulson and S. Roy. © 2010 Blackwell Publishing Ltd.

nonpregnant patient. The evaluation of these complaints seldom requires more than an adequate history, although endoscopy may be a necessary method of evaluating more severe cases in pregnancy. Treatment of these symptoms in the pregnant patient consists primarily of nonpharmacologic interventions, reserving medication for refractory cases. Lifestyle changes such as elevation of the upper body while at rest, and decreasing activity that exacerbates symptoms should be prescribed. If these do not improve the patient's symptoms, antacids may be taken before meals and at bedtime; sucralfate 1 g three times daily may be added. For severe cases, histamine blockers such as cimetidine or ranitidine may be used to alleviate symptoms. Symptoms associated with reflux resolve in most patients in the postpartum period.

Diarrhea

Complaints of diarrhea in pregnancy should be investigated in the same manner as in the nonpregnant state. A careful history should be taken with focus on characteristics of present illness, diet, laxative use, and eating disorders. Acute microbial diarrhea usually is a self-limiting entity, resolving spontaneously within 24–72 hours, and is treated supportively with adequate hydration. If necessary, mild antidiarrheal agents such as kaolin and pectin may be prescribed. Stronger medications should be avoided as they may lead to bacterial overgrowth in the intestines. Care should be taken to ensure that adequate hydration is achieved to prevent preterm labor. For persistent diarrhea, stool culture and examination for ova and parasites should be undertaken and treatment is undertaken accordingly. Endoscopy is safe in pregnancy, and may be employed when necessary for the evaluation of persistent diarrhea.

Irritable bowel disease and constipation

Irritable bowel disease is a constellation of continuous and recurrent abdominal pain, which is relieved with defecation or associated with change in frequency or consistency of stool and/or disturbed defecation with no organic cause. It is a common disorder in the non-pregnant population, and it may often be encountered during pregnancy. Although the etiology is unknown, the decrease in gastrointestinal motility and pressure of the gravid uterus on the large bowel may aggravate symptoms of irritable bowel disease. Treatment of both irritable bowel disease and constipation is conservative. Increased water intake, frequent small meals, and a high-fiber diet are excellent first steps. Stool-bulking agents may be added if necessary, followed by emollient laxatives for more difficult cases.

Peptic ulcer disease

Pregnancy-induced changes in symptoms from peptic ulcer disease may be mediated by a decrease in gastric acid secretion and an increase in mucus secretion. Clark reported that of over 300 women with known peptic ulcer disease, 44% had improvement in symptoms, and an additional 44% became asymptomatic. Pregnant women with symptoms of peptic ulcer disease often have their complaints ascribed to gastroesophageal reflux and are treated accordingly, which often improves ulcer symptomatology. Conventional antiulcer therapy, including antacids after meals and at bedtime, and sucralfate are usually sufficient to ameliorate symptoms encountered during pregnancy. Histamine receptor antagonists should be used if conservative management does not alleviate symptoms. If such measures do not improve patient symptoms, a search for *Helicobacter pylori* infection is indicated and if detected, antimicrobial treatment may be considered. For patients whose symptoms do not improve, or are associated with other "alarm" symptoms such as gastrointestinal bleeding or anemia, endoscopic examination should be undertaken. In the rare event that perforation or hemorrhage complicates ulcer disease, the patient should be managed surgically as in the nonpregnant state. For patients with symptoms that can be managed conservatively during pregnancy, curative surgical therapy should be reserved for the postpartum period.

Inflammatory bowel disease

Inflammatory bowel disease (IBD), although rare, tends to appear most commonly during child-bearing years. In the absence of pelvic surgery, the disease processes do not appear to directly affect fertility. Rates of anomalies, spontaneous abortions, and stillbirths in pregnant women with IBD are similar to those of the general population. Some investigators have described an increase in premature birth, usually related to activity of disease. Although reviews of Crohn's disease have shown a tendency for disease activity to remain static during the course of pregnancy, symptoms of ulcerative colitis may tend to flare earlier in gestation, while Crohn's disease often worsens in the third trimester. Patients trying to conceive should first have their symptoms brought under better control. Medications used to treat IBD such as corticosteroids, sulfasalazine, and antibiotics are safe to use in pregnancy. The route of delivery does not appear to affect the severity of perianal disease.

Hepatitis

The viral hepatitis, except for hepatitis E, do not occur with increased frequency or severity during pregnancy. Systemic symptoms of hepatitis include fever, nausea, vomiting, fatigue, and jaundice. Aminotransferase levels are elevated to greater than 500 units/L. Hepatitis A, transmitted by fecal–oral contact, has a short incubation period followed by the appearance of classic symptoms. Diagnosis is demonstrated by the presence of antihepatitis A IgM antibodies in the serum of acutely or recently ill persons. It is seldom fatal. Good sanitation and hygiene should be emphasized for those in contact with a person acutely infected with hepatitis A.

Hepatitis B is transmitted by contact with blood and bodily fluids (primarily semen and saliva). The mean 12-day incubation period is followed by onset of symptoms of varying severity. In acute illness, HBsAg, HBcAg, and HBeAg are present before the onset of symptoms. HBsAg disappears with recovery from disease, and anti-HBs and anti-HBe rise 2 weeks to 6 months later, marking the end of the illness. The carrier state, present in approximately 5% of immunocompetent adults, is marked by the presence of HBsAg for more than 6 months. All pregnant women should be tested for the presence of HBsAg and if positive, their infants should receive both hepatitis B immune globulin and hepatitis B vaccine after delivery. Hepatitis B vaccination can be given to seronegative mothers during pregnancy.

Hepatitis C has similar risk factors for transmission as hepatitis B. There are no known ways to prevent perinatal transmission of hepatitis C to the fetus. The overall risk of transmission of hepatitis C to the offspring is 4–8%. Diagnosis is made by the presence of antihepatitis C antibody in the serum of affected individuals. δ Hepatitis infection, transmitted in a manner similar to hepatitis B, co-exists with hepatitis B infection. Diagnosis is made by demonstration of viral antigen in serum.

For patients who are carriers of hepatitis B and C, we attempt to avoid any obstetric procedures that will increase the risk of perinatal transmission such as fetal scalp monitors and unnecessary amniotomy. For those patients with hepatitis E, an infection similar to that of hepatitis A, mortality may reach 20% during pregnancy. For the rare case of herpes simplex hepatitis, characterized by oral/vulvar vesicles, mild hyperbilirubinemia, and coagulopathy, examination of liver biopsy for intranuclear inclusions may prompt antiviral therapy, which greatly improves survival. Treatment for acute hepatitis is supportive, encouraging appropriate hygiene and oral intake. Patients with evidence of worsening laboratory values or hepatic failure should be hospitalized and indices of hepatic function followed. The type of hepatitis should be determined by serologic studies and to allow for appropriate immunoprophylaxis of the newborn.

Chronic liver disease

Pregnancy is uncommon in the patient with chronic liver disease, as most of these women are anovulatory, and disease severity tends to correlate with infertility. In general, pregnancy does not worsen hepatic function, although a significant risk of esophageal variceal bleeding may present itself later in gestation, warranting endoscopic examination early in pregnancy to determine the risk.

Intrahepatic cholestasis of pregnancy

Intrahepatic cholestasis of pregnancy (ICP) is the most common liver disorder unique to pregnancy. Usually encountered late in pregnancy, ICP is a condition of total body pruritus and liver dysfunction. Several different measures of liver test abnormalities have been reported in ICP, including elevated transaminases, bilirubin, and serum bile acid concentration. The most commonly accepted laboratory criterion for ICP is an elevated total serum bile acid concentration. The prevalence of this disorder varies throughout the world. There is a high prevalence in Latin America. In Chile, rates have varied from 4% to 22%. The prevalence of ICP in the United States has been reported to be from 0.001 to 0.32%. At the University of Southern California, which has a high Latina population, we have an estimated prevalence of approximately 5.6%. Maternal consequences of the disease include intolerable pruritus and abnormalities of liver function tests. The fetal course may be more complicated. This disease is associated with increased risk for fetal death, meconium passage, and preterm delivery. The fetal deaths are known to cluster at 37 weeks. However, we have observed fetal deaths occurring at earlier gestational ages. Therefore, we currently recommend delivery at 37 weeks with confirmed ICP.

Prior to delivery, it is our practice to administer ursodeoxycholic acid (10–15 mg/kg/day) and this is based on its better tolerability and efficacy in lowering total serum bile acid concentrations, ameliorating pruritus, and improving liver function tests compared to s-adenosylmethione, dexametasone, and cholestyramine. Unfortunately, currently there are no conclusive data that any of the agents used to treat ICP reduce fetal risk. In addition, we place patients with ICP in twice-weekly antepartum testing. However, the use of cardiotocography in this setting is debated, as it is believed that fetal death occurs as an acute event rather than a consequence of chronic hypoxemia. Fetal demises have been reported despite having normal-appearing fetal heart rate testing several days prior and after normalization of total serum bile acid concentrations. On the other hand, concerning fetal heart rate patterns such as prolonged decelerations requiring immediate delivery have been detected with antenatal testing, which is the reason why we use antepartum testing. Patients with ICP should not be prescribed estrogen-containing contraceptives.

Cholecystitis

Cholecystitis is the second most common surgical condition encountered in pregnancy. Acute appendicitis is the most common, and is the subject of Chapter 37 in this textbook. In the great majority of cases, cholecystitis results from cholelithiasis. Symptoms of cholecystitis in pregnancy are similar to those in the nonpregnant patient. Patients complain of colicky epigastric pain, which often radiates to the back, and nausea and vomiting. Murphy's sign (pain on deep palpation in the right upper quadrant) is often absent during pregnancy. Attention should be paid to the presence or absence of jaundice, an indicator of biliary tract obstruction. Fever and tachypnea may be present. The differential diagnosis includes appendicitis, severe pre-eclampsia, and pancreatitis. Evaluation of symptoms and signs suggestive of cholecystitis should include a complete blood cell count, as well as serum levels of alkaline phosphatase, transaminases, amylase, and lipase. Ultrasound imaging of the right upper quadrant may demonstrate the presence of cholelithiasis in the gallbladder or biliary tree, or evidence of gallbladder wall thickening, or dilation of ductal structure indicating obstruction.

Management of cholecystitis in pregnancy involves bowel rest, with suction if needed, along with intravenous fluid therapy and analgesia which generally results in an improvement in symptoms. If symptoms do not resolve or if temperature elevations are suggestive of infection, antibiotic therapy may be necessary, and appropriate consultation with gastroenterology and/or general surgery is obtained. Recurrent episodes of cholecystitis indicating failure of medical management require endoscopic retrograde cholangiopancreatography (ERCP) or surgical intervention.

Pancreatitis

Pancreatitis does not seem to be more or less prevalent during pregnancy. It affects approximately 1 in 1434 pregnancies, and has a slightly higher occurrence during the third trimester. Associated fetal loss rates are between 10% and 20%, and related maternal mortality has been reported to be 3.4%. Causes of pancreatitis in pregnancy do not differ significantly from those in the nonpregnant patient. Obstructive biliary disease is the most common cause, followed by idiopathic causes. Rarely, estrogen-induced hypertriglyceridemia induces pancreatitis during the third trimester. Excessive alcohol consumption, a more common cause of pancreatitis in the nonpregnant patient, occurs less frequently during pregnancy. Common presenting symptoms are epigastric or left upper quadrant pain with radiation to the back associated with nausea, vomiting, ileus, and fever. Characteristic pain is not always present, and pancreatitis should be considered whenever a patient presents with abdominal pain. Confirmation of elevated serum amylase and lipase values are important confirmatory tests. Abdominal ultrasound may demonstrate evidence of pancreatic edema or biliary tract obstruction.

Management is similar to symptomatic cholelithiasis with bowel rest, intravenous fluids, and meperidine analgesia. Nasogastric suctioning may be indicated if ileus and vomiting are prolonged. Oral intake can be gradually introduced with the resolution of symptoms. If the pancreatitis is due to hypertriglyceridemia, oral feeding may have to be completely withdrawn, and a low-fat and low-carbohydrate diet resumed when symptoms improve. Triglyceride levels should be maintained below 1000 mg/dL. Parenteral nutrition may be required. This rare cause of pancreatitis in pregnancy resolves spontaneously after delivery.

Conclusion

With few modifications, most management techniques for the nonpregnant patient with a gastrointestinal disorder can be applied to the pregnant patient. When treated appropriately with attention to maternal and fetal status, morbidity and mortality of most gastrointestinal disorders can be limited for both.

Suggested reading

Alsulyman OM, Ouzounian JG, Ames-Castro M, Goodwin TM. Intrahepatic cholestasis of pregnancy: perinatal outcome associated with expectant management. *Am J Obstet Gynecol* 1996; 175: 957–960.

American Gastroenterological Association Patient Care Committee. Irritable bowel syndrome: a technical review for practice guideline development. *Gastroenterology* 1997; 112: 2120–2137.

Knox TA, Olans LB. Liver disease in pregnancy. *NEJM* 1996; 335: 569–575.

Lee RH, Goodwin TM, Greenspoon J, Incerpi MA. The prevalence of intrahepatic cholestasis of pregnancy in a primarily Latina Los Angeles population. *J Perinatol* 2006; 26(9): 527–532.

Mishra L, Seeff LB. Viral hepatitis, A through E, complicating pregnancy. *Gastroenterol Clin North Am* 1992; 21: 873–887.

Ramin KD, Ramin SM, Richey SD, Cunningham FG. Acute pancreatitis in pregnancy. *Am J Obstet Gynecol* 1995; 173: 187–191.

Scott LD. Gallstone disease and pancreatitis in pregnancy. *Gastroenterol Clin North Am* 1992; 21: 803–815.

Sharp HT. Gastrointestinal surgical conditions during pregnancy. *Clin Obstet Gynecol* 1994; 37: 306–315.

Soll AH, for the Practice Parameters Committee of the American College of Gastroenterology. Medical treatment of peptic ulcer disease. *JAMA* 1996; 275: 622–629.

Chapter 32
Viral Exposures During Pregnancy

Alice M. Stek

Department of Medicine and Obstetrics and Gynecology, Keck School of Medicine, University of Southern California, CA, USA

Introduction

Many viral infections can result in significant adverse maternal and fetal effects if acquired during pregnancy. Some of these adverse outcomes are easily preventable. An overview of the manifestations, prevention and treatment of the more common viral infections during pregnancy is provided below.

Cytomegalovirus

Cytomegalovirus (CMV) is the most common congenital infection, occurring in 0.2–2.2% of neonates. The majority of these infections are asymptomatic; approximately 5% of infected neonates are symptomatic at birth. Congenital CMV is the leading cause of congenital hearing loss. Transmission can occur via transplacental passage of the virus, contact of the fetus with infectious secretions at the time of birth, infected breast milk or blood transfusion.

There is regional variation in the prevalence of primary (0.7–4%) and recurrent (13.5%) infection among pregnant women. CMV is transmitted by contact with infected blood, saliva or urine, or by sexual contact. The mean incubation period is 40 days, with a range of 28–60 days. Primary CMV infection in adults is usually asymptomatic, although a mononucleosis-like syndrome with fever, malaise, myalgias, chills, lymphocytosis, and abnormal liver function tests can occur. Recurrent infection can occur following reactivation of latent virus.

Vertical transmission can occur at any point in pregnancy; the greatest risk is with maternal infection during the third trimester. Maternal CMV infection during the first trimester results in more serious fetal sequelae, should vertical transmission occur. The risk of transmission to the fetus is 30–40% with primary maternal CMV infection; 10% of infants infected *in utero* following primary infection will have signs and symptoms of CMV infection at birth and develop sequelae.

Clinical findings at birth can include jaundice, petechiae, thrombocytopenia, hepatosplenomegaly, intrauterine growth restriction, and nonimmune hydrops. Approximately 30% of infants with symptomatic infection following primary maternal infection die and 80% of surviving infants have severe neurologic sequelae. Vertical transmission after recurrent infection is much lower: 0.15–2%. Infants infected during maternal recurrent infection usually are asymptomatic at birth. Congenital hearing loss is the most common severe sequela of vertical transmission following maternal recurrent infection, and multiple sequelae are unlikely.

Routine serologic screening of women or neonates for CMV is not recommended. The presence of immunoglobulin M (IgM) CMV antibody indicates primary maternal infection. However, both false-positive and false-negative results are possible. Establishing that seroconversion has occurred is the most accurate method for demonstrating maternal primary infection. Detection of the CMV virus by polymerase chain reaction (PCR) from amniotic fluid is the most sensitive test for detecting fetal infection.

There is currently no vaccine for CMV prevention, nor a routinely recommended treatment for maternal or neonatal infection or interventions to prevent vertical transmission.

Parvovirus B19

Parvovirus B19 is the cause of erythema infectiosum, also known as fifth disease. In healthy adults, parvovirus B19 infection is often asymptomatic. Symptoms are generally mild, with a rash on the trunk and peripheral arthropathy, but can rarely include transient aplastic crisis. Transmission occurs through respiratory secretions and hand to mouth contact. Otherwise healthy patients with erythema infectiosum are contagious 5–10 days after

Management of Common Problems in Obstetrics and Gynecology, 5th edition. Edited by T.M. Goodwin, M.N. Montoro, L. Muderspach, R. Paulson and S. Roy. © 2010 Blackwell Publishing Ltd.

exposure, during the week before the onset of the rash, and are not infectious after this. Immunocompromised patients remain contagious from before the onset of symptoms through the period of the rash. Exposure to an infected household member results in approximately 50% risk of acquiring the infection. Over half of pregnant women in the USA are immune to parvovirus B19.

Transplacental transmission occurs in up to 33%. Spontaneous abortion or fetal death occurs in less than 10% of infected pregnancies. Most maternal infections that have resulted in fetal deaths occur between 10 and 20 weeks' gestation, and the spontaneous abortions usually occurred 4–6 weeks after infection. Teratogenicity has not been proven. Parvovirus B19 can infect fetal erythroid precursors and cause anemia, leading to nonimmune hydrops and fetal death. Hydrops is unlikely to develop beyond 8 weeks after maternal infection. Fetal ultrasound examination can easily demonstrate hydrops and the hydropic fetus can be treated by intrauterine transfusions, if severe anemia is demonstrated. Spontaneous resolution may occur, however. There appear to be no long-term sequelae to *in utero* parvovirus B19 infection.

In view of the high prevalence of parvovirus B19 and the relatively low risk of serious harm to the fetus, pregnant women should not be routinely excluded from workplaces where parvovirus B19 is present. Infection control should consist of handwashing, standard precautions and droplet precautions.

Varicella zoster virus (VZV)

Varicella zoster virus causes chickenpox and herpes zoster. VZV is transmitted by respiratory droplets or close contact. The attack rate in nonimmune people is 60–90% after exposure. The incubation period after infection is 10–20 days. The period of infectivity begins 48 hours before the rash appears and continues until the vesicles crust over. Primary infection, chickenpox, is characterized by fever, malaise, and a pruritic rash that develops vesicles. After the primary infection, VZV remains dormant in the sensory ganglia and if reactivated causes herpes zoster. Most people in the United States are immune to varicella, and therefore infection is uncommon in pregnancy, occurring in approximately 0.6 per 1000 pregnant women. While chickenpox is usually a benign and self-limited illness in children, severe complications such as pneumonia and encephalitis are more common in adults. Varicella pneumonia is more serious in pregnant women than in nonpregnant adults, and can be life-threatening. Pregnant women with varicella should be monitored closely for any signs of pneumonia.

Fetal infection after maternal varicella during the first 20 weeks of pregnancy occasionally results in varicella embryopathy, which can include limb atrophy, scarring of the skin of the extremities and central nervous system

and ocular lesions. Congenital varicella syndrome occurs in approximately 2% of exposed fetuses when maternal infection occurs before 20 weeks' gestation.

The neonate is at risk for life-threatening neonatal varicella if the mother develops varicella within 5 days before to 2 days after delivery.

Over 95% of women with a positive history of varicella have serologic immunity; therefore it is unnecessary to perform serologic testing in women with a prior history of varicella. Also, 70–90% of women in the USA with a negative or uncertain history of varicella are immune. A pregnant woman who is exposed to varicella should be tested for immunity if she has no history of prior infection with varicella or vaccination.

Postexposure prophylaxis within 96 hours of exposure with VZV immune globulin (VZIG or VariZIG) is recommended for nonimmune pregnant women with varicella exposure and for infants born to mothers with peripartum varicella. Acyclovir therapy should be considered for pregnant women with chickenpox.

The varicella vaccine contains live-attenuated VZV and should not be given to pregnant women. Women who do not have varicella immunity should receive the first dose of the VZV vaccine post partum prior to hospital discharge.

Rubella

Rubella during pregnancy and congenital rubella are extremely rare in the United States; most cases occur in women born outside the country. All women should be screened for serologic evidence of immunity to rubella at the first prenatal visit. Seropositive women need no further testing.

Recent infection can be demonstrated by detection of rubella-specific IgM antibodies, but false-positive results are common. Demonstration of seroconversion in acute and convalescent serum specimens or isolation of the virus from throat swabs is more reliable.

Fetal structural malformations (serious CNS, cardiac, ocular and skeletal defects) may be caused by rubella infection during embryogenesis. While fetal infection may occur throughout pregnancy, defects are rare if infection occurs after 20 weeks' gestation. If rubella is diagnosed in a pregnant woman, pregnancy termination should be discussed.

Rubella vaccine is a live-attenuated virus, and therefore not recommended during pregnancy. Following immunization, women should be advised to avoid conception for 1 month. However, in a woman who is inadvertently vaccinated during early pregnancy, the teratogenic risk to the fetus is theoretic. Rubella vaccination during pregnancy is not an indication for pregnancy termination.

Women who are not immune to rubella should be offered vaccination post partum prior to discharge from the hospital. Breastfeeding is not a contraindication to rubella vaccination.

Herpes simplex

Herpes simplex virus (HSV) can be differentiated into HSV type 1 (HSV-1) and type 2 (HSV-2). HSV-1 causes labial herpes and gingivostomatitis and keratoconjunctivitis. Most genital infections are caused by HSV-2 but HSV-1 genital infections are becoming increasingly common, particularly among young women; up to 80% of new HSV genital infections among women may be caused by HSV-1.

During initial infection, the incubation period is 2–12 days. HSV replicates in the skin and the virus becomes latent in the sensory ganglia. Reactivation frequently occurs and may manifest clinically as recurrent ulcerative lesions or subclinically as asymptomatic viral shedding.

Most women who are infected with HSV are unaware of this; only approximately 10% of infected women report prior infection. In the United States, approximately 26% of women have serologic evidence of HSV-2 infection. The incidence of new HSV-1 or HSV-2 infection during pregnancy is approximately 2%. Approximately 10% of HSV-2 negative women have partners who are seropositive and are therefore at risk of acquiring HSV-2 during pregnancy. As in nonpregnant women, the majority of new infections in pregnant women are asymptomatic.

Recurrent lesions are common during pregnancy, with 75% of women experiencing this during pregnancy. Approximately 14% of pregnant women will have either prodromal symptoms or lesions at the time of delivery. Because HSV infection is often asymptomatic, approximately 80% of HSV-infected infants are born to women with no reported history of HSV infection.

While neonatal HSV remains a serious infection, mortality has decreased over the past 20 years. Disseminated disease comprises 25% of neonatal HSV infections and mortality for disseminated disease is currently approximately 30%. Central nervous system disease accounts for 30% of neonatal HSV; mortality is currently approximately 4%. About 20% of survivors of neonatal herpes have long-term neurologic sequelae.

A clinical history suggestive of HSV should be confirmed with serologic or viral testing. HSV-2 rarely causes oral infection; therefore detection of HSV-2 antibodies is diagnostic of genital HSV infection. PCR is more sensitive than culture and may replace culture as the standard of care for diagnosis of HSV in the future.

While transplacental infection of the fetus is rare, primary infection with HSV in the first trimester has been associated with microcephaly, chorioretinitis, and skin lesions in the fetus. HSV probably does not increase the risk for spontaneous abortion.

The risk of transmission is highest at the time of delivery. The highest risk is with primary genital herpes infection during pregnancy; the risk of transmission to the neonate with a primary outbreak occurring at the time of delivery is 30–60%. Among women with recurrent lesions at the time of delivery, the rate of transmission with vaginal delivery is 3%. For women with a history of recurrent disease and no visible lesions at the time of delivery, the risk of transmission is 2/10,000.

A primary outbreak in pregnancy can rarely lead to maternal complications such as disseminated HSV, herpes pneumonitis, hepatitis or encephalitis. Antiviral treatment with acyclovir or valacyclovir should be administered orally to reduce the duration and severity of the symptoms of primary infection and to reduce the duration of viral shedding. IV acyclovir may be given intravenously for women with more severe infection.

Women with active recurrent genital herpes should be offered suppressive therapy with acyclovir or valacyclovir, starting at 36 weeks' gestation. Suppressive therapy during late pregnancy decreases viral shedding, the risk of recurrence at delivery and the rate of cesarean delivery for recurrent genital herpes.

All pregnant women should be questioned about a history of genital herpes. However, routine HSV screening of pregnant women is currently not recommended. Women with a history of genital HSV should have a careful examination of the external genitalia at the time of presentation for delivery.

Cesarean delivery is recommended for women with active genital lesions or prodromal symptoms, such as vulvar pain or burning, at the time of delivery, to decrease the risk of neonatal HSV infection. Cesarean delivery does not completely eliminate neonatal herpes. Although the incidence of neonatal herpes is very low when there is recurrent maternal disease, cesarean delivery is recommended because of the life-threatening nature of neonatal herpes infection. In women with active HSV lesions and ruptured membranes, cesarean delivery should be performed without delay, regardless of the duration of ruptured membranes. In women with preterm premature rupture of membranes and active HSV, there is increasing support for continuing the pregnancy and using corticosteroids to decrease the complications of prematurity. There is no consensus regarding the optimal gestational age for delivery in this situation.

Invasive monitoring with fetal scalp electrodes may increase the risk of transmission of HSV.

Unless there is a lesion on the breast, breastfeeding is not contraindicated. Mothers should be instructed in careful hygiene. Mothers or other caregivers with labial HSV lesions should not kiss the baby.

Viral hepatitis A, B, C

Patients with acute hepatitis should be hospitalized if they have encephalopathy, coagulopathy or severe debilitation. Fluid and electrolyte abnormalities and coagulopathy should be corrected. Activity should be limited. Women who are less ill should reduce their level of activity, avoid upper abdominal trauma, and maintain good nutrition. Their household members and sexual partners should receive appropriate prophylaxis and vaccination.

Hepatitis A

The average incubation period of hepatitis A is 28 days (range 15–50 days). Children usually have asymptomatic or unrecognized infection and are often the source of hepatitis A transmission in the home.

Serious complications of hepatitis A infection are uncommon, and there is no chronic carrier state. Breast-feeding is not contraindicated in women with hepatitis A infection, if appropriate hygienic precautions are observed. Although there are few data, hepatitis A vaccination is not contraindicated in pregnancy, and should be considered for women at high risk.

Hepatitis B

Hepatitis B virus (HBV) is the leading cause of chronic liver disease worldwide. HBV is transmitted by parenteral and sexual contact; serum, semen and saliva are infectious. Over 90% of adult patients who become infected with HBV have complete resolution of their infection; 10% or less become chronically infected. Fifteen to 30% of chronically infected patients have continued viral replication and persistence of the hepatitis B e antigen (HBeAg). These individuals are at highest risk of transmission of hepatitis B and of chronic hepatitis and cirrhosis and hepatocellular carcinoma. In contrast, 90% of perinatally infected infants will develop chronic HBV infection and 25% of these will develop cirrhosis or hepatocellular carcinoma.

Serologic testing for HBV infection using hepatitis B surface antigen (HBsAg) should be done in all pregnant women as part of routine prenatal care. Historical information about risk factors fails to identify approximately half of HBV carriers.

Perinatal transmission of HBV generally occurs during labor and delivery; transplacental transmission is rare. Without neonatal prophylaxis, the risk of HBV transmission to the infant is 10–20%, and increases to 70–90% if the woman is HBeAg positive or if acute HBV infection occurs in the third trimester.

The combination of neonatal passive and active immunization is 85–95% effective in preventing perinatal transmission of HBV. Universal active immunization of all infants is the standard of care. Infants of women who are HBsAg positive or whose status is unknown at the time of delivery should receive both passive immunization with HBIG and HBV vaccine within 12 hours of birth. If the neonates receive appropriate prophylaxis, breastfeeding is not contraindicated.

Current research is evaluating the potential benefit of antiviral medications such as lamivudine and HBIG administration to the mother in late pregnancy to further reduce the risk of vertical transmission.

Everyone with risk factors for HBV, including healthcare workers, hemodialysis patients, injection drug users, those with more than one sexual partner during the past 3 months, recent diagnosis of an STI, clients and staff in centers for the developmentally disabled, and international travelers to high or intermediate prevalence areas should be vaccinated for HBV. Pregnancy is not a contraindication for HBV vaccination; pregnant women with these risk factors should be targeted for vaccination.

Hepatitis C

Hepatitis C virus (HCV) is the leading cause of chronic liver disease in the United States. HCV seroprevalence among pregnant women ranges from 0.6% to 6.6%. Risk factors for HCV infection include injection drug use, hemophilia, and the presence of other sexually transmitted infections. Acute HCV infection occurs after a 30–60-day incubation period. Seventy-five percent of patients are asymptomatic but at least 50% of infected adults progress to chronic infection, regardless of the source of infection. At least 20% of chronic HCV infections lead to chronic active hepatitis or cirrhosis and possibly hepatocellular carcinoma.

Vertical transmission of HCV occurs in 2–8%. Risk is increased with maternal viremia, higher HCV viral load, maternal co-infection with HIV, prolonged rupture of membranes during labor, use of internal fetal monitoring, and other sources of increased exposure to maternal blood during delivery.

Routine prenatal screening for HCV is currently not recommended; however, women at higher risk or those with evidence of liver disease should be screened for HCV antibodies.

There are inadequate data on the safety of amniocentesis in women with HCV. Current recommendations are for cesarean delivery based on obstetric indications only, and that breastfeeding is not contraindicated.

Currently treatment with peginterferon and ribavirin is the standard of care for HCV infection. However, ribavirin is contraindicated in pregnancy and treatment with interferon alone will reduce efficacy. The current recommendations are for no treatment for HCV during pregnancy.

There is no vaccination or passive immunization available for HCV.

Human papilloma virus

During pregnancy, genital warts may proliferate, and after pregnancy they often resolve. Treatment may be delayed until post partum, in anticipation of improvement or resolution.

Treatment of genital condylomata during pregnancy can be safely accomplished using cryotherapy, surgical excision or laser treatment. Podophyllin, 5-FU and interferon are not recommended during pregnancy, and there are no data on the safety of imiquimod. Cesarean delivery is not recommended for prevention of transmission of human papilloma virus (HPV) to the neonate. However, rarely genital tract condylomata can be so large that they may obstruct delivery or may lead to extensive lacerations and cesarean delivery may be indicated for this reason. HPV vaccination is not recommended during pregnancy.

Immunizations

Immunization is one of the most important preventive services we can provide.

Ideally, immunizations should be done prior to conception. The benefits of immunization to the pregnant woman and her neonate usually outweigh the potential risks of adverse effects. However, live vaccines are contraindicated during pregnancy because of the theoretical risk of transmission of the vaccine virus to the fetus.

Influenza vaccination using the inactivated vaccine is recommended for all pregnant women. Hepatitis B vaccination is recommended for women at risk. Tetanus and diphtheria vaccination is recommended for previously vaccinated women who have not been vaccinated within 10 years, and women who have not previously been vaccinated. Hepatitis A vaccination should be considered for women at increased risk.

Women who are not immune should be vaccinated for rubella and varicella post partum, prior to discharge from the hospital.

Human papilloma virus vaccination should be delayed until after completion of the pregnancy.

Varicella, rubella, measles, mumps (MMR), vaccinia, yellow fever, and live-attenuated influenza vaccine are contraindicated during pregnancy, as they are live virus vaccines.

Although no adverse effects of polio vaccination have been documented during pregnancy, vaccination of pregnant women should be avoided on theoretical grounds. However, if a pregnant woman is at increased risk for infection, the vaccine can be administered.

Postexposure prophylaxis for rabies is not contraindicated in pregnancy.

Breastfeeding is not a contraindication to any vaccination with the exception of smallpox vaccine.

Updated immunization guidelines are regularly distributed by the Advisory Committee on Immunization Practices and can be found in the MMWR or at the CDC website.

Suggested reading

Advisory Committee on Immunization Practices, US Department of Health and Human Services, Centers for Disease Control and Prevention. *Guidelines for vaccinating pregnant women.* Washington, DC: Advisory Committee on Immunization Practices, 2007.

American Academy of Pediatrics and American College of Obstetricians and Gynecologists. *Guidelines for perinatal care.* Washington, DC: American Academy of Pediatrics, 2007.

American College of Obstetricians and Gynecologists. *Committee Opinion 281: rubella vaccination.* Washington, DC: American College of Obstetricians and Gynecologists, 2002.

American College of Obstetricians and Gynecologists. *Practice Bulletin 20: perinatal viral and parasitic infections.* Washington, DC: American College of Obstetricians and Gynecologists, 2000; reaffirmed 2008.

American College of Obstetricians and Gynecologists. *Practice Bulletin 61: human papilloma virus.* Washington, DC: American College of Obstetricians and Gynecologists, 2005.

American College of Obstetricians and Gynecologists. *Practice Bulletin 82: management of herpes in pregnancy.* Washington, DC: American College of Obstetricians and Gynecologists, 2007.

American College of Obstetricians and Gynecologists. *Practice Bulletin 86: viral hepatitis in pregnancy.* Washington, DC: American College of Obstetricians and Gynecologists, 2007.

American College of Obstetricians and Gynecologists. *Committee Opinion 438: Update on immunization and pregnancy: tetanus, diphtheria, and pertussis vaccination.* Washington, DC: American College of Obstetricians and Gynecologists, 2009.

Chapter 33
HIV in Pregnancy

Alice M. Stek

Department of Medicine and Obstetrics and Gynecology, Keck School of Medicine, University of Southern California, CA, USA

Introduction

In resource-rich settings, we have had remarkable success in preventing mother-to-child transmission of HIV. The overwhelming majority of those infected with HIV live in resource-poor countries. Worldwide, as of December 2007, UNAIDS estimated there were over 33 million people living with HIV/AIDS: 31 million adults and 2.5 million children. Most HIV infections among children are due to mother-to-child transmission. Half of the 31 million HIV-infected adults are women [1].

Prevalence and risk factors in the USA

In the USA, most HIV-infected people do not have AIDS. The Centers for Disease Control and Prevention (CDC) estimated that as of June 2007, the cumulative number of HIV infections in the USA was over 1.6 million [2]. An increase of 40,000 new infections per year is anticipated in the USA. The number of AIDS cases already reported to the CDC is 956,109, and more than 530,000 of these people have died. While worldwide approximately half of adults with HIV are women, this is not the case in the USA. However, HIV among women is increasing; women now constitute 19% of the cumulative reported AIDS cases in the USA, with a total of over 180,000 diagnosed by June 2007, and over 26% of all AIDS cases reported in 2007.

Expanded treatment regimens have improved the prognosis for HIV-positive patients, with a decrease in progression to AIDS and a decrease in deaths due to AIDS. However, AIDS remains an important cause of death in women, especially minority women in the 25–44 years age group. Currently more women with HIV acquired this infection heterosexually (80%) than via their own injection drug use (19%). However, many infections in women can be traced to injection drug use in their sexual partners.

Minority women are disproportionately affected. Black and Hispanic women comprise 24% of the US adult and adolescent female population, but 82% of female AIDS cases.

Seroprevalence varies widely per region. In some cities more than 1% of all pregnant women are HIV positive; in Los Angeles County approximately 0.1%.

Risk factors for acquiring HIV infection include: injection drug use or other needle sharing, cocaine/crack use, commercial sex work, multiple sexual partners, a bisexual male partner, residing in areas of high HIV prevalence such as sub-Saharan Africa, the presence of other STIs, especially syphilis, and blood transfusion in the USA between 1978 and 1985. Any woman with a sexual partner with these risk factors is also at risk; many women are not aware of their partners' risk. All women with active tuberculosis or cervical cancer should be considered high risk.

Diagnosis of HIV infection and AIDS

Voluntary, confidential screening should be offered to all pregnant women. This is the official recommendation by the US Public Health Service, the CDC [3], and also by the American College of Obstetricians and Gynecologists (ACOG) [4].

Several studies have demonstrated that by screening only those pregnant patients acknowledging risk factors such as those listed above, approximately half of HIV infections will be missed; in some populations, up to 70% of HIV-infected pregnant women had no apparent risk factors. Enzyme-linked immunoassay (ELISA or EIA) and confirmatory Western blot to HIV antibodies are used for adult diagnosis. A period of several months between infection and seroconversion is possible, although 2 months or less is typical. Patients undergoing screening must be informed of this "window period" and should have

Management of Common Problems in Obstetrics and Gynecology, 5th edition. Edited by T.M. Goodwin, M.N. Montoro, L. Muderspach, R. Paulson and S. Roy. © 2010 Blackwell Publishing Ltd.

testing repeated in approximately 2 months if they had recent high-risk exposure.

Testing should be repeated in the third trimester in women at increased risk and should be considered in all pregnant women if local seroprevalence among women is > 0.5%. [3,4]

Maternal anti-HIV IgG crosses the placenta and remains in the neonatal circulation for up to 12–18 months and is not useful to diagnose infection in the neonate. Testing the neonate will identify HIV-seropositive mothers and identify infants at risk for HIV. HIV DNA or RNA polymerase chain reaction (PCR) is used to demonstrate HIV infection in the neonate. With these techniques, infants can be diagnosed by 2 months of age.

An HIV-positive patient has AIDS when she develops an AIDS-indicator opportunistic infection such as *Pneumocystis carinii* pneumonia (PCP) or active tuberculosis, wasting, invasive cervical cancer or CD4 count below 200, indicating severe immunocompromise.

Perinatal transmission of HIV

Despite intensive research efforts, many questions remain unanswered.

Half or more of perinatal transmission occurs around the time of delivery. Transmission rarely occurs during the first and second trimesters, but frequently occurs with breastfeeding. In the absence of antiretroviral treatment, reported rates of transmission range from 14% to 40%.

Many factors have been associated with increased transmission, with some studies reporting conflicting results. These include: higher viral load, advanced maternal disease, lower maternal CD4 count, use of scalp electrodes, amniocentesis, prolonged rupture of membranes, chorioamnionitis, concurrent syphilis infection, prematurity, a previous HIV-infected infant, and maternal substance abuse. Nearly all the studies addressing these factors found maternal viral load and/or CD4 count to correlate with perinatal transmission.

Two studies have demonstrated an approximately 50% decreased risk of perinatal HIV transmission with elective cesarean section prior to the onset of labor or rupture of membranes [5,6]. These patients, however, received either no antiretroviral therapy or zidovudine monotherapy. These studies had no data regarding maternal viral load and did not evaluate maternal risk of elective cesarean section. Currently, most HIV-positive pregnant women receiving care at referral centers are using highly active combination antiretroviral therapy (HAART). Studies to date have not demonstrated a benefit of cesarean delivery in women on combination antiretroviral therapy with adequately controlled viral loads.

The May 2000 ACOG Committee Opinion on the use of cesarean delivery in HIV-infected women recommends that women with plasma viral load greater than 1000 copies/mL be offered a scheduled cesarean delivery [7]. If cesarean delivery is chosen, it should be done before rupture of membranes or onset of labor, and scheduled at 38 weeks' gestation. Patients should be counseled that maternal morbidity associated with cesarean delivery may be greater in HIV-infected women. The Committee Opinion also recommends that pregnant women receive appropriate antiretroviral therapy. Increased maternal viral load, usually measured by plasma HIV RNA PCR, has consistently been associated with higher perinatal transmission rates. However, perinatal transmission can occur at any viral load, even with undetectable maternal plasma viremia, although this is infrequent. The risk of transmission is less than 1% if viral load at delivery is < 1000 copies/mL and the woman is on antiretroviral therapy.

The virus is present in breast milk and can infect the nursing infant, increasing the risk of perinatal transmission by an additional 10–20% in women not on antiretroviral treatment.

Role of zidovudine and other antiretroviral medications

The publication of the results of the AIDS Clinical Trials Group (ACTG) Protocol 076 in 1994 had a major impact on the management of HIV infection during pregnancy [8]. This study reported a highly significant reduction in perinatal transmission of HIV by use of zidovudine (ZDV, Retrovir®, AZT) in a selected group of relatively healthy HIV-positive women. They received oral ZDV during the second and third trimesters, IV ZDV intrapartum, and 6 weeks neonatal oral ZDV. ZDV was tolerated well, with no significant side effects. Perinatal HIV transmission was reduced from 23% in the placebo group to 8% in the ZDV group. Since dissemination of these recommendations and increased implementation of prenatal testing and the ZDV regimen, perinatal HIV transmission rates have decreased dramatically throughout the USA.

Several international studies have demonstrated the efficacy of shorter courses of ZDV, although this was not as effective as the "076 regimen" [9]. If the woman received no antiretroviral treatment, intrapartum or neonatal ZDV prophylaxis alone may be of some benefit. An epidemiologic study from the state of New York found that administration of ZDV only to the neonate significantly reduced transmission if initiated within 48 hours of birth [10].

Essentially all studies evaluating ZDV use in pregnancy have demonstrated decreased perinatal transmission with ZDV use; therefore it is recommended that ZDV be offered to all HIV-infected pregnant women regardless of HIV plasma viral load or CD4 count, plus additional antiretrovirals in most cases (see below) [11].

With the increased screening for maternal HIV infection and the widespread perinatal use of ZDV, there has been a dramatic decrease in perinatally acquired HIV in the USA. An estimated < 250 HIV-infected infants are born annually in the USA, while worldwide over 1000 infected infants are born daily.

In the USA, detailed follow-up of hundreds of HIV-negative infants with *in utero* ZDV exposure has found no adverse effects to date [12,13].

Antiretroviral drugs decrease perinatal transmission by lowering maternal viral load and via pre- and postexposure prophylaxis of the infant. Therefore antepartum, intrapartum and neonatal prophylaxis are recommended. Combination antepartum antiretroviral drug regimens are more effective than single-drug regimens in preventing perinatal transmission. Most women should be on combination regimens including at least three drugs during pregnancy, especially if their viral loads are > 1000. Combination regimens are needed to maximally suppress viral replication and to prevent the development of viral resistance.

A large study in Uganda among women not on treatment, HIVNET 012, demonstrated that a single intrapartum oral dose of nevirapine combined with a single oral dose to the infant reduced transmission by nearly 50% compared to ZDV given intrapartum and for 1 week to the neonate [14]. A study in the USA, PACTG 316, evaluating the addition of nevirapine at delivery to an existing antiretroviral regimen, was unable to demonstrate a benefit, owing to the very low rate of transmission in women already receiving appropriate antiretroviral therapy (1.5% in this study) [15].

As ZDV has been proven to decrease perinatal HIV transmission, it is recommended that any antiretroviral regimen the pregnant woman may be receiving include ZDV, unless contraindicated for maternal reasons.

Most experts recommend that women who become pregnant while taking antiretroviral medications should not discontinue them without substituting other drugs. The current standard of care for HIV-positive patients is combination treatment, usually with three medications, to maximally suppress viral replication to < 50 copies/mL, preserve immune function and reduce development of resistance. These medications should not be withheld from pregnant women due to pregnancy *per se*. There are, however, additional concerns regarding potential adverse effects on the fetus/infant and maternal toxicities. Treatment must be individualized and accompanied by extensive counseling.

Several reports of adverse effects of combination antiretroviral therapy with protease inhibitors during pregnancy have raised concern. Two early reports on small cohorts in the USA and in Switzerland found a high rate of prematurity, and in one also congenital and neonatal abnormalities. This has prompted careful evaluation of the experience with combination antiretroviral treatment during pregnancy in the USA. These findings were more reassuring, with no excess anomalies and low rates of prematurity. Several large multicenter retrospective studies of combination antiretroviral therapy during pregnancy found no increased risk of prematurity [16,17].

Nevirapine treatment has been associated with maternal hepatotoxicity in women with higher CD4 counts, although not in women with CD4 < 250 and not with single-dose use. However, in part due to its long half-life, single-dose nevirapine results in HIV mutations conferring resistance to nevirapine and efavirenz in an unacceptably high percentage of women. As this will later result in poor virologic response to two important components of HAART regimens, additional treatment (for example, 3 weeks of zidovudine and lamivudine (Combivir®)) should be provided to cover the nevirapine "tail."

Protease inhibitors may cause glucose intolerance and other metabolic complications, and often have gastrointestinal side effects.

Nucleoside analog drugs may induce mitochondrial dysfunction and can cause lactic acidosis in pregnant women and their neonates. The combination of didanosine (ddI) and stavudine (d4T) is of particular concern and has been associated with several maternal deaths. A French group reported fatal mitochondrial dysfunction in two infants with *in utero* and neonatal exposure to ZDV and 3TC [18]. An extensive review of several much larger cohorts of antiretroviral-exposed infants in the USA identified no deaths attributable to mitochondrial dysfunction [13].

An antiretroviral registry is collecting safety and teratogenicity data on the use of other antiretroviral drugs during pregnancy (Antiretroviral Pregnancy Registry, 800-258-4263, www.APRegistry.com) for voluntary registration of all antiretroviral drug exposures) [19]. To date, no excess birth defects have been reported among prospectively followed pregnancies with first-trimester exposure to zidovudine, lamivudine, abacavir, efavirenz, lopinavir/ritonavir (Kaletra®), nelfinavir, nevirapine, ritonavir, stavudine or tenofovir [19]. The rate of congenital anomalies was nearly doubled with ddI use. Efavirenz (Sustiva®), a non-nucleoside reverse transcriptase inhibitor, has been associated with severe congenital anomalies in pregnant monkeys. Although prospective studies found no increase in anomalies in humans, efavirenz is currently best avoided during the first trimester, along with ddI.

The pharmacokinetics of many drugs are altered during pregnancy and dosing adjustments may be necessary.

The standard doses of lopinavir/ritonavir (Kaletra®) and nelfinavir result in suboptimal blood levels during the third trimester so increased dosing should be considered during this time [20, 21].

Careful counseling regarding the risks/benefits and the lack of adequate data on long-term effects of *in utero* antiretroviral exposure is necessary for each HIV-infected pregnant patient.

With the use of antiretrovirals during pregnancy and in the neonate, in settings of adequate resources, mother-to-child transmission of HIV-1 has been reduced to less than 2%. Because of the importance of preventing mother-to-child transmission, it is recommended that all pregnant women take antiretroviral medications; most should be on a HAART regimen. Many women are taking antiretrovirals during pregnancy for reasons of maternal health, and others for prevention of mother-to-child transmission only. The benefit of antiretroviral therapy during pregnancy in preventing mother-to-child transmission is well documented. Although there are concerns about the safety of antiretrovirals during pregnancy, risk–benefit considerations support the use of antiretrovirals during pregnancy.

This is a rapidly evolving field, becoming more complex, and expert consultation or referral is recommended to optimize maternal health and reduce perinatal transmission.

Pregnancy complications

Other than perinatal transmission, maternal HIV infection has not been conclusively demonstrated to have an adverse effect on pregnancy outcome. However, pregnancy increases the risk of antiretroviral toxicity. An adverse effect of pregnancy on maternal HIV disease has likewise not been conclusively demonstrated, and some investigators have demonstrated a lack of an adverse impact on maternal HIV disease progression.

Rapid testing at labor and delivery

Determining HIV status prior to pregnancy is optimal. While identification of HIV infection during early pregnancy provides more opportunities to intervene and results in lower transmission risk, peripartum interventions can still reduce vertical transmission to the infant.

Standard HIV testing takes several days or weeks, thereby missing the opportunity to intervene. The CDC and ACOG recommend that all pregnant women without documented results when they present for delivery have rapid HIV testing [3,4]. A woman testing positive could be given zidovudine or nevirapine intrapartum; most experts recommend zidovudine and lamivudine and nevirapine

intrapartum with 3 weeks of zidovudine and lamivudine or tenofovir and emtricitabine postpartum to prevent nevirapine resistance.

If not close to delivery, a cesarean could be performed. The woman should not breastfeed, and the infant should receive prophylaxis, starting within hours after delivery. Most experts recommend zidovudine for 6 weeks and lamivudine and nevirapine for a shorter period.

Management of HIV disease and pregnancy

Routine prenatal and peripartum care should include the following.
• Screen all pregnant women for HIV infection. Rapid testing at labor and delivery for those presenting without HIV results.
• Comprehensive psychosocial services.
• Screen for other STIs, especially syphilis and HSV.
• Screen for tuberculosis, toxoplasmosis, CMV, hepatitis B and C.
• Pap test every 6 months, with aggressive follow-up of abnormal results.
• Refer to a tertiary center for enrolment in studies and integrated specialized care: in view of the growing and confusing body of literature and rapidly changing treatment regimens, referral to obstetricians and internists with expertise in the management of HIV disease during pregnancy is strongly recommended and mandated by law in several states.
• Zidovudine and other antiretroviral drugs as indicated to reduce perinatal transmission. Most women should be using HAART.
• Measure CD4 count and viral load at least each trimester and tailor therapy accordingly: strongly consider combination antiretroviral medication with ≥ 3 drugs (HAART), preferably including ZDV, for maximal suppression of viral replication and to prevent resistance. If possible, the antiretrovirals used should be ones about which we have more data on safety, tolerability and pharmacokinetics during pregnancy. The current standard of care at specialized centers is intensive treatment to achieve and maintain undetectable viral load.
• Medications may be discontinued post partum if not needed for maternal health.
• Discuss recommendations regarding the use of antiretrovirals in pregnancy: expert recommendations have been prepared by the US Public Health Service and published on the HIV/AIDS Treatment Information Service website (www.AIDSinfo.nih.gov) [11].
• Prophylaxis for opportunistic infections as indicated by CD4 count and history: pregnant patients should be provided with essentially the same prophylaxis and

treatment of opportunistic infections as nonpregnant patients. The potential risk to the fetus of these medications is outweighed by the risk to the mother of opportunistic infections, which may be more serious during pregnancy.

- Careful monitoring for maternal and fetal toxicities.
- Attention to good nutrition, prenatal vitamins.
- Discuss of mode of delivery: elective cesarean section should be discussed with the patient, but not necessarily recommended, as there is minimal benefit in women on combination antiretroviral therapy with very low viral load.
- Avoid invasive procedures such as chorionic villus sampling (CVS), percutaneous umbilical blood sampling (PUBS), amniocentesis, scalp electrode, scalp pH.
- Avoid artificial rupture of membranes; maintain intact membranes intrapartum.
- Ensure availability of knowledgeable pediatric care for immediate neonatal period. Six weeks neonatal zidovudine; additional medications (lamivudine and nevirapine) if high risk for mother-to-child transmission.
- Counsel against breastfeeding.
- Effective birth control: drug interactions between ethinyl estradiol and antiretroviral drugs limit contraceptive options. Depo-medroxyprogesterone (DMPA) is generally effective and safe [22]. An IUD may be a good option [23].

Prevention

Our goal should be the primary prevention of maternal HIV infection, thereby eventually avoiding the need for managing HIV-infected prenatal patients. Routine obstetric and gynecologic visits provide an ideal opportunity for prevention efforts.

References

1. UNAIDS 2007 AIDS epidemic update. www.unaids.org/en/ KnowledgeCentre/HIVData/EpiUpdate/EpiUpdArchive/2007 default.asp.
2. www.cdc.gov/hiv/topics/surveillance/resources/reports/ 2005report/pdf/2005SurveillanceReport.pdf updated 6.07.
3. Centers for Disease Control and Prevention. Revised recommendations for HIV testing of adults, adolescents, and pregnant women in health-care settings. MMWR 2006; 55(RR14): 1–17.
4. American College of Obstetricians and Gynecologists. *Prenatal and perinatal human immunodeficiency virus testing: expanded recommendations. Committee Opinion No. 418.* Washington DC: American College of Obstetricians and Gynecologists, 2008.
5. Read J, and the International Perinatal HIV Group. The mode of delivery and the risk of vertical transmission of HIV-1: a meta-analysis from 15 prospective cohort studies. *NEJM* 1999; 340: 977–987.
6. European Mode of Delivery Collaboration. Elective cesarean section versus vaginal delivery in prevention of vertical HIV-1 transmission: a randomized clinical trial. *Lancet* 1999; 353: 1035–1039.
7. American College of Obstetricians and Gynecologists. *Committee Opinion No. 234. Scheduled cesarean delivery and the prevention of vertical transmission of HIV infection.* Washington DC: American College of Obstetricians and Gynecologists, 2000.
8. Connor EM, Sperling RS, Gelber R, *et al.* Reduction of maternal–infant transmission of human immunodeficiency virus type I with zidovudine treatment (ACTG 076). *NEJM* 1994; 331: 1173–1180.
9. Shaffer N, Chuachoowang R, Mock PA, *et al.* Short-course zidovudine for perinatal HIV transmission in Bangkok, Thailand: a randomised controled trial. *Lancet* 1999; 353: 773–780.
10. Wade NA, Birkhead GS, Warren BL, *et al.* Abbreviated regimens of zidovudine prophylaxis and perinatal transmission of human immunodeficiency virus. *NEJM* 1998; 339: 1409–1414.
11. Public Health Service, US Department of Health and Human Services, Perinatal HIV Guidelines Working Group. *Public Health Service Task Force recommendations for use of antiretroviral drugs in pregnant HIV-1 infected women for maternal health and interventions to reduce perinatal HIV transmission in the United States.* http://aidsinfo.nih.gov/ContentFiles/PerinatalGL.pdf. Updated April 2009; ongoing updates posted on website at www.aidsinfo.nih.gov.
12. Sperling RS, Shapiro DE, McSherry GD, *et al.* Safety of the maternal-infant zidovudine regimen utilized in the Pediatric AIDS Clinical Trials Group 076 Study. *AIDS* 1998; 12: 1805–1813.
13. Perinatal Safety Review Working Group. Nucleoside exposure in the children of HIV-infected women receiving antiretroviral drugs: absence of clear evidence for mitochondrial disease in children who died before 5 years of age in five United States cohorts. *J Acquir Immune Defic Syndr Hum Retrovirol* 2000; 15: 261–268.
14. Guay LA, Musoke P, Fleming T, *et al.* Intrapartum and neonatal single-dose nevirapine compared with zidovudine for prevention of mother-to-child transmission of HIV-1 in Kampala, Uganda: HIVNET 012 randomised trial. *Lancet* 1999; 354: 795–805.
15. Dorenbaum A, Cunningham CK, Gelber RD, *et al.* Two-dose intrapartum/newborn nevirapine and standard antiretroviral therapy to reduce perinatal HIV-1 transmission: a randomized trial. *JAMA* 2002; 288(2): 189–198.
16. Tuomala RE, Shapiro DE, Mofenson LM, *et al.* Antiretroviral therapy during pregnancy and the risk of adverse pregnancy outcome. *NEJM* 2002; 346(24):1863–1870.
17. Patel K, Shapiro DE, Brogly SB, *et al* for the P1025 team. Prenatal Protease Inhibitor use and the Risk of Preterm Delivery among HIV-infected Women Initiating Antiretroviral Drugs during Pregnancy. JID 2010; 201: 1035–1044.
18. Blanche S, Tardieu M, Rustin P, *et al.* Persistent mitochondrial dysfunction and perinatal exposure to antiretroviral nucleoside analogues. *Lancet* 1999; 354: 1084–1089.
19. Antiretroviral Pregnancy Registry Steering Committee. *Antiretroviral Pregnancy Registry International Interim Report*

for 1 January 1989 through 31 July 2009. Wilmington, NC: Antiretroviral Pregnancy Registry Steering Committee, 2009. www.APRegistry.com.

20. Stek AM, Mirochnick M, Capparelli E, *et al.* Reduced lopinavir exposure during pregnancy. *AIDS* 2006; 20: 1931–1939.

21. Best BM, Stek AM, Mirochnick M, *et al* for the IMPAACT 1026 study team. Lopinavir tablet pharmacokinetics with an increased dose during pregnancy. *J Acquir Immune Defic Syndr* 2010.

22. Cohn SE, Park JG, Watts DH, *et al.,* for the A5093 Protocol Team. Depo-medroxyprogesterone in women on antiretroviral therapy: effective contraception and lack of clinically significant interactions. *Clin Pharmacol Therapeut* 2006; 81(2): 222–227.

23. Stringer EM, Kaseba C, Levy J, *et al.* A randomized trial of the intrauterine contraceptive device vs hormonal contraception in women who are infected with the human immunodeficiency virus. *Am J Obstet Gynecol* 2007; 197: 144e1–144e8.

Chapter 34
Trauma in Pregnancy

Marc H. Incerpi

Department of Medicine and Obstetrics and Gynecology, Keck School of Medicine, University of Southern California, CA, USA

Introduction

Trauma is the leading cause of nonobstetric maternal death, complicating approximately 7% of all pregnancies. Motor vehicle accidents comprise roughly two-thirds of maternal trauma cases, followed by falls and assaults. Regardless of the cause, all pregnant trauma patients must be assessed formally in a medical setting. Evaluation of the pregnant trauma patient presents unique challenges and requires that the obstetrician play an important role in the multidisciplinary approach to the management of trauma in pregnancy.

Blunt abdominal trauma

While the initial assessment of the pregnant patient who has sustained trauma should also take into account the fetus, the patient's welfare and stability are paramount. The rate of fetal mortality after maternal blunt trauma ranges from 3.4% to 38.0%. Most commonly, this results from placental abruption, maternal shock or maternal death. Fetal loss can occur even when the patient has not sustained any abdominal injuries. For this reason, regardless of the apparent severity of injury in blunt trauma, all pregnant women must be evaluated. Given the fact that blunt trauma is relatively common in pregnancy, the pregnant patient should be reminded during prenatal care that if she sustains any form of trauma during pregnancy, she should report this immediately to her physician.

The most important cause of injury to the fetus is abruptio placentae. In one large series of trauma cases, two-thirds of fetal deaths were due to abruption. Abruption complicates 1–5% of minor trauma cases and 20–50% of major accidents. Although abruption may not manifest clinically for several days after the traumatic event, there will almost always be subtle warning signs within hours of the event. These include abdominal and/or uterine tenderness, vaginal bleeding or increased uterine activity. It is vitally important to realize that the diagnosis of placental abruption is a clinical diagnosis based on patient symptoms and abnormalities within the fetal heart rate pattern and/or uterine contraction pattern. Ultrasound misses approximately 50–80% of placental abruption. Therefore, an ultrasound should never be ordered in order to "rule out placental abruption." When placental abruption is severe enough to result in fetal death, clinically evident coagulopathy will be present in 40% of cases. Other placental injuries that have been described after blunt trauma include fracture of the placenta and disruption of fetal vessels on the surface of the placenta.

Direct injury to the uterus is another important risk of abdominal trauma unique to pregnancy. This may manifest as:
- contusion of the uterus with tenderness on examination
- serosal hemorrhage or abrasion
- avulsion of the uterine vasculature resulting in intraperitoneal or retroperitoneal hemorrhage
- uterine rupture with or without extrusion of the fetus or placenta into the abdominal cavity.

The presentation of uterine rupture may vary from mild uterine tenderness and an abnormal FHR tracing with normal vital signs to rapid onset of maternal hypovolemic shock with fetal and maternal death. Direct injury to the fetus is an uncommon but serious complication of blunt abdominal trauma. Fractures of the fetal skull and extremities have been reported. In addition, direct abdominal trauma may result in fetal subdural, sabgaleal, and intracranial hemorrhages.

Fetomaternal hemorrhage (FMH) may occur independently or in association with the above described injuries. In the majority of cases, the FMH is small and without clinical significance. However, large hemorrhages, which result in a severely anemic newborn or fetal death, may

Management of Common Problems in Obstetrics and Gynecology, 5th edition. Edited by T.M. Goodwin, M.N. Montoro, L. Muderspach, R. Paulson and S. Roy. © 2010 Blackwell Publishing Ltd.

occur. The degree of FMH is difficult to predict. Neither the severity of the trauma nor the mechanism of injury correlates well with the incidence or severity of the hemorrhage. The amount of FMH can be roughly calculated by performing a Kleihauer–Betke (KB) test which is used to identify the number of fetal cells that are present in the maternal circulation. Realizing that the average fetal blood volume is approximately 80 cc/kg, it becomes clear that it does not take much of a FMH before the fetus becomes hemodynamically compromised. In this instance there is usually evidence of abnormalities noted on FHR monitoring such as late FHR decelerations or fetal tachycardia. It is recommended that the KB test be performed in all cases of life-threatening abdominal trauma, whenever there is an abnormal FHR tracing after trauma or when the patient is Rh negative. When neither of these factors is present, the likelihood of finding clinically significant trauma is so low that the KB test is not helpful.

Penetrating abdominal trauma

Penetrating abdominal trauma occurs less frequently in pregnancy than blunt trauma. The majority of penetrating trauma is due to gunshots and stab wounds. After mid pregnancy, the uterus is injured more than twice as often as other maternal internal organs. The myometrium, amniotic fluid, fetus, and placenta act as a cushion to protect the other abdominal viscera. However, when the uterus is injured by penetrating wounds, the fetus is injured approximately two-thirds of the time. The damage caused by a bullet is unpredictable and involves many factors. Bullets have a tendency to cause much more intra-abdominal damage that suggested by the small entry wound. Therefore, most authorities recommend exploratory laparotomy for the pregnant patient who sustains a gunshot wound to the abdomen. Stab wounds, on the other hand, do not always require surgical exploration.

Domestic violence occurs more commonly during pregnancy, and is often under-reported for a variety of reasons. Some studies indicate that domestic violence occurs in up to 25% of pregnant women. However, physicians detect only a minority of cases (4–10%). It is important for physicians to screen all patients for domestic violence, and to be familiar with the community resources for assisting patients who experience domestic abuse.

General principles of management

With few exceptions, the treatment of the pregnant trauma patient is no different from that of the nonpregnant patient. While the eventual evaluation and management include the fetus, the initial management scheme is directed toward the mother. If undue attention is drawn to the fetus before the mother is stabilized, serious injuries may be overlooked, decreasing the chances of both maternal and fetal survival. The physiologic changes that occur in pregnancy that may affect trauma management are as follows:

- decrease in systolic and diastolic blood pressure
- increase in maternal blood volume, cardiac output, and heart rate
- decrease in hemoglobin and hematocrit
- increase in white blood cell count
- increase in fibrinogen
- positive D-dimers
- increase in tidal volume
- decreased blood urea nitrogen and serum creatinine
- decreased partial pressure of carbon dioxide
- increase in serum alkaline phosphatase.

In addition, there is decreased gastric emptying, decreased gastrointestinal motility, and increased risk for aspiration. These are important considerations when the gravid patient is given general anesthesia. Lastly, pregnancy is a hypercoagulable state secondary to an increase in clotting factors. Trauma will further increase the risk of thromboembolism. Therefore prophylactic anticoagulation should be judiciously employed.

The initial assessment should include stabilization of the pregnant woman using the standards of assessing and managing airway, breathing, and circulation. Supplemental oxygen should be given when indicated. Large-bore IV lines should be placed as required and the patient should be aggressively hydrated as indicated. Laboratory studies should include a complete blood count, blood type and Rh, coagulation studies, and chemistry profiles, and arterial blood gas measurements as indicated. In order to optimize venous return, the uterus should be displaced laterally of the great vessels.

As soon as the mother is stabilized, a careful assessment of fetal well-being should be undertaken as described below in the case of noncatastrophic trauma. In catastrophic trauma, cardiopulmonary resuscitation (CPR) may be indicated as a life-saving measure. The gravid uterus may impede CPR in the third trimester. Therefore, emergency cesarean delivery should be considered after 3–5 minutes of unsuccessful CPR. Delivery may save the fetus and make the maternal resuscitation mechanically feasible.

Use of open peritoneal lavage to diagnose intraperitoneal hemorrhage has been shown to be safe, sensitive, and specific during pregnancy, particularly in association with abdominal signs and symptoms of intraperitoneal bleeding, altered sensorium, major thoracic injury, unexplained shock, and multiple major orthopedic injuries. This procedure is unnecessary if clinically obvious intraperitoneal bleeding is present or if ultrasound findings are highly suggestive of free blood in the peritoneal cavity.

Much more commonly, the obstetrician becomes involved in cases of noncatastrophic trauma. During the secondary assessment after the patient has been initially stabilized, the patient is examined for nonobstetric injury and treated as necessary. The fetal heart tones are evaluated, and the gestational age is estimated by using history, fundal height, and ultrasound. If fetal heart tones are not detected, and this finding is confirmed by ultrasound, then maternal treatment only is initiated. If fetal heart tones are detected and the fetus is noted to be at least 23–24 weeks' gestation, then the FHR should be continuously monitored. Monitoring should be initiated as soon as possible after maternal stabilization, because most placental abruptions occur shortly after the traumatic incident. If the fetus is estimated to be less than 23 weeks' gestation, there is no need for continuous FHR monitoring.

Most authorities recommend that at least 4 hours of continuous FHR monitoring be employed. However, many institutions monitor the fetus continuously for at least 12–24 hours. The findings which identify the patient who warrants prolonged observation are uterine contractions, vaginal bleeding, spontaneous rupture of membranes, uterine tenderness, abdominal pain, or an abnormal FHR tracing. In addition, when the mechanism of injury is strongly associated with delayed complications (e.g. abruption after a high-velocity motor vehicle accident or automobile versus pedestrian), longer observation is required. While there is no consensus regarding the ideal duration for electronic fetal monitoring, it is reasonable to discharge the patient home after monitoring for 4–6 hours if she remains stable, and if there are no abnormal findings as previously discussed. If any of the above findings are present, then the fetus should be continuously monitored for at least 24 hours. Significant placental abruption, fetal bradycardia or recurrent late decelerations should prompt immediate delivery.

If the patient is Rh negative, 300 μg (one ampoule) of anti-D immune globulin should be given to prevent isoimmunization. This standard dose protects against a hemorrhage of 30 cc of fetal whole blood into the maternal circulation. The KB test should be obtained in Rh-negative patients in order to detect the rare case in which the amount of FMH exceeds that covered by a single ampoule of anti-D immune globulin. For example, if the KB demonstrates a FMH of 43 cc, then the patient would receive two ampoules of anti-D immune globulin. It should be noted that anti-D immune globulin should not be withheld if the KB is negative, since the amount of FMH necessary to sensitize the mother is much less that the lower limit of a positive KB test performed in most clinical laboratories.

An area of concern that often arises in assessing the pregnant trauma patient involves the use of diagnostic imaging and the potential risk to the fetus from radiation exposure. In general, diagnostic imaging should not be withheld if thought to be necessary. The benefit nearly always outweighs the risk. Adverse fetal effects such as impaired fetal growth, mental retardation, microcephaly, and central nervous system defects are not usually observed unless the dose of radiation to the fetus exceeds 5–10 rads. Less than 1% of trauma patients are exposed to more than 3 rads of radiation, making the risk negligible. For example, a CT scan of the entire abdomen is associated with a radiation dose of 2.8–4.6 rads. If multiple studies are required in which the radiation exposure to the fetus is significantly increased, consideration should be given to utilizing MRI imaging.

Prevention

No discussion on trauma in pregnancy would be complete without the mention of prevention. Despite the advances in trauma management, the fetal and maternal mortality rates after traumatic injury have not declined. Therefore, prevention is of great importance. While it would be impossible to prevent all causes of trauma during pregnancy, it does appear feasible to target motor vehicle accidents and domestic violence.

While most motor vehicle accidents cannot be prevented, injury sustained after a motor vehicle accident can be minimized. A very simple modifiable factor for decreasing maternal and fetal injury and mortality is proper seatbelt use. Numerous studies have demonstrated that pregnant women have low rates of seatbelt use. Evidence shows that unrestrained pregnant women are 2.8 times more likely to lose their fetuses than restrained pregnant women. As a preventive measure, it is important to discuss the proper utilization of seatbelts during prenatal care. Patients should be informed regarding the proper usage of the lap and shoulder belt. The lap belt should be placed under the gravid abdomen, while the shoulder belt should be placed to the side of the uterus, between the breast and over the clavicle. It is best to avoid placing the belt directly over the uterus. Airbags have proven to be life-saving. They should therefore not be disabled during pregnancy.

As discussed previously, domestic violence occurs more commonly in pregnancy. Therefore, the provider must have a relatively high index of suspicion. In fact, it is recommended that at the initial obstetric prenatal visit, all patients be screened for domestic violence. Many centers have adopted the use of a simple questionnaire using the acronym SAFE.

• S Does the patient feel safe? At home? At school? In the workplace? If not, whom or what does she fear and why?
• A Has the patient felt abused in a past relationship? Has she felt abused in her present relationship?

• F Does she have friends or family who can help? Who can the pregnant patient turn to for support?

• E Does the patient have an emergency or escape plan? In addition, there is a national domestic violence 24-hour hotline that is available in both English and Spanish (1-800-799-7233). Most communities have shelters or counseling centers available for the abused individual. It must be emphasized that recognition of domestic violence is the first, most important, and most often missed issue. When steps are taken to remove the patient from a hazardous environment, it is reasonable to assume that the likelihood of maternal/fetal morbidity/mortality would be significantly decreased.

Suggested reading

American College of Obstetricians and Gynecologists. *Obstetric aspects of trauma management. Educational Bulletin No. 251.* Washington, DC: American College of Obstetricians and Gynecologists, 1998.

Connolly A, Katz VL, Bash KL, *et al.* Trauma and pregnancy. *Am J Perinatol* 1997; 14: 331–336.

Franger AL, Buschbaum HJ, Peaceman AM. Abdominal gunshot wounds in pregnancy. *Am J Obstet Gynecol* 1989; 160: 1124–1128.

Goodwin TM, Breen MT. Pregnancy outcome and fetomaternal hemorrhage after noncatastrophic trauma. *Am J Obstet Gynecol* 1990; 162: 665–671.

Grossman NB. Blunt trauma in pregnancy. *Am Fam Physician* 2004; 70: 1303–1310.

Patteson SK, Snider CC, Meyer DS, *et al.* The consequences of high-risk behaviors: trauma during pregnancy. *J Trauma* 2007; 62: 1015–1020.

Pearlman MD, Tintinalli JE, Lorenz RP. A prospective controlled study of outcome after trauma during pregnancy. *Am J Obstet Gynecol* 1990; 162: 1502–1510.

Rose PG, Strohm PL, Zuspan FP. Fetomaternal hemorrhage following trauma. *Am J Obstet Gynecol* 1985; 153: 844–847.

Scorpio RJ, Espositio TJ, Smith LG, *et al.* Blunt trauma during pregnancy: factors affecting fetal outcome. *J Trauma* 1992; 32: 213–216.

Williams JK, McClain L, Rosemurgy AS. Evaluation of blunt abdominal trauma in the third trimester of pregnancy: maternal and fetal considerations. *Obstet Gynecol* 1990; 75: 33–37.

Chapter 35
Hypertension in Pregnancy

David A. Miller

Department of Medicine and Obstetrics and Gynecology, Keck School of Medicine, University of Southern California, CA, USA

Introduction

Hypertension is defined as a sustained blood pressure higher than 140/90 mmHg and may be attributable to any of the conditions summarized in Box 35.1. It affects 20–30% of American adults and complicates as many as 5–8% of all pregnancies. Approximately 15% of maternal deaths are attributable to hypertension, making it the second leading cause of maternal mortality in the United States. The classification system of hypertension in pregnancy proposed by the National High Blood Pressure Education Program Working Group is summarized in Box 35.2.

Chronic hypertension

Chronic hypertension complicates as many as 5% of pregnancies and is characterized by a history of high blood pressure before pregnancy, elevated blood pressure during the first half of pregnancy, or elevated blood pressure that persists beyond 12 weeks post partum. Blood pressure is measured in a sitting position with the arm at the level of the heart and multiple measurements are obtained. Other physical findings may include a renal artery bruit, funduscopic abnormalities, an enlarged thyroid gland, diminished peripheral pulses, skin and joint abnormalities.

Laboratory tests include a complete blood count, glucose screen, electrolyte panel, serum creatinine, urinalysis and urine culture. In some cases, additional tests may be needed. In patients with possible renal disease (serum creatinine ≥ 0.8 mg/dL, urine protein > 1 + on dipstick), a 24-h urine collection for creatinine clearance and total protein will provide baseline infor-

> **Box 35.1 Causes of chronic hypertension**
>
> **Idiopathic**
> Essential hypertension
>
> **Vascular disorders**
> Renovascular hypertension
> Aortic coarctation
>
> **Endocrine disorders**
> Diabetes mellitus
> Hyperthyroidism
> Pheochromocytoma
> Primary hyperaldosteronism
> Hyperparathyroidism
> Cushing's syndrome
>
> **Renal disorders**
> Diabetic nephropathy
> Chronic renal failure
> Acute Renal Failure
>   Tubular necrosis
>   Cortical necrosis
> Pyelonephritis
> Chronic glomerulonephritis
> Nephrotic Syndrome
> Polycystic kidney
>
> **Connective tissue disorders**
> Systemic lupus erythematosus

mation that may be helpful in diagnosing the onset of pre-eclampsia later in pregnancy. Additional tests may include antinuclear antibody, thyroid-stimulating hormone, urinary catecholamines, electrocardiogram and chest x-ray.

Fetal assessment in chronic hypertension

Chronic hypertension, regardless of the cause, increases the risk of poor fetal growth. An initial ultrasound

Management of Common Problems in Obstetrics and Gynecology, 5th edition. Edited by T.M. Goodwin, M.N. Montoro, L. Muderspach, R. Paulson and S. Roy. © 2010 Blackwell Publishing Ltd.

examination should be performed as early as possible to confirm the dates and exclude fetal anomalies. Thereafter, fetal growth usually is assessed every 2–4 weeks. Antepartum fetal monitoring is initiated by 32–34 weeks. Doppler velocimetry of the umbilical, uterine and middle cerebral arteries is helpful in optimizing the timing of delivery, particularly in cases of fetal growth restriction.

Management of mild chronic hypertension

In pregnant women with mild hypertension and no evidence of renal disease, serious complications are rare and antihypertensive medication usually is not necessary. Nonpharmacologic therapy includes a healthy diet, moderate exercise and avoidance of alcohol, tobacco and medications that increase blood pressure. A practical management algorithm is summarized in Figure 35.1. Prenatal visits are scheduled every 2–4 weeks until 34–36 weeks, and weekly thereafter. At each visit, blood pressure, urine protein and fundal height are evaluated. Patients are questioned regarding signs and symptoms of pre-eclampsia, including headache, abdominal pain, blurred vision, scotomata, rapid weight gain or marked swelling of the hands and/or face. Antepartum fetal monitoring usually is started around 32–34 weeks and in most cases, delivery is no later than 40 weeks.

Management of severe chronic hypertension

Women with sustained blood pressure ≥ 180/110 mmHg or those with evidence of renal disease may be at higher risk for serious complications such as heart attack, stroke or progression of renal disease and are candidates for antihypertensive medication. As summarized in Figure 35.1, many clinicians use a threshold of 150/100 mmHg for instituting antihypertensive therapy during pregnancy. Fundal height, blood pressure and

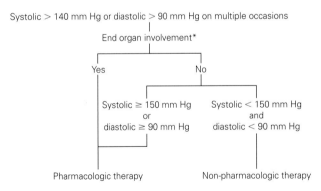

*Abnormal renal function
  Proteinuria (>300 mg/24 hr, >1 + dip, >30 mg/dL)
  Clcr <110 ml/min, serum creatinine >0.8 mg/dL
Cardiac involvement
  Left ventricular hypertrophy
Eye involvement
  Retinopathy

Figure 35.1 Management algorithm for chronic hypertension in pregnancy.

proteinuria are assessed at each visit, and evidence of superimposed pre-eclampsia is aggressively sought. Fetal growth assessment and antepartum testing are performed as described above and delivery usually is accomplished no later than 40 weeks.

Antihypertensive therapy in chronic hypertension

Methyldopa is a centrally acting α-adrenergic agonist that has been studied extensively and is recommended by many as the first-line antihypertensive agent in pregnancy. The total daily dosage of 500 mg to 2 g is administered in 2–4 divided doses. Peak plasma levels occur 2–3 hours after administration and the maximum effect occurs 4–6 hours after an oral dose. Sedation and postural hypotension are the most common side effects. Hemolytic anemia, fever, liver function abnormalities, granulocytopenia, and thrombocytopenia are rare side effects.

Labetalol is an α1-adrenergic blocker and a nonselective β-adrenergic blocker. A large body of clinical evidence suggests that this agent lacks teratogenicity, crosses the placenta in small amounts and is safe during pregnancy. The usual starting dose is 100 mg bid, and the dose may be increased weekly to a maximum of 2400 mg daily. Titration increments should not exceed 200 mg bid.

Nifedipine is a calcium channel blocker that has been used during pregnancy for tocolysis and treatment of hypertension. Several reports suggest that nifedipine is safe during pregnancy. The long-acting formulation (Procardia XL, Adalat cc) can be used once daily and may improve patient compliance. The usual starting dose of 30 mg daily may be increased to 60–90 mg daily. Nifedipine should be used with caution in patients receiving magnesium sulfate. The sublingual route of administration is associated with unpredictable blood levels and should be avoided.

Angiotensin-converting enzyme inhibitors (enalapril, captopril) are associated with fetal hypocalvaria, renal defects, anuria and fetal and neonatal death. These agents are contraindicated in pregnancy. With few exceptions, diuretics (furosemide, hydrochlorothiazide) should be avoided during pregnancy. Fetal bradycardia, growth retardation and neonatal hypoglycemia have been reported in patients treated with β-blockers. Published experience with other agents is limited.

Pre-eclampsia

Pre-eclampsia complicates 5–7% of all pregnancies. Predisposing factors are summarized in Box 35.3. In addition to the classic findings of hypertension and proteinuria, women with pre-eclampsia may complain of scotomata, blurred vision or pain in the epigastrium or right upper quadrant. Examination often reveals brisk patellar reflexes and clonus. Laboratory abnormalities include elevation of the hematocrit, lactate dehydrogenase, serum transaminases and uric acid and occasionally thrombocytopenia.

Management of pre-eclampsia

In the setting of pre-eclampsia, the decision to proceed with immediate delivery versus expectant management is based upon several factors, including disease severity, fetal maturity, maternal and fetal condition and cervical status. Pre-eclampsia is classified as mild or severe, as outlined in Box 35.4.

Mild pre-eclampsia

Women with mild pre-eclampsia are hospitalized for further evaluation and, if indicated, delivery. At 40 weeks and beyond, delivery is indicated regardless of cervi-

---

Box 35.3 Risk factors for pre-eclampsia

Age < 20; > 35
Nulliparity
Multiple gestation
Hydatidiform mole
Diabetes mellitus
Thyroid disease
Chronic hypertension
Renal disease
Collagen vascular disease
Antiphospholipid syndrome
Family history of pre-eclampsia

Box 35.4 Classification of pre-eclampsia

Mild Pre-eclampsia
Blood pressure ≥140/90 but <160/110 on two occasions at least 6 hours apart while the patient is on bed rest
    Proteinuria ≥300 mg/24 hr but <5 gm/24 hr
    Asymptomatic

Severe Pre-eclampsia
Blood pressure of 160 mm Hg systolic or higher or 110 mm Hg diastolic or higher on two occasions at least 6 hours apart while the patient is on bed rest
    Proteinuria of 5 gm or higher in a 24-hour urine specimen or 3 + or greater on two random urine samples collected at least 4 hours apart
    Oliguria of less than 500 mL in 24 hours
    Cerebral or visual disturbances
    Pulmonary edema or cyanosis
    Epigastric or right upper-quadrant pain
    Impaired liver function
    Thrombocytopenia
    Fetal growth restriction

cal status. At 37 weeks and beyond, cervical status is assessed. If the cervix is favorable, induction is initiated. If not, preinduction cervical ripening agents are used as needed. Women with mild pre-eclampsia before 37 weeks usually are managed expectantly with bedrest, frequent antepartum testing, and maternal evaluation as described above. Corticosteroids are administered if the gestational age is < 34 weeks; amniocentesis may be performed as needed to assess fetal pulmonary maturity. Fetal growth is assessed every 2–4 weeks. If the maternal and fetal conditions remain stable, delivery is targeted for approximately 37 weeks. The benefit of prophylactic magnesium sulfate in patients with mild pre-eclampsia has not been demonstrated conclusively in the literature.

Severe pre-eclampsia

Severe pre-eclampsia warrants hospitalization. If the gestational age is ≥34 weeks, fetal pulmonary is confirmed or there is evidence of deteriorating maternal or fetal status, delivery usually is indicated. Hydralazine, labetalol or nifedipine is used as needed to maintain a systolic blood pressure < 160 mmHg and a diastolic blood pressure < 105 mmHg. Overly aggressive control of the blood pressure may compromise maternal perfusion of the intervillous space and adversely impact fetal oxygenation. Hydralazine is a peripheral vasodilator that can be given in doses of 5–10 mg IV. The onset of action is 10–20 minutes and the dose may be repeated in 20–30 minutes if necessary. Labetalol can be administered in doses of 5–20 mg by slow IV push. The dose may be repeated in 10–20 minutes. Nifedipine is a calcium channel blocker that can be used in doses of 5–10 mg orally. The dose may be repeated in 20–30 minutes, as needed.

Management of severe pre-eclampsia before 34 weeks is controversial. At the University of Southern California, delivery is delayed for 24–48 hours whenever possible to permit the administration of corticosteroids. Magnesium sulfate is initiated, fetal status is monitored continuously, and antihypertensive agents are used as needed. Between 32 and 34 weeks, consideration should be given to amniocentesis for pulmonary maturity studies. If mature, delivery is indicated. If immature, corticosteroids are administered and, if possible, delivery is delayed 24–48 hours. Between 24 and 32 weeks, antihypertensive therapy is instituted as indicated, corticosteroids are administered and extensive maternal counseling, including neonatology consultation, is undertaken to clarify the risks and benefits of pregnancy prolongation. The duration of expectant management is determined on an individual basis, taking into account maternal wishes, estimated fetal weight, gestational age and maternal and fetal condition.

When severe pre-eclampsia is diagnosed before 24 weeks of gestation, the likelihood of a favorable outcome is low. Thorough counseling should address the risks and anticipated benefits of expectant management and should include the option of pregnancy termination. If an appropriately informed patient declines the option of pregnancy termination, expectant management should proceed as outlined above.

Intrapartum management of pre-eclampsia

In women with pre-eclampsia without contraindications to labor, vaginal delivery is the preferred approach. During labor, magnesium sulfate is administered for seizure prophylaxis as an intravenous loading dose of 4–6 g over 20–60 min, followed by a maintenance dose of 1–2 g per hour. Urine output and serum creatinine are monitored, and the magnesium dose adjusted accordingly to prevent hypermagnesemia. Patellar reflexes and respiratory rate should be assessed frequently. In the presence of patellar reflexes, serum magnesium levels usually are unnecessary. Therapeutic magnesium levels range from 4 to 8 mg/dL. Loss of patellar reflexes is observed at magnesium levels of 10 mg/dL or higher, respiratory paralysis may occur at levels of 15 mg/dL or above, and cardiac arrest is possible with levels in excess of 25 mg/dL. Calcium gluconate (10 cc of a 10% solution) should be available in the event of hypermagnesemia. To avoid pulmonary edema, intravenous fluid administration is monitored closely. Pain control is achieved with regional anesthesia or with intramuscular or intravenous narcotic analgesics. If cesarean section is required, platelets should be available for possible transfusion for patients with platelet counts < 50,000/mm^3. The use of other blood products is guided by clinical and laboratory findings.

Eclampsia

The estimated incidence of eclampsia is 1–3 per 1000 pre-eclamptic patients. In most cases seizures are self-limited, lasting 1–2 minutes. The first priorities are to ensure that the airway is clear and to prevent injury and aspiration of gastric contents. Diazepam or lorazepam should be used only if seizures are sustained. Most tonic-clonic seizures are accompanied by prolonged fetal heart rate deceleration that resolves after the seizure has ended. If possible, a 10–20 minute period of *in utero* resuscitation should be permitted prior to delivery. Convulsions do not mandate cesarean delivery. However, if vaginal birth is not possible within a reasonable period of time, cesarean delivery is performed in most cases.

HELLP syndrome

The HELLP syndrome is a variant of pre-eclampsia that is characterized by hemolysis, elevated liver enzymes and low platelets. Right upper quadrant pain, nausea, vomiting and malaise are common. Hypertension and proteinuria are variable. The hallmark of the disorder is microangiopathic hemolysis leading to elevation of serum lactate dehydrogenase and fragmented red blood cells on peripheral smear. Transaminases are elevated, thrombocytopenia is present, and disseminated intravascular coagulation may be evident, particularly if HELLP syndrome is accompanied by placental abruption. With few exceptions, the diagnosis of HELLP syndrome constitutes an indication for delivery. Dexamethasone may hasten the improvement of HELLP syndrome following delivery, but not all studies have confirmed this benefit. In one protocol, dexametasone is administered in four doses of 10 mg, 10 mg, 5 mg and 5 mg at 12-hour intervals. If elevated transaminases or thrombocytopenia persist beyond the fourth postpartum day, alternative explanations should be considered, including thrombotic thrombocytopenic purpura, hemolytic uremic syndrome, acute fatty liver of pregnancy, viral or drug-induced hepatitis and systemic lupus erythematosus.

Conclusion

Hypertensive disorders of pregnancy remain among the most common causes of adverse maternal and perinatal outcome. Appropriate management of newly diagnosed chronic hypertension entails a thorough search for an underlying cause. Antihypertensive medications are reserved for women with severe chronic hypertension. Close maternal and fetal surveillance is necessary, and a high index of suspicion must be maintained for the development of superimposed pre-eclampsia.

The management of pre-eclampsia is influenced by many factors, including disease severity, gestational age and fetal condition. Optimal management requires an appreciation of the complexity of the disease process and familiarity with its manifestations in multiple organ systems. Maternal and fetal risks and benefits must be assessed thoroughly. Individualized treatment plans should be formulated and discussed with the patient, and she should be encouraged to participate in major decisions regarding her care. In atypical cases, alternative diagnoses must be considered.

Suggested reading

American College of Obstetricians and Gynecologists. Chronic hypertension in pregnancy. Practice Bulletin No 29. *Obstet Gynecol* 2001; 98: 177–185.

American College of Obstetricians and Gynecologists. Diagnosis and management of pre-eclampsia and eclampsia. Practice Bulletin No 33. *Obstet Gynecol* 2002; 99: 159–167.

Chambers JC, Fusi L, Malik IS, Haskard DO, de Swiet M, Kooner JS. Association of maternal endothelial dysfunction with pre-eclampsia. *JAMA* 2001; 285: 1607–1612.

Duley L. Pre-eclampsia and hypertension. *Clin Evid* 2002; 7: 1296–1309.

Duley L, Gulmezoglu AM, Henderson-Smart DJ. Magnesium sulphate and other anticonvulsants for women with pre-eclampsia. *Cochrane Database Syst Rev* 2004; 3.

Isler CM, Barrilleaux PS, Magann EF, Bass JD, Martin JN. A prospective, randomized trial comparing the efficacy of dexamethasone and betamethasone for the treatment of antepartum HELLP (hemolysis, elevated liver enzymes, and low platelet count) syndrome. *Am J Obstet Gynecol* 2001; 184: 1332–1339.

Lain KY, Roberts JM. Contemporary concepts in the pathogenesis and management of pre-eclampsia. *JAMA* 2002; 287: 3183–3136.

Levine RJ, Maynard SE Qian C, *et al*. Circulating angiogenic factors and the risk of pre-eclampsia. *NEJM* 2004; 350: 672–683.

National High Blood Pressure Education Program Working Group. Report of the National High Blood Pressure Education Program Working Group on high blood pressure in pregnancy. *Am J Obstet Gynecol* 2000; 183: S1–22.

Sibai BM, Ewell M, Levine RJ, *et al*. Risk factors associated with pre-eclampsia in healthy nulliparous women. The Calcium for Pre-eclampsia Prevention (CPEP) Study Group. *Am J Obstet Gynecol* 1997; 177: 1003–1010.

Taylor RN. Review: immunobiology of pre-eclampsia. *Am J Reprod Immunol* 1997; 37: 79.

Chapter 36
Nausea and Vomiting of Pregnancy Including Hyperemesis Gravidarum

T. Murphy Goodwin and Martin N. Montoro
Department of Medicine and Obstetrics and Gynecology, Keck School of Medicine, University of Southern California, CA, USA

Introduction

Nausea and vomiting of pregnancy (NVP) affects about 75% of pregnant women, with 25% reporting nausea alone and 50% reporting both nausea and vomiting. Hyperemesis gravidarum (HG) occurs in 0.3–2% although populations with significantly higher rates have been reported. It is identified by otherwise unexplained intractable vomiting and dehydration. Significant weight loss, usually > 5% of pre-pregnancy weight, confirms the diagnosis.

Maternal mortality was about 10% until the middle of the 20th century. Maternal death is now uncommon but it still does occur, either related directly to HG or to therapeutic interventions. It is the most common cause of hospitalization in the first half of pregnancy and the cost of hospitalization alone is estimated to be more than $500 million annually.

Etiology

Hyperemesis gravidarum is clearly related to a product of placental metabolism since it does not require the presence of the fetus and it occurs commonly in molar gestation. More than 20 studies about hormonal changes in NVP have been published in the last 30 years and despite some conflicting information, the evidence points towards hCG and estradiol as having a role.

There is a strong temporal association between hCG concentrations and the time of peak symptomatology. hCG is also a thyroid stimulator and biochemical hyperthyroidism is commonly seen in HG. It has been difficult, however, to directly link total hCG concentrations with

Management of Common Problems in Obstetrics and Gynecology, 5th edition. Edited by T.M. Goodwin, M.N. Montoro, L. Muderspach, R. Paulson and S. Roy. © 2010 Blackwell Publishing Ltd.

the severity of NVP because its concentrations vary widely in the normal and NVP populations. This occurs because hCG is actually a family of isoforms which differ in their half-life and in their binding potency to the hCG, LH and TSH receptors. Isoforms lacking the carboxyl-terminal portion, for example, are more potent stimulators of the TSH and LH receptor but have shorter half-lives. Hyperglycosylated hCG, on the other hand, has a longer half-life and a longer duration of action.

A link between the action of hCG and estradiol has been suggested because concentrations of hyperglycosylated hCG correlate with estradiol and the severity of nausea and vomiting (NV). It is hypothesized that stimulation of maternal ovarian production of estradiol (and possibly fetal production as well) increases maternal estradiol concentration. NV in women taking the combined oral contraceptive pill increases in direct correlation with the estradiol dose and a history of NV while taking estrogens is a risk factor for the development of HG.

Epidemiologic studies have in general identified some common threads between women with HG and other common NV syndromes such as postoperative and chemotherapy-related NV and include younger age, a history of motion sickness, history of migraines and earlier hour of the day. Of interest is that smoking is associated with decreased concentrations of hCG and estradiol and with less NVP while fetal female gender is associated with greater concentrations of hCG and more severe HG.

Evidence in support of a genetic predisposition to NVP includes the concordance in frequency of nausea and vomiting of pregnancy in monozygotic twins; that siblings and mothers of patients with NVP are more likely to be affected; the variation in the frequency of NVP among different ethnic groups; and the occurrence of NVP in women with inherited glycoprotein hormone receptor defects. The paternal genome may have a role as well since women with HG in one pregnancy for whom there was a different father in the next pregnancy had a 60% lower rate of recurrence HG.

Psychologic factors

For many years it was presumed that women suffering from HG were predisposed by something in their own psychologic make-up or by the circumstances of their lives. Numerous theories, drawn mostly from psychoanalysis, identified these women as rejecting the father of the baby, ambivalent about the pregnancy, rejecting their own feminity and either being too dependent on their mothers … or not dependent enough! One of the most influential studies concluded that women with HG had a hysterical personality type. At present, HG is not believed to be due to any particular psychologic state. In a recent survey, 93 of 96 women believed that HG had a biologic basis and that psychologic problems were secondary to the severe illness. Nevertheless, most of them also reported that friends, family members and caregivers implied that they were somehow in control of their disease state.

The development of food aversions in pregnancy (present in about 50% of women) is closely linked to the onset of nausea. In 64% of cases, the first occurrence of nausea was reported either in the week preceding the first food aversion or in the same week. These findings are consistent with a taste aversion learning mechanism, where foods paired with illness are subsequently avoided. The fact that cravings common in pregnancy do not follow this pattern is supportive of the same concept. Anticipatory vomiting associated with chemotherapy is thought to have a similar mechanism. Interestingly, the food aversions in pregnancy are similar to those that develop with chemotherapy in that they do not generally persist after the acute course of the primary stimulus ends; this is distinct from other conditioned responses which may persist for years. Uncontrolled case series have suggested a benefit of behavioral therapy or hypnosis in treatment of HG.

Embryo protection hypothesis

In the view of evolutionary biology, NVP is a mechanism that has evolved, along with food aversions, to prevent pregnant mothers from ingesting substances that may be harmful to the developing fetus such as infections in the food supply or other toxins. However, even if NVP and HG evolved as a protective phenomenon, this fetal benefit is no longer applicable.

Nausea and vomiting of pregnancy as a syndrome

Nausea and vomiting of pregnancy is better thought of as a syndrome with the final phenotype arising from different pathways. Thus, for example, the stimulus to HG is affected by placental mass (more common in multiple gestation) as well as by aberrant hCG production as in advanced molar gestation or in carriers of trisomy 21

fetuses. The paternal genotype within the placenta must play a role, as is shown by the effect of changing fathers on the recurrence risk of HG. Equally important, the way an individual mother responds to this stimulus is genetically mediated, as is shown by family studies of HG. The susceptibility of the mother varies depending on a number of factors that are recognized as mediating NV in other settings such as postoperative NV and chemotherapy-induced NV.

Clinical presentation

Prospective studies show that virtually all women who develop NVP will have some symptoms by 9 weeks' gestation; 7% have symptoms before the time of the first missed period and 60% are symptomatic by 6 weeks. For the subset of women with HG, there is a tendency for early onset of symptoms and much greater overall duration. The timing of end of symptoms for NVP and HG is shown in Table 36.1.

In addition to NV, associated complaints include excess salivation (ptyalism) in up to 60%. There is a common perception that women with more severe NVP are very sensitive to olfactory stimuli, but it has not been documented in objective studies. Rather, there is a change in the pleasurable (or, rather, lack of pleasurable) rating of odors, something similar to what is seen during chemotherapy-induced nausea.

Recent population-based studies have found that low pre-pregnancy BMI was associated with a higher risk of HG and that the effect was even stronger for women requiring hospitalization. Obesity appeared to decrease the risk of hospital admission for HG.

Laboratory abnormalities

A wide variety of laboratory abnormalities can be seen with HG, including suppressed TSH and/or elevations in free T4, elevated liver enzymes as well as bilirubin,

Table 36.1 Time to cessation of NVP and HG

Weeks	Women (%)	Estimate NVP	(%) HG
<8	8.2		
8–9	9.2		
9–10	9.9	30	10
10–11	15.1		
11–12	17.5	30	15
12–13	8.6		
13–14	11.0		
14–15	7.2		
15–16	4.1	30	20
16+	9.2	10	50

amylase and lipase. These abnormalities resolve when the vomiting stops and do not require specific treatment. There is still insufficient awareness of the spectrum of these transient abnormalities, sometimes resulting in unnecessary antithyroid treatment, cholecystectomy or even termination of pregnancy. Rare cases of hepatic or renal insufficiency have been reported with HG but these are usually transient as well or due to other underlying disease.

Virtually all patients with transient hyperthyroidism related to HG will have a normal TSH after the vomiting stops. In such patients there is no history of symptoms preceding pregnancy, no goiter, no other systemic signs of hyperthyroidism (except occasionally tachycardia) and negative thyroid antibodies.

Maternal complications

Severe metabolic/nutritional maternal complications of HG may include Werrnicke's encephalopathy, beriberi, central pontine myelinolysis, hepatic insufficiency, acute tubular necrosis and peripheral neuropathy. Complications due to the mechanical stress of vomiting may include Mallory–Weiss tear of the esophagus, esophageal rupture, pneumomediastinum, retinal detachment and splenic avulsion.

One of the most serious complications of HG is Wernicke's encephalopathy and more than 40 cases have been reported in the last 25 years. Presenting symptoms may include the classic diagnostic triad of ataxia, nystagmus and dementia but the most common manifestation described in the literature is simply apathy or confusion. No patient has developed this complication with less than 4 weeks of persistent vomiting. More than half of the women reported have died or had permanent neurologic dysfunction. Reflecting the role of thiamine in glucose metabolism, some cases of Wernicke's encephalopathy have been precipitated by infusion of solutions containing dextrose prior to administration of thiamine.

The problem of Wernicke's encephalopathy is best addressed by prevention. All patients with HG should receive the minimum RDA for thiamine (3 mg/day) that is contained in most multivitamins or more. If the vomiting is severe enough to require intravenous hydration, 100 mg thiamine should be administered parenterally on the presumption of thiamine deficiency. It is our practice to administer this daily for 3 days if a patient is in hospital for HG.

Psychologic burden and long-term health consequences

The psychologic burden of severe NVP and HG results from having a disease that has a strong subjective component (nausea) for which the cause is not understood.

The most extreme manifestation of this is termination of an otherwise wanted pregnancy. In one study, 15% of 808 women with HG had at least one termination of pregnancy due specifically to HG. Although women who terminated their pregnancy due to HG did not appear to have more severe disease, they were twice as likely to report that their doctor was uncaring or did not appreciate the severity of the illness.

The long-term health consequences of HG for the women who suffer from it are largely unknown. Two studies suggested an increased risk of breast cancer based on a presumed hyperestrogenic milieu but this has not been confirmed. Post-traumatic stress disorder, depression and a variety of neurologic complaints are commonly reported by these women but there has been no systematic follow-up.

Fetal consequences of hyperemesis

Nausea and vomiting of pregnancy is generally associated with good pregnancy outcome. The problem arises from applying this principle to cases of HG. It is now clear that the vast majority of fetal and maternal complications come from the group of HG women who have sustained weight loss. Although some degree of weight loss is present in many, if not most cases of HG, it is often stabilized with supportive therapy and antiemetic therapy. Women with HG who gain less than 7 kg overall in pregnancy are more likely to have low birthweight and preterm birth than women who gained more than 7 kg. The rate of fetal death is higher in the group with the most weight loss.

Major congenital anomalies appear to be less prevalent in women with NVP and HG, although the data are conflicting. A Swedish population study found that hip dysplasia and Down's syndrome were higher than expected in HG women. Vitamin K deficiency causing fetal coagulopathy or chondrodysplasia has been reported. But apart from these possible anomalies, there is no overall increased rate of birth defects.

The long-term consequences of HG for the offspring are almost entirely unstudied but there is increasing awareness of the fetal origins of many adult diseases (Barker hypothesis). In animal models and in natural experiments such as famine, maternal calorie deprivation, even if limited to a few weeks or months of pregnancy, can have adverse effects on the physical and psychologic well-being of the offspring. Several childhood cancers including testicular cancer and leukemia have been linked to hyperemesis although there are conflicting data.

Differential diagnosis

Gastrointestinal conditions that could be confused with HG include gastroenteritis, gastroparesis, achalasia, biliary tract disease, hepatitis, intestinal obstruction, peptic ulcer disease, pancreatitis and appendicitis. Genitourinary tract conditions include pyelonephritis, ovarian torsion, nephrolithiasis, and degenerating uterine leiomyoma. Metabolic conditions include uremia, diabetic ketoacidosis, porphyria, Addison's disease, severe hyperthyroidism and hyperparathyroidism. Neurologic disorders may include pseudotumor cerebri, vestibular lesions, migraines, intracranial tumors and lymphocytic hypophysitis. Pregnancy-related conditions include acute fatty liver of pregnancy and pre-eclampsia. Other possible causes include drug toxicity or intolerance.

Clinical clues suggesting alternative diagnosis

These include NV antedating pregnancy, nausea beginning after 9 weeks' gestation, abdominal pain, fever, headache, goiter, abnormal neurologic exam, elevated WBC, anemia or thrombocytopenia.

Mild elevations of liver enzymes (usually < 300 U/L) and serum bilirubin (< 4 mg/dL) are encountered in 20–30% of women; serum concentrations of amylase and lipase (up to five times greater than normal levels) are seen in 10–15%. Rarely, significant cholestasis and even liver dysfunction (with a prolongation of the prothrombin time) may be seen. Liver enzyme elevations are much higher with primary hepatitis, and the bilirubin concentration is generally much higher as well. Acute pancreatitis may cause vomiting and hyperamylasemia, but serum amylase concentrations are usually 5–10 times higher than the elevations associated with NVP. Electrolyte abnormalities are found in 15–25% of cases. The most common are hypokalemia, hyponatremia and hypochloremic metabolic alkalosis. With severe volume contraction, a metabolic acidemia may be seen. All the abnormalities have been reported to regress with adequate volume replacement and nutritional support.

Elevated thyroxine and suppressed TSH (see Chapter 24) is noted in 50–70% of women with hyperemesis. It can usually be distinguished from intrinsic thyroid disease in that there is no history of hyperthyroid symptoms preceding pregnancy, no goiter, negative thyroid antibodies, and the tri-iodothyronine is either not elevated or proportionally much less elevated than thyroxine. There are rarely symptoms of hyperthyroidism except occasional tachycardia. The condition, which is due to an effect of hCG on the TSH receptor, is self-limited and does not require specific antithyroid therapy. Because there is an inverse relationship between the severity of NVP and the TSH concentration, a nonsuppressed TSH level suggests that the cause of the NV is something other than NVP. A TSH level greater than 2.5 µU/mL is rare with severe NVP, unless the patient has pre-existing hypothyroidism.

An ultrasound should be performed in cases of HG as it may identify a predisposing factor such as multiple gestation or molar gestation.

Management of hyperemesis gravidarum

Prevention of HG is a subject that arises naturally in a discussion with the patient who has suffered from HG in the past. Until recently, the recurrence risk of HG was not well understood. Two recent studies have shown recurrence risks of 16% and 19%, a 29-fold increase over the primary rate. This is probably an underestimate for the most severe cases since more of these women are unlikely to attempt another pregnancy.

For these women in particular and for HG in general, there is evidence that prevention is possible. Women who are taking a multivitamin at the time of conception and in early pregnancy are less likely to require intervention for HG later in pregnancy. Pre-emptive treatment of HG has been advocated based on the indirect evidence that in women who have NVP sufficient to interfere with their daily routine (30–35% of pregnant women), such treatment is associated with lower rates of hospital admission for HG.

Diet and support

Little is known about what dietary adjustments should be made. Commonsense but unsubstantiated advice is to eat small meals when one feels able. Protein meals rather than carbohydrate, and liquids rather than solids, resulted in less nausea and improved stomach electrical rhythms associated with nausea. Food aversions and changes in the effect of smells are closely linked to the development of nausea, probably through a taste aversion learning mechanism. Besides avoiding the offending foods and odors, there is evidence that behavioral approaches such as relaxation and hypnosis/distracting therapy can diminish nausea and vomiting.

Pharmacologic and alternative therapy

For women who continue to have problematic NV, vitamin B6, 25 mg three times daily, is recommended. Several randomized studies suggest a benefit of B6 in NVP in reducing nausea although the effect on vomiting is less clear. B6 is safe for mother and fetus in doses up to 100 mg daily. If symptoms persist, an antihistamine may be added; antihistamines have proven to be effective and safe.

The combination of B6 and the first-generation antihistamine doxylamine formed the basis of Bendectin which was used by approximately 25% of all pregnant women (33 million) between 1958 and 1982. Several, although small, randomized controlled studies attested to its efficacy but questions about its safety led to its withdrawal from the market, even though the risks have not been substantiated. Because of the scrutiny brought on by the ensuing litigation, Bendectin has been studied extensively. A meta-analysis of studies of Bendectin with more than 14,000 first-trimester exposures found no increase in anomalies above the background rate. Doxylamine itself is only available in the US in the form of Unisom sleep tablets and available over the counter; 25 mg of B6 plus half of a 25 mg Unisom Sleep Tab 3–4 times daily approximates the Bendectin regimen (10 mg B6 and 10 mg doxylamine; B6 is not available in less than 50 mg doses in the United States). The Bendectin formulation can also be obtained from compounding pharmacies, and is available in Canada and several other countries as Diclectin.

For patients who receive no relief from this regimen, the herbal medication Ginger may be added and several randomized controlled studies attest to its efficacy. However, the fetal safety data are limited. Nevertheless, problems have not been seen and theoretical concerns seem adequately addressed in a recent review. Another alternative therapy which has been studied extensively in NVP is acupuncture and acoustic stimulation. Although there are some conflicting data, the weight of evidence suggests some benefit without significant risks.

Other classes of antiemetics include benzamides, phenothiazines, butyrophenones, 5-HT3 receptor antagonists and corticosteroids. While randomized trials of agents in most of these classes have shown some efficacy in NVP overall, there have only been 10 randomized trials of pharmacologic interventions in HG, six involving steroids. Because of their general effectiveness in relieving NV in other states, they have been commonly employed in NVP. Safety data have been limited although in recent years more information has accumulated. Corticosteroids appear to be associated with a slight increase in facial clefts when given in the first trimester.

Since there is not good evidence for the efficacy of any one of the agents among the phenothiazines or benzamides, it is common practice to switch between agents or combine them. One of the main dangers in this regard is the confluence of side effects, in particular extrapyramidal symptoms. Several of these agents have similar side effects and adverse reactions, particularly anxiety, depression and even hallucinations; there is evidence that the extrapyramidal symptoms are commonly overlooked.

Ondansetron and other 5-HT3 receptor antagonists deserve special mention. Most women with HG report that vitamin and herbal remedies and older antiemetics bring little relief. Although these agents may be effective for less severe NVP, more potent interventions appear to be needed for established HG. In this regard, ondansetron has become one of the most widely used antiemetics,

largely by analogy to its demonstrated superiority in chemotherapy-related NV. Although the only randomized controlled study of ondansetron for HG showed that it was not more effective than phenergan, this may be due to selection of patients who were likely to improve with most interventions, a point discussed further below. More safety data have accumulated recently.

Corticosteroids are potent antiemetics in the setting of chemotherapy-induced NV. They have been studied for their effect in HG with conflicting results. Several series described significant diminution or complete resolution of NV with corticosteroid therapy but randomized trials have failed to demonstrate a conclusive benefit. In one study, women discharged on corticosteroids were less likely to be readmitted than those on phenergan but another study did not find such a benefit. There may be a remarkable recrudescence of symptoms with steroid dose lowering which responds immediately to reinstitution of therapy. It has been suggested that the failure to show a benefit from steroids is due to patient selection bias in that less ill patients (those without weight loss in this analysis) are likely to respond to a variety of treatments.

Nutritional support

For a patient who does not respond adequately to therapy and is unable to maintain her weight by oral intake, nutritional support is required. This recommendation is based on several points: higher rates of IUGR in this population, the probability of long-term adverse consequences for the fetus due to changes in programming and, rarely, life-threatening vitamin deficiency. Caloric support may be achieved by either enteral or parenteral nutrition. Probably because of a higher rate of patient acceptance, parenteral nutrition for women with HG has been reported much more often than enteral nutrition. Serious complications of parenteral alimentation can occur, however, including infection, thrombophlebitis, and death due to infection or pericardial tamponade. Peripheral placement of central access was thought to be associated with fewer complications but many of the same complications reported with central access have also occurred.

In a study of 94 women hospitalized with HG, 42 received medication alone, 33 a peripherally inserted central catheter (PICC) line, and 19 a nasogastric or nasoduodenal tube. Of those managed with a PICC line, 66.4% required treatment for infection, thromboembolism or both. In addition, neonatal complications including small for gestational age, admission to neonatal intensive care, termination of pregnancy because of HG, and fetal loss were increased in the women who had a PICC line.

There is little evidence indicating that the better safety record of enteral feeding and comparable efficacy compared with parenteral feeding via a PICC line has led to increased usage. In our own survey of 792 women who

---

Nausea and vomiting of pregnancy: treatment algorithm**,†
(If no improvement, proceed to next step)

↓

Vitamin B$_6$ 10 mg – 25 mg, TID or QID (up to 100 mg daily)

↓

Alternative therapies may be added at any time during the sequence depending on patient acceptance and the familiarity of the attendant: consider P6 acccupressure with Sea Bands® or accustimulation with Relief Band® or Ginger capsules 250 mg 4 times daily

↓

Add:

Doxylamine 12.5 mg, TID or QID[1]
Adjust schedule and dose according to severity of patient's symptoms

↓

Add:

Promethazine (Phenergan®) 12.5 – 25 mg q4h PO/PR
Or
Dimenhydrinate (Dramamine® Oral) 50 – 100 mg q4 – 6h PO/PR
(not to exceed 400 mg per day; not to exceed 200 mg per day if patient is also taking doxylamine)

Stop other medications and substitute:

Metoclopramide (Reglan®) 5 – 10 mg q8h PO
or
Trimethobenzamide (Tigan®) 200 mg q6h – 8h PR
or
Prochlorperzine 25 mg q12h PR

↓

Not tolerating PO

IV fluid replacement and multivitamin and thiamine supplementation[2]

Substitute any of the following (presented here in alphabetical order):
Dimenhydrinate (Dramamine® Injection) 50 mg
(in 50 mL saline, over 20 min) q4–6h IV
or
Metoclopramide (Reglan®) 5–10 mg q8h IV
or
Promethazine (Phenergan®) 12.5–25 mg q4h IV
or
Prochlorperazine 5–10 mg q4h IV (max dose 40 mg/day)

↓

Persistent Vomiting: Substitute:

Ondansetron[3] (Zofran®) 4–8 mg q8h PO/IV.
or
Methylprednisolone[4] (Medrol®) 16 mg q8h PO/IV for 3 days.
Taper over 2 weeks to lowest effective dose.
If beneficial, limit total duration of use to 6 weeks.

---

[1]In the US, doxylamine is available as the active ingredient in Unisom® Sleep Tabs™; one half of a scored 25-mg tablet can be used to provide a 12.5-mg dose of doxylamine.

[2]100 mg thiamine IV daily for 2–3 days (followed by IV multivitamins) is recommended for every woman who requires IV hydration and has vomited for more than 3 weeks.

[3]Less effect on nausea.

[4]Steroids appear to increase risk for oral clefts in first 10 weeks of gestation.

** The use of this algorithm assumes that other causes of nausea and vomiting have been ruled out.

†At any step, consider parenteral nutrition, if dehydration or persistent weight loss is noted.

Figure 36.1 Nausea and vomiting of pregnancy: treatment algorithm.

self-reported HG from 2000 to 2004, 16.7% reported parenteral nutrition, but only 2.3% reported enteral tube feeding.

While there is no doubt that these techniques are less expensive and subject to far fewer complications than parenteral nutrition, the experience is limited to case reports and small series. It is our experience that the nasal tubes are frequently declined by patients; once accepted, they may be difficult to place and are more subject to being vomited up than tubes placed for other reasons. This may be because few disorders requiring enteral nutrition are primarily disorders of vomiting *per se*. A recurring theme in reports of usage of enteral feeding is the presence of a skilled team for replacement and support that is capable of encouraging patients and anticipating their needs.

A schema for an overall approach to prevention and treatment of HG is shown in Figure 36.1.

Suggested reading

Borrelli F, Capasso R, Aviello G, *et al*. Effectiveness and safety of ginger in the treatment of pregnancy-induced nausea and vomiting. *Obstet Gynecol* 2005; 105: 849–856.

Brunetti-Pierri N, Hunter JV, Boerkoel CF. Gray matter heterotopias and brachytelephalangic chondrodysplasia punctata: a complication of hyperemesis gravidarum induced vitamin K deficiency? *Am J Med Genet A* 2007; 143: 200–204.

Buckwalter JG, Simpson SW. Psychological factor in the etiology and treatment of severe nausea and vomiting in pregnancy. *Am J Obstet Gynecol* 2002; 186: S210–214.

Dodds L, Fell DB, Joseph KS, Allen V, Butler B. Outcome of pregnancies complicated by hyperemesis gravidarum. *Obstet Gynecol* 2006; 107: 285–292.

Einarson A, Maltepe C, Navioz Y, *et al*. The safety of ondansetron for nausea and vomiting of pregnancy: a prospective comparative study. *BJOG* 2004; 111: 940–943.

Flaxman SM, Sherman PW. Morning sickness: a mechanism for protecting mother and embryo. *Quart Rev Biol* 2000; 75: 113–148.

Goodwin TM, Hershman JM. Hyperthyroidism due to inappropriate production of human chorionic gonadotropin. *Clin Obstet Gynecol* 1997; 40: 32–44.

Goodwin TM, Montoro M, Mestman JH. Transient hyperthyroidism and hyperemesis gravidarum: clinical aspects. *Am J Obstet Gynecol* 1992; 167: 648–652.

Goodwin TM, Poursharif B, Korst LM, MacGibbon KW, Romero R, Fez MS. Secular trends in the treatment of hyperemesis gravidarum. *Am J Perinatol* 2008; 25(3): 141–147.

Holmgren C, Silver RM, Porter TF, *et al*. Hyperemesis in pregnancy: an evaluation of treatment strategies with maternal and neonatal outcomes. *Am J Obstet Gynecol* 2008; 198: 56e1–4.

Hummela T, von Meringb T, Huchb R, *et al*. Olfactory modulation of nausea during early pregnancy? *BJOG* 2002; 109: 1394–1397.

Kallen B, Lundberg G, Aberg A. Relationship between vitamin use, smoking, and nausea and vomiting of pregnancy. *Acta Obstet Gynecol Scand* 2003; 82: 916–920.

Munch S. Women's experiences with a pregnancy complication: causal explanations of hyperemesis gravidarum. *Soc Work Health Care* 2002; 36: 59–76.

Poursharif B, Korst L, MacGibbon K, Fejzo MS, Romero R, Goodwin TM. Voluntary termination in a large cohort of women with hyperemesis gravidarum. *Contraception* 2007; 76: 451–455.

Safari HR, Alsulyman OM, Gherman RB, *et al*. The efficacy of methylprednisolone in the treatment of hyperemesis gravidarum: a randomized, double-blind, controlled study. *Am J Obstet Gynecol* 1998; 179: 921–924.

Seto A, Einarson T, Koren G. Pregnancy outcome following first trimester exposure to antihistamines: meta-analysis. *Am J Perinatol* 1997; 14: 119–124.

Trogstad L, Stoltenberg C, Magnus P, Skjærven R, Irgens L. Recurrence risk in hyperemesis gravidarum. *BJOG* 2005; 112: 1641–1645.

Yoshimura M, Hershman JM. Thyrotropic action of human chorionic gonadotropin. *Thyroid* 1995; 5: 425–434.

Chapter 37
The Acute Abdomen During Pregnancy: Ovarian Torsion, Appendicitis

Marc H. Incerpi
Department of Medicine and Obstetrics and Gynecology, Keck School of Medicine, University of Southern California, CA, USA

Introduction

Some form of abdominal pain is expected in the majority of pregnant patients. The etiologies vary from benign conditions such as gastroesophageal reflux and constipation to potentially serious conditions including adnexal torsion and appendicitis.

The diagnosis of abdominal pain in pregnancy is confounded by many factors. Symptoms such as nausea and vomiting are essentially ubiquitous in pregnancy, but are cardinal manifestations of many conditions associated with the acute abdomen. Moreover, arriving at a diagnosis on the basis of physical examination is difficult due to the anatomic changes associated with pregnancy. The enlarged uterus can often obscure palpation of the adnexa on pelvic examination. The appendix is displaced from the right lower quadrant to the upper right upper quadrant as pregnancy advances. Finally, clinical laboratory tests that are often used to diagnose causes of abdominal pain are altered in pregnancy. It is not uncommon for a normal pregnant patient to have a white blood cell count of 15,000 per m³.

The practitioner must have an understanding of the normal changes that occur in pregnancy when managing the gravida with abdominal pain. Indeed, determining when surgical intervention is indicated in the pregnant female with abdominal pain can be quite challenging. Ideally, every attempt should be made to avoid nonobstetric surgery during pregnancy, because of the potential risks to the patient and the developing fetus. However, clear situations do exist when nonobstetric surgery is required during pregnancy.

Adnexal masses and ovarian torsion

With the routine use of ultrasound incorporated into obstetric care, the frequency at which adnexal masses are diagnosed during pregnancy ranges from 0.5% to 2.2%. Most adnexal masses are asymptomatic, but the potential for ovarian torsion exists whenever an adnexal mass is detected. Adnexal masses are best assessed via pelvic examination and ultrasound in the first trimester. After the first trimester, identification of the adnexa by either clinical examination or ultrasound examination becomes more difficult as the uterus increases in size. When an adnexal mass is noted during pregnancy, specific information with regard to size, location, presence or absence of pain with palpation, mobility, and ultrasound characteristics such as echogenicity, septations, and nodules should be recorded. Approximately 1% of adnexal masses diagnosed during pregnancy prove to be malignant. Ultrasound characteristics that are used to distinguish benign adnexal masses from malignant masses are: size < 5 cm, unilocular appearance, anechoic appearance, and absence of septa or nodules. The differential diagnosis of pelvic masses during pregnancy is quite extensive, including but not limited to the following: leiomyoma, primary ovarian neoplasm, metastatic ovarian neoplasm, hydrosalpinx, ectopic pregnancy, and infection or abscess.

The management of the adnexal mass during pregnancy is conservative if the mass is small (< 5 cm diameter), and has a benign appearance on ultrasound. If the mass is between 5 and 10 cm and appears benign on ultrasound, serial ultrasound every 2–3 weeks is reasonable. If the mass persists or appears malignant, surgical removal is the treatment of choice. If an adnexal mass is greater than 10 cm regardless of ultrasound appearance, surgery is recommended. Because of the increased risk of spontaneous abortion in the first trimester and the increased risk of preterm labor reported in abdominal surgery after 20 weeks, the optimal time for surgery is between 14 and 20 weeks of gestation. It is important that the patient be counseled regarding the following potential complications

Management of Common Problems in Obstetrics and Gynecology, 5th edition. Edited by T.M. Goodwin, M.N. Montoro, L. Muderspach, R. Paulson and S. Roy. © 2010 Blackwell Publishing Ltd.

that may occur during expectant management of adnexal masses during pregnancy: torsion, rupture, hemorrhage, and delayed diagnosis of a malignancy.

Adnexal torsion has been reported to occur in between 7% and 28% of all pregnancies complicated by adnexal masses. When the pregnant patient presents with an adnexal mass and an acute abdomen regardless of gestational age, surgery is indicated. Ovarian torsion should be diagnosed and treated promptly to avoid the development of ovarian necrosis and peritonitis. Torsion most commonly presents with lower abdominal pain that is usually sudden in onset and colicky in nature. The pain may radiate to the flank, back or groin. Nausea and vomiting are commonly associated with the pain, but are nonspecific findings. Only rarely will patients have evidence of abdominal guarding or rebound tenderness at the time of physical examination.

When adnexal torsion is suspected an abdominal/ pelvic ultrasound is indicated to evaluate for the presence of an adnexal mass. It is rare for a mass less than 5 cm in diameter to undergo torsion. Usually ultrasound will identify a mass larger than 5 cm unless this occurs in the late second or early third trimester when the size of the uterus can obstruct visualization of the adnexae. The addition of Doppler flow studies may help to differentiate a benign ovarian cyst from one that is undergoing torsion. However, if there is a strong clinical suspicion for adnexal torsion, surgery is warranted. In the first trimester, laparoscopy can be used as a diagnostic and therapeutic procedure. In the second or third trimester, laparotomy is the surgical procedure of choice. At the time of surgery, a cystectomy can usually be performed safely. However, if the ovary appears necrotic, an oophorectomy is required.

Appendicitis

Appendicitis occurs in approximately 1/1500 births. It is the most common nonobstetric emergency requiring surgery in pregnancy. While maternal mortality ranges from 0.1% to 4%, the fetal death rate can be as high as 35% when perforation occurs. Preterm labor and delivery can occur in 50% of patients when the diagnosis of appendicitis is made in the third trimester. It is therefore imperative that the diagnosis be made promptly and that surgery be performed without delay so as to avoid these serious complications. Close co-operation between the surgeon and obstetrician is essential in order to minimize fetal and/or maternal morbidity and/or mortality.

Pregnancy does not affect the overall incidence of appendicitis, and the pathophysiology is essentially the same as in the nonpregnant individual. Appendicitis occurs as a result of luminal obstruction, usually resulting from hyperplasia of submucosal lymphoid follicles in response to infection. Sometimes a fecalith, foreign body or parasite will cause obstruction. Continued secretion along with increased bacterial growth in the static lumen causes intraluminal pressure to increase significantly, thereby leading to obstruction of lymphatic drainage and venous outflow. Edema and vascular congestion in the wall of the appendix result. If this process is allowed to continue, arterial insufficiency results, leading to gangrene. Once gangrene has set in, luminal bacteria invade the wall of the appendix where they can potentially migrate to the serosal surface and spread intraperitoneally. Perforation is then likely to follow when appendiceal wall infarction and necrosis develop. Once perforation occurs, the degree to which the omentum and other surrounding structures are able to wall off the infection determines whether or not diffuse peritonitis develops.

The anatomic changes that result in pregnancy are significant. In the nonpregnant or early pregnant state, the appendix is usually located in the right lower quadrant of the abdomen at the inferior tip of the cecum. However, as pregnancy progresses, the appendix is displaced superiorly and laterally by the enlarging uterus. Therefore, abdominal exam is often not as reliable later in pregnancy. It is also believed that the changing position of the appendix limits the ability of the omentum to wall off the inflammation, thus allowing for the bacterial infection to become disseminated and more readily resulting in generalized peritonitis.

The diagnosis of appendicitis in pregnancy is difficult due to the often atypical presentation. Right lower quadrant abdominal pain is the most reliable symptom of appendicitis occurring in pregnancy. The pain, however, is less characteristic than in the nonpregnant state, may be milder, and may be located in the right upper quadrant or right flank. Other common manifestations such as anorexia, nausea, and vomiting are so common during normal pregnancy that they are often discounted. The elevated white blood cell count associated with appendicitis in the pregnant woman may be confounded by the physiologic leukocytosis of pregnancy. In addition, up to 30% of gravidae will have urinary symptoms or an abnormal urinalysis, thus leading to a false diagnosis of urinary tract infection or pyelonephritis. Other differential diagnoses that must be entertained include labor, adnexal torsion, ectopic pregnancy, nephrolithiasis, cholecystitis, pancreatitis, and degenerating uterine myoma.

On physical examination, tenderness may be periumbilical or localized, depending on the stage of infection and uterine size as a result of gestational age. Peritoneal signs including guarding and rebound tenderness are often present, although less often than in the nonpregnant state. Rebound tenderness is present in approximately 55–75% of patients. This finding is not as sensitive in the nonpregnant state, because of the distension of the abdominal wall muscles and the interposition of the gravid uterus between the appendix and the anterior abdominal wall. Fever is not a reliable indicator of appendicitis in pregnancy. Temperature may be normal or only slightly elevated. In short, rarely is the presentation of appendicitis during pregnancy "classic."

If after history, physical examination, and laboratory evaluation the diagnosis of appendicitis remains in doubt, diagnostic imaging is then commonly employed. Graded compression ultrasound is the diagnostic imaging procedure of choice, with high sensitivity and specificity in diagnosing acute appendicitis. It is cost-effective and avoids fetal exposure to radiation. The classic finding is that of an enlarged, tubular, noncompressible structure. In cases in which the appendix is not adequately visualized and no other source for the abdominal pain is found, then other imaging techniques can be used. MRI has been proven to be an excellent modality for use in excluding acute appendicitis in pregnant women who present with acute abdominal pain and whom a normal appendix is not visualized on ultrasound. MRI is felt to be safe for use in pregnancy. In fact, because of the theoretical concerns relating to fetal exposure to ionizing radiation, MRI is preferred over CT scan. CT can be reserved for complicated cases or for locations where MRI is not readily available, or when experience is limited. It should be emphasized that in those situations where a diagnosis of appendicitis is suspected, and sonography is inconclusive or nondiagnostic, and MRI is not available, then CT is a better choice than subjecting the patient to a delayed diagnosis and the risk of appendiceal perforation. While several diagnostic imaging techniques are available, ultrasound should be performed in all pregnant patients presenting with abdominal pain in order to demonstrate fetal viability, gestational age, and possibly rule out other etiologies such as ovarian torsion or a degenerating uterine myoma.

Because of multiple studies demonstrating that the risk of fetal death increases dramatically from 1.5% when the appendix is not perforated to as high as 20–35% when the appendix is perforated, the clinician must have a high index of suspicion when a pregnant patient presents with abdominal pain. In fact, when delay in surgery occurred for greater than 24 hours after presentation, there was a 66% incidence of appendiceal perforation, while there was no case of perforation in patients taken to surgery within 24 hours. Since the diagnosis of appendicitis is more difficult to make during pregnancy, and since delay in diagnosis

can have severe fetal consequences, a higher negative laparotomy rate is acceptable compared to the patient who is not pregnant.

Once the diagnosis of appendicitis has been established, the patient should be prepared for surgery as soon as possible. Careful attention to fluid and electrolyte balance is important because many of these patients are dehydrated, which may lead to uterine contractions and preterm labor. Perioperative antibiotics are frequently given to decrease infectious complications. While a variety of both aerobic and anaerobic micro-organisms have been associated with appendicitis, the most common are *E coli* and *Bacteroides fragilis*. Therefore, patients with acute appendicitis should receive preoperative antibiotics with a cephalosporin and anaerobic coverage. A commonly employed regimen in pregnancy consists of cefuroxime and metronidazole or clindamycin. These have been proven to be safe during pregnancy. Antibiotics should be continued postoperatively until the patient has been afebrile for at least 48 hours. The surgical approach is usually via laparotomy; however, laparoscopy has been used. A variety of incisions can be performed, including McBurney's, Rocky-Davis, subcostal, transverse, and midline. Factors used in determining the most appropriate incision include uterine size, gestational age, type and location of abdominal pain, presence or absence of peritonitis, and surgeon's preference. Uterine manipulation should be minimized at the time of laparotomy. There is no consensus regarding prophylactic tocolysis. Finally, cesarean delivery at the time of appendectomy should be reserved for usual obstetric indications only.

While there are theoretical concerns regarding laparoscopy during pregnancy, pregnancy is not considered to be a contraindication for laparoscopic appendectomy. In fact, multiple published reports have demonstrated laparoscopy to be safe, especially in the first and second trimesters when the uterus is still small. As the pregnancy advances and the uterus increases in size, laparoscopic appendectomy becomes more technically difficult. Most surgeons appear to favor laparotomy in the late second and early third trimesters.

Suggested reading

Augustin G, Majerovic M. Non-obstetrical acute abdomen during pregnancy. *Eur J Obstet Gynecol Rep Biol* 2007; 131: 4–12.

Barloon TJ, Brown BP, Abu-Yousef MM, *et al.* Sonography of acute appendicitis in pregnancy. *Abdom Imaging* 1995; 20: 149–151.

Bider D, Mashiach S, Dulitzky M, *et al.* Clinical, surgical, and pathologic findings of adnexal torsion in pregnant and non-pregnant women. *Surg Gynecol Obstet* 1991; 173: 363–366.

Epstein FB. Acute abdominal pain in pregnancy. *Emerg Med Clin North Am* 1994; 12: 51–65.

Hogston P, Lilford RJ. Ultrasound study of ovarian cysts in pregnancy: prevalence and significance. *BJOG* 1986; 93: 625–628.

Horowitz MD, Gomez GA, Santiesteban R, *et al.* Acute apendicitis during pregnancy. *Arch Surg* 1985; 120: 1362–1367.

Meire HB, Furrant P, Guha T. Distinction of benign from malignant ovarian cysts by ultrasound. *BJOG* 1978; 85: 893–899.

Parangi S, Levine D, Henry A, *et al.* Surgical gastrointestinal disorders during pregnancy. *Am J Surg* 2007; 193: 223–232.

Pastore PA, Loomis DM, Sauret J. Appendicitis in pregnancy. *J Am Board Fam Med* 2006; 19: 621–626.

Pedrosa I, Levine D, Eyvazzadeh AD, *et al.* MR imaging of acute appendicitis in pregnancy. *Radiology* 2006; 238: 891–899.

Reedy MB, Galan HL, Richards WE, *et al.* Laparoscsopy during pregnancy: a survey of laparoscopic surgeons. *J Reprod Med* 1997; 42: 33–38.

Roberts JA. Management of gynecologic tumors during pregnancy. *Clin Perinat* 1983; 10: 369–382.

Tamir IL, Bongard FS, Klein SR. Acute appendicitis in the pregnant patient. *Am J Surg* 1990; 160: 571–576.

Thornton JG, Wells M. Ovarian cysts in pregnancy: does ultrasound make traditional management inappropriate? *Obstet Gynecol* 1987; 69: 717–721.

Witlin AG, Sibai BM. When a pregnant patient develops appendicitis. *Contemp Obstet Gynecol* 1996; 41: 15–30.

Chapter 38
Mood and Anxiety Disorders

Bruce Kovacs and Emily Dossett
Department of Medicine and Obstetrics and Gynecology, Keck School of Medicine, University of Southern California, CA, USA

Mood disorders

Mood disorders are one of the most prevalent types of psychiatric disorders. Clinically mood disorders are classified and defined in *Diagnostic and statistical manual* (DSM) of the American Psychiatric Association [1] and include major depressive disorder, dysthymic disorder, and bipolar disorder.

Clinical depression (also called major depressive disorder or unipolar depression) is relatively common and is characterized by a persistent lowering of mood, loss of interest in usual activities and diminished ability to experience pleasure. While the term "depression" is commonly used to describe a temporary decreased mood when one feels "blue" or "down," clinical depression is a serious illness that involves the body, mood, and thoughts that cannot simply be willed or wished away. It is often a disabling disease that affects a person's work, family and school life, sleeping and eating habits, general health and ability to enjoy life. The course of clinical depression varies widely: depression can be a once in a lifetime event or have multiple recurrences, it can appear either gradually or suddenly, and either last for few months or be a life-long disorder. Having clinical depression is a major risk factor for suicide.

Dysthymic disorder is a milder form of chronic depression. The essential symptom involves the individual feeling depressed almost daily for at least 2 years, but without the more severe symptoms present in a major depressive episode. Low energy, disturbances in sleep or in appetite and low self-esteem typically contribute to the clinical picture as well. Individuals have often experienced dysthymia for many years before it is formally diagnosed. People around them come to believe that the sufferer is "just a moody person," thus delaying or foregoing medical attention altogether.

Bipolar disorder (BPD) is not a single disorder but a category of mood disorders defined by the presence of one or more episodes of abnormally elevated mood, clinically referred to as mania. This condition was formally known as manic-depressive illness, but BPD is now preferred. Having a manic episode is more severe and long-lasting than being "moody" or even having "mood swings." A true mania lasts (include duration and symptoms) at least 1 week. Individuals who experience manic episodes also commonly experience depressive episodes or symptoms, or mixed episodes that present with features of both mania and depression. These episodes are normally separated by periods of normal mood, but in some patients, depression and mania may rapidly alternate, known as rapid cycling. The disorder has been subdivided into bipolar I, bipolar II and cyclothymia based on the type and severity of mood episodes experienced.

Clinical depression is more common in women

In any given year, 10–14 million people experience clinical depression; women 18–45 years of age account for the largest proportion of this group. Clinical depression can develop in anyone, regardless of race, culture, social class, age or gender. However, across virtually all cultures and socio-economic classes, women are more likely than men to experience depression. Underlying this diathesis may be biologic factors, especially hormonal influences, though these have yet to be elucidated. In contrast, bipolar disorder occurs equally in males and females. For many years, pregnancy was believed to be protective against relapse of bipolar episodes. However, recent studies have suggested that relapse rates during pregnancy are significant if the woman chooses to discontinue medication.

Moreover, not surprisingly, sexual and physical abuse are major risk factors for depression. Women are twice as likely as men to have experienced sexual abuse. A recent study found that three out of five women diagnosed with depressive illnesses had been victims of abuse. Clinicians should bear in mind a history of potential abuse when encountering patients with major depression.

Management of Common Problems in Obstetrics and Gynecology, 5th edition. Edited by T.M. Goodwin, M.N. Montoro, L. Muderspach, R. Paulson and S. Roy. © 2010 Blackwell Publishing Ltd.

Pregnancy increases the risk for mood disorders

Recent research reveals that over 10% of pregnant women and approximately 15% of postpartum women experience depression. As many as 80% of women experience the "postpartum blues," a brief period of mood symptoms that is considered normal following childbirth and typically resolves in 2–3 weeks.

However, major clinical depression may be precipitated by the related hormonal and biologic changes associated with pregnancy or the postpartum period and should not be dismissed as "the blues." Postpartum depression includes all the major signs and symptoms of major depressive disorder, and is frequently accompanied by profound anxiety. If there has been a history of mood disorder, there is a threefold increase in risk for depression during or following a pregnancy. Once a woman has experienced an episode of postpartum depression, her risk of having another episode is about 70%. In addition, the first episode of bipolar disorder in women frequently occurs following the birth of a child. Thus pregnancy represents a particularly vulnerable time for the occurrence of mood disorders.

Although technically not a mood disorder, postpartum psychosis is a medical emergency in which the woman may inflict harm upon herself and/or her baby secondary to paranoid delusions. The true risk of postpartum psychosis lies in infanticide, which occurs in roughly 4% of cases. The prevalence of postpartum psychosis itself is about one in 1000 pregnancies. It presents as a manic episode, with excessive agitation, irritability, and decreased need for sleep, as well as psychotic features of paranoia, hearing voices, and delusions.

Anxiety disorders

Anxiety disorders are the most prevalent of the psychiatric disorders. Just as a transient depressed mood is a normal reaction to life events, anxiety is a normal reaction to stress. It helps one deal with a tense situation, focus on a particular task or heighten attention and awareness. In general, it is an adaptive response that helps an individual to deal with particular situations. But when anxiety becomes an excessive, irrational dread of everyday situations, it is a seriously disabling disorder.

Excessive anxiety is an unpleasant emotional state. Anxiety is characterized by worry, doubt and painful awareness that one is powerless to control situations. In contrast to fear, anxiety is irrational. The anxious person is hypervigilant, tense and insecure in most situations. Their heightened negative state leads to some of the bodily complaints that can be particularly prominent. These include excess sweating, trembling, dizziness, heart palpitations, shortness of breath, gastrointestinal upset, hot flashes, dry

mouth, increased urination, fatigue and restlessness. The anxiety episodes can become so intense that individuals believe they are actually "going crazy" or will die.

Anxiety disorders as a class include generalized anxiety disorder (GAD), panic disorder, phobias, post-traumatic stress disorder, social anxiety disorder and obsessive compulsive disorder (OCD). Each of these disorders presents differently, but they all share common symptoms of excessive worry and distressing physiologic sensations.

Panic disorder and OCD appear to be affected by pregnancy. The symptoms of panic disorder appear to worsen in pregnancy and during the postpartum period. It is also suspected that pregnancy and the postpartum period seem to be a particularly vulnerable time for patients with OCD with either new onset or worsening of symptoms. OCD is particularly frightening because the main symptom is intrusive, recurring thoughts of harming the child. These thoughts are "ego-dystonic" or upsetting to the mother, which distinguishes them from the delusions of postpartum psychosis.

Co-morbidity of anxiety and depression is common

Depression and anxiety often occur together. In the National Co-morbidity Survey (2005), 58% of patients diagnosed with major depression were found to have an anxiety disorder; among these patients, the rate of co-morbidity with GAD was 17.2%, and with panic disorder, 9.9%. Patients with a diagnosed anxiety disorder also had high rates of co-morbid depression, including 22.4% of patients with social phobia, 9.4% with agoraphobia, and 2.3% with panic disorder. Patients can also be categorized as having mixed anxiety-depressive disorder, and they are at significantly increased risk of developing full-blown depression or anxiety. Appropriate treatment is necessary to alleviate symptoms and prevent the emergence of more serious disease.

Accumulating evidence indicates that patients with co-morbid depression and anxiety tend to have greater illness severity and a lower treatment response than those with either disorder alone. In addition, social function and quality of life are more greatly impaired. In addition to anxiety and depression being co-morbid, research shows that they often also occur with substance abuse or other conditions associated with stress, such as irritable bowel syndrome.

Diagnosis of mood and anxiety disorders

The diagnosis of mood and anxiety disorders is primarily based on the symptoms described by the patient. There are a number of diagnostic instruments based on structured questions and the responses elicited from the patient which are helpful in establishing the diagnosis. Among the tests which are most well validated and easy to use during pregnancy and the postpartum period are the Edinburgh Postnatal Depression Scale and Postpartum Depression Screening Scale, which both have high sensitivity and specificity. The Patient Health Questionnaire 9, or PHQ9, is also a well-validated test that is user friendly for a prenatal care environment. A positive screen must be followed with a more complete assessment in order to make a diagnosis – the screen alone does not suffice.

Principles of therapy

While medications have become increasingly important in the treatment of anxiety and/or mood disorders, they are best used in combination with ongoing counseling with a mental health professional. Further, there should be a co-ordinated approach to the patient's management involving a mental health professional and obstetrician-gynecologist. Ongoing psychotherapy has been shown to reduce or even obviate the need for medications in many cases, though not all.

Treatment of mood and anxiety disorders during pregnancy and the puerperal period is important but presents unique challenges. Ongoing medication therapy should not be discontinued due to the occurrence of pregnancy and institution of therapy during pregnancy should not be avoided. However, considerations of teratogenicity and potential fetal and infant exposure to psychotropic medications warrant caution in the selection of pharmacologic agent. Agents with clinically established reduced potential for reproductive toxicity should be preferred to medications without a significant history of use during pregnancy. In most cases, single-agent therapy is preferred over multiple medications, even though the dose of the agent may need to be increased. Drugs which are less likely to cross the placenta or be secreted into breast milk are preferred. However, once an agent is selected, it is important to remember that the effect of treatment on anxiety or depression may require weeks to become apparent.

Choice of medication

When it comes to therapeutic agents for depression or anxiety, there is a very large number to choose from, and what works well in one patient may not work well in another. Selection of the correct agent is often empiric and trial and error is not uncommon. Table 38.1 presents a summary of the agents more commonly used

Table 38.1 Agents useful in treating anxiety and depression

Drug name	Comments	Possible risks
Selective serotonin reuptake inhibitors		
Citalopram (Celexa)	Newer SSRI. Limited data in pregnancy. Potential increased excretion in breast milk	Possible withdrawal syndrome when used in third trimester; very slight increase in absolute risk for PPHN
Escitalopam (Lexapro)	An isomer of Citalopram. Limited experience in pregnancy	Possible withdrawal syndrome when used in third trimester; very slight increase in absolute risk for PPHN
Fluoxetine (Prozac)	Good efficacy data in pregnancy. Long half-life less optimal in breastfeeding	Possible withdrawal syndrome when used in third trimester; very slight increase in absolute risk for PPHN
Fluvoxamine (Lovox)	Negligible data in pregnancy and breastfeeding. Many drug interactions. Not first-line choice	Possible withdrawal syndrome when used in third trimester; very slight increase in absolute risk for PPHN
Paroxetine (Paxil)	Avoid use in first trimester unless it is the only medication that worked in past. Highest incidence of NAS at delivery	Possible withdrawal syndrome when used in third trimester; very slight increase in absolute risk for PPHN
Sertraline (Zoloft)	Best for breastfeeding (levels are nondetectable). Relatively safe medication to begin in pregnancy and into postpartum period	Possible withdrawal syndrome when used in third trimester; very slight increase in absolute risk for PPHN
Dual reuptake inhibitors		
Bupropion (Wellbutrin)	Possible slight miscarriage risk; avoid in women with seizure disorder	No data showing risk in pregnancy
Duloxetine (Cymbalta)	Negligible data in pregnancy and breastfeeding	No data showing risk in pregnancy
Venlafaxine (Effexor)	Avoid in women with risk of hypertension	No data showing risk in pregnancy
Mirtazapine (Remeron)	Data for efficacy in pregnancy very limited. Probably not first-line choice	No data showing risk in pregnancy
Tricyclic antidepressants		
Amitriptyline	Second line because of toxicity risk and side effect burden	No data showing risk in pregnancy
Nortriptyline	Second line because of toxicity risk and side effect burden	No data showing risk in pregnancy

in treating anxiety and depression, along with the risk categories based on FDA classification. With respect to safety during breastfeeding, all drugs listed are considered probably safe. In general, among the SSRIs, sertraline (Zoloft), paroxetine (Paxil), and notrytiline are the least detectable in the serum of exposed infants and therefore considered the safest. Detailed information on each can be found online at the LactMed resource in the National Library of Medicine (http://toxnet.nlm.nih.gov/cgi-bin/sis/htmlgen?LACT).

Older agents traditionally used to treat anxiety and depression include benzodiazepines and tricyclic or heterocyclic drugs. Benzodiazapines are effective in treating anxiety but have an associated abuse potential as well as an established adverse effect on the newborn when they are used continuously in the third trimester or immediately prior to delivery. No clear data exist on the longer term effects in early childhood. However, they can be used safely in pregnancy when their beneficial effect on the patient is evident. Tricyclic and heterocyclic agents have a long history of use in pregnancy and are generally effective and safe. Only occasional case reports of fetal abnormalities occurring in patients using these (and other) medications have occurred during the decades of their use.

In the past several years a number of newer antidepressant drugs have been approved for use. These include SSRIs as well as others which work through different pharmacologic mechanisms, such as venlafaxine (Effexor) or bupropion (Wellbutrin). Recently, some concern was raised about the safety of SSRIs and the possibility of birth defects. The most current data suggest that if such a risk exists, either an overall increase of birth defects in general or for specific defects, including cardiovascular malformation, it must be very small. Thus far the only SRRI which is listed as category D is paroxetine because of data suggesting an increased rate of congenital cardiac malformations in infants exposed in the first trimester, though this is currently disputed.

An additional concern with SSRI use is the neonatal abstinence syndrome (NAS), a constellation of symptoms including irritability, respiratory distress, jitteriness, and (very rarely) seizures, that occurs in 10–30% of infants whose mothers were taking SSRIs at the time of delivery. There have been no reported deaths from NAS. It resolves within 48–72 hours (depending on the drug) and it can be managed symptomatically. A more theoretical concern is a suggestion from a retrospective, case–control study linking the use of SSRI's after the completion of the 20th week of gestation with persistent pulmonary hypertension in the newborn (PPHN). The most recent data suggest an increased risk (adjusted odds ratio, 6.1; 95% CI 2.2–16.8); the absolute risk remains tiny (from 0.1% to 0.6%). In contrast, neither the use of SSRIs before the 20th week of gestation nor the use of non-SSRI antidepressant drugs at any time during pregnancy was associated with an increased risk of PPHN. Finally, all SSRIs carry an FDA-mandated warning with regard to increased risk for suicidal thinking and behavior (suicidality) in children, adolescents, and adults less than 24 years of age and should therefore be monitored closely, particularly after treatment initiation. Thus, given the large number of alternatives to SSRIs available, their use in pregnancy should be considered only if other choices are found to be ineffective in a given patient.

Conclusion

There are many choices for the treatment of depression and anxiety. This is because what works in one patient may not work in another. Individual variation in drug response is the rule, not the exception, and the most effective medication with the lowest risk profile should be chosen on a case-by-case basis. It is also important to fully explain the risks and benefits of these medications, including the lack of clear information on use in pregnancy. Overall, the risk of birth defects and other problems for babies of mothers who take antidepressants during pregnancy is very low, thus when there is a need for medication it should not be withheld or discontinued since the risks of no medication may be greater than the risks of use.

Reference

American Psychiatric Association. *Diagnostic and statistical manual of mental disorders: DSM-IV-TR*, 4th edn. Washington, DC: American Psychiatric Association, 2000.

Suggested reading

American Academy of Pediatrics. Edinburgh Postnatal Depression Scale. www.aap.org/practicingsafety/Toolkit_Resources/Module2/EPDS.pdf.

American College of Obstetricians and Gynecologists. *Clinical management guidelines for obstetricians-gynecologist: use of psychiatric medications during pregnancy and lactation*. Washington, DC: American College of Obstetricians and Gynecologists, 2007.

MacArthur Foundation Initiative on Depression and Primary Care. *Patient Health Questionnaire-9*. www.depression-primarycare.org/clinicians/toolkits/materials/forms/phq9/.

Chapter 39
The Older Gravida

Bhuvan Pathak

Department of Medicine and Obstetrics and Gynecology, Keck School of Medicine, University of Southern California, CA, USA

Introduction

Advanced maternal age (AMA) is a term commonly used to describe women who will be 35 years or older at their estimated date of confinement. This distinction has been made given the observation of increased adverse reproductive outcomes in this age group. It should be noted, however, that the adverse changes associated with advancing age occur gradually and are not necessarily an "all or none" effect. Over the last several decades there has been an increase in AMA, given a trend towards delayed child bearing among women living in industrialized nations. This delay has been attributed to multiple factors including, most notably, a greater emphasis on professional development among women. Increasing levels of education, delayed marriage, increasing second marriages, and improved contraceptive options also play a role in delayed child bearing.

The mean maternal age at the birth of a first child in women living in the United States increased from 21.4 years old to 24.9 years old from the 1970s to the 2000s. Similar increases in industrialized European and Asian countries have been reported. Furthermore, the proportion of women giving birth between the ages of 40 and 44 years has also increased from 3.8 to 7.4 per 1000 livebirths between 1981 and 1999. The proportion of women 45 years and older giving birth has increased from 0.2 to 0.4 per 1000 livebirths over the same time period. Much of this increase in maternal age has also been facilitated by assisted reproductive technologies. Finally, not only is the mean maternal age at first birth increasing, but also the overall number of children per family is decreasing.

Although the reproductive outcomes in women of AMA are generally acceptable, difficulties with conception as well as antepartum and intrapartum complications are more common in this obstetric group.

Fertility and conception

With advancing maternal age, fecundity decreases and the time to conception increases. This change is most notable in women older than 35 years of age. This prolongation in conception time is due to poorer oocyte quality and a decrease in the overall number of oocytes (ovarian reserve). Ovulatory dysfunction is also more common with advancing maternal age and contributes to difficulties with conception. Although ovarian factors are most highly associated with decreased fecundity in the AMA group, these women are also more likely to have tubal disease due to either endometriosis or a history of pelvic infections, and are more likely to have fibroids or polyps, which may distort the uterine cavity.

Treatment options for infertility are beyond the scope of this review but include expectant management, ovulation induction, intrauterine insemination, oocyte donation, and assisted reproductive technologies such as *in vitro* fertilization. Of note, maternal age remains the most important prognostic factor in women undergoing *in vitro* fertilization. Pregnancies achieved with the aid of assisted reproductive technologies more often result in multiple gestations and have also been associated with a higher rate of adverse perinatal outcomes, which will be discussed in further detail below.

Given the decline in oocyte quality as well as a potentially suboptimal hormonal and/or physical intrauterine environment, it is not surprising that the risk of spontaneous abortion increases with advancing maternal age. This increased risk of miscarriage is also correlated with the increased proportion of aneuploidies found in the embryos of these women. A large European study examining the reproductive outcomes of over one million pregnancies confirmed this positive correlation between advancing maternal age and the rate of spontaneous abortion. The overall pregnancy loss rate was 13.5% but when stratified by age, women 20–24 years old had

Management of Common Problems in Obstetrics and Gynecology, 5th edition. Edited by T.M. Goodwin, M.N. Montoro, L. Muderspach, R. Paulson and S. Roy. © 2010 Blackwell Publishing Ltd.

a spontaneous abortion rate of 8.9% while women 45 years and older had a rate of 74.7%. Similarly, there was an increasing risk of ectopic pregnancy with advancing maternal age. The overall ectopic rate was 2.3%, with a risk of 1.4% in women aged 21 years at the time of conception versus a risk of 6.9% in women aged 44 years or more at the time of conception.

Risks of congenital anomalies

The risk of aneuploidy increases steadily with advancing maternal age and especially after the age of 35 years. Shuttleworth first described the association between advanced maternal age and trisomy 21, or Down's syndrome, in 1909. This increase is thought to be the result of more common nondisjunction during meiosis, thus leading to oocytes with an abnormal number of chromosomes.

Given this increase in aneuploidy with AMA, invasive genetic testing with amniocentesis has long been advocated in these women, as the risk–benefit balance appears favorable in this group. Specifically, a second-trimester risk of Down's syndrome of 1:270 or a liveborn risk of Down's syndrome of 1:380 has been used as the cut-off at which to offer invasive testing. These numbers correspond to a maternal age of 35 years or greater at the time of delivery. The factors that must be considered when offering invasive testing include the prevalence of the disease in the given age group versus the risks of invasive testing, which include but are not limited to iatrogenic rupture of membranes and miscarriage. Genetic amniocentesis has a diagnostic accuracy of greater than 99%.

There are now a number of noninvasive screening tests which help to refine a woman's risk of carrying a fetus with Down's syndrome or other chromosomal aneuploidies. These tests include several maternal serum biochemical markers, which may be drawn in the first and/or the second trimester of pregnancy, as well as nuchal translucency measurements of the fetus, which are performed in the first trimester. Using maternal age alone, the detection rate for aneuploidy is only 44%. With noninvasive screening tests, the maternal age-related risk of aneuploidy can be refined to give a more accurate adjusted risk. Detection rates as high as 96% with false-positive rates of 5% have been reported for integrated screening methods. A detailed discussion of the various genetic screening tests and their respective detection rates is beyond the scope of this chapter. However, given these much improved detection rates, some authorities no longer recommend maternal age alone as an indication for invasive prenatal genetic diagnosis. At this time the American College of Obstetricians and Gynecologists states that "… all women, regardless of age, should have the option of invasive testing."

In a study examining for birth defects in over 100,000 pregnancies, maternal age of 25 years and older was associated with an increased rate of congenital malformations in chromosomally normal fetuses. More specifically, the risk of cardiac defects was greater in women older than 40 years compared with women 20–24 years old. Clubfoot and diaphragmatic hernia increased with advancing maternal age as well. Interestingly, gastroschisis and polydactyly were both increased with younger women. Another study which also examined the association between maternal age and nonchromosomal birth defects showed correlations with both advanced and young maternal age. AMA was associated with heart defects, hypospadias, other male genital defects, and craniosynostosis. Young maternal age, defined as women aged 14–19 years, had an increased rate of malformations as well. These malformations included anencephaly, hydrocephaly, ear defects, cleft lip, female genital defects, hydronephrosis, polydactyly, omphalocele, and gastroschisis.

Antepartum concerns

Women of AMA have an increased risk of pregnancy-associated complications and adverse pregnancy outcomes. There are several reasons for this which include being of advanced age itself, a greater prevalence of maternal medical conditions, a greater risk of multiple gestation given the increased use of assisted reproductive technologies, and complications associated with increasing parity. It should be emphasized that AMA is an independent risk factor for adverse pregnancy outcomes and is not simply a confounder due to age-related changes.

Hypertension and gestational diabetes mellitus are the two most commonly encountered medical complications affecting pregnancy. Pre-eclampsia affects approximately 3–4% of the general obstetric population and this risk increases to 5–10% in women older than 40 years. Women with pregnancy-associated hypertension have a threefold greater odds of preterm birth, and a 3–4-fold greater odds of having a low-birthweight baby. Gestational diabetes mellitus, which is associated with fetal macrosomia, is found in 3% of the general obstetric population and increases to 7–12% in women older than 40 years. Aside from hypertension and gestational diabetes, older women also have an increased prevalence of diseases antedating pregnancy. Certain pre-existing conditions such as diabetes cause increased congenital abnormalities with an increase in perinatal morbidity and mortality.

Placenta previa is also more commonly seen in women of AMA. While placental abruption is also noted more often in women of AMA, there appears to be no true correlation when parity and hypertension are accounted for. The incidence of placental abruptions is < 1% in primigravidae and 2.5% in grand multiparae. This positive correlation between abruption and parity may reflect some sort of permanent damage to the endometrium after repeated pregnancies.

The number of uncomplicated deliveries is lower in older women when compared with younger women. For example, induction of labor, deliveries complicated by anal sphincter tears, and cesarean section rates are all higher in women of AMA. The odds ratio for maternal mortality has been reported to be as high as 16.2 for women aged 40–44 years when compared to women aged 20–29 years. For women aged 45 years and older, the odds ratio for maternal mortality was 121 when compared with women in the 20–29 age group. It should be noted that absolute risks remain low.

As mentioned above, women of AMA have significantly higher rates of assisted conception. These pregnancies are at increased risk for maternal complications such as pre-eclampsia, gestational diabetes mellitus, placenta previa, placental abruption, and cesarean section. It is not possible to differentiate the risk associated with the assisted reproductive technology itself from the risk due to the underlying cause of infertility. Furthermore, assisted reproductive technologies more often lead to twins and higher-order multiples, which are also associated with higher rates of maternal complications.

Perinatal and neonatal outcomes

Although women of AMA generally have good perinatal outcomes, their rates of very preterm birth (< 32 weeks) and extreme preterm birth (< 28 weeks) are higher. Accordingly, their risk of having neonates with low (< 2500 g), very low (< 1500 g) or extremely low (< 1000 g) birthweights is also increased. These findings are noted even after controlling for potentially confounding factors such as concomitant medical conditions or mode of conception.

Women of AMA are at an increased risk of unexplained intrauterine fetal demise throughout gestation, with the highest rates being between 37 and 41 weeks. This increased risk is noted even when fetuses with congenital anomalies are accounted for. Overall stillbirth rates for women of all ages and at all gestational ages are 4–5/1000. Between 37 and 41 weeks, the relative risk of stillbirth is 1.32 for women aged 35–39 years, compared with women younger than 35 years. The relative risk during the same gestational period is 1.88 for women 40 years and older compared with women younger than 35 years. In studies looking specifically at the obstetric outcomes of women over the age of 40 years, the odds ratio for intrauterine fetal demise was 2.1 in women aged 40–44 years, and 3.8 in women aged 45 years and older when compared with 20–29-year-old women. These odd ratios were calculated after adjusting for pre-existing maternal diseases, significant malformations, and smoking.

Neonatal deaths and therefore perinatal deaths are also increased in women of AMA. In the same studied mentioned just above, in women aged 40–44 years and in those aged 45 years and older, the odds ratio for perinatal mortality was 1.7 and 2.4 respectively when compared to women aged 20–29 years.

Finally, pregnancies conceived with the aid of assisted reproductive technologies have increased risks of perinatal complications including small for gestational age babies, preterm delivery, and perinatal mortality in both singleton and multiple gestations.

Conclusion

Women of AMA have generally good reproductive performances but they remain at elevated risk for certain adverse outcomes. Specifically, they may suffer from subfertility or infertility and therefore may require assisted reproductive technologies, which in and of themselves are associated with an increased risk of adverse pregnancy and perinatal outcomes. Once pregnant, women of AMA have a higher rate of early and/or recurrent pregnancy loss, as well as an increased rate of congenital abnormalities and aneuploidy in their offspring. Finally, gravid women of AMA have elevated risks of medical complications such as hypertension and gestational diabetes, as well as of perinatal complications such as operative deliveries, low-birthweight babies, preterm delivery, intrauterine fetal demise, and neonatal death.

Although the majority of women of AMA have uncomplicated pregnancies, this group should be counseled appropriately regarding their elevated risks of pregnancy-associated complications.

Suggested reading

American College of Obstetricians and Gynecologists. *Practice Bulletin No 77. Screening for fetal chromosomal abnormalities.* Washington, DC: American College of Obstetricians and Gynecologists, 2007.

Anderson AMN, Wohlfahrt J, Christens P, Olsen J, Melbye M. Maternal age and fetal loss: population based register linkage study. *BMJ* 2000; 320: 1708–1712.

Bateman BT, Simpson LL. Higher rate of stillbirth at the extremes of reproductive age: a large nationwide sample of deliveries in the United States. *Am J Obstet Gynecol* 2006; 194(3): 840–845.

Delbaere I, Verstraelen H, Goetgeluk S, Martens G, Backer GD, Temmerman M. Pregnancy outcome in primiparae of advanced maternal age. *Eur J Obstet Gynecol Rep Biol* 2007; 135: 41–46.

Hollier LM, Leveno KJ, Kelly MA, McIntire DD, Cunningham FG. Maternal age and malformations in singletons births. *Obstet Gynecol* 2000; 96(5): 701–706.

Jacobsson B, Ladfors L, Milsom I. Advanced maternal age and adverse perinatal outcome. *Am J Obstet Gynecol* 2004; 104(4): 727–733.

Malone FD, Canick JA, Ball RH, *et al.* First-trimester or second-trimester screening, or both, for Down's syndrome. *NEJM* 2005; 353(19): 2001–2011.

Reddy UM, Ko CW, Willinger M. Maternal age and the risk of stillbirth throughout pregnancy in the United States. *Am J Obstet Gynecol* 2006; 195(3): 764–770.

Reddy UM, Wapner RJ, Rebar RW, Tasca RJ. Infertility, assisted reproductive technology, and adverse pregnancy outcomes: executive summary of a National Institute of Child Health and Human Development workshop. *Obstet Gynecol* 2007; 109(4): 967–977.

Reefhuis J, Honein MA. Maternal age and non-chromosomal birth defects, Atlanta 1968–2000: teenager or thirty-something, who is at risk? *Birth Def Res A Clin Molec Teratol* 2004; 70: 572–579.

Chapter 40
Obesity in Pregnancy

Paola Aghajanian

Department of Medicine and Obstetrics and Gynecology, Keck School of Medicine, University of Southern California, CA, USA

Epidemiology

Obesity has become an epidemic in most parts of the world and its prevalence in the United States has increased by 75% since 1980. Maternal obesity has been defined in various ways, including bodyweight above 80–114 kg (175–250 lb), a weight 50–300% more than ideal pre-pregnancy weight for height, and a Body Mass Index (BMI) of 25 or above. BMI is a measure of body fat calculated as the weight in kilograms divided by the square of the height in meters. The World Health Organization and the National Institutes of Health define normal weight as a BMI of 18.5–24.9. Overweight is defined as a BMI of 25–29.9 and obesity as a BMI of 30 or greater. Obesity is further characterized as class I (BMI 30–34.9), class II (BMI 35–39.9) and class III (BMI greater than 40). Approximately one half of reproductive-aged women are overweight and one-third are obese. The increased prevalence has been especially notable in non-Hispanic black women (48%), Mexican American women (38%) and non-Hispanic white women (31%). The rates of obesity have also increased dramatically in children as young as 2 years old and in adolescents.

Maternal and fetal complications

Maternal pregravid obesity is a significant risk factor for adverse outcomes in pregnancy. Obesity in the nonpregnant woman is a known risk factor for diabetes mellitus, atherosclerosis and certain malignancies and is the second leading cause of preventable death in the United States. The metabolic syndrome is common in obese women and manifests as hypertension, glucose intolerance and hyperlipidemia. In general, obese women are more insulin resistant than nonobese women and are consequently at significantly greater risk for the development of gestational diabetes mellitus (GDM). Gestational hypertension and pre-eclampsia are also more common in the obese gravida. The increase in the latter two conditions may be related to the presence of the metabolic syndrome. Other conditions complicating pregnancies in obese women include sleep apnea, nonalcoholic fatty liver disease, and chronic renal and cardiac dysfunction.

Numerous studies have found associations between obesity and an increased risk of fetal heart defects, neural tube defects, and omphalocele. The mechanisms underlying these anomalies are not well understood and some believe undiagnosed type 2 diabetes may play a role in the etiology. Unexplained intrauterine fetal death also occurs more frequently in overweight and obese women, even after adjustments for maternal age and exclusion of maternal diabetes and hypertensive disorders. Furthermore, obesity is independently associated with an increased risk of large for gestational age infants and this impact on birthweight increases with increasing BMI.

Obstetric complications

An obese woman is at significantly higher risk of early miscarriage and recurrent miscarriage following spontaneous conception compared to a normal-weight woman. Even women undergoing assisted reproductive therapy are at increased risk of pregnancy loss. A higher rate of preterm delivery has also been reported in obese women compared to women of normal weight. However, data from more recent studies are conflicting, showing lower rates of spontaneous preterm birth in the obese group.

Higher rates of failed induction, macrosomia, shoulder dystocia, and operative vaginal delivery are seen in obese women compared to women of normal BMI. Additionally, the likelihood of successful vaginal birth after cesarean delivery decreases and the risk of cesarean delivery increases with increasing BMI. At the time of labor and delivery, the external monitoring of fetal heart rate and

Management of Common Problems in Obstetrics and Gynecology, 5th edition. Edited by T.M. Goodwin, M.N. Montoro, L. Muderspach, R. Paulson and S. Roy. © 2010 Blackwell Publishing Ltd.

uterine contractions in extremely obese women presents a challenge. Anesthesia can pose a particular problem given the difficulty in placement of regional anesthesia and the risk of difficult intubation should general anesthesia be required. Postoperatively, wound complications and respiratory complications are more common in obese patients, as is the incidence of postpartum hemorrhage, postpartum endometritis and deep venous thrombosis (DVT).

Management

When a woman presents for pre-pregnancy counseling, one of the initial steps is assessment of her commitment to behavioral change. Lifestyle measures such as calorie-restricted diets and exercise can together promote meaningful weight loss and long-term maintenance of reduced weight. Given that lifestyle changes are not always successful, alternative treatments such as bariatric surgery may be an option for a select group of women with class III obesity or those with class II obesity and a co-morbid condition. Women who undergo bariatric surgery are at risk of having an unexpected pregnancy after weight loss following surgery and should use a reliable method of birth control for 12–18 months postoperatively until a stable weight is reached. After pregnancy is attained, these women should be followed concomitantly with the bariatric surgeon and receive supplementation with folate, vitamin B12, iron and calcium. In those women with a laparoscopically adjustable gastric band, temporary adjustment or removal of the gastric band may be necessary if nausea and vomiting develop. Unfortunately, most pregnancies in the United States are unplanned, thus precluding preconceptual counseling and weight loss. Women with infertility are more likely to seek preconceptual counseling, and should be encouraged to lose weight prior to undergoing fertility treatment.

Height and weight should be recorded for all women at the initial prenatal visit to allow for calculation of the BMI. Weight gain in pregnancy is the difference between a woman's weight at her most current antenatal visit and her pregravid weight. Although the optimal weight or BMI for women wishing to become pregnant is not known, the Institute of Medicine (IOM) has devised recommendations for weight gain in pregnancy based on a woman's pregravid BMI. For women with a normal BMI, a weight gain of 11.2–15.9 kg (25–35 lb) is suggested. Overweight women should gain between 6.8–11.2 kg (15–25 lb) whereas obese women should gain no more than 6.8 kg (15 lb). This takes into account the fact that the term fetus represents 4–5 kg of weight, the placenta 0.5 kg and the amniotic fluid 0.5–1.0 kg. A referral to a nutritionist and an appropriate exercise regimen in pregnancy should be offered to all overweight and obese women.

An ultrasound evaluation can identify congenital anomalies although visualization of fetal anatomy, especially of the heart and spine, is significantly impaired for BMI greater than 36. Delayed evaluation until after 18 weeks' gestation and the use of a more advanced ultrasound machine may improve the visibility of fetal structures. Glucose screening should be undertaken at the first prenatal visit, preferably in the first trimester. If results are normal, glucose screening should be repeated at 24–28 weeks. The blood pressure should be monitored at each visit. Consideration should be given to obtaining an electrocardiogram, an echocardiogram, sleep studies, renal function tests and liver function tests if clinically indicated. A referral for medical clearance and anesthesia consultation prior to delivery may be warranted.

Antenatal testing in obese women with medical and obstetric complications should be done for routine indications. In the subgroup of obese women without other medical or obstetric problems, close fetal monitoring with fetal kick counts should be employed. The benefit of more extensive fetal monitoring in this setting has not been established.

Because of the increased likelihood of complicated and emergency cesarean delivery, adequate preparation for the day of delivery is prudent. The availability of extra personnel to assist in moving the patient, a large operating table and blood products should be ascertained. The patient should be counseled regarding the fetal and obstetric risks in advance. A cesarean section should be performed for the routine obstetric indications. There are no prospective trials in obese women to determine the optimal type of skin incision during a cesarean section (i.e. vertical or horizontal). Although a low transverse incision carries a lower risk of evisceration, involves less fat dissection and causes less postoperative pain, it potentially increases infection rates due to the warm and moist area underneath the pannus. It can also compromise visualization of the operative field, leading to increased operative time and excessive blood loss. Closure of the subcutaneous layer, if more than 2 cm in depth, has been shown to reduce the incidence of postoperative wound complications. However, the efficacy of subcutaneous drain placement in reducing postcesarean delivery morbidity in this setting is less clear. Early ambulation and compression stockings are beneficial if used properly. Postoperative heparin therapy may prove valuable in obese patients at high risk for DVT but data on the benefits and risks of its universal use in the obese population are insufficient.

Long-term consequences for the mother and infant

The retention of weight post partum is proportional to the weight gained in pregnancy. In general, a weight gain of over 9 kg is more likely to be retained. Postpartum care of the obese patient should involve continued encouragement of healthy eating habits and the establishment of a regular exercise routine. A consultation with a weight loss specialist prior to attempting another pregnancy should be considered.

Long-term consequences of obesity in pregnancy also affect the offspring. Macrosomic infants of obese women are predisposed to developing obesity in adolescence and adulthood. This in turn places them at increased risk for developing type 2 diabetes and the metabolic syndrome. Research in this field is ongoing and will further delineate the long-term risks in offspring of obese women.

Suggested reading

American College of Obstetricians and Gynecologists. Obesity in pregnancy. ACOG Committee Opinion No. 315. *Obstet Gynecol* 2005; 106: 671–675.

Baeten JM, Bukusi EA, Lambe M. Pregnancy complications and outcomes among overweight and obese nulliparous women. *Am J Public Health* 2001; 911: 436–440.

Catalano PM. Management of obesity in pregnancy. *Obstet Gynecol* 2007; 109: 419–433.

Cnattingius S, Bergstrom R, Lipworth L, Kramer MS. Prepregnancy weight and the risk of adverse pregnancy outcomes. *NEJM* 1998; 338: 147–152.

Yu CKH, Teoh TG, Robinson S. Obesity in pregnancy. *BJOG* 2006; 113: 1117–1125.

Chapter 41
Teratogen Exposure in Pregnancy

Bruce Kovacs and Emiliano Chavira

Department of Medicine and Obstetrics and Gynecology, Keck School of Medicine, University of Southern California, CA, USA

Principles of teratology

Teratogens are exogenous agents or factors which have the potential to cause fetal wastage, malformation or organ system dysfunction when exposure occurs during gestation. In general, teratogens can be divided into three broad categories: infectious agents, drugs and chemicals, and physical agents. This chapter will address the more common drug and chemical exposures.

Teratogens affect embryologic development by interfering with cellular growth, differentiation, interaction, and migration, all critical processes in embryogenesis. Considering the vast number of potential teratogens to which the human embryo could be exposed, relatively few are known to cause serious malformations in exposed individuals. The efficacy of a particular teratogen is dependent on the genetic make-up of both mother and fetus, as well as on a number of factors related to the maternal-fetal environment. Most importantly, however, the timing of the exposure during gestation is the primary factor which determines whether or not a teratogenic effect will be seen and which organ system or systems are affected. In humans, the most vulnerable period is between 3 and 8 weeks after the LMP, during the period of organogenesis. Unfortunately, most women do not realize they are pregnant until this critical period of development is well under way, so have not taken precautions to avoid exposure to known teratogenic agents.

Many congenital anomalies caused by teratogenic agents such as oral clefts, congenital heart disease, and neural tube defects, also occur in fetuses not exposed to teratogens. These types of birth defects are thought to be multifactorial or due to a combination of several inherited susceptibility factors and exposures to environmental insults. In this regard, there are probably a number of agents which, given a unique set of circumstances (metabolic status of the mother, a susceptible fetus, an embryologically vulnerable period, and a large teratogenic dose), are capable of producing teratogenic effects. Thus, a number of abnormalities, which are described as multifactorial in etiology, may have a teratology component to their pathogenesis.

Clinical teratology

The US Food and Drug Administration has devised a system for classifying therapeutic drugs for use in pregnancy based on the degree to which risk to the fetus has been ruled out. In most cases, animal studies have been used extensively to determine the possible teratogenic effects of drugs. Although such studies may be helpful, their results do not always reliably predict the response in humans. Because of the uncertainty of applying data from animal studies to humans, the critical value of case reports and human teratogen registries in identifying the teratogenic potential of drugs is obvious. Because there is an empiric background risk of genetic mutation and fetal malformation in any woman using any drug during pregnancy, large and carefully conducted studies are required to prove an agent is a teratogen. Failure to take this concept into account may lead to spurious claims of a causal relationship. Thus, it is important to remind patients that reports in lay literature often ignore these factors.

Potential teratogens

Alcohol

Ethanol is one of the most commonly abused substances in the US. The range and severity of anomalies caused by the prenatal ingestion of ethanol appear to be dose

Management of Common Problems in Obstetrics and Gynecology, 5th edition. Edited by T.M. Goodwin, M.N. Montoro, L. Muderspach, R. Paulson and S. Roy. © 2010 Blackwell Publishing Ltd.

related. Ingestion of one to two drinks per day (1–2 oz) may cause a small reduction in average birthweight, while a complete syndrome is associated with maternal ingestion of 4–6 drinks per day. The incidence of the fetal alcohol syndrome (FAS) is between 1/300 to 1/2000 livebirths depending on the population studied, with 30–40% of the offspring of alcoholic mothers showing the complete syndrome. The three diagnostic criteria for FAS are: prenatal and postnatal growth deficiency for weight, height, and head circumference, distinct craniofacial features, and mild to moderate mental retardation. The average IQ among FAS individuals is 65, but may range from 16 to 105. Although not diagnostic for FAS, renal and cardiac defects and hemangiomas are also present in approximately half of cases. Hypotonia is a frequent finding, along with poor motor coordination. Although full-spectrum FAS probably requires at least moderate exposure to alcohol, adverse effects (e.g. decreased birthweight) have been detected even with light drinking. A safe level of exposure has not been determined, and the most prudent advice is to avoid alcohol consumption during and when planning a pregnancy.

Amphetamines

Teratogenic effects of amphetamine use are difficult to prove because women who abuse amphetamines often use other substances including tobacco, alcohol, and cocaine, and have poor general health and nutrition. Multiple anecdotal associations have been reported including growth restriction, cleft lip, cardiac defects, biliary atresia, hyperbilirubinemia, cerebral hemorrhage, Mongolian spots and undescended testes. Further complicating the analysis is that methamphetamine use has been shown to increase the incidence of premature birth. A withdrawal syndrome has been noted in infants of chronic abusers, and one study found a high incidence of intracranial abnormalities consistent with brain injury. Some studies have shown developmental delay in children exposed to amphetamines *in utero*, but most long-term follow-up studies have failed to identify long-term sequelae.

Antibiotics

Studies on the teratogenicity of most antibiotics have failed to reveal an increased risk to the human fetus. A few, however, appear to have potential for damage. Tetracycline exposure beyond the fourth month of pregnancy has been shown to result in yellow discoloration of the deciduous teeth. The aminoglycosides streptomycin and kanamycin will produce eighth nerve damage with subsequent hearing loss in a small percentage of exposed fetuses. In contrast, ototoxicity has not been reported with gentamicin or vancomycin use. Fluoroquinolones in animal studies have been shown to cause sufficient damage to cartilage to result in lameness. Although no teratogenic effect has been observed in humans, fluoroquinolones are not recommended during pregnancy since other alternatives with well-established safety are available.

Antihypertensive agents

Over the years a number of these agents from various classes have been suspected of causing birth defects. However, until recently no distinct association has been established for any agent despite widespread use. Angiotensin-converting enzyme (ACE) inhibitor use after the first trimester has been associated with oligohydramnios and neonatal anuria. In addition, fetal growth restriction, neonatal hypotension and poor cranial ossification are reported with maternal use of these medications. Recent studies have found an increased risk of cardiac and CNS malformations with first-trimester exposure. For these reasons, ACE inhibitors are contraindicated in pregnancy. Historically, thiazide diuretics have been used in pregnancy to prevent toxemia but no such benefit has been demonstrated. Moreover, thiazide diuretics have been associated with neonatal thrombocytopenia and serious electrolyte disturbances, as well as depletion of maternal intravascular volume. Their use during pregnancy and particularly in the setting of pregnancy-induced hypertension is not recommended.

Antineoplastic agents

Amniopterin and methotrexate, both folic acid antagonists, are proven teratogens. Exposure in the first 6 weeks of gestation is usually lethal to the embryo, while exposure later in the first trimester produces fetal effects which include growth restriction, craniofacial anomalies, abnormal positioning of extremities and mental retardation.

Alkylating agents, including cyclophosphamide, have been associated with severe fetal growth restriction and fetal anomalies such as cleft palate, microphthalmia, limb reductions, digit anomalies and poorly developed external genitalia. The first trimester is a particularly dangerous time for use of these drugs but a number of patients so treated have produced normal offspring. Other agents used for cancer chemotherapy appear to have less risk for teratogenic effects in humans.

Anticoagulants

The use of coumarin derivatives (e.g. warfarin) during the first trimester is associated with an increased risk of spontaneous abortion, growth restriction, central nervous system defects, stillbirth, and a characteristic syndrome of nasal hypoplasia, stippled epiphyses and fetal growth restriction known as the fetal warfarin syndrome. Embryologically, the most vulnerable time appears to be between 8 and 11 weeks after the LMP. There are emerging data that warfarin use even after embryogenesis may produce mild degrees of developmental delay. Because of this teratogenic risk, heparins are generally favored over coumarin derivatives during pregnancy, given that they do not cross the placenta. Patients using coumarin drugs for prophylaxis should be changed to a heparin formulation prior to conception.

Anticonvulsants

The incidence of epilepsy in pregnant women in the US is about 1 in 200. These women have an increased risk for significant fetal abnormalities. It is not clear whether the major proportion of this risk is due to an effect of the underlying convulsive disorder or to a teratogenic effect of the anticonvulsant therapy. It is probably a combined effect as specific patterns of fetal malformations have been associated with different anticonvulsant agents.

For instance, diphenylhydantoin (Dilantin) can produce a specific pattern of malformations known as the fetal hydantoin syndrome. The clinical features of this syndrome include craniofacial abnormalities, limb reduction defects, prenatal-onset growth deficiency, mental retardation, and cardiovascular anomalies. Vitamin K-dependent coagulation factors may also be reduced, causing early hemorrhagic disease of the newborn. Overall, approximately 10% of exposed fetuses have the syndrome, and an additional 30% may have isolated features.

Valproic acid (Depakene) produces congenital malformations similar to those found in the fetal hydantoin syndrome. These infants are also at an increased risk (1–2%) for neural tube defects. Although normal births associated with prenatal valproic acid exposure have been reported, this drug should be avoided during pregnancy.

Carbamazepine (Tegretol) also appears to have a potential for teratogenesis, perhaps as a result of its metabolic breakdown. The malformations reported include minor craniofacial defects, nail hypoplasia and neurodevelopmental delays. There is also an increased risk reported for spina bifida (1%). However, the incidence of malformation is less than that associated with Dilantin.

Phenobarbital may be teratogenic for orofacial clefting, congenital heart disease and peripheral skeletal dysplasia, but reports of the risk are confusing due to simultaneous administration of phenytoin. Use of phenobarbital has also been associated with a reduction in vitamin K-dependent coagulation factors and may result in hemorrhagic disease of the newborn. Prenatal use of this drug may result in neonatal phenobarbital withdrawal symptoms starting on day 7 of life.

Trimethadione (Tridione) and paramethadione (Paradione), used to treat petit mal epilepsy, have been associated with a characteristic pattern of malformations. The features include craniofacial abnormalities, fetal growth restriction, mental retardation and cardiovascular abnormalities. In addition, exposure to these agents has been associated with an increased risk for fetal loss. Taken together, women using trimethadione or paramethadione face an 85% risk of pregnancy loss or major congenital anomalies. In light of the relatively minor nature of petit mal seizures and safer alternatives, these anticonvulsants should not be used during pregnancy.

Cocaine

The actual prevalence of cocaine use in pregnancy is unknown, but is up to 17% in urban areas. Cocaine use is associated with an increased incidence of spontaneous abortion, premature delivery, intrauterine growth restriction, abruptio placentae, microcephaly and maternal and fetal death. There is also evidence of teratogenic effects on CNS structure, including the potential to cause cerebral infarcts in the fetal brain. In addition, there is evidence for genitourinary tract malformations with maternal cocaine use. Although the long-term neurologic outcome of infants exposed to cocaine *in utero* is not yet known, it is prudent to consider it a neurobehavioral teratogen.

Heavy metals

The nonessential metallic elements mercury, lead and cadmium are reproductive and developmental toxicants, but only mercury and lead have proven teratogenic potential. Mercury, especially compounds like methyl mercury, may produce CNS damage and dysfunction, with microcephaly and mental retardation in exposed fetuses. This may lead to cerebral palsy even when exposure occurs in the third trimester. Most exposures occur as a result of the ingestion of fish and grains contaminated with industrial wastes or mercury-containing antifungals. Similarly, lead and lead-containing compounds are neurodevelopmental teratogens, and are responsible for an increased abortion and stillbirth rate. Since both substances are abundant in our industrial society, clinicians need to question patients about potential exposures to these agents in the home or at work.

Organic solvents and compounds

This group of chemicals is diverse and they are widely used in the US. In general, exposure occurs as a result of inhalation of vapors or as absorption through the skin. Fortunately, although there are other adverse effects associated with exposures to these substances, few have any teratogenic effects in humans. However, polychlorinated biphenyls (PCBs) are a notable exception. Ingestion of these chemicals due to contamination of cooking oil has been reported to cause dark skin pigmentation and growth restriction. No pattern of structural malformations was noted, but there was an increase in the incidence of several common malformations.

Psychotropic agents

This group of drugs includes some of the most commonly prescribed drugs in the US, major tranquilizers and antianxiety agents. The data regarding their teratogenicity are conflicting and in general, no specific pattern of teratogenesis is apparent. Exceptions include lithium salts, diazepam (Valium), meprobamate, and impramine, all of which cross the placenta and have been associated with birth defects. However, of these, only lithium is a proven teratogen, with an increased rate of congenital heart disease (principally Ebstein's anomaly). The teratogenic effect is not as significant as early reports suggested.

Steroid hormones

Exposures to progestins and estrogen/progestin combinations in the first trimester occur fairly commonly due to their use in the management of threatened abortion or because women continue taking birth control pills, unaware that they are pregnant. The most consistent abnormality associated with the use of progestins during pregnancy is masculinization of the external genitalia in female fetuses. The magnitude of this risk appears to be between 1% and 2%.

The teratogenicity of estrogen and progestin combinations is more difficult to assess. Potential problems include congenital heart defects, nervous system defects, limb reduction malformations, and modified development of sexual organs. However, except for the latter category, no firm evidence for a causal relationship exists and inadvertent use of low-dose birth control pills in the first trimester has not been associated with teratogenic effects.

Tobacco smoke

Maternal tobacco use reduces the chance for a normal pregnancy outcome, but is not teratogenic. The effects on pregnancy include decreased birthweight, birth length, and head circumference, as well as an increased risk for spontaneous abortion, abruption, prematurity, intrauterine fetal death, and neonatal death. Because of this and its other adverse effects, pregnant women should be counseled to quit smoking, and if unable to, reduce their use as much as possible.

Vitamins

Lack of adequate folate is associated with increased incidence of neural tube defects. Deficiencies of other vitamins and trace elements appear to result in increased pregnancy loss, growth retardation and malformations.

In certain cases large doses of vitamins or their derivatives can be teratogenic. Vitamin A and analogs such as isotretinoin (Accutane), used for treatment of severe acne, are teratogenic. Affected infants demonstrate craniofacial malformations, psychomotor retardation, congenital heart defects, thymic defects and central nervous system malformations. There is also a high spontaneous abortion rate, and loss of pregnancy may be a more common outcome than a liveborn infant with malformations. The critical period of exposure is believed to be 2–5 weeks after conception. Thus, physicians have an important responsibility to discuss these risks with all female patients before beginning treatment. The manufacturer and the FDA recommend that physicians obtain a negative pregnancy test, then wait until the second or third day of the next normal menstrual period to begin therapy. Patients are also strongly encouraged to use contraception. The exact risk for serious defects following exposure during the first trimester has not yet been established, but it appears to be substantial. Etretinate (used for recalcitrant psoriasis) is also a teratogen and is contraindicated during pregnancy and in those planning a pregnancy. Following chronic therapy, detectable serum drug levels have occurred up to 2.9 years after treatment had been stopped, making it difficult to recommend the length of time for which pregnancy should be avoided after completing a course of treatment.

There is no evidence that topical vitamin A (tretinoin) is a teratogen.

Vitamin D may also have teratogenic potential when given in very high doses, but more data are needed to substantiate the validity of this reported association.

Suggested reading

American College of Obstetricians and Gynecologists. *Teratology. Educational Bulletin No. 233*. Washington, DC: American College of Obstetricians and Gynecologists, 1997.

Brent RL. Radiation teratogenesis. *Teratology* 1980; 21: 281.

Briggs GG, Freeman RK, Yaffe SF. *Drugs in pregnancy and lactation*, 6th edn. Philadelphia, PA: Lippincott, Williams and Wilkins, 2002.

Gilstrap LC. Drugs in pregnancy. *Semin Perinatol* 1997; 21(2): 113.

Hanson JL. Teratogenetic agents. In: Emery AE, Rimoin DL (eds) *Principles and practice of medical genetics*. 2nd edn. Edinburgh: Churchill Livingston, 1990: 183.

Chapter 42
Electronic Fetal Monitoring: Definitions and Principles

David A. Miller

Department of Medicine and Obstetrics and Gynecology, Keck School of Medicine, University of Southern California, CA, USA

The evolution of standardized fetal heart rate terminology

In 1997, the National Institute of Child Health and Human Development (NICHD) proposed standardized definitions for fetal heart rate tracings [1]. In 2005 and 2006, the American College of Obstetricians and Gynecologists (ACOG), the Association of Women's Health, Obstetric and Neonatal Nurses (AWHONN) and the American College of Nurse Midwives (ACNM) officially endorsed the NICHD definitions summarized in Table 42.1. The standardized FHR definitions were reaffirmed by a second NICHD consensus report in 2008 [2]. In July, 2009, the definitions were again endorsed in ACOG Practice Bulletin 106 [3].

Evidence-based interpretation of fetal heart rate patterns

This chapter will review standardized FHR terminology and the physiology underlying FHR patterns. Supporting evidence will be stratified according to the method outlined by the US Preventive Services Task Force (Box 42.1) [4]. Level I evidence is considered to be the most robust and level III, the least.

The primary objective of intrapartum FHR monitoring is to assess fetal oxygenation during labor. However, a number of factors can influence the appearance of a FHR tracing via mechanisms unrelated to fetal oxygenation. Some examples are summarized in Table 42.2. If a FHR abnormality is thought to be related to any of these factors, individualized management is directed at the specific underlying process. The following discussion of FHR physiology and interpretation will focus on FHR patterns related specifically to fetal oxygenation.

Management of Common Problems in Obstetrics and Gynecology, 5th edition. Edited by T.M. Goodwin, M.N. Montoro, L. Muderspach, R. Paulson and S. Roy. © 2010 Blackwell Publishing Ltd.

Terminology, physiology and interpretation of specific fetal heart rate patterns

Baseline rate
Baseline FHR is defined as the mean FHR rounded to increments of 5 bpm during a 10-minute segment, excluding accelerations, decelerations and periods of marked variability. Normal FHR baseline ranges from 110 to 160 bpm.

Physiology
Baseline FHR is regulated by cardiac pacemakers and conduction pathways, autonomic innervation, humoral factors (catecholamines), extrinsic factors (medications) and local factors (calcium, potassium). Autonomic input regulates the FHR in response to fluctuations in PO_2, PCO_2 and blood pressure detected by chemoreceptors and baroreceptors.

Tachycardia
Baseline FHR in excess of 160 bpm is defined as tachycardia. There are many potential causes of fetal tachycardia (see Table 42.2). One possible cause is recurrent or sustained interruption of fetal oxygenation leading to metabolic acidemia and blunting of parasympathetic cardiac innervation. If interrupted oxygenation is the cause of fetal tachycardia, other FHR changes may be present, including decelerations, loss of variability and loss of accelerations. The scientific evidence supporting a relationship between fetal tachycardia and interrupted oxygenation primarily is level III.

Bradycardia
According to the definitions proposed by the NICHD, "bradycardia" is a baseline rate below 110 bpm, while a "deceleration" is a periodic or episodic fall in heart rate that interrupts the baseline. Decelerations are common and can reflect interrupted fetal oxygenation. On the other hand, true baseline bradycardia is rare and is not specifically related to fetal oxygenation. Causes of fetal bradycardia are summarized in Table 42.2.

Table 42.1 Standardized FHR definitions

Pattern	Definition
Baseline	Mean FHR rounded to increments of 5 bpm during a 10 min segment, excluding accelerations, decelerations and periods of marked variability The baseline must be at least 2 min in any 10-min segment (not necessarily contiguous) Normal baseline FHR range 110–160 bpm Baseline >160 bpm = tachycardia; baseline <110 bpm = bradycardia
Variability	Fluctuations in the FHR baseline that are irregular in amplitude and frequency Quantitated as the amplitude of peak-to-trough in bpm Absent – amplitude range undetectable Minimal – amplitude range detectable ≤5 bpm Moderate (normal) – amplitude range 6–25 bpm Marked – amplitude range >25 bpm
Accelerations	Abrupt increase (onset to peak <30 s) in the FHR from the most recently calculated baseline At ≥32 weeks, an acceleration peaks ≥15 bpm above baseline and lasts ≥15 s but <2 min At <32 weeks, an acceleration peaks ≥10 bpm above baseline and lasts ≥10 s but <2 min Prolonged acceleration lasts ≥2 min but <10 min; acceleration ≥10 min is a baseline change
Decelerations	
Early	Gradual (onset to nadir ≥30 s) decrease in FHR during a uterine contraction Nadir of the deceleration occurs at the same time as the peak of the contraction
Late	Gradual (onset to nadir ≥30 s) decrease in FHR during a uterine contraction Onset, nadir, and recovery occur after the beginning, peak, and end of the contraction
Variable Prolonged	Abrupt (onset to nadir <30 s), decrease in the FHR ≥15 bpm below the baseline lasting ≥15 s but less than 2 min Deceleration ≥15 bpm below baseline lasting ≥2 min or more but <10 min If a deceleration lasts 10 minutes or longer, it is a baseline change
Sinusoidal pattern	Visually apparent, smooth, sine wave-like undulating pattern in FHR baseline with a cycle frequency of 3–5 per minute which persists for 20 minutes or more

---

Box 42.1 US Preventive Services Task Force stratification of scientific evidence

Level I	Evidence obtained from at least one properly designed randomized controlled trial
Level II-1	Evidence obtained from well-designed control-led trials without randomization
Level II-2	Evidence obtained from well-designed cohort or case–control analytic studies, preferably from more than one center or research group
Level II-3	Evidence obtained from multiple time series with or without the intervention. Dramatic results in uncontrolled experiments also could be regarded as this type of evidence
Level III	Opinions of respected authorities, based on clinical experience, descriptive studies or reports of expert committees

Baseline fetal heart rate variability

Variability is defined as fluctuations in the baseline FHR that are irregular in amplitude and frequency. Variability is quantitated in beats per minute and is measured from the peak to the trough of the FHR fluctuations. There are four categories of variability: absent, minimal, moderate and marked.

Physiology

Fluctuations in PO_2, PCO_2 and blood pressure are detected by chemoreceptors and baroreceptors located in the aortic arch and carotid arteries. Signals from these receptors are processed in the brainstem with regulatory input from higher centers. Autonomic signals from the brainstem modulate the FHR in response to moment-to-moment changes in fetal PO_2, PCO_2 and blood pressure to optimize cardiac output and distribution of oxygenated blood to the fetal tissues.

Absent variability

Variability is defined as absent if the amplitude range of the FHR fluctuations is undetectable to the unaided eye. As summarized in Table 42.2, there are many possible causes of decreased FHR variability. However, when variability is persistently absent, careful evaluation should be undertaken to exclude fetal metabolic acidemia.

Minimal variability

Variability is defined as minimal if the range is detectable but less than or equal to 5 bpm. As summarized in Table 42.2, there are many possible causes of decreased FHR variability. Interrupted fetal oxygenation leading to metabolic acidemia and blunted autonomic regulation of the FHR can result in decreased FHR variability.

Table 42.2 Factors that can influence the appearance of the FHR tracing by mechanisms not directly related to oxygenation

Factor	Reported FHR associations (most evidence level II-3 and III)
Prematurity	Increased baseline rate, decreased variability, reduced frequency and amplitude of accelerations
Sleep cycle	Decreased variability, reduced frequency and amplitude of accelerations
Fever/infection	Increased baseline rate, decreased variability
Medications	Effects depend upon specific medication and may include changes in baseline rate, frequency and amplitude of accelerations, variability and sinusoidal pattern
Hyperthyroidism	Tachycardia, decreased variability
Fetal anemia	Sinusoidal pattern, tachycardia
Fetal heart block	Bradycardia, decreased variability
Fetal cardiac failure	Tachycardia, bradycardia, decreased variability
Maternal hypoglycemia	Bradycardia
Maternal hypothermia	Bradycardia
Fetal tachyarrhythmia	Variable degrees of tachycardia, decreased variability
Congenital anomaly	Decreased variability, decelerations
Pre-existing neurologic abnormality	Decreased variability, absent accelerations

When minimal variability is observed, all possible causes should be considered, including interrupted fetal oxygenation and evolving metabolic acidemia.

Moderate variability
Moderate FHR variability indicates that autonomic regulation of the FHR is not blunted by interrupted fetal oxygenation that has progressed to the stage of metabolic acidemia. One of the central tenets of electronic FHR monitoring is that moderate variability is reliably predictive of the absence of fetal metabolic acidemia at the time it is observed [2,3]. Supporting evidence is level II-2, II-3 and III.

Marked variability
The significance of marked variability is not known. It likely represents a normal variant but may be related to autonomic perturbation in the setting of early hypoxemia. Scientific evidence regarding this pattern is level III.

Sinusoidal pattern

A sinusoidal fetal heart rate pattern is defined as having a visually apparent, smooth, sine wave-like undulating pattern in the FHR baseline with a cycle frequency of 3–5 per minute which persists for ≥ 20 minutes. This pattern classically is associated with severe fetal anemia. Variations of the pattern have been described in association with chorio-amnionitis, fetal sepsis or administration of narcotic analgesics [5]. Scientific evidence regarding etiology of the sinusoidal pattern is level II-2 to level III.

Acceleration

Acceleration is as an abrupt increase in FHR at least 15 bpm above the baseline lasting at least 15 seconds. Before 32 weeks of gestation, an acceleration peaks at least 10 bpm above the baseline and lasts at least 10 seconds. An acceleration lasting at least 2 minutes but less than 10 minutes is defined as a prolonged acceleration. An acceleration lasting 10 minutes or longer is defined as a baseline change.

Physiology
Accelerations occur in association with fetal movement, probably as a result of stimulation of peripheral proprioceptors, increased catecholamine release and changes in sympathetic and parasympathetic stimulation of the heart.

Interpretation
A central tenet of electronic FHR monitoring is that FHR accelerations reliably predict the absence of fetal metabolic acidemia at the time they are observed [2,3]. Accelerations also indicate that autonomic regulation of the FHR is not significantly affected by fetal sleep, tachycardia, prematurity, congenital anomalies, central nervous system depressants or medications [6-9]. Supporting evidence is level II-2, II-3 and III.

Decelerations

Late deceleration
Late deceleration is defined as a gradual decrease in the FHR associated with a uterine contraction. In most cases the onset, nadir, and recovery of the deceleration occur after the beginning, peak, and ending of the contraction, respectively. A late deceleration is a reflex fetal response to transient hypoxemia during a uterine contraction. Myometrial contractions can interrupt maternal perfusion of the intervillous space of the placenta, leading to a decline in fetal PO_2 below the normal range of approximately 15–25 mmHg. Chemoreceptors detect the change and trigger reflex sympathetic outflow, peripheral vasoconstriction and centralization of blood volume to optimize perfusion of the brain, heart and adrenal glands. The resulting rise in blood pressure triggers baroreceptor-mediated parasympathetic outflow and reflex slowing of the heart rate to reduce cardiac output and return the blood pressure to normal [10]. Supporting evidence is level II-1 and II-2.

Early deceleration

Early deceleration is a gradual decrease in FHR associated with a uterine contraction. The onset, nadir, and recovery of the deceleration occur at the same time as the beginning, peak, and end of the contraction, respectively. Early decelerations are thought to represent a fetal autonomic response to changes in intracranial pressure and/or cerebral blood flow caused by compression of the fetal head. They have no known relationship to fetal oxygenation and are considered clinically benign. Supporting evidence is level II-3 and III.

Variable deceleration

Variable deceleration is defined as an abrupt decrease in FHR at least 15 bpm below the baseline lasting at least 15 seconds but less than 2 minutes. Variable decelerations result from transient mechanical compression of the umbilical cord and are not necessarily associated with uterine contractions [11,12]. Initially, compression of the umbilical cord occludes the thin-walled, compliant umbilical vein, decreasing fetal venous return and triggering a baroreceptor-mediated reflex rise in FHR. Further compression of the umbilical cord results in occlusion of the umbilical arteries, causing an abrupt increase in blood pressure. Baroreceptors detect the abrupt rise in blood pressure and trigger an increase in parasympathetic outflow and an abrupt decrease in heart rate. As the cord is decompressed, this sequence of events occurs in reverse. Supporting evidence is level II-1, II-2, II-3 and III.

Prolonged deceleration

Prolonged deceleration is defined as a decrease in FHR at least 15 bpm below the baseline lasting at least 2 minutes. A prolonged deceleration reflects interrupted oxygen transfer from the environment to the fetus. If oxygen transfer is interrupted by mechanical compression of the umbilical cord, the deceleration begins as a reflex autonomic response to fetal hypertension. Alternatively, acute interruption of oxygen transfer (placental abruption, uterine rupture) can cause an abrupt fall in fetal PO_2, reflex peripheral vasoconstriction, centralization of blood volume and increased blood pressure. The resulting deceleration begins as a reflex autonomic response to the rise in blood pressure triggered by falling PO_2. If sustained, interruption of oxygen transfer can lead to direct hypoxic myocardial depression. It is likely that both mechanisms (autonomic reflex and direct myocardial depression) contribute to the pathophysiology of prolonged decelerations. In general, autonomic reflexes appear to predominate initially and direct hypoxic myocardial depression appears to occur late in the process. Supporting evidence is level II-1, II-2, II-3 and III.

Conclusion

Standardized FHR terminology has been endorsed by all major professional organizations in the United States representing providers of obstetric care. Standardized FHR interpretation sets the stage for an evidence-based approach to standardized management.

References

1. National Institute of Child Health and Human Development Research Planning Workshop. Electronic fetal heart rate monitoring: research guidelines for interpretation. *Am J Obstet Gynecol* 1997; 177: 1385–1390.
2. Macones GA, Hankins GD, Spong CY, Hauth J, Moore T. 2008 National Institute of Child Health and Human Development Workshop report on electronic fetal monitoring: update on definitions, interpretation, and research guidelines. *Obstet Gynecol* 2008; 112(3): 661–666.
3. American College of Obstetricians and Gynecologists. Practice Bulletin No. 106: intrapartum fetal heart rate monitoring: nomenclature, interpretation, and general management principles. *Obstet Gynecol* 2009; 114: 192–202.
4. United States Preventive Services Task Force. Guide to clinical preventative services, 2nd edn. Baltimore, MD: Williams and Wilkins, 1996.
5. Hatjis CG, Meis PJ. Sinusoidal fetal heart rate pattern associated with butorphanol administration. *Obstet Gynecol* 1986; 67: 377–380.
6. Hallak M, Martinez-Poyer J, Kruger ML, Hassan S, Blackwell SC, Sorokin Y. The effect of magnesium sulfate on fetal heart rate parameters: a randomized, placebo-controlled trial. *Am J Obstet Gynecol* 1999; 181: 1122–1127.
7. Wright JW, Ridgway LE, Wright BD, Covington DL, Bobitt JR. Effect of MgSO4 on heart rate monitoring in the preterm fetus. *J Reprod Med* 1996; 41: 605–608.
8. Giannina G, Guzman ER, Lai YL, Lake MF, Cernadas M, Vintzileos AM. Comparison of the effects of meperidine and nalbuphine on intrapartum fetal heart rate tracings. *Obstet Gynecol* 1995; 86: 441–445.
9. Kopecky EA, Ryan ML, Barrett JF, *et al*. Fetal response to maternally administered morphine. *Am J Obstet Gynecol* 2000; 183: 424–430.
10. Martin CB Jr, de Haan J, van der Wildt B, Jongsma HW, Dieleman A, Arts TH. Mechanisms of late decelerations in the fetal heart rate. A study with autonomic blocking agents in fetal lambs. *Eur J Obstet Gynecol Reprod Biol* 1979; 9(6): 361–373.
11. Itskovitz J, LaGamma EF, Rudolph AM. Effect of cord compression on fetal blood flow distribution and O2 delivery. *Am J Physiol* 1987; 252: H100–H109.
12. Ball RH, Parer JT, Caldwell LE, Johnson J. Regional blood flow and metabolism in ovine fetuses during severe cord occlusion. *Am J Obstet Gynecol* 1994; 171: 1549–1555.

Chapter 43
Electronic Fetal Monitoring: A Systematic Approach

David A. Miller

Department of Medicine and Obstetrics and Gynecology, Keck School of Medicine, University of Southern California, CA, USA

Introduction

Intrapartum fetal heart rate monitoring is intended to assess the adequacy of fetal oxygenation during labor. To that end, three central concepts of evidence-based FHR interpretation provide the foundation for a systematic approach to the decision-making process underlying FHR management.

All clinically significant FHR decelerations reflect interruption of oxygen transfer from the environment to the fetus at one or more points along the oxygen pathway. Interrupted fetal oxygenation does not result in neurologic injury unless it progresses at least to the stage of significant metabolic acidemia (umbilical artery pH <7.0 and base deficit ≥12 mmol/L) [1].

Moderate variability and/or accelerations reliably predict the absence of metabolic acidemia at the time they are observed [2,3].

Management

General considerations

Reliable information is vital to the success of intrapartum FHR monitoring. Therefore, it is essential to confirm that the monitor is recording the FHR and uterine activity accurately. Ultrasound might be necessary to locate the FHR or to confirm that the observed rate is fetal and not maternal. If external monitoring is not adequate for interpretation, a fetal scalp electrode and/or intrauterine pressure catheter might be necessary.

Evaluate the FHR tracing

After confirming that the monitor is accurately and adequately recording the necessary information, the FHR tracing is evaluated. Thorough evaluation of the FHR tracing includes assessment of five FHR components: baseline rate, variability, accelerations, decelerations, and changes or trends in the tracing over time. If necessary, fetal stimulation should be used to provoke accelerations and/or improve FHR variability.

Evaluation of five FHR components

If all five FHR components are normal, there is a very low probability of interrupted fetal oxygenation. As long as there are no other reasons to review the FHR tracing more frequently (such as pre-eclampsia or fetal growth restriction), routine intrapartum surveillance is appropriate. In low-risk patients, the FHR tracing should be reviewed at least every 30 minutes during the first stage of labor and every 15 minutes during the second stage [3,4]. If one or more of the five FHR components is abnormal, further evaluation is necessary. Corrective measures may be needed before making a decision regarding management. A practical approach can be summarized as follows.

"A" – assess the oxygen pathway

Rapid, systematic assessment of the oxygen pathway from the environment to the fetus can identify possible sources of interrupted oxygenation. This pathway includes the maternal lungs, heart, vasculature, uterus, placenta and umbilical cord.

"B" – begin corrective measures

At each point along the pathway, appropriate corrective measures should be initiated to optimize oxygen delivery. Specific measures are summarized below.

Supplemental oxygen

Fetal oxygenation is dependent upon the oxygen content of maternal blood perfusing the intervillous space of the placenta. Administration of supplemental oxygen by nasal cannula or facemask can increase the PO_2 of inspired air, increasing both the partial pressure of oxygen dissolved in maternal blood and the amount of oxygen bound to

Management of Common Problems in Obstetrics and Gynecology, 5th edition. Edited by T.M. Goodwin, M.N. Montoro, L. Muderspach, R. Paulson and S. Roy. © 2010 Blackwell Publishing Ltd.

hemoglobin. This can increase the oxygen concentration gradient across the placental blood–blood barrier and lead to increased fetal PO_2 and oxygen content. Several studies have reported resolution of FHR abnormalities after administration of supplemental oxygen to the mother, providing indirect evidence of improved fetal oxygenation [5-9]. Fetal pulse oximetry studies have demonstrated increased fetal hemoglobin saturation following maternal administration of oxygen. Available data support the use of a nonrebreather facemask to administer oxygen at a rate of 10 L/min for approximately 15–30 minutes [5,10-12].

Maternal position changes

Supine positioning increases the likelihood that pressure on the inferior vena cava will impair venous return, cardiac output and perfusion of the intervillous space. It also increases the likelihood that pressure on the descending aorta and/or iliac vessels will impede the delivery of oxygenated blood to the intervillous space. Fetal pulse oximetry data confirm that lateral positioning results in higher fetal hemoglobin saturation levels than does supine positioning [5,13,14]. In the setting of suspected umbilical cord compression, maternal position changes may result in fetal position changes and relief of pressure on the umbilical cord.

Intravenous fluid administration

Optimal uterine perfusion depends upon optimal cardiac output and intravascular volume. An intravascular bolus of isotonic fluid can improve cardiac output by increasing circulating volume and increasing venous return, left ventricular end diastolic pressure, ventricular preload and stroke volume. Simpson & James [5] demonstrated a significant increase in fetal oxygen saturation following an intravascular isotonic fluid bolus approximating 10–20% of blood volume (500–1000 cc). Boluses were administered over 20 minutes to normotensive women without evidence of hypovolemia. The maximum effect was achieved with a 1000 cc bolus, and the beneficial impact on fetal oxygen saturation lasted for more than 30 minutes after the bolus.

Correct maternal blood pressure

A number of factors predispose laboring women to transient episodes of hypotension. These include inadequate hydration, insensible fluid losses, supine position resulting in compression of the inferior vena cava, and peripheral vasodilation due to sympathetic blockade during regional anesthesia. Maternal hypotension can reduce uterine perfusion and fetal oxygenation. Hydration and lateral or Trendelenberg positioning usually correct the blood pressure. However, medication may be necessary. Ephedrine is a sympathomimetic amine with weak α- and β-agonist activity. The primary

mechanism of action is displacement of norepinephrine from presynaptic storage vesicles, resulting in release of norepinephrine and stimulation of postsynaptic adrenergic receptors.

Reducing uterine activity

Excessive uterine activity is a common cause of interrupted fetal oxygenation. A number of terms have been used in the past to describe excessive uterine activity. Examples include "hyperstimulation," "hypercontractility" and "tetanic contraction." The 2008 NICHD consensus report stated that the terms "hyperstimulation" and "hypercontractility" are poorly defined and should be abandoned. Normal uterine contraction frequency is defined as five or fewer contractions in 10 minutes averaged over 30 minutes. Contraction frequency in excess of five in 10 minutes averaged over 30 minutes is defined as tachysystole.

For the purposes of FHR management, if an abnormal FHR pattern is thought to be related to excessive uterine activity, options include stopping or reducing uterine stimulants, and/or administering uterine relaxants. If necessary, an intrauterine pressure catheter may help to assess uterine activity.

Alter second-stage pushing technique

During the second stage of labor, maternal expulsive efforts can be associated with recurrent variable or prolonged decelerations. Suggested corrective approaches include fewer pushing efforts per contraction, shorter individual pushing efforts, pushing with every other or every third contraction and, in patients with regional anesthesia, pushing only with perceived urge [15-20].

Amnio-infusion

Intrapartum amnio-infusion involves infusion of isotonic fluid through an intrauterine catheter into the amniotic cavity in order to restore the amniotic fluid volume to normal or near-normal levels. The procedure is intended to relieve intermittent umbilical cord compression that results in variable FHR decelerations and transient fetal hypoxemia and to dilute thick meconium in an attempt to prevent meconium aspiration syndrome. When performed for the indication of oligohydramnios and umbilical cord compression, amnio-infusion reduces the occurrence of variable decelerations and lowers the rate of cesarean delivery [21]. It has no known impact on late decelerations. In a recent large study, amnio-infusion performed for the indication of meconium-stained amniotic fluid alone did not significantly reduce the incidence of meconium aspiration syndrome or perinatal death [22]. The procedure appears to be beneficial in reducing the occurrence of variable decelerations in the setting of oligohydramnios; however, routine amnio-infusion for meconium-stained amniotic fluid without variable decelerations is not recommended by the ACOG [23].

Re-evaluate FHR after corrective measures

After corrective measures, the FHR tracing is re-evaluated. If all five FHR components are normal, there is a very low likelihood of interrupted fetal oxygenation and metabolic acidemia, and routine intrapartum surveillance can be resumed. However, if one or more components is persistently abnormal after corrective measures, further evaluation is necessary.

"C" – clear obstacles to rapid delivery

If conservative corrective measures fail to resolve the FHR abnormalities, it is prudent to plan ahead for the possible need for rapid delivery. This step is frequently overlooked; however, it is a very common area of criticism in the event of an untoward outcome. Planning ahead for a potential emergency does not commit the patient to immediate delivery. However, it can help remove some common sources of unnecessary delay in the event that an emergency arises. Every clinical setting is unique. Therefore, a simple checklist can help ensure that important considerations are not overlooked. A practical, systematic approach takes into account individual characteristics of the facility, staff, mother, fetus and labor.

"D" – decision to delivery time

After clearing obstacles to rapid delivery, it is necessary to estimate the decision to delivery time in the event that emergency delivery becomes necessary. A practical, systematic approach takes into account individual characteristics of the facility, staff, mother, fetus and labor.

The final decision

After "A" assessing the oxygen pathway, "B" beginning conservative corrective measures to optimize oxygen delivery, "C" clearing obstacles to rapid delivery, and "D" determining the decision to delivery interval, a decision must be made. The decision to allow labor to continue or to proceed with delivery balances the perceived benefit of successful vaginal delivery against the perceived risk of evolving fetal metabolic acidemia and potential injury. Clinical circumstance can vary widely but the question is the same in every case: "Is vaginal delivery likely to occur before the onset of significant metabolic acidemia and potential injury?". The answer requires a clinical estimation of two factors: (1) time until vaginal delivery, (2) time until the onset of significant metabolic acidemia. These factors are discussed below.

Time until vaginal delivery

Consider cervical dilation, effacement, station, adequacy of uterine activity and expected rate of progress to estimate the time until vaginal delivery.

Time until possible onset of metabolic acidemia

With recurrent decelerations and minimal-absent variability, fetal metabolic acidemia can evolve over approximately 60–90 minutes (assuming a previously normal FHR tracing and no acute events) [24-27]. This process can progress more slowly or more rapidly, depending upon many factors, including the specific FHR pattern. If vaginal delivery is considered unlikely before the onset of metabolic acidemia and potential injury, the decision process should be documented and the patient counseled regarding the option of operative delivery. If labor is allowed to continue, the decision process should be documented and the FHR tracing reviewed at least every 15 minutes in the first stage of labor and every 5 minutes in the second stage [4]. Periodic documentation should include interpretation of the FHR tracing and the corresponding management plan.

Conclusion

The goal of intrapartum FHR monitoring is to prevent fetal injury that might result from interruption of normal fetal oxygenation during labor. With respect to fetal oxygenation, there are three central concepts in the interpretation of intrapartum FHR tracings.
• All clinically significant FHR decelerations reflect interruption of oxygen transfer from the environment to the fetus at one or more points along the oxygen pathway.
• Interrupted fetal oxygenation does not result in neurologic injury unless it progresses at least to the stage of significant metabolic acidemia (umbilical artery pH <7.0 and base deficit ≥12 mmol/L) [1].
• Moderate variability and/or accelerations are highly predictive of the absence of metabolic acidemia [2,3].
A systematic approach to the decision-making process underlying the management of intrapartum FHR tracings employs these three concepts to decide between three management options: routine intrapartum surveillance, heightened intrapartum surveillance or operative intervention. The decision process uses clinical judgment to weigh the benefit of vaginal delivery against the risk of fetal metabolic acidemia and takes into account the individual characteristics of the facility, staff, mother, fetus and labor. To determine whether vaginal delivery is likely before the onset of significant metabolic acidemia, clinical judgment is used to estimate:
• time until vaginal delivery
• time until possible onset of metabolic acidemia.
After considering these factors, an informed decision can be made with confidence that all key factors have been addressed. This systematic approach does not dictate decisions regarding management. It simply presents a standardized model for the decision-making process

that helps ensure effective communication, thorough documentation and, ultimately, patient safety.

References

1. American College of Obstetricians and Gynecologists' Task Force on Neonatal Encephalopathy and Cerebral Palsy, American College of Obstetricians and Gynecologists, American Academy of Pediatrics. *Neonatal encephalopathy and cerebral palsy: defining the pathogenesis and pathophysiology*. Washington, DC: American College of Obstetricians and Gynecologists, 2003.

2. Macones GA, Hankins GD, Spong CY, Hauth J, Moore T. The 2008 National Institute of Child Health and Human Development workshop report on electronic fetal monitoring: update on definitions, interpretation, and research guidelines. *Obstet Gynecol* 2008; 112(3): 661–666.

3. American College of Obstetricians and Gynecologists. Practice Bulletin No. 106: intrapartum fetal heart rate monitoring: nomenclature, interpretation, and general management principles. *Obstet Gynecol* 2009; 114: 192–202.

4. American Academy of Pediatrics (AAP), American College of Obstetricians and Gynecologists (ACOG). *Guidelines for perinatal care*. Washington, DC: American Academy of Pediatrics (AAP), American College of Obstetricians and Gynecologists, 2002.

5. Simpson KR, James DC. Efficacy of intrauterine resuscitation techniques in improving fetal oxygen status during labor. *Obstet Gynecol* 2005; 105: 1362–1368.

6. Althabe O, Schwarcz RL, Pose SV, Escarcena L, Caldeyro-Barcia R. Effects on fetal heart rate and fetal pO_2 of oxygen administration to the mother. *Am J Obstet Gynecol* 1967; 98: 858–870.

7. Khazin AF, Hon EH, Hehre FW. Effects of maternal hyperoxia on the fetus I. Oxygen tension. *Am J Obstet Gynecol* 1971; 109: 628–637.

8. Bartnicki J, Saling E. The influence of maternal oxygen administration on the fetus. *Int J Gynaecol Obstet* 1994; 45: 87–95.

9. Bartnicki J, Saling E. Influence of maternal oxygen administration on the computer-analysed fetal heart rate patterns in small-for-gestational-age fetuses. *Gynecol Obstet Invest* 1994; 37: 172–175.

10. Haydon ML, Gorenberg DM, Nageotte MP, *et al.* The effect of maternal oxygen administration on fetal pulse oximetry during labor in fetuses with nonreassuring fetal heart rate patterns. *Am J Obstet Gynecol* 2006; 195: 735–738.

11. McNamara H, Johnson N, Lilford R. The effect on fetal arteriolar oxygen saturation resulting from giving oxygen to the mother measured by pulse oximetry. *BJOG* 1993; 100: 446–449.

12. Thorp JA, Trobough T, Evans R, Hedrick J, Yeast JD. The effect of maternal oxygen administration during the second stage of labor on umbilical cord blood gas values: a randomized controlled prospective trial. *Am J Obstet Gynecol* 1995; 172: 46–74.

13. Abitbol MM. Supine position in labor and associated fetal heart rate changes. *Am J Obstet Gynecol* 1985; 65: 481–486.

14. Carbonne B, Benachi A, Leveque ML, Cabrol D, Papiernik E. Maternal position during labor: effects on fetal oxygen saturation measured by pulse oximetry. *Obstet Gynecol* 1996; 88: 797–800.

15. Association of Women's Health, Obstetric and Neonatal Nurses. *Nursing management of the second stage of labor. Evidence-based clinical practice guideline*. Washington, DC: Association of Women's Health, Obstetric and Neonatal Nurses, 2000.

16. Roberts J, Hanson J. Best practices in second stage labor care: maternal bearing down and positioning. *J Midwif Womens Health* 2007; 52: 238–245.

17. Simpson K, James DC. Effects of immediate versus delayed pushing during second-stage labor on fetal well-being: a randomized clinical trial. *Nurs Res* 2005; 54: 149–157.

18. Sameshima H, Ikenoue T. Predictive value of late decelerations for fetal acidemia in unselective low-risk pregnancies. *Am J Perinatol* 2005; 22: 19–23.

19. Williams KP, Galerneau F. Intrapartum fetal heart rate patterns in the prediction of neonatal acidemia. *Am J Obstet Gynecol* 2003; 188: 820–823.

20. Terek MC, Gundem G. Different types of variable decelerations and their effects on neonatal outcome. *Singapore Med J* 2003; 44: 243–247.

21. Hofmeyr GJ. Amnioinfusion for potential or suspected umbilical cord compression in labour. *Cochrane Database Syst Rev* 2007; 3.

22. Fraser WD, Hofmeyr J, Lede R, *et al.* Amnioinfusion for the prevention of the meconium aspiration syndrome. *NEJM* 2005; 353: 909–917.

23. American College of Obstetricians and Gynecologists. *Committee Opinion No 346. Amnioinfusion does not prevent meconium aspiration syndrome*. Washington, DC: American College of Obstetricians and Gynecologists, 2006.

24. Fleischer A, Schulman H, Jagani N, Mitchell J, Randolph G. The development of fetal acidosis in the presence of an abnormal fetal heart rate tracing. I. The average for gestational age fetus. *Am J Obstet Gynecol* 1982; 144: 55–60.

25. Low JA, Galbraith RS, Muir DW, Killen HL, Pater EA, Karchmar EJ. Factors associated with motor and cognitive deficits in children after intrapartum fetal hypoxia. *Am J Obstet Gynecol* 1982; 148: 533–539.

26. Ingemarsson I, Herbst A, Thorgren-Jerneck K. Long term outcome after umbilical artery acidemia at term birth: influence of gender and fetal heart rate abnormalities. *BJOG* 1997; 104: 1123–1127.

27. Parer JT, King T, Flanders S, Fox M, Kilpatrick SJ. Fetal acidemia and electronic fetal heart rate patterns. Is there evidence of an association? *J Matern Fetal Neonatal Med* 2006; 19: 289–294.

Chapter 44
Second- and Third-Trimester Obstetric Ultrasound

Giuliana S. Songster

Department of Medicine and Obstetrics and Gynecology, Keck School of Medicine, University of Southern California, CA, USA

Introduction

Ultrasound imaging has revolutionized obstetrics. The availability of this noninvasive diagnostic study, which produces no known harm on repeated patient exposure, has broadened the ascertainment of information about the condition of the fetus. That information can be used in concert with knowledge of the maternal status for obstetric decision making. This capability has, in the last three decades, significantly enhanced realization of the primary goal of obstetrics: a healthy outcome for both mother and baby.

Obstetric ultrasound imaging in the second and third trimester employs sound waves in the range 2–5 MHz (2–5 million cycles per second), transmitted into the mother's body from a transducer held at her skin surface. Returning echoes are computer analyzed and processed, and the resulting two-dimensional image is displayed on a screen. Rapid data acquisition and processing permit the display of successive images with sufficient rapidity to create the impression that one is observing movement of the imaged structures in real time. The capability to observe movement has led to several important applications. Ultrasound imaging has been used in obstetric practice for fetal measurement, determination of fetal position, assessment of fetal well-being, guidance for procedures, and diagnosis of structural or functional abnormalities. It is well accepted, even requested and enjoyed, by patients.

Standardization of the technique and content of the obstetric ultrasound examination has been developed through clinical research and collective experience for the purpose of optimizing the accuracy of the information obtained from each clinical ultrasound examination. Standards are summarized in publications of professional organizations, for example the American Institute of Ultrasound in Medicine (AIUM): *AIUM practice guideline for the performance of an antepartum obstetric ultrasound examination* [1] (www.aium.org). The clinician is referred to these standards for a greater level of detail.

Content of the standard second- or third-trimester examination

A standard second- or third-trimester examination includes documentation of fetal life, assessment of the intrauterine environment and maternal structures, fetal measurements, and a fetal anatomic survey. A limited examination is applicable to specific circumstances, such as intrapartum management, guidance for certain obstetric procedures, and assessment of fetal well-being after a previous complete standard examination has been performed. A standard examination is expected to include documentation of cardiac activity, fetal movement, number of fetuses and the position of the fetus(es) within the uterus. Maternal structures should be described, noting uterine anomalies, abnormalities of the uterine tissues such as leiomyomata, and the size and appearance of the adnexal structures, if they can be visualized. The intrauterine environment is described, including amount of amniotic fluid, subjective or semi-quantitative using the Amniotic Fluid Index, location and appearance of the placenta, including its proximity to the internal cervical os. Measurement of cervical length may be included if clinically indicated.

The second- and third-trimester ultrasound examination includes, importantly, standard fetal measurements which are used to verify clinical dating or establish gestational age if clinical dating information is absent or inaccurate. Once gestational dating is established, the measurements are used to evaluate fetal growth. Generally, the ultrasound performed earliest in gestation would be expected to be the most accurate predictor of gestational age. A later examiner may occasionally judge that revision of the dating based on a subsequent examination is justified due to unavailability of documentation or the clinical circumstances of the initial examination.

Management of Common Problems in Obstetrics and Gynecology, 5th edition. Edited by T.M. Goodwin, M.N. Montoro, L. Muderspach, R. Paulson and S. Roy. © 2010 Blackwell Publishing Ltd.

Four fetal parameters are routinely measured in the second and third trimesters: biparietal diameter (BPD), head circumference (HC), abdominal circumference (AC) and femur length (FL). Each parameter is measured by a specified technique and compared to a nomogram previously standardized on a well-dated pregnancy population [2-5]. Nomograms provided as charts for bedside comparison with measurement, or programmed into the software of the ultrasound equipment, display a mean ultrasound age associated with each standard measurement. If the mean age associated with each measurement is close to the known gestational age of the pregnancy, within 2 weeks, the gestational age and appropriate fetal growth are confirmed. If the measurements are discrepant with the gestational age or inconsistent with each other, a more detailed analysis is indicated. Measurement variation equivalent to plus or minus 2 weeks is a widely accepted and clinically useful estimate of accuracy applied to measurements in the middle trimester of pregnancy. Greater refinements of the estimates of variance for each parameter, if needed for research purposes, are available in the original literature reports [2-5].

Individual institutions or birth defects screening programs have adopted varying protocols for assignment of gestational age using ultrasound measurements. One method is assignment of the mean gestational age associated with the measured biparietal diameter. Another commonly practiced procedure is use of the average ultrasound age obtained by averaging the mean ultrasound ages associated with each of the four standard measurements, BPD, HC, AC, and FL [6]. Fetal weight estimates are calculated from formulae based on the standard parameters and compared with either nomograms of infant weights measured at birth or of ultrasound estimates [7,8]. The error of the ultrasound fetal weight estimate is in the range of ±18–20%.

Disparities in measurements may be caused by measurement error, congenital anomalies manifested by body asymmetry or fetal growth disorders. Diagnosis of a growth disorder, such as intrauterine growth restriction, requires more than the observation of discrepant mean gestational ages associated with standard measurements. A serial graphic analysis should be carried out, plotting each measurement on its growth curve, thus determining the growth profile of the fetus. The growth profile is then interpreted within the patient's clinical picture.

An anatomic survey is a necessary component of the standard obstetric second- and third-trimester examination. The minimum list of fetal structures to be included are those specified by the AIUM, the American College of Obstetricians and Gynecologists (ACOG), and the American College of Radiology (ACR). These are as follows. In the head, face and neck: cerebellum, choroid plexus, cisterna magna, lateral cerebral ventricles, mid-line falx, cavum septum pellucidum, upper lip; in the chest:

four-chamber heart view, ventricular outflow tracts if feasible; in the abdomen: stomach, kidneys, bladder, umbilical cord insertion into the fetal abdomen, umbilical cord vessel number; in the spine: cervical, thoracic, lumbar and sacral spine; in the extremities: presence or absence of legs and arms; sex: determination is medically indicated in multifetal gestations [9]. The above specified structures should be listed on the report with a comment, and so noted if they are not visualized. The question of whether a repeat examination should be scheduled to image structures that could not be seen on the current examination depends on the indication for the original examination and the relevance of those structures to the clinical question.

A detailed examination of an organ system, with a search for related abnormalities, would be appropriate in the case of an identified abnormality or a known risk for a fetal abnormality. Examination in a referral center with extensive experience in diagnosing anomalies is indicated in this circumstance. Specialized techniques including fetal Doppler sonography, biophysical profile, fetal echocardiogram or three-dimensional ultrasound visualization may be included in such a consultative evaluation.

Efficacy of ultrasound

Major anatomic malformations occur in 2–3% of births. The detection rate for these major structural abnormalities, using ultrasound as a screening tool in low-risk pregnancies, was found to be disappointingly low in the Routine Antenatal Diagnostic Imaging with Ultrasound (RADIUS) trial carried out under the auspices of the National Institute of Child Health and Human Development (NICHHD) between 1987 and 1991 [10]. In this study, encompassing community-based and tertiary referral centers, 71 of 232 (31%) major malformations present in the screened population were identified prenatally. This represented 47% of those types of malformations known to be potentially amenable to visualization by prenatal ultrasound. It should be possible to improve sensitivity modestly by acquiring additional views in the anatomic survey. However, these findings demonstrate the need for caution in the interpretation of ultrasound examination results. It is best to consider the possibility that additional information may come to light after birth, and to counsel patients accordingly.

Indications for a prenatal ultrasound examination

The NICHHD trial did not substantiate the efficacy of ultrasound used as a screening tool for improving neonatal outcome. A list of 28 indications, originally advocated by the NIH Consensus Conference on Diagnostic Ultrasound in Pregnancy, still serves as a useful checklist for prenatal ultrasound. That list includes: 1) gestational age assignment, 2) evaluation of fetal growth, 3) vaginal bleeding in pregnancy, 4) determination of fetal presentation, 5) suspected multiple gestation, 6) adjunct to amniocentesis, 7) size/dates discrepancy, 8) pelvic mass in pregnancy, 9) suspected hydatidiform mole, 10) adjunct to cervical cerclage placement, 11) suspected ectopic pregnancy, 12) adjunct to surgical procedures, 13) suspected fetal death, 14) suspected uterine abnormality, 15) intrauterine contraceptive device localization, 16) biophysical evaluation for fetal well-being, 17) observation of intrapartum events, 18) suspected polyhydramnios or oligohydramnios, 19) suspected abruptio placentae, 20) adjunct to external version from breech to vertex presentation, 21) estimation of fetal weight, 22) presentation in preterm labor and preterm rupture of membranes, 23) abnormal biochemical markers, 24) follow-up observation of identified fetal anomaly, 25) follow-up evaluation of placental location for identified placenta previa, 26) history of previous congenital anomaly, 27) serial evaluation of growth in multiple gestation, and 28) evaluation of fetal condition in late registrants for prenatal care [9]. In fact, one or more of these categories would apply to the majority of obstetric patients.

Documentation of the ultrasound examination

Creating and maintaining documentation of the ultrasound examination is extremely important for patient care and quality assurance. The documentation of an ultrasound examination should include a permanent record of the ultrasound images, including those used for measurements and those of the anatomic structures included in the survey of anatomy, each labeled with the examination date and patient identification. Photographic film, thermal copy, electronic storage and video recording are currently in use for the archiving of images. These image copies should be retained for the number of years consistent with clinical need and institutional policy. A report of the ultrasound findings and interpretation should be included in the patient's medical record.

Conclusion

Ultrasound use for diagnostic imaging has not been associated with clinically recognizable adverse bio-effects. However, some newer diagnostic modalities are associated with slightly higher patient exposures to sound energy. It is possible that effects not now defined might be identified

in the future. For these reasons, professional organizations concerned with diagnostic ultrasound have strongly recommended that patient exposure to ultrasound be limited to only that intensity and duration necessary for a thorough and adequate examination, and that ultrasound be performed only for medical indications. Patient safety is further addressed by attention to proper maintenance of equipment and to infection control. Guidelines to manage these concerns have been developed by the professional organizations who offer accreditation for ultrasound practices, the American Institute of Ultrasound in Medicine and the American College of Radiology.

Diagnostic ultrasound use in obstetrics has developed over the past three decades in terms of available technology and in application. It is a very beneficial adjunct to obstetric care, and has its greatest utility when performed in accordance with standard guidelines. New applications will undoubtedly be forthcoming and will be subjected to similar clinical trials of utility and safety.

References

1. American Institute of Ultrasound in Medicine. AIUM practice guideline for the performance of an antepartum obstetric ultrasound examination. *J Ultrasound Med* 2003; 22: 1116–1120.
2. Hadlock F, Deter R, Carpenter R, *et al.* Fetal biparietal diameter. A critical re-evaluation of the relation to menstrual age by means of real-time ultrasound. *J Ultrasound Med* 1982; 1: 97–99.
3. Hadlock F, Deter R, Harrist R, *et al.* Fetal abdominal circumference as a predictor of menstrual age. *AJR* 1982; 139: 367–371.
4. Hadlock F, Deter R, Harrist R, *et al.* Fetal femur length as a predictor of menstrual age: sonographically measured. *AJR* 1982; 138: 875–878.
5. Hadlock F, Deter R, Harrist R, *et al.* Fetal head circumference: relation to menstrual age. *AJR* 1982; 138: 649–652.
6. Hadlock FP, Deter RL, Harrist RB, *et al.* Estimating fetal age: computer-assisted analysis of multiple fetal growth parameters. *Radiology* 1984; 152: 497–501.
7. Hadlock FP, Harrist RB, Carpenter R, *et al.* Sonographic estimation of fetal weight. The value of femur length in addition to head and abdomen measurements. *Radiology* 1984; 150: 535–540.
8. Shepard MJ, Richards VA, Berkowitz RL. An evaluation of two equations for predicting fetal weight by ultrasound. *Am J Obstet Gynecol* 1982; 142: 47–54.
9. American College of Obstetricians and Gynecologists. *Ultrasonography in pregnancy. Practice Bulletin No. 58.* Washington, DC: American College of Obstetricians and Gynecologists, 2004.
10. Crane JP, LeFevre ML, Winborn RC, *et al.* A randomized trial of prenatal ultrasonographic screening: impact on detection, management, and outcome of anomalous fetuses. *Am J Obstet Gynecol* 1994; 171: 392–399.

Chapter 45
Prenatal Screening for Genetic Disorders

Giuliana S. Songster

Department of Medicine and Obstetrics and Gynecology, Keck School of Medicine, University of Southern California, CA, USA

Introduction

The great majority of birth defects and genetic disorders identified in the newborn period occur in families in which there is no family history of a genetic disease or any identifiable pre-existing risk factor. Genetic screening programs have been developed in an effort to identify pregnancies or couples at increased risk, for whom more definitive testing is warranted.

Carrier screening for autosomal recessive disorders

The American College of Obstetricians and Gynecologists recommends that heterozygote (carrier) screening be offered to members of specific ethnic groups at increased risk for certain well-characterized autosomal recessive disorders that have available highly sensitive and specific prenatal diagnostic tests.

α-Thalassemia occurs most often in individuals of African or Asian descent. It is caused by deletion of one or more of the four α-hemoglobin genes normally present. The most severe form, deletion of all four a genes, results in fetal hydrops and stillbirth. β-Thalassemia occurs most often in individuals of Middle Eastern or Mediterranean descent. The homozygous condition (thalassemia major, Cooley's anemia) renders an individual severely anemic in infancy. Prolongation of life requires frequent transfusions and is complicated by sequelae of iron overload.

The screening test for both types of thalassemia is the mean corpuscular volume (MCV). MCV is routinely included in an automated complete blood count (CBC). A value of 70 fL or less is a positive screening test result. Evaluation of a patient with a low MCV includes iron studies to exclude iron deficiency anemia as the etiology of low MCV, hemoglobin electrophoresis to define or exclude specific hemoglobinopathies, and paternal MCV to assess fetal risk. DNA testing on fetal cells is available for prenatal diagnosis of α- and β-thalassemias when indicated.

Sickle cell disease occurs primarily in individuals of African descent. It is characterized by a tendency of the red cells to become distorted under low oxygen tension. This causes vascular occlusion and infarction in somatic and visceral tissues, and results in painful crises. It may be fatal in early childhood. Sickle cell disease results from a single nucleotide substitution in each of the two β-hemoglobin genes. The mutation is identical in all affected individuals. The screening test for sickle cell disease carrier status is hemoglobin electrophoresis. DNA testing is available for prenatal diagnosis of sickle cell disease using fetal cells. A compound heterozygote, with a sickle hemoglobin gene and a β-thalassemia gene at the two β-hemoglobin loci, can result in a clinical picture similar to sickle cell disease.

Tay–Sachs disease occurs most frequently in individuals of Eastern European Jewish (Ashkenazi) ancestry. It has also been identified at increased frequency in a French-Canadian population. An individual homozygous for Tay–Sachs disease develops normally until the age of 6 months, then undergoes neurologic deterioration and dies in early childhood. Tay–Sachs disease results from deficiency of the enzyme hexosaminidase A. Carrier testing utilizes serum hexosaminidase A measurement. Enzyme levels are altered in pregnancy, requiring use of a leukocyte hexosaminidase measurement in the screening of pregnant patients. Prenatal diagnostic testing for Tay–Sachs disease is available for couples at risk, using a combination of DNA testing with enzyme assay in cultured fetal cells.

Cystic fibrosis (CF) is an autosomal recessive disorder. Manifestations include severe chronic lung disease with onset in early childhood, digestive enzyme deficiencies, and male infertility. The carrier rate for cystic fibrosis is increased in individuals of Northern European descent, and in those of Eastern European Jewish ancestry. Mutation

Management of Common Problems in Obstetrics and Gynecology, 5th edition. Edited by T.M. Goodwin, M.N. Montoro, L. Muderspach, R. Paulson and S. Roy. © 2010 Blackwell Publishing Ltd.

detection is possible with a high rate of sensitivity and specificity in these two groups. A recent NIH consensus conference report on cystic fibrosis screening made a broad recommendation for screening for all couples planning to have children. That recommendation is not supported on a cost–benefit basis for the population as a whole. It is reasonable to offer CF testing to couples with Northern European and Ashkenazi Jewish ancestries or other couples who express the desire to be tested when they present for genetic counseling and prenatal diagnosis. Interpretation and clinical decision making are complicated for couples who have positive CF screening results, due to inexact correlation between the genotype and phenotype and the evolution of treatment for the disorder, which has led to improved health and longevity for affected individuals.

Carrier testing is available for a large number of autosomal recessive and X-linked genetic disorders. It is of undisputed value for individuals with positive family histories. The integration of each proposed carrier test into prenatal screening programs designed for low-risk patients requires extremely careful analysis and judgment regarding costs, accuracy, and prognosis of the subject diseases, ethical and social concerns.

Prenatal multiple marker screening for structural and chromosomal defects

Serum multiple marker screening programs have been implemented throughout the USA and Europe. They are designed to detect fetal abnormalities in a patient's current pregnancy. The American College of Medical Genetics and the ACOG advocate offering this testing program to all women who present for obstetric care before the end of the gestational period for testing. The testing period for first-trimester programs is approximately 10–13 weeks. The testing period for second-trimester programs is in the range 15–20 weeks. Some states, for example California, have health regulations in place that mandate the offering of prenatal screening for birth defects to all pregnant women who present early enough in gestation to undergo screening. The programs are currently designed to detect three types of relatively common serious disorders.

Neural tube defects are present in 1 in 1000 to 1 in 500 births in the USA. They occur as a result of failure of closure of the embryonic neural tube before the end of the fourth week after conception. Anencephaly, a lethal malformation, involves failure of development of the cranium above the brow, and persistence of rudimentary vascularized tissue that represents the remnant of the maldeveloped brain structures. Approximately 97% of anencephalic fetuses in the screened population are detected by the maternal serum α-fetoprotein (MSAFP) screening program. Spina bifida results from failure of closure of the caudal aspect of the embryonic neural tube. The posterior elements of the bony neural canal, as well as overlying connective tissue and epithelium, subsequently fail to form, leaving the neural tissue exposed to the amniotic fluid. Open spina bifida, which comprises about 80% of spina bifida cases, is the form most readily detected, at a rate of approximately 80% using MSAFP and the current screening methodology. Spina bifida, whether open or membrane covered, results in weakness or paralysis of muscles below the spinal level of the lesion, and impairment of bowel or bladder function. Most individuals with spina bifida have associated hydrocephalus, which in many cases also leads to significant intellectual impairment.

High MSAFP, measured in the screening program, suggests an increased likelihood of a fetal open neural tube defect (anencephaly, spina bifida) or abdominal wall defect (gastroschisis, omphalocele). False-positive results may be due to fetal death *in utero*, multifetal gestation or wrong dates. MSAFP elevation confers an increased risk for preterm birth, intrauterine growth restriction or other adverse outcome, even if no sonographic abnormality is found.

Down syndrome is the result of an extra copy of chromosome 21 genetic material. It results in mental retardation, mild to severe, in all affected individuals. Heart defects are present in 40% of affected individuals. Medical illnesses, including thyroid disorders and leukemia, are more frequent. Twenty-eight percent of fetuses with Down syndrome expire *in utero* between the middle trimester and the end of pregnancy.

Second-trimester quadruple marker serum screening for Down syndrome currently uses assays for MSAFP, human chorionic gonadotropin (hCG), unconjugated estriol (UE3), and dimeric inhibin-A (DIA). Approximately 80% of pregnancies with fetal Down syndrome in the screened population are detected using current methods. The typical pattern of four analyses in a pregnancy affected with Down syndrome is MSAFP low, hCG high, UE3 low, and DIA high. Both the screen-positive rate and the detection rate increase with increasing maternal age, since the maternal age-related risk is a major component of the patient-specific risk calculation. A patient is designated screen positive for Down syndrome when the calculated risk yields a chance equal to or greater than the threshold risk (1 in 150 presently in the California program) in the middle trimester for identifying Down syndrome by amniocentesis. Approximately 4.5% of screened individuals in the California quadruple marker program have a screen-positive result for Down syndrome.

Trisomy 18 syndrome is a very severe mental retardation syndrome. Between 80% and 90% of affected individuals have heart defects, 20% have abdominal defects. An affected fetus often has multiple malformations. Seventy percent of fetuses with trisomy 18 syndrome expire *in utero* between the middle trimester and term. Ninety percent of those born alive die in the first year. The typical serum analyte pattern for trisomy 18 is low MSAFP, low hCG, low UE3 and low DIA. A patient-specific risk is calculated for trisomy 18. A patient is designated screen positive if her calculated risk is equal to or greater than the threshold risk (1 in 100 in the California program) for identifying trisomy 18 syndrome by middle-trimester amniocentesis. Approximately 67% of trisomy 18-affected pregnancies are detected by second-trimester serum screening as it is presently designed. About 0.31% of the screened population is referred for genetic services for a positive trisomy 18 screening test in the current California program.

Prenatal screening for fetal chromosomal abnormalities in the first trimester has now been instituted. The first-trimester screening tools include serum assays for pregnancy-associated plasma protein A (PAPP-A) and hCG. In addition, a specifically defined ultrasonic measurement of the thickness of the translucent region at the posterior aspect of the fetal neck (nuchal translucency or NT) may be included in the risk determination. A screen-positive result using these three measured parameters in combination with maternal age may be reported in the first trimester. Alternatively, a program may combine the first-trimester serum results, with or without the NT measurement, with the second-trimester quadruple marker screening results to produce either a full integrated screen result (with NT) or a serum integrated screening result (without NT). Both of the integrated screening tests have higher sensitivity and specificity than either the first-trimester or second-trimester screening tests alone.

Certain medical and demographic facts are necessary for interpretation of serum analyte values, since they differ in various population subgroups. They require the application of correction factors to the test results prior to risk calculation, in order to obtain accurate predictions. These include maternal age, gestational age, maternal weight, and maternal race, number of fetuses, diabetic status, and smoking history.

Maternal serum screening programs are often structured so that the patient undergoes an educational process and gives informed consent or refusal prior to drawing of the serum specimen. For individuals with positive screening tests, follow-up evaluation includes genetic counseling, with family history, consultative ultrasound, amniocentesis if indicated and desired by the patient, and follow-up counseling for abnormal results on diagnostic tests.

The performance parameters of the serum screening program are subject to periodic review. Innovations are regularly introduced to promote improvements. Additional analytes and/or measurements will eventually augment or replace some of those in current use.

The role of second-trimester ultrasound for aneuploidy screening is controversial. Major structural malformations detected by ultrasound confer a significant risk for fetal aneuploidy, and most serve as appropriate indications for offering invasive procedures for chromosome analysis. A variety of minor malformations or biometric variations have been promoted as indicators of fetal chromosome abnormalities. These have included shorter than normal humeri and femurs, nuchal skinfold thickening, choroid plexus cysts, fetal hand position, excess amniotic fluid, and pyelectasis. To date, none of these observed abnormalities has been confirmed to have sufficient sensitivity and specificity to warrant their establishment as screening parameters. At the present time, identification of one or more minor malformations or biometric variants should serve as an indication for a detailed survey of fetal anatomy. The risk for chromosome abnormality should be viewed in the context of all available maternal demographic and medical information, prior to counseling regarding the possible benefit of chromosome analysis.

Suggested reading

American College of Obstetricians and Gynecologists. *Hemoglobinopathies in pregnancy. Practice Bulletin no 78.* Washington, DC: American College of Obstetricians and Gynecologists, 2007.

American College of Obstetricians and Gynecologists. *Screening for fetal chromosomal abnormalities. Practice Bulletin No 77.* Washington, DC: American College of Obstetricians and Gynecologists, 2007.

California Department of Public Health. *The California Prenatal Screening Program prenatal care provider handbook.* Richmond, CA: California Department of Public Health Genetic Disease Screening Program, 2009.

Filly RA. Obstetrical sonography: the best way to terrify a pregnant woman. *J Ultrasound Med* 2000; 19: 1–3.

Gelehrter TD, Collins FS, Ginsburg D, Eds. *Principles of medical genetics,* 2nd edn. Baltimore, MD: Lippincott Williams and Wilkins, 1998.

Kilpatrick SJ, Laros RK. Maternal hematologic disorders. In: Creasy, RK, Resnik, R (eds) *Maternal fetal medicine,* 4th edn. Philadelphia, PA: WB Saunders, 1999: 935–963.

National Institutes of Health. Genetic testing for cystic fibrosis. *NIH Consensus Statement* 1997; 15(4): 1–37.

Sohl BD, Scioscia AL, Budorick NE, *et al.* Utility of minor ultrasonographic markers in the prediction of abnormal fetal karyotype at a prenatal diagnostic center. *Am J Obstet Gynecol* 1999; 181: 898–903.

Chapter 46
Antepartum Testing

David A. Miller

Department of Medicine and Obstetrics and Gynecology, Keck School of Medicine, University of Southern California, CA, USA

Introduction

The goals of antepartum testing are (1) to identify fetuses in jeopardy so that permanent injury or death might be prevented and (2) to identify healthy fetuses so that unnecessary intervention can be avoided. The key measure of an antepartum test is the false-negative rate, usually defined as the incidence of fetal death within 1 week of a normal antepartum test. Another important measure is the false-positive rate. A false-positive test usually is defined as an abnormal test that prompts delivery but is not associated with evidence of acute disruption of fetal oxygenation (meconium, intrapartum "fetal distress" or low Apgar scores) or chronic disruption of fetal oxygenation (fetal growth restriction, oligohydramnios).

Antepartum testing is used primarily in patients at increased risk for disrupted fetal oxygenation. Common obstetric and medical indications for antepartum testing are summarized in Box 46.1. For most medical indications, testing is initiated by 32–34 weeks. Tables 46.1 and 46.2 summarize the usual timing of antepartum testing for medical and obstetric indications.

The contraction stress test (oxytocin challenge test)

The contraction stress test (CST) or oxytocin challenge test (OCT) arose from intrapartum observations linking late decelerations with poor perinatal outcome. The test seeks to identify transient fetal hypoxemia by demonstrating late decelerations in fetuses exposed to the stress of spontaneous (CST) or induced (OCT) uterine contractions. Kubli and associates found that late decel-

---

> **Box 46.1 Indications for antepartum testing**
>
> **Obstetric indications**
> Post-term pregnancy
> Unexplained elevated AFP, hCG
> Cholestasis of pregnancy
> Antiphospholipid syndrome
> Previous unexplained stillbirth
> Suspected fetal growth restriction
> Decreased fetal movement
> Pre-eclampsia
> Multiple gestation (discordant)
> Alloimmunization
> Oligohydramnios
>
> **Medical indications**
> Diabetes
> Chronic hypertension
> Cyanotic cardiac disease
> Renal disease
> Thyroid disease
> Collagen vascular disease
> Pulmonary disease (severe asthma)
> Hemoglobinopathy

erations occurring during spontaneous uterine contractions were associated with increased rates of fetal death, growth retardation and neonatal depression [1]. Similar observations were made by other investigators using oxytocin or nipple stimulation to provoke uterine contractions. The CST is performed weekly and is interpreted as summarized in Box 46.2.

The CST is considered negative if there are at least three uterine contractions in a 10-minute period with no late decelerations on the tracing. In this case, the routine testing schedule is resumed. Unsatisfactory, suspicious or equivocal tests require repeat testing the following day. Usually, a positive CST or OCT warrants hospitalization for further evaluation and/or delivery. Freeman and colleagues tested more than 4600 women with the CST and reported a false-negative rate of 0.4/1000 [2].

Management of Common Problems in Obstetrics and Gynecology, 5th edition. Edited by T.M. Goodwin, M.N. Montoro, L. Muderspach, R. Paulson and S. Roy. © 2010 Blackwell Publishing Ltd.

Table 46.1 Timing of initiation of antepartum testing for medical indications

Medical indications	Timing
Gestational diabetes (diet controlled)	40 weeks
Gestational diabetes (insulin)	32–34 weeks
Type 1 or 2 diabetes	32–34 weeks
Chronic hypertension	32–34 weeks
Cyanotic cardiac disease	32–34 weeks
Renal disease	32–34 weeks
Thyroid disease	32–34 weeks
Collagen vascular disease	32–34 weeks
Pulmonary disease (severe asthma)	32–34 weeks
Hemoglobinopathy	32–34 weeks

Box 46.2 Interpretation of the CST

Negative: No late or significant variable decelerations
Positive: Late decelerations with ≥ 50% or more of contractions (even if the contraction frequency is fewer than three in 10 minutes)
Equivocal-suspicious: Intermittent late decelerations or significant variable decelerations
Equivocal-hyperstimulatory: Fetal heart rate decelerations that occur in the presence of contractions more frequent than every 2 minutes or lasting longer than 90 seconds
Unsatisfactory: Fewer than three contractions in 10 minutes or an uninterpretable tracing

Table 46.2 Timing of initiation of antepartum testing for obstetric indications

Obstetric indications	Timing
Post-term pregnancy	40–41 weeks
Unexplained elevated AFP, hCG	32–34 weeks
Cholestasis of pregnancy	32–34 weeks
Antiphospholipid antibody syndrome	32–34 weeks
Previous unexplained stillbirth	32–34 weeks*
Suspected fetal growth restriction	At diagnosis
Decreased fetal movement	At diagnosis
Pre-eclampsia	At diagnosis
Multiple gestation (discordant)	At diagnosis
Alloimmunization	At diagnosis
Oligohydramnios	At diagnosis

* Or 1 week earlier than previous loss.

Reported false-positive rates range from 8% to 57% with an average of approximately 30% [3]. The advantages of this form of testing include excellent sensitivity and a weekly testing interval. Limitations include a high rate of equivocal results requiring repeat testing, increased expense and inconvenience (particularly if oxytocin is required), and increased time requirement compared to nonprovocative tests. Additionally, the CST is contraindicated in several clinical settings, including preterm labor, placenta previa, vasa previa, cervical incompetence, multiple gestation and previous classic cesarean.

The nonstress test

Fetal heart rate accelerations that occur in association with fetal movements form the basis of the NST. A normal or "reactive" NST usually is defined by two accelerations in a 20-minute period, each lasting at least 15 seconds and peaking at least 15 bpm above the baseline. Before 32 weeks, an acceleration is defined as a rise of at least 10 bpm lasting at least 10 seconds [4,5]. The test usually is repeated once or twice weekly. Boehm reported that the latter approach yielded a threefold reduction in the incidence of fetal death [6]. A FHR acceleration in response to fetal vibroacoustic stimulation (VAS) is highly predictive of normal fetal pH [7,8]. If the FHR tracing is not spontaneously reactive, VAS can be performed by placing an artificial larynx on the maternal abdomen over the fetal head continuously for 1–5 seconds.

Among 1542 women tested weekly with the NST, Freeman reported a false-negative rate of 1.9/1000 [2]. Manning reported an average false-negative rate of 6.4/1000 among nine large clinical trials using the NST as the primary method of surveillance [9]. Decelerations may be observed in 33–50% of patients undergoing weekly NSTs [10-12]. In one study, reactive tests accompanied by variable decelerations were associated with rates of meconium passage and cesarean for fetal indications that were similar to those encountered with nonreactive tests [12]. The authors concluded that FHR decelerations during the NST, regardless of reactivity, warrant consideration of delivery. Reported false-positive rates of the NST vary widely, with an average rate of approximately 50%. A reactive NST with no significant decelerations is considered a normal test and the routine testing schedule is resumed (usually once or twice weekly). A nonreactive NST requires further evaluation. In most cases, a back-up test is performed (contraction stress test or biophysical profile).

Management is guided by the results of the back-up test. When performed twice weekly, the NST alone appears to be an acceptable, though not optimal, method of antepartum testing. Advantages include ease of use and interpretation, low cost, and minimal time requirement. The chief disadvantages include a twice-weekly testing interval, a high false-positive rate, and a higher false-negative rate than achieved with other methods.

The biophysical profile

The BPP assesses five biophysical variables. FHR reactivity, fetal movement, tone and breathing indicate the absence of significant metabolic acidemia, while normal amniotic fluid volume indicates adequate fetal oxygenation and the absence of chronic central shunting [13]. Two points are assigned for each normal variable and zero points for each abnormal variable, for a maximum score of 10 (Table 46.3). A BPP score of 8–10, with normal amniotic fluid volume, is considered normal and the routine testing schedule is resumed. A score of 6 is considered suspicious, and testing usually is repeated the following day. Scores < 6 are associated with increased perinatal morbidity and mortality, and usually warrant hospitalization for further evaluation or delivery. One study reported a false-negative rate of 0.6/1000 among 12,620 women tested weekly with the BPP [14]. Another study reported significantly lower rates of cesarean delivery for fetal distress (3% vs 22%), low 5-minute Apgar scores (1.6% and 3.2% vs 12.5%) and meconium aspiration syndrome when the last BPP before delivery was normal than when it was abnormal [15]. Among 19,221 high-risk pregnancies, Manning reported a false-negative rate of 0.7 per 1000 [16]. The false-positive rate of the BPP ranges from 0% if the last BPP score before delivery was 0 to more than 40% if the last BPP score was 6. Advantages of the BPP include excellent sensitivity, a weekly testing interval, a low false-negative rate and improved detection of structural fetal anomalies. The primary limitation is the requirement for personnel trained in sonographic visualization of the fetus.

The modified biophysical profile

The modified biophysical profile (MBPP) utilizes the NST as a short-term marker of fetal status and the AFI as a marker of longer-term placental function. The AFI is calculated as the sum of the deepest vertical cord-free pockets of amniotic fluid in each of the four uterine quadrants. Normal AFI is ≥ 10 cm. Low normal AFI is > 5 cm but < 10 cm. Low AFI or oligohydramnios is ≤ 5 cm. The upper limit of normal AFI (polyhydramnios) is in the region of 25 cm. Regardless of reactivity, oligohydramnios constitutes an abnormal test. Management of the MBPP is summarized in Figure 46.1.

Nageotte evaluated 2774 high-risk pregnancies with twice-weekly MBPPs and reported a false-negative rate of 0.36/1000 [17]. Miller and colleagues reported a false-negative rate of 0.8/1000, and a false-positive rate of 60% in 15,482 high-risk pregnancies [18]. The fetal death rate in tested "high-risk" patients was nearly sevenfold lower than that in the untested, "low-risk" population. Usually, the AFI is performed with the NST twice weekly. Alternatively, weekly AFI determinations may be reasonable prior to 41 weeks, provided that the AFI remains > 8 cm [19,20]. The MBPP is easier to perform and less time-consuming than the CST or the complete BPP. The sensitivity is superior to that of the NST alone and similar to that of the CST and complete BPP. Limitations include the need for back-up testing in 10–50% of patients, a high false-positive rate and a twice-weekly testing interval.

Fetal movement counts

Maternal perception of normal fetal movement has long been recognized as a reliable indicator of fetal well-being. Cessation of fetal movement in response to hypoxia has been demonstrated in animal studies, but controlled data in human fetuses are lacking. Nevertheless, any acute decrement in the number or strength of fetal movements should prompt further evaluation. Many clinicians recommend routine fetal movement counting, particularly in patients who are considered high risk [21-23]. A common approach is to recommend daily counting of fetal movements for 1 hour. Ten fetal movements in a 1-hour period are considered reassuring. If fewer than 10 movements are

Table 46.3 Biophysical profile scoring

Biophysical variable	Normal (score = 2)	Abnormal (score = 0)
Fetal breathing movements	At least one episode of fetal breathing movements of at least 30-second duration in a 30-min observation	Absent fetal breathing movements or <30 s of sustained fetal breathing movements in 30 min
Fetal movements	At least three trunk or limb movements in 30 min	Fewer than three episodes of trunk or limb movements in 30 min
Fetal tone	At least one episode of active extension with return to flexion of fetal limb or trunk; opening and closing of hand considered normal tone	Absence of movement or slow extension/flexion
AFI	AFI >5 cm or at least one pocket >2 cm	AFI ≥ 5 cm and no single pocket >2 cm
NST	Reactive	Nonreactive

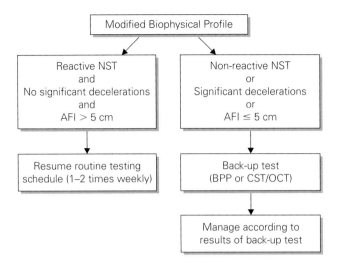

Figure 46.1 Management of the MBPP.

appreciated, counting is continued for another hour. Fewer than 10 movements in a 2-hour period should prompt further evaluation. One study demonstrated a lower rate of fetal death and a higher incidence of intervention for fetal distress in patients using a formalized protocol of fetal movement counting [21].

Umbilical artery Doppler velocimetry

Recent studies have shown significant improvement in perinatal outcome with the use of Doppler ultrasonography in pregnancies complicated by fetal growth restriction [24,25]. Although severe restriction of umbilical artery blood flow, as evidenced by absent or reversed flow during diastole, has been correlated with fetal growth restriction, acidosis and adverse perinatal outcome, the predictive values of less extreme deviations from normal remain undefined. In conditions other than fetal growth restriction, Doppler velocimetry does not appear to be a useful screening test for the detection of fetal compromise. It is not recommended for use as a screening test in low-risk patients. Doppler velocimetry of the middle cerebral artery demonstrates increased diastolic flow in the setting of reduced fetal oxygenation, reflecting the "brain-sparing" effect of hypoxemia [26]. When Doppler velocimetry measurements are used in antepartum fetal surveillance, they should be interpreted in the context of the clinical setting and the results of other tests of fetal condition.

Conclusion

Electronic FHR monitoring is a very sensitive tool for the detection of disrupted fetal oxygenation; truly compromised fetuses rarely fail to exhibit abnormal FHR patterns. The converse, however, is not true. FHR

decelerations, tachycardia and intermittent reduction in variability and/or accelerations frequently are observed in the absence of fetal compromise. The limited positive predictive value is the principal shortcoming of FHR monitoring. Despite the limitations, antepartum testing in "high-risk" pregnancies has been reported to yield a fetal death rate lower than that observed in untested, "low-risk" pregnancies. If this observation is substantiated, future investigation will be needed to address the role of antepartum fetal surveillance in uncomplicated, low-risk pregnancies.

References

1. Kubli FW, Hon EH, Khazin AF, Takemura H. Observations on heart rate and pH in the human fetus during labor. *Am J Obstet Gynecol* 1969; 104: 1190.
2. Freeman RK, Anderson G, Dorchester W. A prospective multi-institutional study of antepartum fetal heart rate monitoring. II. Contraction stress test versus nonstress test for primary surveillance. *Am J Obstet Gynecol* 1982; 143: 778.
3. Lagrew DC Jr. The contraction stress test. *Clin Obstet Gynecol* 1995; 38(1): 11–25.
4. National Institute of Child Health and Human Development Research Planning Workshop. Electronic fetal heart rate monitoring: research guidelines for interpretation. *Am J Obstet Gynecol* 1997; 177: 1385–1390.
5. American College of Obstetricians and Gynecologists. Intrapartum fetal heart rate monitoring. ACOG Practice Bulletin No. 70. *Obstet Gynecol* 2005; 106: 1453–1461.
6. Boehm FH, Salyer S, Shah DM, Vaughn WK. Improved outcome of twice weekly nonstress testing. *Obstet Gynecol* 1986; 67: 566.
7. Elimian A, Figueroa R, Tejani N. Intrapartum assessment of fetal well-being: a comparison of scalp stimulation with scalp blood pH sampling. *Obstet Gynecol* 1997; 89: 373–376.
8. Skupski DW, Rosenberg CR, Eglington GS. Intrapartum fetal stimulation tests: a meta-analysis. *Obstet Gynecol* 2002; 99: 129–134.
9. Manning FA, Lange IR, Morrison I, Harman CR. Determination of fetal health: methods for antepartum and intrapartum fetal assessment. *Curr Prob Obstet Gynecol* 1983; 7: 3.
10. Phelan JP, Platt LD, Yeh S-Y, *et al*. Continuing role of the nonstress test in the management of post-dates pregnancy. *Obstet Gynecol* 1984; 64: 624–628.
11. Meis PJ, Ureda JR, Swain M, Kelly RT, Penry M, Sharp P. Variable decelerations during nonstress tests are not a sign of fetal compromise. *Am J Obstet Gynecol* 1986; 154: 586–590
12. Phelan JP, Lewis PE Jr. Fetal heart rate decelerations during a nonstress test. *Obstet Gynecol* 1981; 57; 228–232.
13. Manning FA, Platt LD, Sipos L. Antepartum fetal evaluation: development of a fetal biophysical profile. *Am J Obstet Gynecol* 1980; 136: 787.
14. Manning FA, Morrison I, Lange I, *et al*. Fetal assessment based upon fetal BPP scoring: experience in 12,620 referred high risk pregnancies. I. Perinatal mortality by frequency and etiology. *Am J Obstet Gynecol* 1985; 151: 343.

15. Johnson JM, Harman CR, Lange IR, *et al*. Biophysical profile scoring in the management of postterm pregnancy: an analysis of 307 patients. *Am J Obstet Gynecol* 1986; 154: 269.

16. Manning FA, Morrison I, Harman CR, Lange IR, Menticoglou S. Fetal assessment based on fetal biophysical profile scoring: experience in 19,221 referred high-risk pregnancies. II. An analysis of false-negative fetal deaths. *Am J Obstet Gynecol* 1987; 157: 880–884.

17. Nageotte JP, Towers CV, Asrat T, Freeman RK. Perinatal outcome with the MBPP. *Am J Obstet Gynecol* 1994; 170: 1672.

18. Miller DA, Rabello YA, Paul RH. The modified biophysical profile: antepartum testing in the 1990's. *Am J Obstet Gynecol* 1996; 174: 812.

19. Lagrew DC, Pircon RA, Nageotte M, Freeman RK, Dorchester W. How frequently should the amniotic fluid index be repeated? *Am J Obstet Gynecol* 1992; 167(4 Pt 1): 1129–1133.

20. Wing DA, Fishman A, Gonzalez C, Paul RH. How frequently should the amniotic fluid index be performed during the course of antepartum testing? *Am J Obstet Gynecol* 1996; 174: 33.

21. Moore TR, Piacquadio K. A prospective evaluation of fetal movement screening to reduce the incidence of antepartum fetal death. *Am J Obstet Gynecol* 1989; 160: 1075–1080.

22. Neldam S. Fetal movements as an indicator of fetal well-being. Dan Med Bull 1983; 30: 274–278.

23. Grant A, Elbourne D, Valentin L, Alexander S. Routine formal fetal movement counting and risk of antepartum late death in normally formed singletons. *Lancet* 1989; 2(8659): 345–349.

24. Alfirevic Z, Neilson JP. Doppler ultrasonography in high-risk pregnancies: systematic review with meta-analysis. *Am J Obstet Gynecol* 1995; 172: 1379.

25. Maulik D. Doppler ultrasound in obstetrics. In: Cunningham G, MacDonald P, Gant N, Leveno K, Gilstrap L (eds) *Williams obstetrics, supplement*. Stanford, CT: Appleton and Lange, 1996.

26. Bahado-Singh RO, Kovanci E, Jeffres A, *et al*. The Doppler cerebroplacental ratio and perinatal outcome in intrauterine growth restriction. *Am J Obstet Gynecol* 1999; 180: 750–756.

Chapter 47
Preconception Counseling and Reproductive Life Planning

Carolina Reyes

Department of Medicine and Obstetrics and Gynecology, Keck School of Medicine, University of Southern California, CA, USA

Introduction

Preparing for a desired pregnancy is a major step towards reducing risks for both mom and baby. For women who do not desire a pregnancy, preconception care can raise awareness about potential health risks and reduce the chance of an unwanted pregnancy. The American Academy of Pediatrics and the American College of Obstetricians and Gynecologists jointly recommend that all health encounters during a woman's reproductive years should include counseling on appropriate medical care and behavior to optimize pregnancy outcomes. Preconception care is recognized not just as a single clinical visit but a process of care tailored to support a woman as she develops a reproductive life plan, identifying factors that can be positively modified to improve maternal and neonatal outcome. A reproductive life plan includes developing a set of personal goals about having (or not having) children based on personal values and resources, and a plan to achieve those goals.

The primary objective of a complete preconception care assessment is to identify factors that can be modified. This includes obtaining a comprehensive medical, periodontal and surgical history, genetic history, reproductive history and family plans, drug history, immunization and infectious disease history, lifestyle and psychosocial history, and a nutrition assessment (Table 47.1).

Preconception counseling

Genetic factors
A three-generation family history of birth defects and inheritable disorders, including race and ethnicity of both parents, can provide significant information about the potential heritability of a disorder. Further testing

Table 47.1 Preconception care: complete risk assessment

Risk factor	Comments
Medical	General health and review of systems, prior diagnosis of chronic condition (diabetes, cancer, cardiovascular, eye disorders)
Genetic	Maternal age, maternal and paternal medical history, a three-generation family history, known genetic disorders, congenital malformations, chromosomal disorders, developmental delay, heart defects, neural tube defects, recurrent miscarriages
Medication and other drugs	Type of medication, frequency, dosing
Family	Medical illness
Environmental	Smoking and alcohol history, home, community and workplace environment
Immunizations and infections	Vaccination and infection history reviewed and updated
Lifestyle	Ideal bodyweight, exercise planning
Nutrition	Nutrition assessment, fish consumption, dietary planning
Reproductive history	Obstetric history, identify modifiable risks
Family planning	Family spacing and contraception

should be recommended when there is a positive family history in the patient or her partner. Common disorders include Tay–Sachs disease (more common in Eastern European Jewish background but also recommended for a French-Canadian or Cajun background); thalassemia (more common in persons of Mediterranean or Asian background); sickle cell anemia (more common among Africans and African Americans); cystic fibrosis (more common in persons of European descent); muscular dystrophy, and Huntington's chorea. With a family history of mental retardation, testing for fragile X syndrome should be considered. Aneuploidy in offspring of women less than 35 years old warrants further testing for paternal or maternal balanced translocations. Women over age 35 should be informed of the increased risk of aneuploidy.

Management of Common Problems in Obstetrics and Gynecology, 5th edition. Edited by T.M. Goodwin, M.N. Montoro, L. Muderspach, R. Paulson and S. Roy. © 2010 Blackwell Publishing Ltd.

Reproductive history

A review of a woman's reproductive history will help identify factors related to a prior pregnancy that may be modifiable and the risk reduced for future pregnancies. With an unexpected pregnancy outcome such as preterm birth, severe pre-eclampsia, stillbirth or cesarean delivery, the patient may not have consulted with her obstetrician after delivery to discuss risks of recurrence in a subsequent pregnancy. Women with a prior preterm birth have a 16% risk of a second preterm birth. The risk increases significantly with two preterm (41%) and three preterm deliveries (67%). Modifiable risk factors associated with recurrent preterm birth include inflammatory changes in the placenta, low maternal pre-pregnancy weight, smoking, short interpregnancy interval (< 12 months), history of cervical insufficiency and periodontal disease, and uterine anomalies.

Women with a history of recurrent spontaneous abortion, three or more consecutive spontaneous abortions, should be offered a work-up to identify a cause. This includes measurement of antiphospholipid antibodies (lupus anticoagulant, anticardiolipin and β2-glycoprotein antibodies), parental karyotyping, and imaging of the uterus. Women with antiphospholipid antibody syndrome can initiate treatment with mini heparin prior to a planned pregnancy. Uterine anomalies and cervical incompetence have the potential to be surgically corrected prior to pregnancy.

Patients with a prior stillbirth have a risk of recurrence increased 2–10-fold over women with no prior stillbirth. A complete medical and obstetric history and a review of the available reports, including fetal autopsy, placental pathology and appropriate testing of the prior stillbirth, can identify potential risk factors and guide the consultation. Previous stillbirth can be associated with genetic disease, chromosomal disorders, and undiagnosed maternal conditions, such as diabetes or antiphospholipid antibody syndrome. A preconception visit should be individualized based on careful questioning and identification of the possible etiology to establish appropriate consultation and a care plan for the next pregnancy. Couples may require additional psychosocial support.

Women planning a subsequent delivery after a previous cesarean can be counseled about the maternal and newborn risks and benefits associated with a trial of labor versus elective cesarean. Family spacing greater than 18 months is recommended since uterine rupture with a trial of labor is reduced with this spacing. A review of potential operative morbidity with multiple cesareans and a risk assessment developing a placenta previa or accreta is warranted.

Chronic medical conditions and any complications associated with a prior pregnancy are important factors to review in preparing a care plan for future pregnancies. There is no substitute for a comprehensive assessment, including review of prior medical records.

Immunization and infectious disease history

A preconception care consultation should include a review of the woman's vaccination history and immunizations should be brought up to date. Table 47.2 identifies recommended immunizations for women of reproductive age. Rubella, poliomyelitis and varicella-zoster vaccinations are live-attenuated and are recommended to be completed 3 months prior to conception. Immunity for rubella and chickenpox should be tested prior to vaccination. Patients should be counseled to use an effective family planning method during this period. A tetanus booster should be given every 10 years and can be given during pregnancy. Vaccination for hepatitis B surface antigen should be provided to seronegative women who are at high risk of exposure, such as healthcare workers, those with multiple

Table 47.2 Vaccinations recommended prior to pregnancy

Vaccination/toxoid	Type	Recommendation	Use in pregnancy
Rubella, MMR	Live-attenuated	Vaccinate all child-bearing nonimmune women	Avoid pregnancy for 3 months
Tetanus	Diphtheria toxoid	Vaccinate all nonimmune or if last booster > 10 years	No contraindication
Hepatitis B	Recombinant	High-risk individuals	No contraindication
Influenza	Inactivated	Immunosuppressed, chronic disease (diabetes, sickle cell, renal disease, SLE, HIV), healthcare workers	Third trimester of pregnancy
Human papilloma virus	Quadrivalent	Women and girls aged 9–26 years	Not in pregnancy
Poliomyelitis	Live-attenuated	All women born after 1956; oral or injected	Oral not recommended IPV-e recommended if high risk for exposure
Pneumococcal	Inactive	Recommend in chronic medical conditions	If chronic medical disease
Varicella-zoster	Live-attenuated	Recommend in adolescents and nonimmune adults	Contraindicated

sexual partners, drug injectors, those with a partner who engages in these behaviors. Vaccination can reduce the risk of perinatal transmission.

Screening for chlamydia, gonococcal infection, syphilis, HPV and HIV should be offered. The HPV vaccine is recommended for women and girls between the ages of 9 and 26 years.

Drug exposure

Drug exposure accounts for 2–3% of birth defects. Medications can be an effective method to control chronic or acute medical conditions prior to pregnancy, such as hypertension, diabetes, mental health disorders, seizures, infections, and hypercholesterolemia. Unfortunately, some commonly prescribed medications are known teratogens. General caution is advised when prescribing medication to women of reproductive age to avoid medication with high teratogenic risk when an alternative medication that poses less risk is available. Women of reproductive age should be counseled about the potential teratogenic risk whether they are planning a pregnancy or not. A thorough history of medication use should include the type of medication, frequency of use, and dosage. The Federal Drug Administration system for classification is provided in Table 47.3. Medications that are known teratogens are listed in Table 47.4.

The most common drug exposures, smoking and alcohol use, are preventable causes of birth defects and developmental disabilities. Tobacco exposure is harmful to both mother and fetus. Fetal exposure can result in intrauterine growth restriction, prematurity, low birthweight, and sudden infant death syndrome. Women who smoke are at increased risk of a range of cancers, cardiovascular disease, and pulmonary disease. Maternal exposure can lead to premature rupture of membranes,

Table 47.3 FDA classification of medication safety during pregnancy

Category	Description
A	Adequate, well-controlled studies in pregnant women have not shown an increased risk of fetal abnormalities
B	Animal studies show no evidence of harm to the fetus, but no adequate and well-controlled studies in pregnant women, or human studies show no risk despite animal studies showing an adverse effect
C	Animal studies have shown an adverse effect and there are no adequate and well-controlled studies in pregnant women; or no animal studies have been conducted and no adequate and well-controlled studies in pregnant women
D	Studies in pregnant women demonstrate a risk to the fetus. However, the benefits outweigh the risk
X	Studies in animals or pregnant women have demonstrated positive evidence of fetal abnormalities. Contraindicated in pregnant women or women who may become pregnant
Undetermined	No pregnancy category from the FDA; other sources are used to assess safety

Table 47.4 Medications that are known teratogens

Medication	FDA code	Fetal risk
Angiotensin-converting enzyme (ACE) inhibitors	D	Fetal renal tubular dysplasia, oligohydramnios, growth restriction, hypoplastic lung
Androgens and testosterone	D	Virilization of female fetus; advanced genital development in male
Folic acid antagonist (methotrexate)	X	Spontaneous abortion, growth restriction, hydrocephalus, cleft palate
Isotretinoin	X	CNS defects, cleft palate, external ear and skull defects, cardiovascular defects
Thalidomide	X	Limb reduction, cardiac and gastrointestinal anomalies
Carbamazepine	D	Neural tube defects, minor craniofacial defects, microcephaly, fingernail hypoplasia, developmental delay
Lithium	D	Cardiac defects, Epstein's anomaly
Phenytoin	D	Cleft lip and palate, growth restriction, microcephaly, dysmorphic cranial features, hypoplasia of distal phalanges, heart defects
Tetracycline	D	Hypoplasia of tooth enamel, permanent yellow-brown discoloration
Trimethadione	D	Cleft lip and palate, microcephaly, growth restriction, mental deficiency, facial appearance characteristic, cardiac defects
Phenobarbital	D	Cleft lip and palate, growth restriction, microcephaly
Valproic acid	D	Neural tube defect, spina bifida, minor facial defects
Diethylstilbestrol	X	Genital tract malformations, vaginal adenosis, clear cell carcinoma
Streptomycin	D	Risk of ototoxicity
HMG-CoA reductase inhibitors (statins)	D	
Aspirin	D	Neonatal hemorrhage, decreased birthweight, prolonged gestation, increased perinatal mortality

placenta previa, and placental abruption. Screening for tobacco in the clinical setting is usually based on patient self-reporting. Referral to intensive counseling and cessation programs should be available. A useful guide for clinicians (*Helping smokers quit: a guide for clinicians*) is available from the US Agency for Health Care Research and Quality. Alcohol is a known teratogen that affects the development of the central nervous system throughout pregnancy. Fetal alcohol syndrome is the most commonly experienced condition of the fetal alcohol spectrum disorder. There is no established safe level of alcohol during pregnancy. Validated screening tools are available, such as TWEAK, T-ACE and AUDIT. Systematic reviews have concluded that brief alcohol interventions are effective in reducing consumption.

Psychosocial history

A psychosocial history can help identify conditions that may have a significant impact on maternal and newborn outcomes. Screening for domestic violence should be a routine part of preconception care. Patients can be referred for safety planning. Depression during pregnancy and post partum can have a severe negative impact on the mother, maternal-fetal relationship and the future mental health of the child. Perinatal depression can have long-term developmental, cognitive and behavioral effects on the child. Depression is also associated with other co-morbidities such as chronic diseases, tobacco, alcohol and illicit drug use. Depression can be treated effectively with psychotherapy, cognitive behavior therapy, and/or medications but it does have a high rate of relapse and should be closely monitored. Screening tools for the primary care provider are available (including the Patient Health Questionnaire-9 and Beck Depression Inventory). Limited data exist on the teratogenicity of psychotropic medications (including selective serotonin reuptake inhibitors and tricyclic antidepressants). Their use should be limited and they should not be employed as a first course of therapy. Patients should be counseled about teratogenic risks. Contraception should be considered until the dosage is minimized or discontinued. Preconception consultation provides time to identify treatment options and reduce risks during pregnancy.

Nutrition

Maternal nutritional status is an important factor in the first weeks of fetal development. The Centers for Disease Control recommends that women capable of becoming pregnant take 0.4 mg of folate beginning at least 1 month before conception, since it has been shown to reduce the risk of neural tube defects by two-thirds. Women with a history of epilepsy, diabetes mellitus or a previous gestation with a neural tube defect may require 4 mg of folate intake daily from 4 weeks prior to conception and

through the first 12 weeks of pregnancy. This dose was demonstrated to reduce the risk of recurrent neural tube defects by 72%.

A low BMI prior to conception is associated with preterm birth and low birthweight. A study by Lam found that infants born to mothers with a pre-pregnancy BMI < 18.1 kg/m^2 were more than three times as likely to have gastroschisis compared with infants of normal-weight mothers. Perinatal morbidity associated with a high BMI includes neural tube defects, preterm delivery, gestational diabetes, hypertensive and thromboembolic disorders. Nutritional assessment and consultation are recommended to help establish goals and a plan of action to achieve appropriate weight. The US Department of Agriculture *Food guide pyramid* and *Dietary guidelines for Americans* provide guidance on food planning and physical activity.

Environmental exposures

An environmental history should include assessment of the home environment, workplace and community. The home and workplace environment may identify exposure to potential teratogens such as heavy metals, organic solvents, oil-based paints, pesticides, and herbicides. Methyl mercury and lead are well-established neurotoxins that can adversely affect fetal development. Identifying exposure to potential teratogens may help a patient modify exposure prior to conception.

Chronic medical conditions

Consultation with a patient with a chronic medical condition who desires to conceive should include information regarding the risk of pregnancy complications associated with her disease and other co-morbidities. A complete medical evaluation is required to establish her disease status and identify co-existing morbidities. Depending on the level of severity, the consultation may require a team of specialists. Ideally, control of the medical condition and maternal health should be accomplished prior to conception. Medication should be reduced to the lowest dosage possible and alternatives considered if it poses a teratogenic risk. A set of goals for medical management should be developed. During this period, the patient should avoid pregnancy and be advised to use an effective contraceptive method based on her medical condition.

Development of a reproductive life plan

Reproductive life planning is based on a set of personal goals on preparing for pregnancy or delaying pregnancy, developed by the patient in co-ordination with her provider and leading to an action plan for the different stages of her reproductive life. Planning includes reviewing a complete preconception checklist; developing pregnancy plans; meeting with healthcare providers on a regular basis to review plans and assess possible changes in lifestyle and relationships; and family planning and spacing. Supporting a woman at different stages in her life to keep an active reproductive life plan is a major step towards optimizing a pregnancy.

Suggested reading

Committee on Perinatal Health. *Toward improving the outcome of pregnancy (TIOP II): the 90s and beyond*. White Plains, NY: March of Dimes National Foundation, 1993.

Dietz PM, Callaghan WM, Cogswell ME, Morrow B, Ferre C, Schieve LA. Combined effects of prepregnancy body mass index and weight gain during pregnancy on the risk of preterm delivery. *Epidemiology* 2006; 17: 170–177.

Fiore MC, Jaen CR, Baker TB, *et al. Treating tobacco use and dependence: update. Clinical practice guideline*. Rockville, MD: US Department of Health and Human Services, Public Health Service, 2008.

Jack B, Atrash HK. Preconception health and health care: the clinical content of preconception care. *Am J Obstet Gynecol* 2008; 199(suppl): S257–395.

Lam PK, Torfs CP, Brand RJ. A low Body Mass Index is a risk factor for an offspring with gastroschisis. *Epidemiology* 1999; 10: 717–712.

US Department of Health and Human Services and US Department of Agriculture. *Dietary guidelines for Americans*. Washington, DC: US Government Printing Office, 2006.

Chapter 48
Fetal Lung Maturation, the Respiratory Distress Syndrome, and Antenatal Steroid Therapy

Emiliano Chavira and T. Murphy Goodwin
Department of Medicine and Obstetrics and Gynecology, Keck School of Medicine, University of Southern California, CA, USA

Introduction

Neonatal respiratory tract disease is a frequent complication following birth, particularly in the preterm infant. In recent decades, advances in the understanding of how the respiratory tract develops and the subsequent emergence of specific therapies such as antenatal corticosteroids and postnatal surfactant have yielded significantly improved outcomes in this area. This chapter provides an overview of fetal lung development, a discussion of the underlying pathophysiology of neonatal respiratory distress syndrome, a review of tests for fetal lung maturity, and finally, a summary of current recommendations regarding the use of antenatal corticosteroid therapy.

Fetal lung development

Fetal lung development occurs in four stages: embryonic, pseudoglandular, canalicular, and saccular/alveolar. During the embryonic stage, the lung begins as a ventral outpouching from the thoracic foregut by about 26 days. The caudal end of this pouch pinches off and separates from the foregut and divides into its first branch point by 33 days. Further branching occurs as the primitive bronchial tree begins to penetrate the mesenchymal tissue that will ultimately become the pulmonary interstitia.

Transition between the embryonic stage and the pseudoglandular stage occurs at around 6–7 weeks. In the pseudoglandular stage, which continues through about the 17th week, the bronchial tree progresses through a series of 15–20 divisions such that the bronchial tree is completed by the 16th week. The glycogen-rich cuboidal epithelium lining the airways begins the process of differentiation into mature pneumocytes in a proximal

to distal direction. Meanwhile, the pulmonary arterial pathways develop in conjunction with the bronchial tree, whereas the venous system develops in a pattern that demarcates lung segments and subsegments.

The next stage, the canalicular stage, spans the period from about 16 weeks to about 25 weeks. It is this period that marks the transformation from a previable organ into one with the potential to function as a gas exchange organ. The key development is the appearance of acini, which are tufts of airways and alveoli that emanate from the terminal bronchioles. The epithelium further differentiates, and type II pneumocytes become distinguishable and begin to synthesize surfactant. The previously cuboidal epithelial cells become flattened and begin to have more lamellar bodies within their cytoplasm. The surfaces, which comprise the future air–blood barrier, begin to take shape as the crude vascular tree coursing through the mesenchyma becomes more intricate and more closely apposed to airway epithelium – the eventual site of gas exchange.

In the final saccular/alveolar stages, which begin around 24 weeks and continue well into childhood, the terminal airway saccules differentiate into alveoli. Alveolarization, which proceeds most rapidly after about 32 weeks, occurs through the formation of septae that divide the saccules into alveoli. These septae contain capillaries as well as collagen and elastin fibers. At term, there are between 50 and 150 million alveoli. Alveoli continue to form after birth up to age 8, when the adult number of 300 million alveoli is attained.

As the fetal lung develops anatomically, it is simultaneously maturing in terms of biochemical function. The primary biochemical activity within the mature lung is the production of surfactant. Surfactant is produced by the type II pneumocytes, stored in cytoplasmic lamellar bodies, and secreted into the alveoli where it decreases surface tension and prevents alveolar collapse. It is composed of about 10% protein, 8% neutral lipids such as cholesterol, and the remainder phospholipids. The proteinaceous portion of surfactant includes many nonspecific proteins as well as surfactant-specific proteins SP-A,

Management of Common Problems in Obstetrics and Gynecology, 5th edition. Edited by T.M. Goodwin, M.N. Montoro, L. Muderspach, R. Paulson and S. Roy. © 2010 Blackwell Publishing Ltd.

SP-B, SP-C, and SP-D. SP-A and SP-D are host defense proteins that bind to micro-organisms and promote their elimination by macrophages. SP-B is necessary for the packaging of surfactant into lamellar bodies, and its absence is lethal. The role of SP-C is not clearly defined, but its absence results in progressive interstitial lung disease.

The phospholipid content of surfactant changes during the second half of pregnancy. The predominant active component of mature surfactant is lecithin or phosphatidylcholine. Other constituents include phosphatidylinositol, phosphatidylethanolamine, phosphatidylserine, phosphatidylglycerol (PG), and sphingomyelin. The changes in concentration of these components can be used to assess fetal pulmonary maturity. One important measure is the ratio of lecithin to sphingomyelin. Following about 24 weeks, both substances begin to increase in concentration, but there is more sphingomyelin than lecithin (L/S ratio less than 1). Lecithin begins to rise sharply in the third trimester such that lecithin and sphingomyelin have equivalent concentrations by around 31–32 weeks (L/S ratio equals 1). Lecithin production continues to increase, and its concentration becomes double that of sphingomyelin by about 34–36 weeks (L/S ratio greater than 2). Concurrent with changes in the L/S ratio is the appearance and rapid rise of PG after about 35 weeks. Both an L/S ratio greater than 2 and the presence of PG signify that the fetus is at low risk for the development of respiratory distress syndrome (RDS) after birth. Both these features of mature surfactant are used in clinical tests of fetal lung maturity, which will be discussed below.

Pathophysiology of the respiratory distress syndrome

If the fetus is born after lung maturity, normal respiration usually ensues. If birth occurs prior to pulmonary viability, death follows. Between these extremes is the premature infant, who has the greatest risk of developing RDS. If there is insufficient surfactant in the terminal bronchioles and alveoli at the time of birth, they collapse. Hypoxia in the collapsed portions of the lung causes local vasoconstriction and a right-to-left shunt. If hypoxemia and shunting are significant, mixed acidosis and hypotension may occur. On chest x-ray a diffuse reticulogranular infiltrate is seen with air in the tracheobronchial tree. Clinically, RDS manifests as tachypnea with nasal flaring, chest wall retractions and grunting. Infants who demonstrate these signs are administered oxygen, which results in vasodilation and reperfusion of the pulmonary vascular bed. The airways may then become filled with an exudate rich in protein, and any necrotic airway epithelium sloughs. On histologic examination of fatal

cases, many alveoli are collapsed while some are widely dilated, and hyaline membranes composed of fibrin-rich protein and cellular debris are seen lining the terminal airways and alveoli. This entity has also been called hyaline membrane disease.

Hyaline membrane disease has decreased as a cause of neonatal death, mostly as a result of antenatal corticosteroid and postnatal surfactant therapy, although RDS still causes significant morbidity and mortality. One reason for this is that there are multiple mechanisms of RDS. Additional causes include meconium aspiration, patent ductus arteriosus, pneumonia, sepsis, hypoxic ischemic encephalopathy, pneumothorax, diaphragmatic hernia, pulmonary hypoplasia, and congenital cardiac malformations. Iatrogenic causes of RDS include oxygen toxicity lung disease as well as injury sustained from mechanical ventilation. Thus, even if the lungs are mature or if steroids and surfactant are used, RDS may still occur. Nevertheless, ensuring that infants are not delivered prior to pulmonary maturity is essential. When this is not possible, such as in cases of intractable preterm labor or severe pre-eclampsia, appropriate use of corticosteroids and surfactant is the mainstay of therapy.

Tests of fetal lung maturity

The lung is thought to be the last fetal organ to mature. Thus, once the lungs mature, the fetus is ready for postnatal life. It is the physician's responsibility to ensure that elective delivery does not occur prior to establishing fetal lung maturity. The ACOG guidelines state that fetal lung maturity can be inferred if any of the following criteria are met:
• fetal heart tones have been present for at least 20 weeks by auscultation or 30 weeks by Doppler
• at least 36 weeks have elapsed since a positive serum or urine hCG pregnancy test was documented by a reliable laboratory
• ultrasound measurement of crown–rump length at 6–11 weeks supports a gestational age of 39 weeks or more
• a clinically determined gestational age confirmed by ultrasound at 12–20 weeks is at least 39 weeks.
If any of these criteria are met, scheduled delivery is appropriate. If delivery is planned at an earlier gestational age and fetal lung maturity cannot be assumed, then testing for fetal lung maturity (FLM) must be considered. On the other hand, according to the ACOG, testing for FLM prior to 33 weeks is rarely warranted because confirmation of FLM at this gestational age is unlikely. In clinical practice, most providers empirically administer corticosteroids if delivery before 34 weeks is either planned or anticipated. Multiple tests for FLM exist, and these are outlined below.

As described earlier, the composition of surfactant changes as the lung matures. Since lung fluid flows into the amniotic cavity, surfactant is accessible for study via amniocentesis. The first reliable test of FLM that was developed was the lecithin to sphingomyelin ratio (L/S ratio). Devised by Gluck and colleagues in 1974 [1], an L/S ratio above 2 has been shown to predict the absence of RDS in 98% of neonates. The converse, however, is not true. When the L/S ratio is less than 2, many of these infants do not develop RDS. Thus, the strength of the L/S ratio lies in its negative predictive value, whereas its ability to positively predict RDS is poor. In pregnancies complicated by maternal diabetes, some have questioned the utility of the L/S ratio, although data on this issue are conflicting.

Because the L/S ratio is widely used, it is critical to understand how blood and meconium can confound the results. Blood itself contains both lecithin and sphingomyelin in a ratio of 1.3/1.5. The presence of blood may therefore raise or lower the amniotic fluid L/S ratio depending on the initial value. Meconium has also been reported to increase the L/S ratio by as much as 0.5 at term. Considering this, an L/S ratio determined from a specimen contaminated with blood or meconium must be interpreted with caution. Heavily contaminated specimens are probably best discarded.

Alternatively, determination of PG can be done via thin-layer chromatography or via the less expensive and more widely available rapid immunologic agglutination tests. Because PG appears late in development, its presence is a reliable indicator of lung maturity. Moreover, the results are not affected by blood or meconium, and results from amniotic fluid collected from a vaginal pool have been found to correlate well with amniocentesis specimens. As with the L/S ratio, the negative predictive value of the presence of PG is high, whereas the positive predictive value is poor. PG tends to appear after the L/S ratio exceeds 2. In cases where PG is not yet present but the L/S ratio is greater than 2, RDS is unlikely. Although controversial, some practitioners consider the presence of PG in diabetic pregnancies to be more reliable than the L/S ratio.

Another widely used test is the TDx test, in which an automated fluorescence polarimeter determines the surfactant to albumin ratio. The second generation of this test uses a value around 55 mg/g as the cut-off for maturity. As with the other tests, it is reliable for predicting the absence of RDS, and has been shown to correlate well with the L/S ratio. It has been found to be reliable in specimens obtained from the vaginal pool in PPROM between 30 and 36 weeks, and is also useful in diabetic mothers.

Lamellar bodies, produced by type II pneumocytes and secreted into the airways, eventually make their way into the amniotic fluid. Being similar in size to platelets, they can be quantified with commercial cell counters. A lamellar body count of less than 8000/μL is 100% predictive of an immature L/S ratio and PG assay, while a count over 32,000/μL correlates with a mature L/S or PG in over 99% of cases. The results are not affected by meconium or blood, but the mature cut-off used by a particular laboratory will depend on the speed of centrifugation and the type of cell counter used.

One final method of FLM testing will be mentioned that tests surfactant function rather than quantity. The Foam Stability Index is a test of the ability of amniotic fluid to stabilize foam when mixed with ethanol. An aliquot of amniotic fluid is added to multiple wells in the test kit containing predetermined quantities of ethanol. The mixtures are then shaken and the highest value well in which a stable ring of foam is seen determines the Foam Stability Index. This test has been shown to be reliable for predicting absence of RDS at birth. It is unreliable in the presence of blood or meconium.

Since these tests share the characteristic of a high negative predictive value, a mature result in any one test obviates the need for further testing. Many laboratories adopt a stepwise approach to FLM testing by beginning with an easily performed and inexpensive screening test such as the TDx. If the test is mature, no further testing is done, whereas an immature test prompts the performance of a second test such as an L/S ratio (indeed, this is the algorithm in place in our own institution). If FLM is confirmed, delivery can proceed with the confidence that RDS is unlikely. If FLM is not confirmed, several options exist including delivery after administration of steroids, repeat testing after a certain time interval has elapsed or simply proceeding with delivery after an appropriate time interval. Which option is best depends on the clinical scenario as well as provider and patient preference.

Antenatal corticosteroid therapy

In 1972, Liggins & Howie conducted the first randomized trial of antenatal corticosteroid therapy in humans [2]. This study showed a decreased incidence of RDS and mortality among those infants delivered before 34 weeks who had received a course of betamethasone. Following this finding, many studies have been performed of different agents and different dosing regimens. Although an exhaustive review of that literature is well beyond the scope of this chapter, a National Institutes of Health Consensus Development Conference was convened in 1994 for this very purpose [3]. The consensus development panel concluded that the benefits of antenatal corticosteroids for fetuses at risk for preterm delivery far outweigh the potential risks. Benefits include decreased mortality (odds ratio 0.6, 95% CI 0.5–0.8), decreased incidence and/or severity of RDS (odds ratio 0.5, 95% CI 0.4–0.6), and decreased intraventricular hemorrhage (odds ratio 0.5, 95% CI 0.3–0.9). Further, follow-up of children so treated up to 12 years of age failed to show any neurodevelopmental deficits that could be attributed to antenatal steroid therapy.

Based on this risk/benefit ratio, the consensus panel recommended that all fetuses from 24 to 34 weeks at risk for preterm delivery be considered candidates for therapy, irrespective of gender, race, availability of surfactant therapy or concomitant tocolytic therapy. The specific regimens endorsed include either two doses of betamethasone 12 mg given intramuscularly every 24 hours or four doses of dexamethasone 6 mg given intramuscularly every 12 hours. Although optimal benefit begins 24 hours after initiation of therapy and lasts for 7 days, some benefit is gained from therapy of less than 24 hours duration. In cases of PPROM, corticosteroid therapy is recommended in pregnancies less than 32 weeks in the absence of chorio-amnionitis because of the protection against IVH at this gestational age.

A second NIH Consensus Development Conference was convened in 2000 to address the issue of repeat courses of antenatal steroids [4]. Data regarding these practices were found to be of poor quality. There were few prospective randomized data, and much more retrospective or observational data. Methodologies varied across the studies, and most did not control for postnatal steroid use, which was commonly practiced at that time. Despite these limitations, there were some legitimate concerns regarding potential adverse maternal and fetal effects of repeat doses. The conclusion of this panel was that while the available data unequivocally support the use of a single course of antenatal steroids, the risk and benefit data are insufficient to recommend routine use of repeat or rescue doses in clinical practice. It was recommended that such practices be limited to the setting of clinical trials. The ACOG Committee Opinion on this topic essentially supports the conclusions and recommendations contained in the two NIH consensus statements.

Conclusion

The fetal lung develops anatomically in four stages: embryonic, pseudoglandular, canalicular, and saccular/

alveolar. As the lung forms anatomically, it simultaneously matures biochemically with respect to its ability to produce surfactant. Delivery of a fetus prior to pulmonary maturity exposes that infant to the risk of hyaline membrane disease or RDS. RDS has several possible etiologies other than surfactant deficiency. In order to avoid surfactant-deficient RDS, tests of fetal lung maturity can be performed to ensure that delivery occurs at an optimal time for the fetus. All the available tests share the common characteristic of a very high negative predictive value. Thus, if any test demonstrates fetal lung maturity, RDS is unlikely. In infants at risk for delivery between 24 and 34 weeks, a single course of antenatal corticosteroids reduces the risks of RDS, IVH, and neonatal mortality.

References

1. Gluck L, Kulovich MV, Borer RC, Keidel WN. The interpretation and significance of the lecithin-sphingomyelin ratio in amniotic fluid. *Am J Obstet Gynecol* 1974; 120: 142–155.
2. Liggins GC, Howie RN. A controlled trial of antepartum glucocorticoid treatment for prevention of the respiratory distress syndrome in premature infants. *Pediatrics* 1972; 50: 515.
3. The effect of antenatal steroids for fetal lung maturation on perinatal outcomes. *NIH Consensus Statement* 1994; 12(2): 1–24.
4. Antenatal corticosteroids revisited: repeat courses. *NIH Consensus Statement* 2000; 17(2): 1–18.

Suggested reading

American College of Obstetricians and Gynecologists. *Assessment of fetal lung maturity. ACOG Educational Bulletin No. 230.* Washington, DC: American College of Obstetricians and Gynecologists, 1996.

American College of Obstetricians and Gynecologists. Antenatal corticosteroid therapy for fetal maturation. ACOG Committee Opinion No. 273. *Obstet Gynecol* 2002; 99: 871-873.

Cunningham FG, Gant NF, Leveno KJ, Gilstrap LC, Hauth JC, Wenstrom KD. *Williams obstetrics,* 21st edn. New York: McGraw Hill, 2001.

Gabbe SG, Niebyl JR, Simpson JL. *Obstetrics. Normal and problem pregnancies,* 4th edn. New York: Churchill Livingstone, 2002.

Chapter 49
Fetal Interventions

Ramen H. Chmait

Department of Medicine and Obstetrics and Gynecology, Keck School of Medicine, University of Southern California, CA, USA

Introduction

The field of prenatal diagnosis has progressed rapidly due to the ubiquitous use of high-resolution ultrasound and the increased sophistication of molecular and genetic testing. Most fetal conditions identified *in utero* are best treated after birth at a tertiary center in the setting of multidisciplinary co-operation. However, there are instances in which delay of treatment until after delivery may result in death or permanent organ damage. A particularly distressing feature of many fetal abnormalities is the lethal secondary complications that may develop during the course of the pregnancy. The goal of fetal therapy is to treat the primary abnormality if possible, or at the very least ameliorate the secondary sequelae, in conditions that would otherwise result in demise or permanent vital organ damage to the fetal patient.

Brief historical perspective

Fetal interventions have undergone three major paradigm shifts over the past several decades related to the invasiveness of the procedure. The landmark work of Liley and others in the 1960s to develop fetal transfusion techniques to treat severe fetal anemia ushered in the possibility of providing *in utero* fetal therapy. The pendulum swung from minimally invasive needle and shunt procedures to the maximally invasive methods of open fetal surgery. The initial enthusiasm for open fetal surgery in the United States of the 1980s waned after realization of the not insignificant rate of maternal morbidity and relatively high rate of prematurity. In the 1990s the pendulum swung back to minimally invasive methods, which included operative fetoscopy. The advantage of operative fetoscopy

Management of Common Problems in Obstetrics and Gynecology, 5th edition. Edited by T.M. Goodwin, M.N. Montoro, L. Muderspach, R. Paulson and S. Roy. © 2010 Blackwell Publishing Ltd.

and other minimally invasive fetal interventions is the relatively nominal violation of the sanctity of the human womb, which has resulted in negligible maternal morbidity and significantly decreased risk of prematurity.

The fetal patient

The concept of the fetus as a patient is a complicated topic that can be addressed from an embryologic, ethical, theologic and/or legal vantage point. It is important as physicians to be cognizant with each of these issues without interjecting personal bias when counseling parents. Once a fetal abnormality has been identified, it is the physician's job to educate the parents about the particular findings, the natural history of the condition, and the spectrum of expected prognoses. The parents should be educated in a nondirective manner regarding all management options. When a mother seeks care from a physician regarding a fetal condition, the fetus should be treated as a patient and be afforded all the opportunities for modern medical care.

Like any patient in medicine, the fetus requires appropriate pain management during invasive procedures. There is controversy in the literature regarding the gestational age at which the fetus has the capacity to perceive pain. Histologic examinations of the spinal cord have identified neurons involved in nociception before 20 weeks' gestational age. Invasive procedures elicit a stress response in fetuses as early as 16 weeks' gestation, while providing fentanyl during fetal interventions has been shown to diminish this stress response. Because of uncertainty over the exact developmental timing at which the fetus may perceive pain, fetal anesthesia and analgesia should be provided during all direct fetal interventions regardless of gestational age.

Open fetal surgery

Open fetal surgery is a fetal intervention in which the gravid uterus is opened to allow direct surgery on the fetus.

The surgery is performed under relatively deep general anesthesia to provide uterine quiescence. Maternal laparotomy and hysterotomy are performed, and the fetus is then partially exposed to allow direct surgical access to the fetal lesion. With minimal manipulation of the umbilical cord, the fetus is maintained on placental support throughout the procedure. After the surgical repair, the fetus is returned into the uterus and the uterine incision and the abutting fetal membranes are sutured closed. The mother is hospitalized for at least 3 days, with often 1 day spent in the intensive care unit. Due to the hysterotomy, the mother will require a cesarean section for that pregnancy and all subsequent pregnancies. Essentially all patients deliver prematurely.

The indications for open fetal surgery have been dwindling over the past decade. Congenital anomalies that have been treated via open fetal surgery include congenital diaphragmatic hernia, pulmonary sequestration, congenital cystic adenomatoid malformation of the lung, sacrococcygeal teratoma, and myelomeningocele. Aside from myelomingocele, all these lesions have been successfully treated via operative fetoscopy or needle/shunt procedures. A study comparing outcomes of myelomeningocele repair by open fetal surgery versus traditional repair after birth should be completed by 2011. Because of the intrusive nature of open fetal surgery and the relatively high risk of maternal and fetal morbidity compared to other fetal interventions, this technique is not expected to play a major role in fetal therapy in the future.

Using several of the surgical techniques developed for open fetal surgery, the *ex utero* intrapartum treatment (EXIT) procedure was developed to treat the term or near term fetus with an extensive airway obstruction. A classic cesarean section is performed and the fetus is partially exteriorized. Without disruption of the placenta and while attempting to maintain blood flow through the intact umbilical cord, surgical access to the airway is obtained. Placental support is discontinued once the airway is secured by clamping and cutting the umbilical cord.

Operative fetoscopy

Operative fetoscopy is a therapeutic modality that strikes a fine balance between surgical access and minimal invasiveness. Using local anesthesia and intravenous maternal sedation, an endoscope that measures up to 3.3 mm in diameter is inserted through the maternal abdomen into the uterus. Intraoperative ultrasound guidance is used to guide trocar insertion. Most surgeries are performed using a single port. The operating channel of the endoscope allows for the use of various surgical instruments. The interlacing muscle fibers of the uterine wall spontaneously seal the uterine insertion site upon removal of the trocar. Recovery for the mother is uncomplicated, and she is usually discharged home after a 1-night hospital stay.

Operative fetoscopy may be performed any time after 16 weeks' gestation. The patient may deliver vaginally in the index pregnancy as well as in all subsequent pregnancies.

The cornerstone of most fetal therapy centers is the treatment of twin–twin transfusion syndrome (TTTS) via operative fetoscopy. TTTS is a condition that develops in 10–15% of monochorionic twins from unbalanced sharing of blood through vascular communications in the shared placenta. A series of pathophysiologic changes ensues from the net shunting of blood from one twin (donor) to the other twin (recipient), resulting in donor twin oligohydramnios, recipient twin polyhydramnios, and characteristic anatomic and arterial/venous flow derangements that can be identified by ultrasound.

The perinatal mortality rate of expectantly managed TTTS approaches 95%. Two treatment modalities, serial amniocentesis and laser therapy, are currently being used to treat this condition. Serial amniocentesis involves drainage of amniotic fluid from the polyhydramniotic recipient sac using vacuum-assisted devices attached to an 18–20 gauge spinal needle. Serial amniocentesis serves to significantly reduce the amount of amniotic fluid volume in the recipient sac, thereby diminishing overall uterine distension. Unlike serial amniocentesis, fetoscopic laser therapy, otherwise known as selective laser photocoagulation of communicating vessels (SLPCV), treats the primary pathogenic cause of TTTS by ablating all vascular communications. The endoscope is used to directly visualize the vessels on the placental surface. Once mapping of the vascular communications has been performed, those vessels are photocoagulated using laser energy that is delivered by quartz fibers through the operating channel of the endoscope.

Controlled nonrandomized trials that compared laser therapy with amnioreduction revealed significantly improved perinatal outcomes in the laser group. A subsequent randomized controlled trial conducted in Europe that compared the two groups was prematurely halted after interim analysis revealed significantly improved perinatal survival in the laser group versus the amnioreduction group. The amniocentesis group had a significantly higher rate of neurologic complications, which persisted at the 6-month follow-up evaluation. The only study that did not show improved perinatal outcomes in the laser group was found to have multiple flaws in study design and surgical technique. Based on the wealth of data showing beneficial outcomes in the laser-treated patients, all patients with mid-trimester TTTS should be offered the option of operative fetoscopic laser therapy at an experienced center.

Other complications of monochorionic twins that can be treated via operative fetoscopy are those that are discordant for the presence of an obligate lethal condition. The classic example is twin reversed arterial perfusion (TRAP) sequence. In this condition, one fetus (often called the "acardiac" twin) is supplied with blood in a reversed fashion, such that the umbilical artery carries deoxygenated blood to the acardiac twin. This leads to severe maldevelopment of cephalic, thoracic, and upper extremity structures, and results in a condition that is not compatible with life outside the womb for that fetus. Because the heart of the other fetus (often called the "pump" twin) must pump blood for both fetuses, there is a 50–75% risk of heart failure and demise in the pump twin, particularly if the acardiac mass is relatively large. In the presence of pump twin heart failure or a large acardiac twin, fetoscopic umbilical cord occlusion of the acardiac fetus is indicated. This can be performed via direct suture ligation or laser photocoagulation of the acardiac twin's umbilical cord or laser photocoagulation of the vascular communications. Other techniques include bipolar coagulation of the acardiac twin's umbilical cord and intrafetal radiofrequency ablation. Infusion of a toxin such as potassium chloride into the acardiac fetus is contraindicated because the substance can traverse the vascular communication and result in death or damage to the pump twin.

Surgical treatments of several congenital malformations have been performed via operative fetoscopy as well. One condition that has received significant attention recently is the fetoscopic treatment of congenital diaphragmatic hernia (CDH). CDH, which affects approximately one in 2500 liveborn infants, is a malformation of the diaphragm that allows abdominal contents to protrude into the thoracic cavity, thereby impairing proper lung development. Infants born with CDH develop respiratory failure due to pulmonary hypoplasia and pulmonary hypertension. This condition is lethal in 30–40% of prenatally diagnosed cases. Mid-gestation ultrasound and MRI have been utilized with variable success to quantify the risk of poor perinatal outcome. One consistent indicator of poor prognosis is the herniation of the liver above the diaphragm. The ultrasound-derived lung-to-head ratio (LHR), calculated by dividing the product of the length and width of the contralateral lung by the head circumference, is an indicator of perinatal survival, particularly in fetuses with liver herniation. In patients with LHR less than 1.0 and with liver herniation into the chest, the perinatal survival is approximately 10%.

The prenatal treatment of CDH has evolved in a similar fashion to fetal surgery as a whole. Early attempts using open fetal surgery to correct the diaphragmatic hernia primarily showed no improvement in outcomes compared to expectantly managed cases. A minimally invasive technique was then sought to ameliorate the secondary complications of the CDH, namely the impaired lung growth induced by mass effect. Animal and human studies showed that purposeful obstruction of the fetal trachea resulted in lung growth. Because the lung continually produces fluid that normally exits the trachea, blockage of the trachea results in expansion of the lung and some reduction of the herniated viscera.

The technique for fetoscopic tracheal occlusion has undergone several modifications over the past dozen years. Fetoscopic tracheal occlusion via direct fetal laryngoscopy was then shown to be technically feasible in humans. Current efforts focus on fetoscopic placement of a device into the trachea at 26–28 weeks' gestation. This device is then removed at 34 weeks' gestation, often via a second fetoscopic procedure, to allow physiologic recovery of the lung. Preliminary data have shown favorable perinatal survival rates compared to historic controls. Further studies are required to delineate surgical criteria and to assess perinatal outcomes compared to matched controls.

Lower urinary tract obstruction (LUTO) is another fetal condition that has been treated by operative fetoscopy. LUTO is a heterogeneous group of disorders that lead to complete obstruction of the lower urinary tract. Common etiologies include posterior urethral valves, urethral atresia, and urethral hypoplasia. Because the vast majority of amniotic fluid arises from fetal micturition during the second and third trimesters, obstruction of the lower urinary tract results in severe oligohydramnios. The resultant high pressure in the urinary collection system leads to renal dysplasia. Also, secondary external compression of the thoracic compartment occurs due to the paucity of amniotic fluid volume. This results in lethal pulmonary hypoplasia.

Ultrasound evaluation reveals characteristic dilation of the urinary collection system. In the case of posterior urethral valves, the massive bladder along with a dilated proximal urethral form a "keyhole" sign. However, ultrasound is a poor predictor of renal damage. Thus, classic work-up includes assessment of renal function via urinary electrolyte assessment via serial vesicocenteses. If renal function is preserved, then urinary diversion is required to relieve the high pressure to the kidneys and restore normal amniotic fluid volume, thereby preventing pulmonary hypoplasia. The traditional method of urinary diversion is placement of a vesicoamniotic shunt. Because shunt dislodgment is not uncommon, patients often must undergo multiple vesicoamniotic shunt placements during the course of the pregnancy. Fetal cystoscopy and direct endoscopic ablation of the posterior urethral valves has been proposed as an alternative to shunting. This approach has several advantages to vesicoamniotic shunting, including the curative nature of the procedure and that it involves only a single intervention.

Amniotic band syndrome is another example of a condition that has been successfully treated via operative fetoscopy. The etiology of this condition remains debatable, although many investigators believe that early rupture of the amnion results in development of bands that criss-cross the uterus. These bands may cause fetal deformations, constrictions, and/or amputations. Many fetuses with amniotic band syndrome have multiple malformations involving multiple organ systems. However, there are cases in which the amniotic bands are restricted to constriction bands involving the fetal extremities and/or umbilical cord. These constriction bands may cause extremity amputation or umbilical cord strangulation and sudden fetal death. Experimental data have shown that release of these constriction bands can restore blood flow and function to a distal extremity. Fetoscopic lysis of amniotic bands has been shown to be technically successful with restoration of blood flow and function to the involved limbs.

Operative fetoscopy is particularly suited to treating vascular tumors that may involve the fetus, such as sacrococcygeal teratoma, or the placenta, such as chorioangioma. Although most tumors are asymptomatic, large tumors may cause high-output heart failure, hydrops, and fetal demise. In the premature fetus, fetoscopic laser ablation of the feeding vessels to these tumors is feasible and may be life-saving.

Needle and shunt procedures

Intrauterine transfusion (IUT) was the first procedure performed to directly treat an underlying fetal condition *in utero*. IUT is currently indicated for the treatment of severe fetal anemia, causes of which include isoimmunization, parvovirus infection, and severe fetal-to-maternal hemorrhage. IUT of platelets is also performed for the treatment of severe alloimmune thrombocytopenia that is recalcitrant to medical management. Because of universal prophylaxis against Rh(D) isoimmunization with Rh(D) immunoglobulin and the rarity of the other conditions, the number of IUTs performed in the United States has declined sharply. Details regarding the pathophysiology, diagnosis, and management of red blood cell isoimmunization are reviewed in Chapter 7.

The early success of IUT ushered in nonvascular fetal needle and shunt procedures. The treatment of lower urinary tract obstruction with vesicoamniotic shunt placement was described above. Another group of disorders amenable to needle drainage and/or shunting is fetal chest abnormalities. Space-occupying lesions in the fetal thorax, whether fluid or solid, may cause underdevelopment of the lung tissue and lethal pulmonary hypoplasia, as well as compression of cardiovascular structures and eventual fetal hydrops. One example of intrathoracic space-occupying pathology is a fetal pleural effusion, an accumulation of fluid in the pleural space caused by a variety of etiologies, such as malformation of the thoracic duct, pulmonary lymphangiectasis, and a variety of genetic syndromes. Pleural effusions may have a variable course from complete spontaneous resolution to fetal hydrops and death. Improved perinatal survival has been shown in fetuses with persistent pleural effusions with hydrops or impending hydrops treated by thoracocentesis or thoracoamniotic shunting.

The two most common intrathoracic masses that can cause fetal hydrops are congenital cystic adenomatoid malformation (CCAM) and pulmonary sequestrations (PS). CCAM is an overgrowth of terminal respiratory bronchioles that form cysts of various diameters. On the other hand, PS consists of nonfunctioning lung tissue that is supported by an anomalous arterial blood supply. Fetal treatment is indicated in those cases with fetal hydrops remote from term gestation. In macrocystic CCAM, thoracoamniotic shunt placement will reverse fetal hydrops. In microcystic CCAM and in PS, needle-delivered sclerotherapy has been shown to reduce the size of the lesion, thereby causing resolution of the hydrops. Laser energy delivered to the feeding arterial vessel of a PS results in similar effect.

Fetal intervention for select cardiac disease is currently in the investigational stage. One area of interest is fetal critical aortic stenosis, which has been documented to evolve into hypoplastic left heart syndrome (HLHS) secondary to hemodynamic changes that occur *in utero*. In newborns with HLHS, the left heart is too small to support the systemic circulation, and affected newborns die without intervention. Surgical repair after birth (staged surgical palliation) results in a 5-year survival rate of 75%. However, survivors face lifelong risks including long-term neurodevelopmental deficits. Aortic stenosis may be relieved *in utero* via aortic balloon valvuloplasty, and has been shown both in animal studies and in human fetuses to promote left ventricular growth, in some cases preventing the development of HLHS. This procedure is performed using a needle that is placed into the fetal heart through which the balloon catheter is passed. Other congenital heart malformations, such as pulmonary stenosis and HLHS with restricted atrial septum, have also been targeted as potentially amenable to fetal intervention.

There is currently much scientific activity regarding the potential for treating fetuses with select genetic disorders using stem cell or gene therapy. The application of these potential treatment strategies has several theoretic advantages in fetuses, although at this time few successful treatments have been performed. Should the potential for these therapeutic modalities become realized in humans, the delivery system would invariably require a fine needle targeted to a specific organ system in a fetus of relatively early gestational age.

Transplacental therapy

Transplacental medical therapy is performed by administering medicines to the mother that are in turn passed to the fetus via the placenta. The most common transplacental treatment in obstetrics is maternal corticosteroid administration in preterm fetuses to promote fetal organ maturation. There are many examples of biochemical and endocrine fetal disorders that can be treated by transplacental therapy. One classic example is 21-hydroxylase deficiency, an inherited enzymatic defect of adrenal steroidogenesis, which results in increased levels of precursor androgens that can lead to virilization of an affected female infant. The masculinization may be reduced or averted by administering corticosteroids before the eighth week of gestation. Transplacental medical therapy is also utilized to treat life-threatening fetal cardiac arrhythmias using antiarrhythmic agents such as digoxin or flecainide. This treatment poses risks to the mother, and should be done in close collaboration with a cardiologist. A final example of a fetal treatment via the transplacental route is maternal administration of intravenous immunoglobulin and steroids for pregnancies complicated by alloimmune thrombocytopenia.

Conclusion

Counseling parents regarding fetal therapy requires candid discussion of the fetal diagnosis and expected prognosis using a nondirective approach. Maternal risks are small when using minimally invasive techniques. The fetal risks of *in utero* interventions, particularly prematurity, must be weighed against the risks of the underlying fetal condition. As surgical equipment advances, prenatal diagnosis becomes more refined, and novel therapeutic modalities are instituted, access to the fetal-placental unit via minimally invasive methods will become ever more important to optimize the care of the fetal patient.

Suggested reading

Kurjak A, Carrera JM, McCullough LB, Chervenak FA. Scientific and religious controversies about the beginning of human life: the relevance of the ethical concept of the fetus as a patient. *J Perinat Med* 2007; 35(5): 376–383.

Quintero R (ed). *Diagnostic and operative fetoscopy*. New York: Parthenon, 2002.

Quintero RA, Chmait RH, Murakoshi T, *et al*. Surgical management of twin reversed arterial perfusion sequence. *Am J Obstet Gynecol* 2006; 194(4): 982–991.

Senat MV, Deprest J, Boulvain M, Paupe A, Winer N, Ville Y. Endoscopic laser surgery versus serial amnioreduction for severe twin-to-twin transfusion syndrome. *NEJM* 2004; 351(2): 136–144.

Chapter 50
Vulvovaginitis

Aaron Epstein and Subir Roy
Department of Medicine and Obstetrics and Gynecology, Keck School of Medicine, University of Southern California, CA, USA

Introduction

Vulvovaginitis is one of the most common problems seen by gynecologists and other primary care practitioners. Due to the nonspecific nature of symptoms, empiric therapy has remained the mainstay of treatment by many physicians despite frequent misdiagnoses. With all the various over-the-counter treatments also available to women, frequent self-diagnosis and therapy have led to inappropriate treatment in many cases. A wide array of microbes, ranging from the normal vaginal flora to sexually transmitted pathogens, cause these genital infections. Bacterial vaginosis, trichomoniasis, and candidal infections are responsible for over 90% of infections. The cardinal symptom is abnormal vaginal discharge. If the vulva is involved, the patient may also complain of pruritus, burning, dysuria, and dyspareunia. The correct diagnosis involves a thorough history and physical examination, vaginal pH, whiff test, and microscopy. Even with all these tools, diagnosis of bacterial vaginosis, trichomoniasis, and candidal infections will be made only 60–90% of the time.

Normal vaginal discharge ranges from 1 to 4 mL per day. The vagina is acidic (pH 3.5–4.5) because of the lactic acid produced by Doderlein's bacillus (*Lactobacillus acidophilus*), which are dominant bacteria in a healthy vaginal ecosystem. Lactic acid, produced by *L. acidophilus*, suppresses the growth of the gram-positive and gram-negative facultative and obligate anaerobes, maintains a normal pH, and inhibits bacteria from adhering to vaginal epithelial cells. In addition, the hydrogen peroxide produced by these organisms is toxic to a wide variety of microbes. Normal vaginal flora consist of many bacterial organisms, including potential pathogens that exist in symbiosis. Cervical mucus, semen, menstrual blood, overgrowth of other organisms of the vaginal flora, and progesterone all raise the vaginal pH and favor the growth of trichomonads and *Gardnerella vaginalis*.

A vaginal discharge can be physiologic when due to mucus secretion from the endocervix at mid-cycle or to desquamation of epithelial cells premenstrually. Other factors that contribute to vulvovaginitis are poorly cornified vaginal epithelium, as seen in prepupertal girls and postmenopausal women, fecal contamination from the anus, sexual intercourse, vaginal douching, pregnancy, and excessive local heat and moisture. In addition, broad-spectrum antibiotic therapy sufficient to destroy the normal bacterial flora, and co-existing systemic disease, such as diabetes, can result in recurrent infections.

In assessing the patient for vulvovaginitis, the history should include accounts of any previous vaginal infections and their treatment, as well as hygienic, contraceptive, and sexual practices. During the pelvic examination, attention should be paid to the appearance of the vulva, as well as the pH, color, consistency, and odor of the vaginal discharge. Abnormal discharge may be white, gray or green-yellow in color; the consistency may be homogeneous, "cottage-cheese" like or frothy in appearance. Microscopic examination of a wet smear will help to differentiate among infections due to fungi, trichomonads, and bacteria. Cultures for *Candida* and trichomoniasis should be done in symptomatic patients who have a negative microscopy due to the low sensitivity of microscopy for *Candida* (22%) and trichomoniasis (62%).

The emotional state of a patient suffering from recurrent vulvovaginitis should not be overlooked, as dealing with these infections can be frustrating. In addition to the symptoms, simply the sense of having a discharge can make sexual activity quite uncomfortable and embarrassing for the woman and may at times lead to stress in personal relationships.

Bacterial vaginosis

Bacterial vaginosis (BV) is the most common type of vulvovaginitis irrespective of age. Various terms have been

Management of Common Problems in Obstetrics and Gynecology, 5th edition. Edited by T.M. Goodwin, M.N. Montoro, L. Muderspach, R. Paulson and S. Roy. © 2010 Blackwell Publishing Ltd.

used in the past to describe this entity, including nonspecific vaginitis (NSV). The term BV has been proposed for this condition since bacteria are involved but without leukocytes. In the majority of these cases, however, the infection is due to a specific, though unidentified, bacterium.

The microbiologic picture of BV consists of the presence of gram-variable coccobacilli, consistent with *G. vaginalis* (found in 40% of women normally), together with numerous anerobic organisms. The latter are thought to be responsible for the production of aromatic amines with names such as putrescine, cadavarine, and trimethylamines, which are volatilized by the addition of 10% potassium hydroxide, resulting in the characteristic fishy odor (positive "whiff test") associated with this disorder. Clue cells (stratified squamous cells with a granular appearance due to a coating of micro-organisms) may be visualized when saline is mixed with the vaginal fluids; however, it is not pathognomonic for this condition.

The diagnosis of bacterial vaginosis requires three of the following:
• a thin, homogeneous, white noninflammatory discharge with the appearance of skim milk
• presence of clue cells on microscopic examination (greater than 20% of epithelial cells)
• pH of vaginal sidewall or fluid > 4.5
• a fishy odor before or after adding KOH (positive "whiff test").
Gram stain of vaginal secretions is also a reliable mode of diagnosing BV (93% sensitive, 70% specific), but it is not commonly used since it requires laboratory processing and delays diagnosis. Cultures for *G. vaginalis* are not useful in diagnosing BV because they are positive in 40–60% of asymptomatic women.

Bacterial vaginosis will resolve spontaneously in up to one-third of women. Treatment should be given to nonpregnant women with symptomatic infection. Numerous drugs (oral vs intravaginal) are available to treat BV. Intravaginal clindamycin (one applicator 2% cream before bedtime for 7 nights or 100 mg vaginal ovule every day for 3 days) and metronidazole (one applicator 0.75% cream before bedtime or twice a day for 5 days) are commonly used, and are comparable in their efficacy in the nonpregnant state. Oral therapies with clindamycin (300 mg twice a day for 7 days) or metronidazole (500 mg twice a day for 5 days) are alternatives as primary treatment or in recurrent infections. A single dose of Clindesse vaginal cream has been shown to be as effective as a 7-day course of Cleocin, which can lead to increased user reliability. Other antibiotic therapies such as ampicillin and erythromycin may eradicate *G. vaginalis* but since they also kill *Lactobacillus*, they raise the vaginal pH and facilitate reinfection. Poor efficacy has been observed also with the use of triple-sulfa creams, tetracycline, and povidone-iodine vaginal douches. Unprotected intercourse has also been shown to predict recurrence after initial improvement, so condoms should be advocated after treatment.

In pregnancy, early infection with BV is a strong risk factor for preterm delivery and spontaneous abortion. This risk can be attributed to BV being linked to chorioamnionitis. However, a Cochrane review of 15 trials [1] reported no clear decrease in the odds of preterm birth with treatment of asymptomatic pregnant women in the general population. But when women with prior preterm birth were looked at separately, a significant reduction in the rate of preterm premature rupture of membranes and low birthweight was seen. Earlier diagnosis and treatment in the first trimester has been shown to be more effective for prevention of preterm birth than in the second trimester and beyond. Therefore, screening and treatment of BV in women with previous preterm birth should be considered at the first prenatal visit. In the first trimester, intravaginal clindamycin treats the infection locally and limits fetal exposure. After the first trimester, oral or intravaginal metronidazole can be used [2].

Causal relations have also been established between BV and upper genital tract infections, postpartum fevers, posthysterectomy vaginal cuff cellulitis, and postabortion infections. If BV is identified in the preoperative evaluation of a patient undergoing hysterectomy, appropriate therapy as listed above should be used to reduce the chance of postoperative surgical site infectious complications.

Candidiasis

Vulvovaginitis due to *Candida* is usually caused by the species *C. albicans*, a dimorphic fungus that forms yeast-like buds, pseudohyphae, and hyphae. This ubiquitous organism is frequently found as a saprophyte on the skin and in the bowel, oropharynx, and vagina. Twenty percent of women are normally colonized with candidal species. Seventy-five percent of women will have at least one episode of vulvovaginal candidiasis during their lifetime. Approximately half experience more than one episode and approximately 5% experience a relapse and recurrence during a period of many years. When the host defenses are impaired, it becomes a pathogen. Certain predisposing conditions are responsible for recurrent candidal infections. These include pregnancy, uncontrolled diabetes, immunocompromised states such as AIDS, and chronic systemic steroid use. In addition, using antibiotics and oral contraceptives with high estrogen levels is associated with recurrent infections in some women. Vulvovaginal candidiasis is not considered a sexually transmitted disease since it occurs in celibate women; however, there is an increased frequency at the time most women begin regular sexual activity.

Candida albicans is currently the most common cause of vaginitis during the reproductive years. However, an increasing frequency of other candidal species, particularly *C. glabrata*, has been reported, possibly due to the widespread use of over-the-counter drugs that are more selective in eradicating *C. albicans*.

The main symptom of this category of vulvovaginitis, in contrast to BV, is vulvar pruritus. A thick vaginal discharge ("cottage-cheese like") is often present. The vulva may be erythematous and edematous, and contain satellite lesions. Burning, particularly with urination, is a common symptom.

The diagnosis of vulvovaginal candidiasis is easily established by the finding of normal vaginal pH (4–4.5) and positive results on saline or 1% potassium hydroxide microscopy. Because of poor sensitivity of these tests and the lack of specificity of clinical signs, the diagnosis of vulvovaginal candidiasis should be obtained by performing a vaginal culture. Either Sabouraud's or Nickerson's medium inoculated with cells from a cotton swab will show evidence of growth in 2 or 3 days. Women with recurrent infections should undergo HIV testing and diabetes screening as indicated.

Treatment involves simple vulvar care measures, such as avoiding the use of harsh soaps and perfumes, and clothing that increases local heat and moisture, such as nylon underwear and tightly fitting garments, and refraining from unprotected intercourse during the treatment period.

Topical agents are the most commonly used initial treatment of uncomplicated vulvovaginal candidiasis. They have few side effects as they have minimal systemic absorption. Among the azoles, tioconazole and teraconazole appear to be the most active *in vitro*. Tioconazole demonstrates activity against *C. albicans* as well as *C. glabrata*, *C. tropicalis*, *C. kruzei* and the other less common species. By contrast, clotrimazole, miconazole, and butoconazole do not seem to be as active against *C. glabrata* and *C. tropicalis* as against *C. albicans*.

Gentian violet, although messy and somewhat irritating, is an effective intravaginal adjuvant therapy that can be applied during an office visit, especially for recurrent cases.

Oral agents are convenient but confer some risk of side effects and drug interactions, particularly with long-term use. A single dose of flucanazole 150 mg has been shown to be as effective as topical antimycotic drugs in treating primary candidal vulvovaginitis, and patients prefer it as first-line therapy over topical agents. For women with severe symptoms, oral fluconazole can be given in two doses, 3 days apart.

Recurrences are common and very frustrating. In these cases, one should consider sending cultures to identify resistant species and treat accordingly. It may also be useful to treat the partners of patients with recurrent infections.

Long-term oral antifungal therapy is sometimes necessary in these patients. Oral fluconazole 150 mg a day for 3 days (days 1, 4, 7), followed by once-a-week suppression is used for chronic vulvovaginal candidiasis. Side effects occur infrequently, but most commonly are gastrointestinal with nausea/vomiting in 3–4% of patients. Hepatotoxicity is also a possible but rare complication. Liver function should be checked after 6 months of therapy. Fluconazole is generally effective against *C. albicans* but not the non-*albicans* species.

Ketoconazole and itraconazole are the other oral agents that can be used for recurrent and chronic infections and routine liver function evaluation should be performed to identify the infrequent hepatic toxicities.

Prophylactic long-term intravaginal treatments may also be considered for recurrent candidal vulvovaginitis, and include clotrimazole 1% cream weekly for 6 months for maintenance, or once a month for prophylaxis, and miconazole twice weekly for 3–4 weeks.

Infection with *C. glabrata* can be treated effectively with a daily 600 mg capsule of intravaginal boric acid, at night for 2 weeks, with a 65–70% success rate. Intravaginal flucytosine cream (5 g a night for 2 weeks) has a higher success rate (> 90%) but is difficult to obtain and must be prepared by a compounding pharmacy.

In pregnancy, vaginal candidiasis is not associated with adverse pregnancy outcomes. Nystatin suppositories and miconazole cream are both category B drugs and can be safely used in the first trimester. After the first trimester, the other topical agents may be used. Oral agents should be avoided due to possible congenital malformations such as craniofacial, cardiac, and skeletal anomalies seen in high doses. Fluconazole, a category C drug, may be used as a single-dose therapy, and it does not seem to increase the risk of congenital abnormalities.

Trichomoniasis

Trichomoniasis is caused by the anaerobic flagellated protozoan *Trichomonas vaginalis*, a sexually transmitted organism found in both men and women. A moderate rise in vaginal pH favors its growth. Another factor encouraging trichomonal infection is local erosion resulting from chemical or mechanical trauma, neoplasm or other forms of vaginal infection.

Approximately 25% of women in the reproductive period harbor *T. vaginalis*, but only one-third of these have symptoms and signs of local inflammation. Trichomoniasis typically presents with a copious yellow-green frothy discharge that may be foul smelling. Trichomonads are identified on microscopic examination of the vaginal discharge. White blood cells are usually present. The vaginal pH is in the range of 5.0–7.0.

The cervix has a strawberry red appearance due to punctate subepithelial microhemorrhages. If the vulva is involved, there may be local tenderness, pruritus, dyspareunia, and dysuria.

In 80% of cases, the diagnosis of trichomoniasis is confirmed by microscopic examination of saline wet mount, with the observation of motile trichomonads; their shape is "football-like" with moving flagella. They also may be identified in both symptomatic and asymptomatic patients by performing a Pap smear, as this method has a sensitivity of 60–70%. Staining methods add little to the diagnosis and cultures are seldom needed. Polymerase chain reaction methods have been developed to aid in the diagnosis with a sensitivity of 90% and a specificity of 99.8%. Because the organism is able to survive outside the vagina, nonsexual transmission may occur.

The treatment of choice is metronidazole, a single dose of 2 g orally. Oral therapy achieves therapeutic levels in the periurethral and urethral tissue and is preferred over vaginal administration. Less than 10% of patients may experience nausea/vomiting with this dose. Alternatively, metronidazole 500 mg orally twice a day for 7 days can be tried. A disulfiram-like reaction is possible with co-administration with alcohol so patients should be counseled to avoid alcohol for 24 hours after treatment. The partner of the patient should also be treated to reduce the incidence of recurrence. Resistant trichomonas infections occur rarely. In these cases, the optimal treatment protocol has not been established but may require high dosages of metronidazole, often combining oral and vaginal dosing. Intravenous metronidazole has a role in treating recurrent severe infection not responsive to the above protocol.

Past evidence of a possible relationship between vaginal trichomoniasis and adverse pregnancy outcomes such as premature rupture of membranes and preterm delivery has led to more aggressive diagnosis and treatment in pregnancy. However, a recent study comparing women randomized to receive either metronidazole 2 g in two doses or placebo for asymptomatic trichomoniasis infection found an increased rate of preterm birth in the treated group [3]. One explanation provided by the authors for this increased risk is that the normal vaginal flora was disrupted by the high dose of metronidazole, possibly leading to opportunistic infections. Due to limitations of the above study and others, treatment of asymptomatic women in pregnancy remains controversial. Metronidazole was previously contraindicated in the first trimester of pregnancy due to its mutagenic properties in bacteria and carcinogenic properties in mice, but recent meta-analysis and other studies have failed to show an association between metronidazole use during pregnancy and teratogenic or mutagenic effects in infants [4].

Recent developments

A self-test for vaginal pH has been studied [5]. This study showed that subjects could correctly read the package insert, read the device and understand its use, especially as an aid in the diagnosis of vaginitis. Moreover, as an over-the-counter (OTC) diagnostic tool, consumers using the vaginal pH device when a vaginal infection was suspected were able to understand when to purchase antifungal medication (pH ≤ 4.5) or seek professional diagnosis from a healthcare provider (pH > 4.5) [6]. Indeed, use of the self-test for vaginal pH could reduce inappropriate use of OTC antifungal medications by approximately 50% and improve the correct diagnosis of vaginitis.

A new point-of-care test for the diagnosis of BV has been reported [7]. This test, called BVBlue (Gryphus Diagnostics, also Genzyme Diagnostics), requiring < 1 minute hands on and 10 minutes to complete, is a chromogenic diagnostic test based on the presence of elevated sialidase enzyme in vaginal fluid samples. Statistical testing comparing BVBlue to gram stain and Amstel criteria showed that it was superior for sensitivity and negative predictive value and similar for specificity and positive predictive value. Thus, this test should be considered, especially when microscopy is not available.

Similarly, another point-of-care test for the rapid detection of *Trichomonas vaginalis* has been reported [8]. This test, called OSOM Trichomonas Rapid Test (Genzyme Diagnostics), uses an immunochromatographic capillary flow (dipstick) assay, providing results in 10 minutes. As compared to a composite reference standard (CRS) composed of wet-mount microscopy and *T. vaginalis* culture, the sensitivity and specificity of OSOM were 83% and 99%, respectively, while for wet mount, they were 71 and 100%, respectively. The sensitivity was significantly better with OSOM than with wet mount (p = 0.004). Culture requires 48–72 hours before becoming positive; therefore, when culture or microscopy is not available, the OSOM for *Trichomonas vaginalis* should be considered. Additionally, the test was not affected by co-infection with *Chlamydia* and *Gonorrhea*.

Viruses

Herpes simplex virus
The most common venereal disease in women in many parts of the world is herpetic infection of the vagina and vulva. This topic is covered in Chapter 52.

Condyloma acuminatum
Condyloma acuminatum is a sexually transmitted infection that produces multiple small papillomatous lesions ("warts"), and is caused by the human papilloma virus (HPV). These lesions are found most often on the vestibule

but may also involve the labia, perianal skin, vagina, and cervix. Large lesions tend to coalesce and become secondarily infected.

Human papilloma virus is now recognized as the major cause of cervical cancer. Among women of reproductive age, the rate of detection of HPV is 6% of those with normal Pap smears to over 60% of those with cervical dysplasia. Infections are subclassified as: latent (asymptomatic), where no visible lesions are present; subclinical, where lesions are seen with acetic acid application and magnification; and clinical, where lesions are obvious on physical examination.

Over 60 HPV types have been identified. They have been subclassified based on their relationship with cervical neoplasia; types 16 and 18 are considered to have the strongest association with cervical and vulvar dysplasia and squamous carcinoma. Vulvar condylomas are usually associated with types 6 or 11.

According to the CDC, genital HPV is the most common sexually transmitted infection in the United States. Clinically, a broad spectrum of findings may be associated with HPV infections. Individuals with evidence of HPV infection in one area of the genital tract have significant risk of having HPV changes in another genital site. A thorough evaluation of the lower genital tract, including magnification if necessary, should be performed to ensure that all lesions are found and treated. Vulvar lesions suspicious for dysplasia or dystrophy should be biopsied. Highly sensitive polymerase chain reaction assays are available for HPV detection and typing.

Treatment of lower genital tract HPV infection is tedious and protracted, with a variety of chemical, mechanical, and ablative techniques being available. Topical concentrated trichloroacetic acid (TCA, 50–85%) works best on moist mucosal lesions. Podophyllin resin (20% in tincture of benzoin) or podofilox (0.5% solution) are applied directly to individual lesions on the vulvar and perianal lesions. These agents should not be used on the vagina or cervix or during pregnancy due to possible myelotoxicity and neurotoxicity. To prevent excessive irritation by podophyllin or TCA, the surrounding skin should be protected with a coating of petroleum jelly, and the skin should be washed 1–2 hours after application. Therapy should be repeated at weekly intervals until all lesions are cleared.

Imiquimod topic 5% cream (Aldara™), a self-administered agent applied to vulvar lesions three times a week over a 16-week treatment course, has shown good success in the treatment of vulvar condyloma. This drug enhances immune competency at a local level by an as yet undetermined mechanism.

Extensive disease or resistant lesions may require cryosurgery, laser therapy or surgical excision under anesthesia.

Pediculosis

An infestation with *Phthirus pubis* will cause chronic vulvar irritation but can easily be missed unless a careful examination is made for this tiny louse. Lindane (Kwell) lotion or shampoo is the treatment of choice. Clothing and linen should be changed frequently during treatment. Repeat treatment in 1 week is commonly required, as is treatment of the sexual partner.

Scabies

Scabies is due to *Sarcoptes scabiei*, which produces small, itchy subcutaneous burrows, papules, and vesicles along the wrists, finger webs, and torso. This condition is highly contagious and is treated in the same way as pediculosis.

Chemicals and allergens

Almost any agent that comes into contact with the vulva or vagina can cause erythema, irritation, ulceration, and/or discharge. The list includes soaps, douche materials, bubble bath, contraceptive preparations, powder, cloth dyes, perfumed or colored toilet paper or sanitary napkins, and local medication. Treatment begins with elimination of the causes listed above, and avoiding contact with the irritant.

Atrophic vaginitis

This topic is covered in Chapter 94.

Prepubertal vulvovaginitis

This topic is covered in Chapter 55.

References

1. Thinkhamrop J, Hofmeyr GJ, Adetoro O, Lumbiganon P. Prophylactic antibiotic administration in pregnancy to prevent infectious morbidity and mortality. *Cochrane Database Syst Rev* 2002; 4.
2. American College of Obstetricians and Gynecologists. *Bacterial vaginosis screening in prevention of preterm delivery. Committee Opinion No. 198.* Washington, DC: American College of Obstetricians and Gynecologists, 1998.
3. Klebanoff MA, *et al.* Failure of metronidazole of prevent preterm delivery among pregnant women with asymptomatic Trichomonas vaginalis infection. *N Engl J Med* 2001 Aug 16;345(7):487–93.
4. Caro-Paton T, *et al.* Is metronidazole teratogenic? A meta-analysis. *Br J Clin Pharmacol* 1997 Aug;44(2):179–82.

5. Roy S, Caillouette JC, Faden JS, Roy T. The role of an over-the-counter vaginal pH self-test device package insert: can subjects learn what the device is for and how to use it? *Am J Obstet Gynecol* 2005; 192: 1963–1969.

6. Roy S, Caillouette JC, Faden JS, *et al*. Improving appropriate use of antifungal medications: the role of an over-the-counter vaginal pH self-test device. *Infect Dis Obstet Gynecol* 2003; 11: 209–216.

7. Myziuk L, Romanowski B, Johnson SC. BVBlue test for the diagnosis of bacterial vaginosis. *J Clin Microbiol* 2003; 41: 1925–1928.

8. Huppert JS, Batteiger BE, Praslins P, *et al*. Use of immunochromatographic assay for rapid detection of *Trichomonas vaginalis* in vaginal specimens. *J Clin Microbiol* 2005; 43: 684–687.

Suggested reading

Baker DA, Douglas JM, Buntin DM, *et al*. Topical podofilox for the treatment of condylomata acuminata in women. *Obstet Gynecol* 1990; 76: 656–659.

Bellina JH. Use of carbon dioxide laser in management of condyloma acuminatum with 8-year follow-up. *Am J Obstet Gynecol* 1983; 147: 375–378.

Carey JC, Klebanoff MA. Is a change in the vaginal flora associated with an increased risk of preterm birth? *Am J Obstet Gynecol* 2005; 192: 1341.

Chen KCS, Forsyth PS, Buchanan TM, *et al*. Amine content of vaginal fluid from untreated and treated patients with nonspecific vaginitis. *J Clin Invest* 1979; 63: 828.

Cotch MF, Pastorek JG 2nd, Nugent RP, *et al*. Trichomonas vaginalis associated with low birth weight and preterm delivery. The Vaginal Infections and Prematurity Study Group. *Sex Transm Dis* 1997; 24: 353.

Gardner HL. *Haemophilus vaginalis* vaginitis after twenty-five years. *Am J Obstet Gynecol* 1980; 137: 385.

Hillier SL, Nugent RP, Eschenbach DA, *et al*. Association between bacterial vaginosis and preterm delivery of a low-birth-weight infant. The Vaginal Infection and Prematurity Study Group. *NEJM* 1995; 333: 1737–1742.

Kaufman RH. The origin and diagnosis of "nonspecific vaginitis". *NEJM* 1980; 303: 637.

Klebanoff MA, Carey JC, Hauth JC, *et al*. Failure of metronidazole to prevent preterm delivery among pregnant women with asymptomatic *Trichomonas vaginalis* infection. *NEJM* 2001; 345: 487–493.

Lugo-Miro VI, Green M, Mazur L. Comparison of different metronidazole therapeutic regimens for bacterial vaginosis. *JAMA* 1992; 268: 92–95.

McCormick WM, Evard JR, Laughlin CF, *et al*. Sexually transmitted conditions among women college students. *Am J Obstet Gynecol* 1980; 139: 130.

Pheifer TA, Forsyth PS, Durge MA, *et al*. Nonspecific vaginitis: role of *Haemophilus vaginalis* and treatment with metronidazole. *NEJM* 1978; 298: 1429.

Sobel JD. Current concepts: vaginitis. *NEJM* 1997; 337: 1896-1903.

Sobel JD, Brooker D, Stein GE, *et al*. Single oral dose fluconazole compared with conventional clotrimazole topic therapy of candida vaginitis. *Am J Obstet Gynecol* 1995; 172: 1263–1268.

Soper DE, Bump RC, Hurt WG. Bacterial vaginosis and trichomoniasis vaginitis are risk factors for cuff cellulitis after abdominal hysterectomy. *Am J Obstet Gynecol* 1990; 163: 1016.

Thin RN, Symonds MA, Booker R, *et al*. Double-blind comparison of a single dose and a five-day course of metronidazole in the treatment of trichomoniasis. *Br J Vener Dis* 1979; 55: 354.

Tidwell BH, Lushbaugh WB, Laughlin MD, *et al*. A double-blind placebo-controlled trial of single-dose intravaginal versus single-dose oral metronidazole in the treatment of trichomonal vaginitis. *J Infect Dis* 1994; 170: 242.

Chapter 51
Sexually Transmitted Diseases

Peyman Saadat and Subir Roy
Department of Medicine and Obstetrics and Gynecology, Keck School of Medicine, University of Southern California, CA, USA

Introduction

The Centers for Disease Control (CDC) estimates that 19 million new cases of sexually transmitted diseases occur each year in the USA, almost half being between the ages of 15 and 24. More than 50% of people worldwide will become affected with an STD in their lifetime. Changes in sexual behavior in the USA and throughout the world have led to an increased incidence of venereal diseases. These behaviors are characterized by decrease in age of coitarche, increased premarital intercourse, increased co-habitation, and increased divorce rate, with divorced individuals having higher rates of sexual activity compared with never married or widowed singles.

Differential diagnosis

There are more than 25 known sexually transmitted diseases, which can be caused by a variety of agents. Bacterial diseases include syphilis, gonorrhea, chancroid, granuloma inguinale, and lymphogranuloma venereum (caused by chlamydia) and chlamydia itself. Viral pathogens including herpes simplex virus, human papilloma virus, human immunodeficincy virus, hepatitis B and C, molluscum contagiosum and human T-lymphocyte virus (HTLV). Trichomonal vaginitis is caused by a protozoan while pediculosis pubis is caused by a louse.

Syphilis

A bacterial agent, *Treponema pallidum*, causes syphilis. This disease affects many organs, including the genitals, skin and mucus membranes, the central nervous system

Management of Common Problems in Obstetrics and Gynecology, 5th edition. Edited by T.M. Goodwin, M.N. Montoro, L. Muderspach, R. Paulson and S. Roy. © 2010 Blackwell Publishing Ltd.

and heart, among other organs. If left untreated, syphilis goes through four stages in the human body. The primary phase is characterized by a chancer, a painless ulcer which appears 10–90 days after incubation (average of 21 days). These ulcers may appear on the mucus membranes (vagina, mouth, and cervix) or on the breast, vulva or anus. Dark-field microscopy will demonstrate the spirochete (*T. pallidum*) if obtained from serum oozing off the chancer. Primary syphilis usually heals in 3–6 weeks. If left untreated, syphilis can lead to serious complications or death, but with early diagnosis and treatment the disease can be successfully treated.

A single chancer is usually typical but there may be multiple sores. Enlarged lymph nodes in the groin may be associated with the chancer. Primary syphilis typically disappears without any treatment, but the underlying disease remains, and may reappear at the secondary or tertiary stage.

The signs and symptoms of secondary syphilis may begin 2–10 weeks after the chancer appears and may include rash marked by red and reddish-brown, penny-size sores over any area of the body, including palms of the hands and soles of the feet, fever, fatigue and feeling of discomfort, soreness and aching, condyloma latum (painful lesion in the anogenital area or a characteristic rash). Dark-field microscopy or biopsy is diagnostic at this stage. In some people a period called latent syphilis, in which no symptoms are present, may follow secondary syphilis. Signs or symptoms may never return or disease may progress to the tertiary stage. The latent stage has two phases: the early latent phase occurs within 1 year after acquiring the infection and the late latent phase if it is more than a year.

Without treatment, the disease may progress to the tertiary stage. During this stage, syphilis bacteria may spread, leading to serious internal organ damage and death years after the original infection. The main organs that may be affected include cardiac, neurologic, ophthalmic, and auditory systems.

The serologic tests for syphilis may be classified into two groups. Nonspecific treponemal antibodies include the Venereal Disease Reseach Laboratory test (VDRL) and rapid plasma reagin (RPR). Treponemal tests, which detect specific treponemal antibodies, include *Treponema pallidum* hemagglutination (MHA-TP), the fluorescent treponemal antibody absorb test (FT-ABS) and most of the new treponemal enzyme immunoassay tests.

An important principle of syphilis serology is the detection of treponemal antibody by screening tests, followed by confirmation of a reactive screening test result by further testing. The confirmatory test or tests should ideally have a lower sensitivity and greater specificity than the screening test and use independent methodology.

The serologic markers usually become positive 4–5 weeks after the initial infection, or 1–2 weeks after the appearance of a chancer. A titer greater than 1:32 is diagnostic, while a titer less than 1:32 should be repeated. A fourfold change in the titer is usually considered clinically significant (e.g. an increase in a titer from 1:4 to 1:16 in a previously treated person might signify reinfection). Most patients' serologic tests will remain reactive once they have become positive. Of those patients treated in the primary stage, only 15–25% might revert to nonreactive serology, while those treated at other stages usually remain positive.

Treatment of syphilis involves a single dose of benzathine penicillin G 2.4 million units IM for patients diagnosed with primary, secondary or early latent stage. Those with a penicillin allergy can be treated with doxycycline 100 mg twice a day for 14 days, or tetracycline 500 mg four times a day for 14 days, or erythromycin 500 mg orally four times a day for 14 days. Tertiary syphilis or the late latent phase can be treated with benzathine penicillin G 2.4 million units IM once a week for 3 weeks (total of 7.2 million units), or doxycycline, tetracycline, and erythromycin taken in the same manner as above for 1 month.

Neurosyphilis can occur at any of the above stages after secondary syphilis and a neurologic examination is prudent prior to initiating therapy. If neurosyphilis is present it may be treated with 12–24 million units of penicillin G administered at 2–4 million units every 4 hours IV for 10–14 days.

Pregnant patients with syphilis need to be desensitized to penicillin, as it is the only effective treatment for the mother and fetus.

Granuloma inguinale (donovanosis)

Granuloma inguinale is caused by a gram-negative bacterium, *Calymmatobacterium granulomatis*. This disease is commonly found in tropical and subtropical areas such as South India, Guinea and New Guinea, but it occurs occasionally in the United States, usually seen in the Southeastern US. There are approximately 100 cases reported each year in the US. The disease is mostly spread through vaginal and anal intercourse. Very rarely, it is spread during oral intercourse. Men are affected more than twice as often as women, with most infection occurring between the ages of 20 and 40. The disease is seldom seen in children and the elderly. Symptoms include small, red bumps that appear on the anus. The skin gradually wears away and the bumps progress into raised beefy red velvety nodules called granulation tissue. They are usually painless but bleed easily if injured and are highly vascular. Tissue biopsy reveals dark-staining Donovan bodies, which are intracellular bacteria (there is no culture medium). The disease slowly spreads and destroys genital tissue. The tissue damage may spread to the inguinal lymph node, where the legs meet the torso.

In the early stages it may be difficult to tell the difference between granuloma inguinale and chancroid. Progression of the disease may cause obstruction of the lymph nodes after lymphatic spread. This may be progressive and followed by formation of pseudobubo and elephantiasis of the lower limbs. Further progression may cause suppuration and sinus formation, which mimics some of the female genital tract carcinomas. Other complications include genital destruction and scarring, loss of skin color in the genital area and permanent genital swelling due to scarring.

Treatment can be difficult and relapses often occur 6–18 months after the initial infection. Treatment options include bactrim DS twice a day for 21 days or doxycycline 100 mg twice a day for 21 days. Alternative regimens include ciprofloxacin and erythromycin. After the treatment course has been completed and the infection has subsided, surgical intervention may be required to correct scarring in the genital area.

Chancroid (soft chancer)

Chancroid is a superficial infection caused by a small gram-negative rod, *Haemophilus ducreyi*. Chancroid is sexually transmitted and is common in tropical countries but rare in other parts of the world. The incidence of chancroid has increased in the United States and it is more commonly seen in men, particularly uncircumcised males. The typical lesion is a painful, shallow, circular vulvar ulcer with an erythematous border and a yellow-to-gray base. Sores are surrounded by narrow red borders, which soon become filled with pus and eventually rupture, leaving painful, open sores. In 50% of the untreated cases, the chancroid bacteria infects the lymph gland in the groin. Within 5–10 days of the appearance of the primary sores, the glands on one and sometimes both sides of the groin become enlarged, hard and painful. The painful swelling may eventually rupture and become suppurative. Dark-field examination eliminates the diagnosis of syphilitic chancer and a gram stain of a smear usually demonstrates the bacilli arranged in a characteristic cluster.

The susceptibility of *H. ducreyi* to antimicrobial agents varies widely; therefore, response to therapy should be carefully monitored and adjusted. Suggested treatments include azithromycin 1 g orally in a single dose, ceftriaxone 250 mg IM using lidocaine as a diluent to minimize pain, ciprofloxacin 500 mg twice a day for 3 days, and erythromycin 500 mg orally four times a day. Chancroid can be cured with early antibiotic treatment in the immunocompetent patient. If it has already progressed to later stages or the host is immunocompromised, it can be more difficult to treat and may have more complications, including scarring, ruptured buboes with severe pain, fistula formation and other complications.

While ulcers generally show improvement within 7 days of instituting therapy, involved lymph nodes take longer to respond. If lymph nodes are fluctuant, needle drainage through dependent healthy skin may speed healing, while incision and drainage of lymph nodes over the most soft fluctuant portion of the mass delays healing and is not advised. A follow-up test for syphilis is advisable.

Lymphogranuloma venereum

Lymphogranuloma venereum is produced by *Chlamydia trachomatis* (serotypes L1, L2, and L3). Transmission is predominately sexual but transmission by nonsexual personal contact and laboratory accidents has been documented. It is a very rare disease in the United States.

The primary stage is marked by the formation of painless herpetiform ulcerations at the site of inoculation, and presents 4–12 days after exposure. Between 1 and 4 weeks later, it progresses by lymphatic spread to the femoral and inguinal lymph nodes associated with systemic symptoms such as fever, headache, myalgia, and arthralgia. Tender inguinal lymphadenopathy is usually unilateral and is the most common clinical manifestation during the secondary stage of the disease. Later, suppurative granulomatous lymphadenitis and perilymphadenitis occur with connection of the lymph nodes; frequently these nodes coalesce and form satellite abscesses. These nodes may separately enlarge on either side of the inguinal ligament, producing a "groove" or "saddle," two terms that have been used to characterize this lesion. Lymphatic buboes with ulceration and drainage are relatively uncommon in women. Lymphatic spread to the perirectal and pelvic nodes produces proctitis, followed by strictures and fistula formation. The urethra can also be involved. About 80% of the patients will have a positive Frei test if injected intradermally with 0.1 mL of the antigen. The diagnosis is usually made serologically and by exclusion of other causes of inguinal lymphadenopathy or genital ulcers.

Doxycycline 100 mg orally twice a day for 21 days or erythromycin 500 mg orally four times a day for 21 days may be used for treatment. The activity of azithromycin has not yet been tested, but it may be as useful against this strain of chlamydia as it is against other strains.

Molluscum contagiosum

Molluscum contagiosum is caused by a pox virus (DNA virus) and is becoming more common secondary to the HIV epidemic. Molluscum contagiosum is a small harmless growth caused by a skin virus. They resemble pimples with a waxy, pinkish appearance and a small central pit. Molluscum is contagious and spread by direct physical contact. It is found most often in children. When found in adults, it is usually as a result of direct sexual contact. In time, the molluscum infection goes away, once the body becomes immune to it. Molluscum is usually asymptomatic, although irritation may lead to secondary infection and localized lymphadenopathy. The umbilicated papule typically appears 2–8 weeks after infection and characteristically contains yellow curd-like material. It can be expressed and stained with gram, Wright or Giemsa stain, revealing large intracellular virions.

Generally, no therapy is required. Although lesions can be sprayed with ethylchloride or frozen with liquid nitrogen, it is normally only necessary to express the contents with curettage of the base. There is some anecdotal evidence that imiquimod 5% cream may facilitate resolution.

Mycoplasma

Mycoplasma hominis and T strains of this genus, which are unique bacteria with no cell wall, frequently inhabit the vagina, are commonly associated with pelvic infections, and can be transmitted sexually.

While *Mycoplasma* and *Ureaplasma* have been commonly implicated as causes of abortion, chorio-amnionitis, low-birthweight infants, bartholinitis, salpingitis, tubo-ovarian abscesses, urinary tract infection, and infertility, especially in men, they appear to have a low rate of virulence. More recently, *Mycoplasma* has been associated with premature rupture of membranes as well as preterm labor.

The antibiotic of choice is doxycycline 100 mg bid for 7 days or erythromycin 500 mg four times a day for 7 days for preterm labor prophylaxis in patients with premature rupture of membranes.

Other diseases

Herpes simplex, condyloma acuminatum, trichomoniasis, pediculosis, scabies, chlamydia, gonorrhea, and HIV are discussed in other chapters.

Suggested reading

Abrams AJ. Lympogranuloma venereum. *JAMA* 1968; 205: 59.

Alergant CB. Chancroid. *Practitioner* 1972; 209: 64.

Centers for Disease Control and Prevention. Sexually transmitted diseases treatment guidelines 2002. *MMWR* 2002; 51(no. RR-6).

Cohen J, Powderly WG. *Infectious diseases*, 2nd edn. New York: Elsevier, 2004: 2053–2056.

Diaz-Garcia FJ, Herrera-Mendoza AP, Giono-Cerezo S, Guerra-Infante FM. *Mycoplasma hominis* attaches to and locates intracellularly in human spermatozoa. *Human Reprod* 2006; 21(6): 1591–1598.

Dohil MA, Lin P, Lee J. The epidemiology of molluscum contagiosum in children. *J Am Acad Dermatol* 2006; 54(1): 47–54.

Lewis DA. Chancroid: clinical manifestations, diagnosis, and management. *Sex Transm Infect* 2003; 79(1): 68–71.

Piot P, Plummer FA. Genital ulcer adenopathy syndrome. In: Holmes KK, March P-A, Sparling PF (eds) *Sexually transmitted disease*. New York: McGraw-Hill, 1990: 71.

Rackel RE, Bope ET. Granuloma inguinale. In: *Conn's Current Therapy 2005*, 57th edn. St Louis, MO: Saunders, 2005: 859.

Ronald A, Alfa M. Chancroid, lymphogranuloma venereum, and granuloma inguinale. In: Gorbach S, Bartlett J, Blacklow N (eds) *Infectious diseases*, 2nd edn. Philadelphia, PA: WB Saunders, 1998: 1012–1013.

Rubiero J. Granuloma inguinale. *Practitioner* 1972; 209: 628.

Sparling PF. Diagnosis and treatment of syphilis. *NEJM* 1971; 284: 642.

Taylor-Robinson D, McCormick WM. The genital mycoplasma. *NEJM* 1980; 302: 1003.

US Department of Health and Human Services, Public Health Service, Division of Sexually Transmitted Diseases. Sexually transmitted diseases treatment guidelines. *MMWR* 1998; 47: 18–41.

US Department of Health and Human Services, Public Heath Service, Division of Sexually Transmitted Diseases. Sexually transmitted diseases treatment guidelines. *MMWR* 2006; 56: RR-11.

Chapter 52
Genital Herpes

Mario J. Pineda and Subir Roy
Department of Medicine and Obstetrics and Gynecology, Keck School of Medicine, University of Southern California, CA, USA

Introduction

Genital herpes is an incurable sexually transmitted infection, whose course is often recurrent in nature. This viral infection is a result of an inoculation of either of two identified serotypes: herpes simplex virus type 1 (HSV-1) or herpes simplex virus type 2 (HSV-2). Although multiple strains of this double-stranded DNA virus have been discovered, approximately 90% of urogenital herpes infections are a result of HSV-2. Recently an increase in the proportion of primary genital herpes infection caused by HSV-1 has been described; genital HSV-1 infections are a result of orogenital contact. Compared to HSV-2 infection, HSV-1 genital herpes results in less frequent recurrences and subclinical shedding.

Transmission often results from direct contact with a herpetic lesion or by exposure to asymptomatic viral shedding. Contact with a herpes lesion will permit the virus to be transmitted through a mucous membrane or an abraded skin surface and subsequently initiate intracellular replication. Furthermore, prospective investigations of sexually active couples with one infected partner demonstrated asymptomatic and unrecognized transmission of HSV-2 infections.

Genital herpes has reached epidemic proportions and according to the Centers for Disease Control at least 50 million persons in the USA have been diagnosed with genital HSV-2 infection based on serologic studies. Risk factors for genital herpes infection include female gender, smoking, abnormal vaginal flora, black race, prior sexually transmitted infection, early age of first intercourse, higher number of lifetime sexual partners, older age, poor socio-economic status and low level of education.

Generally, patients with HSV-2 infection are not diagnosed with genital herpes because the infection is subclinical; only 5–15% of individuals report recognition of their infection. Chronic carriers typically shed this highly contagious virus intermittently in the genital tract. Thus, significant numbers of cases of genital herpes are transmitted annually from persons who are either unaware of their infection or are asymptomatic. While recurrence of genital herpes may be spontaneous, some triggers have been identified. These include fever; exposure to heat, cold, or sunlight; corticosteroid administration; immunosuppression; psychologic stress; fatigue; nerve damage; local tissue trauma; and laser surgery. Symptomatic patients tend to suffer from severe somatic discomfort, which is often associated with psychologic manifestations. As there are no absolute predictors of activation, fear of recurrence often initiates a sense of unwillingness to engage in sexual contact and potentiates feelings of anxiety and depression, and a disruption of routine activities.

Clinical presentation and diagnosis

The primary genital herpes infection tends to have both local and generalized systemic symptomatology. The infection typically presents with multiple, painful, vesicular or ulcerated lesions. Patients may experience parasthesias prior to the appearance of vesicles. Within a few days of sexual contact, vesicles erupt on labia majora, introitus, urethra, and perineum; thighs and buttocks may also be involved. The vesicles are typically superficial, small (1–2 mm in diameter), and have an erythematous border. After approximately 1 week new lesions begin to form. Concomitantly, earlier lesions become more ulcerated and may coalesce. After approximately 2 weeks a dry crust forms and lesions begin to heal without developing a scar. Vulvar herpes is often accompanied by vaginal lesions and, less commonly, cervical lesions. Tender, firm and, often, bilateral inguinal lymphadenopathy may also be present. During the primary infection, 70% of women may experience a "prodrome" of symptoms including fever, malaise, or myalgias. Moreover,

Management of Common Problems in Obstetrics and Gynecology, 5th edition. Edited by T.M. Goodwin, M.N. Montoro, L. Muderspach, R. Paulson and S. Roy. © 2010 Blackwell Publishing Ltd.

symptoms of vaginal or urethral discharge may also be present with herpetic cervicitis or urethritis. The incubation period is 2–12 days and the patient may shed viruses for up to 3 weeks after the appearance of vesicles. The entire primary infection usually resolves within 2–6 weeks but viral shedding may persist for longer.

The diagnosis of genital herpes may be made by clinical history and physical examination with the assistance of laboratory evaluation. One must suspect genital herpes when a sexually active woman presents with the above prodromal symptoms and described genital lesions. Most HSV-2 seropositive individuals do not present with the classic signs and symptoms described above; therefore, history and clinical presentation are insufficient for diagnosis. It is prudent in the work-up of such a patient to rule out other sexually transmitted infections such as syphilis and chancroid, among others. Therefore, cultures for these and other infections should be sent as indicated, in order that the appropriate therapy can be initiated expediently. In addition to sexually transmitted infections, the differential diagnosis should include erosive lichen planus, atopic dermatitis and urethritis.

The laboratory tests that may be useful to confirm the clinical diagnosis of herpes simplex infection include cytology (Tzank smear), direct antibody staining, viral culture, polymerase chain reaction (PCR) and serology. Cytologic specimens that exhibit multinucleated giant cells and intranuclear inclusions may aid in the diagnosis but these tests are neither sensitive nor specific for HSV infection. Direct fluorescent antibody staining or immunohistochemistry may be used to detect type-specific HVS antigen using monoclonal antibodies on viral culture or lesional smear samples; these tests are specific and sensitive, but not widely available. Viral cultures are the "gold standard" diagnostic test. Samples obtained from fresh vesicles with a cotton tip applicator have a high rate of virus isolation but with a higher false-negative rate than PCR analysis, which can detect extremely low concentrations of viral DNA and is thus the most sensitive test. Although this is the laboratory evaluation of choice, it is still not widely available for genital sampling.

Serology is indicated when virologic techniques, antigen detection or PCR are impractical or nondiagnostic, as in patients with healing lesions, recurrent infection or nonactive lesions. Additionally, serologic tests are used to determine serostatus of a patient's partner, thereby identifing transmission risk. Serologic tests are immunometric assays (immunoblot or ELISA) that recognize antibodies that target the HSV glycoprotein. Additionally, a point-of-care test is available for detection of HSV-2 antibodies from blood or serum. Sensitivity of these tests varies from 80–98%, but all have a specificity of $\geq 96\%$. Serology is only useful in detecting whether an individual has been exposed previously to a herpes simplex virus and subsequently categorizing this patient as to the type of infection (primary vs recurrent, HSV-1 vs HSV-2). If a patient presents with an initial genital infection and has no antibodies to HSV, than the patient is considered to have a primary infection. If the patient presents with genital lesions and is IgG antibody positive, the patient is thought to have a nonprimary infection that is caused by reactivation of a latent virus residing in the dorsal root ganglia of sacral nerves 2, 3, and 4. Patients with recurrent genital herpes may or may not have a prior history of a clinical infection. Rate of symptomatic recurrence increases with immunosuppression and decreases with time since primary infection.

Treatment

The aims of therapy are attenuation of the clinical course, viral shedding and complications, and to counsel the patient with respect to the natural course and transmission of genital herpes. It is important that patients understand that the use of antiviral therapy does not eradicate the latent virus. Moreover, antiviral medications do not have any effect on the subsequent frequency or severity of recurrent genital herpes after the termination of therapy. With this in mind, it is of use to determine if the patient is presenting with her first clinical episode of genital herpes or if it is a recurrent episode. Primarily due to the severity and longer duration of the first clinical episode, antiviral therapy tends to be more aggressive than for recurrent episodes.

Oral antiviral agents are nucleoside analogs that inhibit viral replication by interrupting DNA synthesis. Agents approved for use include aciclovir, valaciclovir, which is a valine ester prodrug of aciclovir, and famciclovir, which is the prodrug of penciclovir. The recommended regimens for the treatment of the first clinical episode of genital herpes are:
- aciclovir 400 mg orally three times a day for 7–10 days
- aciclovir 200 mg orally five times a day for 7–10 days
- famciclovir 250 mg orally three times a day for 7–10 days, or
- valaciclovir 1 g orally twice a day for 7–10 days

The antiviral therapy may be continued past 10 days until a satisfactory clinical response has been achieved. Patients who present with first episodes of herpes proctitis, stomatitis or pharyngitis require aciclovir 400 mg orally five times a day. If a patient has severe clinical symptoms requiring hospitalization, such as disseminated infection, pnemonitis, hepatitis, encephalitis or meningitis, aciclovir can be given intravenously at a dose of 5–10 mg/kg of bodyweight every 8 hours for 2–7 days or until there is clinical resolution, followed by oral antiviral therapy to complete at least 10 days of total therapy. Unfortunately, most patients are not aware of their diagnosis and rarely present in their prodromal phase. The majority of patients present with the appearance of genital vesicles. If antiviral therapy is initiated within the first few days of the presentation of symptoms, the median duration of eruptions is shortened and clinical symptomatology is reduced.

Approximately 80–90% of patients with an HSV-2 infection will have an episode of recurrent genital herpes within 12 months. Furthermore, since patients may benefit from episodic and/or suppressive therapy to shorten the duration of lesions and prevent recurrence, it is important to counsel patients to begin therapy with the onset of the prodrome or within 1 day of the onset of lesions. The recommended regimens for episodic recurrent infection are:
- aciclovir 400 mg orally three times a day for 5 days
- aciclovir 800 mg orally twice a day for 5 days
- aciclovir 800 mg orally three times a day for 2 days
- famciclovir 125 mg orally twice a day for 5 days
- famciclovir 1000 mg orally twice daily for 1 day
- valaciclovir 500 mg orally twice a day for 3 days, or
- valaciclovir 1000 mg orally once a day for 5 days

Short-term prophylactic treatment before events that are known to trigger eruption of lesions may decrease frequency and severity of recurrences. Patients with greater than six episodes of genital herpes per year can reduce the frequency of recurrence and subclinical shedding by 80% and 95%, respectively, with daily suppressive therapy. The recommended regimens for daily suppressive therapy after an episode of genital herpes in an immunocompetent host are:
- aciclovir 400 mg orally twice a day
- famciclovir 250 mg orally twice a day
- valaciclovir 500 mg orally once a day, or
- valaciclovir 1000 mg orally once a day (for more than 10 recurrences annually)

Daily suppressive aciclovir has been found to be safe and effective in usage for up to 6 years, and famciclovir and valaciclovir for up to 1 year. There is no indication for intravenous aciclovir in episodic recurrence of genital herpes and topical therapy may only ameliorate symptomatology. The application of topical anesthetics may provide minor relief.

Patient education is extremely important in the management of genital herpes. For all seronegative patients, primary prevention aims at delaying sexual debut and limiting the number of sexual partners. Patients should be counseled at their initial visit and continuously supported and re-educated during routine annual physical evaluations. It is important to emphasize that HSV infection also increases the risk of acquiring other sexually transmitted diseases, including HIV. Annual Pap smears should be stressed, as patients with a history of multiple sexual partners are at an increased risk of

developing cervical cancer. Physicians should also discuss the likelihood of recurrence with patients. It should be stressed that, while use of condoms has been shown to decrease transmission, they do not eliminate transmission as external genital contact between partners with active lesions or asymptomatic viral shedding of highly contagious particles can result in transmission. Therefore, patients should be encouraged to familiarize their partners with this condition, always use condoms, and to avoid sexual contact during the prodomal phase or when lesions are present. Viral transmission is four times more likely from male to female than from female to male. Sex partners of infected persons should be advised that they might be infected even if they have no symptoms. Women of reproductive years should inform their primary care physician and the provider who will care for them during pregnancy of their condition or their partner's. Finally, both partners should be informed of the risks of neonatal transmission, in order that they are aware during the preconceptional period.

Genital herpes and pregnancy

Pregnancy often complicates the clinical management of genital herpes. Moreover, a primary genital herpes infection has approximately a 2% incidence during pregnancy in the general obstetric population. Approximately 10% of women who are HSV seronegative have partners who are HSV seropositive and are at risk for primary infection during pregnancy. It is estimated that one-third of HSV primary infections occur in each trimester. Currently, the availability of point-of-care testing for HSV-2 varies; therefore, physicians often rely solely on their clinical acumen for the diagnosis and acute care of the obstetric patient. In addition, antiviral therapies have not been studied extensively in pregnancy and the safety and efficacy of their use have also not been entirely established. Limited data suggest that there is no increased risk for major birth defects compared to the general population in women treated with aciclovir in the first trimester. While vertical transmission of HSV may occur *in utero*, intrapartum or postpartum, intrapartum transmission predominates.

In addition to supportive maternal care, the focus of management is the prevention of neonatal transmission during labor. It is important to recognize that 80% of HSV infection infants are born to mothers with no reported history of HSV infection. When patients are admitted to labor and delivery, the mother should be asked if she is experiencing any prodromal symptoms. Furthermore, the vulva, the vagina, and the cervix should be thoroughly examined. In the absence of prodromal symptoms and distinguishable lesions, patients should be counseled that the risks of neonatal infection with vaginal delivery are less than 1%. If either prodromal symptoms or lesions are present, cesarean delivery should be recommended. In the most ideal of circumstances, cesarean delivery should be performed prior to rupture of membranes. Regardless, during an active infection abdominal delivery in light of ruptured membranes still decreases the inoculum of virus to which the fetus is exposed in comparison to a vaginal delivery. Cesarean section decreases but does not completely eliminate the risk of HSV transmission to the fetus. Overall, the frequency of neonatal transmission depends on whether the infection is primary or recurrent. A primary infection carries a 30–50% neonatal transmission rate during vaginal delivery. Comparatively, recurrent infections have a neonatal transmission rate of less than 5% during vaginal delivery. However, asymptomatic viral shedding during early labor accounts for 30% of transmission.

Minimal data exist estimating the risks of spontaneous abortion, preterm labor, stillbirths, and intrauterine growth retardation in women with severe primary herpes infections or recurrent infections. A meta-analysis of trials to assess the effectiveness of aciclovir suppression therapy given to prevent clinical recurrence at delivery, cesarean delivery for recurrent genital herpes and the detection of HSV at delivery showed that recurrence was reduced by 75% and rate of cesarean delivery for recurrent genital herpes was reduced by 40% for women who received suppression therapy with dosage schedules of 200 mg four times a day or 400 mg three times a day, after 36 weeks of gestation.

Finally, a significant spectrum of clinical manifestations of neonatal herpes exists, ranging from mucocutaneous lesions to meningitis, encephalitis, jaundice, disseminated intravascular coagulation, and pneumonitis, as well as death.

During the postpartum period, mothers may handle their infants as long as they consciously prevent direct contact of skin lesions with the neonate. Furthermore, breastfeeding is not contraindicated if there are no lesions on the breast or nipple. Treatment with valaciclovir is safe for breastfeeding mothers and while aciclovir is present in breast milk in greater concentration compared to maternal blood, it is only 2% of the therapeutic dose given to infants. It is also advisable that patients, as well as healthcare workers and family members who are in contact with the patient, wash their hands prior to handling the infant. The risk of postpartum infection to the neonate is extremely low when these precautions are implemented and is not of great concern in comparison to intrapartum infection.

Suggested reading

American College of Obstetricians and Gynecologists. *Gynecologic herpes simplex virus infections. Practice Bulletin No 57*. Washington, DC: American College of Obstetricians and Gynecologists, 2004.

American College of Obstetricians and Gynecologists. *Management of herpes in pregnancy. Practice Bulletin No 82*. Washington, DC: American College of Obstetricians and Gynecologists, 2007.

Brown ZA, Wald A, Morrow RA, *et al.* Effect of serologic status and cesarean delivery on transmission rates of herpes simplex virus from mother to infant. *JAMA* 2003; 289: 203–209.

Centers for Disease Control. Sexually transmitted diseases – treatment guidelines 2006. *MMWR Recomm Rep* 2006; 55: 1–94.

Corey L, Hansfield HH. Genital herpes and public health: addressing a global problem. *JAMA* 2000; 283: 791–794.

Fatahzadeh M, Schwartz RA. Human herpes simplex virus infections: epidemiology, pathogenesis, symptomatology, diagnosis, and management. *J Am Acad Dermatol* 2007; 57: 737–763.

Gibbs RS, Mead PB. Preventing neonatal herpes current strategies. *NEJM* 1992; 326: 946.

Sheffield JS, Hollier LM, Hill JB, *et al.* Acyclovir prophylaxis to prevent herpes simplex virus recurrence at delivery: a systematic review. *Obstet Gynecol* 2003: 102: 1396–1403.

Stone KM, Reyes M, Shaik NS, *et al.* Acyclovir-resistant genital herpes among persons attending sexually transmitted disease and human immunodeficiency virus clinics. *Arch Intern Med* 2003; 163: 76–80.

Wald A, Link K. Risk of human immunodeficiency virus infection in herpes simplex virus type 2-seropositive persons: a meta-analysis. *J Infect Dis* 2002; 185: 45–52.

Wald A, Huan ML, Carrell D, *et al.* Polymerase chain reaction for detection of herpes simplex (HSV) DNA on mucosal sureeases: comparison with HSV isolation in cell culture. *J Infect Dis* 2003; 188: 1345–1351.

Chapter 53
Pelvic Infection

Peyman Saadat and Subir Roy
Department of Medicine and Obstetrics and Gynecology, Keck School of Medicine, University of Southern California, CA, USA

Introduction

Each year in the United States, it is estimated that more than one million women experience an episode of upper genital tract infection (UGTI), a term that is more specific, or acute pelvic inflammatory disease (PID), a term that is more widely used, for this condition. More than 100,000 women become infertile each year as a result of PID, and a large number of ectopic pregnancies occurring every year are due to consequences of PID. Annually, more than 150 women die from PID or its complications.

Changes in the sexual behavior of people in the USA and throughout the world are responsible for the increasing rate of pelvic infection among females. These behavioral changes include: earlier age at coitarche, increased premarital intercourse, increased rate of co-habitation (sex is implicit, indeed taken for granted), increase in divorce rate (higher rate of sexual activity compared to those who have never married or widowed singles).

The vagina contains both aerobic and anaerobic organisms (anerobes > aerobes). Pelvic infection may occur as a consequence of the introduction of pathogenic exogenous organisms (e.g. *Neisseria gonorrhoeae* (gonorrhea, GC), *Chlamydia trachomatis* (CT), etc.) and/or by the presence of normal vaginal flora in an abnormal location (e.g. in the endometrium, oviducts, peritoneal cavity, etc.) in sufficient numbers to overwhelm the body's host defense system. The female genital tract has a high concentration of defense cells and immunologic mediators (e.g. T-lymphocytes, macrophages, Langerhans' cells, polymeric immunoglobulin receptor positive cells, plasma cells, etc.). The highest concentration of these mediators is found in the endocervix, including the transformation zone of the cervix. Factors which decrease the host defense mechanism may lead to greater susceptibility to pelvic infections.

Management of Common Problems in Obstetrics and Gynecology, 5th edition. Edited by T.M. Goodwin, M.N. Montoro, L. Muderspach, R. Paulson and S. Roy. © 2010 Blackwell Publishing Ltd.

When an inoculation of mixed (aerobic and anerobic) organisms derived from bowel flora is introduced into an abnormal location (e.g. peritoneal cavity), a biphasic infection pattern may ensue. Initially, peritonitis secondary to the effects of aerobic gram-negative organisms such as *Escherichia coli* precedes abscess formation composed largely of anaerobic organisms, predominantly of the Bacteroides group. Approximately 40% of laboratory animals infected in this manner but not treated with antibiotics have died of peritonitis, while nearly 100% of surviving animals have developed abscesses.

Diagnosis

Pelvic inflammatory disease occurs when bacteria move upward from the woman's vagina or cervix into the reproductive or other organs and can cause PID, but many cases are associated with gonorrhea and chlamydia, two very common bacterial STDs. A prior episode of PID increases the risk of another episode because the reproductive organs may be damaged during the initial bout of infection. Females below the age of 25 are especially at risk, because the cervix of teenage girls and young women is not fully matured, with the squamocolumnar zone on the ectocervix, increasing their sensitivity to STDs and PID.

One out of seven, approximately 14%, of all women will get salpingitis in their lifetime. Pelvic soft tissue infection is more common in blacks than whites. Divorced women are more likely to get salpingitis than currently married women or never married women (19%, 12%, and 6%, respectively). The risk of salpingitis increases with the number of lifetime sexual partners (7% in women with one lifetime partner vs 19% in women with two or more). Other associated risk factors include increased number of sexual partners, people who have sex partners who themselves have more than one sex partner, women who douche frequently, and a slight increased risk at the time of insertion of an intrauterine device (IUD).

Historic information directly correlated with the etiology of a sexually transmitted disease (STD) includes: the time of onset of symptoms relative to the onset of the last menstrual period (LMP), last sexual exposure, number of sexual partners (lifetime but, perhaps more importantly, over the last 2–3 months), history of previous STD (whether treated as an outpatient or as an inpatient), sexual partner with symptoms (complaint of urethral discharge or "drip"), and contraceptive practices. A history of recent instrumentation may elucidate the mechanism by which endogenous flora may gain access to and produce disease of the upper genital tract and includes the following: dilation and curettage (D&C) for diagnosis or elective termination of pregnancy, intrauterine contraceptive device insertion, or hysterosalpinography. Smoking predisposes the patient to more STDs, possibly because smokers are greater risk takers and are more sexually active than nonsmokers and probably because smoking alters the host defense by reducing biologically active estrogens, impairing ciliary activity of oviductal cells, reducing leukocyte action, and reducing immunoglobulin A activity in cervical mucus.

Many signs and symptoms may suggest infection of the pelvic structures. A patient may complain of fever, abdominal or pelvic pain, cervical or vaginal discharge, nausea, vomiting, right upper quadrant pain, etc. Upon examination, she may be found to have a normal temperature or temperature elevation; localized or generalized pain or tenderness with or without evidence of pelvic or abdominal peritonitis; discharge, the source, character and amount of which may be suggestive of the offending pathogen(s), etc. These may be characterized by the presence of "-ors," the classic findings associated with inflammation: color (heat), dolor (pain), rubor (redness), and tumor (mass). Additional findings may be characterized by utilizing the suffixes "-osis," the presence of organisms without histologic changes induced in underlying tissues (e.g. nonspecific vaginosis), and "-itis," the presence of pathogenic organisms with histologic changes induced in the underlying tissues (e.g. vaginitis, endometritis, salpingitis); or abscess, a collection of pus and debris composed of desquamated or necrotic cells, tissues or organisms contained in a circumscribed location (e.g. appendiceal abscess, demarcated by loops of bowel), or by the destruction of organs or tissues (e.g. tubo-ovarian abscess).

In 2006 the CDC set forth the following criteria for diagnosis of PID. The patient must have a minimum of one of the following: lower abdominal pain, adnexal tenderness, and tenderness with cervical motion, and also one or more of the following additional criteria: sign of lower genital tract inflammation, oral temperature more than 101° F, abnormal cervical or vaginal discharge, greatly increased number of white blood cells on saline microscopy of vaginal secretion, elevated erythrocyte sedimentation rate, elevated C-reactive protein levels, laboratory documentation of cervical infection with *C. trachomatis*

or *N. gonorrhoeae*. Additional findings may be present, including: histologic evidence of endometritis at endometrial biopsy, pelvic fluid or tubo-ovarian complex on transvaginal sonogram or images from other modalities, and laparoscopic abnormalities that are consistent with PID, including presence of pus seen exuded through the tube.

Various simple tests may be performed in order to suggest the identity of the pathogenic organisms. A wet-mount smear with sodium chloride may aid in the diagnosis of nonspecific bacterial vaginosis, nonspecific vaginitis or *Trichomonas* vaginalis, while one utilizing potassium hydroxide aids in the diagnosis of *Candida albicans*. Gram stains made of cervical discharge, vaginal discharge, wound infections or from margins of abscesses permit the identification of broad classes of organisms based on their morphologic appearance and gram stain status. Empiric therapy may be selected, accordingly, while results of cultures are pending. These cultures should be obtained from portals or adjacent structures involved in sexual activities. These may include the oropharynx, urethra, cervix, vagina, and rectum. It may be necessary to obtain cultures for aerobic and anerobic organisms, GC, and genital mycoplasmas, as well as tissue cultures for CT. More recently, the availability of ligase chain reaction and polymerase chain reaction has made the screening for GC and CT from cervical or urine specimens more efficient and cost-effective. New tests have emerged that can do screening for both gonorrhea and chlamydia in one culture, which has made the screening process much easier.

Ultrasound of the female pelvis is frequently performed but it has not replaced the pelvic examination. If adnexal masses are visualized by ultrasound, suggesting inflammatory processes, the prudent physician does not aspirate them; instead, a trial of antibiotic therapy is instituted. An x-ray of the abdomen and pelvis may demonstrate gas in soft tissues; air under the diaphragm, suggestive of a perforated viscus; a mass lesion; ileus; etc. A CT or MRI scan may identify masses or a blood-filled collection that are not discernible by other diagnostic studies. A barium enema (BE), upper gastrointestinal tract series (UGI) or intravenous pyelography may be useful in establishing or ruling out the diagnosis of gastrointestinal or genitourinary conditions. Thus, standard diagnostic tests are useful in making the diagnosis of female pelvic soft tissue infections.

An elevated white blood cell count and erythrocyte sedimentation rate may be helpful in making the diagnosis of genital tract infections; however, it is not mandatory that they be elevated in order to make this diagnosis.

Historically, the term "febrile menses" has indicated gonococcal salpingitis. This presumptive diagnosis is made when gram-negative intracellular diplococci organisms are seen on gram stain of a cervical specimen in an individual who has some or all of the following: lower abdominal pain, cervicovaginal discharge, cervical motion tenderness, bilateral adnexal tenderness, elevated white blood cell count, elevated sedimentation rate, and fever. While fever is commonly associated with the presence of GC, it is not essential in order to make the diagnosis. Nongonococcal salpingitis may be suggested with similar findings, except that it may occur at any time during the menstrual cycle (although it could occur with or soon after the onset of the LMP); it may occur in the absence of fever, and is suggestive of CT if the gram stain demonstrates many polymorphonuclear neutrophils and few bacteria ("mucopus"). If the gram stain shows many polymorphonuclear neutrophils and bacteria, generally the patient has fever, and the presumptive diagnosis is based on the morphology of the predominant bacterial species identified.

Pain in the right upper quadrant in a woman with signs and symptoms of salpingitis suggests the Fitz-Hugh–Curtis syndrome in which the spread of pathogenic organisms (originally described with GC but now also reported with CT) along the colic gutters to the liver leads to adhesion formation.

For patients who do not present with the standard signs and symptoms of salpingitis, and provided that they do not have a significant ileus or a large pelvic/abdominal mass, it is advisable to perform diagnostic laparoscopy to clarify the diagnosis. Diagnostic laparoscopy performed in patients with suspected salpingitis has indicated that about 20% of such individuals will have normal-appearing pelvic structures, 3–4% each will be diagnosed as having ectopic pregnancy or appendicitis, and 2–4% will have a variety of other pelvic pathology (e.g. endometriosis, diverticulitis, etc.), while the remainder (about 65–70%) are found to have salpingitis.

Consequences

Prompt and appropriate treatment can help prevent complications of PID. Without treatment, PID can cause permanent damage to the female reproductive organs; infections of chlamydia and gonorrhea may invade into the mucosal layers of the fallopian tube, causing adhesion formation and consequently causing tubal blockage with infertility.

The consequences of infection of the female pelvic soft tissues include a 3–4-fold increase in pelvic pain, a 7–10-fold increase in ectopic gestation, and a 15–60% increase in infertility, proportional to the number of episodes of salpingitis that a patient has suffered. Less well-associated sequelae include adverse pregnancy outcome (e.g. habitual abortion is reported to be associated with *Ureaplasma urealyticum* and postpartum

endomyoparametritis associated with GC, CT, group B streptococcus, etc.).

Effect of birth control

In comparison with patients who use no method of birth control and who are sexually active, barrier method users have half the risk of pelvic infection because of the barrier effect as well as use of nonoxinol-9-containing spermicidal jellies or creams which have been shown to impair the growth of GC or CT or kill HIV. However, if such a jelly or cream is used chronically, it may facilitate rather than reduce the risk of HIV acquisition, as the surface vaginal epithelium may become inflamed or damaged, providing a portal of entry for the HIV. Oral contraceptive users have a reduced risk of pelvic infection by virtue of the thick cervical mucus and, possibly, by the reduced menstrual flow that results from the progestagen component of the combination preparation. Oral contraceptive users have been reported to harbor CT 2–3-fold more frequently in their endocervix than nonusers. It has been suggested, although not proven, that oral contraceptive use in some way makes the squamocolumnar junction tissues of the cervix more susceptible to inoculation by pathogenic organisms such as CT or the human papilloma virus, but decreases the chance of salpingitis secondary to the thickened cervical mucus.

Intrauterine device (IUD) users have the same risk of developing salpingitis as controls, except in those using the Dalkon Shield, or soon after IUD insertion when a small number of organisms are introduced into the endometrial cavity. In addition, it has been shown that the new progesterone IUDs may further decrease the incidence of PID by decreasing menstrual flow and thickening the cervical mucus. The Dalkon Shield had a mutifilament tail enclosed in a sheath which served as a wick, drawing bacterial organisms into the upper genital tract. Modern IUDs have a monofilament tail and their use is not associated with problems generally associated with the Dalkon Shield.

Pathogenic organisms

Pelvic soft tissue infections are polymicrobial, with GC, CT, aerobic and anerobic organisms, endogenous flora, and the genital mycoplasmas comprising the bulk of the community-acquired infections. Some investigators feel that the presence of genital mycoplasma is an indicator of sexual activity and that its presence is not necessarily associated with disease production. Usually, a combination of pathogenic organisms is cultured; however, the failure to culture organisms does not mean that the patient is not infected since, typically, we only have access to the lower genital tract for cultures (vagina, endocervix or endometrium) while the disease may be occurring in the upper genital tract (oviducts or ovary), from which there may be no drainage to the lower genital tract.

In 2003, 877,478 chlamydia infections were reported to the CDC from the 50 US states and the District of Columbia. The reported number of cases of chlamydia infections was more than two times greater than the reported cases of gonorrhea, which was 335,104. From 1987 to 2003 the reported rate of chlamydia infection in women increased from 78.5 cases to 466.9 cases per 100,000 population. This increase in the detected national chlamydia rate may represent increased chlamydia screening, as well as better screening methods for chlamydia. Whereas previously cultures were the only method of screening for chlamydia, the advent of the polymerase chain reaction (PCR) and ligase chain reaction (LCR) has made the screening and diagnosis of CT less time consuming and more accurate compared to the older methods. More recently, rapid over-the-counter tests are becoming available. The tests can be self-administered and physicians can be consulted to treat if the test becomes positive.

The antibody titers to CT (immunoglobulins M and G) are higher in women who have an ectopic gestation when compared to women with an intrauterine pregnancy of the same gestational age or in infertile women when compared to fertile women. In some settings (e.g. Los Angeles County–University of Southern California Medical Center), GC is recovered from around 50% of the women hospitalized for treatment of salpingitis. In most reported series, GC is recovered from 40% to 60% and CT from 5% to 20% of such patients. Our CT recovery, based on endocervical cultures, is around 5–10% from such patients. Both of these pathogens may be recovered simultaneously in high-risk patients.

In studies at the Los Angeles County–University of Southern California Medical Center, *E. coli* was the most frequently recovered aerobic pathogen, slightly more frequently than GC. Among the anerobes, *Bacteroides bivius* and *B. disiens* were more frequently recovered than *B. fragilis* (only 5% of all anerobes).

Both CT and GC are believed to injure the surface epithelium of the female genital tract in an ascending manner (via the endocervix to the oviducts). Subsequent infections with other offending pathogenic organisms may gain access to the underlying tissues (e.g. myometrium, parametrium) or to more remote locations (e.g. the ovary and the broad ligaments). These latter locations may be involved by direct extension or by seeding from hematogenous or lymphatic spread. As a consequence of genital tract tissue injury and because this tissue is generally incapable of complete restoration of structures and function, even after aggressive antibiotic therapy, the sequelae of pelvic infection (pelvic pain, ectopic pregnancy, and infertility) are not surprising.

Treatment

Ambulatory treatment for GC or CT requires therapy for the other pathogen as well. Commonly, a β-lactamase stable second- or third-generation cephalosporin is administered intramuscularly followed by a 7–10-day oral course of tetracycline, a synthetic tetracycline or erythromycin is prescribed. Alternative oral therapy includes azithromycin 1 g (for CT) and cefixime 400 mg (for GC). Ofloxacin and other quinalones are no longer recommended for treatment of gonorrhea in California. The state of California issued new guidelines in 2005, which recommend avoiding the use of fluoroquinolones, including ciprofloxacin, levofloxacin and ofloxacin, to treat gonorrhea in California due to high levels of resistance. Our use of azithromycin (1 g) and cefixime (400 mg), each given once in the emergency room, has been associated with a 22% reduction in admission for inpatient antibiotic administration for salpingitis. Parenteral and oral therapy seem to have similar clinical efficacy when treating women with PID of mild or moderate severity.

Patients should be treated with IV antibiotics if they meet one of the following nine criteria for hospital admissions:
• cannot rule out surgical emergencies such as appendicitis
• pregnant
• outpatient treatment failure
• GI symptoms (nausea and vomiting) or high fevers
• presence of tubo-ovarian abscesses on the ultrasound or clinical examination
• immune deficiency (e.g. HIV infection)
• intrauterine device in place
• history of recent uterine instrumentation
• nulliparous patients

Inpatient therapy for female pelvic soft tissue infection follows a similar philosophy, although there is a greater concern about the ability successfully to treat aerobic gram-negative and anaerobic organisms (both gram negative and gram positive). Parenteral therapy with a β-lactamase stable cephalosporin combined with azithromycin, a synthetic tetracycline or erythromycin is generally recommended for salpingitis without the presence of a mass (on pelvic examination or ultrasound). Alternatively, clindamycin and gentamicin can be used for the same indication. Indeed, recent reports from Patton suggest that therapy with tetracycline, erythromycin or doxycycline may not eradicate CT from the oviduct, because she was able to recover viable CT from extirpated ectopic pregnancies, which occurred following therapy.

If a mass is suspected on the basis of pelvic examination or ultrasound, then therapy should include coverage for anerobes. Gentamicin and clindamycin with or without penicillin can be used for this purpose. Alternatively, a third-generation cephalosporin (cefotaxime and ceftizoxime), a uridopenicillin (piperacillin, ticarcillin, mezlocillin) alone or with a β-lactamase blocker (e.g. unasyn or zosyn) may be used for this indication.

We generally recommend a repeat pelvic examination of the patient 48 hours after she has become afebrile or is clinically improved (pelvic stress test). If the patient has significant resolution of tenderness upon examination and does not spike a fever following the examination while continuing to receive the parenteral therapy during the ensuing 8–24 hours, then she can be considered for change from parenteral to oral antibiotic therapy or for discharge from the hospital. Usually a synthetic tetracycline and oral clindamycin or metronidozole is prescribed to complete a 10–14-day course of antibiotic therapy, although there are no firm data to conclude that oral therapy is beneficial following completion of parenteral therapy provided the woman passes the pelvic stress test. However, if there is no clinical improvement within 48 hours, changing the antibiotic regimen to the alternatives discussed above is usually recommended.

If no clinical improvement is noted by 72 hours, operative intervention must be considered. In addition, if there is a clinical response to antibiotic therapy but persistence of pelvic mass on pelvic examination and an ultrasound study, then surgical intervention is warranted in 6–8 weeks. Approximately 30% of women hospitalized for antibiotic therapy for treatment of end-stage tubal infections will require surgical intervention with extirpation of some or all of the genital tract structures, either during or following the hospitalization, in order to be cured of their infection. There are reports, however, of patients with presumed or actual end-stage tubal disease (e.g. tubo-ovarian abscess on the basis of pelvic examination or ultrasound) who have responded to antibiotic therapy alone or combined with colpotomy drainage (drainage of pelvic abscess via the posterior vaginal fornix, which is relatively safe to perform when the leading edge of the abscess extends below the level of the external cervical os). These patients have had a resolution of the adnexal masses (the larger the mass, the longer the time required for its resolution) and some (generally between 10% and 15%) have conceived with no need for additional corrective surgery of their genital tract structures. It is not mandatory, although sometimes necessary, to remove the uterus when extirpative surgery is required. With the advances of *in vitro* fertilization or embryo transfer, if the uterus can be left *in situ*, then the patient has a chance for future fertility. Also of note is that 30% of postmenopausal females with a presumed diagnosis of tubo-ovarian abscess actually have a pelvic neoplasm.

Actinomyces israeli is a unique organism that may be the cause of tubo-ovarian abscess, especially in patients with an IUD in place, generally in excess of 5 years.

If *Actinomyces* is considered the cause of tubo-ovarian abscess, the patient should be treated with intravenous penicillin (20 million units daily for 14 days), and then switched over to oral penicillin VK (250 mg four times a day for 4 months). In cases of persistent tubo-ovarian abscess secondary to *Actinomyces* (if masses are no longer decreasing in size), surgical intervention should be considered.

Patients who fail antibiotic therapy have successfully undergone ultrasound or CT-guided aspiration of the inflammatory masses, sparing them a laparotomy or extirpative surgery. It should be remembered that such aspirations cannot distinguish between an infected mass and an infected neoplasm. Aspiration of the latter can worsen the patient's prognosis.

Tuberculosis can also be another cause of peritonitis. Typically, cases of tuberculosis causing peritonitis present with pelvic mass and pelvic ascites, which could be diagnosed on ultrasound. Often they are misdiagnosed as pelvic or ovarian cancer. Treatment of pelvic tuberculosis and tubo-ovarian abscess includes a prolonged 9-month course of multiple antituberculosis medications.

Suggested reading

Gaitán H, Angel E, Diaz R, Parada A, Sanchez L, Vargas C. Accuracy of five different diagnostic techniques in mild-to-moderate pelvic inflammatory disease. *Infect Dis Obstet Gynecol* 2002; 10: 171–180.

Ness RB, Hillier SL, Kip KE, *et al*. Bacterial vaginosis and risk of pelvic inflammatory disease. *Obstet Gynecol* 2004; 104: 761–769.

Paavonen J. Pelvic inflammatory disease. From diagnosis to prevention. *Dermatol Clin* 1998; 16: 747–756.

Patton DL, Askienazy-Elbhar M, Henry-Suchet J, Campbell LA. Detection of *Chlamydia trachomatis* in Fallopian tube tissue in women with postinfectious tubal infertility. *Am J Obstet Gynecol* 1994; 171: 95–101.

Peipert JF, Sweet RL, Walker CK, *et al*. Evaluation of ofloxacin in the treatment of laparoscopically documented acute pelvic inflammatory disease. *Infect Dis Obstet Gynecol* 1999; 7: 138–144.

Peipert JF, Ness RB, Blume J, *et al*. Clinical predictors of endometritis in women with symptoms and signs of pelvic inflammatory disease. *Am J Obstet Gynecol* 2001; 184: 856–864.

Roy S, Wilkins J, March CM, *et al*. A comparison of the efficacy and safety of cefizoxime with doxycycline vs. conventional CDC therapies in the treatment of upper genital tract infection with or without a mass. Clinical therapeutics. *Int J Drug Ther* 1990; 12(suppl C): 53–73.

Shafer MB, Pantell RH, Schachter J. Is the routine pelvic examination needed with the advent of urine-based screening for sexually transmitted diseases? *Arch Pediatr Adolesc Med* 1999; 153: 119–124.

Scholes D, Stergachis A, Heidrich FE, Andrilla H, Holmes KK, Stamm WE. Prevention of pelvic inflammatory disease by screening for cervical chlamydial infection. *NEJM* 1996; 334: 1362–1366.

State of California Department of Health Services, Health and Human Services Agency. *Gonorrhea treatment guidelines.* Sacramento, CA: Department of Health Services, 2003: 1–6.

US Department of Health and Human Services, Public Heath Service, Division of Sexually Transmitted Diseases. Sexually transmitted diseases treatment guidelines. *MMWR* 2006; 56: RR-11.

Westrom L, Eschenbach D. In: Holmes K, Sparling P, Mardh P, *et al.* (eds) *Sexually transmitted diseases*, 4th edn. New York: McGraw-Hill, 1999: 771–794 and 855–876.

Zondervan KT, Yudkin PL, Vessey MP, *et al.* The prevalence of chronic pelvic pain in women in the United Kingdom: a systematic review. *BJOG* 1998; 105: 93–99.

Chapter 54
Prevention of Postoperative Surgical Site Gynecologic Infections

Uma Chandavarkar and Subir Roy

Department of Medicine and Obstetrics and Gynecology, Keck School of Medicine, University of Southern California, CA, USA

Introduction

Surgical site infection is perhaps one of the most common complications associated with surgical management of patients and accounts for significant morbidity in 8–10% of gynecologic surgical hospitalizations. Despite vigorous preoperative vaginal cleansing, contamination by endogenous bacteria may occur at the time of gynecologic operations. There are many risk factors for surgical site infections. These include but are not limited to hemostatic sutures around crushed tissue, pooling of blood products in open defects, and bacterial contaminants from the vagina. These may all lead to pelvic cellulitis or pelvic abscesses and often require prolonged hospitalization, medical management with antimicrobials, and surgical debridement.

In general, all surgical procedures can be classified based on the type of procedure and the likelihood of subsequent infection (Table 54.1).

Aerobic and anaerobic bacteria are both represented in cultures from postoperative infections. Gram-positive cocci (streptococci and staphylococci) account for most of the organisms isolated. *Escherichia coli* and Bacteroides are the predominant gram-negative and anaerobic organisms, respectively.

Risk factors and prevention

Several measures may be employed in order to prevent and reduce the rates of infection following gynecology. These include: preoperative showering with an antiseptic soap, shaving of the incision site in the operating room, observation of sterile technique by all operating room personnel, adequate bowel preparation, and the use of prophylactic antibiotics as necessary.

Management of Common Problems in Obstetrics and Gynecology,
5th edition. Edited by T.M. Goodwin, M.N. Montoro,
L. Muderspach, R. Paulson and S. Roy. © 2010 Blackwell
Publishing Ltd.

The criteria for the use of prophylactic antibiotics in gynecology are as follows.
• The operation should involve a significant risk of postoperative site infection.
• The operation should cause bacterial contamination.
• The antibiotic should be targeted to the presumptive microbial contaminants.
• The antibiotic should be present in the target tissue at the time of the initial incision.
• The benefits of prophylactic antibiotics should outweigh the risks of use.

The use of prophylactic antibiotics has decreased operative site infection following vaginal hysterectomy from 32% to 6.3% [1], whereas for abdominal hysterectomies, infection rates with and without antibiotic prophylaxis have been reported to be approximately 9.0–9.8% and 21–23.4%, respectively [2,3].

A study by Burke showed that there was no benefit in using prophylactic antibiotics if they were administered more than 3 hours after bacterial contamination occurred [4]. Preoperative administration of an antimicrobial agent should precede any elective procedure requiring prophylaxis. A short-term course not to exceed 24 hours postoperatively should be employed unless the surgical procedure is prolonged beyond 3 hours or if there is blood loss in excess of 1500 mL. Additional antibiotic administration should be given in either of these events. Several agents have been used: ampicillin, doxycycline, metronidazole, and a variety of cephalosporins. Cephalothin, cephradine, cefazolin, cefoxitin, ceforanide, cefonicid, cefotetan, cefotaxime, ceftizoxime, and moxalactam provide broad-spectrum coverage and allow for a short period of administration. Metronidazole, considered to be effective only against obligate anerobes, is an acceptable prophylactic agent.

The initial dose of antibiotic is usually administered 30–60 minutes before the initial incision is made in order to attain satisfactory serum and tissue levels although administration (IV or IM) in the operating room following induction is acceptable and may be preferable if a short half-life antibiotic is used. Cefoxitin must be diluted

245

Table 54.1 Surgical wound classifications adopted by the American College of Surgeons

Operative procedure	Description	Wound infection rate	Antibiotics	Examples
Clean	Aseptic techniques maintained No mucosal surface is entered	1–3%	Not indicated	
Clean-contaminated	A mucosal surface has been entered Spillage is minimal	10–20%	Greatest benefit from prophylaxis	Abdominal and vaginal hysterectomy
Contaminated	Gross spillage from contaminated site	20–30%	Indicated	
Dirty or infected	Old traumatic wounds Perforated viscera	>30%	Indicated	Ruptured tubo-ovarian abscess, appendix

with lidocaine prior to intramuscular injection to reduce pain at the injection site. A normal prothrombin time or 10 mg vitamin K administration is recommended prior to the use of drugs which are known to lead to hypoprothrombinemia and/or platelet dysfunction with or without clinical bleeding. Such drugs include cefamandole, moxalactam, and cefoperazone.

Other factors such as total operative time, estimated blood loss, regrowth of vaginal flora, and associated procedures performed at the time of hysterectomy have all been studied. Those patients who have the greatest amount of surgery performed (e.g. hysterectomy plus urogynecologic corrective procedures) are at highest risk of a postoperative infection. These infections usually occur more than 72 hours after surgery.

Patients with antibiotic allergies may reduce their risks of infection if their surgeon uses a closed T-tube suction drainage in the space between the peritoneum and vaginal cuff for the 36 hours immediately after surgery [5]. Also, a vaginal pack coated with sterile gel rather than antibiotic cream can reduce the amount of blood and blood products that accumulate between the peritoneum and vaginal cuff, thereby reducing a nidus for infection.

It is not advisable to alter the normal flora of the vagina prior to surgery. Preoperative vaginal douching with an iodophor solution the night before surgery has not been shown significantly to reduce the total number of organisms in the vagina. In fact, the number is reduced from 10^8 to 10^6–10^7. However, thoroughly cleansing the vagina in the operating room just before a vaginal hysterectomy is begun renders the vagina essentially organism free during the time required to perform the surgery. As such, vaginal douching the night before surgery is not recommended.

It is necessary for patients undergoing exploratory laparotomy or abdominal hysterectomy simply to bathe or shower normally the night before surgery. If they use an agent such as iodophor for many days prior to surgery, it could lead to an altered skin flora with predominance of gram-negative organisms, resulting in increased wound infections. The skin preparation immediately prior to surgery will reduce the bacterial count sufficiently during the operative period. Furthermore, Cruse has shown a reduced

postoperative infection rate if the patients are shaved just prior to the operation [6].

In obese patients or those with diabetes mellitus, the peritoneal cavity and subcutaneous layer must be adequately irrigated prior to closure. Placement of a Jackson–Pratt drain subcutaneously, brought out through a different incision, can help reduce postoperative infections.

Management of open wounds

Incisional wounds that are classified as contaminated or dirty should not be closed primarily. These wounds can either be closed by delayed primary closure or left open to granulate secondarily. Delayed primary closure is preferred since it often takes an average of 8 weeks to heal secondarily, with worse cosmetic results. The incision may be packed with moist gauze with a covering dry bandage dressing. After 4 days, the packing can be removed and a delayed primary closure can be performed with sterile tape strips or with supportive monofilament vertical mattress sutures to attain satisfactory approximation of the wound edges.

Late-onset wound infections present with copious serosanguineous or purulent drainage. Prior to opening, these wounds must be probed with a sterile cotton tip to make sure the fascia is intact. If a fascial defect is found, further debridement should be done in the operating room because of the possibility of evisceration, a true surgical emergency. If the fascia is intact, the wound should be opened and necrotic tissue should be debrided with local anesthesia with or without sedation. After appropriate debridement and irrigation, the wound should be packed with moistened Kerlex, and this packing should be changed two to three times per day. Use of a wound V.A.C., a negative pressure wound therapy, may also be considered, especially if there is a large defect, as its use permits granulation tissue to form and skin edges to be drawn closer in a more rapid manner than typical wound care with packing [7]. These wounds may be closed secondarily in 2–3 weeks after good granulation tissue has regenerated. Otherwise, a delayed primary closure can be employed.

Some novel developments

It is generally accepted that chlorhexidine gluconate (CHG) and povidone iodine, two of the most commonly employed active components in preoperative skin preparation antiseptics, have a similar spectrum of antimicrobial activity, fulfilling the proposed FDA rules for antiseptic products [8]; however, chlorhexidine gluconate exhibits superiority by providing prolonged activity on the surface of the skin [9].

A proprietary formulation to seal and immobilize pathogens to help protect against migration of microbes into the incision, InteguSeal, has been marketed recently [10]. This agent is applied to the skin after any preoperative preparation antiseptic is used, before the incision is made, and can be used with any type of skin closure without affecting incision strength.

The role of surgical sutures as a cause of surgical site infections has led to the coating of sutures with triclosan, an antibacterial agent. Significant reduction of attachment to and viability of both gram-positive and gram-negative organisms typically associated with wound infections has been reported with triclosan-coated sutures as compared to noncoated sutures [11]. One study reported that there was less pain associated with the triclosan suture, indicating less "subclinical" infection [12].

Octyl-2-cyanoacrylate (OCA) adhesive for skin closure has been reported to be superior to conventional wound closure in terms of cosmetic and infection rates, following plastic and breast surgery [13,14]. One should insure that the cutaneous edges of the incision are in approximation by using underlying sutures as needed, such as subcutaneous and intradermal sutures. Not all reports favor OCA use over conventional wound closure [15].

Future clinical studies will illustrate whether CHG, InteguSeal, triclosan-coated sutures or OCA, individually or in combination, are associated with reduced surgical site infections.

Diagnosis of surgical site infections

Fever in the postoperative period may have a natural (noninfective) basis with the release of endogenous pyrogens (such as interleukins 1 and 6, tumor necrosis factor, and prostaglandin E2), which may act centrally to produce fever. Fever which persists beyond 4–6 hours (excluding the first 24 hours postoperatively), especially if it is associated with excessive tenderness in the perioperative tissues, or if cellulites or purulent material exude from the operative site, clinches the diagnosis of wound infection and deserves antibiotic therapy. Patients may also have the clinical findings of wound infection without having fever. Although the same antibiotic used for prophylaxis may be used to treat these infections, as usually the pathogenic organisms responsible for the infection may not be resistant, many authors have preferred to use alternative therapy.

If a practice is instituted to treat only those postoperative patients with findings of an operative site infection, with or without fever, especially excluding those who have febrile morbidity alone, then less antibiotic will be utilized, with a reduced chance of altering the microbial flora with resistant organisms. Additionally, the cost of hospitalization will be reduced.

Conclusion

There is no substitute for good operative technique with attention to hemostasis in reducing postoperative infections. No antibiotic or other aids will overcome poor operative technique in reducing surgical site infections.

Patients undergoing contaminated procedures should be treated with therapeutic doses and durations of antibiotics and should not be considered for prophylactic antibiotic administration.

References

1. Sweet R, Gibbs R (eds). *Antibiotic prophylaxis in obstetrics and gynecology*, 3rd edn. Baltimore, MD: Williams and Wilkins, 1995.
2. Mittendorf R, Aronson MP, Berry RE, *et al*. Avoiding serious infections associated with abdominal hysterectomy: a meta-analysis of antibiotic prophylaxis. *Am J Obstet Gynecol* 1993; 169: 1119–1124.
3. Tanos V, Rojansky N. Prophylactic antibiotics in abdominal hysterectomy. *J Am Coll Surg* 1994; 179: 593-600.
4. Burke JF. The effective period of preventive antibiotic action in experimental incisions and dermal lesions. *Surgery* 1961; 50: 161.
5. Swartz WH, Tanaree P. Suction drainage as an alternative to prophylactic antibiotics for hysterectomy. *Obstet Gynecol* 1975; 43: 305.
6. Cruse PJE. Some factors determining wound infection. A prospective study of 30,000 wounds. In: Polle HC Jr, Stone HH (eds) *Hospital-acquired infections in surgery*. Baltimore, MD: University Park Press, 1977: 77–85.
7. www.kci1.com/35.asp
8. Food and Drug Administration. 21 CRF Parts 333 and 369. Tentative final monograph for healthcare antiseptic drug products: proposed rules. Federal Register Part III. 1994;59: 31401–31452.
9. Peterson AF, Rosenberg A, Alatary SD. Comparative evaluation of surgical scrub preparations. *Surg Gynecol Obstet* 1978; 146: 63–65.
10. Kimberly-Clark: Integuseal – Articles and Resources. www.kchealthcare.com.
11. Edmiston CE, Seabrook GR, Goheen MP, *et al*. Bacterial adherence to surgical sutures: can antibacterial-coated sutures reduce

the risk of microbial contamination? *J Am Coll Surg* 2006; 203: 481-489.

12. Ford HR, Jones P, Gaines B, *et al*. Intraoperative handling and wound healing: controlled clinical trial comparing coated VICRYL plus antibacterial suture (coated polyglactin 910 suture with triclosan) with coated VICRYL suture (coated polyglactin 910 suture). *Surg Infect* 2005; 6: 313–321.

13. Silvestri A, Brandi C, Grimaldi L, *et al*. Octyl-2-cyanoacrylate adhesive for skin closure and prevention of infection in plastic surgery. *Aesth Plast Surg* 2006; 30: 695–699.

14. Gennari R, Rotmensz N, Gallardini B, *et al*. A prospective, randomized, controlled clinical trial of tissue adhesive (2-octylcyanoacrylate) versus standard wound closure in breast surgery. *Surgery* 2004; 136: 593–599.

15. Bernard L, Doyle J, Friedlander SF, *et al*. A prospective comparison of octyl cyanacrylate tissue adhesive (Dermabond) and suture for the closure of excisional wounds in children and adolescents. *Arch Dermatol* 2001; 137: 1177–1180.

Suggested reading

Cruse PJ, Foord R. The epidemiology of wound infection. A 10-year prospective study of 62,939 wounds. *Surg Clin North Am* 1980; 60: 27–40.

Dinarello CA. The endogenous pyrogens in host-defense interactions. *Hosp Pract* 1989; 15: 73–90.

Dinarello CA, Cannon JG, Wolff SM. New concepts on the pathogenesis of fever. *Rev infect Dis* 1988; 10: 168.

Kamat AA, Brancazio L, Gibson M. Wound infection in gynecologic surgery. *Infect Dis Obstet Gynecol* 2000; 8: 230–234.

Johnson A, Young D, Reilly J. Caesarean section surgical site infection surveillance. *J Hosp Infect* 2006; 64: 30–35.

Löfgren M, Sundström Poromaa I, Henrik StJerndahl J, Renström B. Postoperative infections and antibiotic prophylaxis for hysterectomy in Sweden: a study by the Swedish National Register for Gynecologic Surgery. *Acta Obstet Gynecol Scand* 2004: 83: 1202–1207.

Muilwijk J, van den Hof S, Wille JC. Associations between surgical site infection risk and hospital operation volume and surgeon operation volume among hospitals in the Dutch nosocomial infection surveillance network. *Infect Control Hosp Epidemiol* 2007; 28(5): 557–563.

Roy S, Wilkins J. Single-dose cefotaxime versus 3-5 dose cefoxitin for prophylaxis of vaginal and abdominal hysterectomy. *J Antimicrob Chemother* 1984; 149(suppl B): 217–221.

Roy S, Wilkins J, Hemsell DL, *et al*. Efficacy and safety of single-dose ceftizoxime vs. multiple-dose cefoxitin in preventing infections after vaginal hysterectomy. *J Reprod Med* 1988; 33: 149–153.

Scardigno D, Lavermicocca T, Magazino MP, Cazzolla A, Lorusso M, Vicino M. A randomized study comparing amoxicillin-clavulanic acid with cefazolin as antimicrobial prophylaxis in laparotomic gynecologic surgery. *Minerva Ginecol* 2006; 58(2): 85–90.

Chapter 55
Prepubertal Vulvovaginitis

Jenny M. Jaque and Claire Templeman
Department of Medicine and Obstetrics and Gynecology, Keck School of Medicine, University of Southern California, CA, USA

Differential diagnosis

Vaginal discharge in a pediatric patient may be physiologic. Estrogen of maternal origin present in the first 2 or 3 weeks of life or in early puberty produces a physiologic leukorrhea which is characterized as a milky-white, yellow or clear mucus discharge without an offensive odor or vulvar involvement. During this interval, under the influence of estrogen, the vaginal epithelium of the newborn is several layers thick and the vaginal pH is acidic. An increase in endogenous estrogen normally occurs in early puberty.

There are several pathologic causes of vulvovaginitis in children (Box 55.1). Poor perineal hygiene may result in the transfer of coliform bacteria and other enteric pathogens to the vagina. Sexually transmitted diseases can occur in prepubertal girls of all ages. A foreign body placed in the vagina may lead to a vaginal discharge and contact irritants can cause vulvar-vaginal symptomatology. Candidiasis, enterobiasis, and shigellosis are infrequent specific causes of vaginal leukorrhea. β-Hemolytic streptococcus and coagulase-positive staphylococcus may be spread manually from their primary site, the nasopharynx, to the vagina. Congenital anomalies of the urogenital system very rarely produce symptoms which may be interpreted as vaginal discharge.

Wiping the perineum in a direction from the anus to the vagina may allow a mixture of enteric organisms to invade the vagina, including gram-negative coliform bacteria, enterococcus and anerobic bacteria secondary to fecal contamination. Mixed enteric organisms, also referred to as nonspecific vulvovaginitis, is the most common cause of leukorrhea in prepubescent girls.

Vaginal discharge may be a clinical manifestation of a sexually transmitted disease (STD) and typically result

> **Box 55.1 Prepubertal vulvovaginitis etiology**
>
> **Physiologic**
> Postnatal
> Premenarchal
>
> **Pathologic**
> Mixed enteric organisms
> Sexually transmitted diseases:
> 1 *Neisseria gonorrhoeae*
> 2 *Chlamydia trachomatis*
> 3 condylomata acuminatum
> 4 herpes simplex
> 5 *Trichomonas vaginalis*
> Foreign body
> Contact irritant
> Candidiasis
> Enterobiasis (pinworms)
> Shigellosis
> Respiratory pathogens:
> 1 β-haemolytic streptococcus
> 2 coagulase-positive staphylococcus
> 3 *Streptococcus pneumoniae*
> 4 *Haemophilus influenzae*
> Congenital anomaly:
> 1 fistula
> 2 ectopic ureter
> 3 meningomyelocele
>
> **Skin disorders**

from sexual abuse. A study of 1538 children known to have been sexually abused reported the following types and frequencies of sexually transmitted infections: *Neisseria gonorrhoeae* (2.8%), *Chlamydia trachomatis* (1.2%), human papilloma virus (1.8%). Members of the immediate family or caregivers should be evaluated and cultured in case the disease was acquired from one of them. When one STD is diagnosed it is possible the child may be co-infected with one or more other STDs and appropriate screening must be conducted. Some infants may acquire these vaginal infections through maternal colonization

Management of Common Problems in Obstetrics and Gynecology, 5th edition. Edited by T.M. Goodwin, M.N. Montoro, L. Muderspach, R. Paulson and S. Roy. © 2010 Blackwell Publishing Ltd.

at the time of delivery. The incubation period for these infections may last up to 2 years. The most reliable diagnostic test for gonorrhea or chlamydia vaginitis in a prepubertal girl is a culture.

Condylomata acuminatum (venereal warts) are dry warty lesions caused by the human papilloma virus (HPV), usually type 6 or 11 in children. These lesions are likely the result of mother-to-child transmission during vaginal birth in children younger than 3 years of age, It is not necessary for the mother to be symptomatic or to report a history of HPV for transmission to occur. Herpes simplex is characterized as small vesicular lesions on an erythematous base caused by the herpes simplex virus, type 2. Examination under magnification of the scrapings taken from the herpetic lesions and prepared with Wright stain demonstrates multinucleated giant cells. *Trichomonas vaginalis* is expressed clinically as a frothy, watery, yellow or green discharge. The motile flagellated parasites are identified in a saline wet-mount preparation. *Trichomonas vaginalis* is very uncommon in prepubertal females.

A foreign body must always be included in the differential diagnosis of a pediatric patient who presents with episodic vaginal bleeding and/or a brown purulent or greenish vaginal discharge. Toilet paper is the most common foreign body found in the vagina of a prepubertal child; small toys, hair ties and paper clips are also common. Most foreign bodies are not radio-opaque and x-rays of the lower abdomen and pelvis are seldom helpful. The foreign object can often be removed with irrigation after the introitus has been treated with a topical anesthetic agent. Examination under sedation may be necessary for removal of larger objects and those that cannot be removed with irrigation.

A long list of contact irritants may inflame the vulvar tissue. Harsh soaps, detergents, disinfectants, bubble baths, powders, perfumes, feminine hygiene sprays, scented or colored toilet paper, cosmetics, chemicals, and topical medications are some of the agents which can act as contact irritants to vulvar tissue. Tight-fitting clothing including leotards, tights, rubber pants, skin-tight jeans, nylon underclothing, and tight-fitting diapers are included in this category. Parents are recommended to avoid use of any contact irritant and rinse the genital area well and gently pat dry.

Vulvovaginal candidiasis is uncommon in the prepubescent female unless she has diabetes mellitus or recent antibiotic use, is immunocompromised or wears diapers. The child with vulvovaginitis due to *Candida albicans* has an inflamed, edematous, pruritic vulva and a thick, white, cheese-like vaginal discharge. It is frequently overdiagnosed and erroneously assumed to be the etiology for patients' symptoms. A potassium hydroxide wet-mount preparation of the discharge demonstrates the characteristic spores and hyphae.

Pinworms can cause vulvar symptoms such as nocturnal perineal pruritus. *Enterobius vermicularis* inhabit the large intestine. Female pinworms emerge from the anus at night to deposit eggs on the perineum. With the aid of a flashlight these worms may be seen around the anus during the night. In the morning the eggs around the anus can be collected on the sticky side of Scotch tape and, following toluene treatment, can be seen with low-power microscopic magnification.

Colonization of the intestinal tract with *Shigella flexneri* or *Shigella sonnei* can cause fever, malaise, diarrhea, and mucopurulent vaginal discharge which sometimes contains blood. The diagnosis of shigellosis is confirmed by positive stool cultures.

Female children may have bacterial spread by manual transmission from the primary ear, nose and throat (ENT) location to the vulvovaginal area, resulting in a vaginal discharge. Children with otitis media, tonsillitis or any upper respiratory tract infection due to streptococcus or staphylococcus species are at increased risk. The diagnosis is confirmed when vaginal cultures are positive for the same organisms identified in the primary infection site.

Congenital anomalies in which a communication exists between the vagina and the rectum or bladder can result in vaginal discharge that has been present since birth. An ectopic ureter, particularly when the ureter drains directly into the vagina or introitus, may be the source of a continuous leakage of urine which is misinterpreted as a vaginal discharge. A meticulous search for the ectopic opening of the ureter is necessary and an intravenous pyelogram may be a useful diagnostic aid.

Lesions affecting the external genitalia of prepubescent girls may be a localized manifestation of a generalized skin disorder. Some skin disorders which affect the vulva include molluscum contagiosum, seborrheic dermatitis, psoriasis, atopic dermatitis, lichen sclerosis, vitiligo, eczema, erythema multiforme, and lichen planus. The treatment of the lesions found on the external genitalia is similar to that given for similar lesions situated anywhere else on the body.

Vaginal discharge is the cardinal symptom of vaginitis. If the vulvar tissue is inflamed, it appears erythematous and edematous and associated symptoms of pruritus, dysuria, frequent urination, and enuresis may be present. A careful history should be obtained and needs to include the character of the discharge, the length of time the discharge has been present, the presence of odor, the presence of blood, the method of perineal hygiene, recent infections that might be streptococcal or staphylococcal in origin, recent venereal disease or parasites among immediate members of the family, nocturnal perianal pruritus, and the placement of a foreign body in the vagina.

Examination

The successful gynecologic examination of the prepubertal female is based on the examiner's ability to place the child at ease and to allow the child to control the examination. Encouraging the child to participate in the history-taking process, a gentle but thorough physical examination, and the presence of a trusted family member all help to establish rapport and confidence between the physician and the young patient.

Selection of the position for the young patient during the gynecologic examination is based on the comfort of the patient and her ability to control the examination. The frog-leg position, the knee–chest position, the dorsal lithotomy position and sitting on a parent's lap have all been advocated for this examination.

Inspection of the external genitalia and introitus may be accomplished by the examiner depressing the perineum on either side of the labia with both thumbs, by the examiner gently grasping each labia between his/her thumb and index finger and separating the labia, or by the examiner placing the index fingers of the child on the labia and separating them. Instructing the child to cough may result in the opening of the hymen and easier exposure of the lower vaginal vault. A swab moistened with saline, a plastic eye dropper or a small plastic tube attached to the tip of an ordinary medicine dropper can be used to collect specimens for wet-mount preparations and cultures. A vaginal lavage may identify a foreign body as the cause of the vulvovaginitis. Xylocaine gel, lidocaine, and prilocaine cream applied to the vulva reduce the chance for discomfort.

An attempt should be made to examine the vagina of every child with prepubertal vulvovaginitis with the child awake. A variety of instruments are available for vaginoscopy of young patients, including fiberoptic vaginoscopes, the Killian nasal speculum, veterinary otoscopes, and urethroscopes. A rectal abdominal examination is an integral part of the gynecologic exam. In addition to palpating a pelvic mass, a vaginal foreign body may be detected and discharge may be directed to the introitus. Any time the discharge is mixed with blood or the patient or her parents indicate that a foreign body has been placed in the vagina, adequate inspection of the vagina must be carried out. In such cases, if vaginoscopy cannot be completed successfully with the patient awake, she should be anesthetized. If the discharge does not contain blood, there is no history of a foreign body, and vaginoscopy is unsuccessful with the patient awake, vaginoscopy under anesthesia need not be performed.

Treatment

There are several nonspecific recommendations which will benefit any prepubertal girl with a vaginal discharge. The child should be instructed that following urination and defecation, she should wipe away from the vulvovaginal area. Scented or colored toilet paper should not be used. The child should switch from tight-fitting clothing and underwear made of wool or nylon to loose-fitting clothing, skirts, and cotton underclothing. The underwear should be changed frequently. The child should be instructed to wash her hands before and after voiding and defecation. Sitz baths once or twice a day with warm water and preferably no soap will provide symptomatic relief. When the child emerges from the tub, the vulvar tissue should be air-dried or at most dried very gently with a soft towel. Topical ointments (A&D ointment, Desitin, Vaseline) or corticosteroid ointments (0.5% or 1.0% hydrocortisone) applied once or twice a day, at least once a day at bedtime, will relieve vulvar symptoms.

Specific treatment is available for prepubertal vulvovaginitis due to *Candida albicans* using topical antifungal creams for 7–14 days. Recurrent vaginal yeast infections may be treated with oral nystatin. Pinworms (enterobiasis) are treated with mebendazole (Vermox) one 100 mg chewable tablet and therapy is repeated in 2 weeks. Shigellosis is treated with trimethoprim/sulfamethoxazole 8–40 mg/kg/day orally for 7 days. Streptococcal and staphylococcal vaginitis is treated with the following oral antibiotics for 7–10 days: penicillin V potassium 125–250 mg four times a day, cephalexin (Keflex) 25–50 mg/kg/day, dicloxacillin 25mg/kg/day, and amoxicillin-clavulanate (Augmentin) 20–40 mg/kg/day.

Sexually transmitted diseases in prepubertal females are treated with regimens appropriate for their body-weight. Gonorrhea cultured from the vaginal discharge of a prepubescent female is treated with a single intramuscular injection with ceftriaxone 125 mg or spectinomycin 40 mg/kg for those children who cannot take ceftriaxone. A positive chlamydia culture from the vaginal discharge is an indication for treatment with oral erythromycin 50 mg/kg/day for 10 days. Children approaching the age of puberty (8 years of age or older) may receive oral doxycycline 100 mg twice a day for 1 week. *Trichomonas vaginalis* is treated with oral metronidazole (Flagyl) 15 mg/kg/day three times a day for 7–10 days. Herpetic lesions may be treated with 5% aciclovir ointment applied every 4–6 hours as needed for relief of symptoms. Imiquimod 5% cream (Aldara) is an immune response modifier which augments the normal immune response to the HPV. It may be applied to the affected areas three times a week for 8–12 weeks. Condylomata acuminata in very young children may be very difficult to treat. For those children with extensive lesions, laser ablation under general anesthesia should be performed. Cryotherapy is an alternative to laser treatment. Podophyllin and trichloracetic acid are used for small lesions only.

Contact irritants should be identified and removed from the perineal area. A foreign body requires removal from the vagina. Vaginal mucosal reactions are frequently noted in pediatric patients found to have a foreign body in the vaginal vault. A 1-week course of topical estrogen cream initiated after the removal of the foreign body helps to resolve these reactions. The application of a local anesthetic ointment to the introitus may aid in the passage of any instrument into the vaginal vault of a prepubertal girl. Congenital anomalies found to be the cause of prepubertal vaginal discharge require surgical correction.

Persistent leukorrhea that fails to respond to therapy is an indication for vaginoscopy even if it requires anesthesia. If a specific etiology is not found by vaginoscopy, persistent vulvovaginitis is treated with estrogen cream applied locally to the vulva for no more than 3 weeks. The estrogen thickens the vaginal mucosa, making it more resistant to infection.

Suggested reading

Arsenault PS, Gerbie AB. Vulvovaginitis in the preadolescent girl. *Pediatr Ann* 1986; 15: 577–585.

Fivozinsky KB, Laufer MR. Vulvar disorders in prepubertal girls: a literature review. *J Reprod Med* 1998; 43: K763–773.

Ingram, DL, Everettm VD, Lyna PR, *et al*. Epidemiology of adult sexually transmitted disease agents in children being evaluated for sexual abuse. *Pediatr Infect Dis J* 1992; 11: 945.

Pokorny SF. Long-term intravaginal presence of foreign bodies in children: a preliminary study. *J Reprod Med* 1994; 39: 931–935.

Vanderen AM, Emans SJ. Vulvovaginitis in the child and adolescent. *Pediatr Rev* 1993; 14: 141–147.

Chapter 56
Dysmenorrhea

Uma Chandavarkar and Subir Roy
Department of Medicine and Obstetrics and Gynecology, Keck School of Medicine, University of Southern California, CA, USA

Introduction

Dysmenorrhea is defined as severe pelvic pain, which may occur during or just before the menstrual cycle. It is commonly associated with nausea, vomiting, sweating, tachycardia, diarrhea, lethargy, dizziness, and breast tenderness. Dysmenorrhea has been classified as primary or secondary. Primary dysmenorrhea is any degree of cramping during menstruation without any attributable pathology and typically affects teenage women who have just established ovulatory cycles. In contrast, secondary dysmenorrhea is due to a pathologic process such as endometriosis, adenomyosis or pelvic masses. For the most part, it develops after menarche and is seen in older women. Dysmenorrhea has been reported to range in prevalence from 3% to 90%. Furthermore, about 15% of women with dysmenorrhea have severe symptoms, which preclude daily activities such as work, school, and child care.

Primary dysmenorrhea

The endometrium of the uterus produces prostaglandin PGF-2α, resulting in contractions of the uterus and smooth muscle in the gastrointestinal tract. In fact, the intensity of the menstrual cramps and associated symptoms of nausea, vomiting, and diarrhea are directly proportional to the amount of PGF-2α released [1].

The treatment of primary dysmenorrhea is directed at blocking the production of prostaglandins with prostaglandin synthetase inhibitors (PGSI). PGSI inhibit cyclo-oxygenase (COX), the enzyme that converts arachidonic acid to endoperoxides. The endoperoxides are then converted to prostaglandins. Nonsteroidal anti-inflammatory drugs (NSAIDs), one class of PGSI, include medications such as ibuprofen, naproxen, and ketoprofen. NSAIDs have been shown to be significantly more effective for pain relief than placebo [2]. In addition to inhibiting endometrial prostaglandin production, NSAIDs have direct analgesic properties at the central nervous system level. Adverse effects of NSAIDs include gastrointestinal symptoms, central nervous system symptoms, hematologic abnormalities, bronchospasm, fluid retention, edema, and toxic effects on the liver and kidney. However, when a 3-day regimen is used in young and healthy women with primary dysmenorrhea, these adverse effects are rare. The fenamates, such as mefenamic acid, belong to a similar class of PGSI and have also been shown to be effective in relieving menstrual-associated pain (Table 56.1).

Other effective treatments include oral contraceptives (OCPs), which prevent ovulation, decrease the production of prostaglandins, and decrease the flow during menstruation. A Cochrane analysis from 2001 gleaned data from four randomized controlled trials and concluded that combined OCPs with medium-dose estrogen and first-/second-generation progestogens were more effective than placebo in relieving primary dysmenorrhea [3]. The relief of pain and reduction in circulating prostaglandins, however, are only confined to the affected cycles; there is no carry-over effect after stopping the OCP.

Alternative pharmacologic treatments for primary dysmenorrhea include rose tea, fennel seeds, vitamin B6, vitamin E, and fish oil (omega-3 fatty acids), which

Management of Common Problems in Obstetrics and Gynecology, 5th edition. Edited by T.M. Goodwin, M.N. Montoro, L. Muderspach, R. Paulson and S. Roy. © 2010 Blackwell Publishing Ltd.

Table 56.1 Common PGSI used for treating dysmenorrhea

Generic name	Trade name	Dosing
Naproxen sodium	Naprosyn	250–500 mg every 6 hours
Ibuprofen	Motrin	400–800 mg every 6–8 hours
Ketoprofen	Orudis	25–200 mg every 6–8 hours
Mefenamic acid	Ponstel	250–500 mg every 6–8 hours
Meclofenamate sodium	Meclamen	100 mg every 8 hours

have all been shown to be more effective than placebo in decreasing perceived menstrual pain [4-7].

A new and effective nonpharmacologic surgical approach in treating primary dysmenorrhea involves transcutaneous electrical nerve stimulation (TENS). TENS works through two principal mechanisms: it sends afferent impulses through large-diameter sensory fibers of the same nerve root and therefore raises the threshold for pain signals, blocking signal reception of uterine hypoxia and hypercontractility along the same root. TENS also stimulates the release of endorphins from the peripheral nerves and the spinal cord, providing further pain relief. Acupuncture, acupressure, heat-wrap therapy, and nerve ablation are other investigated modalities.

Secondary dysmenorrhea

Secondary dysmenorrhea is associated with pathologic conditions in the pelvis. This may cause noncyclic or chronic pelvic pain. These conditions include cervical stenosis, endometriosis, adenomyosis, pelvic congestion, intrauterine devices, and pelvic infections. They can develop at any time during a woman's reproductive age and often are diagnosed simply based on history and physical examination alone. Often, invasive technologies such as ultrasound, hysteroscopy or laparoscopy are employed to aid in diagnosis.

Cervical stenosis is a narrowing of the cervical canal, which prevents menstrual flow egress from the uterus to the vagina. It causes increased pressure in the uterus and may increase pain, cramping, and retrograde flow, resulting in endometriosis. Causes of cervical stenosis include congenital factors, infection, and trauma from prior surgical procedures like conization or cryotherapy. Patients usually complain of light to no menstrual flow with cramping. The diameter of a cotton swab is slightly less than the diameter of the cervical canal in a nulliparous woman. As such, the inability to pass a cotton swab into the cervix helps make this diagnosis. The treatment is directed at dilation of the cervix. This can be accomplished with laminaria, cervical stents, and with hysteroscopy by removing leiomyomata or polyps in the canal. However, there is a chance for recurrence of the stenosis.

Endometriosis is the growth of glands or stroma from the uterus in a heterotopic location. Worldwide, the incidence ranges from 5% to 15% of all women and has contributed to 70–80% of all causes of chronic pelvic pain. Responsible etiologies include retrograde menstrual flow, coelomic epithelial metaplasia, lymphatic and vascular metastasis, genetic causes, and immunologic defects. The true cause of endometriosis has not been elucidated.

Symptoms of endometriosis include pelvic pain often beginning 1–2 days prior to the onset of menses, dyspareunia, dyschezia, diarrhea, dysuria, and urinary frequency.

Often, the severity of symptoms does not correlate with the degree of pathology found at the time of surgery. Physical exam reveals uterosacral nodularity, cervical stenosis, lateral deviation of the cervix, a fixed and tender uterus, and enlarged tender ovaries with limited mobility.

Endometriosis is definitively diagnosed with biopsies demonstrating the pathology after direct visualization with laparoscopy or exploratory laparotomy. Treatment is varied and is aimed at inhibiting ovarian production of estrogen in order to induce amenorrhea. Available agents include OCPs, danazol, GnRH agonists, and Depo-Provera (medroxyprogesterone acetate). Progesterone causes atrophy of the endometriosis lesions. Continuous oral contraceptive pills, thereby not permitting a pill-free interval, induce atrophy of endometrial implants. Approximately 80% of patients will respond to this regimen. Danazol is a testosterone derivative and binds to progesterone and androgen receptors. It induces amenorrhea and atrophic changes in the endometrial implants by decreasing follicular-stimulating hormone (FSH) and luteinizing hormone (LH) surges and inhibiting steroidogenic enzymes in the ovary and adrenal glands. However, danazol has fallen out of favor due to its agonistic action on the androgenic receptor causing untoward side effects such as oily skin, deepening of the voice, weight gain, acne, and hirsutism. GnRH agonists such as Lupron have been used as monthly IM injections for 6 months and can be given every 3 months for two doses. Lupron binds to the GnRH receptors in the hypothalamus, dampening the pulsatility of FSH and LH, inducing amenorrhea and atrophy of implants. The side effects are antiestrogenic: hot flashes, vaginal dryness, insomnia. Depo-Provera ranging from 150 mg every 3 months up to 200 mg every month has also been effective in treatment. Side effects include depression, weight gain, mood changes, and delayed ovulation once fertility is desired. Often, surgical management may be necessary in order to restore normal pelvic anatomy. In severe cases, a total abdominal hysterectomy with bilateral salpingo-oophorectomy may be necessary.

Adenomyosis, traditionally termed endometriosis internii, is the presence of endometrial tissue implants in the myometrium causing severe cramping and heavy menstrual flow. Physical examination reveals an enlarged globular uterus. Adenomyosis is usually treated similarly to endometriosis. Recent data have shown that uterine artery embolization (UAE) is effective in the management of symptomatic adenomyosis [8]. Sometimes, hysterectomy may be necessary.

Pelvic congestion syndrome is caused by dilation of the veins in the broad ligament and ovarian veins. This condition is diagnosed by direct visualization of the engorged vessels by laparoscopy. Pelvic artery embolization has been successful in improving pelvic pain in patients with this syndrome.

Copper-releasing intrauterine devices (Cu-IUDs) may often lead to an increase in prostaglandins after insertion, resulting in heightened cramping and pain. In contrast, levonorgestrol-releasing IUDs (e.g. Mirena IUD) do not increase prostaglandin production after insertion and may, in fact, decrease uterine cramping and pain. Some Cu-IUD users have experienced increased menstrual flow and pain. This can be easily treated with PGSI, as previously mentioned. If bleeding or pain is not significantly improved, the IUD should be removed.

Gonorrheal or chlamydial pelvic infections may lead to abscess or adhesion formation. This pathology may cause pelvic pain and dysmenorrhea and treatment is therefore tailored to remove the pathology both surgically with lysis of adhesions and medically with antimicrobial therapy.

References

1. Dawood MY. Hormones, prostaglandin and dysmenorrhea. In: Dawood MY (ed) *Dysmenorrhea*. Baltimore, MD: Williams and Wilkins, 1981: 20–52.
2. Marjoribanks J, Proctor ML, Farquhar C. Nonsteroidal anti-inflammatory drugs for primary dysmenorrohea (Cochrane Review). Cochrane Library, Issue 4. Oxford: Update Software, 2003.
3. Proctor ML, Roberts H, Farquhar CM. Combined oral contraceptive pill (OCP) as treatment for primary dysmenorrhoea (Cochrane Review). Cochrane Library, Issue 4. Oxford: Update Software, 2001.
4. Tseng YF, Chen CH, Yang YH. Rose tea for relief of primary dysmenorrhea in adolescents: a randomized controlled trial in Taiwan. *J Midwifery Womens Health* 2005; 50: e51–57.
5. Namavar JB, Tartifizadeh A, Khabnadideh S. Comparison of fennel and mefenamic acid for the treatment of primary dysmenorrhea. *Int J Gynaecol Obstet* 2003; 80: 153–157.
6. Wilson ML, Murphy PA. Herbal and dietary therapies for primary and secondary dysmenorrhoea (Cochrane Review). Cochrane Library, Issue 3. Oxford: Update Software, 2001.
7. Ziaei S, Faghihzadeh S, Sohrabvand F, Lamyian M, Emamgholy T. A randomized placebo-controlled trial to determine the effect of vitamin E in treatment of primary dysmenorrhea. *BJOG* 2001; 108: 1181–1183.
8. Kim, MD, Kim S, Kim NK, *et al*. Long-term results of uterine artery embolization for symptomatic adenomyosis. *AJR* 2007; 188(1): 176–181.

Suggested reading

Dawood MY. Primary dysmenorrhea: advances in pathogenesis and management. *Obstet Gynecol* 2006: 108(2): 428–441.

Juang CM, Chou P, Yen MS, Horng HC, Twu NF, Chen CY. Laparoscopic uterosacral nerve ablation with and without pre-sacral neurectomy: a prospective efficacy analysis. *J Reprod Med* 2007; 52(7): 591–596.

Juang CM, Chou P, Yen MS, Twu NF, Horng HC, Hsu WL. Primary dysmenorrhea and risk of preterm delivery. *Am J Perinatol* 2007; 24(1): 11–16.

Kim, MD, Kim S, Kim NK, *et al*. Long-term results of uterine artery embolization for symptomatic adenomyosis. *AJR* 2007; 188(1): 176–181.

Proctor ML, Roberts H, Farquhar CM. Combined oral contraceptive pill (OCP) as treatment for primary dysmenorrhoea. *Cochrane Database Syst Rev* 2001; 4: CD002120.

Proctor ML, Smith CA, Farquhar CM, Stones RW. Transcutaneous electrical nerve stimulation and acupuncture for primary dysmenorrhoea. *Cochrane Database Syst Rev* 2002; 1: CD002123.

Chapter 57
Chronic Pelvic Pain

Judy Chen and Subir Roy
Department of Medicine and Obstetrics and Gynecology, Keck School of Medicine, University of Southern California, CA, USA

Introduction

Pain will bring a patient into the doctor's office. One can even say that the mark of a physician is the ability to differentiate disease processes based upon their pain descriptors. Questions eliciting the quality, time course, location, and associated symptoms of pain complaints may narrow the diagnosis from a vast array of pathologic options. However, what happens when pain becomes only a vague indicator of pathology and not a defining characteristic? How does one treat pain that is no longer an acute presentation of active disease but rather a chronic presence?

By its broadest definition, chronic pelvic pain (CPP) is a noncyclic pain localized to the pelvis and abdomen lasting for greater than 6 months causing functional disability or leading to medical care. Within the US, the estimated prevalence of chronic pelvic pain in the primary care setting ranges from 16% to 39%. Even 10% of all gynecologic referrals are secondary to chronic pelvic pain [1]. Estimations in the UK place the prevalence of CPP equal to that of asthma, back pain, and migraines [2]. Despite the commonality of this disease, about 50% of all CPP have no diagnosed etiology, and 50% of all patients with CPP will remain dissatisfied with their treatment [2,3].

Pathophysiology [4,5]

The anatomy of pain lies within the peripheral nerve, which contains four different neuron axons: A-β, A-δ, C-fiber, and sympathetic axons. Of these four, the A-δ and C-fiber axons fire with painful stimuli, and are labeled as primary afferent nociceptors (pain receptors). A-β fibers

Management of Common Problems in Obstetrics and Gynecology, 5th edition. Edited by T.M. Goodwin, M.N. Montoro, L. Muderspach, R. Paulson and S. Roy. © 2010 Blackwell Publishing Ltd.

exist primarily in the skin and respond to light touch and movement, while sympathetic axons are silent nociceptors (i.e. in the presence of inflammatory mediators they may trigger a pain response). The signals sent by nociceptors reach the somatosensory cortex via the spinal nerves where the brain maps the location, intensity, and quality of pain.

Sensitization and convergence contribute to the primary physiologic cause of chronic pain. In the setting of chronic pain, sensitization of the primary afferent nociceptor pathway occurs with constant or prolonged stimulation of receptors in the presence of damaged or inflamed tissue. Because of the constant stimulation, the threshold of neuron activation decreases while the firing frequency of each neuron increases, thus allowing even innocuous stimuli to cause pain. Convergence contributes to the varied localization of chronic pelvic pain, otherwise known as referred pain. Since each peripheral axon contacts many spinal neurons and each spinal neuron receives input from several peripheral axons, localization of pain often relates to the area covered by a spinal neuron rather than the specific stimulate fiber or receptor.

In reviewing the innervation of the pelvis, the complexity of pelvic pain becomes more evident. Stimulation of the reproductive viscera travels through sympathetic nerves that run through the pelvic plexuses to the hypogastric nerves to end on spinal nerves T11 and T12. At the same time, T11 and T12 receive stimulation from the kidneys, ureters, bowel, and skin dermatomes. Pain fibers (a combination of somatic sensory and autonomic nerves) from the cervix and vagina synapse on spinal nerves S2–4. These same spinal nerves also receive information from the rectum and bladder [4]. Thus, the task at hand is to identify and target therapy at the etiology of the stimulation whether it lies in the reproductive, urinary, gastrointestinal or musculoskeletal organs.

Risk factors

Identifying those patients more prone to chronic pelvic pain has been a difficult task given the amorphous nature of pelvic pain. Latthe *et al.* attempt to list some predisposing factors, which include drug/alcohol abuse, miscarriage, heavy menstrual flow, pelvic inflammatory disease, previous cesarean section, pelvic pathology, abuse, and psychologic co-morbidities [6]. Depending upon the primary complaint, CPP is more often attributed to the urinary or gastrointestinal system, though, 20% of this population will receive a gynecologic diagnosis. Laparoscopic investigation into these 20% of CPP cases reveals that about 33% have endometriosis and 24% have adhesive pathology [2]. A different survey suggests that about 80% of the CPP patients referred to gynecologists may have interstitial cystitis, still most reviews believe inflammatory bowel disease to be a prominent etiologic factor [7]. Pelvic congestion has also been implicated as a cause of CPP. Box 57.1 lists the nongynecologic sources of pelvic pain while Box 57.2 lists common gynecologic etiologies. Here, we will review endometriosis, adhesive pathology, pelvic congestion, interstitial cystitis, and psychosomatic disorders.

Evaluation and examination

Evaluation should begin with a thorough history and physical examination. The site, duration, pattern, quality, intensity, and association with bodily functions or activities add to the differentiation of diagnoses. Physical examination includes a thorough examination of the abdomen and pelvis. Pelvic exam should include inspection of the external genitalia, evaluation of vaginismus, assessment of cervical motion tenderness, notation of uterine mobility/contour/tenderness, enlargement of adnexa with respective tenderness, and finally rectal exam for nodularity/blood/hemorrhoids.

Laboratory testing helpful to the differentiation of possible pathologic processes includes urinalysis, complete

---

Box 57.1 Common causes of pelvic pain not directly associated with the reproductive tract

Appendicitis
Regional enteritis/diverticulitis
Inflammatory bowel disease/syndrome
Urinary tract infection
Renal and bladder calculi
Interstitial cystitis
Mesenteric vascular disease
Rectus hematoma
Aortic aneurysm
Herpes zoster
Porphyria
Sickle cell crisis

Box 57.2 Most common reproductive tract etiologies for pelvic pain

Episodic
Mittelschmerz
Dysmenorrhea
Endometriosis
Adneomyosis
Salpingitis
Ectopic pregnancy
Adnexal torsion
Pelvic venous congestion

Continuous
Adhesions
Pelvic relaxation
Anatomic distortions
(i.e. chronic tubo-ovarian abscess, leiomyomata)

---

blood count, and sedimentation rates. Stool guiaic tests may be helpful in uncovering possible gastrointestinal disorders such as Crohn's disease or ulcerative colitis. Analysis for sexually transmitted infections with a wet mount and/or urinary chlamydia/gonorrhea tests may also delineate the cause of vague pelvic pain.

Radiologic examination with ultrasonography, CT, and MRI may aid diagnosis thorough additional information supporting or refuting clinical suspicions. Transvaginal ultrasound has become an efficient and reliable diagnostic tool in viewing pelvic anatomy, while CT and MRI may add details about other surrounding organs. Depending upon the primary complaint, other more invasive procedures such as endoscopy, cystoscopy, hysteroscopy or laparoscopy, may enhance diagnostic capacity through quintessential physical findings suggestive of pathology as well as provide possible treatment interventions [8].

Treatment

Ideally, treatment modalities target the presumed pathology (see Box 57.3). Infectious etiologies should be treated with appropriate antibiotic treatment. NSAIDs, which decrease inflammatory mediators, help to decrease not only pain sensation but also possible sources of inflammatory aggravation. Modulation of hormonal influences on pain occurs with the administration of oral contraceptive pills or other hormonal anticontraceptives. Surgical interventions vary from directed adhesiolysis to total removal of reproductive organs. Nerve ablation and neurectomy have been proposed as possible surgical solutions to sensitization of a nerve loop. However, large randomized controlled studies between surgical interventions and conservative modalities have yet to be performed.

> **Box 57.3 Targeted treatment for specific pathology**
>
> **Medical therapy**
> *Dysmenorrhea:* oral contraceptives, prostaglandin synthetase inhibitors
> *Endometriosis:* gonadotropin-releasing hormone agonist, oral contraceptives, danazol
> *Salpingitis:* antibiotics
> *Pelvic congestion:* medroxyprogesterone acetate, oral contraceptives
>
> **Surgical herapy**
> Adhesiolysis
> Organ extirpation
> Uterosacral nerve ablation
> Presacral neurectomy

Endometriosis

Pelvic pain is common to patients with endometriosis; however, the extent of their disease has not always correlated to the intensity of pain. Many patients with severe endometriosis are often asymptomatic; in contrast, those patients with mild disease may present with excruciating pain. Endometriosis, otherwise known as heterotopic endometrial tissue under the influence of menstrual hormones, especially estrogen, occurs mainly during the reproductive age. Because of this age group, diagnosis and therapy involve a balance between relief of symptoms and preservation/augmenation of fertility.

Descriptions of symptoms often include a cyclic nature, secondary dysmenorrhea, dyspareunia, and dyschezia. Findings on exam include nodularity of the uterosacral ligaments and/or cul-de-sac, a fixed-retroverted uterus, enlarged and tender ovaries. The gold standard for diagnosis is laparoscopic examination but the positive predictive value of laparoscopic diagnosis, as measured by Stegmann, only approaches 64% [9]. Radiologic exams may also be beneficial. Most frequently transvaginal, transrectal and rectal endoscopic ultrasonography, and MRI are used [10]. Out of these modalities, transvaginal ultrasonography remains the most accurate for evaluation of the pelvis. Variations of transvaginal ultrasonography with a "stand-off" field in order to increase visual acuity of the posterior cul-de-sac appear to augment the sensitivity of ultrasound detection [10].

Consideration of the patient's full picture, including the primary complaint, future fertility, location of disease, extent of disease, and associated pelvic pathology, influences the treatment plan for endometriosis. Surgical therapy focuses upon reducing the burden of disease, while medical therapy seeks to induce amenorrhea or a state of quiescence, thus decreasing symptoms. At the same time diagnosis is established, laparoscopy ablation or excision of disease tissue can be performed. Decreasing nociceptor fiber stimulation by presacral neurectomy or uterosacral nerve ablation can be performed either with laparotomy or under laparoscopy. A Cochrane review by Proctor *et al.* [11] suggests that while evidence reveals the effectiveness of a presacral neurectomy in terms of pain related to endometriosis, more complications occur postoperatively. Uterosacral nerve ablation, however, does not treat the pain of endometriosis as well as a presacral neurectomy. On the other end of the spectrum, symptom suppression through medical amenorrhea can be induced with the use of danazol, GnRH agonists, and hormonal contraceptives. Often a combination of surgical excision and medical amenorrhea extends the symptom-free period of time.

Adhesions

Much debate surrounds the subject of adhesions and pelvic pain. Supporters of the causal relationship between adhesions and pelvic pain state that pain arises from the traction and tension placed upon the peritoneum after adhesion formation. A study done by Kresch *et al.* noted that those individuals with CPP had a greater tendency to have restricted viscera secondary to adhesions compared to those patients without CPP [12]. Immunohistochemistry analysis of adhesive tissue demonstrates the presence of nerve fibers within adhesions, but their presence could be found in patients with or without CPP. Whether or not lysis of adhesions results in decreased pain symptoms varies from study to study [13]. A 2000 Cochrane review states that "there is still uncertainty about the place of adhesiolysis among patients presenting to gynecologists and the conclusion of this review is that there is no evidence of benefit, rather than evidence of no benefit" [14].

Pelvic congestion syndrome

During the reproductive years, some women will complain of deep dyspareunia, postcoital pain, shifting pain, and pain exacerbation after prolonged standing. In the 1940s Taylor labeled this constellation of symptoms as pelvic congestion syndrome (also called pelvic venous incompetence). Current understanding of the pathophysiology highlights dilation of the utero-ovarian venous system coupled with decreased venous return caused by anatomic variations, hormonal influences, and physiologic vasoconstriction [15]. Diagnosis arises from an array of radiologic findings during venography: reduced venous clearance of contrast medium, diameter of the ovarian veins, and distribution of vessels. Medical therapies with medroxyprogesterone acetate or GnRH agonists target possible hormonal effects upon the venous system. Studies in interventional radiology performing ovarian vein embolization suggest effectiveness in relieving symptoms [16]. Surgical intervention with either ligation of vessels or removal of reproductive organs has also treated patients with pelvic congestion syndrome.

Interstitial cystitis

Interstitial cystitis (IC) encompasses not only pelvic pain but also irritative voiding symptoms – frequency, urgency, nocturia – all in the absence of infection or neoplastic diseases. Diagnostic criteria vary depending upon the evaluation tools used. The NIH-NIDDK favored the combination of clinical symptoms with cystoscopy under anesthesia to detect abnormal hydrodistension; however, many clinicians diagnose and treat patients based upon symptomatology only. Another diagnostic tool is the intravesical potassium sensitivity test; however, about 25% of patients with IC will have a false-negative KCl test. Less invasive modalities include the O'Leary-Sant Symptom and Problem Indices and voiding logs, which appear comparable to the favored NIH-NIDDK criteria.

Other diagnostic conundrums surrounding IC lie not only in the varied diagnostic criteria but also in the overlapping symptoms of interstitial cystitis with painful bladder syndrome, frequency-urgency syndrome, overactive bladder syndrome, and other causes of CPP; thus, interstitial cystitis is a diagnosis of exclusion. Variance in diagnostic criteria merely reflects the uncertainty in the etiology of interstitial cystitis. Current hypotheses begin with an insult to the bladder causing epithelial damage and potassium leakage into the bladder, thus instigating a cycle of inflammation and further damage. Targeted therapy attempts to interrupt the cycle of inflammation and further bladder damage by either protecting the bladder epithelium or inhibiting inflammatory factors. Accepted medical therapies include mucosal surface protectants, histamine blockers, neuromodulation with antidepressants or desensitization with detergents [17-19].

Psychosomatic disorder

After an extensive exploration of organic causes of pain yields few answers, the other half of pain pathology should be investigated. Pain, by nature, has a duality; it is not merely a sensation but also an emotion [20]. In addressing the physical sensation of pain, medicine has developed well-organized analyses, but the role of emotion in pain has yet to be clearly elicited. Women with depression and sleep disorders commonly present with chronic pelvic pain. Investigations have also found

a strong association between those who have suffered sexual or physical abuse with pelvic pain, yet the underlying pathology remains unclear.

Undifferentiated somatization disorder as described by the DSM-IV diagnostic criteria [20] include:
- one or more physical complaints
- no known medical cause or direct effect of substance usage
- significant distress/impairment in social and occupational function
- duration for at least 6 months
- symptoms cannot be explained by another mental disorder
- symptoms are unintentionally produced

Given our limited understanding of the interplay between the physical sensation of pain and the emotional quality of pain, diagnosis of a psychosomatic disorder is difficult. Treatment is also time and energy intensive. Patients with psychosomatic disorders firmly believe their medical complaints arise from physical pathology; thus, they become offended and defensive at suggestions that their symptoms are supratentorial. Management techniques often include frequent appointments, undertaking appropriate diagnostic exploration, and co-ordination of medical care.

References

1. Howard FM. Chronic pelvic pain. *Obstet Gynecol* 2003; 101: 595–611.
2. Cheong Y, Stones RW. Chronic pelvic pain: aetiology and therapy. *Best Pract Res* 2006; 5: 695–711.
3. Doyle DF, Li TC, Richmond MN. The prevalence of continuing chronic pelvic pain following a negative laparoscopy. *J Obstet Gynecol* 1998; 3: 252–255.
4. Netter FH. *Atlas of human anatomy*. East Hanover: Novartis, 1997.
5. Braunwald E, Fauci AS, Kasper DL, Hauser SL, Longo DL, Jameson JL. *Harrison's principles of internal medicine*. New York: McGraw-Hill, 2001.
6. Latthe P, Mignini L, Gray R, Hills R, Khalid K. Factors predisposing women to chronic pelvic pain: systematic review. *BMJ* 2006; 332: 728–755.
7. Sant G. Etiology, pathogenesis, and diagnosis of interstitial cystitis. *Rev Urol* 2002; 4(suppl 1): S9-S15.
8. Di Spiezio Sardo A, Guida M, Nappi C, et al. Role of hysteroscopy in evaluating chronic pelvic pain. *Fertil Steril* 2008; 90(4): 1191–1196.
9. Stegmann BJ, Sinaii N, Liu S, et al. Using location, color, size and depth to characterize and identify endometriosis lesions in a cohort of 133 women. *Fertil Steril* 2008; 89(6): 1632–1636.
10. Guerriero S, Ajossa S, Gerada M, et al. "Tenderness-guided" transvaginal ultrasonography: a new method for the detection of deep endometriosis in patients with chronic pelvic pain. *Fertil Steril* 2007; 88(5): 1293–1297.

11. Proctor ML, Latthe PM, Farquhar CM, Khan KS, Johnson NP. Surgicalinterruption of pelvic nerve pathways for primary and secondary dysmenorrhoea (review). Cochrane Library 2007; 4: 1–26.

12. Kresch AJ, Seifer DB, Sachs LB, Barrese I. Laparoscopy in 100 women with chronic pelvic pain. *Obstet Gynecol* 1984; 64: 672–674.

13. Diamond MP, Freeman ML. Clinical implications of postsurgical adhesions. *Human Reprod Update* 2001; 7: 567–576.

14. Stones RW, Mountfield J. Interventions for treating chronic pelvic pain in women. *Cochrane Database Syst Rev* 2000; 2: CD000387.

15. Stones RW. Pelvic vascular congestion – half a century later. *Clin Obstet Gynecol* 2003; 4: 831–836.

16. Kwon SH, Oh JH, Ko KR, Park HC, Huh JY. Transcatheter ovarian vein embolization using coils for the treatment of pelvic congestion syndrome. *Cardiovasc Intervent Radiol* 2007; 30: 655–661.

17. Sant GR, Propert KJ, Hanno PM, *et al*. A pilot clinical trial of oral pentosan polysulfate and oral hydroxyzine in patients with interstitial cystitis. *J Urol* 2003; 170: 810–815.

18. van Ophoven A, Pokupic S, Heinecke A, Hertle L. A prospective, randomized, placebo controlled, double blinded study of amitriptyline for the treatment of interstitial cystitis. *J Urol* 2004; 172: 533–536.

19. Chancellor MB, Yoshimura N. Treatment of interstitial cystitis. *Urology* 2004; 63: 85–92.

20. Ebert MH, Loosen PT, Nurcombe B. *Current diagnosis and treatment in psychiatry*. New York: Lange Medical Books/McGraw-Hill, 2000.

Suggested reading

Chancellor MB, Yoshimura N. Treatment of interstitial cystitis. *Urology* 2004; 63: 85–92.

Cheong Y, Stones RW. Chronic pelvic pain: aetiology and therapy. *Best Pract Res* 2006; 5: 695–711.

Diamond MP, Freeman ML. Clinical implications of postsurgical adhesions. *Human Reprod Update* 2001; 7: 567–576.

Ebert MH, Loosen PT, Nurcombe B. *Current diagnosis and treatment in psychiatry*. New York: Lange Medical Books/McGraw-Hill, 2000.

Katz VL, Lentz GM, Lobo RA, Gershenson DM. *Comprehensive gynecology*. Philadelphia, PA: Mosby Elsevier, 2007.

Proctor ML, Latthe PM, Farquhar CM, Khan KS, Johnson NP. Surgical interruption of pelvic nerve pathways for primary and secondary dysmenorrhoea (review). Cochrane Library 2007; 4: 1–26.

Sant G. Etiology, pathogenesis, and diagnosis of interstitial cystitis. *Rev Urol* 2002; 4(suppl 1): S9-S15.

Stones RW. Pelvic vascular congestion – half a century later. *Clin Obstet Gynecol* 2003; 4: 831–836.

Stones RW, Mountfield J. Interventions for treating chronic pelvic pain in women. *Cochrane Database Syst Rev* 2000; 2: CD000387.

Chapter 58
Abnormal and Dysfunctional Bleeding

Marc J. Kalan

Department of Medicine and Obstetrics and Gynecology, Keck School of Medicine, University of Southern California, CA, USA

Introduction

A normal menstrual cycle occurs once per 21–35 days, lasts <8 days and includes <80 mL of blood loss. Departure from this range is considered abnormal and may be due to a variety of conditions or events. If no causative factor is found, the diagnosis of dysfunctional uterine bleeding (DUB) is applied. This chapter will explore the diagnosis, evaluation, and treatment of abnormal and dysfunctional vaginal bleeding.

Diagnosis

The differential diagnosis of abnormal vaginal bleeding includes pregnancy complications, benign or malignant reproductive tract lesions, and systemic pathologies. Further, urinary and gastrointestinal tract abnormalities can present similarly to reproductive tract pathology. For this reason, urinalysis or stool guiac tests are often a critical step in the work-up of abnormal vaginal bleeding.

Reproductive tract disease

Pregnancy complications
Complications of early pregnancy associated with bleeding include threatened, incomplete or missed abortions, trophoblastic diseases, placental abnormalities and ectopic gestation. Ectopic pregnancy is the leading cause of death in the first trimester and often presents in patients who are unaware they are pregnant. For this reason, abnormal vaginal bleeding in women of childbearing age should be considered an ectopic pregnancy until proven otherwise and should prompt a urine pregnancy test. If positive, transvaginal ultrasound and,

possibly, serial quantitative assays for human chorionic gonadotropin (hCG) should follow.

The combination of ultrasound and hCG is a powerful tool to evaluate for extrauterine pregnancy. A hCG level of 1500 mIU/mL is usually associated with visualization of a gestational sac on ultrasound with a probe of 5.0–7.0 MHz or higher. If the hCG is > 1500 mIU/mL and no sac is seen, suspicion for ectopic gestation must be high. Very rarely (1 in 3000–10,000 pregnancies) combined intrauterine and extrauterine (heterotopic) pregnancy does exist. This risk increases after fertility treatment.

Trophoblastic disease must also be considered in reproductive-age women with abnormal bleeding, especially in those with a recent pregnancy. A sensitive β-hCG assay and sonogram will aid this diagnosis.

Lastly, if intrauterine pregnancy is confirmed, the diagnosis is threatened, inevitable, incomplete or missed abortion. The distinction between these entities depends on history, physical exam and ultrasound findings.

Malignancy
Endometrial cancer, cancer of the cervix, vaginal, vulvar and fallopian tube cancers and estrogen-secreting ovarian tumors may all cause abnormal vaginal bleeding.

The incidence of endometrial cancer increases with age. Approximately 10% of all abnormal uterine bleeding in perimenopausal women and 25% of bleeding in postmenopausal women is due to cancer. Further, women of any age with a long history of oligomenorrhea or anovulatory menstrual cycles are at risk for endometrial carcinoma. Eighty percent of women who develop endometrial carcinoma before age 40 have polycystic ovarian disease (PCOS), an estrogen-dominated syndrome. If abnormal uterine bleeding occurs in the setting of long-standing unopposed estrogen at any age or in the peri/postmenopausal period, the endometrium should be sampled.

Human papilloma virus (HPV) vaccines may decrease the incidence of cervical cancer by up to 70% over the coming decades. Currently, a quadrivalent vaccine against HPV types 6, 11, 16 and 18 is available in the United States. A bivalent vaccine against HPV types 16 and 18 is

Management of Common Problems in Obstetrics and Gynecology, 5th edition. Edited by T.M. Goodwin, M.N. Montoro, L. Muderspach, R. Paulson and S. Roy. © 2010 Blackwell Publishing Ltd.

pending FDA approval. Presently, however, cervical cancer is still a significant cause of abnormal vaginal bleeding and must be considered in the differential diagnosis. This is especially true in women who have never had a Pap smear, as this group makes up more than 50% of cervical cancer cases in the United States.

Benign lesions

Benign lesions such as submucosal myomas or endometrial and cervical polyps may also lead to abnormal bleeding. The mechanisms behind such bleeding are likely related to distorted vascularity and chronic inflammatory processes which accompany these lesions.

Occasionally, a submucosal myoma may protrude completely into the uterine cavity and then dilate the cervix. This is referred to as an aborting myoma and can be associated with copious bleeding. An aborting myoma identified on speculum exam may be twisted off at its base, followed by a sharp curettage. Rarely, carcinoma may present in this fashion. Thus, if suspicion is high, a biopsy and rapid frozen section should be obtained prior to removal.

Smaller endometrial cavity abnormalities, such as polyps, can be more difficult to diagnose. Once bleeding has stopped, hydrosonography or hysterosalpingography are both adequately sensitive to detect the vast majority of lesions.

Infection/vaginitis

Inflammation of the vaginal mucosa can result from a host of causes ranging from bacterial colonization to atrophy. In each of these settings, the inflammatory cascade leads to erythema, vascular fragility and potential bleeding. Consideration of the clinical scenario, a detailed history as well as focused physical exam with wet mount and vaginal pH determination will allow appropriate diagnosis and treatment.

Systemic disease

Anovulation

Anovulation occurs when the hormonal interaction between pituitary, hypothalamus and ovary fails to recruit, stimulate and release an oocyte. In response, the endometrial lining becomes disorganized and sheds in an irregular and unpredictable manner. A host of conditions can lead to anovulatory bleeding, but PCOS is the most common cause.

According to the National Institutes of Health, PCOS is defined by evidence of clinical or biochemical hyperandrogenism, irregular menses and exclusion of other causes of irregular menses (hyperprolactinemia, congenital adrenal hyperplasia, etc.). Treatment for this condition will depend on the patient's wishes and ranges from hormonal contraception to ovulation induction.

Coagulation disorders

Platelet deficiency due to leukemia, severe sepsis, idiopathic thrombocytopenic purpura or hypersplenism as well as platelet dysfunction and conditions like von Willebrand's disease or prothrombin deficiency may all present as abnormal uterine bleeding. Blood dyscrasias usually can be identified by a history of easy bleeding or bruising, a family history of a bleeding disorder, bleeding from other orifices and excessive bleeding associated with minor trauma.

Approximately 20% of adolescent females hospitalized for excessive uterine bleeding are found to have a blood dyscrasia. Therefore, teenage patients with abnormal uterine bleeding, especially that which started with menarche, should be evaluated for a blood dyscrasia.

Liver disease

The liver is central in production of coagulation factors and is also important in estrogen metabolism. Therefore, liver disease could contribute to abnormal bleeding due to impaired coagulation as well as abnormal endometrial proliferation. A history of hepatitis, heavy alcohol ingestion and associated physical findings such as jaundice or hepatomegaly indicate the need to evaluate liver function.

Hypothyroid

Thyroid hypofunction has a variable effect on menstruation. Most hypothyroid patients will not see a change in their periods. Others will notice oligomenorrhea or amenorrhea. A small proportion will have heavier flow. In patients with clinical signs of hypothyroidism such as weight gain, fatigue, cold intolerance, etc., thyroid function should be evaluated.

Trauma

Trauma can cause significant genital bleeding and may occur in settings ranging from motor vehicle accidents to sexual intercourse (consensual or nonconsensual). Because the vaginal mucosa is highly vascular, lacerations often require surgical closure to achieve hemostasis. This is accomplished in a similar fashion to obstetric repairs. One must be suspicious for and inquire about abuse when vaginal lacerations are encountered.

Other causes

Iatrogenic causes of abnormal vaginal bleeding include all hormonal contraceptive methods as well as nonhormonal intrauterine devices (IUDs). Hormone replacement therapy as well as selective estrogen receptor modulators used in cancer therapy or infertility may also cause abnormal bleeding.

Further, digitalis, anticoagulants, hypothalamic depressants, corticosteroids, androgens and anabolic agents all may cause bleeding. A careful history is required to make this diagnosis.

Evaluation

Figure 58.1 graphically represents a step-by-step algorithm to determine the source of abnormal vaginal bleeding. Steps involved with the evaluation are further explained below.

Vital signs and pregnancy test

If the patient is hemodynamically unstable, fluid resuscitation and steps to achieve hemostasis must be concurrent with the diagnostic evaluation. If the patient is hemodynamically unstable and has a positive pregnancy test, the diagnosis is ruptured ectopic pregnancy until proven otherwise.

Pelvic exam and transvaginal ultrasound

A pelvic exam localizes bleeding to the uterus, cervix or vagina. One must be cautious while inserting a speculum into a woman at risk for cervical cancer as a cervical tumor can be extremely friable and trauma from a speculum may cause hemorrhage.

In a stable, pregnant patient, an open cervical os with products of conception (POC) protruding through is consistent with an incomplete abortion. Bleeding with an intrauterine pregnancy on ultrasound and a closed os is consistent with threatened abortion. Bleeding with history of passage of POC is consistent with complete abortion. Finally, bleeding with an adnexal mass and no intrauterine pregnancy on ultrasound is consistent with ectopic pregnancy.

On bimanual exam, an enlarged uterus is consistent with fibroids, adenomas or adenomyosis. Transvaginal ultrasound may display an abnormal endometrium, consistent with hyperplasia or cancer as well as intracavitary lesions such as polyps or myomas. Detection of intracavitary lesions is further enhanced by hydro-sonography or hysteroscopy.

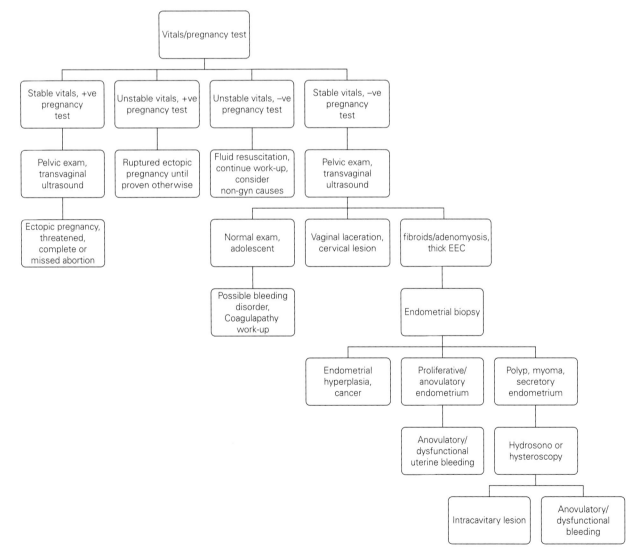

Figure 58.1 Diagnostic algorithm for vaginal bleeding in a reproductive age woman.

Endometrial biopsy

Patients with a history of chronic exposure to unopposed estrogen, such as those with PCOS, anovulatory bleeding, obesity or postmenopausal women taking hormone replacement therapy with breakthrough bleeding, are at increased risk for endometrial hyperplasia or adenocarcinoma. These women should be further evaluated with an endometrial biopsy (EMB).

Hydrosonography, hysteroscopy

If the EMB reveals cancer or hyperplasia, the patient will require medical and/or surgical therapy depending on grade and stage of lesion. If proliferative endometrium is discovered in the absence of other pathology, a diagnosis of DUB or anovulatory bleeding can be applied. If secretory endometrium is encountered, visualization of the endometrial lining is recommended. Visualization can be accomplished by hysteroscopy or hydrosonography. These two techniques share similar sensitivities (80–90%) and specificities (80–90%) for detecting intracavitary lesions. If a lesion is not found, systemic diseases should be excluded.

Coagulopathies

Adolescents with excessive uterine bleeding, especially that which began at menarche, are at significant risk for bleeding disorders. Initial screening should include tests for von Willebrand's disease and platelet dysfunction. If a bleeding disorder is found, consultation with a hematologist may be necessary to identify the specific pathology and initiate treatment. If the coagulation profile is normal, a diagnosis of anovulatory dysfunctional bleeding is assumed and appropriate therapy, usually OCPs, is initiated.

Treatment

Acute

Hemorrhage from the uterus requires utilization of temporizing measures to obtain hemodynamic stability. The overlying principle in this initial step of management is to apply pressure to the source of bleeding. Pressure helps to slow or stop bleeding via three mechanisms. First, tissue compression decreases vascular and capillary volume and promotes clot formation. Second, clot formation leads to a tamponade effect within the endometrial cavity, further slowing bleeding. Third, transvaginal pressure raises the uterus out of the pelvis and applies tension to the uterine vessels which will subsequently deliver less blood to the uterus. This step can be accomplished in a number of ways. A sponge stick can be employed to apply direct pressure to the cervix or lower uterus. Vaginal packing with sterile gauze can be used to fill the vagina and compress the lower uterine segment. Finally, an inflatable balloon (30 cc Foley or Bakri balloon) may be placed into the endometrial cavity and filled with sterile liquid to tamponade the uterus. One must ensure that during this process, a catheter is also placed into the bladder to monitor renal function and prevent urinary retention.

Once hemodynamic stability is obtained, treatment options, either medical or surgical, can be considered in a less frenetic environment.

High-dose estrogen is the cornerstone of medical treatment for abnormal vaginal bleeding. Estrogen promotes platelet plug formation as well as rapid regrowth of the endometrium. Conjugated equine estrogen (CEE) can be given orally (10 mg daily in four divided doses) or intravenously (25 mg every 3–4 h). If bleeding is not controlled within the first 24 hours, the oral dose may be doubled (20 mg/day). If still ineffective, a D&C or a hysteroscopically directed curettage should be considered. If CEE is successful, once the bleeding has stopped, two more intravenous doses should be administered and then the patient should be switched to oral therapy. A progestin such as medroxyprogesterone acetate (MPA) 10 mg/day should be given concomitantly for the last 7–10 days of treatment. The estrogen and progestin are then discontinued to allow withdrawal bleeding. Subsequently, the endometrium should be supported for the next three cycles with cyclic oral contraceptives.

Another regimen employs OCPs. Three or four active tablets of monophasic OCPs containing 35 μg of ethinylestradiol are administered daily in divided doses. Treatment is continued for at least 1 week after the cessation of bleeding. Following the first withdrawal bleed, hormonal support for the endometrium should continue with cyclic OCPs for the next 3–4 cycles.

Dilation and curettage is a surgical option to stop acute heavy uterine bleeding. The procedure is both therapeutic and diagnostic in that it not only stops bleeding, but provides a tissue diagnosis. Unfortunately, D&C is rarely curative. In the absence of long-term therapy, heavy blood loss often returns within two menstrual cycles following the procedure.

Chronic

Long-term treatment of DUB depends on the clinical scenario, the patient's history, presence or absence of concurrent pathology, and the patient's wishes. Structural abnormalities such as pelvic relaxation may make surgical treatments more attractive, while desire for future fertility or concurrent medical conditions may push one towards medical therapy. We will now explore medical and surgical treatments for DUB.

Medical

Approximately 85% of cases of DUB are the result of anovulatory menstrual cycles. In the absence of progesterone production by the corpus luteum, an unpredictable, disorganized shedding of the endometrium occurs. Administration of a progestin leads to an organized desquamation of the endometrium and subsequent cessation of uterine bleeding.

Treatment regimens include oral MPA 10 mg per day for 10–12 days per month. Oral norethindrone acetate 5 mg twice a day or micronized progesterone 300 mg a day for 10–12 days may also be used. Additionally, the conventional administration of combination OCPs is similarly effective.

Alternatively, direct administration of progestin to the endometrial tissue can be accomplished using an IUD. The levonorgestrel-releasing intrauterine system (LNG-IUS, Mirena), which releases 20 μg of levonergesterol per day, significantly decreases menstrual bleeding in 60% of users and 30% experience amenorrhea within 2 years. Further, comparisons of conservative surgery and the LNG-IUS find similar patient satisfaction rates and fewer complications associated with the LNG-IUS after 1 year of use.

Nonsteroidal anti-inflammatory drugs are also effective in controlling heavy menstrual flow, especially in subjects with ovulatory DUB. In this setting, NSAIDs reduce menstrual blood loss by 20–50%. Mefenamic acid 500 mg tid, ibuprofen 400 mg tid, meclofenamate sodium 100 mg tid and naproxen sodium 275 mg q 6 h after a 550 mg loading dose have all been successfully used to treat ovulatory DUB. Treatments are administered daily until bleeding ceases or for the first 3 days of menses. Not only can NSAIDs be used as monotherapy, but when used in combination with oral contraceptives or progestins, greater reduction in blood loss is often achieved compared to either therapy alone.

Antifibrinolytic agents, danazol and ergot derivatives have also been used to control DUB. However, due to their side effects and presence of equally or more effective alternatives, their use has become limited in recent years.

Lastly, gonadotropin-releasing hormone (GnRH) agonists may be used in selected patients to control heavy bleeding. GnRH agonists create a premenarchal hormonal environment with profound suppression of ovarian steroidogenesis which effectively stops uterine bleeding for the duration of the treatment. GnRH agonists cannot be used indefinitely due to associated bone loss from postmenopausal estrogen levels. For this reason, they should be used in patients who are awaiting definitive treatment such as surgery or are on the verge of natural menopause. In the absence of definite treatment, once GnRH agonists are discontinued, blood loss returns to pretreatment levels.

Surgical

Surgical options for the treatment of DUB include endometrial ablation and hysterectomy.

Endometrial ablation is the process of selectively destroying endometrial tissue using electric radiofrequency, thermal or laser energy applied via a transcervical route. This procedure is reserved for women who have failed medical therapy, do not desire future fertility, have normal cervical cytology and endometrial histology and do not have associated pelvic pathology which would be better treated with hysterectomy. Advantages of endometrial ablation over hysterectomy include shorter operating times, less blood loss, lower complication rates, shorter hospitalization, reduced morbidity and lower cost.

First-generation endometrial ablation techniques include laser photovaporization using a neodymium–YAG laser (Nd:YAG laser) under hysteroscopic visualization and electrocautery using a resectoscope or a ball-end electrode. Electrocautery is less costly than the Nd:YAG laser. The rollerball electrode has a larger contact area, provides easier access to the cornual areas of the endometrial cavity, offers easier contact with the endometrial tissue and requires less time to master than the resecting loop. Some surgeons use both the resectoscope and the rollerball electrode when performing endometrial ablation.

A second generation of endometrial ablation techniques became available in the mid-1990s. These techniques do not require hysteroscopic guidance and have the advantage of decreased operative time. Second-generation techniques include radiofrequency, microwave, heated water, cryotherapy and the thermal balloon. A meta-analysis comparing first- and second-generation techniques found no significant difference in patient satisfaction or amenorrhea rates between the techniques.

Reported rates of amenorrhea following endometrial ablation vary from 25% to 85%. Rates of a satisfactory response defined as amenorrhea, oligomenorrhea or return to normal menstrual flow vary between 80% and 95%.

Hysterectomy is appropriate for patients with DUB who also have concomitant pelvic disease such as leiomyomata and uterine prolapse. DUB manifested by these patients should be unresponsive to medical therapy and be severe enough to cause anemia if untreated. In addition, uterine artery embolization (UAE) is a minimally invasive procedure employed to stop bleeding due to fibroids. UAE is not considered a therapy for DUB.

Conclusion

There is no one medical or surgical intervention which is appropriate or successful in the treatment of all cases of DUB. Management must be individualized to the specific patient with consideration of her unique physical findings, medical history and personal desires.

Suggested reading

Abbott JA, Garry R. The surgical management of menorrhagia. *Hum Reprod Update* 2002; 8: 68–78.

Centers for Disease Control and Protection. Ectopic pregnancy – United States, 1990–1992. *MMWR* 1995; 44: 46–48.

Dueholm M, Lundorf E, Hansen ES, Ledertoug S, Olesen F. Evaluation of the uterine cavity with magnetic resonance imaging, transvaginal sonography, hysterosonographic examination, and diagnostic hysteroscopy. *Fertil Steril* 2001; 76: 350–357.

Jensen JT. Contraceptive and therapeutic effects of the levonorgestrel intrauterine system: an overview. *Obstet Gynecol Surv* 2005; 60: 604–12.

Lethaby A, Hickey M, Garry R. Endometrial destruction techniques for heavy menstrual bleeding. *Cochrane Database Syst Rev* 2005; 4: CD001501.

Leyden WA, Manos MM, Geiger AM, *et al.* Cervical cancer in women with comprehensive health care access: attributable factors in the screening process. *J Natl Cancer Inst* 2005; 97: 675–683.

Marjoribanks J, Lethaby A, Farquhar C. Surgery versus medical therapy for heavy menstrual bleeding. *Cochrane Database Syst Rev* 2006; 2: CD003855.

Villa LL, Costa RL, Petta CA, *et al.* Prophylactic quadrivalent human papillomavirus (types 6, 11, 16, and 18) L1 virus-like particle vaccine in young women: a randomised double-blind placebo-controlled multicentre phase II efficacy trial. *Lancet Oncol* 2005; 6: 271–278.

Zawadski JK, Dunaif A. Diagnostic criteria for polycystic ovary syndrome: towards a rational approach. In: Dunaif A, Givens JR, Haseltine F (eds) *Polycystic ovary syndrome*. Boston: Blackwell Scientific, 1992: 377–384.

Chapter 59
Premenstrual Syndrome

Sara Twogood and Jennifer Israel
Department of Medicine and Obstetrics and Gynecology, Keck School of Medicine, University of Southern California, CA, USA

Introduction

Premenstrual disease (PMD) occurs from menarche to menopause, approximately ages 14–51. Severe symptoms in women with premenstrual dysphoric disorder (PMDD), usually last 6–7 days/cycle. In general, US women with PMDD will experience ~8 years of severe symptoms during their reproductive years. Causes may include genetic vulnerability where complex altered interactions between central nervous system, gonadal hormones, and other modulators are responsible for unpleasant symptoms. Ovulation/gonadal hormones likely contribute to the symptoms; increased frequency and decreased amplitude of luteal-phase progesterone and luteinizing hormone pulses may be a cause. Neurotransmitters and neurohormonal systems contribute as well; serotonin abnormalities (abnormal 5-HT actions), g-aminobutyric acid (GABA) abnormalities, or the renin-angiotensin-aldosterone system (impaired interaction between estrogen and progesterone) may be at fault.

Symptoms

Practically every unpleasant symptom has been attributed to premenstrual syndrome (PMS). Symptoms should be distinguished from typical moliminal symptoms. The most commonly reported symptoms appear in Box 59.1.

Diagnosis

The clinician's task is complicated by the fact that many if not most patients arrive with a self-diagnosis or an

---

> **Box 59.1 Common symptoms of premenstrual syndrome**
>
> - Anger
> - Anxiety
> - Bloating or weight gain
> - Breast swelling or tenderness
> - Depression, sadness, hopelessness
> - Decreased alertness or concentration
> - Decreased self-esteem
> - Decreased interest in usual activities
> - Fatigue or lethargy
> - Food craving or overeating
> - Gastrointestinal complaints
> - Headache or migraine
> - Impulsivity
> - Irritability, agitation or listlessness
> - Mood swings
> - Muscle and joint pain
> - Sleep disturbances (insomnia, hypersomnia)
> - Tension

unevaluated referral diagnosis. Patients and clinicians often misconstrue dysmenorrhea as a component of PMS. A prospective symptom calendar is perhaps the best way to differentiate common maladies from those which are specific to the luteal phase of the otherwise normal menstrual cycle.

Two months of charting on any of the widely available self-reporting scales often used as research tools (e.g. Calendar of Premenstrual Experiences, University of California, Department of Reproductive Medicine) will allow the patient and physician to differentiate PMS from normal fluctuations in well-being. These tools can also help to differentiate those affective disorders which the patient may prefer to attribute to hormonal fluxes. Prospective diaries for 2–3 consecutive months should

Management of Common Problems in Obstetrics and Gynecology, 5th edition. Edited by T.M. Goodwin, M.N. Montoro, L. Muderspach, R. Paulson and S. Roy. © 2010 Blackwell Publishing Ltd.

show≥1 affective or somatic symptom consistent with PMS and restriction of symptoms to the luteal phase. Exclusion of other disorders is necessary.

The persistence required to complete this task will help the clinician to establish the extent to which the patient is interested in treatment.

There are two methods of diagnostic assessment. One, used primarily by nonpsychiatrists, is described by the *International classification of diseases 10* (ICD-10) as PMS and requires just a single symptom. The other more stringent diagnostic criteria are used mainly by mental health workers and require five of 11 defined symptoms and are associated with social dysfunction. Prospective charting is also required to achieve the diagnosis called PMDD in the *Diagnostic and statistical manual of mental disorders IV* (DSM-IV). Less than 5% of PMS sufferers are estimated to have this more severe form of the condition.

The American College of Obstetricians and Gynecologists (ACOG) diagnostic criteria for PMS included affective and somatic symptoms. The affective symptoms are:
• irritability, which is considered to be the hallmark affective symptom for premenstrual syndrome
• depression
• angry outbursts
• anxiety
• confusion
• social withdrawal
The somatic symptoms include:
• breast tenderness
• abdominal bloating
• headache
• swelling of extremities
Premenstrual dysphoric disorder is the most severe form of PMS.

The DSM-IV diagnostic criteria for PMDD also include both affective and somatic symptoms. For the DSM-IV diagnosis of PMDD, a patient must meet a minimum of five symptoms. One of the four core symptoms must be included. Any/all somatic symptoms count as one. The symptoms must be persistent for more than 1 year, and remit within a few days of the follicular phase. Symptoms are absent the week following menses. Symptoms are confirmed with prospective cycle diaries for at least two consecutive menstrual cycles. These symptoms must not be an exacerbation of any other disorder.

The core affective symptoms are:
• marked sadness, depressed mood, feelings of hopelessness, self-deprecating thoughts
• marked anxiety, tension, feelings of being "on edge"
• marked affective lability
• marked or persistent irritability or anger, or increased interpersonal conflicts
Other affective symptoms are:
• decreased interest in usual activities
• sense of difficulty concentrating
• marked lack of energy, lethargy or easy fatiguability
• marked change in appetite, overeating or specific food cravings
• hypersomnia or insomnia
• sense of being overwhelmed or out of control
Somatic symptoms include:
• breast tenderness or swelling
• headaches
• joint or muscle pain
• abdominal bloating
• extremity swelling
• weight gain
• interferes with work, social activities or relationships
The women experiencing these symptoms must suffer from identifiable dysfunction in social or economic performance. The symptoms must be present in the absence of any pharmacologic therapy, hormone ingestion or drug or alcohol use.

Premenstrual syndrome is a diagnosis of exclusion. It is necessary to rule out other causes of physical and psychologic distress before assigning the label. Common psychiatric conditions, especially major and minor depressive disorders, bipolar disease and panic/anxiety disorders, can masquerade as PMS. Medical conditions exacerbated by menses include anemia, thyroid disease, and endometriosis.

A careful history should be directed toward exclusion of common causes of specific complaints. A history of regular menses without the use of hormonal contraception is required for the diagnosis, because ovulation is necessary for diagnosis. Adverse symptoms occur only during the luteal phase of ovulatory cycles and disappear soon after the onset of menses.

A self-diagnosis of PMS is also a marker for risk of co-existent psychiatric disease. One report found 30% of PMS patients to have a psychiatric diagnosis.

The physical examination should reveal no evidence of disease. Laboratory tests should include a complete blood count (CBC) and thyroid-stimulating hormone (TSH) with additional testing as indicated by specific symptomatology.

Treatment

Patient education about the nature of PMS is the first line of therapy. The commonly held belief that hormonal imbalance is the cause of PMS should be corrected and the patient encouraged to make healthy lifestyle changes as part of the first line of therapy.

Lifestyle modification
A 3-month trial of increased aerobic exercise, decreased saturated fat intake, and calcium supplementation with calcium carbonate 1500 mg twice a day should sufficiently reduce symptoms in a large proportion of patients.

Decreased caffeine should also be encouraged when anxiety is a complaint.

The decline in endorphin levels that normally occurs in the late luteal phase of the menstrual cycle has been suggested as an underlying mechanism for premenstrual symptoms in some women. Regular aerobic exercise leads to the release of endorphins in the central nervous system. It is recommended that women perform at least 20–30 minutes of aerobic exercise per day on at least 3 days each week.

A number of dietary modifications have been used to treat premenstrual symptoms. Limited data indicate a possible benefit for a beverage containing complex and simple carbohydrates in reducing premenstrual symptoms. Reductions in salt, sugar, alcohol, and caffeine intake are often recommended for premenstrual symptoms. Vitamin B6 may have some minimal benefit in reducing premenstrual symptoms, but doses in excess of 100 mg/day may potentially cause permanent neurologic damage. Primrose oil may possibly decrease the symptom of breast tenderness.

Oral contraceptive pills

For those patients whose symptoms continue to be troublesome, especially if they require contraception, a trial of monophasic low androgenic oral contraceptives may be tried. This is especially useful when local pelvic symptoms predominate. Most formulations have not been studied for treatment of PMS or PMDD. New formulations and altered regimens of hormonal contraceptives, e.g. increasing the number of consecutive days of hormone use, have been shown to reduce the severity of premenstrual symptoms compared to placebo. Studies of an OC formulation containing drospirenone 3 mg plus ethinylestradiol 20 μg administered for 24 days in a 28-day cycle have found percent response rates comparable to those found for continuous and intermittent sertraline in clinical studies.

Selective serotonin reuptake inhibitors

The SSRIs fluoxetine hydrochloride (Serafem®), sertraline hydrochloride (Zoloft®), and paroxetine hydrochloride (Paxil®) are currently the only pharmacologic agents with an FDA indication for premenstrual dysphoric disorder. SSRIs interact primarily with serotonin 5-HT reuptake receptors.

Fluoxetine 20 mg can be used daily, intermittently or as a single dose in mid-cycle. Side effects include anxiety, nausea, insomnia or lethargy. Intermittent and prn dosing has been shown to be as effective as continuous therapy and is better tolerated. A reasonable initial trial of therapy would therefore be a single dose of 20 mg of fluoxetine at mid-cycle. If this results in an inadequate response after an appropriate period of evaluation, an increase in the duration of therapy to cover the entire luteal phase with fluoxetine 20 μg/day should be instituted.

Sertraline 50–150 mg daily has also been shown to be effective, and the side effects are similar to fluoxetine.

Tricyclic antidepressants

Tricyclic antidepressants (e.g. clomipramine 25–75 mg/day) have been shown to be more effective than placebo in controlled studies. The side effect profile includes dry mouth and vertigo. SSRIs have been shown to be more effective than tricyclic antidepressants.

Spironolactone

Spironolactone was originally given only for premenstrual fluid retention. However, it has also been shown to relieve other symptoms associated with the premenstrual phase of the cycle. Spironolactone is an aldosterone receptor antagonist derived from 17α-spirolactone, that acts as a potassium-sparing diuretic. The usual dose is 50–100 mg per day.

GnRH angonists

The use of GnRH analogs can be effective in severe cases. GnRH agonists inhibit follicle-stimulating hormone and luteinizing hormone, suppress ovarian steroid hormone production, and prevent ovulation, in effect inducing medical oophorectomy. Their use is limited by both the increase in symptoms associated with initiation of therapy and side effects such as hot flushes and decreased libido. Longer-term use (> 6 months) would theoretically put the patient at increased risk for osteoporosis, heart disease, and even CNS disease. Since GnRH agonists induce medical menopause, either estrogen and progestin must be added back for symptom relief. Bone-sparing therapy, such as a bisphosphonate, may be used to preserve bone density. GnRH agonists are indicated only for patients with severe premenstrual symptoms who are unresponsive to other treatments.

Anxiolytics

Alprazolam is sometimes used to treat premenstrual symptoms, especially when anxiety is the prominent affective symptom. The typical dose is 0.25 mg once or twice daily during the luteal phase; the dose should be tapered at menses. Studies of alprazolam in women with premenstrual symptoms have had inconsistent results. Use of this drug is contraindicated in women with a history of drug abuse or dependence. Alprazolam causes sedation in some women.

Danazol

Given in the luteal phase, danazol has been reported to decrease catamenial migraine. Its use is limited by side effects including amenorrhea, weight gain, acne, and moodiness. Lower doses (200 mg/day) may have a therapeutic effect and FDA approval for the treatment and prevention of mastalgia. This dose does not prevent ovulation and should not be used by women at risk of pregnancy. Danazol, however, is classified as pregnancy category X and should not be used by women at risk of becoming pregnant.

Bilateral salpingo-oopherectomy

Bilateral salpingo-oopherectomy (BSO) has been considered in the most severe forms of intractable disease, as a last resort. Such treatment is controversial due to its irreversibility and a cause of therapeutic failure may be due to an incorrect diagnosis. Strict diagnostic criteria must be met. Prior to BSO, a 3-month trial of GnRH agonist is appropriate to determine if BSO will be effective and if the patient can tolerate hormone replacement therapy.

Other treatments

Whole PMS industries have been built on the use of progesterone suppositories. Topical "progesterone creams" continue to be sold in the retail market for PMS symptoms. Controlled studies have failed to show progesterone to be superior to placebo and higher doses actually exacerbate symptoms in many women. The use of progesterone suppositories, oral or topical micronized progesterone is not scientifically justifiable.

Conclusion

If the recommendations outlined above are insufficient to control symptoms or if the therapies exacerbate the condition, treatment specifically directed at the most troublesome complaint can be offered. By definition, PMS sufferers are ovulating and therefore at risk for pregnancy.

It should be noted that the patient needs to be advised of the unknown fetal effects of many of the pharmacologic interventions discussed.

Premenstrual syndrome is a common chronic recurrent condition which is best approached with information and lifestyle changes after appropriate evaluation.

For the small number of women for whom these interventions are not sufficient, therapies directed at the specific chief complaint are likely to be successful.

Suggested reading

American College of Obstetricians and Gynecologists. *Compendium 2007. Practice Bulletin No 15*. Washington, DC: American College of Obstetricians and Gynecologists ,2000: 917–923.

American Psychiatric Association. *Diagnostic and statistical manual of mental disorders*, 4th edn. Washington, DC: American Psychiatric Association, 1994: 715–718.

Dimmock PW, Wyatt KM, Jones PW, O'Brien PMS. Efficacy of selective serotonin-reuptake inhibitors in premenstrual syndrome: a systematic review. *Lancet* 2000; 356: 1131–1136.

Freeman E, Rickels K, Sondheimer SJ, Polansky M. Ineffectiveness of progesterone suppository treatment for premenstrual syndrome. *JAMA* 1990; 264: 349–353.

Moline ML. Pharmacologic strategies for managing premenstrual syndrome. *Clin Pharm* 1993; 12; 181–196.

Pearlstein TB, Frank E, Rivera-Tovar A, *et al*. Prevalence of axis I and axis II disorders in women with late luteal phase dysphoric disorder. *J Affect Disord* 1990; 20: 129–134.

Physicians' desk reference. Montvale, NJ: Medical Economics Company, 2000.

Thys-Jacobs S, Starkey P, Bernstein D, Tian J. Calcium carbonate and the premenstrual syndrome: effects on premenstrual and menstrual symptoms. Premenstrual Syndrome Study Group. *Am J Obstet Gynecol* 1998; 179: 444–452.

World Health Organization. Mental, behavioral and developmental disorders. In: *International classification of diseases*, 10th revision (ICD-10). Geneva: World Health Organization, 1996.

Chapter 60
Adnexal Masses

Judy Chen and Lynda D. Roman
Department of Medicine and Obstetrics and Gynecology, Keck School of Medicine, University of Southern California, CA, USA

Introduction

Accurately diagnosing an adnexal mass has become a challenge given the vast diagnostic possibilities. Adnexal masses may arise from infections, ovulation abnormalities, mullerian defects or pelvic organs. Unlike other pathologies, these masses do not have a common etiologic pathway. Depending upon the underlying cause, an adnexal mass may be benign or malignant. Characteristics that increase the likelihood of malignancy include age (prepubescent versus postmenopausal females), transvaginal ultrasound (TVUS) appearance, genetic predisposition, ascites, and tumor marker levels.

Differential diagnosis

Childhood years

Childhood presentation of adnexal masses rarely occurs. In the neonatal period, functional ovarian cysts may be present secondary to stimulation by maternal hormones. Other possible abdominal masses are Wilms' tumors or neuroblastomas. However, if an adnexal neoplasm does appear, it tends to be a germ cell tumor such as dysgerminomas or teratomas.

Adolescent years

During adolescence, the most common adnexal pathology is a functional cyst, which can vary in size from 3 to 10 cm. As the name suggests, functional cysts arise from the physiologic follicle maturation process associated with ovulation. These cysts are either follicular or corpus luteum cysts and will eventually disappear with subsequent menstrual cycles.

One of the most common presentations of an adnexal mass in this age group is adnexal torsion. Under torsion,

Management of Common Problems in Obstetrics and Gynecology, 5th edition. Edited by T.M. Goodwin, M.N. Montoro, L. Muderspach, R. Paulson and S. Roy. © 2010 Blackwell Publishing Ltd.

the blood supply to the ovary decreases or subsides, placing the ovary at risk of death. The risk of ovarian death and altered fertility makes torsion a surgical emergency in this age group. Benign teratomas in this age group will frequently present under torsion.

Malignant ovarian tumors, in this age group, tend to be germ cell cancers. About 70% of ovarian tumors found during childhood and adolescence originate from germ cells [1].

Reproductive years

A variety of pelvic masses arise during the reproductive years. Pedunculated myomas of the uterus and, rarely, the cervix may appear to arise from the adnexa. Abnormal placentation of an embryo, an ectopic pregnancy, will also appear as an adnexal mass on transvaginal ultrasound. Remnants of the mesonephric ducts may resemble cystic pelvic masses. Endometriomas are also described as adnexal masses. Polycystic ovary syndrome also causes abnormal ovarian morphology. Untreated or undertreated pelvic inflammatory disease may progress to formation of an intrapelvic abscess; when associated with the ovary it is known as a tubo-ovarian abscess.

Despite the varied possible diagnoses in this age group, about 13% of women during their reproductive years will have a malignant ovarian neoplasm [2]. Histologically, the majority of malignant ovarian neoplasms are epithelial. A substantial percentage of these neoplasms will fall into the category of low malignant potential (borderline) tumors. These types of tumors separate themselves from invasive ovarian carcinoma by their often indolent behavior. Subsequently, a diagnosis of a borderline tumor has an excellent prognosis. Other cell types include germ cell and sex cord stromal. Benign ovarian neoplasms include serous and mucinous cystadenomas, which can vary in size from 5 cm to over 20 cm. Mucinous cystadenomas are known for their large size on presentation. Still, the most common adnexal masses between the ages of 20 and 40 are functional ovarian cysts, and the most common neoplasms are benign teratomas.

Perimenopausal/menopausal years

As with all neoplastic processes, advancing age places a woman at higher risk for developing both benign and malignant ovarian carcinomas. About 80–90% of all ovarian cancers, including borderline tumors, will occur after the age of 40 [1]. The majority of these diagnoses are epithelial ovarian cancers with a serous histologic type. Twenty percent of epithelial ovarian cancers are mucinous, endometrioid, clear cell, Brenner or undifferentiated histology types [1]. Simple benign cysts still occur in 18% of postmenopausal women [3]. Germ cell tumors are extremely rare in women over the age of 40.

Risk factors

Reproductive and genetic factors influence the incidence of ovarian cancer. In an epidemiologic study by Adami *et al.* in Sweden [17], it was noted that increasing parity resulted in a subsequent decrease in relative risk for invasive ovarian cancer. They also noted a decrease in odds ratio between the age of uniparous women and ovarian cancer: women who gave birth at age 35 + had a lower odds ratio than those who gave birth at 20. However, the protective effects of parity did not alter the incidence of borderline tumor. Oral contraceptive pill (OCP) usage has also been proven to decrease the relative risk of ovarian cancer by about 40%, although the maximal protective effects occur after 5 years of usage [4].

While the majority of ovarian cancer cases arise from sporadic mutations, about 10% have an autosomal dominant inheritance related to three genetic mutations [5]. The most commonly known are the BRCA 1 and 2 mutations on chromosome 13 and 17; the third mutation is a mutation in the DNA mismatch repair genes associated with hereditary nonpolyposis colon cancer. BRCA mutations cause about 90% of all inherited ovarian cancer. The increased risk associated with the BRCA gene mutations ranges from 30% with BRCA 2 to 60% with BRCA 1. Despite the increased risk, evidence suggests an improved survival rate for these patients. Patients with these associated mutations may undergo prophylactic bilateral salpingo-oophorectomies in order to prevent occurrence of disease.

Etiology

Our current understanding of ovarian epithelial carcinoma roots itself in the hypothesis that unhindered ovulation causing rupture of the ovarian epithelium and subsequent activation of molecular repair mechanisms gives rise to mutations leading to ovarian cancer. Although chemopreventive data from OCPs support this theory, further analysis reveals that OCPs decrease ovulation only by 15% but the risk for ovarian cancer falls by 50% with OCP usage. Epidemiologic studies on the protective effects of parity also lend credence to the ovulatory hypothesis of ovarian cancer.

Recent investigations demonstrate that 90% of epithelial ovarian carcinomas arise from a monoclonal mutation suggesting that a premalignant lesion occurs within the ovary or fallopian tube after accumulation of multiple mutations [4]. The difficulty lies in finding a premalignant lesion within either organ. A commentary by Dubeau questions the old adage that epithelial carcinoma of the ovarian arises from unhindered ovulation by pointing out two inconsistencies: (1) the mullerian-like histology of epithelial ovarian carcinoma and (2) rare occurrence of preneoplastic changes of the ovarian epithelium. He proposes that epithelial ovarian carcinomas originate from the secondary mullerian system that contributes to the formation of paraovarian/paratubal cyst, rete ovarii, and endometriosis [18].

Diagnosis

One of the difficulties of ovarian carcinoma is early detection. Only 19% of epithelial ovarian cancers are diagnosed while still confined to the ovary; the majority are found after abdominal and extra-abdominal spread occur [6]. Efforts have been concentrated on finding effective screening tools, currently with little success. Women complaining of increasing abdominal girth, decrease in appetite, decrease in weight, early satiety or persistent abdominal/pelvic pain deserve an investigation into the source. These nonspecific gastrointestinal complaints often lead to endoscopic evaluation; however, in women over 40 years old a transvaginal ultrasound may aid in diagnostic investigations.

Transvaginal ultrasonography

Transvaginal ultrasonography (TVUS) has a higher efficacy in delineating soft pelvic organs as well as their physical characteristics than computed tomography or plain film radiography. When compared to MRI, TVUS has similar rates of differentiation of adnexal masses to contrast-enhanced MRI, while it has increased sensitivity and specificity over noncontrast-enhanced images [7]. Given the affordability and availability of ultrasonography, it is the currently favored radiologic modality.

Augmentation of ultrasonography with color Doppler does not clearly increase the sensitivity and specificity of distinguishing malignancy. Buy *et al.* report a 95% accuracy rate, 88% sensitivity rate, and 97% specificity rate when using color Doppler in distinguishing adnexal masses. However, additional information provided by spectral Doppler, including the Resistive Index (RI) and Pulsatility Index (PI), has not shown an increase in sensitivity/specificity of the TVUS technique [8,9]. Overlap between the RI and the PI of benign and malignant masses complicates the correlation of these values with disease state.

Physical characteristics of adnexal masses on TVUS are the mainstay of evaluating malignancy potential. The Morphology Index (MI) described by DePriest *et al.* examines the malignancy potential of an adnexal mass evaluated on TVUS by a scoring system of ovarian volume and ovarian structures such as septations, papillations, and percent solid tissue. Ovarian volumes, determined by using the prolate ellipsoid formula: length [mult] width [mult] height [mult] 0.523, of > 20 cm^3 in premenopausal women and > 10 cm^3 in postmenopausal women are considered abnormal. Results from using the MI reveal a risk of malignancy of 0.3% for tumors with a score less than 5 and 84% with a score 8 or greater [10]. In general, ovarian masses over 5 cm with solid components, multiple septations or papillations strongly suggest the presence of a malignancy.

Serum tumor markers

At its inception, it was hoped that CA 125 would be as effective a screening tool for ovarian cancer as Pap smears were for cervical cancer. CA 125 can be found on a high molecular weight glycoprotein produced primarily by tissue of mullerian origin. Elevated CA 125 occurs in about 80% of patients with ovarian cancer, but it is also elevated in women with endometriosis, menses, and pregnancy [11]. Elevated levels of CA 125 in postmenopausal women carry the most significance with regard to an adnexal mass. In combination with the physical exam and TVUS, CA 125 increases specificity for a malignant tumor to 92% for postmenopausal women [12]. The negative predictive value of all three values (physical exam, TVUS, and CA 125) approaches 100%. Other usages of CA 125 include monitoring the chemotherapeutic response, detecting disease recurrence or enhancing research protocols. About 20% of epithelial ovarian cancers do not produce CA 125 in substantial amounts; thus, the search for more sensitive markers or possible proteomic markers continues.

In patients with germ cell ovarian tumors, levels of α-fetoprotein (AFP), lactate dehydrogenase (LDH), and human chorionic gonadotropins (hCG) help to monitor the progression or regression of disease. AFP tends to be elevated in endodermal sinus tumors while LDH increases with dysgerminoma and hCG rises with nongestational choriocarcinoma [13].

Management

Definitive diagnosis of an adnexal mass requires a tissue diagnosis upon surgical intervention. However, the types of surgical intervention can range from a simple cystectomy for benign disease to total abdominal hysterectomy with bilateral salpingo-oophorectomy, lymph node dissection, omentectomy, peritoneal and diaphragm biopsies, and peritoneal washings for malignant disease. Given the wide range of surgical approaches, careful counseling and clear diagnostic parameters help to determine the appropriate management.

Consideration of age, risk factors, TVUS results, and tumor markers helps to guide counseling of patients and planning for operative intervention. Any complex mass greater than 4 cm deserves thorough investigation into its malignant potential. In a young reproductive age group, where the majority of adnexal masses are functional cysts, a mass that is simple, unilocular, and less than 10 cm in diameter can be followed with serial TVUS every 6 weeks for 6 months to a year [13,14]. The greatest risk for disease in this group is the potential for torsion. Patients must be counseled on the possibility of torsion, the implications of torsion, and the signs of undergoing torsion. In a postmenopausal group, a mass with a diameter greater than 3–5 cm requires surgical intervention, especially a mass with complex features. However, about 60–70% of simple unilocular cysts measuring 5 cm or less in diameter in postmenopausal women will resolve asymptomatically; thus, for such patients monitoring with serial TVUS every 3–6 months may be a viable option [3,15]. Despite the varied management options, most women, at any age, with an adnexal mass greater than 4 cm and any complex feature (solid components, papillations, thickened septations, etc.) suggestive of malignancy require pathologic diagnosis with surgery.

Adnexal masses during pregnancy [16]

Evaluation of adnexal masses during pregnancy is the same as in the nonpregnant state. The transvaginal ultrasonic appearance, genetic predisposition, ascites, and tumor marker levels all contribute to increased suspicion for malignancy. Aside from the concerns for malignancy, pregnancy also increases the risk for torsion and/or rupture of adnexal masses. As the pregnant uterus grows above the pelvic brim, the ovaries no longer have the same restrictions in the abdomen as in the pelvis.

The incidence of adnexal masses found during pregnancy is approximately 1 in 1000. Of these masses, about 3% will have malignant potential. However, of the adnexal masses detected during early pregnancy, only 26% will still be present after 16 weeks of gestation.

Multiloculated, septated cysts greater than 8 cm should be evaluated surgically. Surgical intervention usually occurs during the second trimester, after organogenesis. Since the majority of adnexal masses during pregnancy resolve by the second semester, observation is an option. Although pregnancy is not an absolute contraindication to laparoscopic surgery, one must consider the amount of space available with a gravid uterus as well as compromise of fetal blood supply during abdominal insufflation. Often these two issues of operating space and fetal well-being favor exploratory laparotomy over laprascopic surgery.

References

1. Berek JS, Hacker NF. *Practical gynecologic oncology.* Philadelphia, PA: Lippincott Williams and Wilkins, 2005.

2. Koonings PP, Campbell K, Mishell DR, Grimes DA. Relative frequency of primary ovarian neoplasms: a 10-year review. *Obstet Gynecol* 1989; 74: 921–926.

3. McDonald JM, Modesitt SC. The incidental postmenopausal adnexal mass. *Clinical Obstet Gynecol* 2006; 49: 506–516.

4. Ozols RF, Daly MB, Klein-Szanto A, Hamilton TC, Bast RC, Brewer MA. Specific keynote: chemoprevention of ovarian cancer: the journey begins. *Gynecol Oncol* 2003; 88: S59–S66.

5. Karlan BY, Boyd J, Strong L, Garber J, Fountain J, Beller U. Discussion: hereditary ovarian cancer. *Gynecol Oncol* 2003; 88: S11–S13.

6. Bhoola S, Hoskins WJ. Diagnosis and management of epithelial ovarian cancer. *Obstet Gynecol* 2006; 107: 1399–1410.

7. Yamashita Y, Torashima M, Hatanaka Y, *et al.* Adnexal masses: accuracy of characterization with transvaginal US and pre-contrast and postcontrast MR imaging. *Radiology* 1995; 194: 557–565.

8. Jain KA. Prospective evaluation of adnexal masses with endovaginal gray-scale and duplex and color doppler US: correlation with pathologic findings. *Radiology* 1994; 191: 63–67.

9. Stein SM, Laifer-Narin S, Johnson MB, *et al.* Differentiation of benign and malignant adnexal masses: relative value of gray-scale, color doppler, and spectral doppler sonography. *AJR* 1995; 164: 381–386.

10. Van Nagell JR, DePriest PD. Management of adnexal masses in postmenopausal women. *Am J Obstet Gynecol* 2005; 193: 30–35.

11. Jacobs I, Bast RC. The CA 125 tumour-associated antigen: a review of the literature. *Human Reprod* 1989; 4: 1–12.

12. Schutter EMJ, Kenemans P, Sohn C, *et al.* Diagnostic value of pelvic examination, ultrasound, and serum CA 125 in postmenopausal women with a pelvic mass: an international multicenter study. *Cancer* 1994; 74: 1398–1406.

13. Hoffman MS. Overview of the evaluation and management of adnexal masses. www.utdol.com/utd/content/topic.do?topicKey=genwomen/3056&view=print>.

14. Modesitt SC, Pavlik EJ, Ueland FR, DePriest PD, Kryscio RJ, van Nagell JR. Risk of malignancy in unilocular ovarian cystic tumors less than 10 centimeters in diameter. *Obstet Gynecol* 2003; 102: 594–599.

15. Bailey CL, Ueland FR, Land GL *et al.* The malignant potential of small cystic ovarian tumors in women over 50 years of age. *Gynecol Oncol* 1998; 69: 3–7.

16. Hermans RHM, Fischer DC, van der Putten HWHM, *et al.* Adnexal masses in pregnancy. *Onkologie* 2003; 26: 167–172.

17. Adami H, Hsieh C, Lambe M, *et al.* Parity, age at first childbirth, and risk of ovarian cancer. *Lancet* 1994; 344: 1250–1254.

18. Dubeau L. The cell of origin of ovarian epithelial tumors and the ovarian surface epithelium dogma: does the emperor have no clothes? *Gynecol Oncol* 1992; 72: 437–442.

19. Roman LD, Muderspach LI, Stein SM, Laifer-Narin S, Groshen S, Morrow CP. Pelvic examination, tumor marker level, and gray-scale and Doppler sonography in the prediction of pelvic cancer. *Obstet Gynecol* 1997; 89: 493–500.

20. Buy JN, Ghossain MA, Hugol D, *et al.* Characterization of adnexal masses: combination of color Doppler and conventional sonography compared with spectral Doppler analysis alone and conventional sonography alone. *AJR* 1996; 166: 385–393.

21. Finkler NJ, Benacerraf B, Lavin PT, Wojciechowski C, Knapp RC. Comparison of serum CA 125, clinical impression, and ultrasound in the preoperative evaluation of ovarian masses. *Obstet Gynecol* 1988; 72: 659–664.

22. Strigini FAL, Gadducci A, del Bravo B, Ferdeghini M, Genazzani AR. Differential diagnosis of adnexal masses with transvaginal sonography, color flow imaging, and serum CA 125 assay in pre- and postmenopausal women. *Gynecol Oncol* 1996; 61: 68–72.

Suggested reading

Adami H, Hsieh C, Lambe M, *et al.* Parity, age at first childbirth, and risk of ovarian cancer. *Lancet* 1994; 344: 1250–1254.

Berek JS, Hacker NF. *Practical gynecologic oncology.* Philadelphia, PA: Lippincott Williams and Wilkins, 2005.

Bhoola S, Hoskins WJ. Diagnosis and management of epithelial ovarian cancer. *Obstet Gynecol* 2006; 107: 1399–1410.

Hermans RHM, Fischer DC, van der Putten HWHM, *et al.* Adnexal masses in pregnancy. *Onkologie* 2003; 26: 167–172.

Jacobs I, Bast RC. The CA 125 tumour-associated antigen: a review of the literature. *Human Reprod* 1989; 4: 1–12.

Karlan BY, Boyd J, Strong L, Garber J, Fountain J, Beller U. Discussion: hereditary ovarian cancer. *Gynecol Oncol* 2003; 88: S11–S13.

McDonald JM, Modesitt SC. The incidental postmenopausal adnexal mass. *Clinical Obstet Gynecol* 2006; 49: 506–516.

Ozols RF, Daly MB, Klein-Szanto A, Hamilton TC, Bast RC, Brewer MA. Specific keynote: chemoprevention of ovarian cancer: the journey begins. *Gynecol Oncol* 2003; 88: S59–S66.

Stein SM, Laifer-Narin S, Johnson MB, *et al.* Differentiation of benign and malignant adnexal masses: relative value of gray-scale, color doppler, and spectral doppler sonography. *AJR* 1995; 164: 381–386.

Yamashita Y, Torashima M, Hatanaka Y, *et al.* Adnexal masses: accuracy of characterization with transvaginal US and precontrast and postcontrast MR imaging. *Radiology* 1995; 194: 557–565.

Chapter 61
Ectopic Pregnancy: Diagnosis and Management

Vanessa Sun and Donna Shoupe
Department of Medicine and Obstetrics and Gynecology, Keck School of Medicine, University of Southern California, CA, USA

Introduction

Ectopic pregnancy occurs when an embryo implants outside the uterine cavity. Ninety-five percent of ectopic pregnancies implant in the fallopian tube, while the other 5% occur elsewhere, such as the ovary, cervix, abdominal cavity, uterine myometrium or cesarean section scar. The danger of having an ectopic pregnancy is that it may rupture the fallopian tube or other organ where it is implanted, causing severe pain, blood loss, tissue damage and occasionally death. Today, the diagnosis of ectopic pregnancy is associated with a more favorable outcome due to more sensitive and rapid pregnancy tests, sophisticated ultrasound, and advances in surgical and medical management. The mortality rates in the USA decreased from 35.5 to 3.8 deaths per 10,000 women from 1970 to 1989. Though deaths from ectopic pregnancies still occur, they are often in patients who fail to seek timely medical advice. The aim of treatment has shifted from an immediate life-saving intervention to the development and implementation of conservative methods directed at preserving fertility and reducing morbidity.

The classic symptoms of ectopic pregnancy are abdominal pain, delayed menses, and vaginal bleeding. However, these are not specific for the diagnosis of ectopic pregnancy, as a spontaneous or threatened abortion may present in a similar way. To further complicate the diagnosis, one-third of affected women have no clinical signs or symptoms. An ectopic pregnancy must be suspected in any sexually active, reproductive-age woman with abdominal pain or abnormal uterine bleeding. Risk factors include tubal damage caused by infection or surgery, smoking, failed contraception, previous ectopic pregnancy, and diethylstilbestrol exposure.

Management of Common Problems in Obstetrics and Gynecology, 5th edition. Edited by T.M. Goodwin, M.N. Montoro, L. Muderspach, R. Paulson and S. Roy. © 2010 Blackwell Publishing Ltd.

Incidence

Ectopic pregnancies are relatively common, accounting for 1.3–2% of all reported pregnancies in the USA. This represents a fourfold increase since 1948 when the reported incidence of ectopic pregnancy was only 0.4%. Suggested reasons for continued increases include the greater presence of risk factors in the general population, improvements in diagnostic methods, and the delay in childbearing until later reproductive life, at which time ectopic pregnancy rates are increased.

Seventy-five percent of deaths in the first trimester and 9–13% of all pregnancy-related deaths in the first trimester are associated with extrauterine pregnancies. However, the mortality rates are on the decline. The case–fatality rate is now approximately 3.8 deaths per 10,000 cases of ectopic pregnancies, a decline of 90% from the 35.5 death per 10,000 reported in 1970.

Risk factors

Identifying risk factors can lead to early diagnosis, allowing for conservative management. A previous history of salpingitis, previous or current sexually transmitted disease, infertility, tubal surgery (including tubal ligation), a history of ectopic pregnancy, past abdominal surgery, and *in utero* exposure to diethylstilbestrol are risk factors. Others include advanced maternal age, progestin-only contraceptives, postcoital estrogen contraceptives, progesterone-containing intrauterine devices, ovarian hyperstimulation, smoking, and prior *in vitro* fertilization and embryo transfer.

One-third of ectopic pregnancies are associated with tubal damage due to surgery or infection, while another one-third is seen with smoking. Women who have undergone assisted reproduction have a risk for an extrauterine pregnancy twice that of women who spontaneously conceive.

Women who experience failure of their method of contraception (especially progestin-only oral contraceptives, progestin-only implants, an IUD or permanent surgical sterilization) should be evaluated for an ectopic pregnancy. These methods of contraception reduce the overall rate of ectopic pregnancy because they reduce the rate of all pregnancies. However, the pregnancies that do occur are often implanted outside the uterus.

Clinical findings

The clinical presentation of ectopic pregnancy ranges from asymptomatic to acutely ill. About 50% of patients present with abdominal pain, usually localized to the affected side, and vaginal bleeding after a late or missed period. To complicate the diagnosis, one-third of patients may have no signs or symptoms. Generally, in the early part of the disease course, patients are asymptomatic except possibly for symptoms of pregnancy. As time progresses, symptoms of unilateral pain, vaginal spotting or bleeding generally begin. In the more advanced stages, patients may exhibit syncopal episodes, dizziness, severe pain, orthostatic changes, tachycardia, shock, and/or a distended, rigid abdomen. The ectopic pregnancy generally causes at most a slight temperature elevation or a slight rise in the white blood cells.

Making the diagnosis

The clinical presentation of an ectopic pregnancy is not specific and can often present a challenge to the clinician. The differential for ectopic pregnancy includes threatened or incomplete abortion, ruptured ovarian cyst or a normal intrauterine pregnancy. Refer to Box 61.1 for a more complete list of differential diagnoses.

Making the diagnosis of ectopic pregnancy consists of taking a thorough history, investigating risk factors, doing a physical examination, a pregnancy test (serum or urine), and a transvaginal ultrasound. Serial quantitative serum β-human chorionic gonadotropin (β-hCG) is particularly helpful in making the diagnosis in women

uncertain of their last menstrual period or when the diagnosis is not certain.

Transvaginal ultrasound can identify an intrauterine pregnancy by the presence of a yolk sac, embryo or embryonic cardiac activity. An intrauterine pregnancy almost always excludes the presence of ectopic pregnancy, although a heterotopic pregnancy occurs in every 30,000 pregnancies. Heterotopic pregnancies, a simultaneous ectopic and intrauterine pregnancy, are more common following assisted reproduction techniques. Ultrasound can also identify a complex adnexal mass with or without cardiac motion and free fluid in the cul de sac, all of which are highly suggestive of ectopic pregnancies.

Understanding the predictable pattern of β-hCG change in pregnancy can help make the diagnosis of ectopic pregnancy. The quantitative serum β-hCG is positive as early as 8 days after conception. During the first 6 weeks of gestation in the majority of normal intrauterine pregnancies, the doubling time of β-hCG is 1.4–2.2 days. Helpful guidelines are shown in Table 61.1. Serial β-hCG levels that do not double in an appropriate pattern signify an abnormal gestation and demand that the clinician determine the implantation site. Most ectopic pregnancies have a much slower rise in β-hCG levels, often reaching a low-level plateau.

The specific level of β-hCG can also be used in conjunction with ultrasound findings. Specific findings on transvaginal ultrasound correspond to specific levels of β-hCG (Table 61.2). In a patient with a β-hCG level of 1500–2000 IU/L, transvaginal ultrasound should show the presence of a gestational sac. Alternatively, if the level is greater than 1500 IU/L and no gestational sac is seen, an ectopic pregnancy should be suspected. However, there are exceptions to this guideline such as multiple gestations where the β-hCG level may be higher than 1500 IU/L with no ultrasound findings. Following serial ultrasounds and β-hCG levels can further clarify the diagnosis.

If the β-hCG is less than 1500 IU/L and there are no clear ultrasound findings, a repeat blood test in 3 days can be used to follow the rate of rise. If the repeat value does not follow the normal intrauterine pattern of rise, the diagnosis of ectopic pregnancy or nonviable intrauterine pregnancy is considered.

Other less popular diagnostic tests include measuring serum progesterone, curettage, laparoscopy, culdocentesis, and MRI.

Box 61.1 Differential diagnosis of ectopic pregnancy

Appendicitis
Ruptured ovarian cyst
Ruptured corpus luteal cyst
Salpingitis
Threatened, missed or incomplete abortion
Urinary tract disease, kidney stone
Degeneration/torsion of a uterine leiomyoma
Torsion of the ovary or tube
Normal intrauterine pregnancy
Blighted ovum

Table 61.1 Guidelines for β-hCG radio-immunoassay

Days from last menstrual period	Gestation (weeks)	β-hCG miU/mL
28	4	100
35	5	1000
42	6	10,000

Table 61.2 Ultrasound findings to correspond to β-hCG values

β-hCG miU/mL	UTZ findings
500	Gestational sac
1000	Crown–rump length
15,000	Cardiac motion

Management

Ectopic pregnancies can be managed expectantly, with medicine or with surgery. The clinician must evaluate the patient and her clinical presentation to determine the appropriate treatment.

Expectant management
Expectant management or nonintervention may be considered when:
- β-hCG titers are falling or they are less than 1000 IU/L
- there is no active bleeding
- there is no evidence of rupture on TVUS or physical exam
- there is an adnexal mass of less than 3 cm
- there is no cardiac activity

Approximately 60–90% of small ectopic pregnancies undergo spontaneous resolution. These patients should be followed with serial β-hCG levels until they return to normal (< 2). The patient must be amenable to using some form of birth control until her levels return to normal, as a new pregnancy can confound the management. Following successful expectant management, tubal patency is maintained in over 80% and subsequent pregnancy rates are over 50%. These rates are similar to those obtained following conservative surgical management. The advantages of expectant management include lower cost and avoiding the risks of surgery. However, it requires close supervision and patient compliance.

Medical management
Medical management can be used in women who are stable, not in excessive pain, and have no evidence of rupture. The most common form of medical management is methotrexate, a folinic acid antagonist that interrupts DNA synthesis and cell division. Methotrexate targets rapidly dividing cells that includes a fetus or trophoblastic tissue. General criteria for successful medical management are: hemodynamic stability, pretreatment β-hCG less than 5000 IU/L, adnexal mass less than 3.5 cm, and no fetal cardiac activity. There are two commonly used regimens for administration – the multidose regimen and the single-dose regimen.

The multi-dose regimen entails administering methotrexate (1mg/kg IM on days 1, 3, 5, 7) and leucovorin (0.1 mg/kg IM on days 2, 4, 6, 8) on alternate days until there is a drop in β-hCG of ≥ 15% in 48 hours or four doses of methotrexate have been given. A repeat course can be given if the β-hCG has not dropped to less than 40% of the initial value by day 14.

The single-dose regimen calls for one dose of methotrexate (50 mg/m² IM, on day 1). A repeat dose is given if the β-hCG is not < 15% between days 4 and 7. Up to four subsequent doses can be given if β-hCG does not decline by 15% every week. There is evidence that suggests the multidose regimen is more efficacious (92% vs 88%), but patients who receive the single-dose regimen and any necessary subsequent doses according to protocol experience similar efficacy to the multidose protocol and have fewer side effects.

A novel "double-dose" regimen of methotrexate has recently been introduced as a hybrid between the single- and multiple-dose treatments. Its goal is to increase efficacy while streamlining the treatment process. This regimen delivers one dose of methotrexate (50 mg/m² IM) on day 0 and day 4. β-hCG is measured on day 4 and day 7, and if there is a decline greater than 15%, the treatment is successful. Additional doses of methotrexate are given on day 7 and/or day 11 if the β-hCG does not fall by over 15%. If by the fourth dose the drop is not greater than 15%, the treatment has failed. Success rates of 87% and patient satisfaction rates of 90% are reported with this regimen.

Another medical management strategy is direct injection of low-dose methotrexate into the ectopic pregnancy by ultrasound guidance. This is not recommended as a routine first-line therapeutic treatment.

The most common side effects of methotrexate are stomatitis and conjunctivitis. Less common effects are gastritis, enteritis, dermatitis, pneumonitis, alopecia, elevated liver enzymes, and bone marrow suppression. Prior to administration of methotrexate, the patient should have her liver function tests and creatinine evaluated. Contraindications to methotrexate include breastfeeding women, immunodeficiency, active pulmonary disease, peptic ulcer disease, hypersensitivity to drug, significant hepatic, renal or hematologic disease, and co-existent viable intrauterine pregnancy. Patients who undergo medical management should be reliable and amenable to postponing subsequent pregnancies until their β-hCG hormone is undetectable.

Surgical management
Surgical management is indicated when:
- the patient has severe pain
- the patient is hemodynamically unstable or the ectopic pregnancy is ruptured
- the patient has a contraindication to use of methotrexate
- the patient is unreliable (poor compliance)
- medical therapy fails
- the patient desires permanent contraception
- the patient has had a previous tubal sterilization

• the patient has known tubal disease with planned *in vitro* fertilization for future pregnancy
• the patient has co-existing intrauterine pregnancy
Surgical management is also considered if any of the factors that make medical treatment success unlikely are present (β-hCG > 5000, cardiac motion, adnexal mass > 3.5cm).

The usual treatment is operative laparoscopy with linear salpingostomy, segmental resection or salpingectomy. Salpingostomy is preferred, but salpingectomy is usually performed when:
• there is uncontrolled bleeding from the implantation site
• the case is a recurrent ectopic pregnancy in the same tube
• the tube is severely damaged
• the tubal pregnancy is large
• the patient has completed childbearing or will be treated with *in vitro* fertilization
Future fertility is the same in women who have salpingostomy compared to salpingectomy as long as the contralateral tube is normal. If the unaffected tube is diseased, there is greater future fertility for women after a salpingostomy. Segmental resection is recommended for the treatment of a ruptured isthmic or ampullary gestation when future fertility is an issue. If the tube is preserved, serial β-hCG titers should be obtained every 3–7 days until levels are undetectable.

Laparotomy is recommended in cases of unstable hemodynamics, uncontrolled bleeding or inaccessibility of the tube. In the rare instance of an interstitial (corneal) pregnancy, a cornual resection is preferred over a hysterectomy. In some cases of ruptured cornual pregnancy or cervical pregnancy, hysterectomy may be necessary to control bleeding.

Interstitial pregnancies (where the ectopic is embedded in the segment of tube embedded in the myometrium) are treated similarly to the tubal ectopic pregnancy by the multiple-dose methotrexate regimen. However, if the patient presents with increasing abdominal pain, surgery should be considered. Treatment involves an exploratory celiotomy with corneal resection.

In a heterotopic pregnancy, surgery is the standard of care since methotrexate is contraindicated due to the intrauterine component. One can avoid surgery in an unruptured ectopic by injecting 5 mEq of potassium chloride directly into the extrauterine sac. This is usually done by ultrasound guidance.

Cervical pregnancies, a rare form of ectopic pregnancy, can cause severe hemorrhage leading to hysterectomy. There are no clear guidelines for management of a cervical pregnancy. If the patient is asymptomatic, multidose methotrexate is appropriate. If there is cardiac motion seen in the pregnancy, potassium chloride can be injected into the gestational sac in addition to methotrexate therapy.

If the patient is not hemodynamically stable, she may require a dilation and curettage/evacuation. Due to the possibility of extreme blood loss, uterine artery embolization prior to the D&C can be considered.

Ovarian pregnancies are usually treated surgically although methotrexate has been used successfully in some case reports. Abdominal pregnancies have variable symptomatology and findings that include abdominal pain, vaginal bleeding, painful fetal movement, oligohydramnios, persistent unusual fetal lie, and labor abnormalities. Rarely do these pregnancies continue to term. The difficulty in their management is related not to the fetus but to the placenta. Primary methotrexate therapy has generally not been successful. Surgery is the mainstay of treatment. Delivery of the fetus is uncomplicated, but surgical removal of the placenta should be done with care as it can result in massive hemorrhage. There is evidence to support leaving the placenta in place, and treating postoperatively with methotrexate is a safer approach.

Ectopics rarely occur in hysterotomy scars. They often present the same way as a tubal pregnancy. Again, there is no clear management. Some authors suggest methotrexate therapy with direct administration of potassium chloride if cardiac motion is present. Resolution may take several months. Surgical options include wedge resection of the scar by celiotomy or hysteroscopy.

Conclusion

The diagnosis of ectopic pregnancy is associated with a more favorable outcome than in the past due to the use of newer, more sensitive and rapid pregnancy tests, sophisticated ultrasound, and advances in surgical and medical management. Women today have less morbidity and mortality than their past counterparts. The diagnosis of ectopic pregnancy can be a clinical dilemma. Successful treatment requires good communication between the physician and the patient as well as good patient compliance.

Suggested reading

Barnhart K, Hummel AC, Sammel MD, *et al*. Use of "2-dose" regimen of methotrexate to treat ectopic pregnancy. *Fertil Steril* 2007; 87(2): 251–256.

Farquhar C. Ectopic pregnancy. *Lancet* 2005; 336: 583–591.

Lipscomb GH, Givens VM, Meyer NL, Bran D. Comparison of multi-dose and single-dose methotrexate protocols for the treatment of ectopic pregnancy. *Am J Obstet Gynecol* 2005; 192: 1844–1848.

Erdem M, Erdem A, Arslan M, *et al*. Single-dose methotrexate for the treatment of unruptured ectopic pregnancy. *Arch Gynecol Obstet* 2004; 270; 201–204.

NCHS. *Advanced report of final mortality statistics, 1992*. Hyattsville, MD: US Department of Health and Human Services, Public Health Services, CDC, 1994.

Chapter 62
Endoscopic Surgery

Allan S. Lichtman and Claire E. Templeman
Department of Medicine and Obstetrics and Gynecology, Keck School of Medicine, University of Southern California, CA, USA

Introduction

Most gynecologic procedures can be performed utilizing laparoscopic guidance. Although the term "minimally invasive" has been applied to these procedures, "minimal access surgery" is more accurate and reminds us that these procedures are often just as complex as those done by laparotomy.

Electrosurgery

Safe use of electrosurgery is essential to any surgery, including laparoscopic surgery. Electrosurgical units are the most common piece of surgical equipment in the operating room. A clear understanding of the principles of electrosurgery will allow the operating surgeon to avoid inadvertent injury to their patient [1].

Electric current is the movement of electrons and voltage is the force that causes this movement. The electric current is proportional to the voltage and resistance (impedance) in the circuit. Electrosurgical units are composed of the generator, an active electrode and the dispersive pad. The generator transforms the electricity from the power source into electrical energy. The active electrode delivers the electrical energy to the surgical site and can be monopolar or bipolar in nature.

Monopolar electrodes have a single electrode that delivers current that travels to the return electrode through the patient. These electrodes can be in many forms such as scissors, hooks or spatulas. Bipolar electrosurgery utilizes an electrical current that passes through two parallel poles, one of which is positive and the other negative. The flow of current is between the two poles, which are typically graspers. Bipolar energy uses a lower energy waveform because the poles are in close proximity to each other.

Management of Common Problems in Obstetrics and Gynecology, 5th edition. Edited by T.M. Goodwin, M.N. Montoro, L. Muderspach, R. Paulson and S. Roy. © 2010 Blackwell Publishing Ltd.

The return electrode is commonly known in the operating room as the grounding pad. This provides a large surface area for the current to move from the patient's tissue back to the electrosurgical generator. This prevents the current from heating and damaging the patient's skin. Perfect contact between the pad and the patient's skin is essential to prevent burns. An understanding of the cutting and coagulation settings on the electrosurgical generator is important. Cutting uses a continuous wave form where the energy is concentrated in a small area, resulting in heating of the cells. Coagulation utilizes an intermittent current that produces less heating than the cutting current but produces dehydration of tissue, coagulation of vessels and more lateral spread than the cutting current.

The specific electrosurgical dangers associated with laparoscopic surgery arise when there is transfer of current from instrument to tissue within the abdominal cavity outside the direct view of the surgeon. Whilst operating, the surgeon must pay particular attention to the location of the active electrode (instrument) and the location of other metal instruments in the abdomen. Direct coupling is a phenomenon that occurs when the active electrode comes into contact with another instrument in the surgical field, resulting in transfer of current (and potentially injury) to remote tissue.

Trocar placement

Endoscopic surgery requires transabdominal placement of small metallic or plastic hollow tubes, known as trocars, to enable passage of a variety of operative instruments into the intra-abdominal operative site. The first instrument placed is the Verres needle that allows passage of carbon dioxide to establish a pneumoperitoneum. The Verres needle is approximately 2 mm in diameter. It has a sharp point with a spring-activated retractable blunt protective cover that moves back and forth over the needle. A small skin incision is created either vertically intraumbilically or horizontally infraumbilically to allow insertion of the needle. Once the incision has been created, the surgeon and assistant elevate the abdominal wall. The Verres needle is grasped in its entirety and the tip is placed into the inferior portion of the incision at a point where even in patients with large BMIs, the peritoneum is just a few millimeters away. The needle is advanced through the various layers of the umbilical abdominal wall into the peritoneal cavity. During this blind needle placement, maximum effort is utilized to prevent injury to underlying bowel and vasculature. The needle is advanced and the popping sound and sensation of fascia and peritoneum being pierced are heard and felt by the operator. The needle advancement is then halted. The operator then tests to determine if intra-abdominal placement has been achieved by placing some saline at the outer end of the needle. Lifting the abdominal wall creates a negative pressure and this will draw the saline drop into the abdominal cavity, thus reflecting that a direct, clear connection has been established. Once this process is completed, tubing from the carbon dioxide insufflator is attached to the needle, allowing carbon dioxide to flow into the peritoneal cavity. Percussion of the abdomen will then indicate that the cavity is distended and full of carbon dioxide, again reaffirming the proper placement of the Verres needle.

A second and completely different technique to establish a pneumoperitoneum is to place a trocar under direct vision. An approximate 2 cm intraumbilical incision is created, allowing the operator to tunnel down through the fascia and open the peritoneum directly. Hasson first described this technique [3] and as such, a Hasson trocar is placed into the peritoneal cavity that then allows maintenance of the pneumoperitoneum.

The pneumoperitoneum, independent of technique, allows placement of the laparoscope and the larger diameter trocars that are required for the operative procedures to be performed.

Laparoscopes, with cameras attached, vary in diameter and the trocars used for them must be of similar size. The two traditional scopes used are either 5 mm or 10 mm in diameter. The trocar that houses the camera is usually placed intraumbilically, in a blind fashion, utilizing the sense of pressure release that one feels when the trocar successfully enters the abdominal cavity. Once this trocar is placed, the laparoscope with attached camera may be placed through the hollow trocar into the peritoneal cavity to establish full-magnified vision of the entire cavity. Additional trocars, varying in number and also in diameter, can then be placed under direct vision. The usual trocar diameter for these accessory instruments is 5 mm. These trocars are placed as far lateral as possible from the umbilicus at the level of the umbilicus. Placement of the accessory instrument trocars in this manner allows the instruments to have the best mechanical advantage when operating on the adnexa and the upper uterus. Additional instruments may need to be utilized for retraction, grasping, and gaining access to the cul de sac or the lower retroperitoneum. For these instruments, one or more

trocars can be inserted inferiorly at any portion of the lower abdomen that enhances access. Some surgeons have utilized specific anatomic guidelines for the placement of the trocars but in most instances, the additional sites of placement are better dictated by the particular surgical need.

Two most important rules for trocar placement are, first, that one should transilluminate the abdominal cavity to attempt to avoid injuring a major abdominal wall vessel when inserting the trocar, and second, that the camera should be utilized to view the trocar tip completely as it enters the abdominal wall. This is the most successful way of avoiding damage to vascular, bowel or other underlying structures. Occasionally, accessory instruments are used that have 10–12 mm or even 18 mm diameters and there will need to be an expansion of one or more trocar sites to accommodate these larger instruments.

Emergency needle

Whenever laparoscopy is performed, the trocar placement may induce abdominal wall bleeding. Several methods are available to suture this arterial or venous bleeding quickly that allows the safe continuation of the endoscopic procedure. One of the most effective emergency needle systems is the Carter–Thomasen system [4]. This needle can be used for suturing as large a vessel as the inferior epigastric artery and can be effectively utilized even if there is only one accessory trocar placed. This system is also extremely useful for closing the peritoneum and fascia of trocar sites that are 10 mm or greater in diameter. This closure is sufficient to reduce the risk of trocar site hernias.

Laparoscopy

The laparoscopic approach is being used for a wide range of gynecologic surgeries including, infertility, hysterectomy, adnexal pathology, and myomectomy. During laparoscopy, there is decreased tissue drying and less exposure to environmental contaminants. The magnification afforded by the laparoscope permits the pinpoint application of energy sources and allows access to some areas with less trauma than by laparotomy. Thus, laparoscopic surgery has many other advantages in addition to more rapid recovery and less pain during the postoperative period.

Infertility

In infertile women, the reported incidence of endometriosis is between 5% and 48%. Among patients with severe pelvic pain, endometriosis may be found in up to 80% of cases. Laparoscopic surgery remains the treatment of choice for the diagnosis of endometriosis, especially in its milder forms. Several modalities have been advocated for the treatment of endometriosis: medical therapy, surgery, combined medical and surgical therapy, and *in vitro* fertilization. Patients with mild disease may conceive without treatment. Therefore, it is more difficult to prove any benefit in these patients. In the surgical treatment of endometriosis, laparoscopy is preferable to laparotomy. Several studies have shown comparable pregnancy rates when laparoscopy is compared to laparotomy. There is no place for medical suppressive therapy alone in the treatment of patients with moderate and severe endometriosis, most of whom have adhesive disease. In these cases, restoration of the normal pelvic architecture is the primary goal of laparoscopic surgery.

The surgical treatment of endometriosis may be divided into three areas: removal of implants, lysis of adhesions, and the excision of endometriomas. Compared to vaporization and coagulation, excision of lesions offers the advantages of providing a histologic diagnosis and assuring complete removal of the disease. In addition, if lesions are vaporized or if coagulation is employed, the char induced may not be distinguished with certainty from the characteristic blue-black implants.

Endometriomas should be excised. Following aspiration, recurrences are common. Suture closure of the ovary is usually not necessary because the edges fall together spontaneously. However, if needed, sutures should not encompass the ovarian cortex in order to reduce the incidence of adhesion formation. After hemostasis has been secured, the ovary is wrapped in Interceed.

Second-look laparoscopy (SLL) following conservative infertility surgery has been performed only after an extended period has elapsed without a pregnancy. Early SLL, performed 1–8 weeks after the initial procedure, is recommended because the early postoperative period is when adhesions that have begun to form or reform are filmy and avascular, making adhesiolysis easy.

In order to assess the impact of adhesions upon fertility, Tulandi *et al.* used life-table analysis to assess the cumulative pregnancy rates among infertile patients with adnexal adhesions of similar extent [2]. These were 32% and 45% at 12 and 24 months after adhesiolysis but only 11% and 16% at the same time periods in patients who elected not to undergo surgery.

Tubal surgery

There are five laparoscopic procedures. Fimbrioplasty is the deagglutination of the fimbria or a broadening of a phimotic tubal opening. Salpingostomy (neosalpingostomy) is the opening of a tube that had complete distal obstruction. Salpingo-ovariolysis applies to the lysis of adhesions surrounding the fallopian tube and ovary that may prevent ovum pick-up. This is usually necessary prior to fimbrioplasty or salpingostomy. The fourth category is tubal resection and reanastomosis and the last is treatment of proximal tubal obstruction by simultaneous laparoscopy and hysteroscopy with tubal cannulation. Fimbrioplasty is a relatively simple technique that is easy to accomplish. Sharp dissection or incision by laser or an electrosurgical microelectrode or even a "bougie" technique is employed. Forceps are passed through the stenotic opening and the agglutinated fimbriae are separated. Pregnancy rates are excellent.

Salpingostomy is more complex. The tube is grasped with atraumatic forceps near the occluded distal end and the lumen of the distal tube is distended by hydrochromopertubation. After identifying the "dimple" at the site of the former tubal ostium, a cruciate incision is made starting at the dimple and extending proximally along the avascular planes of fimbrial closure. Care must be taken to avoid extending the incisions too far into the proximal ampulla. Finally, the edges are everted in order to prevent reclosure of the tube. Pregnancy rates are similar to those following microsurgery at laparotomy. Most pregnancies occur within 1–2 years of surgery.

Because laparoscopy is performed prior to tubal reanastomosis in order to evaluate the distal tubal segment, it is advantageous to complete the operation without having to resort to laparotomy. This approach is feasible but the learning curve is steep. The same steps utilized for tubal resection and reanastomosis by laparotomy are employed.

Ovarian surgery

Bassil and colleagues followed 43 patients after laparoscopic treatment of benign ovarian cysts [5]. The fecundity rate for these patients after surgery was 7.8%. There was no difference in pregnancy rates whether aspiration of functional cysts or resection of neoplasm was performed. There was also no difference in pregnancy rates after the treatment of large (> 6 cm) or small cysts.

If ovarian torsion has occurred and the ovary appears viable, the mass is untwisted. The risk of embolization is small. If normal blood flow and color return to the ovary, a cystectomy is performed. The ovarian ligament is shortened using a nonreactive, fine permanent suture. This procedure may reduce the risk of recurrent torsion.

Laparoscopic procedures to induce ovulation in polycystic ovary syndrome have been introduced as an alternative to ovarian wedge resection. Gjönnaess demonstrated high rates of ovulation and pregnancy after laparoscopic unipolar diathermy [6]. The mechanism for resumption of ovulation following ovarian cortical injury is unknown. Based on the above evidence, the goal of surgery should be to drain the multiple peripheral cysts and destroy ovarian stroma. This technique has been variously termed ovarian drilling, photocoagulation or multiple ovarian cystotomy. Ovulation rates of 67–97% have been reported.

Uterine surgery
Hysterectomy
Laparoscopy has also been utilized by the gynecologic surgeon to perform hysterectomy [7] and, in some

instances, oncologic staging procedures that result in reducing some morbidity of the operative procedure. Patients undergoing laparoscopically aided hysterectomy may enjoy shortened postoperative recovery time, enhanced quality of life by reducing postoperative pain, allowing return of gastrointestinal function more quickly and generally enabling reduced time to full recovery.

The surgical route that is the method of choice for hysterectomy is vaginal hysterectomy. This technique has the least morbidity and mortality and quickest recovery time. If vaginal hysterectomy is not technically possible, if a clear view of the abdominal cavity is required or if the surgery dictates the absolute need for adnexectomy or other intra-abdominal procedure, the next best alternative route is laparoscopically assisted vaginal hysterectomy (LAVH) [8,9]. Further, if the access to the vagina is doubtful or impossible, a choice of total laparoscopic hysterectomy (TLH) may have advantage over an abdominal hysterectomy for the same reasons as already mentioned. The total laparoscopic approach is an alternative only for those surgeons trained in that approach [10].

The LAVH may be accomplished using three trocar ports and an assortment of other instruments such as a variety of cautery instruments, endoloop, harmonic scalpel, and/or argon beam. Completion of the hysterectomy begun abdominally is accomplished through the traditional vaginal hysterectomy technique. Total laparoscopic hysterectomy is completed entirely laparoscopically, with the uterus being removed vaginally and the vaginal cuff closed endoscopically. An alternative to this is the laparoscopic subtotal hysterectomy where, when indicated and appropriate, the cervix may be left in place. In that instance, the uterus is removed utilizing the laparoscopically directed morcellator [11-13].

Myomectomy

The value of myomectomy in order to restore fertility remains controversial. However, most surgeons would agree that the presence of submucous myomas and those that distort the architecture of the uterine cavity or cause tubal blockage might be a factor. Most intramural and subserosal myomas can be removed laparoscopically. Most surgeons reserve the laparoscopic approach for the smaller tumors. In general, the principles are the same as for laparotomy.

Myoma resection is accomplished with three or four abdominal punctures. A dilute (10 units in 20 mL of saline) vasopressin solution is introduced into the uterus with a 20 gauge spinal needle. The pedicle of a pedunculated myoma may be ligated (if small) with an endoloop or it may be transected with a laser, harmonic scalpel, unipolar electrode or bipolar forceps. After transection, hemostasis is secured. For broad-based subserosal myomas and all intramural myomas, the surgery begins with incision of the overlying myometrium. Once exposed,

traction on the myoma is essential to facilitate dissection. The dissection is carried down to the base and all "feeder vessels" are sealed. After separation, the myoma may be removed by morcellation and extraction through a trocar sleeve. Alternatively, enlargement of a trocar incision or a colpotomy incision may be utilized. Although the risk of infection and adnexal adhesion formation may be small, we prefer to avoid colpotomy in patients who wish to conceive in the future.

We advocate closure of the uterine defect in multiple layers for all intramural and most subserosal myomas in order to maintain uterine wall integrity during a subsequent pregnancy. Postoperative evaluation of uteri closed without myometrial repair has shown large defects. In addition, uterine dehiscence at the site of myomectomy in which only the serosa was closed has been reported during the third trimester.

Hysteroscopy

Most surgical procedures for the diagnosis and management of intrauterine pathology can be managed hysteroscopically. This technique enhances diagnostic and therapeutic modalities of the "minimal access" type.

The hysteroscopic armamentarium has dramatically advanced in recent years. New instrumentation enables diagnostic procedures to be performed in office settings utilizing instruments with diameters as small as 3 mm [14]. In addition to the increased ease and accuracy of diagnostic hysteroscopy, definitive treatment for many intrauterine submucosal masses utilizing an operative hysteroscopic technique allows for the successful resection of the intrauterine pathology. In many cases, this may avoid hysterectomy [15-18]. Additional hysteroscopic advances include: new modalities for endometrial ablation for the treatment of severe menorrhagia [19,20]; a very successful technique for sterilization as an alternative to laparoscopic tubal sterilization [21,22]; and continued moderate success of transcervical hysteroscopic balloon tuboplasty [23,24].

Diagnostic hysteroscopy

Diagnostic hysteroscopy is used to definitively diagnose and establish the existence and type of intrauterine pathology. Examples of these abnormalities include intrauterine adhesions, submucous leiomyomata, endometrial polyps, congenital anomalies, and embedded intrauterine devices [25,26].

Absolute contraindications to hysteroscopy are acute pelvic infection and invasive cervical cancer. Acute uterine bleeding, pregnancy, a recent uterine perforation, and uterine cancer are relative contraindications [27–29].

Complications of diagnostic hysteroscopy are rare and mild. The most common are abdominal pain, bleeding, and shoulder pain. Occasional acute vasovagal episodes occur that are distressing, but are almost always self-limited, treated by utilizing the Trendelenburg position and supportive care. Rarely, intravenous atropine may be required to support the heart rate while waiting for the vasovagal response to diminish.

The most common medium utilized for outpatient diagnostic procedures is carbon dioxide. If carbon dioxide is used as the distension medium, a proper insufflator will reduce the incidence of acidosis and arrhythmias to only theoretic possibilities. In recent years, mini-hysteroscopes have been developed with outer diameters of 3 mm, that utilize saline for distension. These instruments are very well tolerated, since they do not require cervical dilation and provide unusually excellent diagnostic fields of vision.

Operative hysteroscopy

Various abnormalities may be treated utilizing an operative hysteroscopic approach. The more common uses for operative hysteroscopy are menorrhagia, sterilization and tuboplasty. A variety of instruments are available for ablation of the endometrial surface. This is utilized as an alternative treatment of severe menorrhagia. The placement of tubal implants under direct hysteroscopic vision has recently become available to perform outpatient sterilization procedures. Infertility secondary to proximal tubal obstruction may be alleviated with hysteroscopic transcervical balloon tuboplasty.

Problems occurring in operative hysteroscopic procedures are also infrequent and for the most part very mild. On rare occasions, a serious complication can occur in operative hysteroscopy. Mild complications include pain, bleeding, infection, uterine perforation and cervical lacerations [30-32]. The rare but more serious complications are usually related to the medium utilized to distend the uterine cavity. The most common media utilized are hypertonic solutions of which sorbitol or glycine is the most common. If a large amount of any hypertonic material enters the venous circulation, generally in excess of 1000 cc, circulatory overload accompanied by severe hyponatremia is possible. The most serious consequences of this are congestive heart failure, cardiac arrhythmia, adult respiratory distress syndrome and death [33]. Instruments utilizing normal saline as the distending medium have recently been introduced that will, theoretically, reduce the hyponatremic effect of absorption of hypertonic solutions. Large volumes of glycine may cause ammonia retention in patients with limited hepatic function. Careful monitoring of the intake and output of the fluid media is required during any operative hysteroscopic procedure.

Intrauterine adhesions

Intrauterine adhesions (IUAs) are found frequently in patients with reproductive problems and after various types of uterine trauma. The most common symptoms of this abnormality are amenorrhea and infertility. Although injury to the pregnant or recently pregnant uterus is the most common antecedent factor, any uterine injury can cause endometrial sclerosis and/or adhesion formation. Hysteroscopic lysis of adhesions is the treatment of choice for this lesion and it has proven to be very successful for alleviating these issues [34-36].

Congenital anomalies

Obstetric problems such as first-trimester abortions, premature labor and abnormal fetal presentations are common in patients with uterine anomalies. Abortion has been reported to occur in as many as 30% of pregnancies in women with septate uteri.

Hysteroscopy has been used to assess the size, length and breadth of the septum. The hysteroscope also enables treatment of this lesion by providing direct visualization for incision of the septum [37]. Simultaneous laparoscopy is needed to verify that the uterus is unified externally and also to provide guidance for the hysteroscopist. Scissors are passed through the operating channel of the hysteroscope, and the central portion of the septum is incised. The fibroelastic band of tissue retracts immediately and does not bleed. The dissection is carried cephalad until the septum is incised completely and the uterine architecture is normalized. If the cervix is also septate, the incision is begun at the level of the internal os and carried cephalad. The cervical portion of the septum is "spared" in order to reduce the risk of hemorrhage and cervical incompetence.

In order to epithelialize the area over the incised septum, conjugated estrogens, 1.25 mg, are prescribed for 25 days. Medroxyprogesterone acetate, 10 mg daily, is given during the last 5 days of the estrogen treatment. Office hysteroscopy should be performed after the withdrawal menses to assess healing. If normal, the patient may attempt to conceive immediately thereafter.

Abnormal uterine bleeding

The hysteroscopic management of abnormal bleeding varies with the particular underlying pathologic process. The hysteroscopic resectoscope is employed to remove submucosal masses such as leiomyomas and/or polyps, utilizing a traditional unipolar wire electrode with either saline or sorbitol for distension [38,39]. A hysteroscopic morcellator that uses mechanical energy for the resection and saline as the distending medium may also be employed. In many instances, the abnormal bleeding may be completely eradicated utilizing this procedure [40]. After endometrial hyperplasia and/or carcinoma are eliminated as a possible etiology, and in the absence of any observable submucosal lesions, hysteroscopic endometrial ablation may be employed to decrease menorrhagia [41]. A variety of instruments are available for this treatment. Rollerball requires hysterscopic visualization utilizing the resectoscope. Nonresectoscopic instruments recently introduced utilize freezing, heating or radiofrequency electricity to accomplish the same endpoint. These ablative techniques have a high level of patient satisfaction by producing amenorrhea or oligomenorrhea in 90% of cases for at least 3 years [20].

Sterilization

Hysteroscopic tubal occlusion for the purposes of sterilization which has recently been introduced may provide an acceptable alternative to laparoscopic sterilization [42]. The technique utilizes direct hysteroscopic visualization facilitating placement of plugs into the tubal ostia bilaterally. The results appear promising.

Proximal tuboplasty

Obstruction of the proximal fallopian tubes is observed in 10–20% of hysterosalpingograms (HSG) performed because of infertility. If an HSG indicates proximal tubal occlusion, it is reasonable to proceed to laparoscopy with hydrotubation. Should this confirm bilateral patency, no further procedures need to be carried out unless the patient requires hysteroscopy. In patients with proximal tubal obstruction whose distal fallopian tubes appear normal, transcervical tuboplasty is indicated to restore patency and has had some degree of success. Significant lesions, such as salpingitis isthmica nodosa, severe fibrosis, endosalpingiosis or previous reconstructive surgery, have a significantly lower chance of being corrected by the transcervical hysteroscopic balloon tuboplasty approach [43].

References

1. Broadman M. Electrocautery devices: the way they work. *Contemp Ob/Gyn* 2007(8): 52: 85–93.
2. Tulandi T, Collins JA, Burrows E, *et al.* Treatment-dependent and treatment-independent pregnancy among women with periadnexal adhesions. *Am J Obstet Gynecol* 1990; 162: 354–357.
3. Hasson HM. A modified instrument and method for laparoscopy. *Am J Obstet Gynecol* 1971; 110: 886–887.
4. Carter JE. A new technique of fascial closure for laparoscopic incisions *J. Laparoendosc Surg* 1994; 4: 143–146.
5. Bassil S, Canis M, Pouly A, *et al.* Fertility following laparoscopic treatment of benign adnexal cysts. In: Donnez J, Nisolle M (eds) *An atlas of laser operative laparoscopy and hysteroscopy.* New York: Parthenon Publishing, 1994: 165.
6. Gjönnaess H. Polycystic ovarian syndrome treated by ovarian electro-cautery through the laparoscope. *Fertil Steril* 1984; 41: 20–25.
7. Reich H, Decaprio J, McGlynn F. Laparoscopic hysterectomy. *J Gynecol Surg* 1989; 5: 213–216.
8. American College of Obstetricians and Gynecologists. *Appropriate use of laparoscopically assisted vaginal hysterectomy. Committee Opinion No 311.* Washington, DC: American College of Obstetricians and Gynecologists, 2005.
9. Carter JE, Jisun R, Katz A. Laparoscopic assisted vagianl hysterectomy: a case control comparative study with total abdominal hysterectomy. *J Am Assoc Gynecol Laparosc* 1994; 1: 116.
10. Harkki P, Kurki T, Sjoberg J, Titinen A. Safety aspects of laparoscopic hysterectomy. *Acta Obstet Gynecol Scand* 2001; 80: 383–391.
11. Garry R, Fountain J, Mason S, *et al.* The eVALuate study: two parallel randomized trials, one comparing laparoscopic with abdominal hysterectomy, the other comparing laparoscopic with vaginal hysterectomy. *BMJ* 2004; 328: 129.
12. Munro MG, Parker WH. A classification system for laparoscopic hysterectomy. *Obstet Gynecol* 1993; 82: 624–629.
13. American College of Obstetricians and Gynecologists. *Laparoscopic sub-total hysterectomy. Committee Opinion No. 388.* Washington, DC: American College of Obstetricians and Gynecologists, 2007.
14. Cicinelli E, Parisi C, Galantino P, *et al.* Reliability, feasibility, and safety of minihysteroscopy with a vaginoscopic approach: experience with 6000 cases. *Fertil Steril* 2003; 80(1): 199–202.
15. Neuwirth RS. A new technique for and additional experience with hysteroscopic resection of submucous fibroids. *Am J Obstet Gynecol* 1978; 135: 91–94.
16. DeCherney A, Polan ML. Hysteroscopic management of intrauterine lesions and intractable uterine bleeding. *Obstet Gynecol* 1983; 61(3): 392–397.
17. Clark TJ, Mahajan D, Sunder PK, Gupta JK. Hysteroscopic treatment of symptomatic submucous fibroids using a bipolar intrauterine system:a feasibility study. *Eur J Obstet Gynecol Reprod Biol* 2002; 100: 237–242.
18. Song AH. Global endometrial ablation devices: minimally invasive surgical alternatives to hysterectomy. *Female Patient* 2007; 32: 46–50.
19. Shushan A, Revel A, Laufer N, Rojansky N. Hysteroscopic treatment of intrauterine lesions inpremenopausal and postmenopausal women. *J Am Assoc Gynecol Laparosc* 2002; 9(2): 209–213.
20. American College of Obstetricians and Gynecologists. Endometrial ablation. Practice Bulletin No 81. *Obstet Gynecol* 2007; 109: 1233–1248.
21. Duffy S, Mars F, Rogerson L, *et al.* Female sterilisation: a cohort controlled comparative study of ESSURE versus laparoscopic sterilisation. *BJOG* 2005; 112: 1522–1528.
22. Levie MD, Chudnoff S. Office hysteroscopic sterilization compared with laparoscopic sterilization: a critical cost analysis. *J Minim Invas Gynecol* 2005; 12: 318–332.
23. Risquez F, Confino E. Transcervical tubal cannulation, past, present, and future. *Fertil Steril* 1993; 60: 211–226.
24. Deaton JL, Gibson M, Riddick DH, *et al.* Diagnosis and treatment of cornual obstruction using a flexible tip guidewire. *Fertil Steril* 1990; 53: 232–236.
25. Farquhar C, Ekeroma A, Furness S, Arroll B. A systematic review of transvaginal ultrasonography, sonohysterography, and hysteroscopy for the investigation of abnormal uterine bleeding in postmenopausal women. *Acta Obstet Gynecol Scand* 2003; 8: 493–504.
26. Pal L, Lapensee L, Toth TL, Isaacson KB. Comparison of office hysteroscopy, transvagianl ultrasonography and endometrial biopsy in evalation of abnormal bleeding. *J Soc Laparoendosc Surg* 1997; 1: 125–130.
27. Paschopoulos M, Polyzos N P, Lavasidis LG, *et al.* Safety issues of hysteroscopic surgery. *Ann NY Acad Sci* 2006; 1092(1): 229–234.

28. Bradley WH, Boente MP, Brooker D, *et al*. Hysteroscopy and cytology in endometrial cancer. *Obstet Gynecol* 2004; 104(5): 1030–1033.

29. Obermair A, Geramou M, Gucer F, *et al*. Does hysteroscopy facilitate tumor cell dissemination? *Cancer* 2000; 88: 139–143.

30. Cooper JM, Brady RM. Intraoperative and early postoperative complications of operative hysteroscopy. *Obstet Gynecol Clin North Am* 2000; 27: 347–366.

31. Agostini A, Cravello L, Shojai R, *et al*. Postoperative infection and surgical hysteroscopy. *Fertil Steril* 2002; 77: 766–768.

32. Propst AM, Liberman RF, Harlow BL, Ginsburg ES. Complications of hysteroscopic surgery: predicting paients at risk. *Obset Gynecol* 2000; 96: 517–520.

33. Kim AH, Keltz MD, Arici A, Rosenberg M, Olive DL. Dilutional hyponatremia during hyteroscopic myomectomy with sorbitol-mannitol distention. *J Am Assoc Gynecol Laparosc* 1995; 2(2): 237–242.

34. March CM, Israel R, March AD. Hysteroscopic management of inauterine adhesions. *Am J Obstet Gynecol* 1978; 130(6): 653-657.

35. Capella-Allouc S, Mrsad F, Rongieres-Bertrand C, Taylor S, Fernandez H. Hysteroscopic treatment of severe Asherman's syndrome and subsequent fertility. *Human Reprod* 1999; 14(5): 1230–1233.

36. Magos A. Hysteroscopic treatment of Asherman's syndrome. *Reprod Biomed Online* 2002; 4(3): 46–51.

37. Israel R, March CM. Hysteroscopic incision of the septate uterus. *Am J Obstet Gynecol* 1984; 149(1): 66–73.

38. Townsend DE, Fields G, McCausland A, Kaufman K. Diagnostic and operative hysteroscopy in the management of persistent postmenopausal bleeding. *Obstet Gynecol* 1993; 82(3): 419–421.

39. Batra N, Khunda A, O'Donavan P J. Hysteroscopic myomectomy. *Obstet Gynecol Clin North Am* 2004; 31(3): 669–685.

40. Emanuel MH. Hysteroscopic morcellation, a new technique for the removal of endometrial polyps and submucous myomas. *J Min Invas Gynecol* 2005; 12(5,1): 90.

41. Loffer FD, Grainger D. Five-year follow-up of patients participating in a randomized trial of uterine balloon therapy versus rollerball ablation for treatment of menorrhagia. *J Am Assoc Gynecol Laparosc* 2002; 9(4): 429–435.

42. Ubeda A, Labastida R, Dexeus S. Essure: a new device for hysteroscopic tubal sterilization in an outpatient setting. *Fertil Steril* 2004; 82: 189–196.

43. Confino E, Tur-Kaspa I, DeCherney A, *et al*. Transcervical balloon tuboplasty. A multi-center study. *JAMA* 1990; 264: 2079–2082.

Chapter 63
Postsurgical Adhesion Formation and Prevention

Claire E. Templeman, Joseph D. Campeau and Gere S. diZerega
Department of Medicine and Obstetrics and Gynecology, Keck School of Medicine, University of Southern California, CA, USA

Introduction

Adhesion formation is the leading cause of failed therapy following gynecologic surgery [1-3]. Postsurgical adhesions may be characterized as either filmy, avascular adhesions or as dense and/or vascular adhesions. New adhesions developing at sites that did not have pre-existing adhesions are known as *de novo* adhesions and may form at the site of surgery or at another site in the peritoneal cavity remote from the surgical field. Adhesions may also reform after adhesiolysis and there is good evidence that the physiology of *de novo* and reformed adhesions is different as adhesive tissue contains higher levels of growth factors, suggesting the greater likelihood of adhesion reformation. Since these factors depress fibrinolytic activity and induce tissue fibrosis, it is not surprising that reformed adhesions tend to be more dense and severe than *de novo* adhesions.

While laparoscopic procedures are commonly believed to be less adhesiogenic and cause fewer *de novo* adhesions to form, the incidence of adhesion formation following gynecologic laparoscopy has been shown to range from 70% to 100% [4,5]. For many procedures, the risk of associated complications of postsurgical adhesions following open and laparoscopic gynecologic surgery is comparable [6]. Adhesiolysis remains the main treatment, despite the fact that adhesions reform in 85% of patients regardless of the method of adhesiolysis or the type of adhesions being lysed [7]. The rate of recurrence does not differ following laparotomy compared to laparoscopy. The ovaries, fallopian tubes, uterus, bowel, omentum, broad ligaments, side wall, and other pelvic surfaces are often involved.

Adhesions are now the most frequent complication of abdominopelvic surgery, yet many surgeons are still not aware of the extent of the problem and the serious consequences of postsurgical adhesions [8]. Although most patients will have no apparent problems associated with adhesions, in a considerable proportion of cases there are major short- and long-term consequences, most notable of which are small bowel obstruction (SBO), secondary infertility in women and chronic pelvic pain. Even where there are no apparent problems associated with adhesions, they cause serious reoperative complications with a considerable mortality risk.

Adhesion formation

The peritoneum is the most extensive serous membrane in the body. It minimizes friction and facilitates free movement of abdominal viscera, resists and localizes infections and stores fat. It is not, however, an inert container but an organ in its own right. It comprises a single-cell layer of mesothelium lying on a submesothelial connective tissue matrix containing numerous capillaries and lymphatic channels opening into the mesothelial cell monolayer.

The pathogenesis of adhesion formation is complex, with many factors involved. The process of postsurgical adhesion formation commences from the moment of peritoneal injury during surgery, as a result of which the inflammatory cascade is triggered and fibrin is deposited at the damaged surfaces as a result of bleeding and post-traumatic inflammation. Thus the process of adhesion formation commences during surgery. While the severity and extent of adhesions may change over weeks or months, the question of whether or not an adhesion develops is determined in the 3–5 days after peritoneal trauma takes place, i.e. after surgery has been carried out. During this postsurgical period the fibrin layer is reduced through fibrinolysis and the peritoneal membrane either becomes fully re-epithelialized or not. If fibrinolysis does not occur, an irreversible tissue bridge (adhesion) develops, which strengthens in the following weeks and months with the ingrowth of blood vessels and nerve fibers.

Management of Common Problems in Obstetrics and Gynecology, 5th edition. Edited by T.M. Goodwin, M.N. Montoro, L. Muderspach, R. Paulson and S. Roy. © 2010 Blackwell Publishing Ltd.

Epidemiology of adhesions

The initial evidence for the extent of the problem of adhesions came largely from single-center practice-based research. However, the Surgical and Clinical Adhesions Research (SCAR) group quantified the epidemiology and burden that adhesions pose to patients, surgeons and health systems. The trilogy of studies focused on the adhesion-related hospital readmissions of the entire population of Scotland. The initial study followed up adhesion-related hospital readmissions over a period of 10 years in a cohort of patients undergoing open abdominal or gynecologic surgery [9]. This showed that over the 10-year study period, up to one in three patients were readmitted at least twice for adhesion-related problems or other surgery that would potentially be complicated by pre-existing adhesions and, moreover, that the readmissions continued steadily throughout the 10 years.

Patient rights

Adhesion-related complications are increasingly the subject of forensic and medicolegal debate. There is evidence that medicolegal litigation resulting from complications secondary to postoperative adhesion formation is adding to the healthcare costs and the clinician's burden [10]. Careful surgical consent advising patients of the reasons for and nature of the procedure, along with the risks, benefits and consequences of not undergoing the procedure, is important. With a risk of a direct adhesion-related hospital admission of 1:50 following open tubal or ovarian surgery and 1:80 following similar laparoscopic surgery, this is considerably higher than the risk of complications normally discussed during the consent process – including general anesthesia risks (~1:100) and general complications after laparoscopy such as pain, bleeding, infection or damage to bowel/bladder/urethra (1:1000 in sterilizations and 1:500 for other procedures) [11].

With published evidence demonstrating that the long-term risk of adhesion-related complications is high in the majority of gynecologic procedures, there is a clear need for gynecologists to consider the potential for medicolegal action if patients are not routinely informed of the risk of adhesions and active strategies initiated to reduce the risk.

Minimizing adhesion formation

The main approaches to minimize the deleterious effects of adhesions include minimizing tissue damage with good surgical technique, and the use of preventive barriers such as instilled solutions (Adept) or locally applied physical barriers (Interceed, Seprafilm).

The key fundamental is meticulous surgical technique adopting the principles of microsurgery, which need re-emphasizing in laparoscopic surgery and in the treatment of endometriosis where there is heightened inflammatory response and angiogenesis with an associated increased risk of adhesion formation.

A conflicting problem is that many of the traumas that cause adhesions are a routine part of surgery. Meticulous hemostasis is a fundamental of adhesion prevention but to achieve this while limiting use of cautery which causes adhesions is problematic. Therefore, while surgeons should adopt the adhesion reduction steps listed in Box 63.1 as a routine part of good surgery, all the evidence highlights that these steps alone will not be sufficient to prevent adhesion formation.

Importantly, surgical adhesiolysis remains the main treatment for adhesions and yet the high rate of reformation (mean 85%) as well as the development of *de novo* adhesions is a key limiting factor [8]. Reformed adhesions are also more dense and severe [3]. The use of antiadhesion adjuvants should be actively considered.

Adhesion reduction agents

Pharmacologic agents

The pathophysiology of adhesion formation provides various opportunities for pharmacologic intervention aimed at affecting the fibrin formation/degradation balance. These include antibiotics, NSAIDs, corticosteroids and fibrinolytics but to date no clinical studies have shown adhesion reduction benefits using pharmacologic regimens and there have been safety concerns with some agents [12]. Research continues on a range of pharmacologic agents

---

Box 63.1 Key adhesion reduction steps

- Carefully handle tissue with field enhancement (magnification) techniques
- Perform diligent hemostasis and limit use of cautery
- Reduce cautery time and frequency and aspirate aerosolized tissue following cautery
- Excise tissue – reduce fulguration
- Reduce duration of surgery
- Reduce pressure and duration of pneumoperitoneum in laparoscopic surgery
- Reduce risk of infection
- Reduce drying of tissues (limit heat and light)
- Use frequent irrigation and aspiration in laparoscopy and laparotomy
- Limit use of sutures and choose fine nonreactive sutures and small knots
- Avoid foreign bodies, such as materials with loose fibers
- Minimal use of dry towels or sponges in laparotomy

including incorporation into antiadhesion films, gels and solutions but their approval for clinical use is some way off.

Physical barriers

Physical barriers are the only available adjuncts to reduce adhesion formation. To be effective, they must effectively separate traumatized peritoneal surfaces during the critical period of adhesion development in the 3–5 days after surgery during which peritoneal healing occurs. This separation can broadly be achieved by site-specific films and gels or by the use of broad coverage fluid agents to keep surfaces apart during the healing process. While a number of these have been investigated, only a minority have received FDA approval. Currently, there are three devices approved by the FDA specifically for use as adhesion reduction adjuvants in abdominopelvic surgery – two site-specific agents (Interceed® and Seprafilm®) and one broad coverage fluid (Adept®). Key steps to increase the effectiveness of these three adhesion reduction devices are given in Box 63.2.

Interceed® (oxidized regenerated cellulose)

This was the first resorbable barrier to be approved and has been available since 1990. It forms a viscous

---

Box 63.2 Procedures recommended for FDA-approved adhesion reduction devices

Use of Interceed absorbable adhesion barrier
1. Apply at the end of the procedure
2. Hemostasis must be achieved before application
3. Place patient in reverse Trendelenburg position and remove as much of the irrigation fluid as possible from the cul de sac (< 10 mL)
4. Cut to size to allow at least 5 mm margin around area at risk
5. If Interceed turns black upon application, then blood is present and may reduce efficacy. Remove Interceed and achieve hemostasis. Then apply a new piece of Interceed
6. If more than one piece is required, allow the pieces to overlap by a margin of 3–5 mm to ensure contiguous coverage of the area at risk
7. No sutures needed
8. Moisten with up to 2 mL of irrigant per 7.6 cm × 10.2 cm piece

The ovary may be completely wrapped with Interceed by:
1. Lifting the ovary away from the ovarian fossa and placing a corner of Interceed (one-half piece) up into the ovarian fossa
2. Allowing the ovary to return to the normal position, thereby holding the Interceed in place
3. Lifting the opposite corner laterally over the ovary, then moistening with a few drops of irrigating solution to ensure adherence of the barrier to the ovary

---

For tubal surgery, the Interceed barrier is suspended by two grasping instruments and brought into contact with the salpingostomy site. The barrier is then folded over the surgical site until the four corners of the barrier are in contact with the isthmic portion of the fallopian tube. Irrigating solution (3–5 mL) is placed over the Interceed, thereby "sealing" an Interceed bag around the fimbria. If the surgeon prefers the fimbria not to come into contact with the barrier, the fimbria should be wrapped with a "cuff" of Interceed followed by moistening of the cuff to ensure that the Interceed covers the outer portion of the ampulla.

Use of Seprafilm bioresorbable membrane
1. Apply at the end of the procedure
2. Membrane and surgical field must be kept dry before application
3. Open the pouch immediately before application, cut membrane and holder with scissors to desired size and shape
4. The membrane should be handled gently with dry instruments and/or gloves
5. Expose 1–2 cm of the membrane through the open end of the holder
6. When necessary, facilitate entry into the abdominopelvic cavity by slightly curving or arching the membrane/holder
7. When applying, avoid contact with tissue surfaces until directly at the site of application. If contact occurs, moderate application of standard irrigation solution may be used to gently dislodge membrane from unintended tissue surfaces
8. Allow exposed membrane to first adhere to desired position on the tissue or organ by gently pressing down the membrane with a dry gloved hand or instrument and then withdrawing the holder
9. Allow sufficient overlap of individual membranes to ensure complete, continuous coverage of traumatized tissue surface

Use of Adept adhesion reduction liquid
1. Remove the outer wrap from the 1 L Adept bag and hang the sterile bag of solution on a stand
2. Remove the twist-off tab from the spike port and insert a standard IV infusion set for connection to a laparoscope/irrigation cannula or an IV set for dispensing the solution directly into the abdominal cavity in the case of laparotomy
3. Adept should be used intraoperatively as an irrigant solution, and postoperatively as an instillate. The solution will flow through an IV infusion set (and through a laparoscope/irrigation cannula) or it can be dispensed into a sterile basin and applied using a syringe and cannula
4. When used as an intraoperative irrigant solution, at least 100 mL of Adept should be introduced into the cavity every 30 minutes
5. Remove remaining fluid before introducing the final instillation
6. For the final instillation of Adept, prior to closure of the abdominal cavity or removal of the laparoscope, at least 1 L should be used. Direct the solution at the operative sites initially then distribute the remainder throughout the cavity

gel when it comes into contact with fluids and is completely resorbed within 4 weeks. It was approved for use in gynecologic laparotomy only. Interceed can be used at most intraperitoneal locations and in Europe has been used in laparoscopic as well as open surgery. Meticulous hemostasis is important, as the efficacy of the product is reduced in the presence of active bleeding. There is substantial literature on the use of Interceed in gynecologic surgery and the product has been shown to reduce adhesion formation without affecting healing. More recent work with Interceed reported its effect on reducing adhesions results in improved pregnancy outcomes in infertile patients [13].

Seprafilm® (hyaluronic acid/carboxymethylcellulose)

Seprafilm is a barrier film which is usually placed over a suture line, as in myomectomy. It persists during the period of re-epithelialization and is absorbed spontaneously. Seprafilm does not conform to the shape of the pelvic organs as well as Interceed and is usually used as a barrier placed between the bowel or omentum and the anterior abdominal wall at the time of wound closure, where it can prevent adherence and, potentially, reduce the risk of enterotomy at subsequent surgery. It has been approved for use in the USA in general surgery and gynecologic surgery via laparotomy but not laparoscopy. Alongside the main pivotal studies, there is mounting literature on its use and it is the only agent to have been investigated for the reduction of SBO [14,15]. The study highlighted that the use of Seprafilm at the site of anastomosis should be avoided, due to increased anastomotic leaks.

Adept® (4% icodextrin solution)

Adept has been approved in Europe since 2000 as an adhesion reduction agent in open and laparoscopic gynecologic and general surgery. It was approved by the FDA in 2006 for use as an irrigant and postoperative instillate in gynecologic laparoscopy with adhesiolysis. It is the first antiadhesion agent to be granted approval for use laparoscopically and is the only broad coverage agent approved as an antiadhesion device.

Adept is a nonviscous, iso-osmotic, clear solution which handles like normal saline. It requires no change to surgical practice nor any special training or equipment. Adept works by having a sufficiently long intraperitoneal residence to provide coverage throughout the peritoneal cavity, keeping tissues and organs apart through the critical 3–5-day period of adhesion formation.

Crystalloids

Administering crystalloid instillates at the end of surgery has long been suggested as a useful adhesion reduction technique. However, while saline, lactated Ringer's

---

Box 63.3 Consensus proposals: actions to reduce adhesions

1. Adhesions need to be recognized as the most frequent complication of abdominal surgery
2. Surgeons, other healthcare workers, budget holders and policy makers need to increase their awareness and understanding of adhesions and the associated healthcare burden costs and take active steps to reduce this
3. Patients need to be informed of the risk of adhesions, given that adhesions are now the most frequent complication of abdominal surgery
4. Surgeons who do not advise of the risk of adhesions may put themselves at risk of claims for medical negligence
5. Surgeons have a duty of care to protect patients by providing the best possible standards of care, which should include taking steps to reduce adhesion formation
6. Surgeons should adopt a routine adhesion reduction strategy, at least in surgery at high risk for adhesions, such as ovarian surgery, endometriosis surgery, tubal surgery, myomectomy and adhesiolysis.
7. Good surgical technique is fundamental to any adhesion-reduction strategy – see Box 63.1
8. Surgeons should consider the use of adhesion reduction agents as part of their adhesion reduction strategy, giving special consideration to agents with data to support safety in routine abdominal pelvic surgery and efficacy in reducing adhesions. The practicality and use of agents, as well as the cost of any agent, will influence their acceptability in routine practice
9. Further research to understand the impact that adhesion reduction agents have on clinical outcomes will be important
10. Research towards more effective preventative agents should be encouraged, including the use of combinations of agents to prevent the formation of *de novo* adhesions, as well as adhesion reformation
11. Surgeons need to act now to reduce adhesions and fulfill their duty of care to patients

---

solution and Hartmann's solutions have all been used, these crystalloid solutions may not significantly reduce adhesion formation and are rapidly absorbed from the peritoneal cavity at the rate of 30–50 mL/h so that by 24 hours after surgery, little if any solution is left in the pelvis.

Proposals for surgical action

The European Society of Gynaecological Endoscopy has published consensus proposals on actions that surgeons should now take given the weight of evidence of the problem of adhesions and particularly that postoperative adhesions are now the most frequent complication of abdominopelvic surgery [8,16]. Their proposals are detailed in Box 63.3 to facilitate consideration of local adoption in surgical practices.

References

1. Holmdahl L, Risberg B, Beck DE, *et al*. Adhesions: pathogenesis and prevention – panel discussion and summary. *Eur J Surg* 1997; 163: 56–62.
2. Menzies D, Ellis H. Intestinal obstruction from adhesions – how big is the problem? *Ann R Coll Surg Engl* 1990; 72: 60–63.
3. Monk BJ, Berman ML, Montz FJ. Adhesions after extensive gynecologic surgery: clinical significance, etiology and prevention. *Am J Obstet Gynecol* 1994; 170: 1396–1403.
4. Canis M, Chapron C, Mage G, *et al*. Second-look laparoscopy after laparoscopic cystectomy of large ovarian endometriomas. *Fertil Steril* 1992; 58: 617–619.
5. Operative Laparoscopy Study Group. Postoperative adhesion development after operative laparoscopy: evaluation at early second-look procedures. *Fertil Steril* 1991; 55: 700–704.
6. Lower AM, Hawthorn RJS, Clark D, *et al*. Adhesion-related readmissions following gynaecological laparoscopy or laparotomy in Scotland: an epidemiological study of 24,046 patients. *Hum Reprod* 2004; 19: 1877–1885.
7. Diamond MP, Freeman ML. Clinical implications of postsurgical adhesions. *Hum Reprod Update* 2001; 7: 567–576.
8. DeWilde RL, Trew G, on behalf of the Expert Adhesions Working Party of the European Society of Gynaecological Endoscopy (ESGE). Postoperative abdominal adhesions and their prevention in gynaecological surgery. Expert consensus position. *Gynecol Surg* 2007; 4: 161–168.
9. Ellis H, Moran BJ, Thompson JN, *et al*. Adhesion-related hospital readmissions after abdominal and pelvic surgery: a retrospective cohort study. *Lancet* 1999; 353: 1476–1480.
10. Ellis H. Medicolegal consequences of adhesions. *Hosp Med* 2004; 65: 348–350.
11. Trew G. Postoperative adhesions and their prevention. *Rev Gynaecol Perinat Pract* 2006; 6: 47–56.
12. Metwally M, Watson A, Lilford R, Vandekerckhove P. Fluid and pharmacological agents for adhesion prevention after gynaecological surgery. *Cochrane Database Syst Rev* 2006; 2: CD001298.
13. Sawada T, Nishizawa H, Nishio E, Kadowaki M. Postoperative adhesion prevention with an oxidized regenerated cellulose adhesion barrier in infertile women. *J Reprod Med* 2000; 45: 387–389.
14. Fazio VW, Cohen Z, Fleshman JW, *et al*. Reduction in adhesive small-bowel obstruction by Seprafilm adhesion barrier after intestinal resection. *Dis Colon Rectum* 2006; 49: 1–11.
15. McLeod R. Does Seprafilm really reduce adhesive small bowel obstruction? *Dis Colon Rectum* 2006; 49: 1234–1238.
16. Parker MC, Wilson MS, Menzies D, *et al*. The SCAR-3 study: 5-year adhesion-related readmission risk following lower abdominal surgical procedures. *Colorectal Dis* 2005; 7: 551–558.

Suggested reading

diZerega GS (ed). *Pelvic surgery*. New York: Springer-Verlag, 1997.

diZerega GS (ed). *Peritoneal surgery*. New York: Springer-Verlag, 2000.

diZerega GS, Rodgers KE. *The peritoneum*. New York: Springer-Verlag, 1992.

diZerega GS, Tulandi T. Prevention of intra-abdominal adhesions in gynecologic surgery. *Reprod BioMed* 2008; 17: 303–306.

Chapter 64
Uterine Leiomyomata

Brendan Grubbs and Robert Israel
Department of Medicine and Obstetrics and Gynecology, Keck School of Medicine, University of Southern California, CA, USA

Introduction

Uterine leiomyomata are benign muscle tumors, and the most common female pelvic tumors. Prevalence estimates range from 30% to 70% of women, with higher rates in African Americans and women over the age of 40. The pathogenesis of leiomyomata is multifactorial, with genetics, sex hormones, and growth factors linked to their development. The majority of patients with myomata are asymptomatic. They may be diagnosed on routine physical exam, incidentally found on pelvic imaging or discovered when associated symptoms are investigated. Their clinical importance is usually limited to the reproductive years. They tend to enlarge during pregnancy and shrink after menopause.

Leiomyomas range in size from microscopic lesions to huge tumor masses filling the entire abdomen. They can be single or multiple, and are classified according to their location as submucous, intramural or subserous. Occasionally, they can be found between the leaves of the broad ligament, in the cervix or associated with the round ligaments. They are surrounded by a pseudocapsule of areolar tissue from which they derive their blood supply. The tumors themselves consist of tightly compacted muscle and fibrous tissue arranged in a whorled pattern that is relatively avascular. On rare occasions, a leiomyoma can undergo sarcomatous change. As there are no laboratory or imaging studies to screen or predict malignant change, sudden growth of the tumor may be the only clue. Generally, subserous myomata are asymptomatic, but may be confused with an adnexal mass; intramural tumors may also be asymptomatic, but can cause pressure and pain as they enlarge; and the submucous ones often stimulate heavy bleeding with menses. Other symptoms associated with leiomyomatous uteri include urinary frequency and increased abdominal girth secondary to external bladder pressure and increased tumor growth.

Evaluation

History

If the patient is symptomatic, it must be determined how and to what degree these symptoms affect her life. Any co-existing medical problems must be elucidated to determine if they are contributing to her symptoms, and to what extent they might influence treatment choices. Pelvic pain and pressure are very common complaints, so it must be determined whether the leiomyomata are the cause of these symptoms or just coincidental to other pathology. Timing of the pain, especially in relation to menses, the effectiveness of any prior therapy for this pain, any previous pelvic surgeries, rapid growth of the tumors or any associated gastrointestinal or urinary symptoms might point towards or away from the leiomyomata being the source of the symptomatology.

Abnormal vaginal bleeding, usually menorrhagia, is another common symptom of the leiomyomatous uterus, especially if submucous myomata are present, and its evaluation should include a detailed menstrual history with any documentation of prior anemia or blood transfusions. In multiple studies, patient self-evaluation of actual menstrual blood loss has been found to be inaccurate. However, changes noted in the menstrual pattern are generally reliable.

Obstetric history, including future fertility desires, as well as any history of recurrent spontaneous abortion strongly influence treatment decisions.

Physical exam

As any co-existing condition may influence symptoms or treatment, a complete physical exam should be performed on any patient presenting for evaluation of leiomyomata. A speculum exam will reveal any vulvar, vaginal or cervical lesions, as well as any pelvic prolapse. The bimanual examination should evaluate uterine size, position, and

Management of Common Problems in Obstetrics and Gynecology, 5th edition. Edited by T.M. Goodwin, M.N. Montoro, L. Muderspach, R. Paulson and S. Roy. © 2010 Blackwell Publishing Ltd.

mobility, and the location and size of any palpable leiomyomata. Other causes of uterine enlargement and asymmetry, such as pregnancy, adenomyosis, and congenital anomalies, must be considered. Additionally, other pelvic masses, such as solid or cystic ovarian tumors, hydrosalpinges, and endometriosis, can be confused with myomata.

Laboratory findings

Laboratory abnormalities associated with leiomyomata depend on the symptoms. Each patient should have a complete blood count and metabolic panel to assess any anemia, as well as any other conditions which might influence treatment. Additionally, women who are over the age of 35 with any type of abnormal bleeding should have an endometrial biopsy to determine the presence of hyperplasia or cancer. Women under 35 years with an irregular menstrual pattern should also be considered for an endometrial lining biopsy.

Imaging

Transvaginal ultrasound is the best imaging procedure for evaluating uterine anatomy. On occasion, transabdominal ultrasound may be needed to visualize uteri which have grown out of the pelvis. Broad ligament leiomyomata may be difficult to differentiate from adnexal masses, and a CT or MRI may be beneficial. With a central, globularly enlarged uterus, especially if myomectomy is planned, an MRI can differentiate myomata, a surgically resectable condition, from adenomyosis, a nonsurgically resectable lesion.

Evaluation of the uterine cavity may be achieved with office hydrosonography and/or with hysteroscopy. Both permit visualization of intracavitary polyps and leiomyomata, and indicate the potential for hysteroscopic resection. Further characterization of the uterine cavity can be gained by performing hysterosalpingography, which has the added benefit of evaluating fallopian tube patency. These three modalities have their greatest value when uterine preservation is being considered.

Treatment

Due to the low risk of malignancy with leiomyomata, treatment decisions are based on symptoms, leiomyoma location, the fertility wishes of the patient, and any co-existing medical problems. Treatment options currently available are no treatment, medical treatment, surgical treatment, and uterine artery embolization.

Asymptomatic leiomyomata are most common and only require annual exams. If the tumors become symptomatic or by sudden growth a concern for malignancy is raised, intervention is indicated. Suspicion for leiomyosarcoma is raised with rapid growth of a solitary leiomyoma, especially after menopause. Other causes for worry include failure of existing leiomyomata to regress after menopause, withdrawal of hormone replacement therapy or following medical treatment. Malignancy risk is also higher with prior pelvic radiation. In some cases, MRI may be suggestive of malignancy, but no studies have shown MRI to be definitive.

While the exact pathogenesis of uterine leiomyomata is unknown, their observed responsiveness to different hormonal states has supported the use of steroids to control symptoms in preparation for, or as an alternative to, surgery. While estrogen may be the most obvious candidate, it may stimulate or suppress leiomyomata growth, so interaction with progesterone, locally elevated aromatase levels and, possibly, FSH and LH may all play a role in influencing leiomyomata growth and/or suppression.

A trial of oral contraceptives may be of some benefit in leiomyoma management, especially when dysmenorrhea is the dominant symptom, or with menorrhagia, if there is not a significant intracavitary component. However, their usefulness may be limited secondary to the estrogen component stimulation of the myomata.

Leuprolide acetate, a gonadotropin-releasing hormone (GnRH) agonist, is currently the mainstay of treatment for leiomyomata. It may be used preoperatively to shrink uterine volume in order to perform a vaginal, rather than an abdominal, hysterectomy; as a means of inducing amenorrhea in order to build up hemoglobin prior to surgery; and/or a way to decrease blood flow to the leiomyomata in order to minimize blood loss at myomectomy. In some instances, surgery can be avoided altogether by using the GnRH agonist as a bridge to menopause in women with abnormal perimenopausal bleeding. The major drug side effects are menopausal symptoms and osteoporosis. If used for longer than 6 months, add-back therapy, with some combination of estrogen and/or progesterone use, is recommended to prevent these complications. Maximum leiomyomata shrinkage occurs within 3 months of the onset of therapy.

However, as a sole therapeutic modality, a GnRH agonist is of limited value because, within 6 months of discontinuing the medication, the myomata will return to their original size, unless menopause has occurred.

Other medical modalities being studied for the treatment of leiomyomata include mifepristone, as well as GnRH antagonists and aromatase inhibitors. All are in varying stages of evaluation, and are not yet recommended for treatment, other than in well-controlled, IRB-approved trials.

The definitive treatment for symptomatic leiomyomata is hysterectomy. Removal of the uterus prevents recurrence of the tumors and their symptoms but, obviously, is not the procedure of choice in a patient wishing to preserve fertility. The decision as to an abdominal or a vaginal approach is dependent on the size, mobility, and degree of uterine prolapse, adequacy of the pelvic arch, and prior surgical history. As previously noted, medical treatment of leiomyomata prior to surgery may accomplish a sufficient reduction in uterine size to permit vaginal hysterectomy. The presence of obscuring leiomyomata may require intraoperative myomectomy before the uterus itself can be removed. With a large broad ligament myoma, preoperative placement of ureteral stents may aid in identifying their course, thus preventing injury.

Myomectomy reduces leiomyoma symptoms and preserves fertility. The location, size, and symptomatology of the leiomyomata will determine the surgical approach. Aborting myomas may cause significant menorrhagia and anemia but, with a narrow stalk, they can be twisted off with little difficulty. Removal allows for normal uterine contractions and resolution of the bleeding. Subserosal and intramural myomectomies may be performed laparoscopically or via celiotomy. Even large leiomyomata, unless there is limited visibility, may be removed laparoscopically, with or without the robotic DaVinci system. The approach is dependent on myomata size and operator skill.

Whatever surgical route is selected, blood loss will be higher with myomectomy than with hysterectomy. Transfusion may be required in up to 20% of myomectomies. Effective strategies to reduce surgical blood loss include injection of dilute vasopressin into the myometrium, a pericervical tourniquet, and vascular clamps placed over the infundibulopelvic ligaments. Use of a cell-saver also lessens the risk of blood transfusion. With abdominal myomectomy, intraoperative blood loss can be reduced further with vertical uterine incisions that, if possible, are confined to the anterior uterine wall to reduce subsequent bowel and adnexal adhesions to the uterine surface. To minimize the total number of myometrial incisions, as many myomata as possible should be removed through each uterine incision. Postoperative adhesions are higher with myomectomy than with hysterectomy, which might be counterproductive to the patient wishing future fertility. Close attention to hemostasis throughout the operation, and use of an adhesion prevention barrier in the pelvis at the conclusion of the myomectomy will also help reduce subsequent pelvic adhesions.

Postoperatively, the recurrence rate of clinically significant myomas in one large study was 10%, with a third of the patients requiring hysterectomy.

Intracavitary leiomyomas may be identified with hydrosonography or hysteroscopy. These two modalities, unlike hysterosalpingography, permit assessment of how much of the submucous myoma is in the uterine cavity and how much of it is in the uterine wall. With 80–90% of the myoma in the endometrial cavity, successful hysteroscopic resection can be carried out, thus reducing uterine bleeding with an operative approach that has significantly lower morbidity than hysterectomy or myomectomy. Newer, more accurate fluid management systems allow better estimation of the fluid deficit that can occur with uterine distension during hysteroscopic surgery, thus reducing the risk of electrolyte abnormalities associated with this procedure.

Uterine artery embolization (UAE), while not recommended for those wishing future fertility, is a viable alternative for patients with symptomatic myomata, who are either poor surgical candidates or do not desire hysterectomy. The FIBROID Registry study looked at a 12-month follow-up for 1701 women who had undergone UAE and found that, subjectively, 82% had improved quality of life following the procedure. Of this group, only 2.9% required hysterectomy during the period. A different study compared UAE to surgical management and found little difference between satisfaction at 1 year post intervention. Surgery was associated with immediate postprocedural pain and a longer hospital stay, whereas the embolization group required more frequent interventions for recurrent symptoms and more hospitalizations throughout the study period. The longest follow-up study is a series of 182 patients from Georgetown University Hospital followed for 5 years after their UAE. At 5 years, 146 (80%) had continued symptom control and 36 (20%) had failed or recurred. Of the 36, 25 patients had undergone hysterectomy (25/182, 13.7%), eight myomectomy (8/182, 4.4%), and three repeat UAE (3/182, 1.6%). UAE is not recommended for women desiring future fertility. A 10–15% risk of amenorrhea and early menopause has been reported, especially in women undergoing UAE who are younger than 40–45 years of age. In a series of 50 patients who became pregnant after UAE, there was an increased rate of malpresentation, small for gestational age fetuses, premature delivery, cesarean sections, and postpartum hemorrhage. All patients who wish subsequent fertility should be informed of these risks reported with UAE.

The link between uterine leiomyomata and fertility is tentative. Obviously, myomata that block passage of sperm through the cervical os or passage of ova through the fallopian tubes will hinder conception. Although submucous myomata, or intramural ones that distort the endometrial cavity, have been thought to increase the rate of late first- or early second-trimester spontaneous abortions, no definitive prospective studies have been reported. However, if no other cause for these early gestational losses can be identified, resectable submucous myomata should be removed hysteroscopically and intramural lesions that distort the uterine cavity can be removed by laparoscopy or celiotomy.

In obstetrics, uterine leiomyomata can be associated with malpresentation, obstruction of labor, abruption, and first-trimester bleeding. Except for the occasional pedunculated myoma causing pain, degenerating myomas should be treated conservatively. Attempting myomectomy during pregnancy can result in massive hemorrhage and pregnancy loss. In patients with a prior myomectomy, where the myometrium was entered, uterine rupture may occur before labor and should be managed as for a patient with a prior classic cesarean section.

Each generation would fain believe itself the acme; each succeeding generation disproves the belief, and so the advance goes on, and the amazement of today becomes the commonplace of tomorrow. We surgeons form one small group of a great host whose marching cry is "something better," and therein lies our certainty of the future; for, even while we sit talking here, somewhere or other in the world, minds are at work plotting discoveries to astonish the coming years …. and in today already walks tomorrow. (Victor Bonney MD, 1946)

Suggested reading

Bazot M, Cortez A, Darai E, *et al*. Ultrasonography compared with magnetic resonance imaging for the diagnosis of adenomyosis: correlation with histopathology. *Hum Reprod* 2001; 16: 2427–2433.

Coronado GD, Marshall LM, Schwartz SM. Complications in pregnancy, labor and delivery with uterine leiomyomas: a population-based study. *Obstet Gynecol* 2000; 95: 764.

Edwards RD, Moss JG, Lumsden MA, for the Committee of the Randomized Trial of Embolization versus Surgical Treatment for Fibroids. Uterine-artery embolization versus surgery for symptomatic uterine fibroids. *NEJM* 2007; 356: 360–370.

Fauconnier A, Chapron C, Babaki-Fard K, Dubuisson JB. Recurrence of leiomyomata after myomectomy. *Hum Reprod Update* 2000; 6: 595.

Goldberg J, Pereira L, Berghella V. Pregnancy after uterine artery embolization. *Obstet Gynecol* 2002; 100: 869–872.

Kongnyuy EJ, Wiysonge CS. Interventions to reduce haemorrhage during myomectomy for leiomyomata. *Cochrane Database Syst Rev* 2007; 1: CD005355.

LaMote AI, Lalwani S, Diamond MP. Morbidity associated with abdominal myomectomy. *Obstet Gynecol* 1993; 82: 897–900.

Schwartz LB, Zawin M, Carcangiu ML, Lange R, McCarthy S. Does pelvic magnetic resonance imaging differentiate among the histologic subtypes of uterine leiomyomata? *Fertil Steril* 1998; 70: 580–587.

Shozu M, Sumitani H, Segawa T, Yang HJ, Murakami K, Inoue M. Inhibition of in situ expression of aromatase P450 in leiomyoma of the uterus by leuprorelin acetate. *J Clin Endocrinol Metab* 2001; 86(11): 5405–5411.

Spies JB, Bruno J, Czeyda-Pommersheim F, Magee ST, Ascher SA, Jha RC. Long-term outcome of uterine artery embolization of leiomyomata. *Obstet Gynecol* 2005; 106: 933–939.

Spies JB, Myers ER, Worthington-Kirsch R, *et al.*, for the FIBROID Registry Investigators. The FIBROID Registry: symptom and quality-of-life status 1 year after therapy. *Obstet Gynecol* 2005; 106(6): 1309–1318.

Chapter 65
Breast Disorders

Heather R. Macdonald

Department of Medicine and Obstetrics and Gynecology, Keck School of Medicine, University of Southern California, CA, USA

Introduction

As specialists in the female reproductive system, obstetrician gynecologists are sought frequently by patients for breast complaints. Resolving these complaints, ruling out underlying malignancy, providing reassurance and symptom relief, estimating a woman's individual risk of breast cancer and counseling her regarding her screening and preventive options are among the most challenging tasks that face our specialty. In an increasingly hostile medicolegal climate, these activities can also cause clinicians anxiety. This chapter will provide guidelines to clinicians to appropriately identify those patients with a malignancy and reassure and treat those with symptomatic but benign conditions. We will address breast cancer screening, genetic testing, palpable masses, mastalgia, nipple discharge and breast inflammation.

Documentation scheme for clinical breast exam

Breast cancer mortality has improved in the past several decades in developed countries in large part due to increased breast cancer screening. Because it has an 85% sensitivity of detecting cancer, screening mammography has allowed clinicians to identify malignancies at an earlier size and stage when therapy is more likely to result in cure. Large series have confirmed that patients with screen-detected cancers have improved survival when compared to those with symptomatic cancers. The American Cancer Society and the American College of Obstetricians and Gynecologists agree that women over the age of 50 should undergo annual screening mammography. Screening between the ages of 40 and 50 is still the subject of some controversy but most experts agree that

Management of Common Problems in Obstetrics and Gynecology, 5th edition. Edited by T.M. Goodwin, M.N. Montoro, L. Muderspach, R. Paulson and S. Roy. © 2010 Blackwell Publishing Ltd.

women aged 40–49 should undergo screening mammography every 1–2 years. Women with first-degree relatives with breast cancer younger than 50 should begin their annual screening mammography 10 years younger than the youngest woman in their family to be diagnosed and should be considered for genetic counseling. Because over 10 years of screening, 50% of women will be called back for additional imaging and 25% for tissue biopsies but less than 10% (or 3/10 patients undergoing breast biopsy) will be diagnosed with breast cancer, research into ever better breast screening modalities continues.

Breast MRI has an equal or better sensitivity to mammography in detecting breast cancer but is not very specific. The American Cancer Society and American College of Radiology recommend screening breast MRI only for patients at a lifetime risk of breast cancer of 20–25% or greater. The combined sensitivity and specificity of mammogram and MRI in high-risk women approaches 95%.

Clinical breast exam (CBE) by contrast has a 64% sensitivity of detecting cancer, self breast exam (SBE) 25%. Thus, while CBE continues to be an important part of women's annual health maintenance, SBE has not been shown to increase cancer detection. SBE has been shown to raise anxiety while increasing detection of benign lesions.

To estimate a patient's lifetime risk of breast cancer, several calculators are available: the Gail model, the Claus model and the NCI calculator. They incorporate patient's age, family history, ethnicity, reproductive history, number of breast biopsies and number of atypical breast biopsies in varying degrees. However, it is important to counsel a patient that these are population risk indicators and are difficult to apply to individual patients. These models have been validated in only narrow populations of patients. Estimating a patient's individual breast cancer risk as it changes over time remains difficult and is the subject of much research.

Genetic testing

One of the strongest predictors of a breast cancer risk is family history. Approximately 10% of breast cancer patients will be found to have an inheritable genetic condition that caused their disease. These include BRCA 1, BRCA 2, pTen and p53 mutations. Each of these mutations carries risks for additional malignancies as well as breast so their identification in both affected and unaffected patients is paramount. The BRCA mutations are the most commonly identified (Box 65.1). All patients should be screened with a family history. If family members are identified with any malignancies, the age of diagnosis, treatment received, survivorship and numbers and health conditions of siblings and children should be recorded. Families in whom a genetic cancer syndrome pattern is suspected should be referred to a certified genetic counselor for quantification of risk of inherited cancer syndrome as well as elucidation of which gene mutations is most likely to be present. The genetic counselor will guide testing recommendations and interpretation of results. Additionally, genetic counselors are trained to address the psychosocial aspects of family genetic testing and to address fears and anxieties provoked by testing. If at all possible, the family member who carries the cancer should be the first person tested. If they test positive, unaffected family can be tested in a directed approach.

Palpable mass

One of the most anxiety-provoking complaints a patient can bring to her physician is a palpable breast mass. In large series the incidence of breast cancer in a palpable mass has ranged from 15% to 60%. Therefore any palpable mass deserves a careful evaluation that includes physical examination, imaging and tissue biopsy.

A palpable mass that exhibits three dimensions and has a distinct texture different from the surrounding breast tissue should be documented by its clock face position (12:00 superior to the nipple, 6:00 inferior, etc.) and distance from the nipple. The mass's texture (firm, soft, etc.) and size should also be included. Physical exam characteristics suspicious for underlying malignancy include skin tethering, erythema, fixation to underlying or overlying structures, new nipple inversion or retraction, associated nipple discharge and associated axillary lymphadenopathy and should be documented as well.

If the patient is older than 30, a diagnostic mammogram should be ordered to image the area as well as screen the breast for additional lesions. A diagnostic mammogram will include the standard two-view mammogram, additional mammographic views as deemed necessary by the radiologist and a targeted ultrasound at the area of the abnormality. If the patient is less than 30, the density of the breast tissue will make mammogram difficult to interpret and a targeted ultrasound of the palpable area should be ordered. The characteristic of the mass on imaging will provide important information regarding the solid or cystic nature of the mass as well as give a mammographic estimation of the possibility of malignancy as stated in the BIRADS score (Box 65.2).

Tissue biopsy can be obtained by fine needle aspiration (FNA), image-guided core needle biopsy and open surgical biopsy. Fine needle aspiration is the least invasive biopsy method. It does not leave a scar and can be performed in the office at the time of initial examination. If the lesion is cystic and disappears completely to palpation with the withdrawal of clear or green fluid, the diagnosis of simple cyst is made and the patient is reassured. She should be re-examined in 6 weeks for reaccumulation. Any material other than clear fluid should be sent for cytology. For a patient who has barriers to being compliant with follow-up visits, a FNA allows the clinician to see and treat at the initial visit. The drawbacks to FNA are its nondiagnostic rate (varies by operator but up to 60% in large series) and the absence of physical or radiologic scar, making it difficult to identify the area where the biopsy was performed if additional work-up is required. FNA also does not provide architecture of the tissue being sampled. For example, it can diagnose a ductal malignancy but not distinguish between ductal carcinoma *in situ* and infiltrating ductal carcinoma.

Image-guided core needle biopsy can be performed under either ultrasound or mammographic guidance as an office procedure under local anesthesia. A 2–3 mm nick is made in the overlying skin and cores of tissue are removed. A minute inert clip is then placed in the biopsy site to mark the area on future imaging studies. Core needle biopsy can definitively diagnose malignant lesions as well as benign but leaves a skin scar and causes more discomfort to the patient.

Once a needle biopsy (FNA or core) has been performed, it is critical that a concordance test be applied to ensure appropriate treatment. The concordance test (or

---

Box 65.1 BRCA mutation: high-risk family history

Two or more close relatives with breast or ovarian cancer
Breast cancer diagnosed < 50 years of age
Bilateral breast cancer in a close relative
Breast and ovarian cancer in the same family
Breast and ovarian cancer in the same family member
Male family member with breast cancer

Box 65.2 Breast Imaging and Reporting System (BIRADS)

1 Negative study
2 Benign finding
3 Short-interval follow-up; likely benign
4 Suspicious abnormality: biopsy should be considered
5 Highly suggestive of malignancy
6 Known malignancy identified
0 Needs additional imaging

triple test) compares the physical exam impression, the imaging impression and the results of the needle biopsy. When all three agree and are benign, the false-negative rate (or risk that an occult malignancy has been missed) is less than 1:1000 in large series. If all three agree and are malignant, the positive predictive value (the chance that a lesion that has been called malignant is truly malignant) is 100%. If all three elements are not in agreement, the lesion must be further evaluated and may warrant surgical excision.

Open surgical biopsy is the removal of a palpable abnormality for diagnosis and treatment simultaneously. However, many benign masses do not require surgical removal and malignant lesions require more extensive surgery than open biopsy. Diagnosis of a breast mass is best made by one of the needle approaches described above. Surgical biopsy for diagnosis should be a procedure of last resort, employed usually for a nonconcordant triple test.

Most palpable masses are benign and once a definitive diagnosis is secured, require nothing further than a 6-month follow-up exam and ultrasound (Box 65.3). However, any patient who desires surgical excision should be given one. A benign mass should be removed with as little normal breast tissue as possible to prevent a resulting breast distortion. Any mass that shows atypia should be excised to rule out an underlying malignancy.

Mastalgia

As many as two-thirds of women will complain of breast pain over their reproductive life. Pain can be cyclic, associated with menstrual cycles, or constant (noncyclic). Cyclic mastalgia occurs in approximately half of menstruating women. Because breast cancer is the most commonly diagnosed cancer in American women, women overestimate their breast cancer risk. Often a woman who presents with complaints of breast pain has a second question she may be afraid to verbalize: could this be how cancer announces itself? She deserves a thorough

evaluation and reassurance (when appropriate) in addition to symptom relief.

All patients with mastalgia should be evaluated by a careful history, review of symptoms and physical exam to rule out underlying pathology (Box 65.4). Many other causes of chest and upper abdominal pain can present as mastalgia, and breast specialists frequently diagnose costochondritis, reflux and gallstones, among others. Any woman with breast pain and a missed menses should undergo pregnancy testing as breast pain may be the first symptom of pregnancy. Women over 35 years should also undergo screening mammography. Cysts too deep to palpate on exam may be the cause of the woman's pain and are easily treated with image-guided aspiration.

Mastalgia is a diagnosis of exclusion and once other causes have been ruled out, patients should be reassured that breast cancer rarely presents with pain. A properly fitted supportive bra will ameliorate some patients' symptoms. NSAIDs are often adequate pain relief. Contrary to popular belief, there is no randomized placebo-controlled data proving the benefit of caffeine restriction for pain reduction. Case–control studies similarly have shown no benefit. Vitamin therapy too has not proven to be effective. In fact, the levels of vitamin E studied have recently been shown to have harmful collateral effects, including thromboembolism and hypertension. Evening primrose oil has shown benefit for some although may be due to placebo effect. For women with cyclic mastalgia, low-dose birth control pills have long-term efficacy in pain reduction, although breast pain may increase at the start of therapy.

Between 5% and 20% of patients with mastalgia experience moderate to severe pain and require pharmacologic intervention for symptom control. Endocrine manipulation offers the best treatment for breast pain although it has significant side effects. Danazol is the only FDA-approved medication for breast pain, although masculinizing side effects limit its usefulness. Bromocriptine can be used to decrease prolactin levels and thus reduce breast stimulation and pain but studies of low-dose bromocriptine have shown low efficacy and higher doses have been associated with intolerable side effects such as dizziness, headache and nausea. Use of short-term (3 months) tamoxifen both 10 mg and 20 mg daily has been shown to decrease cyclic breast pain by 90% and noncyclic breast pain by

Box 65.3 Differential diagnosis of a breast mass

Cyst
Fibrocystic change
Fibroadenoma
Lipoma
Carcinoma
Phyllodes (benign or malignant)
Hamartoma
Adenoma (tubular, lactating)
Galactocele
Fat necrosis
Pseudoangiomatous hyperplasia (PASH)

Box 65.4 Differential diagnosis of mastalgia

Cyclic breast pain
Noncyclic breast pain
Costochondritis (Tietze's syndrome)
Reflux disease
Peptic ulcer disease
Gallstones
Shoulder arthritis/musculoskeletal pain
Cardiogenic
Mondor's disease

50%. Tamoxifen, a selective estrogen receptor modulator, reduces estrogen stimulation of the breast. Its side effects include menopausal symptoms and a < 1% risk of serious adverse events, including thrombosis and uterine cancer. In clinical trials, similar numbers of patients responded to a low-dose short-term regimen with fewer side effects and theoretically lower risks of adverse events.

In summary, patients with breast pain in whom pathologic causes of pain have been ruled out should be offered reassurance that symptoms are not related to an undiagnosed breast cancer. If NSAIDs are not enough to control a woman's pain, she can be offered danazol, bromocriptine and tamoxifen with a thorough discussion of the side effects of each, as often it is the side effects rather than treatment efficacy that will guide her therapy.

Nipple discharge

While nipple discharge can be an early symptom of breast malignancy or underlying endocrinopathy, it more frequently is unrelated to serious pathology and is often physiologic (Box 65.5). Discharge associated with endocrinopathies is usually spontaneous, bilateral and milky, consistent with galactorrhea. Discharge suspicious for underlying breast pathology is usually spontaneous, unilateral, involving only one duct and serous or bloody. Discharge that is present only with expression, involving many ducts and green or black is physiologic. It may involve one or both breasts.

As the differential diagnosis of nipple discharge involves various systemic disorders a history, review of systems and physical exam should encompass symptoms and signs of thyroid, reproductive and neurologic disorders. Specifically, signs of hypothyroidism and pituitary disease should be queried. As medications can interfere with dopamine-prolactin metabolism, a careful list of medications including start and stop dates and dose changes should be recorded (Box 65.6). Patients should be asked if discharge is uni- or bilateral, one or multiduct, spontaneous or expressed, and color of fluid. Pregnancy can also cause galactorrhea in multiparous women so a pregnancy test should be ordered on any woman presenting with nipple discharge and amenorrhea. All patients should be counseled to stop examining their breasts for discharge. Continued breast exams and pressure will encourage galactorrhea and milk production.

On physical examination, the clinician should note which breast is involved, whether the discharge is present on clothing (more likely spontaneous), if it is expressible, how many ducts are involved, and what color it is. Special attention should be paid to any masses present or if the discharge is expressed with pressure at any particular area of the breast. If present, both should be noted to guide the mammographer's imaging efforts. If the discharge is consistent with a physiologic condition, the woman should

---

Box 65.5 Differential diagnosis of nipple discharge

Physiologic
Lactation
Stimulation
Infection
Medication
Trauma
Pituitary disease
Thyroid disease
Chronic renal failure
Herpes zoster
Papilloma (serous, bloody)
Cancer (serous, bloody)
Thoracic neoplasms

Box 65.6 Medications known to cause galactorrhea

Opiates
Oral contraceptives
Tricylic antidepressants
Methyldopa
Metoclopramide
Phenothiazines
Calcium channel blockers
Prochlorperazine
Butyrophenones
Amphetamines
Cimetidine

---

be reassured and counseled regarding compliance with mammographic screening recommendations.

If the patient's history and exam are more consistent with an underlying endocrinopathy, she should be worked up with appropriate lab testing: TSH and prolactin levels, and others as clinical signs and symptoms dictate, and treated appropriately. She should also be counseled to begin her mammographic screening at an appropriate age (40; if family history contains breast cancer younger than 50, then 10 years younger than the youngest affected family member).

If galactorrhea is associated with oligo- or amenorrhea and frequent headache, a prolactinoma should be suspected. Visual field testing should be included in the physical examination and a head MRI should be obtained, with instructions to the radiologist to examine the sella turcica. Most prolactinomas are benign microadenomas (< 1 cm) and remain stable or regress. The presence of headache raises the suspicion of a larger lesion. Any patient with hyperprolactinemia should be treated as osteoporosis can occur. In a patient with infertility, normalizing prolactin levels can achieve pregnancy. Either bromocriptine or cabergoline can be used, although in women hoping to achieve pregnancy, bromocriptine is preferred due to its safety profile. Any patient with a macroadenoma in the pituitary should be referred for specialty care.

Any patient with abnormal breast findings or discharge that is suspected to be pathologic should undergo a diagnostic mammogram regardless of age. Often a targeted retroareolar ultrasound will also be performed. If an abnormality is identified, the patient should undergo an image-guided core needle biopsy for diagnosis. If her mammogram and ultrasound are nonfocal and the discharge is persistent, a ductogram can be considered to rule out underlying ductal pathology. Alternatively, a breast MRI may identify the abnormality. If all imaging attempts are negative and the discharge persists, the patient should be referred for a terminal duct excision to both diagnose and treat the underlying abnormality. The duct should not be excised before the imaging work-up is completed, however, as transection of the ducts will "cure" the discharge without ruling out an occult underlying pathology.

The most common pathologic cause of nipple discharge is a benign ductal papilloma. Traditionally, these are excised to exclude an intrapaillary carcinoma. Nipple discharge is ofen associated with benign duct ectasia and dilated ducts. Bloody or serous nipple discharge can be associated with DCIS or an invasive ductal cancer. The risk of malignancy is higher when discharge is associated with a palpable breast mass. Any patient diagnosed with malignancy should be referred for appropriate specialty care.

A cytologic smear is not indicated in the work-up of nipple discharge. In large series of patients, nipple discharge cytology is neither sensitive nor specific in the diagnosis of breast malignancy. Approximately half of patients with an underlying malignancy will have a negative cytologic smear, and a large proportion of patients with abnormal cytology will never have a malignancy identified.

Mastitis

When evaluating a woman with an inflamed breast, the following differential should be kept in mind: mastitis vs abscess vs inflammatory carcinoma.

Mastitis, or infection of the breast parenchyma and overlying skin, presents with a 1–2-week history of breast erythema and tenderness. Patients are often post partum or lactating but mastitis can occur at any age. Fever may be present. On exam, localized erythema is present with smooth margins without fluctuance or a palpable mass. Axillary lymph nodes are usually enlarged and tender. The patient should be treated empirically with antibiotics that cover *Staph. aureus* and other skin pathogens, the most common bacteria associated with breast infections. An ultrasound should be obtained to rule out a deep abscess. If the patient is nursing, she should be counseled to continue to drain the breast as milk stasis will cause persistent infection and abscess formation. The patient should be reassured that her infant can continue to nurse from the affected side if appropriate antibiotics are given. If she is too uncomfortable to allow the infant to nurse, she should manually express the milk.

A breast abscess presents much like mastitis although a palpable fluctuant mass will be present. The patient should be imaged with ultrasound to determine the size of the abscess. Ultrasound will reveal a complex cystic mass filled with debris. Abscesses less than 3 cm in diameter can be drained completely by a large-bore needle. All fluid should be sent for culture and sensitivity to guide antibiotic therapy. The patient should be placed on empiric antibiotics and re-examined in 1 week to rule out reaccumulation. Abscesses larger than 3 cm can be drained by a small skin incision or by placement of a pigtail catheter by ultrasound guidance. Larger skin incisions for either drainage or catheter placement increase the risk of breast distortion and poor cosmetic outcome after treatment so consideration should be given to incision size and placement.

A patient with a breast infection refractory to antibiotic treatment should raise concern regarding the following underlying conditions: undiagnosed diabetes or other immune compromise, antibiotic-resistant infection, untreated galactorrhea or inflammatory breast cancer. Patients who fail to respond within 1 week of therapy should be reassessed with ultrasound, repeat cultures, tissue biopsy and appropriate blood work.

Inflammatory breast cancer (IBC) presents at any age as an indurated erythematous breast for weeks to months, sometimes treated with several failed courses of antibiotics. The breast is firm and often lifted, with generalized induration and nipple retraction. Axillary lymph nodes are enlarged and often nontender. The erythema present has irregular margins. A discrete breast mass is usually not palpable. Targeted ultrasound usually demonstrates a solid mass and markedly abnormal axillary lymph nodes. Diagnosis is made by ultrasound-guided core needle biopsy. If an expedited core biopsy is not available, the diagnosis can be made by skin punch biopsy of indurated erythematous skin. Tumor infiltration of the dermal lymphatics will make the diagnosis of IBC. Inflammatory breast cancer is a malignancy with a poor prognosis and the patient should be referred immediately to an oncologist for systemic chemotherapy.

Suggested reading

Breast Care, William Hindle (ed.). Springer-Verlag, New York NY, 1998.

Diseases of the Breast, 4th edition. Jay Harris (ed.). Lippincott Williams & Wilkins, Philadelphia PA, 2010.

Image Detected Breast Cancer: State of the Art Diagnosis and Treatment. Melvin J Silverstein, Abram Recht, Michael D. Lagios, *et al. Am College Surg* 2009; 209.

Chapter 66
Rectovaginal Injuries

Brendan Grubbs and Subir Roy

Department of Medicine and Obstetrics and Gynecology, Keck School of Medicine, University of Southern California, CA, USA

Perineal wound breakdown

Patients with perineal wound breakdown typically present within several days to 2 weeks post partum. Fever, wound swelling, discharge, and pain are often the inciting complaints that cause patients to present to their physician. Evidence of wound separation, purulent discharge, edema, and erythema is often present. Endometritis, operative vaginal delivery, episiotomy, and shoulder dystocia are significant risk factors associated with perineal morbidity.

The successful surgical correction of rectovaginal injuries depends on healthy tissues at the site of injury and good surgical technique, as well as the avoidance of postoperative infection. Under adverse circumstances, even the simplest of operative repairs can fail. Several simple techniques should be employed prior to the surgical approximation of a perineal wound dehiscence, as the majority of these lacerations heal well by secondary intention. First, a thorough irrigation of the wound with normal saline should be performed. Next, devitalized and necrotic tissue should be thoroughly debrided under local anesthesia. If the patient has a cellulitis of the perineum, cultures should be collected, followed by intravenous oxacillin 1–2 g every 4–6 hours or cefazolin (Ancef) 1 g every 6–8 hours during hospitalization. If there is suspicion of MRSA, then vancomycin 1 g IV every 12 hours should be used until cultures and sensitivities are available. Upon resolution of cellulitis, intravenous therapy can be changed to oral dosing based on culture results for a 10-day total course of therapy. In addition, twice-daily irrigation of the wound with normal saline should be performed in order to augment secondary healing.

If a wound does not approximate by secondary intention, consideration should be given to closure in the operating room. If the wound is the result of a recent trauma or the breakdown of a surgical repair, the operation must be delayed until the injured tissues are free of edema and induration or other evidence of residual infection. Traditionally, this has been thought to be at least 4 weeks and often longer. Multiple studies have questioned the necessity of this waiting period and have shown excellent results with much shorter waiting periods. Arona *et al.* used initial debridement of the wound, outpatient wound care, and surgical repair when the wounds were free of infection and demonstrated healthy granulation tissue. A total of 23 secondary repairs were performed from day 4 to day 10 (average 7 days) and all were successful with no need for subsequent reoperation [1].

Preoperative preparation of patients with either perineal tears or rectovaginal fistulae is an important part of the total management of these injuries. Preparation should first begin with mechanical evacuation of the bowel by instituting a variety of measures, beginning with a clear liquid diet 3 days prior to surgery. Furthermore, on the day before surgery the patient should ingest 4 L of Golytely (each liter containing 105 g of polyethylene glycol plus electrolytes) over 4 hours and one 10 oz (25 g) bottle of magnesium citrate (at a concentration of 1.745 g/oz) at 23:00 hours. Fleets enemas should be administered until clear at bedtime. Reglan 10 mg IV or given orally should be given prior to the ingestion of Golytely, and then every 6 hours as needed for nausea.

In addition, the patient should receive an antibiotic bowel preparation and a regimen of antibiotic prophylaxis to cover the intraoperative and postoperative periods. Although the perfect method of antibiotic bowel preparation has yet to be devised, one antibiotic bowel preparation consists of metronidazole (Flagyl) 1 g IV at 12:00 and 23:00 hours with neomycin 1 g taken orally at 12:00, 18:00, and 23:00 hours the day prior to surgery. The antibiotic prophylaxis that is instituted should give broad aerobic and anaerobic coverage such as provided by cefoxitin (Mefoxin) 2 g IV on call to surgery and then 2 g IV every 6 hours twice, then 1 g every 6 hours for 3–5 days. Other antibiotic regimens give similar results.

Management of Common Problems in Obstetrics and Gynecology, 5th edition. Edited by T.M. Goodwin, M.N. Montoro, L. Muderspach, R. Paulson and S. Roy. © 2010 Blackwell Publishing Ltd.

The use of antibiotics is extremely important because of the considerable risk of postoperative infection, leading to operative failure.

Under anesthesia, a rectal examination should be performed. If any stool or fecal liquids are encountered, they should be removed and the patient should be treated with povidone enemas until clear before beginning the repair procedure.

Complete perineal tear

A recent randomized trial by Duggal, *et al.* demonstrated a decreased rate of wound complications at two week follow up of third and fourth degree perineal lacerations (8.2% vs. 24.1%, p = 0.037) when a single dose of a second generation Cephalosporin was given IV prior to repair. Unless a contraindication exists these antibiotics should be strongly considered [2]. A complete perineal tear can be effectively repaired by a layer closure. Nonabsorbable sutures should be avoided because they can form a nidus of infection and lead to secondary fistula formation. Either chromic catgut or polyglycolic sutures are satisfactory. It does not matter whether a submucosal or through-and-through stitch is used to close the rectal mucosa; what is important is that the muscular coat of the rectum and its fascia be reapproximated with a second layer of sutures. Repair of the rectal sphincter usually requires that some time be devoted to recovering the well-retracted torn ends. It is important that the entire sphincter is repaired and not just the portion closest to the anus. Some controversy exists regarding whether to use an end to end or an overlapping technique while repairing external anal spincters; a recent randomized trial suggests that an overlapping technique results in a lower incidence of incontinence, urgency, and perineal pain [3]. The use of a paradoxic incision, partial or complete, in the reapproximated sphincter is occasionally necessary so that the repaired sphincter admits a single digit tightly. The pubococcygeal muscles should be reapproximated because they contribute to fecal continence.

Rectovaginal fistula

A rectovaginal fistula can be repaired either by excision with a three-layer closure of the rectal mucosa, rectal muscular coat, and vagina or by laying open the fistulous tract by means of an episioproctotomy, followed by excision of the tract and a three-layer closure. The latter technique is usually preferred whenever the fistula involves the perineal body or multiple fistulous tracts are suspected. But with either procedure, as with repair of a complete perineal tear, careful approximation of the muscular coat of the rectum is the single most important step. Irrespective of the location of the rectovaginal fistula, the use of a diverting colostomy is not indicated as a primary procedure.

Reoperation

When the first operation for correction of a rectovaginal injury has failed, the success of a second or third operation can be greatly enhanced by the use of a Martius graft to reinforce the area of closure. A Martius graft consists of a flap of bulbocavernous muscle and its surrounding fat that has been isolated through a longitudinal incision in the labia majora, detached at its anterior pole, brought through a tunnel under the lateral vaginal wall, and fixed in place between the rectum and posterior vagina. The Martius graft should always be used whenever healing is uncertain because of previous scarring or multiple operative failures. The use of a diverting colostomy is never indicated as a primary procedure and is rarely needed following operative failures. Before resorting to colostomy, a repair incorporating a Martius graft should first be attempted.

Fecal incontinence

Aside from childbirth, there are several neuroanatomic causes of fecal incontinence in women, including Crohn's disease, ulcerative colitis, scleroderma, diabetes, and pelvic irradiation. In this chapter attention will be focused on the mechanisms surrounding childbirth. Abnormalities of the anal sphincter mechanism are predominantly a result of pudendal neuropathy as well as anatomic disruption of the anal sphincter musculature. Traction injury to the pudendal nerves during labor and delivery is responsible for the neuropathy associated with this phenomenon. Furthermore, the obstetric injury commonly associated with midline episiotomy, operative vaginal delivery, macrosomia, and shoulder dystocia results in an anatomic disruption of the anal sphincter mechanism, which may lead to fecal incontinence. There is some evidence that primary repair of the external anal sphincter with an overlapping technique rather than end-to-end results in improved continence [3].

A thorough history during the evaluation of a woman with fecal incontinence should begin with any prior medical problems, medications the patient is taking and prior surgeries, including hemorrhoidectomy, fistula repair or pelvic fracture repair, in addition to a complete obstetric history. Severity may be assessed by the frequency of symptomatology, the need for a pad, consistency of the stool, the timing of incontinence, and its impact upon the patient's lifestyle.

Physical examination of the perineum should begin with an external inspection of the vagina, the perineal body, and the anus. The clinician should note any gross anatomic deformities, mass lesions, prolapse, hemorrhoids or obvious fecal soilage on the perineum. A digital examination of the external anal sphincter should assess resting tone and tone upon contracting effort of the anus.

Further, the cutaneous reflex of the external anal sphincter, commonly referred to as the "anal wink," should be assessed by stroking the perineal skin adjacent to the anus and observing a constriction of the musculature of the anal sphincter. Deficiency in this test is suggestive of pudendal neuropathy. Additional tests including endoscopic evaluation of the anorectum, electromyography of the anal sphincter, and endoanal sonography routinely assist in the diagnosis and management of fecal incontinence. Ultrasound is able to detect small defects which may be functionally significant but unable to be detected on digital rectal exam [4].

Dietary modifications, pelvic floor muscle exercises, and biofeedback have been invaluable in the management of fecal incontinence. Conservative management directed toward sustaining formed stools and rehabilitating tone of the pelvic floor musculature can improve symptoms in approximately half of patients. Increasing dietary fiber and performing regular Kegel exercises significantly helps patients with fecal incontinence. Of those patients whose symptoms are not ameliorated with medical management, surgical sphincteroplasty should be offered. Sphincteroplasty may also be offered to patients with pudendal neuropathy who fail medical management. However, patients should be counseled that the success rate of this procedure is lower than those achieved for patients who require correction of an anatomic defect.

Postoperative care

The postoperative care of these patients requires some special measures in order to minimize the likelihood of operative site infection with subsequent failure of the surgery. Generally, particulate matter in the surgical field is undesirable because of the relatively poor blood supply in this region. Therefore, a variety of strategies can be adopted in an attempt to keep the bowel empty until the operative tissues have had a chance to heal. One can institute clear liquids with Vivonex and a low-residue diet for up to several weeks or the administration of peripheral intravenous total parenteral nutrition for 5–7 days. Should any loose stools occur during the first few days, Lomotil can be used. Alternatively, simply prescribing stool softeners until normal bowel function has been restored has also been recommended. Finally, for patients who have undergone surgical correction for any of the previously discussed indications, cesarean delivery should be strongly considered in order to prevent further morbidity.

References

1. Arona AJ, al-Marayati L, Grimes DA, Ballard CA. Early secondary repair of third- and fourth- degree perineal lacerations after outpatient wound preparation. *Obstet Gynecol* 1995; 86: 294–296.

2. Duggal N, Mercado C, Daniels K, *et al.* Antibiotic Prophylaxis for Prevention of Postpartum Perineal Wound Complications. *Obstetrics & Gynecology* 2008; 111(6): 1268–1273.

3. Fernando RJ, Sultan AH, Kettle C, Radley S, Jones P, O'Brien PM. Repair techniques for obstetric anal sphincter injuries: a randomized controlled trial. *Obstet Gynecol* 2006; 107: 1261–1268.

4. Dobben AC, Terra MP, Deutekom M, *et al.* Anal inspection and digital rectal examination compared to anorectal physiology tests and endoanal ultrasonography in evaluating fecal incontinence. *Int J Colorect Dis* 2007; 22: 783–790.

Suggested reading

Allen RE, Hosker GL, Smith AR, *et al.* Pelvic floor damage and childbirth: a neurophysiological study. *BJOG* 1990; 97: 770–779.

Brantley JT, Burwell JC. A study of fourth degree perineal lacerations and their sequalae. *Am J Obstet Gynecol* 1960; 80: 711–714.

Goldaber KG, Wendel PJ, McIntire DD, *et al.* Postpartum perineal morbidity after fourth-degree perineal repair. *Am J Obstet Gynecol* 1993; 168: 489–493.

Green JR, Soohoo SL. Factors associated with rectal injury in spontaneous deliveries. *Obstet Gynecol* 1989; 73: 732–738.

Harris RE. An evaluation of median episiotomy. *Am J Obstet Gynecol* 1970; 106: 660–665.

Hibbard LT. Surgical management of rectovaginal fistulas and complete perineal tears. *Am J Obstet Gynecol* 1978; 130: 139–141.

Kiff ES, Swash M. Slowed conduction in the pudendal nerves in idiopathic (neurogenic) faecal incontinence. *Br J Surg* 1984; 71: 614–616.

Kok AL, Voorhorst FJ, Burger CW, *et al.* Urinary and faecal incontinence in community-residing elderly women. *Age Aging* 1992; 21: 211–215.

Legino LJ, Woods MP, Rayburn WF, McGoogan LS. Third and fourth degree perineal tears: 50 years' experience at a university hospital. *J Reprod Med* 1988; 33: 423–426.

Martius M. *Martius' gynecologic operations.* Boston: Little Brown, 1956: 328.

McIntosh LJ, Frahm JD, Mallett VT, *et al.* Pelvic floor rehabilitation in the treatment of incontinence. *J Reprod Med* 1993; 38: 662–666.

Miller NF, Brown W. The surgical treatment of complete perineal tears in the female. *Am J Obstet Gynecol* 1937; 34: 196–209.

O'Leary JL, O'Leary JA. The complete episiotomy. Analysis of 1224 complete lacerations, sphincterotomies, and episioproctotomies. *Obstet Gynecol* 1965; 25: 235–240.

Russell TY, Gallagher DM. Low rectovaginal fistulas. *Am J Surg* 1977; 134: 13–18.

Shiono P, Klebanoff MA, Oarey JC, *et al.* Midline episiotomies: more harm than good? *Obstet Gynecol* 1990; 75: 765–770.

Snooks SJ, Setchell M, Swash M, *et al.* Injury to innervation of pelvic floor sphincter musculature in childbirth. *Lancet* 1984; ii: 546–550.

Snyder RR, Hammond TL, Hankins GD, *et al.* Human papillomavirus associated with poor healing of episiotomy repairs. *Obstet Gynecol* 1990; 76: 664–667.

Thomas TM, Egan M, Walgrove A, *et al.* The presence of faecal and double incontinence. *Community Med* 1984; 6: 216–220.

Womack NR, Morrison JFB, Williams NS, *et al.* The role of pelvic floor denervation in the etiology of idiopathic faecal incontinence. *Br J Surg* 1986; 73: 404–407.

Chapter 67
Prepubertal Vulvar Lacerations and Hematomas, Labial Adhesions, and Prolapse of the Urethra

Jenny M. Jaque and Claire E. Templeman
Department of Medicine and Obstetrics and Gynecology, Keck School of Medicine, University of Southern California, CA, USA

Vulvar lacerations

Vulvar lacerations may arise from accidental trauma or from physical or sexual abuse. Frequently, on physical exam, a single vessel is identified as the source of the bleeding. It is very tempting to secure hemostasis and repair the child's vulvar laceration using local anesthesia. However, repair can seldom be accomplished under these conditions. Most children do not remain sufficiently immobile for the sutures to be properly placed and the operative field kept sterile. Vulvar lacerations in prepubertal children should be repaired under general anesthesia, even when the laceration is small and a single pumping vessel is identified as the source of the bleeding. The laceration should be debrided and irrigated, all bleeding vessels identified and ligated, and the wound closed with fine absorbable suture material. If the location of the laceration suggests that the vagina, urethra, bladder or rectum might be involved in the injury, these structures are examined while the patient is anesthetized. Lacerations involving the posterior fourchette not involving the hymen must be differentiated from dehisced labial adhesions or failure of midline fusion. Skin suturing should be avoided in the treatment of vulvar lacerations. Sutures, if necessary, should be placed with the child under general anesthesia or conscious sedation to decrease additional trauma for the child. A vulvar abrasion may be the source of bleeding which can be controlled with the application of absorbable gelatin sponge (Gelfoam) or absorbable hemostat of oxidized regenerated cellulose (Surgicel).

Vulvar hematomas

The most common cause of vulvar hematomas in children is "straddle" injuries. Straddle injuries occur when a child straddles an object as he or she falls, striking the urogenital area with the force of his or her bodyweight. Injury is the result of compression of soft tissues against the bony margins of the pelvic outlet. These injuries occur most often during bicycle riding, falls, and playing on monkey bars.

The prepubertal child with a vulvar hematoma presents with a swollen, ecchymotic, tender labial lesion. Vulvar hematomas are usually small in size, well localized, and do not present a life-threatening event nor require special treatment. Most hematomas will resolve spontaneously. Small hematomas can be controlled by bedrest and applying pressure with an ice pack. Treatment with ice is recommended during the first 12–24 hours after injury to reduce edema. The ability to urinate should also be assessed because large hematomas may obstruct the urethra. If the hematoma has not expanded after a minimum of 4 hours of observation, the patient has spontaneously voided clear urine, and the hematoma is not large enough to cause her undue distress, a nonsurgical approach may be used. A hematoma that enlarges, causes considerable pain, and/or obstructs the urethra must be treated surgically. The hematoma should be incised, the blood clots evacuated, and actively bleeding vessels identified and ligated. The use of a drain is not necessary if complete hemostasis is secured. The cavity is then closed in layers. If the bed of the hematoma continues to ooze then the use of a pack and drain for 24 hours may be considered.

Inspection and palpation of the vulva, along with a rectal examination, must be performed in order to identify the lesion's full extent and to identify any collection of concealed blood.

Labial adhesions

Labial fusion or labial agglutination can occur in young girls at any age prior to puberty. The labia can become fused as the result of adhesions. Fusion may be partial or it may completely occlude the vaginal orifice. Fusion usually starts at the posterior fourchette and progresses

Management of Common Problems in Obstetrics and Gynecology, 5th edition. Edited by T.M. Goodwin, M.N. Montoro, L. Muderspach, R. Paulson and S. Roy. © 2010 Blackwell Publishing Ltd.

towards the clitoris. The adhesions may be so extensive that only a small opening remains for the passage of urine. Identifying this opening upon initial inspection of the perineum may be difficult. Usually a pale, translucent vertical raphe is present in the midline demarcating the site of fusion. The etiology of labial adhesions is usually unknown, but they may be the result of local inflammation and chronic irritation to hypoestrogenized vulvar tissue. Symptoms include genital irritation and slight genital bleeding. Infrequently the child may report postvoid urinary dribbling, urinary tract infections and even urinary retention.

Treatment is based on the patient's ability to void spontaneously. As long as the child can urinate without discomfort and is free of urinary tract symptoms, there is no need to initiate therapy. The patient and parents should be counseled that in most cases the labia separate spontaneously in early puberty as the concentration of endogenous estrogen in the peripheral circulation increases. Attempts to separate the labia manually are rarely indicated and these manipulations are guaranteed to cause both physical and emotional trauma. Occasionally, when the line of fusion is very thin, the adhesions may be separated by use of a blunt probe following the administration of a local anesthetic ointment. These attempts should be terminated if they cause the child any discomfort.

Treatment must be started if the labial adhesions cause problems in voiding, recurrent urinary tract infections or pain with activity. Improved perineal hygiene and the topical application of estrogen cream to the labia once or twice a day for 10–14 days is almost always successful in bringing about separation of the labia. Once the labia separate, the estrogen cream is continued for another 7 consecutive days at bedtime so that the new edges of the labia have a chance to re-epithelialize. This reduces the chance that the labia will fuse again when the estrogen cream has been discontinued. Application of topical emollient after each voiding episode may also prevent the reformation of the labial adhesions.

Labial adhesions may be confused with vaginal agenesis or congenital fusion. When the vagina is congenitally absent, the vulva appears normal except for the absence of an opening into the vagina. The urethra has a normal anatomic location and appearance and the urethral meatus is easily identifiable. With vaginal agenesis, the opening to the vagina is replaced by vulvar tissue which has some minor folds. As opposed to congenital fusion, labial adhesions are not present at birth due to estrogen being present.

Prolapse of the urethra

Prolapse of the urethra results in the urethral mucosa protruding through the external urethral orifice as an annular mass that is reddish or reddish-blue in color. Urethral prolapse tends to occur in hypoestrogenized females and more frequently in children of African descent. The tissue may be friable or even necrotic in nature. Urethral prolapse is usually first noted after a sudden increase in intra-abdominal pressure from crying, coughing or straining. This disorder most commonly occurs in childhood with a peak incidence observed between the ages of 5 and 9 years. Children with prolapse of the urethra may complain of vulvar pain, bleeding, dysuria or even urinary retention. Diagnosis is usually made by recognizing the urethral orifice in the center of the mass, which to some degree may be friable. Passage of a catheter into the urinary bladder will confirm the diagnosis. At times, the diagnosis may be more difficult, especially when the mass of prolapsed tissue is quite large and edematous. Examination under anesthesia, vaginoscopy and even biopsy may rarely be necessary to distinguish a prolapse of the urethra from a mesodermal mixed tumor, condylomas, papilloma, periurethral cyst, and periurethral abscess.

Prolapse of the urethra usually responds to nonsurgical treatment. Sitz baths, topical application of estrogen, antibiotics, and saline compresses have all been successfully used to reduce the edema and return the prolapsed tissue to its normal anatomic location. Indications for surgical intervention include the presence of necrotic prolapsed tissue, failure of nonsurgical methods to achieve return of the prolapsed tissue to its normal site, and frequent recurrence. Surgery involves excising the redundant prolapsed mucosa and suturing the mucosal edge to the skin using fine sutures, followed by short-term indwelling catheterization. Cauterization is not recommended as a treatment for prolapse of the urethra. The procedure requires anesthesia and carries the risk of bleeding, urethral stenosis, and recurrence.

Suggested reading

Adducci JE, Fischbach AL, Adducci CJ. Microsurgical repair of pediatric vulvar trauma. *J Reprod Med* 1985; 30: 792–794.

Berkowitz CD, Elvik SL, Logan MK. Labial fusion in prepubescent girls: a marker for sexual abuse? *Am J Obstet Gynecol* 1987; 156: 16–20.

Bond GR, Dowd MD, Landsman I, Rimsza M. Unintentional perineal injury in prepubescent girls: a multicenter, prospective report of 56 girls. *Pediatrics* 1995; 95: 628.

Dowd MD, Fitzmaurice L, Knapp JF, Mooney D. The interpretation of urogenital findings in children with straddle injuries. *J Pediatr Surg* 1994; 29: 7.

Fernandes ET, Dekermacher S, Sabadin MA, Vaz F. Urethral prolapse in children. *Urology* 1993; 41: 240–242.

Gianini GD, Method MW, Christman JE. Traumatic vulvar hematomas: assessing and treating nonobstetric patients. *Postgrad Med* 1991; 89: 115–118.

Jenkinson SD, Mackinnon AE. Spontaneous separation of fused labia minora in prepubertal girls. *Br J Med* 1984; 289: 160–161.

Johnson CF. Prolapse of the urethra: confusion of clinical and anatomic characteristics with sexual abuse. *Pediatrics* 1991; 87: 722–725.

Khanam W, Chogtu L, Mir Z, Shawl F. Adhesion of the labia minora – a study of 75 cases. *Obstet Gynecol Surv* 1978; 33: 364–365.

McCann J, Voris J, Simon M. Labial adhesions and posterior fourchette injuries in childhood sexual abuse. *Am J Dis Child* 1988; 142: 659–663.

Muram D. Genital tract injuries in the prepubertal child. *Pediatr Ann* 1986; 15: 616–620.

Propst AM, Thorp JM Jr. Traumatic vulvar hematomas: conservative versus surgical management. *South Med J* 1998; 91: 144–146.

Rimsza ME. Gonorrheal vulvovaginitis, labial fusion; imperforate hymen. *Am J Dis Child* 1989; 143: 381–382.

Rudin JE, Geldt VS, Alecseev EB. Prolapse of urethral mucosa in white female children: experience with 58 cases. *J Pediatr Surg* 1997; 32: 423–425.

Starr WB. Labial adhesions in childhood. *J Pediatr Health Care* 1996; 10: 26–27.

Wheeler RA, Burge DM. Urinary obstruction due to labial fusion. *Br J Urol* 1991; 67: 102.

Williams TS, Callen JP, Owen LG. Vulvar disorders in the prepubertal female. *Pediatr Ann* 1986; 15: 588–605.

Chapter 68
Female Sexual Function and Dysfunction

Lauren Rubal

Department of Medicine and Obstetrics and Gynecology, Keck School of Medicine, University of Southern California, CA, USA

Introduction

Sexuality plays an integral role throughout a woman's life. Multiple disparate factors influence sexuality and sexual health, including general health, psychologic status, interpersonal relationships, anatomy, hormonal patterns, and cultural mores.

Female sexual function

Physiology

There are several basic models that form the foundation of our current knowledge of the female sexual response. Masters & Johnson established the classic paradigm with the publication of *Human sexual response* in 1966. In it, they observed the sexual activity of 700 subjects, and delineated four stages of sexual response: excitement, plateau, orgasm, and resolution (Figure 68.1).

As noted in Figure 68.1, female sexual response patterns may differ from woman to woman and from one sexual encounter to another. This is typically considered a linear model and one pattern (A) corresponds the most with the male sexual response, but with a longer plateau phase and the possibility of multiple orgasms (without the male refractory period). Another pattern (B) has no orgasm stage but instead, a prolonged plateau phase with several peaks and troughs, finally culminating in the resolution stage. The final pattern (C) has a rapid shift from the excitement phase to orgasm, followed by quick resolution.

Excitement is the first stage and can be initiated via external or internal stimuli (Figure 68.2). This phase is mediated initially by the central nervous system, via stimulation of the parasympathetic autonomic nervous system. This in turn increases blood flow and smooth muscle relaxation throughout the body. There is generalized vasocongestion, hyperventilation, hypertension, and tachycardia. The labia majora increase to 2–3 times their nonaroused size in all women. In nulliparous women, the labia majora become tauter and thinner. The established and extensive vascular channels in multiparous women cause the labia majora to swell. The clitoris also engorges during the excitement phase. Both the clitoral glans and the shaft (also known as the prepuce) increase in diameter. The deep tissues of the vagina begin producing a clear transudate within 10–30 seconds after the initiation of sexual arousal. This fluid not only facilitates intercourse but also neutralizes vaginal pH, thereby assisting in

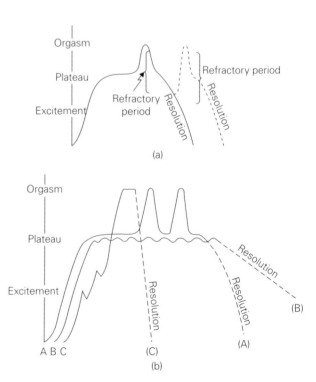

Figure 68.1 The sexual response in (a) men and (b) women. The curves represent degrees of sexual arousal. The three different female cycle patterns in (b) are discussed in the text. Reproduced from Jones RE. *Human reproductive biology*, 2nd edn. San Diego: Academic Press, 1997.

Management of Common Problems in Obstetrics and Gynecology, 5th edition. Edited by T.M. Goodwin, M.N. Montoro, L. Muderspach, R. Paulson and S. Roy. © 2010 Blackwell Publishing Ltd.

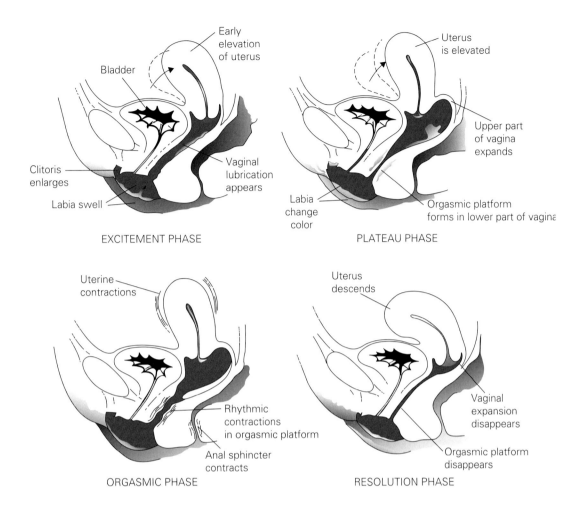

Figure 68.2 Changes in the female sex organs during the sexual response cycle. Adapted from Masters WH, Johnson VE, Kolodny RC. *Biological foundations of human sexuality.* New York: Harper Collins College Publishers, 1993.

survival of sperm. Skin flushing may occur over the body, especially the face, neck, back, and breasts. The breasts enlarge, as does the areola. Nipple erection is an early sign of sexual excitement.

The plateau phase is the peak of the excitement phase. The parasympathetic system continues to dominate throughout this time. Further changes take place in the proximal vagina – specifically, expansion of the posterior fornix. This occurs in preparation for the volume of semen deposited with ejaculation. The entire vagina lengthens during this phase. In the lower vagina, an orgasmic platform is formed through vasocongestion of the perineal, bulbocavernosus, and pubococcygeus muscles. This platform decreases the transverse vaginal diameter, leading to increased friction during intercourse. The uterus becomes engorged during both the excitement and plateau stages. It lifts upward during the plateau phase. This tenting of the uterus possibly is due to Valsalva maneuvers during intercourse.

Orgasm represents the third stage of sexual response and is regulated by the sympathetic autonomic nervous system. It is the peak of sexual pleasure and is described as the release of sexual tension. Physiologically, the uterus, orgasmic platform, and anal sphincter rhythmically contract. These spasms commence about 2–4 seconds after the woman senses the orgasm, and occur on average at 0.8-second intervals (although this period becomes longer at the end of the orgasm). Usually, there are 3–15 contractions noted. The contractions are initially intense and gradually become weaker as the orgasm subsides. Associated generalized myotonic contraction may also occur. The proximal vagina continues expanding during orgasm. The clitoris retracts under its hood behind the symphysis pubis and flattens. In 10–40% of women fluid may be expelled from the Skene's glands.

Resolution represents the final phase in the sexual response cycle and involves the return of the genitopelvic anatomy to the nonaroused state. Mental and physical relaxation predominate, and the woman experiences a sense of euphoria and well-being. Women may not experience a refractory period, and thus can be stimulated to experience several sexual orgasms in repeated cycles in one session.

The second theory of female sexual response adds the concept of sexual desire and it was first introduced by Helen Kaplan Singer. Desire is a common prelude to sexual response, though not a necessary stage. Kaplan's triphasic model encompasses desire, excitement and orgasm phases, each distinct in its physiology, pathology and therapies for dysfunction.

Rosemary Basson discussed the circular model of female sexual function (Figure 68.3). In this concept, the reaction to sexual stimuli is not spontaneous but rather represents a complex interaction of biology, psychology, sociocultural influences, and interpersonal relationships. This biopsychosocial model proposes that sexual response does not necessarily occur in a linear, automatic fashion but rather is dependent on several emotional, physical, and environmental components. The phases of sexual response can occur at overlapping or varying times. The motivation for sexual function may be from a variety of different facets including an innate desire, the need for intimacy or because the woman is genitally aroused. The goal of the sexual experience is personal and relationship satisfaction, and orgasmic release is not necessary. This novel model therefore implies that treating sexual dysfunction must address all mechanisms of sexual response, not solely the physical one.

Recent research by Michael Sands and colleagues demonstrated that women demonstrate the Masters & Johnson model, the Kaplan model and the Basson Model. They may shift from one model to the next during a sexual experience or between experiences. Women with sexual complaints may more often identify with the Basson model of female sexual function.

Physiology of female sexual function

The physiology of the female sexual response does not solely involve the genital pelvic organs and the internal

pelvic structures. The spinal and central nervous system are also major contributors to female sexual response as well as many areas of the brain, including the hippocampus, hypothalamus, limbic system, and medial preoptic area. Many neurotransmitters and secondary modulators have also been implicated in the response cycle. This includes the neuropeptides serotonin, dopamine, norepinephrine, and epinephrine, opioids, nitric oxide, acetylcholine, and vasoactive intestinal peptide. Sex steroids are essential in the female genital response, and estradiol and testosterone have been clearly implicated in the normative functioning of the response cycle. Sex steroids are one of many components in the complex and multifaceted cycle, but they are one of its critical mediators. They translate stimulus-triggered neurologic impulses into physical responses, such as altered vascular blood flow.

Estrogens

Estrogens have a beneficial effect on sexual function. They can act centrally as well as in the periphery to increase blood flow to both the brain and genitals. The hypothalamus, one of the primary regulators of both mood and sexual function, contains many estrogen receptors. Estrogen increases vasoactive substances in the blood vessels. For example, estrogen is partially responsible for the increased nitric oxide in endothelial cells during arousal. Nitric oxide, in turn, contributes to the vasodilation that is so important to the sexual response. Estrogens may also enhance vibratory sense in the periphery. They facilitate neuronal growth and transmission. Estrogens are critically important to the health of the vaginal lining, not only the suppleness of the mucosa but also the normal vaginal acidic pH. These actions of estrogen can affect a woman's sexual health.

Estrogen declines gradually in the perimenopause, with a sharp drop after menopause. Vulvar, clitoral, and vaginal atrophy are changes seen after estrogen depletion. The initial alterations in the epithelium manifest as fewer superficial cells, more parabasal cells, with decreased support and elasticity of the tissue. The vaginal pH becomes more basic, thereby providing a more conducive environment for vaginal infections via growth of different types of bacteria. After long-term estrogen deficiency, there is atrophy of the vessels, muscles, and stroma of the vagina. This results in less blood flow to the area and more advanced signs of atrophy, such as a decrease in vaginal length and constriction of the vagina. The urinary system is affected by lower estrogen levels, with similar changes in the mucosa. This can manifest as urinary urgency, frequency, dysuria, nocturia, and incontinence. The clitoris also undergoes atrophy. It can decrease in size by up to half of its premenopausal diameter. There is decreased blood flow to the clitoris, and it may manifest by increased latency to orgasm or decreased orgasmic intensity. With decreased estrogen,

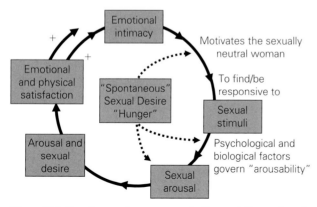

Figure 68.3 Female sexual response cycle: Basson intimacy-based model. Adapted from Basson R. Female sexual response: the role of drugs in the management of sexual dysfunction. *Obstet Gynecol* 2001: 98(2): 350–353.

there is diminished nerve impulse conduction, with decreased touch and vibratory sensation. These changes may culminate in sexual dysfunction, not only secondary to dyspareunia but because of decreased blood supply to the genitals. This manifests as decreased engorgement of the genitals, decreased proximal vaginal expansion, and even pain with orgasmic contractions (thought to be due to a mechanism similar to ischemia).

It has been challenging to elucidate the definitive etiology behind the decline in sexual function in peri- and postmenopausal women. The Melbourne Women's Midlife Health Project delineated the effects of advancing age versus menopausal status. This is a prospective, observational study that followed 438 women (aged 45–55 at baseline) over 8 years with validated questionnaires regarding sexual function. It examined the differences between women who went through natural menopause during the study period and the control group, who did not experience any of those hormonal changes. The results demonstrate that sexual responsivity declines with age (shown in both the menopausal and control groups). However, menopause specifically affects libido, frequency of intercourse, and vaginal dyspareunia. It is important to note that relationship factors have a major influence on the sexual functioning of the postmenopausal woman.

Estrogen therapy has been studied in the short term, with acknowledged benefit for postmenopausal women with sexual dysfunction. One report by Sarrel examined the symptoms of vaginal dryness, pain with penetration, and burning sensation in 93 women, and found these symptoms correlated to a serum estradiol level less than 50 pg/mL, with resolution of these complaints when estradiol rose above 50 pg/mL. This study showed that, per the subjects' reports, there was an increase in orgasm frequency, clitoral sensitivity, libido, and sexual activity after oral estrogen therapy. Estrogen levels affect a variety of facets for female sexual function. Estrogen works both centrally and in the periphery to maintain vaginal health.

Some studies have linked long-term estrogen therapy with breast cancer risk.

Androgens

Androgens are important precursors for estrogen synthesis. They also are necessary for bone metabolism, cognition, and ovarian follicular development. Many tissues in the body have androgen receptors, including the central nervous system, bone, and ovaries. Androgens have a role in sexual function but this remains to be elucidated. There is conflicting evidence correlating serum androgen to sexual desire. Some studies report an association, while others do not. A cross-sectional study by Davis *et al.* of 1021 women aged 18–75 years measured serum concentrations of testosterone, free testosterone, androstenedione, and DHEA-S. These authors also administered a validated questionnaire. The group found no correlation between low serum androgen levels and low sexual function. However, there are other studies that demonstrate utility in restoring sexual desire in the woman who suffers from low libido. Testosterone treatment remains experimental, since it is not FDA approved in the United States and treatment remains off label. There are continued concerns about long-term safety effects, including effects on the cardiovascular system, lipid changes and its role in breast cancer. At supraphysiologic levels, testosterone can have some serious side effects. Hair growth, changes in lipid functions, and mood changes may be common at high doses. Clitoromegaly and voice changes may be irreversible.

Progestins

All progestins decrease estrogen receptors in the body, not only in the pelvic region but also in the brain, heart, and bone. Progestins have been associated with a depressive central nervous system effect with regard to mood. Several studies have demonstrated that effects of progestins include diminished sexual desire and decreased blood flow.

The effect of progestins on sexual function is still under investigation. This is in part due to the varied subtypes of progestins, each with different actions and effects. For example, medroxyprogesterone acetate (a C-21 progesterone derivative), the most potent progestin available, does not significantly alter sex hormone binding globulin levels. A study by Sherwin showed that 48 naturally menopausal women reported decreased sexual function measurements after being given combination estrogen/medroxyprogesterone acetate, as opposed to estrogen alone. However, another progestin subtype, norethindrone acetate (a 19 nortestosterone derivative, along with norgestimate), is more androgenic. Norethindrone acetate thus decreases sex hormone binding globulin levels, as well as increasing bone density. Decreased sex hormone binding globulin is desirable because it translates into more bio-available hormones, such as estrogens and androgens, which can then positively influence sexual function.

Female sexual dysfunction

Sexual function depends on multiple aspects of a woman's life, including her emotional and psychologic state, anatomy and hormones, concurrent medical problems, and medications. Thus, there are myriad causes for sexual dysfunction.

Epidemiology

The National Health and Social Life Survey was a probability sample performed in 1999. It studied sexual behavior in a demographically representative population of American men and women – specifically, 1749 persons aged 18–49 years. Interestingly, in those who reported at least one partner in the past 12 months, sexual dysfunction was present in 43% of women (as opposed to 31% of men). Predictors of sexual dysfunction included marital status, age, education, and ethnicity. Women who are younger, unmarried, have less than a college education, or are Caucasian or African American reported sexual dysfunction more frequently.

In Shifren's recent study "Sexual problems and distress in the United States: women prevalence and correlates," 31,581 female respondents aged 18 years and older from 50,002 households were polled. The study demonstrated that any distressing sexual problem (defined as reporting a sexual problem and sexually related personal distress) occurred in 12.0% of respondents and was more common in women aged 45–64 years (14.8%) than in younger (10.8%) or older (8.9%) women. Correlates of sexual problems included poor self-assessed health, low education level, depression, anxiety, thyroid conditions, and urinary incontinence.

Etiology

The etiology of female sexual complaints is known to be multifactorial. There are clear medical conditions that can contribute to sexual complaints. Psychosexual problems and interpersonal conflicts can also influence a woman's response and interest in sexual activities.

Some of the biologic factors implicated in sexual functioning include chronic medical diseases, cardiovascular and coronary arterial disease, diabetes, autoimmune syndromes and neurologic impairment. Neuropathies lead to decreased sensation, and vascular insufficiency will impede genital vasocongestion. These manifestations can arise from medical diseases, such as diabetes mellitus. Also, nerve damage from pelvic or spinal surgery or trauma may affect sensation. Blood flow to the area may also be affected by trauma. Malignancy, urogynecologic problems and endocrinopathies can also affect sexual anatomy, physiology, and the normative response. Some of the causes of estrogen depletion include natural, surgical or chemically induced menopause, and premature ovarian failure. Young women who have either anorexia or exercise-induced amenorrhea, bulimia, or who have had chemotherapy or radiation may also experience vaginal atrophy and sexual dysfunction. Lactation-induced amenorrhea is common in women exclusively breastfeeding and these postpartum women may also suffer from hypoestrogenemia, vaginal dryness, and atrophic complaints.

Interpersonal conflicts such as marital infidelity or psychiatric illnesses such as depression, anxiety or substance abuse can also affect sexual function. Past history of sexual abuse or physical violence can also present as female sexual dysfunction. Marital discord, poor partner health, cultural conflicting mores, guilt and shame about sex, lack of privacy, and poor relationship trust and quality can also contribute to sexual problems. Poor technical skills in the partner and sexual naiveté about anatomy and orgasmic response may also be issues.

Many medications can detrimentally affect sexual responsivity. The treatment of medical disorders can also cause sexual dysfunction. Anticholinergic medications will decrease vaginal lubrication. Antidepressants, especially selective serotonin reuptake inhibitors (SSRIs), are notorious in their adverse sexual effects, including diminished desire and orgasm. Even over-the-counter medications can result in decreased desire: diphenhydramine (Benadryl), naproxen, and ranitidine have been associated with reduced desire. Other common culprits include psychotropic medications, antipsychotic drugs, many cardiovascular agents, mood stabilizers, histamine receptor blockers, and oral contraceptives, as well as other medications.

Classification of sexual complaints

There are several subclasses in the diagnosis of sexual dysfunction (Table 68.1). The term refers to a persistent or recurring sexual dysfunction that results in personal distress to the patient. Each of the categories is subtyped as lifelong versus acquired, generalized versus situational, and by the etiology (such as organic, psychogenic, mixed or unknown).

Sexual desire disorders

Hypoactive sexual desire disorder (HSDD) is defined as the persistent or recurrent deficiency (or absence) of sexual fantasies, thoughts and/or desire for, or receptivity to, sexual activity, which causes personal distress. This is a complex disorder because many factors can transiently interfere with sexual desire, and couples also have to synchronize their libidos in a partnership. However, once a person demonstrates decreased ability to become aroused or has no sexual interest, this disorder must be considered. An important consideration in the diagnosis of HSDD is to differentiate it from a generalized psychiatric disorder, such as depression or bipolar disorder.

Table 68.1 Consensus classification system

Main division	Subdivision
Sexual desire disorders	Hypoactive sexual desire disorder
	Sexual aversion disorder
Sexual arousal disorders	Subjective arousal disorder
	Genital arousal disorder
	Combined arousal disorder
	Persistent genital arousal disorder
Orgasmic disorders	
Sexual pain disorders	Dyspareunia
	Vaginismus
	Noncoital sexual pain disorders

Hypoactive sexual desire disorder

Absent or diminished feelings of sexual interest or desire, absent sexual thoughts or fantasies, and a lack of responsive desire. The lack of interest is considered to be beyond a normative lessening with life cycle and relationship duration.

Sexual aversion disorder

Persistent or recurrent extreme aversion to, and avoidance of, all or almost all genital sexual contact with a partner. Axis I Disorders OCD or major depression have been ruled out.

Sexual arousal disorders

This subgroup is defined by a recurrent inability to reach or sustain sufficient sexual excitement, which causes personal distress. This includes deficiencies in either subjective excitement or genital/somatic responses.

Subjective sexual arousal disorder

Absence of or markedly diminished feelings of sexual arousal, excitement, and sexual pleasure from any type of sexual stimulation. Vaginal lubrication or other physical responses still occur.

Genital sexual arousal disorder

Persistent or recurrent partial or complete failure to attain or maintain lubrication, swelling response of sexual excitement until completion of sexual activity. Subjective excitement still occurs.

Combined sexual arousal disorder

Absence of or markedly diminished feelings of sexual arousal (sexual excitement and pleasure) from any type of sexual stimulation as well as reports of absent or impaired genital sexual arousal (vulvar swelling and lubrication).

Persistent genital arousal disorder

Spontaneous, intrusive, and unwanted genital arousal (tingling, throbbing, pulsating) in the absence of sexual interest and desire. Any awareness of subjective arousal is typically, but not invariably, unpleasant. Arousal is unrelieved by one or more orgasms and the feelings of arousal persist for hours or days.

The physical response includes abnormal vaginal lubrication, decreased clitoral or labial sensation or engorgement, and lack of vaginal smooth muscle relaxation. Women can have subjective arousal disorder, genital arousal disorder or both subtypes.

Orgasmic disorders

These disorders are characterized by difficulty, delay or absence of attaining orgasm after sufficient sexual stimulation and arousal, causing personal distress to the patient. Primary anorgasmia refers to a patient who has never experienced an orgasm. Secondary anorgasmia occurs when a woman had orgasms in the past, but now does not. Situational anorgasmia is diagnosed when a patient is able to orgasm during certain types of stimulation, but not with others.

Sexual pain disorders

Vaginismus

Recurrent or persistent difficulties in allowing vaginal entry of a penis, finger or object despite the woman's expressed wish to do so. There is often phobic avoidance, anticipation/fear and pain, along with variable and involuntary pelvic muscle contraction. Structural and other physical abnormalities must be ruled out.

Dyspareunia

Recurrent or persistent genital pain with attempted or complete vaginal entry and/or penile vaginal intercourse.

Dyspareunia is pain with intercourse, and is a common endpoint for a variety of different conditions and even symptoms. Assessing when and where the pain occurs (for example, only with deep thrust versus only with penetration and deep in the middle abdomen versus on the perineum) may help with the diagnosis. The most common cause of dyspareunia varies by age (and by hormonal status). Women under 50 years old most frequently have dyspareunia secondary to vulvar vestibulodynia, while those over 50 years old report vulvovaginal atrophy. Table 68.2 shows the multiple etiologies for dyspareunia, and diagnostic tools for the clinician.

Evaluation and treatment of female sexual complaints

The mainstay of sexual medicine evaluation is a comprehensive detailed medical and psychosexual history combined with a detailed physical and pelvic examination. Often laboratory assessment of hormonal levels and other advanced assessment techniques can be utilized to help the professional discern the differential diagnosis.

History

A detailed history is critical for correct assessment of female sexual complaints. Characterizing the complaint in the patient's own words is often helpful. In addition, sometimes, structured formalized interview scales and checklists can be incorporated into the work-up of the patient with sexual complaints. Some of the more popular screening and assessment tools include the Female Sexual Function Index (FSFI) and the Brief Sexual Symptom Checklist.

Physical examination

A complete physical examination should be done in order to assess general health and rule out possible chronic diseases that may affect the sexual response cycle. It is

Table 68.2 Common differential diagnoses for painful sexual intercourse

Diagnosis	Clues	Etiology	Physical findings	Evaluation*
Dyspareunia	Pain at entry, vaginal or deep	Unknown; may be associated with other diagnoses listed in this table	No findings to suggest alternate diagnoses listed in this table	Consider psychologic evaluation.
Vulvodynia	Well-defined entry pain; vulvar pain, burning, irritation; poor response to prior treatments, symptoms with activities that put pressure on vulva (sitting or bicycle riding)	Frequently unknown; possibly infections or irritants	Unremarkable or mild erythema; markedly tender; leukoplakia, ulcerations, pigmented lesions or nodules are suspicious	Visual inspection; colposcopy and biopsy of suspicious area; apply acetic acid to highlight areas.
Vulvar vestibulitis (subset of vulvodynia)	Well-defined entry pain; painful inflammation of vulvar vestibular area; dull ache, burning or pruritus	Unknown	Flat, non-ulcerated erythema, intensity varies; margins distinct or vague; exquisite tenderness on touch of cotton-tipped applicator	Same as above
Vaginismus	Well-defined entry pain; involuntary spasm of introital muscles; difficulty with insertion of penis, tampons or digit	Unknown; conditioned response of musculature versus psychologic	Palpable spasm of vaginal musculature; difficulty inserting speculum	Physical; consider psychologic evaluation based on history.
Atrophic tissue or impaired lubrication	Well-delineated entry pain; vaginal pain; vaginal dryness, friction, irritation; difficulty and pain with penetration	Estrogen deficiency; arousal-phase difficulty; decreased lubrication and impaired vaginal barrel distention; surgery	Visual inspection of pubic hair, labial fullness, integrity of vaginal mucosa, vaginal depth; vaginal mucosal friability, fissures	Based on physical examination; discussion of foreplay, arousal-phase mechanics and expected sensations
Endometriosis and pelvic adhesions	Deep pain; cyclic pain with menses; complaint of "something being bumped into"	Unknown for endometriosis; prior surgery/infections for pelvic adhesions	Nodules; fixed uterus or adnexa	Laparoscopy
Adnexal pathology	Deep pain; may be localized to one side	Cysts; infections	Enlarged adnexa, tenderness or fixed	Laparoscopy
Retroverted uterus; pelvic relaxation; uterine fibroids	Deep pain	Anatomic position	Uterus retroverted, prolapsed or enlarged	Trial of position changes
Chronic cervicitis; pelvic inflammatory disease; endometritis	Deep pain	Infections	Discharge, lesions; cervical friability; uterine tenderness or cervical motion tenderness	Colposcopy; culture; laparoscopy
Pelvic congestion	Postcoital ache; deep pain; pelvic pain	Unknown	Unremarkable	Based on history
Urethral disorders; cystitis; interstitial cystitis	Suprapubic pressure, frequency, nocturia, urgency	–	Palpation tenderness along urethra or bladder	Urinalysis and urine culture (negative in interstitial cystitis)

*—*Psychologic factors may be a part of the continued pain cycle and should be explored with all diagnoses.*
Adapted from Heim LJ. Evaluation and differential diagnosis of dyspareunia. *American Academy of Family Physicians* 2001; 63: 1535.

important to assess whether atrophy, stenosis or prolapse is present. Palpation of the vulva and vagina can identify specific areas of pain. The clinician must rule out any vaginitis that may be contributing to the pain.

Treatment

The treatment of female sexual health concerns is a complex process encompassing treatment of both underlying medical issues and of psychologic or psychosexual barriers. Often many healthcare providers are involved in the dynamic treatment process and the provider should have access to many specialists in their community. Psychosocial counseling is critical in the treatment process. The use of hormone replacement therapy should be considered to treat genitourinary atrophy. Testosterone treatments remain experimental.

Future directions

Although the awareness of both normal sexual physiology and dysfunction is growing, there are still many questions to be elucidated regarding the basic mechanisms of disease and possible treatment modalities. Important areas of research include determining the prevalence, predictors, and outcome of female sexual dysfunction, clarifying the hormonal effects on sexuality and establishing reproducible measurement devices and instruments for evaluating female sexual response. The silence concerning the lack of communication between patient and healthcare provider must be broken. Sexual health and wellness is an integral part of the human experience and many are troubled by their sexual complaints. Physicians and healthcare providers must continue to become informed regarding the diagnosis and treatment of female sexual health, wellness, and dysfunction.

Suggested reading

Barrett-Connor E, Young R, Notelovitz M, *et al*. A two-year, double-blind comparison of estrogen-androgen and conjugated estrogens in surgically menopausal women: effects on bone mineral density, symptoms, and lipid profiles. *J Reprod Med* 1999; 44:1012–1020.

Basson R. Female sexual response: the role of drugs in the management of sexual dysfunction. *Obstet Gynecol* 2001: 98(2): 350–353.

Basson, R. Clinical practice. Sexual desire and arousal disorders in women. *NEJM* 2006: 354(14): 1497–1506.

Berman JR, Berman LA, Werbin TJ. Clinical evaluation of female sexual function: effects of age and estrogen status on subjective and physiologic sexual responses. *Int J Impot Res* 1999: 11(suppl 1): S31–38.

Davis SR, Davison SL, Donath S, Bell RJ. Circulating androgen levels and self-reported sexual function in women. *JAMA* 2005: 294(1): 91–96.

Dennerstein L, Dudley E, Hopper J, Burger H. Sexuality, hormones, and the menopausal transition. *Maturitas* 1997: 26(2): 83–93.

Keil K. Urogenital atrophy: diagnosis, sequelae, and management. *Curr Women's Health Rep* 2002: 2(4): 305–311.

Laumann EO, Paik A, Rosen RC. Sexual dysfunction in the United States: prevalence and predictors. *JAMA* 1999: 281(6): 537–544.

Margo K, Winn R. Testosterone treatments: why, when, and how? *Am Fam Physician* 2006; 73: 1591–1598.

Masters WH, Johnson VE. *Human sexual response*. Boston: Little, Brown, 1966.

Masters WH, Johnson VE, Kolodny RC. *Biological foundations of human sexuality*. New York: Harper Collins College Publishers, 1993.

Chapter 69
Endometriosis

Lauren Rubal and Robert Israel

Department of Medicine and Obstetrics and Gynecology, Keck School of Medicine, University of Southern California, CA, USA

Introduction

In 1921, J.A. Sampson described endometriosis as "the presence of ectopic tissue which possesses the histological structure and function of the uterine mucosa." Since his classic contribution, there has been a growing appreciation of the frequency, pathology, and clinical characteristics of this enigmatic gynecologic disorder. Endometriosis is marked by variability in its symptoms, manifestations, effects, and therapies. The current literature on endometriosis is vast, but there is still much contradictory or insufficient information. In many ways, endometriosis remains a mystery.

Incidence and distribution

The characterization of endometriosis has not changed much since Sampson first formally described it. It is the presence of endometrial glands and stroma outside the endometrial cavity and uterine musculature.

Since endometriosis is dependent on ovarian steroids for its existence and proliferation, its occurrence and clinical importance are confined generally to the reproductive years. Although endometriosis has been reported in premenarchal and postmenopausal women not using exogenous hormones, the mean age at diagnosis is 25–29 years [1].

The prevalence of endometriosis is difficult to establish. Different authors have suggested a prevalence of 3–10% in reproductive-aged women. A precise determination of prevalence is hard because definitive diagnosis requires laparoscopy with possible biopsies, and even the presumptive diagnosis may be skewed by symptoms, access to care, and cultural attitudes towards pain. However, studies have shown an association between endometriosis and delayed childbearing, lower BMI, and Caucasian race [2]. The prevalence of documented endometriosis at time of surgery ranges from 1% found in all gynecologic procedures to higher values (9–50%) when the surgery is performed to evaluate pelvic pain or infertility [3].

Pathophysiology

While the exact etiology of endometriosis is still unclear, there are several proposed theories.

The coelomic (peritoneal) cavity has undifferentiated cells that may undergo metaplastic transformation to endometriosis. Support for this hypothesis resides in cases of endometriosis in men, premenarchal girls, and those with congenital absence of the uterus. However, this theory remains problematic. Although the endometriosis cases mentioned above do occur, they represent a rare presentation of the disorder. Also, even though the coelomic membrane overlies the thoracic and abdominal cavities, the vast majority of endometriosis resides in the pelvis. Furthermore, metaplasia in general increases with older age, but endometriosis first presents at a relatively young age [4].

The transplantation theory holds that the endometrium is actively disseminated to an ectopic location. This can occur via mechanical, lymphatic or vascular mechanisms. Retrograde menstruation (mechanical transport) is widely accepted as a causative factor in endometriosis. Lending credence to this are several studies demonstrating lower endometriosis rates with later menarche, irregular menstrual cycles, more deliveries, and longer oral contraceptive use [5]. The fact that endometriosis is primarily a disease of menstruating women, especially those with regular menses, also sustains this theory.

The induction theory combines the above two hypotheses. It suggests that shed endometrium secretes a biochemical substance that causes differentiation of peritoneal cells.

Altered immunity, both humoral and cell mediated, appears to play a role in endometriosis as well. First,

Management of Common Problems in Obstetrics and Gynecology,
5th edition. Edited by T.M. Goodwin, M.N. Montoro,
L. Muderspach, R. Paulson and S. Roy. © 2010 Blackwell
Publishing Ltd.

impaired immune detection of ectopic endometrial nests has been demonstrated. In women with endometriosis, there may be alterations in their human leukocyte antigen (HLA) class I expression, which affects immune recognition [6]. Second, a decreased immune response contributes to the persistence of the ectopic endometrium. Decreased natural killer cell activity in women with endometriosis reduces cytotoxicity to the endometriosis cells [7]. Apoptosis may be inhibited, both by an increased amount of antiapoptotic factors and by resistance to interferon-γ-induced apoptosis [8]. Compared to a nonendometriosis group, a survey demonstrated a higher association between women with endometriosis and other autoimmune inflammatory diseases, such as hyperthyroidism, fibromyalgia or chronic fatigue syndrome [9].

Recent research has focused on the adhesion and proliferation of endometriosis implants. One theory ties together altered immune response with growth factors that appear to be vital in the development of endometriosis, suggesting that increased peritoneal leukocytes and macrophages, together with endometriotic nests, secrete cytokines and growth factors. The cytokines, such as specific interleukins and tumor necrosis factor, stimulate implant growth, angiogenesis, and a greater inflammatory milieu [10].

Hormones may affect endometriosis. There is increased aromatase activity in women with endometriosis, which increases estrogen levels in the implants.

In some women, a genetic component of endometriosis has been established, probably via a multifactorial, polygenic inheritance pattern. First-degree relatives of women with endometriosis have a 7% chance of developing endometriosis compared to 1% chance in controls, i.e. unrelated persons [11]. A combination of different theories, plus alterations in immunity, expression of different growth factors, and possible genetic influences likely represent the complex etiology of endometriosis.

The most frequent pelvic locations for endometriosis are the ovaries (involved in 66% of cases), uterine ligaments (round, broad, uterosacral), pelvic peritoneum, and the rectovaginal septum. Other sites include the umbilicus, laparoscopy/laparotomy scars, hernial sacs, liver, appendix (involved in 2–4% of cases), small intestine, sigmoid, rectum, bladder, ureters, vulva/vagina/cervix, lymph nodes, extremities, pleural cavity, and lung. The multiplicity and widespread distribution of these sites make acceptance of one histogenetic theory difficult.

Like everything else connected with endometriosis, the gross pathology is characterized by variability. Endometriotic lesions classically appear as "powder-burn," black or blue-ish areas. However, they may be clear, red, yellow or white. The different manifestations of endometriosis may depict the various phases of the disease, with clear or reddish lesions signaling active proliferation and darker lesions or fibrotic areas indicative of quiescence. At times, the only evidence of endometriosis is a peritoneal window. With diagnostic uncertainty, including areas of suspected nonpigmented endometriosis, laparoscopic biopsy will help establish the histologic diagnosis. When biopsy specimens of grossly normal peritoneum are taken, 25% of patients demonstrate microscopic endometriotic foci.

Endometrial islands may occur anywhere on the pelvic peritoneum, initially involving just the serosal surface but, with progression, possibly infiltrating deeply (>5–6 mm) into the retroperitoneum. Women presenting with endometriosis and pelvic pain usually have this type of deep penetration. Occasionally, invasion and penetration occur in the sigmoid. Progressive submucosal scarring can result in luminal constriction. However, mucosal involvement with associated rectal bleeding is a late phenomenon.

More significant ovarian involvement means the formation of unilateral or, commonly, bilateral endometrial cysts (endometriomas, "chocolate" cysts). Even when quite small, the cysts show a strong tendency to perforate with escape of menstrual blood and subsequent ovarian adherence to any adjacent structure, usually the posterior surface of the broad ligament or uterus.

Definitive diagnosis requires microscopic demonstration of endometrial tissue, preferably both glands and stroma. However, a wide range of patterns may occur, from normal-appearing to completely denuded endometrium, secondary to repeated menstrual bleeding and desquamation, with hemorrhage and pigment-laden macrophages the only microscopic clues. In one-third of clinically typical endometriotic cases, a specific histologic diagnosis cannot be made.

Malignant changes occurring in endometriomas are rare and almost always histologically low grade (adenoacanthoma). Although 10% of endometroid ovarian carcinomas are associated with ovarian endometriosis, it is unusual for malignant transformation of the endometriosis to be demonstrable.

Diagnosis

The symptomatology associated with endometriosis can be as variable as anything else connected with this disorder. Many women are asymptomatic, with an incidental diagnosis of endometriosis made during surgery for other causes. Otherwise, women usually present complaining of pain, gastrointestinal or genitourinary issues, or infertility.

Pain is a common symptom, with dysmenorrhea, dyspareunia and dyschezia presenting individually or as a classic symptom complex. However, even with extensive, but noninfiltrating endometriosis, pain may not be a significant clinical entity. Unless rupture occurs, ovarian endometriomas can expand painlessly. However, incapacitating dysmenorrhea and pelvic pain may be associated with minimal amounts of active, but invasive, surface endometriosis. Thus, the degree of endometriotic involvement and spread bears no constant relationship to the presence or absence of subjective discomfort.

Over 50% of patients with endometriosis complain of dysmenorrhea. Usually, it is the secondary variety although if primary dysmenorrhea is present, endometriosis can worsen it. The dysmenorrhea may be secondary to either secretory changes in the endometriotic islands, with subsequent bleeding in areas encapsulated by fibrous tissue, or the release of prostaglandins from aberrant endometrium. With involvement of the rectovaginal septum or uterosacral ligaments, the dysmenorrhea is often referred to the rectum or the lower sacrococcygeal area, and dyspareunia becomes a concomitant complaint. Dyschezia results from endometriotic bleeding in the rectosigmoid muscularis or serosa with subsequent fibrosis. Chronic pelvic pain may also result from endometriosis, due to the mechanisms outlined above, with possible exacerbation by chronic pelvic nerve irritation from the endometriosis. Occasionally, abnormal uterine bleeding, such as premenstrual spotting or menorrhagia, may occur.

Infertility is another frequent complaint. Although endometriosis does not appear to prevent conception, 30–40% of patients with endometriosis have concomitant infertility. This percentage may be skewed because of selection bias in this group. Advanced-stage disease (moderate and severe endometriosis) probably leads to infertility due to adhesion formation and, possibly, lessened ovarian reserve. Early endometriosis (minimal and mild stage) results in decreased fecundability (the probability of becoming pregnant in one menstrual cycle). The biochemical and hormonal changes that occur in endometriosis may have an effect on sperm motility and tubal peristalsis.

Although the diagnosis may be suggested by the history, it cannot be made with any certainty on symptoms alone. Even a pelvic examination, which at times can be quite distinctive, cannot be considered pathognomonic. Tender, nodular uterosacral ligaments combined with a fixed, retroverted uterus are findings highly suggestive of endometriosis, but inflammation and cancer cannot be ruled out by bimanual examination.

CA-125, the antigenic determinant of the monoclonal antibody OC-125, is found on the surface of coelomic epithelium and can be elevated in some patients with moderate and severe endometriosis. However, it may be elevated with multiple benign and malignant conditions that cause peritoneal inflammation. Although the low specificity of the assay rules it out as a screening test for endometriosis, in the future other cell surface proteins, specific for endometriosis tissue, may be found and detected by immunoassay techniques.

Standard radiography, ultrasonography, CT scans, and MRI have had little or no impact on improving the diagnosis of endometriosis. Ultrasound imaging is currently used to aid in the diagnosis of endometriomas.

For definitive diagnosis, endoscopic visualization of the pelvis can be carried out prior to therapy. When lesions are identified and doubt still remains, confirmatory transendoscopic biopsy should be performed. A complete laparoscopic pelvic and peritoneal cavity inspection should be carried out. One of several available instruments for uterine manipulation and transuterine tubal dye instillation should be secured in the cervical canal. The palpating probe can be used to run over various structures, e.g. the uterosacral ligaments, to detect subperitoneal implants. Each ovary must be lifted to visualize the undersurface adjoining the broad ligaments. The appendix and the serosa of any bowel in the pelvis should be carefully inspected for endometriotic implants.

Uniformity in classification has helped categorize and analyze the success or failure of the various endometriosis therapeutic modalities. The most widely accepted classification, utilizing the degree of active disease or adhesions involving the peritoneum, ovaries, and tubes, is from the American Society for Reproductive Medicine (ASRM), which uses four stages: I (minimal), II (mild), III (moderate), and IV (severe). Points are assigned based on dimensional spread in three categories: 1 cm, 1–3 cm, and 3 cm. Although the classification fails to address the very important area of depth of invasion, it does permit an immediate operating room recording of the general spread of active disease and adhesions.

Therapy

The therapeutic approach to endometriosis must be individualized according to the patient's current reproductive status and desires: infertility, symptoms in a patient wishing to retain future fertility, or symptoms in a patient with severe disease with no desire to preserve reproductive function.

Infertility

When therapy is indicated, conservative surgery and ovarian stimulation or assisted reproductive technology (ART) are the treatments of choice. As all medical therapies for endometriosis prevent conception, they should not be utilized in the infertility patient with endometriosis. Initially, a complete infertility work-up is indicated in these women with identification and treatment of all reversible causes of infertility. A randomized controlled trial has demonstrated higher fecundability in women who underwent laparoscopic endometriosis excision compared to a similar group of women with stage I/II endometriosis, who had no laparoscopic therapy of their implants [12]. After laparoscopy, to improve fecundability, ovarian stimulation combined with intrauterine insemination (IUI) should be utilized. If pregnancy has not occurred, *in vitro* fertilization (IVF), should be considered. With significant stage III/IV endometriosis, conservative surgery is the therapeutic choice with, at best, a postsurgical pregnancy rate of 25–45% prior to the consideration of ART.

These surgeries should only be carried out by a highly trained, skilled operator. Even in experienced hands, endometriosis with large adnexal masses, extensive adhesions, and/or intestinal involvement may not be safely amenable to endoscopic surgery.

If no pregnancy occurs postoperatively, even with ovarian stimulation and IUI, IVF remains the best chance for pregnancy in those women with severe endometriosis.

Desire to retain reproductive function + symptoms

After laparoscopic diagnosis, staging, and initial resection, the woman with symptomatic endometriosis who is not infertile but wishes to retain reproductive potential should be treated with hormonal suppression. If operative laparoscopy was used and visible endometriosis eliminated, the patient may become symptom free. If endometriosis and symptoms still exist after laparoscopy, or recur after operative laparoscopy, hormonal suppression should be utilized. As rupture while on therapy may occur, these regimens are not recommended in the presence of significant ovarian endometriomas, which should be surgically excised. The patient should be informed that any hormonal therapy of endometriosis is suppressive rather than curative and, after an interval of nontreatment, repeat therapy may be indicated for recurrent symptomatology. Multiple treatment courses with one or another therapeutic agent may have to be interspersed between months or years of pain-free, therapy-free intervals.

Ectopic endometrium responds to steroid hormones in the same way as intrauterine endometrium. The hypothalamic-pituitary-ovarian axis is suppressed, so the implants lose central stimulation and, with menstrual cessation, further implant seeding is prevented. The drugs may also act directly on the implants to inhibit growth and aid resolution. Any type of medical therapy improves symptoms in the majority of patients. So, the therapeutic choice depends on the side-effect profiles, long-term use, and cost. There is no evidence that any of the current methods affect long-term future fertility.

Oral contraceptive pills (OCPs) are effective in reducing dysmenorrhea, especially in early-stage disease, when used in conjunction with nonsteroidal anti-inflammatory drugs (NSAIDs). This fact, combined with their low rate of side effects, makes OCPs a good choice in mild-to-moderate dysmenorrhea. Any low-dose monophasic combination pill with a high progestin/estrogen ratio used continuously (daily) for 6–9 months can be effective in treating symptomatic endometriosis. If breakthrough bleeding occurs, the dose can be doubled or tripled, and continued until the bleeding has stopped, when the dose can be incrementally dropped back to the original. Any contraindications to OCPs should be ascertained prior to the start of therapy.

Progestin-only therapy can relieve pelvic pain. In randomized trials, intramuscular depo-medroxyprogesterone acetate (DMPA) was as effective as GnRH agonists in symptom reduction [13]. While there is some bone density loss during prolonged DMPA treatment, it is completely reversible after DMPA cessation. Common side effects include irregular bleeding, which may occur in 30% of patients, and prolonged, post-therapy amenorrhea, which will adversely affect any immediate attempts at fertility. The most studied oral agent, medroxyprogesterone acetate (MPA), is effective in relieving pain starting at a dose of 30 mg/day (10 mg three times a day), which can be increased depending on clinical response and bleeding patterns. Trials have demonstrated efficacy in symptom relief with the levonorgestrel-releasing intrauterine device.

GnRH agonists have been approved for use in endometriosis. The most commonly used drug is leuprolide acetate, 3.75 mg IM per month, or 11.25 mg, depot, every 3 months. In downregulating and desensitizing the pituitary to produce low levels of circulating estrogen, the GnRH agonist produces a medical oophorectomy. The three most common side effects are associated with estrogen deprivation: hot flushes, vaginal dryness, and insomnia, but, as GnRH agonists have no effect on sex hormone-binding globulin, no significant changes occur in free testosterone, total serum cholesterol or HDL/LDL levels. Although a decrease in bone mineral density of the trabecular bone in the lumbar spine results in a 2–7% decrease of bone mass over the usual 6 months of therapy, complete recovery occurs 12–24 months after discontinuing therapy. Ideally, if a pregnancy test is negative, GnRH agonist therapy should be started in the luteal phase rather than the follicular because serum estradiol levels are reduced faster and amenorrhea occurs within 3–4 weeks instead of 6–8 weeks. After 6 months of GnRH agonist treatment, ovarian function will return to normal in 6–12 weeks. To reduce or eliminate the common GnRH agonist side effects, add-back hormonal replacement therapy with doses similar to menopausal treatment can be used simultaneously. Add-back doses are not high enough to interfere with the GnRH inhibition of endometriotic growth.

Severe disease with no desire to preserve reproductive function

For the woman with moderate or severe pelvic pain who has completed her family, a total abdominal hysterectomy is the therapeutic choice. If the ovaries are involved or other endometriotic areas remain, a bilateral salpingo- oophorectomy could be considered. Any remaining endometriosis will become fibrotic and scar without endogenous ovarian stimulation. When the ovaries are preserved, for example in a young woman or by patient desire, and residual endometriosis is present, postoperative hormonal suppression for 3–6 months will suppress any residual disease. After hysterectomy and bilateral salpingo- oophorectomy, estrogen replacement therapy can be used. However, as low a dose as possible should be prescribed. If residual endometriosis remains after removal of the uterus and ovaries, oral contraceptive therapy or DMPA, rather than estrogen alone, could be given for 3–6 months. Theoretically, estrogen-only therapy might activate any residual disease but, other than case reports, there are no hard data suggesting that this would happen. Ovarian conservation at the time of hysterectomy for severe endometriosis has a relative risk (RR) for pain recurrence of 6.1 and a RR for reoperation of 8.1 compared to bilateral oophorectomy, but removing both ovaries requires the patient to use hormonal replacement therapy (HRT) [14]. Without the use of HRT, bothersome menopausal symptoms and a significant risk for osteoporosis will occur. Although HRT may reduce these events, long-term HRT use has low patient compliance rates, so the risks and benefits of bilateral oophorectomy require careful preoperative consideration by both the patient and her physician.

It were not best that we should all think alike; it is the difference of opinion that makes horse races. (Mark Twain, 1889)

References

1. Olive DL, Schwartz LB. Endometriosis. *NEJM* 1993; 328: 1759.
2. Missmer SA, Hankinson SE, Spiegelman D, *et al*. Incidence of laparoscopically confirmed endometriosis by demographic, anthropometric, and lifestyle factors. *Am J Epidemiol* 2004; 160: 784.
3. Sangi-Haghpeykar H, Poindexter,AN. Epidemiology of endometriosis among parous women. *Obstet Gynecol* 1995; 85: 983.
4. Laufer MR, Goitein L, Bush M, *et al*. Prevalence of endometriosis in adolescent girls with chronic pelvic pain not responding to conventional therapy. *J Pediatr Adolesc Gynecol* 1997; 10: 199.
5. Eskenazi B, Warner M. Epidemiology of endometriosis. *Obstet Gynecol Clin North Am* 1997; 24: 235–258.
6. Ishii K, Takakuwa K, Mitsui T, Tanaka K. Studies on the human leukocyte antigen-DR in patients with endometriosis: genotyping of HLA-DRB1 alleles. *Hum Reprod* 2002; 17: 560.
7. Oosterlynck DJ, Cornillie FJ, Waer M, *et al*. Women with endometriosis show a defect in natural killer activity resulting in a decreased cytotoxicity to autologous endometrium. *Fertil Steril* 1991; 56: 45.
8. Nishida M, Nasu K, Ueda T, Fukuda J, Takai N, Miyakawa I. Endometriotic cells are resistant to interferon-gamma-induced cell growth inhibition and apoptosis: a possible mechanism involved in the pathogenesis of endometriosis. *Hum Reprod* 2005; 11: 29.
9. Sinaii N, Cleary SD, Ballweg ML, *et al*. High rates of autoimmune and endocrine disorders, fibromyalgia, chronic fatigue syndrome and atopic diseases among women with endometriosis: a survey analysis. *Hum Reprod* 2002; 17: 2715.
10. Dmowski W, Gebel H, Braun D. The role of cell-mediated immunity in pathogenesis of endometriosis. *Acta Obstet Gynecol Scand* 1994; 159(suppl): 7.
11. Simpson J, Elias S, Malinuk L, *et al*. Heritable aspects of endometriosis in genetic studies. *Am J Obstet Gynecol* 1980; 137: 327.
12. Olive D, Lee K. Analysis of sequential treatment protocols for endometriosis-associated infertility. *Am J Obstet Gynecol* 1986; 154: 613.
13. Crosignani P, Luciano A, Ray A, Bergquist A. Subcutaneous depot medroxyprogesterone acetate versus leuprolide acetate in the treatment of endometriosis-associated pain. *Hum Reprod* 2006; 21: 248.
14. Namnoum AB, Hickman TN, Goodman SB, *et al*. Incidence of symptom recurrence after hysterectomy for endometriosis. *Fertil Steril* 1995; 64: 898.

Chapter 70
Urinary Incontinence

John Klutke and Begüm Özel
Department of Medicine and Obstetrics and Gynecology, Keck School of Medicine, University of Southern California, CA, USA

Introduction

Urinary incontinence is defined by the International Continence Society (ICS) as the involuntary loss of urine. The condition is very common among women. Even among young, nulliparous women, there are reports that half have experienced incontinence at one time or another and 16% suffer from this problem daily. Established risk factors include pregnancy, obesity, aging, and functional impairment. Family history may also be a risk factor. Data regarding ethnicity and urinary incontinence are conflicting. Previous definitions of urinary incontinence included the requisite that the involuntary loss of urine be "socially embarrassing." However, this is no longer part of the ICS definition. While any amount of incontinence is abnormal, only when the incontinence has progressed to the point where it is bothersome to the patient does it require treatment.

Urinary incontinence can be caused by lowered urethral resistance (stress urinary incontinence), inappropriate elevation of bladder pressure (urge urinary incontinence) or when anatomic urethral resistance is bypassed (such as a fistula, diverticulum or ectopic ureter). Accurate diagnosis of urinary incontinence is crucial, since treatment depends on the underlying etiology. A fourth cause, overflow incontinence, is uncommon in women, although obstruction of the urethra due to leiomyomata, a gravid uterus or severe prolapse has been reported. Neuropathy resulting from diabetes mellitus, multiple sclerosis or other neurologic lesions can also present with bladder overflow.

The medical morbidity associated with urinary incontinence includes skin breakdown and infections from constant skin moisture and irritation from incontinence pads, falls and fractures from slipping on urine or falling during attempts to reach the bathroom quickly, urinary tract infections and possible urosepsis from urinary retention and catheter use, and sleep disruption from nocturia. In addition, women often suffer from poor self-esteem, social withdrawal, isolation, sexual dysfunction and depression as a result of their incontinence. Urinary incontinence remains one of the leading reasons for nursing home placement.

Stress incontinence

Definitions

Stress urinary incontinence (SUI) is the complaint of involuntary loss of urine on effort or physical exertion (e.g. sporting activities) or on sneezing or coughing. Urodynamic stress incontinence (USI) is the involuntary leakage of urine during filling cystometry, associated with increased intra-abdominal pressure, in the absence of a detrusor contraction.

Diagnosis

The diagnosis may be established in three phases. The first two phases should provide enough information to establish the diagnosis in most patients. Phase III requires sophisticated urodynamic testing and is required only for certain women with risk factors such as previous surgical failures, combined SUI and urge urinary incontinence (UUI) symptoms, following radical pelvic surgery or radiation therapy, or when a negative Q-Tip test is identified.

Phase I
History and physical examination
A detailed questionnaire completed by the patient, followed by history taking, can guide the physician, but history alone is unreliable for establishing a diagnosis. Studies have shown that the history of "pure" SUI was urodynamically confirmed in 70–75% of cases, while the history of "pure" urge incontinence was urodynamically confirmed in only 50% of cases.

Management of Common Problems in Obstetrics and Gynecology, 5th edition. Edited by T.M. Goodwin, M.N. Montoro, L. Muderspach, R. Paulson and S. Roy. © 2010 Blackwell Publishing Ltd.

The physical examination should include the neurologic evaluation of the S2–S4 lower micturition center, since urinary incontinence may be secondary to central nervous system lesions. This evaluation includes testing the sensation in the inner thighs, perirectal, and vulvar areas (sensory dermatomes representing S2–S4). The bulbocavernous reflex, a gentle squeeze or tap to the clitoris resulting in reflex contraction of the perirectal muscle, confirms an intact motor component of S2–S4, where the lower micturition center is located; however, it is not often used in common practice due to patient discomfort. The anal wink reflex, a reflex contraction of the anal sphincter in response to stroking the perianal skin, is more commonly applied clinically but may be absent in 20% of neurologically intact women.

Postvoid residual

Although overflow incontinence is unusual in women, it is essential to rule it out in the initial phase of diagnosis. Measurement of postvoid residual (PVR) urine volume is useful in this respect. The volume of urine remaining in the bladder after spontaneous voiding is measured by catheterization or ultrasound. To be useful, the volume voided should be greater than 200 cc. There is no consensus as to what is considered a normal PVR, but most specialists in the field define it as either less than 50 mL and/or less than 20% of the total voided volume. Isolated elevations of PVR should be confirmed by repeat evaluation. If the PVR is consistently greater than 200 mL, overflow incontinence is suspected.

Urinalysis, urine culture and sensitivity

A midstream urine culture should be taken at the time of initial evaluation. Urinary infection can masquerade as any lower urinary tract pathology, including SUI or UUI. Diagnosis of incontinence made at the time of unsuspected urinary tract infection is inaccurate in at least half of patients.

Bladder diary

Bladder diaries are patient recordings of the time and volume of all fluid intake as well as continence and incontinence voids. Clinically, 3-day diaries are most commonly used. Diaries can provide information on the usual timing and circumstances of urinary incontinence, amount of urine per void, voiding frequency, and urinary incontinence frequency, and the total daytime and nocturnal urine output.

Phase II

Cystourethroscopy

Cystourethroscopy may be performed in the clinic using either carbon dioxide or a fluid medium, although fluid medium is fairly standard. The cystourethroscope is used to examine the urethra, trigone and bladder for gross pathology. The urethrovesical junction (UVJ) is examined dynamically. The response to "hold urine," in the absence of peripheral neuropathy, should be that the UVJ will close. The response to cough and the Valsalva maneuver should also be that the UVJ should close as a reflex mechanism; in SUI and weak urethral sphincter, the UVJ often funnels and opens with cough or Valsalva. The cystourethroscope is slowly withdrawn along the urethra while it is distended, allowing a thorough examination for diverticula, which may simulate SUI or exudate, since urethritis may simulate UUI.

Cotton-tipped swab (Q-Tip) test

A sterile cotton-tipped swab, lubricated with lidocaine jelly, is introduced into the urethra and advanced to the UVJ. Using the orthopedic goniometer, the resting and straining angles of the Q-Tip to the horizontal are measured. There is no consensus as to what defines a positive Q-Tip test, but a starting angle greater than 45° or a change of greater than 30° is generally indicative of poor support of the UVJ. A negative Q-Tip test should raise doubt about the diagnosis of SUI and more sophisticated urodynamic tests should then be ordered.

Stress test or simple (single channel) cystometry

For women with isolated SUI symptoms without other risk factors such as prior incontinence surgery, negative Q-Tip, a history of radiation therapy or a history of radical pelvic surgery, a stress test or simple cystometry may be sufficient. The stress test is performed by asking the patient to stand and cough with a full bladder.

Simple cystometry is performed with a single catheter in the bladder, in the standing position, with periodic cough provocations. The bladder is usually filled with a fluid medium (saline or sterile water), and the intravesical (bladder) pressures are measured during the procedure. An increase in intravesical pressure >15 cm H_2O above baseline suggests detrusor overactivity (DO). Increased intra-abdominal pressure, such as with Valsalva, will also result in an increase in intravesical pressure and cannot be differentiated from DO on simple cystometry. DO should always be ruled out before the diagnosis of SUI is established since bladder contractions induced by cough can result in symptoms and clinical findings of SUI. If simple cystometry suggests DO, then multichannel urodynamics is indicated.

In cases of pure SUI where cystourethroscopy demonstrates a weak sphincter and no other pathology, the Q-Tip test demonstrates poor support to the UVJ, and the stress test or simple cystometry does not suggest DO, the diagnosis of SUI can be established, and the phase III evaluation is not required. If any of these tests is inconsistent with SUI, phase III urodynamic evaluation is necessary.

Phase III
Multichannel urodynamics
Concomitant pressures in the bladder, urethra, and abdomen are recorded with catheters placed in the bladder, urethra and vagina or rectum, respectively, while filling the bladder with fluid medium. Detrusor pressures (pressure generated by the detrusor muscle of the bladder) can be calculated by subtracting abdominal pressure from intravesical pressure. If a rise in intravesical pressure is seen, these multiple recordings allow for determination as to whether this rise is due to DO or an increase in intra-abdominal pressure such as with Valsalva. A detrusor contraction is defined as a rise in detrusor pressure > 15 cm H_2O above baseline or > 10 cm H_2O above baseline with associated urgency.

Multichannel urodynamics will detect small detrusor contractions as well as urethral relaxation incompetence ("urethral instability"), which is leakage due to urethral relaxation in the absence of raised abdominal pressure or a detrusor contraction. The test performed in the supine position will diagnose 85% of patients with DO, while the test performed in the standing position with cough provocation will diagnose 98% of patients with DO.

Abdominal leak point pressure (LPP)
This is defined as the lowest value of the intentionally increased intravesical pressure that provokes urinary leakage in the absence of a detrusor contraction. The increase in pressure is usually induced by Valsalva (Valsalva LPP). LPP values might also be affected by many other factors such as the technique to confirm urine loss, catheter size, bladder volume, and patient position. These should all be standardized. A low abdominal LPP is suggestive of poor urethral function although it has not been correlated with failure of specific surgical procedures.

Urethral pressure profiles
Urethral pressure profiles are performed along the urethra, while bladder and abdominal pressures are concomitantly recorded. A diagnosis of SUI and low maximum urethral closure pressure on resting urethral pressure profile (< 20 cm H_2O) is associated with high failure rates for the Burch or Marshall–Marchetti–Kantz (MMK) colposuspension and thus requires a sling procedure.

Voiding cystometry or pressure flow study
This is the pressure volume relationship of the bladder during micturition. Measurements to be recorded are the intravesical, intra-abdominal and detrusor pressures and the urine flow rate. This testing is useful in women with symptoms or signs of voiding dysfunction.

Urge incontinence

Definitions
Urge incontinence is the complaint of involuntary loss of urine associated with urgency. Urgency is a sudden, compelling desire to pass urine which is difficult to defer. Detrusor overactivity is when involuntary detrusor muscle contractions occur during filling cystometry. Overactive bladder (OAB) syndrome is urinary urgency, usually accompanied by frequency and nocturia, with or without urgency urinary incontinence, in the absence of urinary tract infection or other obvious pathology.

Pathophysiology
Detrusor overactivity may sometimes be secondary to a central nervous system lesion. If a primary central nervous system lesion is identified, the bladder condition is defined as neurogenic detrusor overactivity. If no neurologic abnormality can be identified, the condition is defined as idiopathic detrusor overactivity, which accounts for 90% of cases. Neurologic screening tests of S2–S4 lower micturition center (sensory dermatomes of lower extremities and the bulbocavernous and anal wink reflexes as described earlier) are essential to rule out central neuropathy that may result in DO.

Extraurethral ("bypass") incontinence

Extraurethral incontinence refers to the observation of urine leakage through channels other than the urethral meatus, for example through a fistula or an ectopic ureter. When attempting to make a diagnosis of a fistula into the vagina, a "cotton ball test" (rather than a "tampon test") can be performed by packing the vagina with several cotton balls and filling the bladder with methylene blue-tinted fluid. The patient is asked to ambulate for a few minutes and then the cotton balls are removed. If only the most distal cotton ball is blue, then loss of urine may be due to urethral incontinence rather than a fistula, but a careful exam for an urethrovaginal fistula must be performed. If the more proximal cotton balls are blue, a fistula between the bladder and vagina is likely to be present. Once the diagnosis is established, the treatment is surgical closure of the fistula. Urethral diverticula may be diagnosed by careful exam and/or urethroscopy and confirmed by urethrography (using a Trattner catheter). A surgical correction is needed for symptomatic diverticula.

Treatment of urinary incontinence

Stress urinary incontinence
Weight loss
There are several studies suggesting that weight loss can decrease episodes of SUI. Weight loss should be

recommended to all obese (BMI > 30 kg/m^2) women during their initial evaluation for urinary incontinence.

Pelvic floor (Kegel's) exercises

Pelvic floor exercises promote hypertrophy and thickening of the striated periurethral muscle and thus strengthen the muscular components of the urethral closure mechanism. The patient tightens her pubococcygeus muscle (which she learns to identify by starting and stopping her urine stream without moving her legs). The basic recommended regimen is three sets of 8–12 slow-velocity contractions sustained for 6–8 seconds each, performed daily and continued for at least 15–20 weeks. Significant improvement or cure is reported in > 50% of patients who remain compliant with the therapy.

Biofeedback

Biofeedback is used as an adjunct to pelvic floor exercises to teach correct muscle contraction. It is generally performed under the direct supervision of a therapist trained in the technique.

Electrical stimulation

Electrical stimulation of the pudendal nerve through the vagina or rectum causes a contraction of the striated periurethral muscle. The mechanism of action and treatment duration are similar to pelvic floor exercises.

Vaginal pessary

A vaginal pessary mechanically supports the bladder base and restores the urethra to an intra-abdominal position. It also increases urethral resistance to prevent the loss of urine associated with increases in abdominal pressure.

Surgical therapy for stress incontinence

Although many different surgical procedures for stress incontinence have been developed through the history of pelvic surgery, the most common surgical procedures performed today are the retropubic (Burch) colposuspension, proximal (bladder neck) slings and midurethral (retropubic or transobturator) slings.

Risks of surgery

Although surgery for stress incontinence is frequently necessary, it should be chosen as a last resort since it is an invasive therapy. Surgery for stress incontinence offers, at best, a compensatory abnormality. Even when restoring stress continence, it has the potential to alter other aspects of pelvic function, including the ability to empty the bladder, normal bladder sensation and sexual function. In addition to the risks of anesthesia, infection, and bleeding, there are certain risks associated with all anti-incontinence procedures that must be reviewed with the patient in the preoperative counseling. These risks include the potential for failure of the procedure, urinary retention, prolonged catheterization, the development of *de novo* urge incontinence, dyspareunia, and other negative effects on sexual function.

Retropubic colposuspension

A retropubic colposuspension, such as the Burch procedure, is often used when an abdominal incision is already planned, such as concomitant to an abdominal hysterectomy or sacral colpopexy. It is also an option in a patient who refuses mesh placement or has had a mesh complications in the past. In the Burch procedure, the endopelvic fascia adjacent to the mid and proximal urethra is attached to the pectineal (Cooper's) ligaments on the posterior surface of the superior pubic ramus on both sides. The Burch procedure has been shown to be more effective than the MMK procedure, in which the periosteum of the posterior pubic symphysis is used rather than Cooper's ligament, and is thus the preferred approach. In addition, the MMK procedure has been associated with osteitis pubis in 1% of cases. The Burch colposuspension has the best documentation of long-term success of any anti-incontinence procedure, in the range of 70–90%. The Burch procedure has been shown to have a high failure rate in women with a maximum urethral closure pressure of less than 20 cm H$_2$O and should not be used in these women.

Proximal (bladder neck) slings

In the bladder neck sling, a hammock of tissue is placed beneath the proximal urethra via a vaginal incision. The two ends are then passed behind the pubic bone to the anterior abdominal wall, where they are secured to the rectus fascia. This hammock may be composed of autografts (rectus fascia or fascia lata), allografts, xenografts and synthetic mesh. The bladder neck slings have been shown to be highly efficacious and more effective than the Burch colposuspension in one large, multicenter, randomized controlled trial. However, these slings are associated with higher rates of voiding difficulty, urinary tract infections, and *de novo* urge incontinence. They are generally reserved for women who have failed other surgical therapies.

Midurethral slings

The midurethral slings are minimally invasive slings first introduced in 1998 with the tension-free vaginal tape (TVT) procedure. The TVT introduced several modifications to the bladder neck slings and resulted in a revolutionary change in how stress incontinence is surgically managed. These modifications were midurethral placement, no suture fixation of the sling mesh, no tension placed on the urethra, and minimal dissection. In addition, mobility of the proximal urethra is now understood to be normal and, in fact, important for the initiation of voiding. Surgery should avoid interference with the mobility of the urethra. The use of a cough stress test intraoperatively can minimize the potential to cause voiding disturbance by providing a physiologic feedback that guides the surgeon in applying outlet resistance.

The concept of surgical wounding and its effect on the nervous system, which has been explored in the anesthesia literature, has been applied in the arena of anti-incontinence surgery, through the use of local anesthetic as a means of pre-emptive block to reduce negative neurologic consequences.

It is appropriate to attribute much of the recent improvement in surgical therapy to the work of Ulf Ulmsten. Ulmsten's original concepts and his insistence on scrutinizing them with rigorous scientific methodology are laudable and represent a milestone in the evolution of surgical practice. Even so, more than 10 years after introduction of the TVT procedure, technical limitations are apparent. Although serious complications associated with the procedure are uncommon, stress incontinence is an exceedingly common condition. With experience totaling hundreds of thousands of women, it has become apparent that serious complications can result from the TVT procedure and the other retropubic midurethral slings that copy it. Injuries in the colon, small bowel, urethra, bladder vasculature, fallopian tube and ovary have been associated with the procedure, as have erosions of the sling material into the vagina, bladder, and urethra. Bleeding, hematoma, abscess formation, retention and voiding dysfunction can occur. The most feared of these complications is bowel perforation. Not only is it potentially fatal, but also the injury occurs blindly and recognition is usually not immediate. The TVT is a blind procedure, with needle passage occurring in proximity to the bowel, and even experienced, well-trained surgeons may encounter this complication.

A frank discussion should be undertaken with the patient regarding realistic expectations of anti-incontinence surgery. Connective tissue abnormalities are recognizable in women with incontinence, and these are abnormalities that surgery does not address. Midurethral slings result in a dense, collagen-rich structure in the anterior vagina, rather like a ligament, which is not normally present in the vagina. Although an effective compensatory procedure, anti-incontinence surgeries do not correct the underlying defect responsible for stress incontinence, thus surgical therapy is not perfect. As with surgery for prolapse, recurrence of incontinence symptoms because of an ongoing connective tissue problem is always possible. This connective tissue defect is time dependent and difficult to predict.

In the continuing effort to evaluate and improve surgical therapy for incontinence, the transobturator (TOT) approach has recently reached mainstream clinical practice.

It is a type of midurethral sling and incorporates the concepts of midurethral placement, the use of local anesthesia and an intraoperative cough stress test. We use TOT as a first-line surgical treatment for stress incontinence in the majority of women. In most respects, the transobturator and retropubic midurethral sling procedures are identical. Both use a hammock-like strip of polypropylene placed beneath the midurethra for support. The main difference is in technique: with transobturator placement, the introducer needle passes through the obturator foramen and remains superficial to the urogenital diaphragm. By avoiding blind retropubic needle passage, there is less potential for injury to bowel, bladder or large vessels. One systematic review found that the transobturator approach was associated with a lower overall risk of complications (OR 0.40, 95% CI 0.19–0.83), including perioperative hematoma, infection, vascular or bladder injury. There are some data to suggest that women with maximum urethral closure pressure less than 42 cmH$_2$O and abdominal LPP less than 60 cmH$_2$O might not do as well with the TOT and might benefit from a retropubic sling procedure.

Urge urinary incontinence/detrusor overactivity
Anticholinergic medications
Tolterodine, oxybutinin, solifenacin, and other similar anticholinergic agents have been shown to be more effective than placebo in the treatment of women with urge urinary incontinence, although the absolute benefit over placebo is small; compared to placebo, these medications result in 40% higher rate of cure or improvement. Side effects often limit the use of these medications. Dry mouth may affect up to 70–80% of women, and constipation can also be a significant problem. Dosing should be titrated according to the response and side effect tolerance of the individual patient. An initial trial of at least 4 weeks is recommended before abandoning treatment.

Vaginal estrogen therapy
Vaginal estrogen therapy may benefit postmenopausal women with UUI who also have symptoms or signs of vaginal atrophy.

Behavior modification (bladder drills)
The aim of this treatment is to regain cortical inhibitory control over the bladder. These treatments are effective in > 70% of patients but require prolonged treatment, a motivated patient, and dedicated personnel.

Electrical stimulation
Electrical stimulation of the pudendal nerve through the vagina or rectum causes reflex inhibition of the pelvic nerve (which innervates the detrusor muscle) through inhibition of the lower micturition center.

Sacral neuromodulation (sacral nerve stimulation)

Sacral nerve stimulation is a minimally invasive procedure that involves implanting a modulator in the patient's buttock area, much like a pacemaker, and has been shown to be effective in some women with refractory cases of detrusor overactivity. The exact mechanism is uncertain.

Botulinum toxin

This therapy is currently under investigation. Botulinum toxin A is injected directly into the detrusor muscle via cystoscopy. Urinary retention is the major complication. Repeated courses of the treatment are usually necessary as the effect of the toxin is only temporary. Studies have been small, and dosage and safety have not yet been established.

Extraurethral incontinence
Fistula

Urethrovaginal or vesicovaginal fistulas, which are not secondary to irradiation or tumor, can be corrected vaginally or abdominally.

Ectopic ureter

The collecting system can be connected end-to-side to the other ureter. An intravenous pyelogram is required prior to such a procedure.

Urethral diverticula

Diverticula are usually treated only if they are symptomatic. If the diverticulum is small and distal to the area of maximal urethral pressure, a simple Spence procedure (marsupialization) may be adequate.

Suggested reading

Anast JW, Skolarus TA, Yan Y, Klutke CG. Transobturator sling with intraoperative cough test is effective for patients with low valsalva leak point pressure. *Can J Urol* 2008 ; 15(4): 4153–4157.

Bergman A. Office work-up of lower urinary tract dysfunctions and indications for referral for urodynamic testing. *Obstet Gynecol Clin North Am* 1989; 16: 787.

Bergman A, Bhatia NN. Effect of urinary tract infection upon urethral and bladder function. *Obstet Gynecol* 1985; 66: 366.

Bergman A, Ballard CA, Koonings PP. Comparison of three different surgical procedures for genuine stress incontinence: prospective randomized study. *Am J Obstet Gynecol* 1989; 160: 1102.

Bullock TL, Ghoniem G, Klutke CG, Staskin DR. Advances in female stress urinary incontinence: mid-urethral slings. *BJU Int* 2006; 98(suppl 1): 32–40; discussion 41–42.

Castillo OA, Bodden E, Olivaries RA, Urena RD. Intestinal perforation: an infrequent complication during insertion of tension-free vaginal tape. *J Urol* 2004; 172: 1364.

Cindolo L, Salzano L, Rota G, *et al*. Tension-free transobturator approach for female stress urinary incontinence. *Minerva Urol Nefrol* 2003; 55: 89–98.

Costa P, Grise P, Droupy S, *et al*. Surgical treatment of female stress urinary incontinence with trans obturator tape (T.O.T.) Uratape: short term results of a prospective multicenter study. *Eur Urol* 2004; 46(1): 102–106.

Delorme E. Transobturator urethral suspension: mini-invasive procedure in the treatment of stress urinary incontinence in women. *Prog Urol* 2001; 11(6): 1306–1313.

Delorme E, Droupy S, de Tayrac R, Delmas V. Tranobturator tape: a new minimally invasive procedure to treat female urinary incontinence. *Eur Urol* 2004; 45: 203–207.

Karram MM, Bhatia NN. The Q-tip test: standardization of the technique and interpretation in women with urinary incontinence. *Obstet Gynecol* 1988; 71: 807.

Klutke C, Siegel S, Carlin B, *et al*. Urinary retention after tension-free vaginal tape procedure: incidence and treatment. *Urology* 2001; 58(5): 697–701.

Minaglia S, Ozel B, Klutke C, Ballard C, Klutke J. Bladder injury during transobturator sling. *Urology* 2004; 64(2): 376–377.

Minaglia S, Ozel B, Hurtado E, Klutke CG, Klutke JJ. Effect of transobturator tape procedure on proximal urethral mobility. *Urology* 2005; 65(1): 55–59.

Petros PEP, Ulmsten UI. An integral theory of female urinary incontinence: experimental and clinical considerations. *Acta Obstet Gynecol Scand* 1990; 69(suppl 153): 7–31.

Tamussino KF, Hanzal E, Kolle D, *et al*. Tension-free vaginal tape operation: results of the Austrian registry. *Obstet Gynecol* 2001; 98(5 Pt 1): 732–736.

Ulmsten U, Johnson P, Rezapour M. A 3 year follow-up of TVT for surgical treatment of female urinary stress incontinence. *BJOG* 1990; 106(4): 345–350.

Ulmsten U, Henriksson L, Johnson P, Varhos G. An ambulatory surgical procedure under local anesthesia for treatment of female urinary incontinence. *Int Urogynecol J Pelvic Floor Dysfunct* 1996; 7(2): 81–85.

Chapter 71
Urinary Tract Injuries

Micheline Wong and Begüm Özel
Department of Medicine and Obstetrics and Gynecology, Keck School of Medicine, University of Southern California, CA, USA

Introduction

Hysterectomy is the most common gynecologic surgery performed worldwide, with 500,000–600,000 hysterectomies performed in the United States each year. Hysterectomy is also one of the most common causes of iatrogenic urinary tract injury because of the frequency with which the surgery is performed and the close proximity of the upper female genital tract to the urinary tract. Historically, gynecologic surgery accounted for most cases of urinary tract injury, but this has changed over the years with fewer hysterectomies and more procedures in urology, vascular, colorectal, and orthopedic surgery being performed. In one recent review, gynecologic surgery accounted for 34% of ureteral injuries, still coming second to urologic procedures, which accounted for 42% of such injuries. Minimally invasive urologic surgery has now become the most common cause of iatrogenic urinary tract injury.

Urinary tract injury during gynecologic surgery requires longer operative time for repair, longer hospital stay, prolonged bladder catheterization, and repeat surgery if unrecognized at the time of initial procedure. Women with urinary tract injury during abdominal hysterectomy were found to have greater blood loss, more febrile morbidity, and more frequent transfusions. There may be complications of the repair, such as fistula formation, ureterovesical reflux or ureteral stricture, which can result in further surgery for the patient. These may all result in more pain, days lost from work, anxiety, depression, and worsening quality of life for the patient.

In a study published in 2005 in which universal cystoscopy was performed, among 471 hysterectomies (abdominal, vaginal and laparoscopic), the total urinary tract injury rate was 4.8% (1.7% ureteral injury, 3.6%

bladder injury); no difference in rate of injury by type of hysterectomy was identified. However, a recent meta-analysis of 30 studies found that urinary tract injuries are more common during laparoscopic hysterectomy (OR 2.61, 95% CI 1.22–5.60), although much of that is believed to be due to operator inexperience rather than to the approach itself. The rate of ureteral injury was lowest with vaginal hysterectomy (0.2 per 1000), followed by supracervical abdominal hysterectomy (0.5 per 1000), total abdominal hysterectomy (0.9 per 1000), and laparoscopic hysterectomy (7.3 per 1000). For bladder injury, the rates were 2.7, 0.3, 2.1, and 6.0 per 1000 for vaginal, supracervical abdominal, total abdominal, and laparoscopic hysterectomy, respectively. There does not appear to be a significant difference in rates of total urinary tract injury between total abdominal and vaginal hysterectomy, but ureteral injury may be more common with the total abdominal hysterectomy and bladder injury more common with vaginal hysterectomy. Possible predisposing factors for urinary tract injury are pelvic adhesions, distortion of normal pelvic anatomy, previous radiation, and history of previous pelvic surgery.

Bladder injury

Between 1968 and 1998, 155 incidental cystotomies occurred at Los Angeles County-University of Southern California (LAC-USC) Medical Center, with a rate of 1.2% for vaginal hysterectomy and 0.7% for abdominal hysterectomy.

Bladder injury during hysterectomy may be avoided by using sharp instead of blunt dissection when operating near the vesicouterine space. Utilizing the intrafascial rather than extrafascial technique of hysterectomy also aids in avoiding bladder injury. Many bladder injuries are easily identified at the time of surgery due to efflux of urine or visualization of the Foley catheter. However, if there is any suspicion of bladder injury, it is crucial for the surgeon fully to evaluate the bladder and ureters. Injury to the bladder can be confirmed by filling the bladder through a transurethral catheter with methylene blue dye.

Management of Common Problems in Obstetrics and Gynecology,
5th edition. Edited by T.M. Goodwin, M.N. Montoro,
L. Muderspach, R. Paulson and S. Roy. © 2010 Blackwell
Publishing Ltd.

Cystotomies can occur at the dome of the bladder when entering the peritoneum abdominally, near the base of the bladder when dissecting the vesicouterine space on an abdominal hysterectomy, when entering the peritoneum anteriorly on a vaginal hysterectomy, or during anterior colporrhaphy. Fortunately, most cystotomies heal rapidly if they are identified in a timely manner and repaired appropriately. Cystotomies can be repaired using 2-0 delayed absorbable suture in two to three layers. The first layer should be closed using continuous nonlocking or interrupted stitches through the mucosa and muscularis. A second continuous nonlocking imbricating stitch reinforces this first layer. A third layer is sometimes necessary; this layer may comprise the peritoneum. If the cystotomy is large or irregular, the bladder should be filled with fluid with or without methylene blue in order to confirm that the closure is watertight. Cystotomies that occur at the bladder dome can be drained for 3–5 days.

Injuries that occur at the base of the bladder are more complex because they are more frequently unrecognized, healing may be impaired due to contamination from vaginal flora, there is an increased likelihood of ureteral compromise, and a greater likelihood of fistula formation. The most common cause of injury to the bladder base is during entry into the anterior peritoneum during vaginal hysterectomy. A 2–3-layer closure as previously described should be performed, followed by cystoscopy with intravenous indigo carmine dye to confirm patent ureters. If the injury is large or lateral, assessment of ureteral patency and possible ureteral stent placement should precede any attempted repair. Whenever ureteral injury is suspected or if the injury is large or inaccessible, an abdominal approach should be considered for the repair. Because the bladder base is a dependent area, postoperative bladder drainage should be continued for 10–14 days.

In cases where the cystotomy is adjacent to the vaginal cuff, as commonly occurs during a hysterectomy, the bladder suture line should be covered with peritoneum to separate it from the vaginal suture line; alternatively, an omental graft may be placed. This serves to separate the two suture lines and prevent fistulization; the omental graft also brings in blood supply to the area to improve healing. Vaginally, a bulbocavernosus fat pad graft serves the same purpose but is relatively more involved; however, it should be considered in cases where there is extensive bladder injury.

Ureteral injury

Between 1968 and 1998, there were 44 ureteral injuries at the LAC-USC Medical Center, of which 33 were associated with total abdominal hysterectomy (TAH) and only

three were associated with total vaginal hysterectomy (TVH). Of the 44 ureteral injuries, there were 38 ureteral transections, three crush injuries, and three partial obstructions. Risk factors associated with ureteral injury include a large uterus, high-grade cystocele, ectopic insertion of the ureter into the bladder, endometriosis, ovarian neoplasm, distorted anatomy, cervical myomas, and previous pelvic surgery.

Injury to the ureter during hysterectomy most often occurs during ligation of the uterine arteries and cardinal ligaments. Other possible sites of injury are at the level of the ovarian vessels when ligating the infundibulopelvic ligaments if the course of the ureter is not completely visualized or if the dissection comes too close to the lateral side wall. The ureters may also be injured when closing the vaginal cuff, such as when placing angle stitches or performing a McCall's culdoplasty.

If the surgeon suspects that it may be difficult to identify the ureters, such as in cases of severe endometriosis or tubo-ovarian abscess, ureteral stents may be placed in the operating room prior to starting the case. However, if there are extensive adhesions and distorted anatomy, the ureter may not be palpable despite the presence of the stents. Familiarity with the retroperitoneal anatomy and confident ability to identify the course of the ureter are important for preventing inadvertent injury. Adequate surgical exposure of the operating field is also essential.

Outcomes following ureteral injury depend on a timely diagnosis of the injury. Repairs are most successful when performed immediately at the time of surgery. Immediate diagnosis also spares the patient a repeat trip to the operating room. Unfortunately, studies have reported recognition of ureteral injury at the time of initial surgery to be between 11% and 50%; at LAC-USC, only one-third of ureteral injuries have been detected at the time of surgery. Surgeons must always have a high index of suspicion and fully evaluate any potential injury. If there is any suspicion of ureteral injury, intraoperative cystoscopy should be performed at the time of hysterectomy. Alternatively, an extraperitoneal cystotomy at the dome of the bladder can facilitate direct visualization of the ureteral orifices. Intravenous indigo carmine dye is usually given and jets of blue from the ureteral orifices confirm patency. If no efflux of indigo carmine is seen, a fluid bolus or a diuretic such as furosemide can be given. After about 15–20 minutes, if still no efflux is seen, the surgeon may attempt to pass a 4 or 5 French ureteral stent through the ureteral orifice on the side where there is no ureteral jet. This should be performed only by a surgeon experienced with ureteral stenting due to the risk of ureteral perforation. Having the patient in the dorsal lithotomy position for all cases allows for easy access if cystoscopy is necessary for suspected ureteral injury.

Universal cystoscopy at the time of surgery has not been a common practice because of the fairly low incidence of urinary tract injuries. The cost-effectiveness of routine intraoperative cystoscopy depends on the rate of ureteral injury. If that rate exceeds 1.5% for abdominal hysterectomy and 2% for vaginal or laparoscopically assisted vaginal hysterectomy, then routine cystoscopy is considered cost-effective.

Unfortunately, ureteral injury is often not recognized until 1–2 days postoperatively. Most injuries are asymptomatic, but potential symptoms include flank pain, abdominal pain, fever, ileus, hematuria or urinary tract infection. An asymptomatic increase in creatinine is the first sign of an injury in some cases, and any increase in creatinine of more than 0.5 mg/dL above baseline without other known etiology should raise concern. However, in many cases there is no increase in creatinine above baseline; thus a normal creatinine does not rule out ureteral injury. Intravenous pyelogram (IVP) is the most commonly utilized study to detect ureteral injury, but it can only be performed if the creatinine is no more than mildly elevated (usually < 1.5–2.0 mg/dL). A renal ultrasound can detect hydroureter or hydronephrosis, but a negative study is not helpful since ureteral dilation may not always be present. Therefore, a retrograde pyelogram is recommended when the creatinine is too high to safely give intravenous contrast for an IVP; stent placement can be performed at the same time, if appropriate. Other studies that may be useful in selected cases are nuclear renal scan with furosemide, noncontrast computed tomography, and magnetic resonance urography.

The management of ureteral injuries depends on the location and extent of the injury. Intraoperative management of ureteral injuries is dependent upon the location and type of injury. If the ureter has been crushed or tied with suture, but not transected, it must be carefully inspected. Ureteral stents may be warranted during healing of the injured area. Ureteral kinking is usually best managed by releasing the suture causing the obstruction. Passage of ureteral stents may be indicated to confirm full patency. Ureteral transection is the most devastating injury, and its management depends upon the location of injury and length of ureter damaged. If the injury is in the lower third of the ureter, it should be reimplanted into the dome of the bladder. If the injury is in the mid and upper third of the ureter, an uretero-ureteral anastomosis is indicated. The retroperitoneum should be drained via flank drain (a Jackson–Pratt or Blake drain), and ureteral catheters should be left in place for 14–21 days. The drain should not be removed until complete resolution of drainage occurs. When necessary, tension on the anastomosis should be reduced with a psoas hitch.

If the injury is recognized early in the postoperative period, repair can be attempted as soon as the diagnosis is made. Immediate repair is contraindicated in patients at risk of sepsis or who are unstable and poor surgical candidates. Ureteral stent placement can be attempted if partial transection or ligation is suspected and, if successful, obviates the need for surgical repair. If the diagnosis has been delayed, repair is postponed for 1–3 months. Percutaneous nephrostomy is usually needed to maintain renal function during this time.

Suggested reading

Gilmour DT, Das S, Flowerdew G. Rates of urinary tract injury from gynecologic surgery and the role of intraoperative cystoscopy. *Obstet Gynecol* 2006; 107(6): 1366–1372.

Hurt G. Gynecologic injury to the ureters, bladder, and urethra. In: Walters MD, Karram MM (eds) *Urogynecology and pelvic reconstructive surgery*, 3rd edn. Philadelphia, PA: Mosby, 2006: 436–444.

Selzman AA, Spirnak JP. Iatrogenic ureteral injuries: a 20-year experience in treating 165 injuries. *J Urol* 1996; 155(3): 878–881.

Vakili B, Chesson RR, Kyle B, *et al*. The incidence of urinary tract injury during hysterectomy: a prospective analysis based on universal cystoscopy. *Am J Obstet Gynecol* 2005; 192(5): 1599–1604.

Visco AG, Taber KH, Weidner AC, *et al*. Cost-effectiveness of universal cystoscopy to identify ureteral injury at hysterectomy. *Obstet Gynecol* 2001; 97(5 Pt 1): 685–692.

Chapter 72
Fistulae

Micheline Wong and Begüm Özel
Department of Medicine and Obstetrics and Gynecology, Keck School of Medicine, University of Southern California, CA, USA

Introduction

Fistulae involving the female pelvic organs consist of abnormal connections between the bladder and vagina, vagina and bowel, or bladder and bowel. A urinary tract fistula is an abnormal opening between the urinary and genital tracts that results in continuous and unremitting urinary incontinence. Types of urinary tract fistulae include vesicovaginal, ureterovaginal, urethrovaginal, vesicouterine, and ureterouterine. Vesicovaginal fistulae are by far the most common type of urinary tract fistula. Colorectal fistulae include colovesical, colovaginal, rectovaginal, and anovaginal fistulae, the last two being the most common types of fistulae involving the bowel.

Fistulae are severely devastating and debilitating conditions. Prior to the development of modern obstetrics, obstructed labor was the most common cause of fistula formation, and it remains so in developing countries where there is little, if any, access to obstetric care. In more developed countries, the most common cause of a urogenital fistulae is gynecologic surgery. Colorectal fistulae, particularly rectovaginal and anovaginal fistulae, are most commonly seen as a consequence of vaginal delivery in both developed and underdeveloped countries. Other common causes for pelvic fistulae include malignancy and radiation therapy.

Vesicovaginal fistulae

In developed countries, gynecologic surgery is the most common cause of urinary tract fistulae; abdominal hysterectomy accounts for more than 50% of urinary tract fistulae

Management of Common Problems in Obstetrics and Gynecology, 5th edition. Edited by T.M. Goodwin, M.N. Montoro, L. Muderspach, R. Paulson and S. Roy. © 2010 Blackwell Publishing Ltd.

associated with gynecologic surgery. Vesicovaginal fistulae are the most common type of urinary tract fistula. The incidence of vesicovaginal fistula is estimated at 1 in 1000 hysterectomies.

Bladder injury and devascularization is often the underlying etiology in the development of vesicovaginal fistulae. Suture erosion, hematoma formation, and infection may also play a role. In a rabbit model, the simple placement of a suture through the bladder and vaginal walls did not lead to fistula formation, suggesting that accompanying tissue necrosis and devascularization are necessary for the development of a urinary tract fistula. A history of pelvic irradiation, prior pelvic surgery, prior cesarean delivery, presence of pelvic infection, diabetes mellitus, chronic steroid use, and tobacco use increase the risk of fistula formation.

The most common symptom associated with urinary tract fistulae is continuous urinary incontinence and constant leakage of urine per vagina. Symptoms are often worse with positional changes, such as moving from supine to upright position. Other symptoms include vaginal discharge, hematuria, and recurrent cystitis. Postoperative fistulae usually become symptomatic 1–2 weeks after surgery but may become apparent any time in the postoperative period. Radiation-induced fistulae can take years to develop. On exam, urine is often present on the vulva and can be seen as a fluid collection in the posterior vagina. There may be evidence of skin irritation from constant contact with urine. Careful inspection with a speculum will often locate the fistula. However, it is sometimes too small to visualize on speculum exam. In these cases, a "tampon test" may help confirm a vesicovaginal or ureterovaginal fistula. To perform this test, three cotton balls are placed in the vagina, and approximately 250 mL of water or saline containing a blue dye, such as methylene blue, is instilled into the bladder via a catheter. If there is concern for an ureterovaginal fistula, the patient may be given oral pyridium or intravenous indigo carmine. The use of pyridium will allow the practitioner to distinguish between a vesicovaginal and ureterovaginal fistula by looking at the color of the cotton balls. The patient should be asked to ambulate for at least 20–30 minutes. The cotton balls are then removed and inspected for color change and wetness. Cotton balls are preferred to a tampon because they allow the physician to distinguish the level at which the staining occurs. Tampons act as a wick, drawing fluid up through the tampon regardless of the level at which the fluid exposure occurs. If the cotton ball does not change color, a fistula is less likely. Staining of the lowermost cotton ball may suggest other forms of incontinence. A cystogram may also be helpful in the diagnosis of a vesicovaginal fistula.

Cystourethroscopy is essential to determine the exact anatomic location of the fistula in the bladder and its relation to the ureteral orifices. The condition of surrounding tissues can also be evaluated with cystoscopy. Intravenous pyelogram or retrograde pyelography is recommended for all cases of vesicovaginal fistula as well as all suspected cases of ureterovaginal fistula to evaluate ureteral involvement.

When the diagnosis of vesicovaginal fistula is confirmed, bladder drainage should be accomplished. If the fistula is less than 2 cm, continuous bladder drainage with an indwelling catheter alone may allow for spontaneous closure of the fistula. Prompt diagnosis and institution of bladder drainage increases the chances of spontaneous healing. In one study, 15–20% of fistulae closed spontaneously with up to 6 weeks of bladder drainage. To maximize the chances for a successful surgical repair, a waiting period of at least 3 months is usually indicated to allow maturation of the fistulous tract and minimize the associated inflammation. This waiting period is somewhat controversial; the basic principle is that the repair should be timed such that surrounding inflammation and edema are minimized. It is generally recommended that continuous bladder drainage be maintained until the time of surgical repair. Antibiotic prophylaxis is controversial in this setting. In general, it is not recommended that patients receive continuous antibiotic prophylaxis with prolonged catheterization as it only leads to the development of antibiotic resistance and does not reduce the incidence of symptomatic infections. Bacterial colonization of the catheter is nearly universal after 30 days; therefore, only symptomatic infections should be treated. However, a course of antibiotics is indicated perioperatively to sterilize the urine when surgical intervention is planned.

Vesicovaginal fistulae may be repaired vaginally or abdominally. The choice of surgical route is dependent upon several factors; when the fistula is small, easily accessible, and does not involve the ureters, the vaginal route is preferred. Most fistulae can be successfully repaired with a vaginal approach. Ureteral stents should be used when the fistula is close to the ureteral orifices.

Box 72.1 lists the basic principles of fistula repair that should be adhered to in all repairs.

The Latzko procedure is the most commonly used method of vesicovaginal fistula repair. In this procedure, the bladder and vaginal epithelium are mobilized carefully. A pediatric (10 French) Foley catheter may be inserted through the fistulous tract in order to better identify the edges of the fistula. Excision of the fistulous tract is indicated only in order to remove extensive fibrotic tissue or areas of tissue necrosis. The fistula should be freed completely from the surrounding tissues so that the edges can be coapted easily. All sutures should be placed so that they are tension free. The bladder epithelium is closed with 3-0 delayed absorbable suture, such as polyglactin suture, in two or more layers of interrupted sutures, and the endopelvic fascia and vaginal epithelium are closed with 2-0 delayed absorbable suture in a running fashion. A bulbocavernosus (Martius) fat pad graft can be utilized to provide reinforcement to closures in women with risk factors for poor wound healing. The integrity of the closure is tested for watertightness by filling the bladder with blue dye or sterile milk. The sites of leakage can be oversewn with interrupted 3-0 delayed absorbable suture. Bladder drainage is continued for 10–14 days to prevent bladder distension. Success of surgical repair of vesicovaginal fistulae depends on the amount of scar tissue present and adherence to general principles of fistula repair. If careful surgical techniques are used, success rates are 80–90% for first repairs.

The abdominal approach should be taken in cases of ureteral involvement or close proximity, size greater than 4 cm, poor visualization, multiple fistula, vesicocervical fistula or complex fistula involving other organs such as the uterus or bowel. The vesicovaginal component of the fistula is reached by sagittal cystotomy in order to access the fistula. The fistulous tract is excised and widely dissected. The vaginal epithelium is closed in two layers using 3-0 polyglactin, and the bladder is closed in three layers using 3-0 polyglactin. The first layer approximates

---

Box 72.1 Basic principles of fistula repair

- Obtain good surgical exposure
- Use sharp dissection
- Maintain hemostasis
- Minimize tissue trauma
- Widely mobilize tissue layers
- Use multilayer, tension-free closure
- Use vascular grafts when indicated

the bladder epithelium and the second two are placed to imbricate the adjacent muscularis. A layer of peritoneum or omentum may be placed to separate the vaginal and bladder repairs. An omental graft will both serve to separate the two suture lines and supply additional blood to the area.

Urinary diversion may be the only option in cases of multiple failed procedures and in fistulae that result from radiation therapy.

Ureterovaginal fistulae

Ureterovaginal fistulae have symptoms identical to vesicovaginal fistulae, and the evaluation is essentially the same. If a ureterovaginal fistula is identified, immediate ureteral stenting should be attempted. If successful, the stent should be maintained for 6–8 weeks. In one series, 82% of ureterovaginal fistulae diagnosed within the first month resolved with stent placement. Ureterovaginal fistulae that have not healed by 8 weeks will require surgical repair.

Ureterovaginal fistulae must be repaired abdominally. Injury or fistula involving the distal one-third (distal 4–5 cm) of ureter is treated by ureteroneocystotomy (ureteral reimplantation into the bladder). A psoas hitch may be necessary to maintain the anatomic position of the bladder and reduce tension of the ureter and bladder. A fistula involving the middle and upper thirds of the ureter must be repaired by resecting the involved area and reanastomosing the two ends of the ureter (ureterouretorostomy). This is usually done over ureteral stents. The retroperitoneum should be drained with a Jackson–Pratt or Blake drain postoperatively.

Other urinary tract fistulae

Urethrovaginal fistulae can occur as a complication of excision of a urethral diverticulum and incontinence procedures. They are repaired vaginally with wide mobilization of the tissues and layered closure with 4–0 delayed absorbable sutures. The urethra should be closed vertically to minimize the risk of urethral shortening. Whenever possible, care should be taken to avoid overlapping suture lines. Martius graft placement is often helpful in these types of fistulae. Transurethral drainage with a Foley catheter is indicated postoperatively for at least 14 days. Stress urinary incontinence can develop postoperatively if the normal continence mechanism of the urethra has been affected.

Vesicouterine and ureterouterine fistulae are rare fistulae usually associated with cesarean delivery; other reported causes include vaginal birth after cesarean, placement of intrauterine contraceptive device, dilation and curettage, myomectomy, and uterine artery embolization. Cyclic hematuria is sometimes seen in women with vesicouterine fistulae, and many women will actually be completely continent. Some women will present solely for infertility evaluation. A hysterosalpingogram may be helpful if a vesicouterine fistula is suspected. Repair of vesicouterine and ureterouterine fistulae is similar to vesicovaginal and ureterovaginal fistulae, respectively. The abdominal approach is required. Hysterectomy in women not desiring future fertility may facilitate the repair.

Rectovaginal and anovaginal fistulae

Rectovaginal and anovaginal fistulae as a result of obstetric lacerations are not uncommon in developed countries. Most often, these occur as a result of vaginal lacerations involving the rectal mucosa that are either not identified or the repair breaks down. Repairs complicated by infection may be more likely to fistulize. Other causes of these types of fistulae include colorectal surgery, pelvic radiation, malignancy, inflammatory bowel syndrome, and, rarely, gynecologic surgery, such as a posterior vaginal repair. These women will report fecal incontinence, stool or flatus per vagina, and foul-smelling vaginal discharge. Fistulae that result from obstetric injury are usually located at the distal third of the vagina and are easy to identify on vaginal exam. Fistulae distal to the dentate line are classified as anovaginal. If there is suspicion of a fistula not clearly seen on exam, the rectum can be filled with normal saline containing a few drops of methylene blue dye and the vagina examined for blue dye. A barium enema may be useful for identifying the fistula. Often, there is associated perineal breakdown and disruption of the anal sphincter; therefore, evaluation should include endoanal ultrasonography to diagnose anal sphincter defects.

Rectovaginal and anovaginal fistulae can be repaired as soon as they are identified as long as there is no local infection or extensive inflammation. The basic principles of repair include wide mobilization of the tissues, complete excision of the fistulous tract, and multilayer closure without tension using delayed absorbable suture. The rectal mucosa should be repaired using 3–0 or 4–0 delayed absorbable suture. The subsequent layers may use 2–0 or 3–0 delayed absorbable suture, such as polyglactin. Usually, at least four layers are required. A Martius (bulbocavernosus) fat pad graft may be used in recurrent fistulae and in patients with inflammatory bowel disease or history of radiation. This graft serves to separate the two suture lines and also brings in vascular supply to the healing tissues. In recurrent fistulae, radiation-induced fistulae, and fistulae due to inflammatory bowel disease, diverting colostomy may be necessary to allow for healing. The colostomy is then taken down about 3 months after the fistula repair, once healing is complete.

Other colorectal fistulae

Colovesical and colovaginal fistulae can occur as a consequence of pelvic surgery, malignancy, radiation, diverticular disease, and inflammatory bowel disease. Women with colovaginal fistulae have symptoms similar to women with rectovaginal fistulae. Women with colovesical fistulae will present with recurrent urinary tract infections, pneumaturia or fecaluria. Repair of these types of fistulae usually requires an abdominal approach and should be performed in consultation with a colorectal surgeon.

Obstetric fistulae in developing countries

Fistulae due to obstetric injury occur primarily in sub-Saharan Africa and South Asia. These include vesicovaginal, urethrovaginal, rectovaginal or anovaginal fistulae. Large and complex fistulae involving multiple sites are not uncommon. The mechanism of injury in obstetric fistulae almost always involves obstructed labor. When labor is obstructed, the fetal vertex places pressure on the soft vaginal tissues, leading to tissue necrosis and, eventually, fistula formation. Labor is prolonged, with women spending up to 4–5 days in labor. The infant rarely survives. There are 33,000–130,000 reported cases of fistulae annually in Africa alone. However, the true incidence of obstetric fistulae is unknown due to under-reporting because few women actually seek medical care for this problem. It is estimated that there are at least 2–3.5 million women in the developing world with unrepaired fistulae.

Obstetric fistulae are more common in countries where there is poorly supervised labor, lack of emergency obstetric care, and inaccessibility of medical care in rural areas. Fistula formation in developing countries has also been attributed to malnutrition, young age at marriage and child bearing, sexual abuse, coital injury, and female genital cutting. In one study of women with obstetric fistulae, the average age of marriage was 15.6 years, and the average age of first pregnancy was 17.1 years. These girls often become pregnant before they have achieved full pelvic growth. Many young women who develop obstetric fistulae in this manner are ostracized by their communities and abandoned by their husbands and families. Obstetric fistulae in developing countries are often highly complex in nature, difficult to repair successfully without additional sequelae, and result in social isolation and suffering for the afflicted women and girls. Prevention of these types of injuries through education and providing access to healthcare is critical.

Suggested reading

Ahmed S, Holtz SA. Social and economic consequences of obstetric fistula: life changed forever? Int J Gynaecol Obstet 2007; 99(suppl 1): S10–15.

Bahadursingh AM, Longo WE. Colovaginal fistulae. Etiology and management. J Reprod Med 2003; 48(7): 489–495.

Elkins TE, Delancey JO, McGuire EJ. The use of modified Martius graft as an adjunctive technique in vesicovaginal and rectovaginal fistula repair. Obstet Gynecol 1990; 75(4): 727–733.

Evans DH, Madjar S, Politano VA, et al. Interposition flaps in transabdominal vesicovaginal fistula repairs: are they really necessary? Urology 2001; 57: 670–674.

Garcea G, Majid I, Sutton CD, et al. Diagnosis and management of colovesical fistulae: six-year experience of 90 consecutive cases. Colorectal Dis 2006; 8(4): 347–352.

Grissom R, Snyder TE. Colovaginal fistula secondary to diverticular disease. Dis Colon Rectum 1991; 34(11): 1043–1049.

Homsi R, Daikoku NH, Littlejohn J, Wheeles CR Jr. Episiotomy: risks of dehiscence and rectovaginal fistula. Obstet Gynecol Surv 1994; 49(12): 803–808.

Hurt WG. Vesicovaginal and ureterovaginal fistulae. In: Ostergard DR, Bent AE, Cundiff GW, Swift SE (eds) Ostergard's urogynecology and pelvic floor dysfunction, 5th edn. Philadelphia, PA: Lippincott, Williams and Wilkins, 2003: 433–446.

Iselin CE, Aslan P, Webster GD. Transvaginal repair of vesicovaginal fistulae after hysterectomy by vaginal cuff excision. J Urol 1998; 160: 728–730.

Jozwik M, Jozwik M. Spontaneous closure of vesicouterine fistula account for effective hormonal treatment. Urol Int 1999; 62: 183–187.

Karram MM. Lower urinary tract fistulae. In: Walters MD, Karram MM (eds) Urogynecology and pelvic reconstructive surgery, 3rd edn. Philadelphia, PA: Mosby, 2006: 445–460.

Kleeman SD, Vasallo B, Segal J, Margolis T, Mercer LJ. Vesicovaginal fistula. Obstet Gynecol Surv 1994; 49(12): 840–847.

Meyer L, Ascher-Walsh CJ, Norman R, et al. Commonalities among women who experienced vesicovaginal fistulae as a result of obstetric trauma in Niger: results from a survey given at the National Hospital Fistula Center, Niamey, Niger. Am J Obstet Gynecol 2007; 197(1): 90.

Miklos JR, Sze E, Parobeck D, Karram MM. Vesicouterine fistula: a rare complication of vaginal birth after cesarean. Obstet Gynecol 1995; 86: 638–689.

Mondet F, Chartier-Kastler EJ, Conort P, Bitker MO, Chatelain C, Richard F. Anatomic and functional results of transperitoneal-transvesical vesicovaginal fistula repair. Urology 2001; 58: 882–886.

Murphy JM, Lee G, Sharma SD, et al. Vesicouterine fistula: MRI diagnosis. Eur Radiol 1999; 9: 1876–1878.

Park BK, Kim SH, Cho JY, et al. Vesicouterine fistula after cesarean section: ultrasonographic findings in two cases. J Ultrasound Med 1999; 18: 441–443.

Rangnekar NP, Imdad Ali N, Kaul SA, Pathak HR. Role of the Martius procedure in the management of urinary-vaginal fistulae. J Am Coll Surg 2000; 191: 259–263.

Solkar MH, Forshaw MJ, Sankararajah D, et al. Colovesical fistula – is a surgical approach always justified? Colorectal Dis 2005; 7(5): 467–471.

Sullivan CJ, Goldberg J, Aizenman L, Chon JK. Vesicouterine fistula after uterine artery embolization: a case report. Am J Obstet Gynecol 2002; 187: 1726–1727.

Tancer ML. Vesicouterine fistula – a review. Obstet Gynecol Surv 1986; 41(12): 743–753.

Wall LL. Obstetric vesicovaginal fistula as an international public-health problem. Lancet 2006; 368(9542): 1201–1209.

Wall LL, Arrowsmith SD, Lassey AT, Danso K. Humanitarian ventures or 'fistula tourism?': the ethical perils of pelvic surgery in the developing world. Int Urogynecol J Pelvic Floor Dysfunct 2006; 17(6): 559–562.

Wiskind AK, Thompson JD. Transverse transperineal repair of rectovaginal fistulae in the lower vagina. Am J Obstet Gynecol 1992; 167(3): 694–699.

Wittman AB, Wall LL. The evolutionary origins of obstructed labor: bipedalism, encephalization, and the human obstetric dilemma. Obstet Gynecol Surv 2007; 62(11): 739–748.

Chapter 73
Pelvic Organ Prolapse

Micheline Wong and Begüm Özel
Department of Medicine and Obstetrics and Gynecology, Keck School of Medicine, University of Southern California, CA, USA

Introduction

Pelvic organ prolapse (POP) is the descent of the pelvic organs (bladder, uterus, bowel) into the vagina as a result of defects in pelvic support. POP significantly affects the quality of life of women affected by the condition. The prevalence of POP varies by definition and the population of women being examined but is estimated at about 2% in the general population. POP is closely linked in pathophysiology to urinary and fecal incontinence, and many women suffer from all three disorders.

Anatomy

The role of the pelvic floor is to support and assist in the function of the bladder, uterus, vagina, and rectum. The pelvic organs rest on the band of muscles and fascia that make up the pelvic floor. The muscular component of the pelvic floor consists of the coccygeus muscle; the levator ani complex, which is composed of the iliococcygeus and pubovisceral muscles; the external anal sphincter; the striated urethral sphincter; and the superficial perineal muscles. The iliococcygeus attaches the pelvic side wall to the arcus tendineus fascia pelvis (ATFP). The pubovisceral muscles are a U-shaped band running from the pubic bone to the lateral wall of the vagina and rectum, condensing on the ATFP. This muscular complex forms a sling-like band that supports the pelvic organs. The iliococcygeus and pubovisceral muscles work together to maintain tone in the levator hiatus, keeping it closed against intra-abdominal pressure.

There are three levels of connective tissue support as described by DeLancey. Level I consists of the uterosacral and cardinal ligaments. Level II support is made up of the paravaginal attachments of the vagina to the ATFP. Level III support describes the most distal support of the vagina and includes the endopelvic fascia and perineum. The muscular and fascial components of the pelvic floor work together to support the pelvic organs and prevent their descent into the levator hiatus.

Pathophysiology

There are data to suggest that genetic factors predispose some women to developing POP. European American and Latina women appear to have a higher incidence of prolapse compared to African American women. Increasing prevalence of POP is also seen with increasing age. Pregnancy, vaginal delivery, operative vaginal delivery and the delivery of larger infants are all associated with increased risk of POP. However, nulliparity and cesarean delivery do not preclude the development of prolapse. Data from the Women's Health Initiative indicated that among women aged 50–79, 5% of nulliparous women have vaginal wall descent to the hymen or beyond. However, among younger women, vaginal delivery appears to be a significant factor in the development of POP.

There are modifiable risk factors for POP. According to data from the Women's Health Initiative, a BMI of greater than 30 kg/m^2 increases the risk of prolapse by 40–75%. Anything that causes chronically increased intra-abdominal pressure may increase the risk of POP; these include chronic cough from smoking, asthma, bronchitis or gastroesophageal reflux; chronic constipation; and chronic straining, such as with repetitive heavy lifting.

Diagnosis

Symptoms of POP are subjective. What may be bothersome to one patient may be asymptomatic in another. While early stages of prolapse are often asymptomatic, it is common for women with prolapse beyond the hymenal ring to have some degree of bother.

Management of Common Problems in Obstetrics and Gynecology, 5th edition. Edited by T.M. Goodwin, M.N. Montoro, L. Muderspach, R. Paulson and S. Roy. © 2010 Blackwell Publishing Ltd.

The most common symptom is the sensation of a vaginal bulge or the complaint of vaginal pressure. This symptom has been found in epidemiologic studies to be most closely associated with the presence and degree of prolapse. Anterior compartment prolapse sometimes leads to urinary hesitancy, frequency and incomplete bladder emptying. Patients may report a need to reduce their prolapse in order to void. If the patient is unable to reduce her prolapse, elevated postvoid residual volumes are common with severe anterior prolapse. Stress incontinence is often decreased or absent with severe anterior prolapse due to the kinking of the urethra by the prolapse. Patients with posterior compartment prolapse often have difficulties with defecation, including constipation, straining, incomplete emptying and needing manually to reduce the prolapse in order to have a bowel movement. Other symptoms include difficulty with sexual intercourse and avoidance of sexual intercourse due to embarrassment.

Physical exam confirms the diagnosis and assesses the degree of prolapse. On speculum exam the practitioner should look for erosions and ulcers in the vaginal and cervical epithelium.

Clinically, POP is graded according to the Baden Walker system: stage 1 refers to prolapse that extends to halfway to the introitus; stage 2 extends to a level from the lower half of the vagina to the introitus; stage 3 is prolapse extending past the hymenal ring or introitus, and stage 4 is complete eversion of the vaginal walls. A more comprehensive method of measuring degree of prolapse was developed by the International Continence Society in 1995 and is called the Pelvic Organ Prolapse Quantification (POP-Q) system (Box 73.1). Using the posterior blade of a Graves speculum and ring forceps or disposable ruler, nine points on the vagina and vulva are measured relative to the hymenal ring. This system defines prolapse as stage 1–4 based on the point of prolapse extending the furthest (Box 73.2).

Assessment of paravaginal defects is not part of the standard POP-Q evaluation. On clinical exam, the existence of paravaginal defects can be determined by placing ring forceps in the lateral vaginal fornices. If the prolapse is reduced with this maneuver, a paravaginal defect may be present. However, the reliability of preoperative clinical exam for paravaginal defect has been questioned. The diagnosis of a paravaginal defect is definitively made at the time of surgery.

During physical exam, assessment of the pelvic muscles should also be performed by palpation on bimanual and rectal exam. Grading of pelvic muscle strength is done on the Oxford rating scale, where 0 indicates no strength and 5 indicates maximal strength. The examiner should assess both resting muscle tone and voluntary muscle contraction. This may aid in selecting patients who may benefit from focused exercises to strengthen the pelvic floor.

Box 73.1 Pelvic Organ Prolapse Quantification (POP-Q) points

- PB: length of perineal body
- GH: length of genital hiatus
- TVL: total vaginal length (without Valsalva)
- D: location of pouch of Douglas during Valsalva
- C: most distal edge of cervix or cuff during Valsalva
- Aa: point on anterior vagina 3 cm proximal to hymen in absence of prolapse (range – 3 cm to + 3 cm)
- Ba: most dependent portion of anterior wall
- Ap: 3 cm proximal to hymen on posterior wall in absence of prolapse (range – 3 cm to + 3 cm)
- Bp: most dependent portion of posterior wall

All women with POP should be screened for urinary and anal incontinence. The postvoid residual (PVR) urine volume should also be measured to determine if the patient is able to void completely. A PVR less than 50 mL is generally considered normal assuming a voided volume greater than 150 mL. Urodynamics may be indicated even in the absence of incontinence symptoms in cases of severe prolapse that may mask incontinence. This is true regardless of the site of prolapse; even severe posterior vaginal wall prolapse has been shown to result in masking of incontinence. The prolapse should be reduced during the urodynamics study. However, this must be done with care in order not to put too much pressure on the urethra. There is no optimal method for prolapse reduction; options include using the posterior blade of a speculum, cotton balls, pessary, vaginal packing or manual reduction. Radiologic imaging, such as defecography and pelvic MRI, may be useful in some cases but is not routinely necessary in the evaluation of POP.

Treatment

The indication for treatment is patient symptoms. Asymptomatic prolapse can generally be managed expectantly.

Box 73.2 Staging of POP-Q

- Stage 0: no prolapse
- Stage I: leading edge of prolapse < –1 cm
- Stage II: most distal edge of prolapse ≥ –1 cm but ≤ + 1 cm
- Stage III: most distal edge ≥ + 1 cm, but less than total vaginal length – 2 cm
- Stage IV: total eversion of genital tract (distance relative to hymenal ring)

Stage 1–2 prolapse is often asymptomatic. Occasionally women with stage 3 and 4 prolapse will deny symptoms. Observation may not be appropriate in such a patient who has advanced prolapse if it causes urinary retention due to the risk of recurrent urinary tract infections, urosepsis, and hydronephrosis. In addition, exposed vaginal epithelium is prone to ulcerations and infection. These risks should be considered and discussed with the patient when deciding on treatment modality.

Nonsurgical treatment

All women should be offered nonsurgical therapy as first line. Women with stage 1–2 prolapse may be instructed to practice pelvic floor exercises. The effectiveness of pelvic muscle training for improvement of prolapse has not been studied, but it may potentially prevent worsening of the prolapse. If the patient's chief complaints are related to gastrointestinal symptoms such as splinting, excessive straining or constipation, she may be counseled on dietary and behavioral changes to improve stool consistency.

Pessaries may be used to delay or avoid surgery. Patients with severe medical conditions who are poor candidates for surgery or women who would prefer nonsurgical therapy may choose to have a pessary. Women treated with a pessary must be compliant with follow-up and pessary care; frequent clinic visits are often necessary. Pessaries are prescribed with lubricating gel and/or vaginal estrogen therapy which decreases the risk of vaginal erosion. The use of vaginal estrogen is especially important for postmenopausal women who are unable to remove the pessary at home. Ideally the patient will be able to remove and wash the pessary with soap and water nightly, then replace it in the morning. However, many elderly or debilitated women are unable to remove the pessary and do not have someone who can help them with its removal at home. In this case pessaries can usually be left in place for a maximum of 12 weeks. Closer follow-up in the first few months of use is recommended, with subsequent increase in visit intervals to a maximum of 12 weeks.

There are various shapes and sizes of pessaries, and they should be selected according to location and stage of POP. Most pessaries are made of silicone, plastic or medical-grade rubber, and are classified into either space filling or supportive. A ring pessary with or without support is a good initial choice for most women with prolapse regardless of stage. The doughnut and Gellhorn pessaries are space filling and are usually used for stage 3 and 4 prolapse. The pessary should fill the vagina from side wall to side wall with enough space to pass a finger between the pessary and vaginal wall. It should fit securely behind the pubic symphysis anteriorly and posteriorly in the vaginal fornix behind the cervix (if present). A Gellhorn pessary has a disk that fills the upper vagina and a knob on a stem that should point downward behind the perineal body. The patient should not feel the pessary in place. If she feels too much pressure or tightness, it may be too big and the next smaller size should be tried. If she is aware of the pessary in the introitus, it has slipped out of position and is probably too small. She should be asked to move around and Valsalva to ensure that the pessary does not fall out or change position. She should also be asked to void to make sure that the pessary does not cause urinary retention. When fitting a pessary, the clinician should observe the patient removing and replacing the pessary to ensure that she will be able to manage it on her own.

Women who menstruate may find it inconvenient to wear a pessary. They can remove and clean their pessary daily or refrain from wearing the pessary during menstruation. The ring pessary can often be left in during intercourse, but space-filling pessaries must be removed. Some women may find it bothersome and embarrassing to remove the pessary prior to intercourse.

Surgical management

The goal of surgery for prolapse is to alleviate symptoms. Women who are sexually active require surgery to reconstruct the normal vagina and to restore and maintain vaginal function. Women who are no longer sexually active are candidates for obliterative surgery to relieve symptoms of prolapse.

Surgical procedures for POP are generally divided into the vaginal and abdominal approaches. The advantages to vaginal surgery compared to the abdominal approach include less pain, decreased hospital stay, more rapid recovery, and lower costs; however, success rates tend to be lower with the vaginal approach. The choice of surgical treatment of POP depends on surgeon experience and patient preferences, as well as the patient age and risk of undergoing major surgery. A recent survey of Society of Gynecologic Surgeons found that many prefer the vaginal approach with their older patients and an abdominal approach in younger women.

The anterior vaginal defect may be repaired vaginally with anterior colporrhaphy, vaginal paravaginal repair, with or without a mesh or graft augmented repair. In the traditional anterior colporrhaphy, the vaginal muscularis is plicated in the midline with U-stitches of braided delayed absorbable suture. The abdominal approach primarily consists of the abdominal paravaginal repair. In paravaginal defect repairs, the anterior lateral vaginal sulcus is reattached to the ATFP using permanent suture. Surgeons recently have started to modify the abdominal sacral colpopexy to correct anterior vaginal wall prolapse in cases where there is also apical prolapse; in these cases, the bladder is dissected off the anterior vagina to the level of the bladder trigone and the colpopexy mesh is placed between the bladder and vagina. There are limited data on the efficacy of any of these procedures, and anterior vaginal wall prolapse is accepted as the most difficult defect to repair satisfactorily. Recurrences are common and occur in as many as 50% of women.

Using a graft to reinforce the repair of anterior prolapse from the vaginal approach is a variation on the traditional repairs. The graft or mesh is placed over the midline plication or used without midline plication. Usually it is attached laterally to the ATFP similar to an abdominal paravaginal repair. Cure rates have been shown to be improved with polyglactin mesh, which is an absorbable mesh, or with porcine dermis graft to reinforce the repair, but the long-term benefits of mesh or graft placement over traditional repair have not been proven. *De novo* dyspareunia and mesh erosion into the vagina or bladder are known complications associated with graft or mesh use. We reserve the use of mesh or graft for carefully selected women who have failed prior surgery and who have been extensively counseled regarding associated risks.

Posterior vaginal prolapse is usually repaired vaginally. The rectovaginal fascia is either plicated in the midline or a site-specific repair is performed in which the isolated defects in the rectovaginal fascia are identified and closed with interrupted stitches using delayed absorbable suture. Both procedures have around a 90% success rate, but the site-specific approach is associated with less dyspareunia postoperatively and is preferred for sexually active women. Some surgeons also plicate the levator ani, but this technique has been associated with dyspareunia and should be avoided in sexually active women. A perineorrhaphy, in which the bulbocavernosus and transverse perinei muscles are plicated in the midline, is commonly performed at the time of posterior repair. Many colorectal surgeons favor the transanal approach to posterior vaginal wall prolapse, but the vaginal approach has been proven to have higher success rates compared to the transanal approach. Given the high success of primary repair, there is little role for graft or mesh in the primary repair of posterior vaginal wall prolapse.

Apical prolapse can be approached vaginally or abdominally. The abdominal sacral colpopexy (ASC) has been shown to have a lower rate of recurrent vault prolapse and less dyspareunia and a trend towards a lower reoperation rate for vaginal prolapse at any site compared with the vaginal sacrospinous ligament suspension (SLS). However, the SLS is quicker and cheaper to perform and women have an earlier return to activities of daily living. The uterosacral ligament suspension (USLS) is another vaginal approach that has not been compared to the ASC or SLS but appears to have satisfactory success rates.

In the ASC, the vaginal apex is suspended to the anterior sacral ligament at the level of the sacral promontory.

Permanent mesh is associated with lower failure rate, and polypropylene is the mesh of choice for most surgeons due to the low rate of mesh complications with this type of material. The ASC requires laparotomy and should be reserved for good surgical candidates who can tolerate a lengthy procedure. There is a small risk of hemorrhage due to laceration of sacral veins during dissection over the sacrum. These veins easily retract into the bone and bleeding can be difficult to control. As with any laparotomy, complications include risk of infection, adhesions, and small bowel obstruction. About 1% of women will require reoperation for a small bowel obstruction. Mesh erosion and infection most often occur in the immediate postoperative period, but also can present years after surgery. Mesh erosion may be more common if the vaginal cuff is opened, as in the case of a concomitant hysterectomy. The overall rate of mesh erosion is around 3.4%. A prophylactic Burch colposuspension in women without stress incontinence is recommended due to the risk of *de novo* stress urinary incontinence. A mid-urethral sling may be performed in women with urodynamic stress incontinence. The ASC has a success rate of 78–100% in published studies.

The SLS and USLS are both vaginal approaches to apical prolapse. In the SLS, the vaginal cuff is suspended to the sacrospinous ligaments. This is usually performed unilaterally, but some surgeons prefer bilateral suspension. The SLS results in an exaggerated posterior deflection of the vaginal cuff and is associated with high recurrence of anterior vaginal prolapse. Potential complications include buttock pain, pudendal nerve or vessel injury, and rectal injury. Gluteal pain is reported in 3% of women. Massive hemorrhage from laceration of the hypogastric venous plexus or the pudendal vein has been reported. Published success rates for the SLS range from 63% to 97%. The USLS involves the suspension of the vaginal apex to the uterosacral ligaments bilaterally. The most common complication of USLS is ureteral kinking or obstruction; this is reported to be as high as 11%. Surgeons performing this procedure must be comfortable identifying the pelvic anatomy vaginally, and routine cystoscopy to confirm ureteral patency is indicated in all cases. Success of the procedure is reported to be as high as 97% at 5 years of follow-up, but there are few published studies.

The laparoscopic repair of POP is gaining popularity, especially with the use of robotic assistance. The laparoscopic sacral colpopexy, uterosacral suspension, and paravaginal repair are the most common prolapse procedures performed laparoscopically. There is decreased morbidity and hospital stay with laparoscopic procedures, but they require a high level of operator skill. Additionally, there are no long-term data investigating the success and comparing complication rates of these procedures.

Obliterative procedures

Colpocleisis or colpectomy is performed to alleviate prolapse symptoms in women who are no longer sexually active and do not plan to be in the future. Obliterative procedures require less operative time than reconstructive procedures, and can be done under sedation, regional or local anesthesia. There is usually less blood loss and risk of bowel, bladder or nerve injury. In the LeForte colpocleisis the vaginal epithelium is removed in a rhomboid shape over the anterior and posterior vagina up to the prolapsed cervix. The cervix is inverted and the vaginal walls are sutured together, closing the vaginal vault with the cervix and uterus inside. Since the cervix will no longer be assessable, the patient should have normal cervical cytology preoperatively and an evaluation of the endometrial cavity by ultrasound or biopsy is recommended. A midurethral sling may be placed at the time of colpocleisis, since up to 30% may develop *de novo* stress urinary incontinence following the procedure. Colpectomy is performed for posthysterectomy prolapse and involves excision of the vaginal walls and closure of the vaginal epithelium, permitting a single finger immediately below the urethra to the level of the introitus. A perineorrhaphy with levator plication is often performed at the same time.

Suggested reading

Bo K, Finckenhagen HB. Vaginal palpation of pelvic floor muscle strength: inter-test reproducibility and comparison between palpation and vaginal squeeze pressure. *Acta Obstet Gynecol Scand* 2001; 80(10): 883–887.

Brubaker L, Cundiff GW, Fine P, *et al*. Abdominal sacrocolpopexy with Burch colposuspension to reduce urinary stress incontinence. *NEJM* 2006; 354(15): 1557–1566.

Bump RC, Mattiasson A, Bo K, *et al*. The standardization of terminology of female pelvic organ prolapse and pelvic floor dysfunction. *Am J Obstet Gynecol* 1996; 175: 10.

Culligan PJ, Blackwell L, Goldsmith LJ, *et al*. A randomized controlled trial comparing fascia lata and synthetic mesh for sacral colpopexy. *Obstet Gynecol* 2005; 106(1): 29–37.

Cundiff GW, Amundsen CL, Bent AE, *et al*. The PESSRI study: symptom relief outcomes of a randomized crossover trial of the ring and Gellhorn pessaries. *Am J Obstet Gynecol* 2007; 196(4): 405.

Fitzgerald MP, Richter HE, Siddique S, *et al*. Colpocleisis: a review. *Int Urogynecol J Pelvic Floor Dysfunct* 2006; 17(3): 261–271.

Kobak WH, Walters M, Rosenberger K. Interobserver variation in the assessment of pelvic organ prolapse. *Int Urogynecol J Pelvic Floor Dysfunct* 1996; 7(3): 121–124.

Jelovsek JE, Maher C, Barber MD. Pelvic organ prolapse. *Lancet* 2007; 369(9566): 1027–1038.

Maher CF, Qatawneh AM, Dwyer PL, *et al*. Abdominal sacral colpopexy or vaginal sacrospinous colpopexy for vaginal vault prolapse: a prospective randomized study. *Am J Obstet Gynecol* 2004; 90(1): 20–26.

Maher C, Baessler K, Glazener CM, Adams EJ, Hagen S. Surgical management of pelvic organ prolapse in women. *Cochrane Database Syst Rev* 2007; 3: CD004014.

Meschia M, Pifarotti P, Bernasconi F, *et al*. Porcine skin collagen implants to prevent anterior vaginal wall prolapse recurrence: a multicenter, randomized study. *J Urol* 2007; 177(1): 192–195.

Nygaard IE, McCreery R, Brubaker L, *et al*. Abdominal sacrocolpopexy: a comprehensive review. *Obstet Gynecol* 2004; 104(4): 805–823.

Paraiso MF, Barber MD, Muir TW, Walters MD. Rectocele repair: a randomized trial of three surgical techniques including graft augmentation. *Am J Obstet Gynecol* 2006; 195(6): 1762–1771.

Rogers RM. Anatomy of pelvic support. . In: Ostergard DR, Bent AE, Cundiff GW, Swift SE (eds) *Ostergard's urogynecology and pelvic floor dysfunction*, 5th edn. Philadelphia, PA: Lippincott, Williams and Wilkins, 2003: 19–42.

Silva WA, Pauls RN, Segal JL, *et al*. Uterosacral ligament vault suspension: five-year outcomes. *Obstet Gynecol* 2006; 108(2): 255–263.

Swift SE. Epidemiology of pelvic organ prolapse. In: Ostergard DR, Bent AE, Cundiff GW, Swift SE (eds) *Ostergard's urogynecology and pelvic floor dysfunction*, 5th edn. Philadelphia, PA: Lippincott, Williams and Wilkins, 2003: 35–50.

Sze EH, Karram MM. Transvaginal repair of vault prolapse: a review. *Obstet Gynecol* 1997; 89(3): 466–475.

Weber AM, Walters MD, Piedmonte MR, Ballard LA. Anterior colporrhaphy: a randomized trial of three surgical techniques. *Am J Obstet Gynecol* 2001; 185(6): 1299–1306.

Chapter 74
Infections of the Lower Urinary Tract

Christina Dancz and Begüm Özel

Department of Medicine and Obstetrics and Gynecology, Keck School of Medicine, University of Southern California, CA, USA

Introduction

Acute lower urinary tract infections (UTI, also called acute bacterial cystitis) are responsible for 3.6 million office visits in the US each year, accounting for $1.6 billion in direct costs. Acute bacterial cystitis in the otherwise healthy nonpregnant adult woman is termed an uncomplicated UTI. A complicated UTI is any infection in the setting of anatomic urinary tract abnormalities, indwelling catheters, recent urinary tract instrumentation, pregnancy, recent antimicrobial administration, immunosuppression (including diabetes mellitus), atypical symptoms or symptoms lasting more than 7 days. If any of these factors are present, it increases the likelihood of treatment failure and warrants consideration of parenteral treatment, culture-based treatment or empiric treatment with broad-spectrum antibiotics.

Urinary tract infections develop when bacteria from the gastrointestinal tract colonize the vagina and enter the urethra. In a meta-analysis of 3108 women with acute cystitis, 78.6% were caused by *Escherichia coli*, followed by *Staphylococcus saprophyticus* (4.4%), *Klebsiella pneumoniae* (4.3%), and *Proteus mirabilis* (3.7%). *Citrobacter*, *Enterococcus* and *Pseudomonas* are occasional causes of UTI. Sexual activity is the most important risk factor for development of UTI.

The primary symptoms of acute cystitis are dysuria, frequency, urgency, suprapubic pain, and/or hematuria. Suprapubic urine aspiration and culture is the gold standard for diagnosis of urinary tract infection; however, patient discomfort, cost and delay in culture results have led clinicians to look for more convenient and rapid diagnostic techniques. In most patients with symptoms of acute cystitis (dysuria, frequency or

urgency), urine culture is not necessary as these symptoms in an otherwise healthy individual are highly sensitive for a UTI. Evaluation of mid-stream urine for pyuria has a high sensitivity (95%) but a relatively low specificity (71%) for infection; its absence strongly suggests a noninfectious cause for the symptoms. The presence of visible bacteria on microscopic examination is less sensitive but more specific. Urine dipstick testing has largely supplanted microscopy and urine cultures, because the dipstick method is cheaper, faster and more convenient. Dipsticks are most accurate when the presence of nitrite or leukocyte esterase is detected. The presence of gross or microscopic hematuria is helpful since it is common in women with UTI but not in women with urethritis or vaginitis. Hematuria is not a predictor for complicated infection and does not warrant extended therapy. In patients with a complicated infection, atypical symptoms, recurrent symptoms (less than 1 month after prior treatment) or failure to respond to initial therapy, urine culture is indicated and should guide treatment choice.

When obtaining a clean voided urine sample for urine dipstick testing or urine culture, patients should be given clear instructions on urine collection. The urethral meatus should be cleansed with a nonfoaming antiseptic solution. The labia should be held apart to minimize local contamination from skin flora. The first part of the stream is likely to be contaminated and should be discarded before collection of a mid-stream sample in a sterile container. Samples should be taken rapidly to the laboratory or placed on ice, as bacterial replication in the sample container may result in elevated bacterial counts. The first voided specimen in the morning is likely to demonstrate higher bacterial counts but is impractical in the clinical setting. Patients with indwelling catheters should have sampling directly from the catheter with a sterile needle and syringe. Samples taken directly from the catheter bag are usually contaminated.

Bacteriuria is defined as the culture from a voided urine specimen greater than 10^5 cfu/mL of a single

Management of Common Problems in Obstetrics and Gynecology, 5th edition. Edited by T.M. Goodwin, M.N. Montoro, L. Muderspach, R. Paulson and S. Roy. © 2010 Blackwell Publishing Ltd.

micro-organism. The isolation of less than 10^5 cfu/mL in an asymptomatic woman has a low positive predictive value for UTI and therefore is not an indication for antibiotic treatment. However, in patients with symptoms, a culture greater than or equal to 10^2 cfu/mL has a positive predictive value of 0.88. Therefore, in patients with symptoms of UTI, a culture of greater than 10^2 cfu/mL can be considered positive. Additionally, in patients who are already on antimicrobial therapy, lower colony counts may represent true infection rather than contamination. Likewise, lower colony counts of atypical organisms (*Klebsiella, Pseudomonas, Enterobacter, Serratia,* and *Moraxella* spp.) are more likely to represent true infection.

The US Preventive Services Task Force recommends against screening asymptomatic women for bacteriuria, as it has not been shown to be associated with any long-term sequelae. Women with asymptomatic bacteriuria (two consecutive specimens with greater than 10^5 cfu/mL of the same species) are more likely to develop symptomatic cystitis; these patients should be followed and treated only if symptomatic. Some groups of patients are at increased risk of developing asymptomatic bacteriuria, including patients with diabetes, spinal cord injuries and indwelling urinary catheters. These patients should be followed more closely but should not be treated for asymptomatic bacteriuria. Suppression with antibiotics is not indicated for indwelling catheters because it does not reduce the risk of infection and only results in the development of bacterial resistance. Nearly 100% of indwelling catheters will become colonized by 30 days. Whenever possible, the indwelling catheter should be removed and the patient should receive clean intermittent catheterization to reduce the risk of symptomatic cystitis. Pregnant patients with asymptomatic bacteriuria are at increased risk for developing pyelonephritis and should be treated.

Some patients may present with dysuria with a negative urine culture. False-negative urine cultures may be seen in patients who have been treated or are self-treating with antibiotics, or if the bladder has been irrigated or diluted. Patients with dysuria without frequency and urgency may have urethritis or vaginitis, and in these patients careful attention must be paid to evaluation for urethritis caused by *Neisseria gonorrhoeae* or *Chlamydia trachomatis*. Patients with a past history of sexually transmitted infections (STIs), recent change in sexual partner or symptoms of a gradual onset should be carefully evaluated for STIs. Patients should also be evaluated for signs and symptoms of vaginitis, particularly if dysuria is accompanied by symptoms of pruritus, dyspareunia, vaginal dryness or discharge. In postmenopausal women, atrophic vaginitis can be a cause of dysuria with negative urine cultures.

Symptomatic women without complicating factors can be treated with 3 days of trimethoprim/ sulfamethoxazole (TMP-SMX) double strength (DS) twice daily or trimethoprim 100 mg twice daily. Patients allergic to sulfa drugs or trimethoprim may be treated with nitrofurantoin 100 mg twice daily for 7 days or ciprofloxacin 250 mg twice daily for 3 days. In areas with high levels (> 20%) of *E. coli* resistant to TMP-SMX, first line should be either nitrofurantoin or ciprofloxacin. Increasing resistance to TMP-SMX is a growing concern and is being monitored closely. Local resistance patterns should be reviewed prior to prescription. Increases in quinolone resistance are being seen internationally and underscore the need to reserve ciprofloxacin use for serious infection. Caution should be used with both sulfa drugs and ciprofloxacin, which can increase INR values in patients on warfarin. Ciprofloxacin should not be used in patients who are pregnant or breastfeeding. In patients with severe urgency and dysuria, phenazopyridine (200 mg orally every 8 hours for up to 2 days) can be offered for analgesia, although it should not be used long term because of risks of toxicity. Additionally, patients should be warned that orange-red urinary discoloration is a common effect of this medication.

Sexual intercourse and spermicide use, especially with a diaphragm, have been shown to increase the risk of developing a UTI. Patients should be counseled and offered other forms of birth control and STI prevention. Increased fluid intake and postcoital voiding are reasonable strategies to dilute bacterial colonization of the bladder and urethra and are unlikely to be harmful, though neither strategy has been shown to improve outcomes in controlled trials. Cranberry juice has been embraced as a natural remedy for UTI and has been shown in some studies to decrease the adherence of bacteria to the uroepithelial cells, though clinical studies have had mixed results on the efficacy of cranberry juice. Several studies suggest that 300–750mL daily reduces the risk of recurrence. Capsules or tablets of nutritional supplements of cranberry juice might be preferred for patients to decrease the caloric load of high volumes of cranberry juice.

Recurrent UTI can be frustrating for patients and for clinicians. Most recurrent UTIs represent reinfection, and urine culture can help delineate whether or not the infection is from the same organism. Multiple recurrences with the same organism may necessitate further urologic evaluation for anatomic abnormalities or stones. Either continuous or postcoital prophylaxis is effective at preventing recurrent cystitis. Prophylaxis may be initiated after eradication of the active infection. Continuous prophylaxis is an option for women with two or more symptomatic infections during one 6-month period or three symptomatic infections over a 12-month period. Prophylaxis with nitrofurantoin, trimethoprim, TMP-SMX or ciprofloxacin may be considered, though studies have lacked power to suggest one agent over another. Prophylaxis is usually attempted for a 6-month period, though limited data suggest it may be continued for 2–5 years. In women who note a clear association of symptoms with sexual activity, postcoital prophylaxis may be a good option. Typical regimens to be taken within 2 hours after sexual intercourse include: TMP-SMX (80/400) half to one tablet, nitrofurantoin 50–100 mg or ciprofloxacin 250 mg. Another option for motivated, reliable patients is intermittent self-treatment. Women should be given a prescription for a 3-day course of antibiotics to start at the onset of symptoms, though they should be instructed to seek medical attention if symptoms do not resolve within 48 hours of the completion of antibiotics. Some postmenopausal women not on estrogen therapy may suffer from recurrent infections, presumably from the preferential growth of pathogenic organisms when the vaginal pH is > 4.5. Such patients respond to antibiotic treatment to eradicate the infection and estrogen therapy to restore vaginal epithelium integrity (thickening) and to restore a normal vaginal pH (< 4.5) and a normal balance of organisms.

Suggested reading

American College of Obstetricians and Gynecologists. ACOG practice bulletin No. 91. Treatment of urinary tract infections in nonpregnant women. *Obstet Gynecol* 2008; 111(3): 785–794.

Avorn J, Monane M, Gurwitz JH, Glynn RJ, Choodnovskiy I, Lipsitz A. Reduction of bacteriuria and pyuria after ingestion of cranberry juice. *JAMA* 1994; 271: 751–754.

Colgan R, Nicolle LE, McGlone A, Hooton TM. Asymptomatic bacteriuria in adults. *Am Fam Physician* 2006; 74: 985–990.

Fihn S. Acute uncomplicated urinary tract infection in women. *NEJM* 2003; 349: 259–266.

Hooton TM, Scholes D, Hughes JP, *et al.* A prospective study of risk factors for symptomatic urinary tract infection in young women. *NEJM* 1996; 335: 468–474.

Warren JW, Abrutyn E, Hebel JR, Johnson JR, Schaeffer AJ, Stamm WE. Guidelines for antimicrobial treatment of uncomplicated acute bacterial cystitis and acute pyelonephritis in women. Infectious Diseases Society of America (IDSA). *Clin Infect Dis* 1999; 29: 745–758.

Chapter 75
Voiding Dysfunction

Rebecca Urwitz-Lane and Begüm Özel

Department of Medicine and Obstetrics and Gynecology, Keck School of Medicine, University of Southern California, CA, USA

Introduction

Female voiding dysfunction is poorly understood and has no official definition. The term can be used to describe any number of voiding difficulties. According to the International Continence Society, "normal voiding is achieved by a voluntarily initiated continuous detrusor contraction that leads to complete bladder emptying within a normal time span, and in the absence of obstruction." Therefore, female voiding dysfunction can be presumed to be any condition that falls outside this definition.

Voiding dysfunction affects as many as 62% of women being referred to a urogynecologist or urologist for lower urinary tract symptoms (LUTS). The prevalence increases with age, and many women are asymptomatic. Often, urinary urgency and frequency are the only symptoms, and women are treated for urinary tract infections or overactive bladder without diagnosis of the voiding dysfunction.

Physiology of urine storage and voiding

The normal storage and emptying of urine depend on co-ordinated control at the level of the brainstem, spinal cord and peripheral nerves. The pontine micturition center controls voluntary voiding by co-ordinating relaxation of the urethral sphincter and contraction of the detrusor (bladder wall) muscle. This center receives inhibitory input from suprapontine centers including the cerebral cortex, cerebellum and basal ganglia, and stimulatory input from the anterior pons and posterior hypothalamus. It then relays efferent input to the bladder and urethral sphincter. There is another micturition center in the sacral spinal cord at the level of S2–4.

Management of Common Problems in Obstetrics and Gynecology, 5th edition. Edited by T.M. Goodwin, M.N. Montoro, L. Muderspach, R. Paulson and S. Roy. © 2010 Blackwell Publishing Ltd.

This center allows for bladder contraction without pontine or suprapontine input. The lower urinary tract gets its peripheral innervation from the pelvic, hypogastric and pudendal nerves. The bladder receives parasympathetic efferent innervation from S2–4 via the pelvic nerve; the bladder and urethra get sympathetic efferent innervation from T10–L2 via the hypogastric nerve; and the striated external urethral sphincter receives sympathetic innervation from S2–4 via the pudendal nerve.

Bladder filling and distension cause firing of sensory afferent nerves, which travel up the spinal cord to the pontine micturition center. If it is time to void, this center will relay that message via efferent output down the spinal cord to the pelvic plexus at spinal cord segments S2–4. From there, the pelvic nerve stimulates the detrusor muscle to contract. This is co-ordinated with the pudendal nerve signaling the urethral sphincter to relax and allow the passage of urine. If, on the other hand, it is not an appropriate time to void, suprapontine centers will send inhibitory input to the pontine micturition center and prevent voiding until the time is appropriate.

Patient evaluation

Patient history should focus on symptoms related to the lower urinary tract. Symptoms of voiding dysfunction include urinary urgency, frequency, hesitancy, a sense of incomplete bladder emptying, straining to void, decreased force of stream, and urinary retention. A complete medical and surgical history will often identify the underlying etiology. Relevant history includes symptoms of pelvic organ prolapse, neurologic symptoms, medical history such as diabetes mellitus, history of stroke or other neurologic injury, and surgical history, including surgery for incontinence or prolapse, any pelvic surgery, especially radical hysterectomy or colectomy, and neurologic or orthopedic spine surgery.

On exam, particular attention should be paid to the pelvis. The urethra should be examined for any lesions, such as obstructing masses. The vagina should be examined for prolapse of the anterior vaginal wall, vaginal apex or cervix, and the posterior vaginal wall, all of which can obstruct the urethra. On bimanual exam, the presence of any pelvic masses, such as leiomyomas, should be determined. Cervical and lower uterine myomas may sometimes lead to obstruction of the bladder outlet.

Urinary symptoms can often be the presenting symptoms of neurologic disease in young women. It is therefore crucial to perform a thorough neurologic evaluation of all patients with LUTS. The neurologic history focuses on mental status changes, upper and lower extremity weakness or sensory defects, as well as gait. Physical examination assesses these same functions. The Mini Mental Status Examination is a reliable tool for the evaluation of mental status. Having the patient extend and flex the hip, knee and ankle and invert and evert the foot tests muscle strength of the lower extremities. These tests assess sacral spinal cord integrity. Patellar, ankle and plantar deep tendon reflexes are also tested. Upper motor neuron lesions may be associated with hyper-reflexia, whereas lower motor neuron lesions may demonstrate diminished reflexes. Light touch and pinprick are used to test sensory function along the sacral dermatomes on the perineum and thighs. The anal reflex can assess the function of spinal cord segments L5–S5. When this reflex is intact, stroking the skin adjacent to the anus will elicit a reflex contraction of the external anal sphincter muscle. This reflex can be difficult to evaluate and is not always present in neurologically intact individuals. Cerebellar function can be evaluated by observing the patient's gait or by testing finger-to-nose or heel-to-shin co-ordination. In addition to inhibiting the pontine micturition center, the cerebellum also maintains pelvic floor tone.

Urinalysis must be performed in any patient presenting with LUTS to rule out infection. A postvoid bladder volume should also be measured to assess for retention. A postvoid residual bladder volume (PVR) of less than 25% of the total bladder volume is considered to be within the normal range; however, regardless of bladder volume, the PVR should always be less than 100 mL.

Filling cystometry and pressure flow voiding studies and uroflowmetry are used to further investigate bladder function during the filling and emptying phases. Filling cystometry assesses the ability of the bladder to fill and store urine. The bladder muscle (detrusor) should be quiescent during bladder filling. Women with voiding dysfunction may have contractions of the bladder muscle (detrusor contractions) during the filling phase or they may have decreased or absent bladder sensation during filling. These women may hold large volumes of fluid in their bladder without any urge to void. On uroflowmetry and pressure flow voiding studies, the voiding phase of bladder function can be assessed. The relationship between detrusor pressure and flow rate can help in identifying the underlying mechanism of voiding dysfunction.

Types of voiding dysfunction

There are two basic types of voiding dysfunction in women: neurogenic and non-neurogenic. Non-neurogenic voiding dysfunction refers to bladder outlet obstruction and is more common in men as a result of prostatic hypertrophy.

Non-neurogenic voiding dysfunction

Non-neurogenic voiding dysfunction is due to obstruction of the bladder outlet. This can be a functional problem in which the patient has developed a habit of dysfunctional voiding or an anatomic problem in which the bladder outlet and urethra are obstructed, such as by a urethral diverticulum, a urethral myoma, vaginal prolapse or prior incontinence surgery.

Dysfunctional voiding is the presence of external urethral sphincter contraction during voluntary voiding in a neurologically intact individual. This most commonly occurs in children who will present with enuresis and recurrent urinary tract infections, but it is also seen in adults. This is a learned behavior. It is normal to contract the pelvic floor muscles and urethral sphincter in order to defer voiding. This voluntary contraction is common in people who need to delay voiding due to work or other reasons, or who want to avoid voiding due to associated pain from inflammation, infection or other causes. If pelvic floor contraction becomes the body's response to a desire to void, it may also happen when the patient actually wants to empty her bladder. If this occurs during volitional voiding, the result is incomplete emptying and urinary retention. Electromyography evaluation of these patients will reveal increased pelvic floor activity during the voiding phase. These patients can be successfully managed with behavioral therapy or physical therapy aimed at relaxing the pelvic floor. α Blockade or diazepam may also help to decrease urethral tone. Sacral neuromodulation has also been shown to be effective in these cases and is FDA approved for the treatment of nonobstructive urinary retention.

Prolapse of the anterior vaginal wall can cause kinking of the urethra and resultant urgency, frequency and urinary retention. Sometimes apical or uterine prolapse and posterior vaginal wall prolapse will also be sufficiently great as to obstruct the urethra. This can be demonstrated by performing a urodynamic evaluation both with and without reduction of the prolapse. If the obstructive symptoms are due to the prolapse, they will resolve with the prolapse reduced. Pessary placement or surgical correction of the prolapse will treat the lower urinary tract symptoms in these cases. Reduction of prolapse can also unmask potential stress incontinence. It is therefore recommended that preoperative urodynamic evaluation be performed on all women who will be undergoing surgical correction of severe prolapse.

Urinary retention is a known complication of all surgeries aimed at correcting stress urinary incontinence. Most such cases of urinary retention resolve within the first week, but all patients should be counseled pre-operatively regarding the potential need for postoperative catheterization. In the rare case that urinary retention does persist, surgical correction may be required. Mid-urethral slings may be adjusted by pulling down the sling. This is a simple procedure that must be performed in the first 2–3 weeks before tissue ingrowth renders the sling material immobile. Post-sling retention diagnosed after this time can be treated by vaginally incising the sling. This will relieve the obstruction in 70–80%, while still retaining continence in up to 75% of women. Urinary retention following retropubic suspension procedure can be relieved in 65–93% of cases by performing urethrolysis. This involves surgical takedown of the periurethral scar tissue which can be performed suprapubically or transvaginally.

Acute urinary retention can develop postoperatively following any pelvic surgery or vaginal delivery. This can be due to pain, edema, hematoma or narcotic pain medication. It is important to diagnose acute urinary retention promptly and institute bladder drainage immediately to minimize overdistension of the bladder, which may result in potential injury to the bladder muscle and neurogenic bladder. Radical hysterectomy can lead to urinary retention due to denervation of the bladder. While most of these cases of urinary retention resolve with time, the injury may become permanent.

Neurogenic voiding dysfunction

Neurogenic voiding dysfunction can result from lesions at any level, and symptoms differ according to the location of the lesion. Suprapontine lesions, such as brain tumors, Parkinson's disease, multiple sclerosis, and cerebrovascular disease, usually result in uninhibited detrusor contractions. This condition is called detrusor hyper-reflexia or neurogenic detrusor overactivity. Affected individuals usually have urinary frequency, urgency and urge incontinence. Urinary retention is less common.

Spinal cord lesions or injuries cause uninhibited detrusor contractions as well as a dysco-ordination between the bladder and external sphincter, called detrusor–external sphincter dyssynergia (DESD). A properly functioning external sphincter relaxes when the detrusor muscle contracts to allow passage of urine. In DESD, the external sphincter and detrusor muscles contract simultaneously, resulting in bladder outlet obstruction and urinary retention. This is the most severe form of voiding dysfunction,

and can eventually lead to high bladder storage pressure, vesicoureteral reflux, and resultant damage to the upper urinary tract. Since high bladder pressures may result in vesicoureteral reflux and damage to the upper urinary tract, including hydronephrosis, it is important to evaluate the upper urinary tract in these women. Renal ultrasound to look for hydronephrosis, and BUN and creatinine to evaluate renal function should be obtained.

Infrasacral spinal cord lesions and peripheral nerve lesions can impair sensation and contractility of the bladder and external urethral sphincter, resulting in a hypotonic bladder. Common conditions that lead to this type of dysfunction include radical pelvic surgery, acute overdistension of the bladder, diabetic neuropathy, lumbar disk prolapse, sacral cord lesions, and spina bifida.

Treatment of voiding dysfunction in women with neurogenic causes primarily consists of clean intermittent catheterization (CIC). Indwelling catheters are not recommended because of the associated risks of infection, stone formation, and erosions. In women who cannot perform CIC, suprapubic catheterization may be considered. Anticholinergic medication may be used concomitantly for detrusor contractions. Injection of botulinum toxin into the urethral sphincter has also been shown to improve the ability to void.

Suggested reading

Ahmed HU, Shergill IS, Arya M, Sha PJ. Management of detrusor-external sphincter dyssynergia. *Nat Clin Pract Urol* 2006; 3(7): 368–380.

Chai AH, Wong T, Mak HL, *et al.* Prevalence and associated risk factors of retention of urine after caesarean section. *Int Urogynecol J Pelvic Floor Dysfunct* 2008; 19(4): 537–542.

Dörflinger A, Monga A. Voiding dysfunction. *Curr Opin Obstet Gynecol* 2001; 13(5): 507–512.

Germain MM. Urinary retention and overflow incontinence. In: Ostergard DR, Bent AE, Cundiff GW, Swift SE (eds) *Ostergard's urogynecology and pelvic floor dysfunction*, 5th edn. Philadelphia, PA: Lippincott, Williams and Wilkins, 2003: 285–291.

Glavind K, Bjørk J. Incidence and treatment of urinary retention postpartum. *Int Urogynecol J Pelvic Floor Dysfunct* 2003; 14(2): 119–121.

Lazarou G, Scotti RJ, Mikhail MS, *et al.* Pessary reduction and postoperative cure of retention in women with anterior vaginal wall prolapse. *Int Urogynecol J Pelvic Floor Dysfunct* 2004; 15(3): 175–178.

Musselwhite KL, Faris P, Moore K, *et al.* Use of epidural anesthesia and the risk of acute postpartum urinary retention. *Am J Obstet Gynecol* 2007; 196(5): 472.

Nitti V, Fleishmann N. Voiding dysfunction and urinary retention. In: Walters MD, Karram MM (eds) *Urogynecology and pelvic reconstructive surgery*, 3rd edn. Philadelphia, PA: Mosby, 2006: 390–401.

Olujide LO, O'Sullivan SM. Female voiding dysfunction. *Best Pract Res Clin Obstet Gynaecol* 2005; 19(6): 807–828.

Özel B. Incarceration of a retroflexed, gravid uterus from severe uterine prolapse: a case report. *J Reprod Med* 2005; 50(8): 624–626.

Özel B, Minaglia S, Hurtado E, *et al.* Treatment of voiding dysfunction after transobturator tape procedure. *Urology* 2004; 64(5): 1030.

Sokol AI, Jelovsek JE, Walters MD, *et al.* Incidence and predictors of prolonged urinary retention after TVT with and without concurrent prolapse surgery. *Am J Obstet Gynecol* 2005; 192(5): 1537–1543.

Swinn MJ, Wisemann OJ, Lowe E, Fowler CJ. The cause and natural history of isolated urinary retention in young women. *J Urol* 2002; 167(1): 151–156.

Van Kerrebroeck PE, van Voskuilen AC, Heesakkers JP, *et al.* Results of sacral neuromodulation therapy for urinary voiding dysfunction: outcomes of a prospective, worldwide clinical study. *J Urol* 2007; 178(5): 2029–2034.

Chapter 76
Painful Bladder Syndrome/ Interstitial Cystitis

Begüm Özel

Department of Medicine and Obstetrics and Gynecology, Keck School of Medicine, University of Southern California, CA, USA

Introduction

Painful bladder syndrome/interstitial cystitis (PBS/IC) is characterized by a constellation of symptoms including pelvic pain, urinary urgency and frequency, pain with bladder filling, and dyspareunia. Painful bladder syndrome (PBS) and interstitial cystitis (IC) are two names for the same disorder. PBS is the term preferred by the International Continence Society, but since the term IC is so familiar to most physicians, its use remains widespread. Therefore, we will refer to the condition as PBS/IC.

Painful bladder syndrome/interstitial cystitis is generally considered in the context of chronic pelvic pain (CPP). CPP is defined as noncyclic pain lasting longer than 6 months and affects an estimated 15% of women in the United States. About 10% of gynecology referrals are for CPP. A large analysis of multiple studies indicated that 37% of cases of CPP are gastrointestinal in origin, with urologic conditions accounting for an estimated 31% of cases, and gynecologic causes occurring in 20% of cases. Other causes include musculoskeletal and psychologic.

Urologic conditions that account for CPP in women include bladder neoplasm, chronic or recurrent urinary tract infection, radiation cystitis, urethritis, urolithiasis, uninhibited bladder contractions, urethral diverticulum, chronic urethral syndrome, and PBS/IC. A thorough evaluation to rule out these other causes is recommended before giving a woman the diagnosis of PBS/IC. Since there is no way to diagnose PBS/IC definitively, the diagnosis is largely one of exclusion. In women with overactive bladder refractory to medical management, PBS/IC should be considered.

The mean age at onset of PBS/IC is 42 years, although 30% of those diagnosed are younger than 30 years of age. The disorder also affects men but is more common in women, with a female-to-male ratio of 10:1. The estimated prevalence among women in the US is 0.5%.

Symptoms

The most common symptoms of PBS/IC are urinary urgency and frequency, often associated with nocturia; 92% of patients report these symptoms. Suprapubic pelvic pain, often associated with bladder filling and relieved with voiding, is found in 70% of patients. Dyspareunia occurs in 50% of women with the diagnosis. Less common symptoms include vulvar, rectal or low back pain. Dysuria is not common. Symptoms tend to wax and wane, with flare-ups followed by periods of relative quiescence. Frequently women with this condition will be diagnosed with recurrent urinary tract infections. The symptoms will appear to have resolved with antibiotic treatment, but the transient resolution of symptoms is simply part of the natural history of the disorder. There is significant overlap between PBS/IC and other diagnoses, especially overactive bladder, which is characterized by urinary urgency and frequency without pelvic pain, and endometriosis, which can present with suprapubic pelvic pain and pain with bladder filling but usually lacks the urgency and frequency that are hallmarks of PBS/IC. There have been some reports noting an association between PBS/IC and vulvodynia and irritable bowel syndrome.

Several questionnaires exist for quantifying symptoms in PBS/IC. It is important to note that none of these questionnaires has been sufficiently studied for establishing the diagnosis. The most commonly used questionnaires are the O'Leary–Sant Interstitial Cystitis Symptom Index and Problem Index questionnaire and the Pelvic Pain and Urgency/Frequency symptom scale. The Pelvic Pain and Urgency/Frequency symptom scale has also been validated in US Spanish. These questionnaires can be useful in following the course of the disorder and the response to treatment.

The diagnosis of PBS/IC is determined by the presence of symptoms consistent with PBS/IC and the

Management of Common Problems in Obstetrics and Gynecology,
5th edition. Edited by T.M. Goodwin, M.N. Montoro,
L. Muderspach, R. Paulson and S. Roy. © 2010 Blackwell
Publishing Ltd.

exclusion of other possible etiologies based on physical exam and diagnostic testing. Certain historical factors such as a history of pelvic radiation and chemical cystitis due to cyclophosphamide use probably excludes the diagnosis. Other exclusion criteria for the diagnosis set by the National Institute of Diabetes and Digestive and Kidney Diseases/National Institutes of Health (NIDDK/NIH) for research purposes include bacterial cystitis within the last 3 months, history of bladder calculi, genital herpes in the last 12 weeks, history of uterine, cervical, vaginal or urethral cancer, urethral diverticulum, history of tuberculous cystitis, history of benign or malignant bladder tumors, and active vaginitis.

Pathophysiology

It is important to remember that there is no way to diagnose PBS/IC definitively. There is no proven etiology or pathognomonic features. Leading theories of pathogenesis include neurogenic inflammation and urothelial dysfunction. Neurogenic inflammation is a normal response to injury and involves the activation of peripheral sensory nerves. This results in a release of substance P and neuropeptides from unmyelinated C fibers, mast cell and vascular smooth muscle activation, and sensory nerve fiber proliferation. There is thought to be an altered or increased sensory neuropeptide and inflammatory mediator expression and increased sympathetic innervation in patients with PBS/IC. Urothelial dysfunction refers to the absence or deficiency of the glycosaminoglycan (GAG) layer that is believed to protect the urothelium from urinary toxins. This layer is thought to be deficient in patients with PBS/IC. However, this has not been conclusively demonstrated. It is also possible that deficiency of the layer may be the result of neurogenic inflammation rather than an independent etiology of PBS/IC. Furthermore, some studies have found no difference in the GAG layer in the bladders of women with PBS/IC compared to controls.

Evaluation

An evaluation of a patient with PBS/IC begins with a thorough history including a voiding diary, physical exam, urinalysis, urine culture, urine cytology, and cystoscopy. If there is evidence of infection, this should be treated, and successful treatment confirmed by a urine culture for test-of-cure. Cystoscopy is recommended for most women with these symptoms to rule out bladder lesions such as malignancy, benign bladder tumors or bladder stones. The presence of microscopic or gross hematuria has poor sensitivity for detecting bladder lesions; therefore, cystoscopy is indicated regardless of the urinalysis findings. Many women with these symptoms

will be unable to tolerate office cystoscopy, so cystoscopy under anesthesia may be required. Cystoscopy under general or regional anesthesia can be performed with or without hydrodistension. Cystoscopy with hydrodistension under general or regional anesthesia is one of the diagnostic criteria for NIDDK/NIH-funded studies, but many clinicians have abandoned it due to its poor specificity. In bladder hydrodistension, the bladder is filled to a pressure of 80 cmH$_2$O with the patient under anesthesia to determine the patient's maximum anesthetized bladder capacity. In normal women, anesthetized bladder capacity is usually about 1000 mL; in women with PBS/IC it is often less than 800 mL. After the bladder is drained, repeat cystoscopy is performed to examine the bladder epithelium for petechiae, glomerulations, which represent broken submucosal capillaries, submucosal hemorrhage, and Hunner's ulcers. The presence of a Hunner's ulcer on cystoscopy is not common but is the most specific finding that is diagnostic of PBS/IC. Some studies have found that there is little difference in bladder lesions between women with and without symptoms consistent with PBS/IC; for this reason, many physicians have abandoned the use of this technique.

The potassium sensitivity test (PST) is also highly controversial, and most experts in the field consider its use still investigational. The PST is based on the premise that a deficient GAG layer is responsible for PBS/IC and aims to diagnose women with deficient GAG layers through the use of a hypertonic potassium solution that is instilled in the bladder. However, even in the hands of the proponents of the test, only 71% of those clinically diagnosed with PBS/IC had a positive test. Among women with other diagnoses, 55% of women with urethral syndrome, 78% with laparoscopically proven endometriosis, and 81% with CPP had a positive test, suggesting that the test indicates generalized hypersensitivity rather than the diagnosis of PBS/IC. Since it does not improve diagnostic yield, causes the patient extreme pain, and is unable to differentiate between causes of CPP, it is not recommended for clinical practice.

Urinary markers are the future of PBS/IC, but currently remain investigational. Antiproliferative factor is the best studied of urinary markers and has been shown to normalize with treatment. Further studies in this area are under way.

Treatment

There are very few effective therapies for PBS/IC, and none that has been proven to alter the course of the disease. Patients given this diagnosis should be counseled regarding the chronic nature of the disease and the absence of a cure, and referred to support groups for PBS/IC. Dietary instructions are often given that exclude certain bladder irritants, such as alcohol, citrus fruits and other acidic foods, and caffeine, from the diet. Oral agents that have been proven to be effective in the syndrome in randomized controlled trials include amitriptyline and pentosan polysulfate (PPS). Amytriptyline is commonly used for pain syndromes and may modify pain sensitivity. PPS is the only FDA-approved oral agent for the treatment of PBS/IC. While it is more effective than placebo, success as determined by greater than 50% improvement is seen in no more than 50% of patients taking the drug. Improvement in urinary frequency occurs in 54% of patients while improvement in pain occurs in only 37% of those affected. Common side effects include reversible alopecia, diarrhea, nausea, and headache, although it is generally well tolerated. PPS is a weak heparinoid and is believed to work by restoring the GAG layer in patients affected with the condition. Maximal benefit with PPS is seen at 3–6 months; therefore, the duration of use should be at least 3–4 months before it is deemed ineffective.

Other oral agents that are used in treating PBS/IC include hydroxyzine 25–75 mg daily, gapapentin 300–2100 mg daily, and anticholinergics, such as oxybutynin and tolterodine, for treating the urgency and frequency associated with the condition.

Dimethyl sulfoxide (DMSO) is currently the only FDA-approved intravesical therapy. It is a chemical solvent with anti-inflammatory, analgesic, muscle relaxation, mast cell inhibition, and collagen dissolution properties and is given in weekly or biweekly treatment. It is commonly associated with garlic-like odor and taste as well as transient bladder instability in those receiving the treatment. The mechanism of action is not determined but may involve depletion of sensory neuropeptides or mast cell inhibition. Other intravesical therapies that are used include intravesical instillation of methylprednisone 500–1000 mg in 10–20 mL of normal saline, heparin 10,000–20,000 units in 5–20 mL, and 20–30 mL of lidocaine 1% or marcaine 0.5%. Often these three are combined into one "cocktail" and administered intravesically through a urethral catheter. The patient is asked to wait at least 20–30 minutes or as long as she can tolerate before emptying her bladder. The treatment is given 1–3 times per week for 6–8 weeks. Some patients may be able to instill the solution into their bladder at home. Unfortunately, there are currently limited data on the efficacy of these instillations.

Other effective therapy includes passive bladder hydrodistension which provides symptomatic temporary relief in up to 50% of patients, making it both a therapeutic as well as a diagnostic test. However, the mechanism of action is not understood and is thought to involve injury to nerve endings in the bladder, making it an unattractive option for many clinicians. Physical therapy and psychologic counseling may be beneficial in some patients. Sacral nerve stimulation, pudendal nerve stimulation, and intravesical botulinum toxin may be other potential therapies. Multimodal therapy is beneficial in most patients, since no one therapy is likely fully to relieve symptoms.

In summary, PBS/IC is a complex and poorly understood disorder. It is one of the many causes of CPP and is a diagnosis of exclusion. Urinary urgency and frequency accompanied by pelvic pain and pain with bladder filling should raise suspicion for the disorder and prompt further evaluation of the lower urinary tract in these patients. FDA-approved treatments include PPS and DMSO, although amitryptyline and bladder hydrodistension have also been proven to be effective in small randomized trials.

Suggested reading

Chai TC. Interstitial cystitis. In: Ostergard DR, Bent AE, Cundiff G, Swift S (eds) *Ostergard's urogynecology and pelvic floor dysfunction*, 5th edn. Philadelphia, PA: Lippincott Williams and Wilkins, 2003: 245–260

Clemons JL, Arya LA, Myers DA. Diagnosing interstitial cystitis in women with chronic pelvic pain. *Obstet Gynecol* 2002; 100(2): 337–341.

Dawson TE, Jamison J. Intravesical treatments for painful bladder syndrome/interstitial cystitis. *Cochrane Database Syst Rev* 2007; 4: CD006113.

Dimitrakov J, Kroenke K, Steers WD, *et al*. Pharmacologic management of painful bladder syndrome/interstitial cystitis: a systematic review. *Arch Intern Med* 2007; 167(18): 1922–1929.

Lubeck DP, Whitmore K, Sant GR, Alvarez-Horine S, Lai C, Psychometric validation of the O'Leary–Sant Interstitial Cystitis Symptom Index in a clinical trial of pentosan polysulfate sodium. *Urology* 2001; 57: 62.

Minaglia SM, Özel B, Bizhang R, Mishell DR Jr. Increased prevalence of interstitial cystitis in women with detrusor overactivity refractory to anticholinergic therapy. *Urology* 2005; 66(4): 702–706.

Minaglia SM, Özel B, Nguyen JN, Mishell DR Jr . Validation of Spanish version of Pelvic Pain and Urgency/Frequency (PUF) patient symptom scale. *Urology* 2005; 65(4): 664–669.

Nickel JC, Barkin J, Forrest J, *et al*. Randomized, double-blind, dose-ranging study of pentosan polysulfate sodium for interstitial cystitis. *Urology* 2005; 65(4): 654–658.

O'Leary MP, Sant GR, Fowler FJ Jr, *et al*. The Interstitial Cystitis Symptom Index and Problem Index. *Urology* 1997; 49(5A suppl): 58–63.

Parsons CL, Dell J, Stanford EJ, *et al*. Increased prevalence of interstitial cystitis previously unrecognized urologic and gynecologic cases identified using a new symptom questionnaire and intravesical potassium sensitivity. *Urology* 2002; 60: 573–578.

Rosamilia A. Painful bladder syndrome/interstitial cystitis. *Best Pract Res Clin Obstet Gynaecol* 2005; 19(6): 843–859.

Van de Merwe JP, Nordling J, Bouchelouche P, *et al*. Diagnostic criteria, classification, and nomenclature for painful bladder syndrome/interstitial cystitis: an ESSIC proposal. *Eur Urol* 2008; 53(1): 60–67.

Van Ophoven A, Pokupic S, Heinecke A, Hertle L. A prospective, randomized, placebo controlled, double-blind study of amitriptyline for the treatment of interstitial cystitis. *J Urol* 2004; 172(2): 533–536.

Chapter 77
Urethral Disorders

Rebecca Urwitz-Lane and Begüm Özel

Department of Medicine and Obstetrics and Gynecology, Keck School of Medicine, University of Southern California, CA, USA

Normal urethral anatomy

The female urethra is a muscular tube approximately 4 cm long and 6 mm wide. It derives embryologically from the urogenital sinus. It lies within the adventitia of the anterior vagina, extending from the bladder base to the external meatus, which opens into the vestibule. The wall of the urethra is made up of four layers. The innermost layer is stratified squamous epithelium, which becomes transitional near the bladder. This epithelium is surrounded by a submucosa with a rich vascular supply and multiple glands, which open into the urethra. The largest of these are the Skene's glands, adjacent to the distal urethra. Surrounding the submucosa are two layers of smooth muscle: an inner longitudinal layer and an outer circular layer. The outermost layer of the urethra, the striated urogenital sphincter muscle, is made up of slow-twitch fibers which maintain the constant resting tone of the urethra and can contract to provide additional pressure when needed. The anterior urethral and the pubourethral (posterior urethral) ligaments form a sling that suspends the urethra behind the pubic symphysis.

Urethral diverticula

Urethral diverticula are epithelium-lined sacs pouching out from the urethral lumen. They lie within the periurethral fascia and have no surrounding muscular wall. They generally range in size from 3 mm to 3 cm in diameter. It is believed that repeated infection of the periurethral glands leads to ductal obstruction and eventual rupture into the urethral lumen. This rupture tract will eventually epithelialize and become a diverticulum. A noncommunicating diverticulum can occur if the diverticular neck becomes obstructed. As these glands are present throughout the urethra, a diverticulum can occur anywhere along the length of the urethra, but is most commonly located posteriorly. Diverticula are prone to urine stasis and infection. Inflammation and chronic irritation can rarely lead to malignant degeneration.

Urethral diverticula most commonly present in women in their 20s to 40s. Their reported incidence is 0.6–6%, but the actual incidence may be higher as the diagnosis can be missed. Symptoms are often nonspecific. Some women complain of a suburethral vaginal mass, but many do not. Other common symptoms include dyspareunia, recurrent urinary tract infections, postvoid dribbling, urinary urgency and frequency, and symptoms of stress incontinence. The classic symptom triad of dysuria, dyspareunia, and dribbling is rarely seen. A urethral diverticulum should be ruled out in all women with recurrent refractory urinary tract infections.

Physical exam may reveal a suburethral cyst, but is often unremarkable. In these cases, additional studies are needed. Positive pressure urethrography (PPUG) was described in 1958 as a method of diagnosing diverticula. In this procedure, a double-balloon catheter blocks the urethra at both ends as it fills with contrast. If present, a diverticulum will be seen to fill with dye in up to 90% of cases. Transvaginal or transperineal ultrasonography is equally effective in making the diagnosis and is simpler to perform and more comfortable for the patient. Pelvic MRI has better sensitivity and better positive predictive and negative predictive value than PPUG for the diagnosis of urethral diverticula. MRI also has the advantage of delineating the extent of a diverticulum, which can aid in surgical planning. Urethroscopy may identify diverticular openings up to 90% of the time. Voiding cystourethrogram can be performed, but only has a diagnostic accuracy of 65–70%.

The risks of surgery include hemorrhage, infection, wound breakdown and development of a urethral stricture or urethrovaginal fistula. For this reason, nonsurgical management is preferred for asymptomatic diverticula and for those identified during pregnancy

Management of Common Problems in Obstetrics and Gynecology, 5th edition. Edited by T.M. Goodwin, M.N. Montoro, L. Muderspach, R. Paulson and S. Roy. © 2010 Blackwell Publishing Ltd.

or in any woman who is not a good surgical candidate. These patients can be managed conservatively with antibiotics and decompression or aspiration. Aspiration is performed by inserting an 18 gauge needle into the diverticulum and aspirating its contents with a syringe.

The details of surgical removal of a urethral diverticulum are beyond the scope of this chapter. But it is important to know that when a diverticulum is excised surgically, the urethra is repaired in layers, with nonoverlapping suture lines. The goal of the repair is a tension-free watertight anastomosis. Bladder drainage is continued for 2 weeks postoperatively. A voiding cystourethrogram is obtained 2 weeks postoperatively. If there is no extravasation, bladder drainage can be discontinued.

Atrophic urethritis

The urethra is estrogen sensitive and a lack of estrogen can lead to atrophic changes. The symptoms of atrophic urethritis include urgency, frequency, dysuria, dyspareunia, and recurrent urinary tract infections. Physical examination reveals an atrophic vagina and urethral meatus, which may appear pale and friable. An elevated vaginal pH > 4.5 is consistent with a lack of estrogen. Treatment is with vaginal estrogen replacement, which restores the vaginal pH to < 4.5 usually within several weeks.

Acute urethritis

Acute infection of the urethra is usually the result of a sexually transmitted infection, most commonly gonorrhea or chlamydia. Symptoms include dysuria, urgency and frequency. The differential diagnosis therefore includes urinary tract infection as well as any infection that could cause vulvovaginal inflammation. A pelvic exam, wet mount and urine cultures should be performed to rule out vaginal and urinary tract infection. Urethral swabs looking for gonorrhea and chlamydia should be taken.

Nongonococcal urethritis should be treated with azithromycicn 500 mg daily for 6 days or a 2-week course of doxycycline 100 mg twice daily. Gonorrhea should be treated with a single dose of cephalosporin with either a single dose of azithromycin or a 1-week course of doxycycline to cover chlamydia.

Urethral pain syndrome

Urethral pain syndrome is defined by the International Continence Society as "the occurrence of recurrent episodic urethral pain usually on voiding, with daytime frequency and nocturia, in the absence of proven infection or other obvious pathology." Symptoms must persist for a minimum of 6 months. Patients often give a history of recurrent urinary tract infections or recurrent yeast infections, which do not respond to treatment. There is a bimodal distribution for the incidence of this syndrome with women most commonly affected in their 20s or their 50s. The cause is not known, but some theories include hypersensitivity dysfunction, allergy, early interstitial cystitis and response to stress. It is possible that this syndrome is brought on by an initial infection with poor resolution of symptoms, which leads to a hypersensitization of the nerves of the urethra and pelvic floor. In order to make the diagnosis, one must rule out vaginal and urinary tract infections, acute urethritis, atrophic urethritis, urethral pathology and interstitial cystitis.

Patient education is the first and crucial step in the treatment of this syndrome. Treatment often takes a long time and will include oral and local medication, physical therapy and dietary and lifestyle modifications. Each patient will need to experiment with diet to determine which foods exacerbate her particular symptoms. It is generally believed that caffeine, alcohol and spicy or acidic foods should be avoided. A course of doxycycline or azithromycin should be given to treat any possible subacute or undiagnosed infection.

There is a wide variety of pharmacologic agents available for the treatment of urethral pain syndrome. Amitryptyline is a tricyclic antidepressant with pain-modulating effects that has been used successfully in various chronic pain syndromes including interstitial cystitis and urethral pain syndrome. Selective serotonin reuptake inhibitors have also been used with good results. Urethral smooth muscle relaxants (such as prazosin or terazosin) and skeletal muscle relaxants (such as diazepam) have also been shown to improve the symptoms of urethral pain syndrome. None of these therapies takes effect immediately, and it is important to explain this to patients. Anti-inflammatory medications are helpful in controlling symptoms while waiting for definitive therapy to have its effect. Courses of antispasmodics such as phenazopyridine can also be given for 1–3 days for acute flares. Bladder retraining and sacral neuromodulation may help with symptoms of urinary frequency. Pelvic floor exercises can help to relax overactive pelvic muscles, thereby relieving pain. Accupuncture can also be considered, although data are lacking.

Urethral caruncle

A caruncle appears as a 5–10 mm red inflammatory lesion on the posterior aspect of the urethral meatus. They are commonly seen in postmenopausal women. These may be asymptomatic or may cause pain and bleeding. Treatment is with sitz baths and local estrogen, and surgical excision may be necessary if this fails.

Urethral prolapse

Urethral prolapse is a circumferential eversion of urethral mucosa protruding beyond the urethral meatus. There is a separation of the smooth muscle layers that leads to prolapse of the mucosal layer. The condition is usually painless unless the mucosa becomes strangulated; bleeding may be the presenting symptom. The condition appears most often in premenarchal girls and postmenopausal women. There are several reports of the condition after periurethral injections of bulking agents. Treatment is with topical estrogen and sitz baths. Surgical excision is reserved for symptomatic women if conservative treatment fails. Complications of surgical excision include recurrence and urethral stricture.

Suggested reading

Bent A. Disorders affecting the urethra. In: Ostergard DR, Bent AE, Cundiff G, Swift S (eds) *Ostergard's urogynecology and pelvic floor dysfunction,* 5th edn. Philadelphia, PA: Lippincott Williams and Wilkins, 2003: 245–260.

Delancey JOL. Anatomy of the female bladder and urethra. In: Ostergard DR, Bent AE, Cundiff G, Swift S (eds) *Ostergard's urogynecology and pelvic floor dysfunction,* 5th edn. Philadelphia, PA: Lippincott Williams and Wilkins, 2003: 3–18.

Fortunato P, Schettini M, Gallucci M. Diagnosis and therapy of the female urethral diverticula. *Int Urogyn J* 2001; 12(1): 51–57.

Özel B, Ballard C. Urethral and paraurethral leiomyomas in the female patient. *Int Urogynecol J Pelvic Floor Dysfunct* 2006; 17(1): 93–95.

Özel B, Urwitz-Lane R, White T. Patient characteristics and pathology of surgically treated periurethral masses. *J Pelvic Med Surg* 2007; 13(3): 141–143.

Palma PC, Riccetto CL, Martins MH, et al. Massive prolapse of the urethral mucosa following periurethral injection of calcium hydroxylapatite for stress urinary incontinence. *Int Urogyencol J Pelvic Floor Dysfunct* 2006; 17(6): 670–671.

Prasad SR, Menias CO, Narra VR, et al. Cross-sectional imaging of the female urethra: technique and results. *Radiographics* 2005; 25(3): 749–761.

Valerie E, Gilchrist BF, Frischer J, et al. Diagnosis and treatment of urethral prolapse in children. *Urology* 1999; 54(6): 1082–1084.

Vasavada SP. Urethral diverticula. In: Walters MD, Karram MM (eds) *Urogynecology and pelvic reconstructive surgery,* 3rd edn. Philadelphia, PA: Mosby, 2006: 461–471.

Chapter 78
Anal Incontinence

Ticaria Jackson and Begüm Özel
Department of Medicine and Obstetrics and Gynecology, Keck School of Medicine, University of Southern California, CA, USA

Anatomy

The anus is composed of an external anal sphincter, an internal anal sphincter, and an anal canal. The anal canal is the terminal end of the gastrointestinal tract. It is composed of a mucosa and submucosa surrounded by the lamina propria, an internal circularly oriented muscle layer, and an external longitudinal layer. The dentate (or pectineal) line is the visually identifiable mucocutaneous junction that divides the anal canal. Above the dentate line, the mucosa is composed of columnar epithelium. Below the dentate line, the anal canal is lined by squamous epithelium. The external anal sphincter (EAS) is 0.6–1.0 cm in thickness, composed of striated muscle and innervated by the pudendal nerve. The EAS is divided into superficial and deep portions. The superficial portion attaches to the coccyx posteriorly and sends fibers into the perineal body anteriorly. The deep portion encircles the rectum and blends into the puborectalis muscle. The EAS provides 25–30% of the resting tone. The internal anal sphincter (IAS) is a continuation of the inner circular smooth muscle of the bowel wall. It is 0.3–0.5 cm thick and lies just deep to the EAS. The IAS can be identified just beneath the anal submucosa and provides 50–80% of the resting tone of the anal wall. It is innervated by the intrinsic autonomic system of the gastrointestinal tract and is in a continuous state of maximal contraction. The anal canal is 2.5–4 cm in length. The blood supply to the upper half of the anal canal is from the superior hemorrhoidal artery, a distal branch of the inferior mesenteric artery.

The puborectalis is part of the pubococcygeus muscle and is the most medial portion of the levator ani complex. It arises from the inner surface of the pubic bones, passes the urethra without attaching to it, and inserts into the rectum. Some fibers insert into the EAS. The puborectalis forms a sling around the rectum, creating the anorectal angle at the anorectal junction. The anorectal angle is 90° at rest, 70° with squeezing, and 110–130° during defecation.

The pudendal nerve provides sensory and motor function to the pelvis. It arises from the sacral plexus (S2–S4). The labial nerve and inferior rectal nerve, both branches of the pudendal nerve, innervate the perineum. The pudendal nerve also innervates the EAS and perianal skin via the inferior hemorrhoidal branch.

Maintenance of continence

As colonic contents move into the rectum, the rectum distends. The IAS relaxes, allowing rectal contents to come into contact with specialized sensory epithelium in the anal canal. This is called anorectal sampling. The EAS contracts via a parasympathetically mediated reflex. The EAS exerts a greater percentage of the anal tone in the presence of rectal distension. If evacuation of the rectum is not appropriate, sympathetically mediated inhibition of the smooth muscle of the rectum and voluntary contraction of the EAS and puborectalis musculature occur. The bolus of material is pushed back up the rectum to the rectal reservoir. Contraction of the puborectalis increases the anorectal angle and keeps the bolus above the IAS.

Prevalence of anal incontinence

Anal incontinence (AI) is the involuntary loss of flatus, liquid or solid stool; fecal incontinence (FI) is the involuntary loss of liquid or solid stool. Among women aged 18–65, anal incontinence is reported by 28.4% and fecal incontinence by 15.9%. In women over the age of 40, fecal incontinence is reported by 24%. Women are affected 8:1 over males. Less than 20% of patients with fecal incontinence actually report it to their physician. In a study of 200 women seen in our urogynecology clinic, we found that women were more likely to report

Management of Common Problems in Obstetrics and Gynecology, 5th edition. Edited by T.M. Goodwin, M.N. Montoro, L. Muderspach, R. Paulson and S. Roy. © 2010 Blackwell Publishing Ltd.

this symptom in a written questionnaire when compared to direct questioning by the physician.

Etiology of anal incontinence

The most important risk factors for fecal incontinence include increasing age, increasing BMI and irritable bowel syndrome. Other risk factors are diabetes mellitus, history of stroke, spinal cord trauma, degenerative nervous system disorders, history of pelvic and/or anorectal surgery, and inflammatory diseases of the bowel.

Childbirth is a common predisposing factor to fecal incontinence in younger women; however, the effect of childbirth on rates of fecal incontinence disappears with age. Besides disruption of the internal or external sphincter by a third- or fourth-degree perineal laceration, which has been shown to increase the risk of postpartum fecal incontinence, damage to the pudendal nerve through overstretching and/or prolonged compression and ischemia may play a role. Fecal incontinence in the postpartum period is more common after a fourth-degree than a third-degree perineal laceration. As many as 50% of women who sustain a third- or fourth-degree obstetric tear experience some impairment of anorectal function after primary repair. Obstetric risk factors predisposing to anal sphincter lacerations include episiotomy, use of forceps or vacuum assistance, occiput posterior presentation, fetal weight > 4000 g, and prolonged second stage of labor.

History and physical examination

It is important to obtain a thorough history, including the onset, frequency, type of stool lost, history of obstetric tears, trauma, surgery, and medical conditions predisposing to incontinence. A careful physical exam including a vaginal exam, evaluation of the perineum, and a neurologic exam should be performed. Resting tone represents the IAS and squeeze pressure represents the EAS. The EAS is palpable as a 1.5–2 cm moderately firm doughnut-shaped mass within the perineal body. Usually one index finger is inserted rectally and the thumb of the same hand or the other index finger is used to identify the anal sphincter and to determine if there are any defects.

Imaging and diagnostic studies

Endoanal ultrasound

Sensitivity and specificity of ultrasound for detecting sphincter defects are 98–100% for the EAS and 95.5% for the IAS. Normal thickness of the EAS is 7.5–9 mm and it appears as a hyperechoic circumferential ring. The IAS has a normal thickness of 6–7 mm and appears as a hypoechoic or sonolucent ring that is medial to the EAS.

Endoanal ultrasonography is the single most important study for determining treatment options for a patient with fecal incontinence because it identifies the presence of sphincter defects that may be amenable to surgical repair.

Anal manometry

Anal manometry is used to evaluate both resting and squeeze pressures of the anal sphincter, as well as rectal capacity and rectal compliance. The average sphincter length is 3 cm. Normal resting rectal pressure is 10 mmHg, resting anal pressure is 40–80 mmHg, and maximum squeeze anal pressure is 80–160 mmHg. The normal minimal sensory volume within the rectum is 10 mL. Mean resting and squeeze pressures are lower in women who have had a vaginal delivery regardless of sphincter disruption.

Electromyography (EMG)

Electromyography helps evaluate the electrical activity generated by muscle fibers during rest, voluntary muscle contraction, and Valsalva-type activities. Results can be used to map normal muscle fibers. Abnormal EMG findings are present in over 90% of patients with fecal incontinence.

Pudendal nerve terminal motor latency (PNTML)

Pudendal nerve terminal motor latency helps to evaluate the length of time required for a fixed electrical stimulus to travel along the pudendal nerve from the ischial spine to the anal verge. Normal latency is less than 2 ms. In one study, the only predictor of the development of the anal incontinence at 2–4 years post partum in women with disruption of the anal sphincter was an abnormal PNTML. Many investigators have suggested PNTML as the most significant predictor of the outcome of sphincteroplasty. Prolonged PNTML may increase the likelihood of failure of surgical therapy, and this should be discussed with the patient. However, if a sphincter defect is present, sphincteroplasty may at least improve the patient's symptoms and should be offered.

Treatment

Nonsurgical therapy

Patients should be encouraged to maintain regular bowel habits and to make a conscious effort to have bowel movements after eating in order to take advantage of the gastrocolic reflex. Fiber intake should be 25–35 g/day. If patients have loose stools, increasing fiber alone will help "bulk up" stools, leading to better control over bowel movements. If fiber is recommended for constipation, the patients should also drink sufficient amounts of water to ensure that fiber will be effective.

For chronic loose stools, diphenoxylate and atropine (Lomotil) or loperamide (Imodium) 4 mg before meals may be used. For fecal impaction, lactulose 10 mL is recommended twice daily. For neurogenic anal incontinence, codeine phosphate should be given 30–60 mg/day to constipate the patient, followed by Fleet enemas every other day to have predictable bowel movements.

Biofeedback

Efferent training involves enhancing the voluntary contraction of the EAS through training. Afferent training involves improving sensation in the anorectal canal. Three modalities have been described.
• Use of an intra-anal electromyographic sensor, a probe to measure intra-anal pressure or perianal surface electromyographic electrodes to teach the patient how to exercise the anal sphincter.
• Use of a three-balloon system to train the patient to correctly identify the stimulus of rectal distention and to respond without delay.
• Use of a rectal balloon to retrain the rectal sensory threshold, usually with the aim of enabling the patient to discriminate and respond to smaller rectal volumes.
The use of biofeedback has been studied in only a few well-designed randomized trials. One RCT of 171 patients comparing biofeedback versus biofeedback plus home biofeedback versus pelvic floor exercises versus standard care found no benefit to any of these treatments compared to standard care alone. One prospective study of 94 patients, 60 of whom completed 1-year follow-up, found that 63% were continent, with increase in anal resting and squeeze pressure, squeeze duration and decreased sensory thresholds. Another small study found that biofeedback in addition to anal sphincteroplasty improved quality of life compared to anal sphincteroplasty alone.

Surgical therapy
Anal sphincteroplasty

Anal sphincteroplasty is indicated when there is an identified EAS defect. However, the outcome of anal sphincteroplasty is poor, with long-term cure of incontinence of liquid or solid stool of 5–51%. Pudendal nerve neuropathy is associated with a higher failure rate. No consensus exists as to the best pre- and postoperative management of anal sphincteroplasty. Full mechanical bowel preparation is probably unnecessary; a bowel prep with magnesium citrate and Fleet enema is probably sufficient. Oral antibiotics have not been shown to have any additional benefit; however, a parenteral dose of antibiotics given immediately preoperatively has been shown to decrease infection rate by 75%.

Postoperative management is highly varied among surgeons. Postoperative antibiotics are probably not necessary. Stool softeners with docusate sodium are generally recommended to avoid constipation. However, diarrhea should generally be avoided also. A clear liquid or low-residue diet is recommended for 3–7 days postoperatively. Sitz baths are not recommended. Pain is a common complication of this procedure and usually resolves over time. Other complications include infection (3–5%), fistula formation (< 1%), and superficial separation of the skin and subcutaneous tissues (25%). Hematoma formation, bleeding, and anal strictures occur, but these are rare events.

Graciloplasty

Graciloplasty is indicated when there is severely damaged or absent EAS. It works by increasing passive resistance of the anal canal by the bulk of the encircling muscle. If an implanted neurostimulator is used, this maintains tonic contraction around the anus. To defecate, the patient interrupts the stimulation. This is called "dynamic graciloplasty."

A medial thigh incision is made and the gracilis muscle is mobilized. The insertion of the muscle to the medial tibia is divided. The muscle is delivered through a transperineal tunnel and wrapped around the anal canal. The distal tendon of the muscle is then anchored to the ischial tuberosity. Roughly 50–75% of patients have at least 50% improvement at long-term follow-up after dynamic graciloplasty. Reoperation is needed in as many as 50% of patients.

Artificial sphincter

An artificial anal sphincter is indicated when there is severely damaged or absent EAS. It is composed of three parts: Silastic inflatable cuff that encircles the anal canal, reservoir balloon, and patient-activated valve placed in the labia majora that permits defecation. In a multicenter prospective trial of Actinon artificial bowel sphincter implanted in 115 patients, 46% required revision. Twenty-five percent of artificial sphincters became infected and needed surgical revision. Thirty-seven percent of patients had the device explanted. An intention-to-treat analysis showed a 53% success rate at 12 months and an 85% success in patients with functional devices. Outcomes from other smaller series from single institutions are similar.

Sacral nerve stimulation (neuromodulation)

Sacral nerve stimulation works by stimulating sacral spinal nerves, allowing additional residual function of an inadequate pelvic floor musculature to be recruited. The stimulation also modulates normal anorectal reflexes and stimulates the sacral nerve motor outflow. There are limited published data on sacral nerve stimulation but the results are promising, and fecal incontinence is the number one indication for sacral neuromodulation in Europe. Evidence of EAS disruption does not preclude treatment with this modality. In one small double-blind randomized cross-over study of sacral neuromodulation implanted in 27 subjects, there was a significant improvement in fecal incontinence episodes and enhanced ability to postpone defecation when the modulator was on. In a prospective study of 59 patients, 46 (78%) were implanted after test stimulation; at a median of 12 (range 1–72) months follow-up, 96% showed improvement. Fecal incontinence episodes significantly reduced from median 7.5 to 1 episode per week, and the ability to defer defecation significantly improved from 1 to 10 minutes. Maximum squeeze pressure and rectal sensation also increased significantly. In another prospective study of 75 patients, 62 (83%) had implantation after test stimulation. Fecal incontinence episodes significantly reduced from median 7.5 to 0.7 episodes per week.

Diversion

A colostomy is a procedure in which a part of the colon is connected to the anterior abdominal wall, creating what is known as a stoma. A colostomy may be the last option for some patients suffering from debilitating fecal incontinence.

Suggested reading

Barisic GU, Krivokapic ZV, Markovic VA, Popovic MA. Outcome of overlapping anal sphincter repair after 3 months and after a mean of 80 months. *Int J Colorectal Dis* 2006; 21: 52–56.

Boreham MK, Richter HE, Kenton KS, *et al*. Anal incontinence in women presenting for gynecologic care: prevalence, risk factors, and impact upon quality of life. *Am J Obstet Gynecol* 2005; 192(5): 1637–1642.

Bravo Gutierrez A, Madoff RD, Lowry AC, *et al*. Long term results of anterior sphincteroplasty. *Dis Colon Rectum* 2004; 47(5): 727–732.

Chapman AE, Geerdes B, Hewett P, *et al*. Systematic review of dynamic graciloplasty in the treatment of faecal incontinence. *Br J Surg* 2002; 89(2): 138–153.

Cook, TA, Brading AF, Mortensen NJ. The pharmacology of the internal anal sphincter and new treatments of ano-rectal disorders. *Aliment Pharmacol Ther* 2001; 15(7): 887–898.

Davis KJ, Kumar D, Poloniecki J. Adjuvant biofeedback following anal sphincter repair: a randomized study. *Aliment Pharmacol Ther* 2004; 20: 539–549.

Gordon PH. Anorectal anatomy and physiology. *Gastroenterol Clin North Am* 2001; 30(1): 1–13.

Halverson AL, Hull TL. Long-term outcome of overlapping anal sphincter repair. *Dis Colon Rectum* 2002; 45(3): 345–348.

Hull TL, Zutshi M. Fecal incontinence. In: Walters MD, Karram MM (eds) *Urogynecology and pelvic reconstructive surgery*, 3rd edn. Philadelphia, PA: Mosby, 2006: 309–319.

Jarrett ME, Mowatt G, Glazener CM, *et al*. Systematic review of sacral nerve stimulation for faecal incontinence and constipation. *Br J Surg* 2004; 91: 1559–1569.

Jarrett ME, Varma JS, Duthie GS, *et al*. Sacral nerve stimulation for faecal incontinence in UK. *Br J Surg* 2004; 91: 755–761.

Karoui S, Leroi AM, Koning E, *et al*. Results of sphincteroplasty in 86 patients with anal incontinence. *Dis Colon Rectum* 2000; 43(6): 813–820.

Leroi AM, Parc Y, Lehur PA, *et al*. Efficacy of sacral nerve stimulation for fecal incontinence: results of a multicenter double-blind crossover study. *Ann Surg* 2005; 242(5): 662–669.

Malouf AJ, Norton CS, Engel AF, *et al*. Long-term results of overlapping anterior anal-sphincter repair for obstetric trauma. *Lancet* 2000; 355: 260–265.

Matzel KE, Kamm MA, Stosser M, *et al*. Sacral spinal nerve stimulation for faecal incontinence: multicentre study. *Lancet* 2004; 363: 1270–1276.

Minaglia SM, Ozel B, Gatto NM, *et al*. Decreased rate of obstetrical anal sphincter laceration is associated with change in obstetric practice. *Int Urogynecol J Pelvic Floor Dysfunct* 2007; 18(12): 1399–1404.

Mundy L, Merlin TL, Maddern GJ, Hillier JE. Systematic review of safety and effectiveness of an artificial bowel sphincter for faecal incontinence. *Br J Surg* 2004; 91: 665–672.

Norton C, Chelvanayagam S. Wilson-Barnett J, Redfern S, Kamm MA. Randomized controlled trial of biofeedback for fecal incontinence. *Gastroenterology* 2003; 125(5): 1320–1329.

Ozturk R, Niazi S, Stessman M, Rao SS. Long-term outcome and objective changes of anorectal function after biofeedback therapy for faecal incontinence. *Aliment Pharmacol Ther* 2004; 20: 667–674.

Peschers UM, Delancey JO, Fritsch H, Quint LE, Prince MR. Cross-sectional imaging anatomy of the anal sphincters. *Obstet Gynecol* 1997; 90(5): 839–844.

Rasmussen OO, Buntzen S, Sorensen M, *et al*. Sacral nerve stimulation in fecal incontinence. *Dis Colon Rectum* 2004; 47(7): 1158–1163.

Rao SS. Diagnosis and management of fecal incontinence. *Am J Gastroenterol* 2004; 99(8): 1585–1604.

Tan JJ, Chan M, Tjandra JJ. Evolving therapy for fecal incontinence. *Dis Colon Rectum* 2007; 50(11): 1950–1967.

Uludag O, Koch SM, van Gemert WG, *et al*. Sacral neuromodulation in patients with fecal incontinence: a single center study. *Dis Colon Rectum* 2004; 47(8): 1350–1357.

Vaizey CJ, Norton C, Thornton MJ, *et al*. Long-term results of repeat anterior anal sphincter repair. *Dis Colon Rectum* 2004; 47(6): 858–863.

Varma MG, Brown JS, Creasman JS, *et al*. Fecal incontinence in women older than aged 40 years: who is at risk? *Dis Colon Rectum* 2006; 49(6): 841–851.

Chapter 79
Preinvasive Disease of the Lower Genital Tract

Amy D. Brockmeyer and Laila I. Muderspach

Department of Medicine and Obstetrics and Gynecology, Keck School of Medicine, University of Southern California, CA, USA

Vulvar intraepithelial neoplasia

Background

Vulvar intraepithelial neoplasia (VIN) is a common vulvar lesion with malignant potential if left untreated. While named for uniformity with the more common cervical intraepithelial neoplasia (CIN), differences in clinical behavior do exist. First, the biologic continuum from VIN I to VIN III to invasive cancer has not been proven. Second, the association with the human papilloma virus is significant but it is not universal, as in CIN. Even though MORE than 30% of women with VIN present with pruritis, pain, a palpable mass or dysuria, the diagnosis is often delayed. Routine examination, high suspicion, and low threshold for biopsy are essential to appropriate management of this condition. Factors that put patients at highest risk are cigarette smoking, immunocompromised conditions such as those requiring steroids, poor hygiene, and pregnancy.

Evaluation

Evaluation consists of careful inspection of the entire vulva and perineum. Appearance can vary widely depending on the degree of keratinization, the patient's race or complexion, and the type of lesion. The most common locations are the labia minora and the introitus between 3 and 9 o'clock. While disease involving the anal canal and intergluteal cleft can occur in up to 30% of cases, VIN of the glans clitoris and urethra is rare.

Whereas colposcopic examination can aid in defining the extent of VIN, acetic acid (vinegar) staining is also useful. Multiple biopsies may be required to define the extent of the disease and to exclude invasion. Squamous dysplasia and carcinoma tend to involve all organs of the lower genital tract sequentially or simultaneously.

Consequently, the cervix and vagina must also be evaluated for squamous neoplasia whenever the vulva is involved.

Treatment

The treatment of VIN has undergone major changes in the past two decades. The most important difference is the general recognition that total or even simple vulvectomy is seldom warranted and usually is contraindicated. In addition, treatment planning must take into consideration that spontaneous regression can occur, especially if the dysplasia is low grade. In general, women with mild vulvar dysplasia can be followed with close examination every 6 months, assuming compliance is not an issue. If the patient is very bothered by the lesion (either because of pruritis or for esthetic reasons), treatment can be offered. Patients with moderate or severe vulvar dysplasia should be offered treatment as these lesions have a greater potential for progression than low-grade lesions. An exception is the woman who is either pregnant or in the puerperium. Even severe vulvar dysplasia may regress once the immune-inhibiting effects of pregnancy dissipate.

The two options for treatment for VIN are laser ablation and wide local excision. The former is generally preferred as it gives excellent cosmetic results in an area where preservation of appearance is important. It is essential to rule out invasive disease before laser ablation is performed. As invasive disease in association with VIN is more likely to occur in a postmenopausal patient than a younger woman, the preferred treatment method has been excision for the older woman and laser ablation for the younger woman. However, there is room for individualization. Though rare, invasive cancer of the vulva has been reported even in very young women (less than 25 years old), where it has frequently been misdiagnosed as condyloma. It is essential to thoroughly biopsy, if not excise, suspicious vulvar lesions (markedly papillary, ulcerated or indurated) in young women prior to laser ablation. In postmenopausal women, laser ablation may be used in conjunction with excision to allow primary

Management of Common Problems in Obstetrics and Gynecology, 5th edition. Edited by T.M. Goodwin, M.N. Montoro, L. Muderspach, R. Paulson and S. Roy. © 2010 Blackwell Publishing Ltd.

closure and to avoid excision at problematic sites such as the urethral or clitoral areas. It should also be kept in mind that the sites most likely to harbor invasive disease are the posterior perineal and perianal areas; both should be thoroughly examined prior to laser treatment. The failure rate of both excision and laser in the treatment of VIN ranges from 15% up to 40%.

Vaginal intraepithelial neoplasia

Etiology

Preinvasive lesions of the vaginal squamous epithelium occur in only 1–3% of the patients with cervical neoplasia. The majority of women with this lesion, however, have had CIN. In a series of over 50 cases of vaginal intraepithelial neoplasia (VAIN) reviewed at our institution, 40% had prior and 15% co-existing cervical or vulvar neoplasia. As discussed earlier, human papilloma virus is thought to be a major etiologic factor in VAIN, as well as in CIN and VIN. Other predisposing causes of VAIN are radiation and immunosuppressive therapy. It has been suggested that postmenopausal atrophy of the vagina is also conducive to the development of VAIN; however, it is more likely that exfoliated cells from the atrophic vaginal epithelium often are interpreted incorrectly as intraepithelial neoplasia, exaggerating the true association of these factors.

Detection and evaluation

The Papanicolaou (Pap) smear is the single most important means of bringing the preinvasive vaginal lesion to the attention of the physician. A spatula or brush is used for cytologic sampling of the vaginal mucosa as the speculum is withdrawn and rotated.

Colposcopy is helpful in evaluating the patient with VAIN. Before performing colposcopy, a Pap smear is obtained and the vaginal tube is then moistened thoroughly with vinegar. To provide an end-on view of the tissues, the speculum is withdrawn and rotated, causing the vaginal mucosa to fold over the end of the speculum blades. Biopsies of lesions that appear to be invasive (raised, ulcerated) are taken immediately. Intraepithelial lesions are generally white, sharply bordered, and finely granular, often with areas of punctation. Mosaic structure is rarely seen.

Another useful adjunct for evaluation of the vagina is aqueous Lugol's solution. Lugol's iodine is placed into the vagina, taking care not to let excessive iodine spill on to the vulva. Again, the speculum is withdrawn and rotated. The most significant lesions usually stain a light yellow and have sharp borders, in contrast to the mahogany color of the normal mucosa. Less significant lesions have a variegated iodine uptake with indistinct borders.

After the number and distribution of the lesions are determined, biopsies are taken of representative areas. These can be painful and if multiple biopsies are required, consideration should be given to the use of a local anesthetic. The patient with postmenopausal or postradiation atrophy of vaginal mucosa should use intravaginal estrogen cream daily for 2 weeks before colposcopy, as the atrophic epithelium is often difficult to interpret colposcopically and does not stain well with Lugol's solution. Moreover, if the abnormal cytology is due to atrophic cells, topical estrogen cream will convert the cytology to normal.

The most common location of VAIN is the upper third of the vagina; the middle and lower thirds are involved less than 10% of the time. The lesions are often multifocal and may be found within the vaginal folds. The posthysterectomy recesses at the 3 and 9 o'clock "corners" are especially common sites for VAIN. In this situation, the fold can be everted with an iris hook or exposed with an endocervical speculum to obtain a satisfactory view.

Treatment

For limited focal VAIN, surgical excision is an effective means of treatment. Shortening of the vagina can result, however, if the excision is very large and the defect is closed. An excisional biopsy is recommended for those patients with only one or two lesions in whom invasion is suspected. For many cases of vaginal dysplasia, however, the CO_2 laser provides a simple and effective means of treatment.

The posthysterectomy patient may present a difficult management problem if the VAIN lesions involve the corners of the vaginal cuff. When this situation exists, surgical excision is the treatment of choice, although the laser can be used successfully in favorable situations. Excision of lesions in this location must take into account the close proximity of the ureter. In the postmenopausal patient, intravaginal estrogen for 3–4 weeks can reverse early VAIN lesions in about 50% of cases. As a consequence, a trial of intravaginal estrogen cream is warranted in postmenopausal women after invasive cancer has been ruled out.

Perhaps the most challenging clinical problem among women with VAIN is multifocal disease that involves many levels of the vagina. Total vaginectomy and skin grafting have been used with success, as has radiation therapy. Laser ablation is difficult to use in this situation, as it is extremely hard to encompass the entire vagina. Also, diffuse lasering of the vagina may lead to adherence of the vaginal walls during healing, resulting in a shortened vagina. Topical 5% 5-fluorouracil (Efudex) has gained popularity for use in cases of diffuse VAIN because it offers a relatively simple and effective method of eradicating the dysplastic lesions on an outpatient basis without compromise of vaginal function. Approximately 80% can expect to have all clinical and cytologic evidence of vaginal dysplasia remit after one or two courses of local therapy. Several regimens have been tried, ranging from half an applicator nightly for 7 days to half an applicator nightly once a week for 10 weeks. While both regimens appear to be equally effective, the latter may cause less vulvitis. The perineum is protected by applying a coat of zinc oxide paste before each treatment and every morning. Because of its simplicity, we recommend topical 5-fluorouracil as the treatment of choice for this group of patients. Laser therapy may be tried when the 5-fluorouracil treatment is unsuccessful.

Cervical intraepithelial neoplasia

Background
The detection of CIN has changed dramatically in the past decades due to the recognition and understanding of the causal role of the human papilloma virus (HPV) and cervical cancer. This knowledge, along with the use of liquid-based Pap smears, has allowed for both improved detection precursor lesions and prevention via vaccine development and implementation.

Detection
While there have been at least 100 different types of HPV identified, the vast majority of cervical cancers in the United States are caused by certain high-risk types including 16 and 18. Other low-risk types are not carcinogenic but are related to benign conditions like genital warts. Infection with high-risk HPV has been shown to be a necessary but not sufficient cause of cervical cancer, so its detection by Hybrid Capture 2 technology has allowed for improved and focused intervention and treatment for cervical dysplasia. While use of liquid-based cytology alone has improved screening sensitivity, it has also allowed for the combination of cytology and HPV detection in one screening test, improving ease of use for physician and patients. By combining these modalities, dysplastic cervical lesions associated with high-risk HPV types can be identified and treated while those with low-risk or no HPV infection can avoid additional unnecessary interventions.

Screening for cervical dysplasia in women should begin at age 21, or 3 years after the onset of sexual activity. Yearly liquid-based Pap, without HPV testing, is recommended until the age of 30 when reflex HPV testing should be added to cytologic screening in cases where atypical squamous cells are diagnosed. After a woman has had negative cytology with negative high-risk HPV testing, screening can be completed every 3 years. It is important to note that cytologic diagnoses of low- and high-grade intraepithelial lesions are not equivalent to the histologic diagnosis of CIN I, II, and III. Also, the diagnosis and treatment of cervical dysplasia in special populations, including adolescents, postmenopausal, and pregnant patients, differ from standard guidelines and in some cases are treated differently. In particular, the investigation and treatment of abnormalities in adolescence are simplified and less invasive. Current guidelines should be reviewed prior to treatment of adolescents.

Atypical squamous cells (ASC)
The diagnosis of ASC on Pap can either be of undetermined significance (ASC-US) or equivocal to high-risk intraepithelial lesion (ASC-H). Women with an ASC-US Pap have a 0.1% chance of having a malignancy at the time of screening and require follow-up in one of the following three ways: repeat cytology in 6 months until two negative paps are obtained, colposcopy with endocervical curettage (ECC) and biopsies and, if negative, return to yearly screening, or Hybrid Capture 2 HPV testing for high-risk HPV with return to yearly screening if negative and colposopy with endocervical curettage if positive. Of these options, the preferred method is reflex HPV testing, or testing for HPV in the original liquid-based Pap specimen if ASC-US is diagnosed. This allows only the most high-risk patients to be referred for coloposcopy while those without high-risk HPV have routine yearly screening, and prevents women from having to return for a second office visit for separate HPV testing. Those women with ASC-H paps should be treated as those with a high-grade intraepithelial lesion (HSIL).

Low-grade intraepithelial lesions (LSIL) and high-grade intraepithelial lesions (HSIL)
Low-grade intraepithelial lesions and HSIL are associated with infection with high-risk HPV in the vast majority of the cases, and therefore HPV testing is not recommended. LSIL and HSIL are associated with CIN II or higher in 12–15% and 53–66% of cases respectively and require further diagnositic testing with colposcopy with ECC and biopsy.

Atypical glandular cells (AGC)
Atypical glandular cells is an uncommon cytologic diagnosis that can be associated with reactive/benign cervical changes but also malignancies of the cervix, endometrium, and ovary. This diagnosis in women over the age of 35 should include HPV testing, colposcopy with ECC and biopsies, endometrial biopsy, and pelvic examination. Even in patients where these tests are negative, suspicion for neoplasia should remain high and screening with Pap should be repeated in 6 months even if all other testing is negative.

Cervical intraepithelial neoplasia I
Cervical intraepithelial neoplasia I confers a 13% risk of CIN II–III at 2 years but can also remit spontaneously over time, especially in patients less than 23 years of age. No intervention is necessary at the time of diagnosis,

but cytology should be repeated at 6 and 12 months or at 12 months if reflex HPV testing is employed. Triage based on these results at follow-up is appropriate.

Cervical intraepithelial neoplasia II–III

Cervical intraepithelial neoplasia II–III are pathologically difficult to distinguish and are both recognized as cancer precursors that do not spontaneously remit as often as CIN I lesions. Treatment includes removal of the transition zone by a trained provider with conization or loop electrosurgical excision procedure.

A note on colposcopy

Colposcopy is an important office technique in the evaluation of women with an abnormal Pap smear, an abnormal-looking cervix, and any abnormalities of the vulva, vagina or anus. It permits the physician to determine easily the precise nature of most squamous lesions of the lower genital tract, and up to 95% of the time it will eliminate the need for diagnostic conization of the cervix. The colposcopic examination uses up to 15-fold magnification combined with a green filter and vinegar (acetic acid) to accentuate the colposcopic findings. The standard examination consists of the following.

1. Gross examination of the vulva, vagina, and cervix.
2. Repeat cytology if there is no access to preceding abnormal Pap smear.
3. Cleaning the cervix with vinegar (2–5% acetic acid).
4. Colposcopic examination.
5. Endocervical curettage (not performed in pregnant patients).
6. Colposcopically directed punch biopsies of the most suspicious lesions.

Colposcopy is considered to be satisfactory in patients in whom the entire limits of the dysplastic lesion and the squamocolumnar junction are visible. In patients with an adequate colposcopic examination, ECC should be performed routinely, as assessment errors have been documented repeatedly.

Chapter 80
Vulvar Carcinoma

Merieme Klobocista and Laila I. Muderspach
Department of Medicine and Obstetrics and Gynecology, Keck School of Medicine, University of Southern California, CA, USA

Introduction

Vulvar carcinoma accounts for 4% of all gynecologic malignancies. Squamous cell carcinoma is the most common histologic subtype of vulvar carcinomas, which is not surprising since 40% of all vulvar cancers are associated with the human papilloma virus (HPV). Malignant melanoma is the second most common cancer of the vulva and accounts for 8–10% of all vulvar malignancies. Other subtypes include basal cell carcinoma, adenocarcinoma (Bartholin gland, eccrine sweat glands, Paget's disease or ectopic breast tissue), soft tissue sarcomas and metastatic lesions to the vulva.

Pathophysiology

Squamous cell carcinoma accounts for approximately 90% of all vulvar carcinomas. The HPV-related vulvar carcinomas are warty or basaloid and found in younger aged women (mean age 40 years), are associated with preinvasive disease, and have similar risk factors as that for cervical cancer. Keratinizing squamous cell carcinoma occur in older women (mean age 70 years) and are more likely to be HPV negative, and are associated with lichen sclerosis or epithelial hyperplasia. The lymphatic channels of the vulva course anteriorly through the labia majora, turn laterally at the mons pubis and drain primarily to the superficial inguinal lymph nodes, then to the deep inguinal lymph nodes, then drain superiorly into the external iliac nodes and then upward to the pelvic and aortic lymphatics. Lateralized lesions drain to the ipsilateral inguinal lymphatics. Mid-line lesions or lesions within 1 cm of the mid-line can drain to either side.

Malignant melanoma of the vulva is a disease of the elderly with the median age of diagnosis of 66 years.

Management of Common Problems in Obstetrics and Gynecology, 5th edition. Edited by T.M. Goodwin, M.N. Montoro, L. Muderspach, R. Paulson and S. Roy. © 2010 Blackwell Publishing Ltd.

It occurs more commonly in white women. Signs and symptoms are similar to other vulvar malignancies and the most common complaint is a vulvar mass. It most commonly arises from the labia minor, the labia majora or the clitoris. There are three subtypes of vulvar melanoma: superficial spreading melanoma (66%), nodular melanoma (24%), and acral lentiginous melanoma (10%). There are many different systems used to stage vulvar melanoma. The AJCC system and the Breslow microstaging system are superior for determining prognosis.

Diagnosis

Initial symptoms of vulvar carcinoma include pruritus, irritation, pain, mass or lesion that does not resolve. Occasionally the patient presents with bleeding or spotting and drainage from the tumor. The delay between initial symptoms and diagnosis can be due to the patient's hesitation to see a physician or the physician who may prescribe various topical therapies without a careful physical examination. Initial assessment includes a comprehensive history and physical exam, with measurements of the tumor and evaluation for extension to adjacent mucosal or bony structures and inguinal lymphadenopathy. Evaluation of the vagina and cervix, including a Pap smear of the cervix, should be performed in all women with a vulvar neoplasm. The lesions may be raised, flat, ulcerated and endophytic, exophytic or plaque-like. All suspicious lesions should be biopsied in the office. The biopsy should include the lesion and the underlying stroma so that depth of invasion of the carcinoma can be assessed. If the lesion is small, excisional rather than incisional biopsy is preferred. For malignant melanoma, the biopsy should include the underlying subcutaneous tissue to assess the full thickness of the lesion.

Treatment

Radical *en bloc* resection of the vulva and bilateral groins used to be the standard treatment for all invasive squamous cell carcinoma of the vulva. Over the years the standard has changed to a more conservative and individualized approach. For lesions confined to the vulva, a radical excision of the vulvar lesion (a hemi-vulvectomy or less) to achieve a 1–2 cm gross margin and ipsilateral inguinal node dissection through a separate incision is performed. Bilateral inguinal node dissection is performed if the ipsilateral nodes are positive or if the lesion is mid-line or less than 2 cm from the mid-line. Ipsilateral pelvic lymphadenectomy should be considered if the inguinal lymph nodes are positive. In addition, metastatic groin nodes are treated with postoperative radiation therapy to the ipsilateral groin and hemipelvis. Inguinal lymphadenectomy is superior to superficial groin node dissection or radiation alone. For lesions that are locally advanced and/or clinically positive groin nodes, treatment should be individualized. The patient may require chemoradiation alone as treatment or preoperative chemoradiation for local control.

Microinvasive vulvar carcinoma is defined as a lesion that measures 2 cm or less and depth of invasion is no greater than 1 mm (stage IA). This subgroup of patients has excellent survival and a low recurrence rate. This information has allowed less radical surgery and therefore these early lesions are treated with wide deep local excision without inguinal lymphadenectomy.

Prognosis

Approximately 70% of all patients present with early-stage disease and the 5-year survival rate is 85–90%. The 5-year survival rate for patients with stage III disease is 60% and for stage IV disease is 15%. The predominant site of recurrence is the vulva. Approximately 75% of vulvar recurrence can be salvaged with excision of the recurrence. Groin recurrences tend to occur sooner and the prognosis is poor. Distant recurrences occur less often and treatment is often palliative. Most recurrences are diagnosed within 2 years after treatment.

Local recurrence of vulvar melanoma is 30–50%. The most common site of recurrence is the groin. Widespread metastatic disease most commonly involves the lungs, liver and brain. The 5-year survival rate is 8–55% with a mean of 36%.

Complications

The rate of complications is proportional to the radicality of the surgery. Complications associated with vulvar cancer surgery include wound dehiscence and infection, although the incidence has decreased with the advent of less radical surgical procedures. Other complications include necrosis of flaps used during surgery, pelvic floor defects, osteomyelitis pubis (2%), urinary incontinence, lymphocysts, lymphedema, and venous thromboembolism. The rate of venous thromboembolism can be decreased by using sequential compression devices and/or prophylactic low-dose heparin or lovenox. Radiation complications can range from local desquamation, to ulcerative lesions of the vulva, lower extremity edema, and femoral head toxicities/fractures.

Suggested reading

Hoskins WJ, Perez, CA, Young RC, Barakat RR, Markman M, Randall ME. Vulva. In: *Principles and practice of gynecologic oncology*. Philadelphia: Lippincott Williams and Wilkins, 2005: 665.

Irvin WP Jr, Legallo RL, Stoler MH, *et al*. Vulvar melanoma: a retrospective analysis and literature review. *Gynecol Oncol* 2001; 83(3): 457–465.

Moore DH, Thomas GM, Montana GS, *et al*. Preoperative chemoradiation for advanced vulvar cancer: a Phase II study of the Gynecologic Oncology Group. *Int J Radiat Oncol Biol Phys* 1998; 42(1): 79–85.

Morrow CP, Curtin JP. Surgery for vulvar neoplasia. In: *Gynecologic cancer surgery*. New York: Churchill Livingstone, 1996: 381.

Saraiya M, Watson M, Wu X, *et al*. Incidence of in situ and invasive vulvar cancer in the US, 1998–2003. *Cancer* 2008; 113(10 suppl): 2865–2872.

Stehman FB, Bundy BN, Thomas G, *et al*. Groin dissection versus groin radiation in carcinoma of the vulva: a Gynecologic Oncology Group study. *Int J Radiat Oncol Biol Phys* 1992; 24(2): 389–396.

Chapter 81
Vaginal Carcinoma

Huyen Q. Pham

Department of Medicine and Obstetrics and Gynecology, Keck School of Medicine, University of Southern California, CA, USA

Introduction

Due to its proximity to other pelvic structures, the vagina is a site of frequent metastasis by direct extension from locally advanced primary carcinomas arising in the cervix, uterus, ovary, urinary bladder and colorectal tract. Primary vaginal carcinoma, on the other hand, is an uncommon malignancy of the female pelvic reproductive tract that occurs in the absence of cervical or vulvar cancer in at least the preceding 5 years. Annual cases in the US amount to 2210 with 760 deaths, numbers that account for only 1–2% of all malignancies in the female reproductive tract. The age-adjusted incidence in the US is 0.69 per 100,000 women with median age of 68 years.

Clinical presentation

Generally, affected women may not have any symptoms. The first sign of disease may be an abnormal Papanicolaou smear done for routine cytologic screening. Symptoms may also include abnormal vaginal discharge and irregular vaginal bleeding as part of menses, coitus or postmenopausal state. In addition, depending on the location and stage of the tumor, there may be associated pelvic pressure, pelvic pain, back pain, urinary discomfort, urinary urgency, dyschezia and bloody bowel movement.

Most vaginal cancer lesions occur at the upper third of the posterior vaginal wall. Early disease may not be readily evident on examination, especially since the blades of the bivalve speculum routinely obscure the anterior and posterior vaginal walls. However, if close inspection continues as the speculum is slowly withdrawn from the vaginal canal, then a tumor plaque, ulcer, friable lesion or mucosal nodule may be detected. More advanced lesions can present as large tumors felt on palpation that may extend to the pelvic supportive structures, pelvic side walls, urethra, urinary bladder or rectum. Diagnosis is confirmed with a biopsy of any suspicious lesions in the vaginal canal with or without the aid of colposcopy.

Etiology

The cause of vaginal cancer is unknown but is thought to mirror those for the vulva and cervix such as immunosuppression, smoking, early age of coitarche, having multiple sexual partners, history of previous pelvic radiation, history of cervical cancer, or human papillomavirus infection. Vaginal dysplasia (vaginal intraepithelial neosplasia or VAIN) is thought to precede frank invasive cancer. Persistent infection of oncogenic HPV leads to the development of cervical dysplasia and invasive cancer when the dysplasia is left untreated. Although the relationship between vaginal cancer and oncogenic HPV infection is not as well described, it is generally believed that the same linear relationship holds true for the vaginal tract. Published data have described similar detection of HPV in vaginal cancer compared to vulvar and cervical cancer. History of previous pelvic malignancy also increases risk of vaginal cancer. Retrospective data from a large series of vaginal cancers show that one-third of these patients had history of previous gynecologic malignancy.

Histology

Squamous cell carcinoma (SCCA) makes up around 80% of malignant vaginal histology. The behavior of vaginal SCCA is similar to SCCA detected at other body sites. Verrucous carcinoma is a variant of SCCA that tends to be exophytic and disfiguring but has an indolent course. Adenocarcinoma accounts for 15% of primary vaginal cancer and is more likely for women with history of diethystilbestrol (DES) exposure *in utero*. Among sarcomas of the vagina, embryonal rhabdomyosarcoma and sarcoma botryoides are most common. As a group, sarcomas

Management of Common Problems in Obstetrics and Gynecology, 5th edition. Edited by T.M. Goodwin, M.N. Montoro, L. Muderspach, R. Paulson and S. Roy. © 2010 Blackwell Publishing Ltd.

tend to be more aggressive with poorer prognosis and require multimodality therapy. Melanoma can also arise in the vagina from the mucosal melanocytes. Melanoma makes up only 3% of vaginal cancer and typically occurs in the lower third of the vagina in the anterior vaginal wall.

Staging and pattern of disease spread

Vaginal cancer is staged clinically using physical examination, biopsy, x-ray radiography, cystoscopy or proctoscopy. The staging system follows guidelines established by the American Joint Committee on Cancer (AJCC) and correlates well with the International Federation of Gynecology and Obstetrics (FIGO). Vaginal cancer stages are summarized as follows.

- Stage I   Tumor confined to the vaginal mucosa
- Stage II   Tumor involving submucosal tissue (IIA) or parametrium (IIB)
- Stage III   Tumor extension to pelvic side wall
- Stage IV   Tumor extension to urinary bladder or rectal mucosa (IVA) or to distant site (IVB)

Vaginal cancer spreads by direct extension into adjacent structures, by hematogenous or lymphatic spread. Depending on its location, the tumor can invade the urinary bladder, rectum, parametria or pelvic bones. The upper two-thirds of the vagina follow the lymphatic drainage of the cervix and lower uterus in the pelvis. The lower one-third of the vagina first drains into the groin lymphatic channels before emptying into the pelvic lymphatics. Therefore, depending on the location of vaginal tumor, treatment is tailored to include the fields of lymphatic drainage to ascertain that the local site of tumor involvement is adequately covered.

Management

Due to its rarity, there is no established standard of care for vaginal cancer. Treatment decisions are usually determined by the location and extent of tumor, relationship to other pelvic organs and the patient's psychosexual function and medical co-morbidities.

Surgery is usually reserved for stages I and IIA, especially if the tumor is found in the upper vagina. For superficial tumors, it is possible to treat with partial vaginectomy followed by vaginal brachytherapy. For a tumor up to 2 cm, pelvic lymphadenectomy with either radical hysterectomy or radical vaginectomy for patients with history of previous hysterectomy is acceptable. Surgery potentially avoids the long-term side effects of radiotherapy which can significantly affect the patient's quality of life.

For patients with larger tumors, stage IIA tumor in the lower vagina, poor medical health, or tumor extension to other pelvic structures (stages IIB to IVA), radiotherapy is the treatment of choice. Typically prescribed treatment consists of external pelvic radiotherapy to total doses of 40–50 Gy and additional intracavitary or interstitial brachytherapy to a total dose of 75 Gy. Bulky para-aortic lymphadenectomy warrants extended-field radiotherapy in addition to pelvic treatment.

For the last decade, the mainstay of primary treatment for locally advanced cervical cancer has been chemoradiotherapy. Specifically, the addition of chemosensitizing cisplatin has improved the overall survival in this group of patients. Since the scarcity of vaginal cancer makes any meaningful randomized trial unlikely, the success of chemoradiotherapy has been met with extrapolation of cervical cancer treatment to that for vaginal cancer. There are small series that show efficacy of chemotherapy in vaginal cancer treatment.

Bulky vaginal tumor or tumor involving the bladder or rectal mucosa may not be treated with radiotherapy alone. In the case of the former, the sheer size of the tumor increases the likelihood that not all of the tumor is uniformly susceptible to treatment. Thus, some of the cancer tissue will survive at the end of radiotherapy. For the latter, completion of radiotherapy means formation of urinary bladder and/or rectal fistulae which pose special management issues and significantly affect patients' quality of life. Therapy, therefore, has to employ combination treatment modalities. To overcome the challenges mentioned above, selected patients may require some radiotherapy to shrink the tumor followed by pelvic exenterative surgery. The completion of the operation means the removal of pelvic viscera and construction of new urinary and/or lower gastrointestinal outlets for waste disposal.

Chemotherapy is reserved for widely metastatic disease (stage IVB) or for recurrent vaginal cancer not amenable to surgical treatment. Because vaginal cancer is not considered a chemotherapy-sensitive tumor, the intention of this treatment modality is palliative in most settings. There are mostly case reports of response to chemotherapeutic agents but no good data from clinical trials verifying the efficacy of these agents.

Prognosis

Using population-based cancer registries, the 5-year disease-specific survival rates are reported to be 84% (stage I), 75% (stage II), and 57% (stages III and IV).

Suggested reading

American Joint Committee on Cancer. *Cancer staging manual*, 6th edn. Philadelphia: Lippincott Raven, 2002.

Creasman WT. Vaginal cancers. *Curr Opin Obstet Gynecol* 2005; 17: 71–76.

Creasman WT, Phillips JL, Menck HR. The National Cancer Data Base report on cancer of the vagina. *Cancer* 1998; 83: 1033.

Daling JR, Madeline MM, Schwartz SM, *et al*. A population-based study of squamous cell vaginal cancer: HPV and cofactors. *Gynecol Oncol* 2002; 84: 263–270.

Dalrymple JL, Russell AH, Lee SW, *et al*. Chemoradiation for primary invasive squamous carcinoma of the vagina. *Int J Gynecol Cancer* 2004; 14: 110–117.

Faaborg LL, Smith ML, Newland JR. Uterine cervical and vaginal verrucous squamous cell carcinoma. *Gynecol Oncol* 1979; 8: 104–109.

Goodman A. Primary vaginal cancer. *Surg Oncol Clin North Am* 1998; 7: 347–361.

Herbst AL, Robboy SJ, Scully RE, Poskanzer DC. Clear-cell adenocarcinoma of the vagina and cervix in girls: analysis of 170 registry cases. *Am J Obstet Gynecol* 1974; 119: 713–724.

Herbst AL, Ulfelder H, Poskanzer DC. Adenocarcinoma of the vagina. Association of maternal stilbestrol therapy with tumor appearance in young women. *NEJM* 1971; 284: 878–882.

Insinga RP, Liaw KL, Johnson LG, Madeleine MM. A systematic review of the prevalance and attribution of human papillomavirus types among cervical, vaginal, and vulvar precancers and cancers in the United States. *Cancer Epidemiol Bio Prev* 2008; 17: 1611.

Jemal A, Siegel R, Ward E, *et al*. Cancer statistics, 2008. *CA Can J Clin* 2008; 58: 71–96.

Kirkbride P, Fyles A, Rawlings GA, *et al*. Carcinoma of the vagina – experience at the Princess Margaret Hospital (1974–1989). *Gynecol Oncol* 1995; 56: 435–443.

Merino MJ. Vaginal cancer: the role of infectious and environmental factors. *Am J Obstet Gynecol* 1991; 15: 1255–1262.

Morris M, Eifel PJ, Lu J, *et al*. Pelvic radiation with concurrent chemotherapy compared with pelvic and para-aortic radiation for high-risk cervical cancer. *NEJM* 1999; 340: 1137–1143.

Perez CA, Gersell DJ, McGuire WP, *et al*. (eds). *Principles and practice of gynecologic oncology*, 3rd edn. Philadelphia, PA: Lippincott Williams and Wilkins, 2000: 811–840.

Piura B. Management of primary melanoma of the female urogenital tract. *Lancet Oncol* 2008; 9: 973–981.

Rose PG, Bundy BN, Watkins EB, *et al*. Concurrent cisplatin-based radiotherapy and chemotherapy for locally advanced cervical cancer. *NEJM* 1999; 340: 1144–1153.

Sedlis A, Robboy SJ. Diseases of the vagina. In: Kurman JR (ed) *Blausteins's pathology of the female genital tract*. New York: Springer 1987: 98–140.

Shah CA, Goff BA, Lowe K, Peters WA, Li CI. Factors affecting risk of mortality in women with vaginal cancer. *Obstet Gynecol* 2009; 113: 1038–1045.

Stock RG, Chen ASJ, Seski J. A 30-year experience in the management of primary carcinoma of the vagina: analysis of prognostic factors and treatment modalities. *Gynecol Oncol* 1995; 56: 45–52.

Tjalma WA, Monaghan JM, de Barros Lopes A, Naik R, Nordin AJ, Weyler JJ. The role of surgery in invasive squamous carcinoma of the vagina. *Gynecol Oncol* 2001; 81: 360–365.

Wu X, Matanoski G, Chen VW, *et al*. Descriptive epidemiology of vaginal cancer incidence and survival by race, ethnicity and age in the United States. *Cancer* 2008; 113(10 suppl): 2873–2882.

Chapter 82
Cervical Cancer

Lynda D. Roman

Department of Medicine and Obstetrics and Gynecology, Keck School of Medicine, University of Southern California, CA, USA

Introduction

Cervical cancer is the third most common gynecologic malignancy in the United States. However, it is the most common gynecologic cancer in the world, with less developed countries bearing the brunt of this disease. Cervical cancer screening via Papanicolaou (Pap) smear has led to a significant reduction in the incidence and mortality from this malignancy. Screening has increased the diagnosis and treatment of preinvasive disease.

Epidemiology

Cancer of the cervix has long been known to be related to sexual activity. Early age at coitarche and multiple sexual partners are known risk factors. In addition, women who are partners with males who had a previous partner with cervical cancer are at higher risk themselves for this disease. The causative agent of the vast majority of cervical precancerous and cancerous lesions is the human papilloma virus (HPV). Certain high-risk genotypes of HPV, most commonly types 16 and 18, are more frequently associated with cancer of the cervix, while other types, such as types 6 and 11, are usually associated with condyloma and nonprogressive mild dysplasia. Cigarette smoking is also associated with an increased risk of cervical cancer, although the exact causal factor is still unknown.

Signs and symptoms

Postcoital bleeding has been considered to be a frequent finding with cervical cancer; however, patients are more likely to present with either postmenopausal bleeding or irregular menses than a specific complaint of bleeding after intercourse. Patients may also complain of an abnormal vaginal discharge. Only about 20% of women are asymptomatic at the time of diagnosis. Pain, urinary symptoms, leg edema, and weight loss are symptoms of advanced disease.

The general physical examination is usually normal with cervical cancer, particularly with early-stage disease. Cervix cancer spreads most frequently by local extension and contiguous nodal spread to the pelvic, then aortic lymph nodes. Occasionally a patient will have an enlarged scalene lymph node at the time of diagnosis which is palpable on physical examination. Other signs of advanced disease may include ascites, enlarged inguinal nodes, leg edema or pleural effusion. The speculum examination may reveal a lesion with any of the following characteristics: ulcerative, endophytic, exophytic, papillary, necrotic or friable. Occasionally, the exocervix may appear completely normal if the cancer is endocervical in origin. In this situation, the Pap smear might also be normal. However, on examination, the cervix is often very firm or the endocervix might be expanded. It is not uncommon in this situation for a diagnosis of cervical fibroids to be erroneously made. The speculum examination also notes if there is disease spread onto the vaginal mucosa. The bimanual examination is important for determining the dimensions of the cervical tumor; however, the rectovaginal examination is critical for the clinical staging of cancer of the cervix. The rectovaginal examination evaluates the lateral support tissue of the cervix, the parametria, as this is the most likely area of local spread. Differentiation between disease into the parametria (stage IIb) versus disease to the pelvic sidewall (IIIb) has prognostic and therapeutic significance.

Diagnosis

As with any type of cancer, cervical carcinoma is a histologic diagnosis. The Pap test is a screening procedure only, and false negatives in the presence of invasive cancer may be as high as 20%. Because of this, all lesions of the cervix require biopsy. Biopsies should be taken

Management of Common Problems in Obstetrics and Gynecology, 5th edition. Edited by T.M. Goodwin, M.N. Montoro, L. Muderspach, R. Paulson and S. Roy. © 2010 Blackwell Publishing Ltd.

from the center of an ulcerative lesion, as this is the area most likely to yield adequate tumor for diagnosis. Cone biopsy is contraindicated in the presence of overt carcinoma. Whenever the endocervix is palpably abnormal, even in the presence of a normal pap smear, it is advisable to perform an endocervical curettage or core biopsies of the endocervix prior to assuming that the diagnosis is cervical fibroids.

Histology

Squamous cell carcinoma is the most frequent histologic type of cervical cancer, comprising 75–80% of all cases. Adenocarcinomas of the cervix are increasing in frequency, comprising 20–25% of cases. Adenosquamous cancer accounts for about 25% of the adenocarcinomas. Clear cell and small cell neuroendocrine cancers of the cervix are quite rare.

Microinvasive (FIGO stage Ia) cervical cancer is defined as a clinically occult tumor that invades less than 5 mm into the cervical stroma and is less than 7 mm in width. It is a diagnosis which requires a cone biopsy specimen with clear margins. Stage Ia1 is a subset of microinvasive cancer where the lesion has no more than 3 mm of cervical stromal invasion and is less than 7 mm wide. Women with such tumors that also have no lymph-vascular space involvement can be managed conservatively, especially if the histology is squamous. Cone biopsy with negative margins is sufficient if future fertility is desired or simple hysterectomy may be performed otherwise. For adenocarcinomas meeting these criteria, conservative management has not been as well established. However, there is an emerging body of data suggesting that similar conservative management might be in order for adenocarcinomas as well. In the latter case, it is very important that the histopathology slides are evaluated by a pathologist with expertise in cervical cancer, as the measurement of depth of invasion in cervical cancer is frequently difficult to determine. For tumors with a depth of invasion between 3 and 5 mm or in the presence of lymph-vascular space invasion (LVSI), a modified radical hysterectomy with lymph node dissection is the preferred management. Last, for women desirous of future fertility who have stage Ia1 cancers with LVSI, stage Ia2 cancers or small (2 cm or less) stage IB1/IIa cancers, radical trachelectomy with pelvic lymphadenectomy is an option.

Staging work-up

Cervical cancer is staged clinically (Box 82.1). The most important aspect of staging cervical cancer beyond histologic confirmation is the pelvic examination and particularly the rectovaginal examination. Radiologic studies are generally not useful for early-stage disease. The exception is the stage Ib2 bulky cervical cancers; these have an increased risk of nodal disease which may

---

Box 82.1 Staging of cervical carcinoma (clinical)

- **Stage 0:** carcinoma *in situ*
- **Stage I:** carcinoma confined to the cervix
- Ia: invasive cancer identified only microscopically, invasion limited to measured stromal invasion with a maximum depth of 5.0 mm and no wider than 7.0 mm
- Ia1: stromal invasion not >3.0 mm deep, not >7.0 mm wide
- Ia2: stromal invasion 3.0–5.0 mm deep, not >7.0 mm wide
- Ib: clinical lesions confined to the cervix or preclinical lesions larger than Ia
- Ib1: clinical lesions not >4.0 cm in size
- Ib2: clinical lesions >4.0 cm in size
- **Stage II:** carcinoma extends beyond the cervix but has not extended to the pelvic wall; carcinoma involves the vagina but not as far as the lower third
- IIa: no obvious parametrial involvement
- IIb: obvious parametrial involvement
- **Stage III:** carcinoma has extended onto the pelvic wall; on rectal examination there is no cancer-free space between the tumor and the pelvic wall; the tumor involves the lower third of the vagina; all cases with a hydroureter or nonfunctioning kidney should be included unless they are due to another cause
- IIIa: no extension onto the pelvic wall but involvement of the lower third of the vagina
- IIIb: extension to the pelvic wall or hydronephrosis or nonfunctioning kidney
- **Stage IV:** carcinoma has extended beyond the true pelvis or has clinically involved the mucosa of the bladder or rectum
- IVa: spread of the growth to adjacent organs
- IVb: spread to distant organs

---

be detected on CT scan. Cystoscopy and proctoscopy are warranted only if the tumor palpably encroaches upon these organs. If there is disease spread into the parametria, an intravenous pyelogram or CT scan with contrast will detect if there is evidence of ureteral occlusion or hydronephrosis.

It has long been known that large-volume stage I cervical cancer, so-called barrel or bulky cervical cancer, has a worse prognosis than small lesions confined to the exocervix. The International Federation of Gynecology and Obstetrics (FIGO) staging reflects this difference by designating stage Ib cervical cancer as Ib1 for those tumors less than or equal to 4 cm in greatest diameter and Ib2 for those tumors greater than 4 cm. This designation has important implications for treatment as well as for prognosis.

Treatment

For early-stage cervical cancer, stages Ib and selected IIa, treatment may be either surgery (radical hysterectomy with pelvic lymphadenectomy) or radiation therapy. Survival results in stage Ib1 tumors are identical for the two modalities. The advantages to surgery are the ability to evaluate the lymph nodes, preservation of the ovaries, better preservation of vaginal function, and fewer late complications. Radiation avoids the necessity for surgery, and therefore avoids the potential blood loss, infection, thromboembolic or anesthetic complications associated with surgery. With bulky cervical lesions, stage Ib2, the ideal treatment is somewhat controversial. Some prefer chemoradiation (a combination of radiation accompanied by weekly cisplatin used as a chemosensitizer) followed by extrafascial (adjuvant) hysterectomy for these patients while others recommend chemoradiation alone, and still others prefer radical surgery followed by radiation, depending on the surgical findings. The addition of chemotherapy to radiation has been shown to lead to a lower rate of recurrence, and the use of adjuvant hysterectomy has been shown to lead to a reduced rate of local recurrence than that seen with chemoradiation alone.

For higher stage disease, radiation remains the treatment of choice if the tumor is localized. Chemotherapy (usually cisplatin given weekly) is given as a radiation sensitizer. Randomized trials have documented that chemoradiation is superior to radiation alone in locally advanced cervix cancers. If disease is metastatic outside the radiation fields, chemotherapy is given; however, chemotherapy alone remains in most circumstances a palliative therapy and continued research is necessary to uncover better treatment regimens. In order to assess if there is disease spread to the lymphatic chain outside the pelvis, a staging procedure may be performed to assess the para-aortic lymph nodes. Sampling of the para-aortic lymph nodes is accomplished by either a retroperitoneal or a laparoscopic approach. Open transperitoneal removal of lymph nodes places the patient at high risk for intestinal adhesions within the radiation field, which increases the likelihood of radiation bowel complications. The retroperitoneal or laparoscopic approach greatly reduces production of intestinal adhesions. The radiation field can be altered to incorporate the para-aortic chain if these nodes should be involved with cancer.

Prognosis

Prognosis is most closely related to stage of disease at the time of diagnosis. For early-stage cervical cancer, there are recognized factors which place the patient at higher risk for either lymph node metastases or recurrence. In a Gynecologic Oncology Group study, increased tumor size, increased depth of cervical stromal invasion, and presence of LVSI in stage Ib cervical cancer correlated with increased risk of lymph node metastasis and decreased disease-free interval. Patients with a combination of high risk factors listed above are often treated adjuvantly with radiation therapy. Patients with involved margins, parametria or pelvic lymph nodes benefit from the addition of chemotherapy to pelvic radiation. Typically, whole-pelvis radiation is delivered via an external beam. If para-aortic lymph nodes are involved, radiation should incorporate the aortic chain as well as the pelvis.

Adenocarcinoma of the cervix has been reported to have a worse prognosis than squamous cell carcinoma. Evaluation of the literature reveals that prognosis is indeed poor for poorly differentiated adenocarcinoma or for women with metastases to the lymph nodes. However, when one controls for tumor volume and grade, there does not appear to be a significant difference in prognosis compared with squamous carcinoma. Adenosquamous cancer is reported by some to have a poorer outcome than either pure adenocarcinoma or squamous cancer. Small cell neuroendocrine cervical carcinoma is an especially aggressive subtype with a predilection for distant metastases. In such cases, combination chemotherapy, usually with an etoposide/cisplatin regimen, is combined with either radical hysterectomy (in early cases) or radiation (in more advanced cases).

Surveillance

The majority of women who have a recurrence of cervical cancer will do so in the first 2 years after completing therapy. During that period, close observation is warranted with regular examinations and Pap smears. Particular attention is paid to the vaginal cuff and the remainder of the lower genital tract. After 2 years, visits can occur at longer intervals, and most women who are cancer free at 5 years are cured of their disease. Therefore, yearly evaluations in the absence of any symptoms may be adequate once the patient is 5 years from treatment completion. CT scans are warranted in women with symptoms suggestive of recurrence or with metastatic disease which has previously been treated. On follow-up visits, patients should be questioned about any vaginal bleeding, leg pain, leg edema, changes in weight, changes in bowel or bladder habits, and cough as possible indicators of disease recurrence.

Recurrent disease

The prognosis for recurrent cervical cancer remains poor, with the exception of central pelvic recurrence which is amenable to either local radiation or surgical therapy. For patients with prior radiation therapy who develop a central recurrence, pelvic exenteration remains an option. This procedure removes the central tumor and adjacent organs such as the bladder, vagina, and rectum. Reconstructive surgery is a critical portion of the procedure, with options including colon reanastomosis, continent urinary diversion, and myriad neovaginal procedures. In some series as many as 50% of women who are able to have an exenteration are cured of their cancer. For recurrences which are not amenable to either local radiation or surgical resection, chemotherapy remains an option, although generally it is only palliative. The most active compound in cervical cancer to date is cisplatin.

Special circumstances

Cervical cancer removed inappropriately by simple hysterectomy

Simple hysterectomy performed for an unknown cervical cancer occurs when the patient has been incompletely evaluated prior to her surgery. Most frequently, the preoperative diagnosis is cervical dysplasia, but it may also occur with uterine myomas, dysfunctional bleeding or tubo-ovarian abscess. The prognosis in this situation correlates with the extent of disease found. For a small lesion, the use of chemoradiation or radical parametrectomy and pelvic lymphadenectomy can be curative. Larger lesions (particularly those in which the surgical margins are involved with cancer) do less well, particularly if gross residual disease remains. Chemoradiation is the treatment of choice, but complete responses occur less commonly than when the cervix is *in situ* due to limitations in brachytherapy dosimetry. If localized disease remains after chemoradiation, consideration should be given to exenterative surgery.

Cervical cancer in pregnancy

Cancer of the cervix appears to have a similar prognosis when diagnosed during pregnancy as when diagnosed in the nongravid patient. In early pregnancy, there appears to be a higher proportion of tumors diagnosed as stage I, perhaps reflecting asymptomatic women receiving cervical screening for the first time or with a long interval since prior Pap smear and examination. The classic recommendation when cervical cancer is diagnosed prior to viability is to offer therapy to the woman at that time. However, in recent years, many papers have been published suggesting that early lesions can be safely followed in pregnancy, even when diagnosed in the first trimester, as long as they do not progress. Diagnosis of early cervical cancer later in pregnancy warrants delay of treatment until fetal viability is achieved. We recommend women be delivered via classic cesarean section when the cervix is cancerous to avoid excessive blood loss and the possibility of metastasis of tumor to the episiotomy site and other distant sites.

Future directions

The recent development of a vaccine which prevents infection by HPV types 6, 11, 16, and 18 will hopefully have an impact on the incidence of cervical cancer worldwide; however, only time will elucidate the degree of this impact. Investigative work is ongoing involving development of a more comprehensive preventive vaccine, as well as development of a therapeutic vaccine for women already infected with HPV. Successful development of such vaccines could lead to eradication of cervical cancer.

Chapter 83
Endometrial Hyperplasia: Diagnosis and Management

Huyen Q. Pham
Department of Medicine and Obstetrics and Gynecology, Keck School of Medicine, University of Southern California, CA, USA

Introduction

Endometrial hyperplasia is a spectrum of proliferative changes ranging from simple crowding of glands to a malignant precursor lesion. The over-riding cause of endometrial hyperplasia is prolonged exposure to estrogen in the absence of progesterone.

Classification

The World Health Organization classification system for endometrial hyperplasia relies on changes to glandular architecture and nuclear changes within the endometrium [1]. Diffuse glands with normal gland-to-stroma ratio denote simple hyperplasia while irregular glands with increased gland-to-stroma ratio are designated complex hyperplasia. The presence of nuclear atypia gives rise to simple hyperplasia with atypia and complex hyperplasia with atypia, respectively. Since simple hyperplasia with atypia is rare, for all practical purposes, atypical hyperplasia refers mostly to atypical complex hyperplasia [2].

Malignant potential

Besides compartmentalizing the spectrum of endometrial hyperplasias, the WHO classification also confers a tendency for malignant transformation. A classic study found that the risk of endometrial cancer was significantly greater when nuclear atypia was present [3]. In the study cohort, the authors reported the risk of endometrial cancer at 1% for simple hyperplasia, 3% for complex hyperplasia, 8% for simple hyperplasia with atypia and 23% for complex hyperplasia with atypia. More recent data for patients found to have atypical complex hyperplasia undergoing hysterectomy within 12 weeks found that the risk of concurrent endometrial cancer was 42.6% [4]. In summary, the malignant potential for complex hyperplasia with atypia approaches 50% and is reported to be from 23% to 43% in the literature.

Risk factors and clinical presentation

Briefly, the stimulatory effects of unopposed estrogen are thought to promote hyperplasia and subsequent carcinoma [5]. Thus, the risks for endometrial hyperplasia are very similar to those of endometrial cancer. Chronic unopposed estrogen replacement, anovulation, marked obesity, and estrogen-secreting tumors containing granulosa and theca cells are some of the causes of an excess estrogenic state.

Premenopausal patients can present with heavy or prolonged menstrual flow, irregular vaginal bleeding or a Papanicolaou smear showing atypical glandular or endometrial cells. Postmenopausal patients may present with postmenopausal bleeding or a Pap smear showing endometrial or atypical endometrial or glandular cells. A detailed history may reveal a history of unopposed estrogen, whether it be physiologic or pharmacologic. Pelvic examination may be normal or may reveal the presence of an enlarged uterus or mass. Pelvic ultrasound may show a thickened endometrial echo complex for the menstrual history. Diagnosis is confirmed by obtaining endometrial tissue for histologic examination either in the office using an outpatient sampling device or by endometrial curettings completed in the operative room.

Treatment

Since the risks of malignancy are low for simple hyperplasia and complex hyperplasia without atypia, medical therapy is recommended as an initial treatment. The goal is to regulate menstrual flow to prevent onset of significant anemia and progression to endometrial lesions

Management of Common Problems in Obstetrics and Gynecology, 5th edition. Edited by T.M. Goodwin, M.N. Montoro, L. Muderspach, R. Paulson and S. Roy. © 2010 Blackwell Publishing Ltd.

with higher malignant potential. Progestins are effective treatment and have been shown to result in high rates of complete regression of hyperplasia [6]. Progestins exist in oral pills, vaginal ointments or intrauterine device. Though all progestin preparations have been shown to be effective, the oral treatment has the longest track record with the most information. Typical oral treatment is medroxyprogesterone acetate (MPA) 10 mg daily for 14 days each month to continue for 3–6 months. Repeat endometrial sampling is performed to document regression of the hyperplasia. Persistent hyperplasia or inability to tolerate progestin treatment would be an indication for surgical treatment which is hysterectomy with thorough pathologic evaluation.

Since lesions with nuclear atypia are associated with significant risk (approaching 50%) of having concurrent endometrial cancer, medical treatment is usually not recommended for this group of patients. The most controversial aspect with the diagnosis of atypical endometrial hyperplasia remains the lack of its reproducibility among pathologists [4,7,8]. And, surgery confers 100% cure rate for endometrial hyperplasia with atypia. Thus, it is understandable that the case for surgery is compelling. Surgery usually comprises hysterectomy and possible removal of ovaries. Surgery may be performed by more than one technique and may be approached laparoscopically, vaginally or abdominally, depending on the patient's specific medical condition and needs. In the event that endometrial malignancy is detected, appropriate surgical staging should be completed, depending on the risk nature of the primary tumor.

There are premenopausal women with the diagnosis of atypical endometrial hyperplasia who wish to preserve their fertility. These patients should first have the histology reviewed or have additional endometrial tissues obtained by curetting procedure to ascertain absence of frank endometrial malignancy. If uterine malignancy is ruled out, then medical therapy can be prescribed. There is no standard progestin agent or optimal dosing schedule for medical therapy of atypical complex hyperplasia [9]. Usual treatment is high-dose progestins (megesterol acetate 80–320 mg/day or MPA 600 mg/day) on a continuous basis. Alternatively, the use of progestin-containing IUDs has been described in selected patients. The endometrial cavity should be sampled at regular intervals (every 3 months is recommended) to document regression of the lesion within 6–9 months. Once the lesion has regressed, the patient should continue progestin suppression indefinitely with periodic sampling of endometrial tissue for continued surveillance. However, despite medical therapy, one-quarter of treated patients may have persistence or progression of the original atypical hyperplasia [11]. Patients failing medical therapy should be counseled to undergo surgical treatment.

There may be postmenopausal patients with atypical endometrial hyperplasia who are not surgical candidates or who decline surgery. An option of using medical treatment as outlined above should be considered although there is arguably less efficacy in treating the atypical hyperplasia than with surgical intervention. Medical treatment may be a temporizing measure until surgical intervention becomes a viable option.

References

1. Scully RE, Bonfiglio TA, Kurman RJ, Silverberg SG, Wilkinson EJ. Uterine corpus. In: *World Health Organization: histological typing of female genital tract tumors*. New York: SpingerVerlag, 1994: 13–31.
2. Lacey JV, Chia VM. Endometrial hyperplasia and the risk of progression to carcinoma. *Maturitas* 2009; 63:3 9–44.
3. Kurman RJ, Kaminski PF, Norris HJ. The behavior of endometrial hyperplasia. A long-term study of "untreated" hyperplasia in 170 patients. *Cancer* 1985; 56: 403–412.
4. Trimble CL, Kauderer J, Zaino R, *et al.* Concurrent endometrial carcinoma in women with a biopsy diagnosis of atypical endometrial hyperplasia: a Gynecologic Oncology Group study. *Cancer* 2006; 106: 812–819.
5. Gusberg S. Precursors of corpus carcinoma: estrogens and adenomatous hyperplasia. *Am J Obstet Gynecol* 1947; 54: 905–927.
6. Gambrell RD. Progestogens in estrogen-replacement therapy. *Clin Obstet Gynecol* 1995; 38: 890–901.
7. Zaino RJ, Kauderer J, Trimble CL, *et al.* Reproducibility of the diagnosis of atypical endometrial hyperplasia: a Gynecologic Oncology Group study. *Cancer* 2006; 106: 804–811.
8. Allison KH, Reed SD, Voigt LF, Jordan CD, Newton KM, Garcia RL. Diagnosing endometrial hyperplasia: why is it so difficult to agree? *Am J Surg Pathol* 2008; 32: 691–698.
9. Lethaby A, Suckling J, Barlow D, Farquhar CM, Jepson RG, Roberts H. Hormone replacement therapy in postmenopausal women: endometrial hyperplasia and irregular bleeding. *Cochrane Database Syst Rev* 2004; 3: CD000402.
10. Marsden DE, Hacker NF. Optimal management of endometrial hyperplasia. *Best Pract Res Clin Obstet Gynaecol* 2001; 15: 393–405.
11. Reed SD, Voigt LF, Newton KM, *et al.* Progestin therapy of complex endometrial hyperplasia with and without atypia. *Obstet Gynecol* 2009; 113: 655–662.

Chapter 84
Endometrial Carcinoma: Evaluation and Management

Melissa Moffitt and Laila I. Muderspach

Department of Medicine and Obstetrics and Gynecology, Keck School of Medicine, University of Southern California, CA, USA

Incidence

Endometrial carcinoma is the most common malignancy of the female genital tract in the USA. Among all malignancies in women, it is exceeded in frequency only by breast, lung, and colorectal cancer. The median age at the time of diagnosis is 62 years. A total of 40,100 new cases were estimated to be diagnosed in 2008. Only 7470 deaths from the disease occurred in 2008. The death rate for endometrial cancer is low because 85–90% are diagnosed early, while the tumor is still confined to the uterus. White women have higher incidence rates of endometrial carcinoma than black women, Asian women, American Indian women and Hispanic women, but black women have a much higher mortality rate from this disease than white women do. This is thought to be due to black women having a higher incidence of more aggressive histology types than white women, as well as less access to healthcare.

Risk factors

There appear to be two types of endometrial carcinoma: one which is estrogen related and one which is not. Factors associated with estrogen-related endometrial carcinoma include obesity, hypertension, diabetes mellitus, nulliparity, infertility, endogenous or exogenous estrogen, tamoxifen use and precursor lesions such as endometrial hyperplasia. Most estrogen-related endometrial carcinomas are diagnosed early and have a good prognosis, with an overall 5-year survival rate of 80%. Oral contraceptives, combined estrogen and progesterone postmenopausal hormone replacement therapy and cigarette smoking are protective factors.

Nonestrogen-related endometrial carcinoma tends to be seen more often in older, nonobese, parous women. These cancers tend to be more aggressive and are classified histologically as papillary serous and clear cell endometrial cancer. They have overall 5-year survival rates of 54% and 63% respectively.

There are also familial endometrial cancer syndromes such as Lynch II syndrome and hereditary nonpolyposis colorectal cancer syndrome.

Symptoms

The first sign of endometrial carcinoma is usually abnormal vaginal bleeding occurring after or around the time of the menopause. Any woman with abnormal perimenopausal or postmenopausal bleeding requires a careful evaluation for genital tract cancer.

Common presumptions regarding postmenopausal bleeding that can lead to a delay in diagnosis are that the bleeding is:
• due to supplemental estrogens in women receiving such therapy
• of vaginal origin in women with atrophic vaginitis
• from the endometrium, when it may be arising from cervical, vaginal or ovarian carcinoma
• not sufficient to require evaluation

Less commonly, the patient with endometrial carcinoma may present with enlargement of the uterus without bleeding or with chronic vaginal discharge (pyometra).

Prognostic factors and spread pattern

Prognosis and therefore survival are related to the histologic degree of differentiation, the extent of disease at the time of diagnosis, the quality of the therapy, and the patient's medical status. Pretreatment evaluation is directed toward the definition of these factors.

The histology of endometrial carcinoma is often not straightforward. Pathologists frequently have difficulty

Management of Common Problems in Obstetrics and Gynecology, 5th edition. Edited by T.M. Goodwin, M.N. Montoro, L. Muderspach, R. Paulson and S. Roy. © 2010 Blackwell Publishing Ltd.

distinguishing between severe atypical hyperplasia and very well-differentiated adenocarcinoma. At the other end of the spectrum, it can also be difficult to distinguish between poorly differentiated endometrial carcinoma and endometrial sarcoma. As with many cancers, the degree of histologic differentiation may vary from one area of tumor to another. If the tumor is not adequately sampled, an error in assessing the histologic grade may occur. In addition to poor differentiation of the typical endometrioid pattern of endometrial carcinoma, other more aggressive histologic types, such as papillary serous carcinoma, clear cell carcinoma or mixed mesodermal sarcoma, may occur.

Endometrial carcinoma usually arises in the upper corpus and tends to remain localized. Initially, it spreads by extension within the endometrium and then invades the myometrium, advancing towards the isthmus and cervix. Pelvic node, aortic node, and adnexal metastases are common. It can disseminate within the peritoneal cavity after invading the full thickness of the uterine musculature or by transtubal spread. Other patterns of spread are parametrial invasion, metastases to the vagina, particularly the suburethral area, and lung metastases.

Work-up and diagnosis

Based on the preceding information, the preoperative evaluation should include a general physical examination with special attention to the supraclavicular nodes, inguinal nodes, abdominal masses, the suburethral area, vaginal walls, and the cervix. On bimanual rectovaginal examination, the uterus, adnexa, and parametria are evaluated. An endometrial biopsy or fractional curettage is performed, submitting the endocervical and endometrial specimens separately. (This can often be carried out in the office.) A chest x-ray is a sufficient metastatic survey unless the patient has a poorly differentiated cancer or evidence of extrauterine spread. In these cases CT or MRI of the abdomen and pelvis is recommended. Many of these patients have medical problems related to age and obesity; evaluation for diabetes, hypertension, and renal disease is required.

Management of clinically localized cases

The cornerstone in management of endometrial carcinoma apparently confined to the uterine corpus is total hysterectomy and bilateral salpingo-oophorectomy. This procedure can be performed laparoscopically or abdominally. The vaginal approach is generally not useful as it inhibits thorough evaluation for extent of disease. Cytologic washings are taken from the pelvis, and the abdomen is carefully explored. Enlarged or suspicious pelvic and aortic nodes should be removed or biopsied.

Removal of the adnexa is part of the therapy, as they may be sites of occult metastases. In addition, the ovaries may contain an occult ovarian tumor or produce estrogen that might stimulate residual, occult disease. It is not necessary to remove a margin of vaginal cuff, nor does there appear to be any benefit in freeing up the ureters and taking extra parametrial tissue in the typical case. The entire cervix, however, should be excised with the uterus.

The pathologist's evaluation of the specimen is very important. He/she must identify the least differentiated area of the tumor, the greatest depth of myometrial invasion, vascular space invasion, and the proximity of the tumor to the isthmus or cervix. Each of these factors has prognostic as well as therapeutic implications. In addition, accurate study of the peritoneal cytology, lymph nodes, and adnexa is crucial.

If the lesion is grade 2 or 3, or is grade 1 with more than 50% myometrial invasion or extension to the isthmus on frozen section, pelvic lymphadenectomy should be performed with selective para-aortic lymph node dissection.

Postoperatively, all patients with deep (greater than one-third) myometrial invasion or a poorly differentiated cancer should have consideration for adjunctive therapy, which may include local or whole-pelvis radiation, hormonal therapy or chemotherapy.

Special management problems

Postoperative diagnosis of endometrial cancer
Occasionally endometrial cancer is an unexpected finding in the hysterectomy specimen. This situation may arise after a vaginal or abdominal hysterectomy if the uterus is not routinely evaluated in the operating suite by the pathologist. Reoperation is recommended to remove the adnexa and surgically stage the patient when the lesion is deeply invasive or is poorly differentiated. These procedures may be done laparoscopically.

The surgically inoperable patient
Morbid obesity and severe cardiopulmonary disease are the most common reasons a patient with endometrial carcinoma is deemed medically inoperable. Clinical judgment will vary a great deal in these cases. Nevertheless, in everyone's experience there will be patients for whom the risks of anesthesia and surgery exceed the likely benefits of hysterectomy. For the patient with a grade 1 lesion and a temporary contraindication to general anesthesia or who is altogether unsuited to radiation therapy or surgery, high-dose progestin is the treatment of choice.

Most other cases will be candidates for radiation therapy. If the uterus is small, intracavitary brachytherapy alone may be used, otherwise external beam pelvic radiation therapy is standard. Whether radiation or hormonal therapy is administered in this situation, endometrial biopsy or curettage should be performed after 3 months. If the cancer is still present, the contraindications to surgery must be reassessed.

The young woman

The diagnosis of endometrial carcinoma during the reproductive years should always be viewed with skepticism since the malignancy is uncommon and confusion with hyperplasia is frequent. The histologic distinction between atypical hyperplasia, which can be treated hormonally, and well-differentiated carcinoma, which should be treated surgically, is to some extent subjective. When preservation of fertility is a significant clinical factor, the diagnosis of well-differentiated carcinoma should be based on endometrial curettings, and consultation with a recognized authority in the field of endometrial pathology is recommended. Equivocal lesions should be managed in the same manner as atypical hyperplasia, i.e. continuous high-dose progestin (such as medroxyprogesterone acetate, MPA, 20–40 mg by mouth once or twice daily) should be administered for 3 months. Endometrial biopsy is performed at that time to demonstrate that the lesion is responding. If the lesion has been reversed within 6 months (based upon D&C), ovulation induction can proceed.

Vaginal hysterectomy

Surgical staging and appropriate surgical therapy can be accomplished in many patients with endometrial carcinoma by means of laparoscopic or laparoscopic-assisted vaginal hysterectomy. Without laparoscopy, however, the vaginal approach to hysterectomy for endometrial carcinoma must be reserved for special circumstances: in the obese, parous woman with a well-differentiated carcinoma, in the young woman with significant pelvic relaxation and grade 1 endometrial carcinoma, and in the case of the patient who for medical reasons may tolerate vaginal hysterectomy but not abdominal hysterectomy. Otherwise, the operation will compromise surgical staging and often surgical treatment as well. Removal of the adnexa is more difficult through the vagina, exploration of the pelvis and abdomen cannot be performed, nor can peritoneal cytology and node sampling be carried out.

Estrogen replacement

Many women after treatment for endometrial cancer will suffer the effects of estrogen insufficiency, such as hot flashes, dyspareunia from vaginal dryness, and rapid loss of calcium from bone. Such women also are concerned about recurrent cancer and reasonably exhibit fear with respect to taking estrogens. There are, however, limited data on the safety of estrogen replacement following endometrial cancer surgery. The risks and benefits should be discussed with each patient and management individualized.

Chapter 85
Ovarian Carcinoma: Management

Lynda D. Roman

Department of Medicine and Obstetrics and Gynecology, Keck School of Medicine, University of Southern California, CA, USA

Introduction

Ovarian carcinoma ranks fourth among all cancers as a cause of death in women in the United States and is responsible for more deaths than any other gynecologic cancer. The risk at birth of eventually developing ovarian cancer is approximately 1 in 70, and approximately 1 woman in 100 will die of this disease. In 2006, it was estimated that 20,180 women will develop this disease, and that 15,310 women will die of it. Since 1980, the age-adjusted death rate from ovarian cancer has been slowly decreasing. Epidemiologically, ovarian carcinoma is predominantly a malignancy of industrialized countries. Women at greatest risk are those of low parity and high social status. Approximately 10% of the ovarian cancer burden is due to a familial syndrome, the most common of which are due to mutations in the BRCA 1 or BRCA 2 genes (both are also associated with a marked increase in risk of developing breast cancer). No means of early detection has been discovered; consequently, more than two-thirds of ovarian malignancies are widely metastatic when first diagnosed. The overall 5-year survival rate for women with ovarian cancer has been increasing. It was reported to be 36% in the 1970s and had increased to 53% by 1998. However, this rate ranges from less than 5% to greater than 90%, depending on the stage, histology, and treatment.

Operative treatment

Surgery is an important phase of treatment for all types of ovarian cancer and should be undertaken as soon as the diagnostic survey has been completed, assuming the patient's condition allows it. A low transverse incision is inappropriate with a presumptive diagnosis of ovarian carcinoma. The surgeon selecting this incision should forewarn the patient that an upper abdominal incision may be required if carcinoma is encountered. Upon entering the abdomen, the surgeon performs a thorough exploration to evaluate the extent of disease. Ovarian carcinoma spreads predominantly by intraperitoneal implantation and retroperitoneal lymphatic metastasis. The undersurface of the diaphragm, surface of the liver, omentum, retroperitoneal nodes, paracolic gutters, parietes, pelvic peritoneum, pelvic cul-de-sacs, and small and large bowel surfaces are inspected and palpated for signs of spread. Findings suggestive of malignancy include: bilateral ovarian tumors, ascites (especially bloody ascites), surface papillations, and a cystic/solid tumor. None of these is, however, diagnostic of malignancy.

After exploration of the abdomen and in the absence of ascites or obvious extraovarian spread, cytologic specimens (washings) should be obtained from over the liver, the posterior cul-de-sac, and both paracolic gutters. The surgeon must guard against rupturing a malignant cyst if intraperitoneal spread is not already apparent, as spillage of fluid from a malignant mass increases the stage, and may worsen prognosis.

The surgical procedure most appropriate for epithelial ovarian carcinoma depends largely on the patient's age, the tumor histology, and the extent of disease. Premenopausal women with borderline tumors in whom there is no evidence of metastatic disease can be managed with cystectomy in the case of a unilocular cyst that shells out easily, or unilateral salpingo-oophorectomy otherwise. Generally, hysterectomy and bilateral salpingo-oophorectomy are only indicated if the patient is postmenopausal or if there is widespread involvement of the pelvic organs.

In the case of a frankly invasive ovarian carcinoma, if the patient is desirous of future fertility and the carcinoma is limited to one adnexa, unilateral salpingo-oophorectomy is appropriate. In all other cases, total abdominal hysterectomy and bilateral salpingo-oophorectomy is considered the standard of care. An exception is the young woman with a germ cell tumor, in whom a unilateral salpingo-oophorectomy cn be considered even in the face of metastatic disease, given the marked chemosensitivity of these tumors. If there is no evidence of extrapelvic disease, multiple peritoneal biopsies

Management of Common Problems in Obstetrics and Gynecology,
5th edition. Edited by T.M. Goodwin, M.N. Montoro,
L. Muderspach, R. Paulson and S. Roy. © 2010 Blackwell
Publishing Ltd.

(including pelvic, right and left paracolic gutters, and right diaphragmatic), greater omentectomy, and bilateral pelvic and aortic nodal sampling should be performed. If the disease is widespread the goal is to remove as much of the tumor as possible. Ideally, the patient should be left with no residual disease. If this is not possible, leaving less than 1 cm of tumor (optimal debulking) results in an improved disease-free survival. If it is clear at surgery that the patient cannot be adequately debulked, then biopsy for diagnosis followed by closure of the abdomen is in order.

At times, the malignancy is so extensive, or the patient's condition is so poor, that initial surgical management is not feasible. In such instances, diagnosis is established via aspiration of pleural or peritoneal effusions, or fine needle aspirate of metastatic tumor.

Pathologic study of the surgical specimen(s) is a very important phase in the evaluation of ovarian neoplasms. Both epithelial malignancies and germ cell tumors are notorious for the histologic variability within a single tumor. Without adequate sampling, the most malignant portion of the tumor may remain undiagnosed, which may lead to undertreatment. Consultation with a pathologist who is knowledgeable in this area is recommended whenever there is a diagnosis of a benign solid teratoma, a germ cell tumor in a woman over age 30, a poorly differentiated carcinoma in a woman under age 30, or a granulosa cell tumor. The 1985 International Federation of Gynecology and Obstetrics (FIGO) staging scheme for ovarian cancer is given in Box 85.1.

Postoperative management

Borderline ovarian carcinoma is managed surgically because neither chemotherapy nor radiation therapy has proved to be of therapeutic value. Thus, surgery is the primary therapy and the preferred treatment for recurrence. In the face of unresectable, progressive disease, chemotherapy with paclitaxel and carboplatinum is recommended (Table 85.1).

For a patient with a frankly invasive carcinoma (serous, mucinous, endometrioid), no postoperative therapy is required if the patient has a stage Ia/b grade 1 or 2 lesion. For all other stage I and all II cases, three to six cycles of chemotherapy with paclitaxel and carboplatinum are recommended. For patients with optimally resected stage III epithelial ovarian cancer, the incorporation of intraperitoneal platinum-based chemotherapy as part of the front-line treatment has been shown to lead to a significantly improved survival in at least three prospective randomized studies. For all other cases, a total of eight cycles of paclitaxel and carboplatinum is recommended. Though intraperitoneal chemotherapy has not been well studied in patients with suboptimally resected disease, it has been our practice to consider laparoscopy after 4–5 cycles in women with suboptimal stage III disease who appear to be

Box 85.1 FIGO staging of ovarian carcinoma*

- **Stage I**: growth limited to the ovaries
- Ia: growth limited to one ovary; no ascites. No tumor on the external surface; capsule intact
- Ib: growth limited to both ovaries; no ascites. No tumor on the external surface; capsules intact
- Ic**: tumor either stage Ia or Ib but with tumor on surface of one or both ovaries; or with capsule ruptured; or with ascites present containing malignant cells or with positive peritoneal washings
- **Stage II**: growth involving one or both ovaries with pelvic extension
- IIa; extension and/or metastases to the uterus and/or tubes
- IIb: extension to other pelvic tissues
- IIc**: tumor either stage IIa or IIb, but with tumor on surface of one or both ovaries; or with capsule(s) ruptured; or with ascites present containing malignant cells or with positive peritoneal washings
- **Stage III**: tumor involving one or both ovaries with peritoneal implants outside the pelvis and/or positive retroperitoneal or inguinal nodes. Superficial liver metastasis equals stage III; tumor is limited to the true pelvis but with histologically proven histologically malignant extension to small bowel or omentum
- IIIa: tumor grossly limited to the true pelvis with negative nodes but with histologically confirmed microscopic seeding of abdominal peritoneal surfaces
- IIIb: tumor of one or both ovaries with histologically confirmed implants of abdominal peritoneal surfaces not exceeding 2 cm in diameter. Nodes are negative stage IIIc. Abdominal implants greater than 2 cm in diameter and/or positive retroperitoneal or inguinal nodes
- **Stage IV**: growth involving one or both ovaries with distant metastases. If pleural effusion is present, there must be positive cytology to allot a case to stage IV. Parenchymal liver metastasis equals stage IV

* Stages are based on findings at clinical examination and/or surgical exploration. The histology is to be considered in the staging, as is cytology concerning effusions. It is desirable that a biopsy be taken from suspicious areas outside the pelvis.
** To evaluate the impact on prognosis of the different criteria for allotting cases to stage Ic or IIc, it would be valuable to know: 1) if rupture of the capsule was a) spontaneous or b) caused by the surgeon; or 2) if the source of malignant cells detected was a) peritoneal washings or b) ascites.

responding well to chemotherapy. If there is only minimal residual disease, we have completed the eight cycles using intravenous paclitaxel and intraperitoneal cisplatin.

It is prudent to begin chemotherapy as soon as the patient is reasonably recovered from surgery, ideally within 2 weeks from the date of operation. If multiagent chemotherapy is contraindicated or the patient is unwilling

Table 85.1. Ovarian carcinoma chemotherapy regimen

Drug	Dosage	Frequency
Paclitaxel	175 mg/m^2	every 3 weeks
Carboplatinum	AUC 5–6	every 3 weeks

AUC = area under the curve.

to accept such rigorous therapy, treatment with single-agent carboplatinum is appropriate.

Consolidation therapy

While most patients with advanced ovarian cancer have a complete response to front-line treatment, most will also eventually recur. Consolidation chemotherapy (given after primary treatment in women with complete responses) has been studied to evaluate whether it could affect the rate of recurrence. In a large randomized trial, the use of 12 monthly cycles of paclitaxel consolidation therapy lead to an improved disease-free survival as compared to the use of three monthly cycles. However, the trial was discontinued before any conclusion could be made regarding survival. Thus, while there is evidence that such consolidation therapy delays recurrence (at the cost of increased toxicity), there is no proof that it prevents it.

Second-line treatment

Patients with recurrent ovarian cancer are categorized regarding the length of their remission. Patients who have disease progression while receiving front-line chemotherapy have "platinum-refractory" disease and a poor prognosis. Investigational therapies are a consideration for these patients, as are therapies containing biologic agents such as bevacizumab, an inhibitor of vascular endothelial growth factor (VEGF). Patients who have a disease-free period of less than 6 months have "platinum-resistant" disease. There are various agents that can be utilized for these patients, including liposomal doxorubicin, topotecan, gemcitabine, and weekly paclitaxel. In this patient population, the likelihood of response is less than 15%, though a fair number of women may have stable disease. A bevacizumab combination is also a consideration, as are investigational therapies. Patients who have had a disease-free period of 6 months or greater have "platinum-sensitive" disease. In these women, secondary surgical cytoreduction is a consideration. The longer the disease-free interval (especially if 2 years or more) and the less the disease, the greater the potential benefit of this surgery. For example, a woman who has had a disease-free period of 2 years who recurs with a unifocal lesion is an ideal candidate for this surgery, while a woman who has had a disease-free period of 6 months who recurs with carcinomatosis is not a good candidate. Women with platinum-sensitive disease are frequently treated with a platinum combination. The likelihood of response is directly related to the length of the disease-free period.

Serous effusion

Ascites and pleural effusion commonly are associated with ovarian carcinoma. Preoperative removal of these fluids is not recommended unless the patient is experiencing respiratory embarrassment or pain. This policy minimizes the likelihood of rupturing a large, malignant ovarian cyst. Often ascites formation is a problem in the immediate postoperative period. In this circumstance, intravenous chemotherapy is initiated promptly to stop the loss of fluid and protein into the abdominal cavity. This also helps to avert the complications related to abdominal distension and oliguria. When pleural effusions are refractory to systemic chemotherapy, insertion of a chest tube and pleurodesis may be therapeutic.

Follow-up

Follow-up evaluation for ovarian carcinoma should be frequent (every 2–3 months) during the first 2 years; the majority of recurrences will appear during this time. Long-term follow-up is also recommended, as this malignancy may recur 5 or more years after treatment.

The follow-up evaluation consists of a history and physical examination at each visit, as well as serum CA 125 measurements, assuming this marker was elevated at initial diagnosis. A rising CA 125 titer is almost universally associated with recurrence, and will usually precede symptoms. A progressive rise in CA 125 should be evaluated with computed tomography (CT). Positron emission tomography (PET), in combination with CT scanning, is a promising technique for detection of recurrence. The abnormal metabolism detectable by PET may detect recurrence before clear-cut morphologic changes occur.

Suggested reading

Colgan TJ, Norris HJ. Ovarian epithelial tumors of low malignant potential: a review. *Int J Gynecol Pathol* 1983; 1: 367.

Gershenson DM, Copeland LJ, Wharton JT, *et al*. Prognosis of surgically determined complete responders in advanced ovarian cancer. *Cancer* 1985; 55: 1129.

Markman M, Liu PY, Wilczynski S, *et al*. Phase III randomized trial of 12 versus 3 months of maintenance paclitaxel in patients with advanced ovarian cancer after complete response to platinum and paclitaxel-based chemotherapy: a Southwest Oncology Group and Gynecologic Oncology Group trial. *J Clin Oncol* 2003; 21: 2460.

Ozols RF, Bundy BN, Greer BE *et al*. Phase III trial of carboplatin and paclitaxel compared with cisplatin and paclitaxel in patients with optimally resected stage III ovarian cancer: a Gynecologic Oncology Group study. *J Clin Oncol* 2003; 21: 3194.

Schroder W, Zinny C, Rudlowski C, *et al*. The role of 18F-fluorodeoxyglucose positron emission tomography (18F-FDG PET) in diagnosis of ovarian cancer. *Int J Gynecol Cancer* 1999; 9: 117.

Trimble EL, Christian MC. Intraperitoneal chemotherapy for women with advanced epithelial ovarian carcinoma. *Gynecol Oncol* 2006; 100: 3.

Chapter 86
Special Tumors of the Ovary

Annie A. Yessaian

Department of Medicine and Obstetrics and Gynecology, Keck School of Medicine, University of Southern California, CA, USA

Germ cell tumors

Proper management of germ cell tumors of the ovary is important because many are malignant and occur in young women. It is possible to treat many of these tumors without loss of fertility. The mature cystic teratoma (dermoid cyst) may be the most common ovarian neoplasm while the malignant germ cell tumors are distinctly uncommon: immature teratoma, dysgerminoma, endodermal sinus tumor, and choriocarcinoma.

Teratoma

More than 95% of teratomas are benign mature cystic teratomas, commonly referred to as dermoid cysts. These tumors can occur throughout a woman's reproductive life and frequently give rise to symptoms of an acute abdomen secondary to either torsion or rupture. Most commonly, dermoid cysts are detected on routine pelvic examination or during the investigation of minor complaints. More than half can be diagnosed by ultrasonography or x-ray through the identification of calcifications, tooth formation, a specific fat-halo sign on x-ray or the characteristic density appearance on ultrasound.

In a young woman, the surgical procedure of choice for a dermoid cyst is cystectomy or enucleation with preservation of as much ovarian tissue as possible. The opposite ovary should also be evaluated by inspection and palpation for the presence of a dermoid tumor. Dermoid cysts have an overt bilateralism rate approaching 15%. However, bilateralism is not always expressed at the time of surgery and may not be detected until months or years later. If the contralateral ovary is normal to inspection and palpation and normal on preoperative ultrasound, no further evaluation is necessary.

Management of Common Problems in Obstetrics and Gynecology,
5th edition. Edited by T.M. Goodwin, M.N. Montoro,
L. Muderspach, R. Paulson and S. Roy. © 2010 Blackwell
Publishing Ltd.

Approximately 1% of dermoid cysts will contain a malignancy. Usually these malignancies occur in postmenopausal women and are squamous cell carcinomas. However, a variety of other malignancies also may occur. These tumors usually are found in the solid papilla on the inside of the cyst, the so-called Rokitansky protuberance.

Malignant ovarian teratomas are called "immature teratomas" because their malignant behavior is exhibited by tissues that are embryonic or fetal in appearance. The more immature the tissue, the more malignant its behavior. These immature elements are usually composed of immature neuroepithelial tissue. A microscopic grading system for immature teratomas has been proposed by Norris and seems to correlate well with prognosis.

Most immature teratomas occur in adolescent girls and involve only one ovary. In these patients, the operative treatment consists of unilateral salpingo-oophorectomy. Bilateral extension requires bilateral salpingo-oophorectomy and metastasis requires as much cytoreduction as possible.

A patient with higher grade or metastatic immature teratoma needs additional treatment after surgery with chemotherapy. Radiotherapy has not been proven beneficial and causes sterility. Impressive results have been obtained with combination chemotherapy using bleomycin, etoposide, and cisplatin, or BEP.

Dysgerminoma

The dysgerminoma is the most common malignant germ cell tumor of the ovary. It usually occurs before age 30, often in females with dysgenetic gonads. Most often, it is confined to one ovary at the time of diagnosis. In 15% of cases, the dysgerminoma is not a pure tumor or possesses other germ cell types as well. Therefore, it is important that it is extensively sampled microscopically, particularly in areas of hemorrhage or necrosis, to rule out the presence of a more malignant element.

A suggested treatment plan for dysgerminoma is as follows. If a patient is young and desirous of future childbearing, the dysgerminoma involves only one ovary, is less than 10 cm in diameter, unruptured, and without malignant ascites or positive peritoneal cytology, a unilateral salpingo-oophorectomy should be performed. A "slice" or "wedge" biopsy of the opposite, normal-appearing ovary should be performed, as there is a 15% bilaterality rate and there may be a subclinical focus of tumor. At surgery, particular attention should be paid to pelvic and para-aortic lymph nodes, as this is the primary route of metastasis. Any enlarged lymph nodes should be removed. The performance of peritoneal washings and omental biopsy is indicated. A karyotype should be obtained to rule out the presence of a Y chromosome. The presence of a uterus and a nonstreak gonad does not necessarily rule out the presence of a Y chromosome and dysgenetic gonads. If a Y chromosome is found, bilateral gonadectomy is indicated because prospects for fertility are nonexistent and malignant risk is present in both gonads.

If the tumor is bilateral, larger than 10 cm or accompanied by rupture or malignant ascites, the likelihood of metastasis mandates performance of pelvic and para-aortic lymph node biopsies, omental biopsy, peritoneal washings, and target biopsies. Surgery should be followed by chemotherapy when fertility is desired. The chemotherapy is similar to the BEP regimen (bleomycin, etoposide, and cisplatin) described above for immature teratomas. If chemotherapy were to fail, radiation therapy is an option for treatment.

Follow-up of patients with ovarian dysgerminoma should include physical examination every 3 months with annual chest x-ray, and consideration of CT scan of the abdomen and pelvis. Serum lactic dehydrogenase (LDH) may be elevated with dysgerminomas and can subsequently be followed as a tumor marker. Essentially, all recurrences become manifest within 5 years.

Endodermal sinus tumor

The endodermal sinus tumor (or yolk sac carcinoma) is a very malignant neoplasm. It is rare, occurring usually in female children or young adults (age 10–30). Rapid growth, production of α-fetoprotein (AFP), and a propensity to rupture characterize these tumors.

When only one ovary is involved, a unilateral salpingoo-ophorectomy is appropriate. When intra-abdominal metastases are encountered, cytoreduction is performed. The ultimate fate of these patients, whether the tumor seems confined to one ovary or not, rests on the success of chemotherapy. Intensive combination chemotherapy with the BEP regimen is indicated. Serial assays of AFP levels should be included in the treatment and follow-up of patients to confirm tumor progression, regression or recurrence.

Choriocarcinoma

Pure choriocarcinoma arising in the ovary is a very rare tumor. It is virulent and is reported to have a high mortality rate. These tumors secrete human chorionic gonadotropin (hCG), which should be used as a tumor marker. Most patients have been treated postoperatively with chemotherapy regimens similar to those used for gestational choriocarcinoma. The most common regimen is EMA/CO: etoposide, methotrexate, dactinomycin, cyclophosphamide, and vincristine.

Gonadoblastoma

The gonadoblastoma occurs almost exclusively in dysgenetic gonads. The affected females usually have a Y chromosome. The gonadoblastoma is included here because nearly 30% are associated with the development of malignant germ cell tumors. The gonadoblastoma is a benign tumor composed of two cell types: primitive germ cells and a sex cord stromal element. There also may be cells resembling luteinized theca cells or Leydig cells. Because of the high risk of dysgerminomas, endodermal sinus tumors, etc. developing into gonadoblastomas, the appropriate therapy is bilateral gonadectomy.

Mixed germ cell tumors

Not uncommonly, malignant germ cell tumors contain more than one histologic cell type. Usually, routine examinations of the primary tumor and sampling of metastases, if present, will make the mixture apparent. However, the detection of elements may be difficult due to the presence of only small foci in a large tumor mass. Therefore, it is recommended that thorough and painstaking microscopic investigation be carried out for all germ cell malignancies.

The detection of a mixed germ cell tumor may be indirect. The presence of an elevated hCG or AFP level in the serum of a patient presumed to have an immature teratoma or a dysgerminoma is evidence for the presence of choriocarcinoma or endodermal sinus tumor elements as well. These components confer a worse prognosis and mandate more aggressive treatment than might otherwise be considered.

Sex cord stromal neoplasms

Approximately 5% of ovarian neoplasms are derived from the ovarian stroma. Neoplasms of the stroma unique to the ovary are called "specialized" gonadal stromal tumors and are known clinically as granulosa cell, theca cell tumors (alone or in combination), and Sertoli–Leydig tumors (arrhenoblastomas). The only common neoplasm of the nonspecialized ovarian stroma is the fibroma.

Granulosa theca cell tumors

Granulosa and theca cell tumors as pure cell types occur in equal numbers. It is more common, however, to find them combined in a neoplasm. Neoplastic granulosa cells are malignant, whereas the theca cell tumor component is invariably benign. Both granulosa and theca cells are capable of autonomous production of sex steroids, usually estrogens but occasionally androgens. Therefore, at times, these neoplasms can present with symptoms of precocious z, between 5% and 15% of granulosa–theca tumors have been associated with endometrial adenocarcinoma.

Granulosa cell tumors usually are confined to one ovary and represent a low-grade malignant risk. Of the cases that recur, a significant percentage relapse 10 or even 20 years after diagnosis. When confined to one ovary in a young woman, removal of the ovary is sufficient; however, in a woman near menopause or older, removal of both ovaries and the uterus is recommended. If conservative surgery is performed, the uterus should be sampled to rule out endometrial pathology. If the tumor has spread beyond one ovary, removal of both ovaries and the uterus, together with postoperative chemotherapy, is indicated. The BEP regimen is generally employed.

Theca cell tumors are unilateral and benign. Treatment is surgical, usually unilateral oophorectomy in the young woman in whom fertility is to be retained. In the woman at or near menopause, hysterectomy and bilateral oophorectomy are generally recommended.

Sertoli–Leydig cell tumor (arrhenoblastoma)

The term "arrhenoblastoma" is being replaced by the more informative designation of Sertoli–Leydig cell tumor. Classically, the Sertoli–Leydig cell tumor produces testosterone, which in turn produces defeminization, then virilization. Rarely, these neoplasms produce estrogen instead. In young women with the neoplasm confined to one ovary, unilateral salpingo-oophorectomy is sufficient treatment. In women at or near menopause, hysterectomy and bilateral salpingo-oophorectomy are indicated. If heterologous elements or high cellular grade are present, postoperative chemotherapy is warranted with the BEP regimen.

Fibroma

The fibroma is the most common neoplasm of the non-specific mesenchyme of the ovary. Not uncommonly, it is found incidentally in ovaries removed for other reasons. Occasionally, these tumors are bilateral. Fibromas frequently cannot be distinguished easily from theca cell tumors, and vice versa. The fibroma of the ovary is well known as the prime causative factor for Meig's syndrome: benign ovarian tumor larger than 6 cm, ascites, and hydrothorax. These findings of ascites and pleural effusion usually indicate advanced metastatic ovarian cancer, but in the case of an ovarian fibroma resolve with surgical removal.

Most fibromas do not produce effusions, however, and are treated by unilateral oophorectomy in the young woman and bilateral salpingo-oophorectomy and hysterectomy in the woman at or near menopause.

Chapter 87
Trophoblastic Neoplasia: Diagnosis and Management

Annie A. Yessaian

Department of Medicine and Obstetrics and Gynecology, Keck School of Medicine, University of Southern California, CA, USA

Definition

Molar pregnancy and gestational trophoblastic neoplasia (GTN) are rare human tumors that originate from placental tissue. They are characterized by gross vesicular swelling of the placental villi and the absence of a fetus or embryo.

Categories

Each of these categories has a different propensity for invasion and metastasis:
- complete mole
- partial mole
- invasive mole
- choriocarcinoma
- placental site trophoblastic tumor

Epidemiology

The incidence varies widely in different parts of the world. The disease incidence is influenced by socio-economic and nutritional factors. Maternal age, prior spontaneous miscarriage and infertility have all been shown to increase the risk of a molar gestation. In the USA, the incidence is 1/1500 livebirths.

Diagnosis

Clinical features

- *Vaginal bleeding*: this could be significant and prolonged, leading to significant anemia. The patient may occasionally experience the passage of the pathognomonic grape-like vesicles.

Management of Common Problems in Obstetrics and Gynecology, 5th edition. Edited by T.M. Goodwin, M.N. Montoro, L. Muderspach, R. Paulson and S. Roy. © 2010 Blackwell Publishing Ltd.

- *Uterine size larger than gestational age*: it is important to rule out other causes of an enlarged uterus, such as multiple gestations, leiomyomas, and polyhydramnios.
- *Toxemia*: this is classically associated with hypertension, proteinuria, and hyper-reflexia. When it happens in early pregnancy, GTN should be ruled out as the underlying cause.
- *Hyperemesis*: this can occasionally be severe enough to require treatment with intravenous fluid. This is more likely to happen in patients with markedly elevated levels of hCG.
- *Hyperthyroidism*: this can be associated with its classic signs of tachycardia, tremor and warm skin.
- *Theca lutein ovarian cysts*: these are related to the elevated levels of hCG. They do not require surgical intervention and resolve spontaneously after the successful treatment of the GTN.

Imaging studies

Ultrasound remains a sensitive modality for diagnosing molar pregnancy. Due to its widespread use, molar pregnancies are being diagnosed earlier and earlier. This will help rule out multiple gestations, confirm the large uterine size and document the presence of the theca lutein ovarian cysts. The characteristic vesicular sonographic pattern is known as the "snowstorm."

Laboratory work-up

- *Serum hCG*: markedly elevated levels of serum hCG are suggestive of complete hydatidiform mole. However, patients with partial hydatidiform mole are less likely to present with very high levels of hCG. Patients with placental site trophoblastic disease can actually have a normal hCG level.
- *Urine hCG*: in the past, the measurement of urinary hCG was used to help identify patients with molar pregnancies. Its current use is limited to evaluating cases with "false-positive" or "phantom" serum hCG. This is caused by a circulating heterophilic antibody that can produce a false elevation in serum hCG. Therefore, serum and urine samples should be collected simultaneously. Patients

Box 87.1 FIGO staging of gestational trophoblastic tumors (GTT)

Stage I: disease confined to the uterus
- IA: disease confined to the uterus with no risk factors
- IB: disease confined to the uterus with one risk factor
- IC: disease confined to the uterus with two risk factors

Stage II: GTT extends outside the uterus but is limited to the genital structures (adnexa, vagina, broad ligament)
- IIA: GTT involving genital structures without risk factors
- IIB: GTT extends outside the uterus but limited to the genital structures with one risk factor
- IIC: GTT extends outside the uterus but limited to the genital structures with two risk factors

Stage III: GTT extends to the lungs with or without known genital tract involvement
- IIIA: GTT extends to the lungs with or without genital tract involvement and with no risk factors
- IIIB: GTT extends to the lungs with or without genital tract involvement and with one risk factor
- IIIC: GTT extends to the lungs with or without genital tract involvement and with two risk factors

Stage IV: all other metastatic sites
- IVA: all other metastatic sites without risk factors
- IVB: all other metastatic sites with one risk factor
- IVC: all other metastatic sites with two risk factors

Notes:
1. The following factors should be considered and noted in reporting: prior chemotherapy; placental site tumors should be reported separately; histologic verification of disease is not required.
2. Risk factors affecting staging including the following: hCG >1,000,000 mIU/mL; duration of disease more than 6 months from termination of the antecedent pregnancy.

with "phantom" hCG will have no measurable hCG in their urine sample.

- *Thyroid function test*: elevated serum levels of free thyroxine (T_4) and tri-iodothyronine (T_3) can commonly be detected in asymptomatic patients with hydatidiform mole. These levels will rapidly normalize after the evacuation of the molar gestation.
- *Type and screen*: after the evacuation of the molar gestation, it is recommended that RhoGAM be given to Rh-negative mothers, although hydatidiform mole has not been documented as a cause of Rh sensitization.

Tissue diagnosis

The pathologic examination of the evacuated tissue remains an important part of the diagnosis. This will help differentiate between the different entities of complete, partial or invasive mole and rule out choriocarcinoma or placental site trophoblastic disease.

Treatment

As soon as the diagnosis of molar gestation is confirmed, the patient should be evaluated for the presence of complications including anemia, electrolyte imbalance, hyperthyroidism and pre-eclampsia. Once she is stabilized, the route of evacuation should be decided. The desire for future fertility is an important factor in making this decision.

Evacuation-termination

The molar pregnancy should be evacuated by suction curettage. This remains the preferred method when fertility preservation is desired. Conventional sharp curettage is adequate in patients who have spontaneously evacuated part of the mole so that the uterus is less than 12 weeks' gestational size. Oxytocin or prostaglandin induction is indicated only in the patient with a co-existent fetus. Suction curettage is carried out under general anesthesia in the operating room. If the patient is bleeding heavily on admission, an oxytocin infusion is started at the time; otherwise, none is given until the curettage is under way or completed.

Hysterectomy

This is an excellent choice in women who do not desire future fertility. This should be done with the mole *in situ* to minimize blood loss. The ovaries can be preserved despite the presence of theca lutein cysts.

Postevacuation prophylactic chemotherapy

The indications for treatment are:
- the presence of metastases
- β-hCG titer rising or plateau over a 3-week period
- rise in titer after remission

It is not necessary to obtain a tissue diagnosis prior to initiating therapy. The diagnosis is based on clinical history and hCG titer. Early detection based on postevacuation serial hCG titers assures a virtually 100% cure rate of these potentially lethal growths.

Follow-up after treatment

Serial serum hCG

The importance of follow-up cannot be overemphasized. Patients should have weekly serum hCG until undetectable (5 mIU/mL) for 3 weeks. Thereafter, monthly hCG for 6 months. If no rise occurs, no further follow-up is necessary.

During the period of surveillance with serial hCG titers, no other test or examinations need be carried out unless the patient develops symptoms or the hCG titer fails to fall. The most common associated problem is vaginal bleeding which may require curettage. In the absence of vaginal bleeding or an enlarging uterus, uterine curettage is not indicated and is of neither diagnostic nor therapeutic value.

Rule out metastasis

The patient who develops stable or rising hCG titers should be evaluated for evidence of metastasis by physical examination and chest x-ray. In the case of rising hCG titers, an intrauterine pregnancy should be excluded by ultrasonography. The most common sites of metastases are the lungs and lower genital tract. If metastases are noted on these studies, additional work-up is necessary. The work-up and the management of metastatic disease are discussed later in this chapter.

Contraception

Pregnancy should be prevented with hormonal contraception during follow-up to avoid difficulties in interpreting a rise in hCG titer. Intrauterine devices should be avoided for fear of uterine perforation.

Complications

- Hemorrhage
- Sepsis
- Acute pulmonary crisis
- Thyroid storm
- Eclampsia
- Ovarian cysts with torsion

During the immediate postoperative period, the most common and important complications are sepsis and acute pulmonary crisis. The latter is due to trophoblastic embolization or fluid overload with heart failure. This syndrome appears within a few hours post evacuation and is characterized by dyspnea, tachycardia, and hypotension. Rarely, heart failure appears prior to evacuation. This complication may be life-threatening.

Unilateral or bilateral enlargement of the ovaries due to multiple theca lutein cysts is clinically detectable in approximately 30% of patients with hydatidiform moles. In some cases, they are not noted until the first or second week after evacuation. These cysts apparently result from the high levels of hCG. They regress slowly as the hCG titer diminishes post evacuation. The presence of these cysts should not lead to surgical intervention or the mistaken belief that they represent an ovarian neoplasm.

Nonmetastatic trophoblastic neoplasia

The treatment of choice for postmolar nonmetastatic disease is simple hysterectomy for those women who wish to be sterilized. The ovaries need not be removed. Patients treated by hysterectomy must still be monitored postoperatively by monthly hCG titers until the titers have been normal for 12 months. Titer remission, as this is called, must be confirmed by β-hCG serum measurement which has a sensitivity of at least 5 mIU/mL.

Most women with a molar pregnancy wish to retain their childbearing capacity, and the treatment of choice is systemic chemotherapy. Chemotherapy should be carried out only by an experienced physician who is also knowledgeable in the treatment of trophoblastic disease. Single-agent therapy, using weekly methotrexate intravenously or intramuscularly or biweekly actinomycin-D, is the treatment of choice.

Chemotherapy is continued to one course past the first normal hCG titer. The average number of treatments required to induce titer remission is four. Patients must use an effective means of contraception during treatment to avoid the confusion of a rising hCG titer due to an intercurrent pregnancy. Following titer remission, patients are monitored by monthly hCG assays until a minimum of 1 year of remission has been observed.

Chemotherapy has not been associated with a detectable increase in congenital anomalies in subsequent pregnancies, but these women may have a higher probability of spontaneous abortion. However, patients with a history of molar gestation have a greater frequency of infertility and spontaneous abortions than women without such a history. Any woman who has had one molar pregnancy has an approximately 2% risk of having another molar pregnancy during her reproductive life.

Metastatic trophoblastic neoplasia

In contrast to trophoblastic neoplasia confined to the uterus, metastatic trophoblastic disease is, in the great majority of cases, choriocarcinoma rather than invasive mole. Because of the important differences in prognosis and management, these two clinical situations are presented separately.

Metastatic trophoblastic neoplasia usually has a latency period of several months following the culpable pregnancy. During this time, the patient invariably has low but detectable levels of hCG, which neither cause symptoms nor interfere with normal cyclic menstruation. She may, in fact, ovulate and conceive during this latency period. Occasionally, metastases from choriocarcinoma appear during a molar or nonmolar gestation, particularly a normal intrauterine pregnancy.

Metastatic choriocarcinoma is a great mimic, often presenting with symptoms entirely unrelated to the genital tract. It must be considered in women of reproductive age who have any of the following presumptive diagnoses: stroke, intracerebral hemorrhage, brain or spinal cord tumor, hepatitis, gastrointestinal bleeding, hematuria, nodular or diffuse pulmonary disease, and any malignancy of uncertain histology and origin. It is good policy to screen all women admitted with these diagnoses using a sensitive pregnancy test.

The patient with choriocarcinoma also may have signs and symptoms of eclampsia, hemoperitoneum, threatened or missed abortion, ectopic pregnancy or delayed postpartum hemorrhage. The patient with intrauterine choriocarcinoma presenting with the symptoms of threatened or missed abortion has a typical history of amenorrhea followed by uterine enlargement, vaginal spotting, and a positive pregnancy test. A high suspicion should be aroused if there is a history of molar pregnancy. The diagnosis is made when the uterus fails to enlarge further; curettage is performed, and trophoblast without fetal or placental tissue is obtained.

Hemoperitoneum may be secondary to a ruptured liver, bleeding ovarian metastases, ruptured theca-lutein cysts or perforation of the uterus by tumor. Understandably, these patients often undergo laparotomy, with a presumptive diagnosis of ruptured ectopic pregnancy. Every patient with delayed postpartum bleeding should be screened for choriocarcinoma by pregnancy testing, even though the yield will be small.

The importance of the hCG titer in the diagnosis of choriocarcinoma cannot be overemphasized. This test and the medical history are sufficient to make the diagnosis in virtually every case. Tissue diagnosis is almost always unnecessary, sometimes dangerous, and often misleading.

On physical examination, special attention is given to the genital tract, as choriocarcinoma often metastasizes to the cervix, vagina, urethra, and vulva. There may be parametrial extension and ovarian metastases. In addition to a chest x-ray, CT scan of the brain, abdomen and pelvis should be performed as a part of the work-up. If the chest x-ray is negative, a CT scan of the thorax is warranted in the presence of a high hCG titer or other metastases.

Management

The management of metastatic choriocarcinoma will depend to some extent upon the site of the metastases. Patients with metastases only in the lung have the most favorable prognosis; those with metastases in the liver are the most difficult to cure. All cases with metastases should receive combination chemotherapy, usually employing the EMA/CO regimen (etoposide, methotrexate, actinomycin-D, cyclophosphamide, and vincristine). When the patient with metastatic choriocarcinoma presents in poor condition, combination drug therapy may not be feasible. In this situation, it has been our practice to initiate treatment with actinomycin-D alone.

The most common reason for treatment failure is bone marrow and gastrointestinal toxicity, rather than drug resistance. Toxicity can result in a prolonged interval between treatment courses, during which the tumor recovers along with the normal tissues. If the EMA/CO regimen cannot be given more frequently than every 3 weeks, cure is unlikely.

To monitor tumor response, hCG titers are obtained weekly. The drugs are continued on an every-other-week schedule until three consecutive weekly β-hCG serum values of less than 1 mIU/mL are reported. Because of an approximately 10% relapse rate after titer remission, continuing treatment is recommended for a minimum of three courses after the first normal titer.

The presence of central nervous system (CNS) metastases requires special management because of the threat of intracranial hemorrhage. The brain is also thought to be a sanctuary for cancer, because the blood–brain barrier protects it from cytotoxic agents. Although choriocarcinoma is sometimes initially diagnosed at craniotomy, surgery usually can be avoided if the diagnosis is made earlier. Nevertheless, decompression craniotomy may be a necessity.

As soon as the presence of brain metastases has been demonstrated by clinical symptoms, physical examination or CT scan, whole-brain irradiation should be initiated. A total dose of 2000–3000 cGy is given over 2 weeks. This has the immediate effect of preventing hemorrhage, and it is therapeutic as well.

Liver metastases are a most difficult problem. To prevent hemorrhage and eradicate tumor, some authorities have recommended whole-liver irradiation to approximately 2000 cGy. However, this has not been proved effective, and we reserve it for cases with extensive or subcapsular metastases. We recommend chemotherapy alone for all other cases with liver involvement.

The prognosis is excellent for patients with lung metastases only. Approximately 90% can be expected to have a sustained remission. For those with CNS metastases, a 50% cure rate can be anticipated. Those with liver metastases have a significantly poorer prognosis – perhaps 25% of them survive.

The curability of metastatic choriocarcinoma is to a great extent dependent on the therapist's understanding of this cancer, the role of surgery, radiation, and chemotherapy in its management, and the nuances of hCG testing. Consequently, referral to a treatment center is advisable. Metastatic trophoblastic disease is so extraordinarily uncommon that few physicians, even specialists, have the experience required to manage this malignancy optimally.

Suggested reading

Bagshawe KD. Risks and prognostic factors in trophoblastic neoplasia. *Cancer* 1976; 38: 1373–1385.

Berkowitz RS, Goldstein DP. Chorionic tumors. *NEJM* 1996; 335: 1740–1748.

Berkowitz RS, Goldstein DP. Current management of gestational trophoblastic disease. *Gynecol Oncol* 2009; 112: 654.

Dubuc-Lissoir J, Zweizig S, Schlaerth JB, Morrow CP. Metastatic gestational trophoblastic disease. A comparison of prognostic classification system. *Gynecol Oncol* 1992; 45: 40.

Fisher RA, Hodges MD, Newlands ES. Familial recurrent hydatidiform mole: a review. *J Reprod Med* 2004; 49: 595–601.

Hammond CB, Soper JT. Poor-prognosis metastatic gestational trophoblastic neoplasia. *Clin Obstet Gynecol* 1984; 27: 228.

Hammond CB, Weed JC Jr, Currie JL. The role of operation in the current therapy of gestational trophoblastic disease. *Am J Obstet Gynecol* 1980; 136: 844.

Kovacs BW, Shahbahrami B, Tast DE, Curtin JP. Molecular genetic analysis of complete hydatidiform moles. *Cancer Gent Cytogenet* 1991; 54(2): 143–152.

Lathrop JC, Lauchlan S, Nayak R, Ambler M. Clinical characteristics of placental site trophosblastic tumor (PSTT). *Gynecol Oncol* 1988; 31; 32–42.

Lurain JR, Brewer JI, Torok EE, *et al.* Gestational trophoblastic disease: treatment results at the Brewer Trophoblastic Disease Center. *Obstet Gynecol* 1982; 60: 354.

Lurain JR, Brewer JI, Torok EE, *et al.* Natural history of hydatidiform mole after primary evacuation. *Am J Obstet Gynecol* 1983; 145: 591.

Lurain JR, Singh DK, Schink JC. Primary treatment of metastatic high-risk gestational trophoblastic neoplasia with EMA-CO chemotherapy. *J Reprod Med* 2006; 51: 767–772.

Morrow CP. Postmolar trophoblastic disease. Diagnosis, management and prognosis. *Clin Obstet Gynecol* 1984; 27: 211.

Morrow CP, Schlaerth JB. Recent advances in trophoblastic disease. In: Morrow CP, Bonnar J, O'Brien TJ, *et al* (eds). *Recent clinical developments in gynecologic oncology.* New York: Raven Press, 1983: 532–567.

Muller CY, Cole LA. The quagmire of hCG and hCG testing in gynecologic oncology. *Gynecol Oncol* 2009; 112: 663–672.

Newland ES, Bagshawe KD, Begent RHJ, *et al.* Developments in chemotherapy for medium and high-risk patients with gestational trophoblastic tumors (1979–84). *BJOG* 1986; 93: 63.

Schlaerth JB. Methodology of molar pregnancy termination. *Clin Obstet Gynecol* 1984; 27: 192.

Schlaerth JB, Morrow CP, Kletzky OA. Prognostic characteristics of serum human chorionic gonadotropin titer regression following molar pregnancy. *Obstet Gynecol* 1981; 58: 478.

Szulman AE, Surti U. The syndromes of partial and complete molar gestation. *Clin Obstet Gynecol* 1984; 27: 199.

Weed JC Jr, Hammond CB. Cerebral metastatic choriocarcinoma. Intensive therapy and prognosis. *Obstet Gynecol* 1980; 55: 89.

Yordan EL, Schlaerth JB, Gaddis O, *et al.* Radiation in the management of gestational choriocarcinoma metastatic to the central venous system. *Obstet Gynecol* 1987; 69: 627.

Chapter 88
Precocious Puberty

Marsha B. Baker[1] *and Mitchell E. Geffner*[2]

[1]Department of Medicine and Obstetrics and Gynecology, Keck School of Medicine, University of Southern California, CA, USA
[2]Saban Research Institute, Childrens Hospital Los Angeles, Keck School of Medicine, University of Southern California, CA, USA

Introduction

Precocious puberty is defined as the onset of any component of pubertal development and accelerated growth that occurs ≥2.5 standard deviations (SD) below the mean age for normal children.

Historically, the average age of onset of puberty in girls was approximately 10 years of age, and pubertal changes occurring before the age of 8 years (−2 SD) were considered precocious. However, the definition of precocious puberty has been contested by recent studies. The 1997 Pediatric Research in Office Settings (PROS) Network evaluated the timing of puberty in approximately 17,000 healthy young female patients. While the mean age of onset of breast development was 10.0 years in Caucasian girls, it was 8.9 years in African American girls. The National Health and Nutrition Examination Survey III (NHANES III) also reported that the average age of puberty showed notable variation among ethnic groups, with Caucasian, African American, and Mexican American girls showing pubertal changes beginning at the mean ages of 10.4, 9.5, and 9.8 years, respectively. That said, the findings of the PROS study have also been challenged because breast development was determined visually (not by palpation), mean BMI of the subjects favored overweight (increasing the likelihood of labeling fat in the chest area as true breast tissue), and no testing was performed to rule out pathologic causes in borderline cases. Furthermore, the reported time of menarche in this study was unchanged from prior data, suggesting an unexplained longer duration of puberty.

Thus, it remains unclear whether or not girls may be starting puberty earlier than previously thought, so that most authorities in the field still recommend an evaluation if changes begin prior to the age of 8 years, with careful individualization between 6 and 8 years depending on race, weight, and rate of progression of pubertal changes. While the evaluation of precocious puberty is primarily conducted by pediatric endocrinologists, the practicing obstetrician-gynecologist may be called upon to make the diagnosis. This discussion will be focused on the essentials of recognition of this condition, and its diagnosis and management.

Classification of precocious puberty

Precocious puberty is classified into two types: 1) complete, central or gonadotropin-releasing hormone (GnRH) dependent, and 2) incomplete, peripheral or GnRH independent.

Central precocious puberty

Central precocious puberty (CPP) has also been referred to as GnRH-dependent precocious puberty. Ninety percent of all female children with precocious puberty have the central form in which there is premature activation of hypothalamic GnRH pulses causing release of gonadotropins. The etiology of CPP always involves the central nervous system (CNS). CPP is divided into two diagnostic subgroups: idiopathic and organic.

An idiopathic basis is the most common etiology for female CPP, accounting for 70% of cases. The underlying etiology for the premature activation of the hypothalamic-pituitary-ovarian axis is unknown but, regardless, the endocrine events that occur are advanced with respect to the child's chronologic age. Children with pathologic forms of precocious puberty have a growth spurt which is early, rapid, and of shorter duration than normal. At first, they are much taller than their peers but if untreated, they may end up very short as adults due to premature epiphyseal closure. Their skeletal maturation will be reflected by a bone age that is significantly older than their chronologic age. In general, the earlier the process begins, the shorter the adult height. The onset of symptoms may occur at any age prior to 8 years, but is quite uncommon in the first few years of life.

Management of Common Problems in Obstetrics and Gynecology, 5th edition. Edited by T.M. Goodwin, M.N. Montoro, L. Muderspach, R. Paulson and S. Roy. © 2010 Blackwell Publishing Ltd.

The rate of progression and the sequence of symptoms can vary greatly. Spontaneous remissions occur, but are relatively uncommon. The general health of children with idiopathic CPP is not impaired, but the pubertal changes may create emotional conflicts for both the child and her family. These children may have an increase in minor psychopathologic symptoms, but do not manifest an increase in severe psychiatric disorders. Children with idiopathic CPP may have functional follicular ovarian cysts identified by a pelvic ultrasonographic examination which are the result, not the cause, of their early puberty. Problems of infertility and premature ovarian failure are not increased in children with a history of idiopathic CPP. The diagnosis is made by excluding all other causes of precocious puberty.

Central nervous system disease is responsible for 30% of the children with CPP. The development of high-resolution imaging modalities has resulted in an increase in the identification of organic brain disease which includes hypothalamic hamartomas, congenital mid-line defects, tumors, cysts, postinfectious lesions, neurofibromatosis, and post-traumatic brain injury. Hypothalamic hamartoma is the most common CNS tumor observed in young children with CPP. The hamartoma is a benign congenital malformation typically attached to or suspended from the floor of the third ventricle, and may, on occasion, be associated with gelastic (laughing) or other seizures. Mechanisms by which hamartomas are thought to cause precocious puberty include the production of TGF-α which, in turn, stimulates GnRH release and the "ectopic" production of GnRH itself by the tumor, but in general, the cause is unknown.

All children with CPP must have a thorough evaluation, including a complete neurologic examination and magnetic resonance imaging (MRI) scan before CNS disease can be excluded. CT scans provide poor resolution of the suprasellar region and are not recommended in the evaluation of CPP. A newly recognized genetic cause of CPP involves an activating mutation of the GPR54 receptor, the ligand for which is known as kisspeptin, and the normal function of which is the activation of GnRH.

Peripheral precocious puberty

Peripheral precocious puberty (PPP) has also been referred to as GnRH-independent precocious puberty. Children with PPP do not attain cyclical function of the reproductive axis, follicular maturation, and ovulation. PPP is divided into the following diagnostic subgroups:
- ovarian tumors or cysts
- human chorionic gonadotropin (hCG)-producing tumors
- adrenal tumors
- exogenous sources of sex steroids
- primary hypothyroidism
- McCune–Albright syndrome

One of the major causes of PPP in the female patient is an estrogen-producing ovarian granulosa-theca cell tumor (also commonly known as a granulosa cell tumor). These tumors are almost always palpable on rectal-abdominal examination and can be identified by ultrasonography. Most granulosa-theca cell tumors are benign and are confined to one ovary. The usual treatment is unilateral salpingo-oophorectomy. Estrogen-secreting ovarian cysts may also be a cause of PPP. Germ cell tumors, in girls, may rarely secrete hCG which stimulates ovarian estrogen secretion and causes precocious puberty.

An estrogen-secreting adrenal tumor is a very rare cause of precocious puberty. Clinically virilizing symptoms and signs usually precede or accompany the clinical manifestations of excess estrogen.

Exogenous administration of sex steroids or gonadotropins may cause peripheral precocious puberty. A complete history and careful review of all possible external sources of estrogen in the home (medications, creams, cosmetics, powders, etc.) are the only means of identifying exogenous sources of estrogen. A similar approach in search of androgenic compounds needs to be taken when solely virilizing symptoms are present.

Children who are markedly hypothyroid lose the central negative feedback of thyroxine and develop early puberty in the setting of enlarged pituitary glands often misclassified as adenomas. One purported explanation for this phenomenon is that thyrotropin-releasing hormone (TRH) secretion is increased by the hypothalamus, resulting in a concomitant indiscriminate increase in gonadotropins (the so-called "overlap" syndrome). The increase in gonadotropins produces clinical signs of precocious puberty and may stimulate the growth of ovarian cysts. With thyroid replacement therapy, the children will become euthyroid and the ovarian cysts will regress. Children with primary hypothyroidism are typically short in stature and their bone age is delayed; however, the concomitant presence of sexual precocity may change the reliability of these findings. Hypothyroidism as a cause of precocious puberty is limited almost entirely to girls.

McCune–Albright syndrome is composed of the triad of precocious puberty, multiple areas of fibrous dysplasia of bone, and irregularly shaped *café-au-lait* spots of the skin (described as "coast of Maine" in shape). Facial asymmetry and/or skeletal deformities are pathognomonic of polyostotic fibrous dysplasia. The diagnosis can be suspected from the identification of dysplastic lesions of bone seen on x-ray. This rare disease is found more frequently in girls. The associated precocious puberty, typically presenting as isolated menarche in girls < 3 years of age, is due to the autonomous production of estrogen by the ovaries, caused by an activating G-protein mutation. Early in life, children with McCune–Albright syndrome have widely fluctuating estrogen levels and low gonadotropin concentrations which are independent of GnRH stimulation. Other autonomous endocrinopathies associated with McCune–Albright syndrome include hyperthyroidism, growth hormone excess, and Cushing's syndrome.

Combined peripheral and central precocious puberty

Children initially presenting with PPP may, over time, shift to a pattern of central puberty. As the primary process progresses, the central reproductive hormonal axis is activated and GnRH-dependent precocious puberty ensues. Congenital adrenal hyperplasia is the most common cause of combined precocious puberty. Other causes include McCune–Albright syndrome and virilizing adrenal tumors.

Incomplete precocious puberty

Precocious puberty is incomplete if only one pubertal change, premature adrenarche (pubic hair) or premature thelarche (breast development), is clinically apparent without any evidence of a systemic sex steroid effect. Failure of the bone age seen at x-ray to exceed 2 SD beyond the chronologic age is suggestive for the absence of a systemic hormonal effect. The remaining pubertal events typically occur at a normal age.

Premature thelarche

Premature thelarche is the appearance of breast development prior to the age of 8 years without the presence of any other pubertal change or evidence of systemic estrogen effect. This condition is benign and therapy is not required. It may manifest in a unilateral or bilateral form, with little darkening or widening of the areola. Premature thelarche occurs most commonly between 1 and 2 years of age, but may begin at birth. Long-term follow-up of young girls with premature thelarche reveals that most have no progression of their breast development, one-third have regression of their breast changes, and one-tenth have progressive breast enlargement. Young girls with premature thelarche have prepubertal levels of both estradiol (as measured in an ultrasensitive assay (< 10 pg/mL)) and luteinizing hormone (LH), along with a moderate increase in serum follicle-stimulating hormone (FSH), but not LH, following GnRH stimulation.

Premature adrenarche

Premature adrenarche is the appearance of pubic hair and/or axillary hair, with associated body odor and acne, prior to the age of 8 years (precocious pubarche), along with a rise in serum levels of dehydroepiandrosterone sulfate (DHEAS). By definition, it occurs without the presence of any other pubertal changes or evidence of systemic estrogen effect. Premature adrenarche is the result of a functional increase in the production of adrenal androgens. An adrenocortical enzyme deficiency is infrequent in these patients, although it must be considered in certain high-risk populations (e.g. Ashkenazi Jews, Yugoslavs, Hispanics, and Italians), especially if signs of virilization and/or rapid growth are present. In these situations, an ACTH stimulation test should be performed, but, in simple pubarche, it is usually not indicated. Girls with premature adrenarche may find themselves at increased risk for anovulation during their reproductive lives, which may eventually evolve into polycystic ovary syndrome.

Diagnosis

All children with suspected precocious puberty should have a thorough history and physical examination. The degree of pubertal development is assessed by the method of Tanner staging. The child's height should be determined accurately using a stadiometer at each visit. The child's growth chart should be reviewed to determine the age of onset of any increase in rapid growth velocity. Bone age assessment by radiograph of the left hand and wrist should be performed to determine the degree of skeletal maturation. Diagnostic laboratory testing should include basal ultrasensitive LH, FSH, and estradiol. The incomplete forms of precocious puberty (premature thelarche and premature adrenarche) are diagnosed when serial observations at least 6 months apart reveal that only one pubertal change has occurred, the change is slowly progressing, and the bone age corresponds with the chronologic age or is only slightly advanced. Girls with CPP typically have increased circulating concentrations of estradiol above the prepubertal range, elevated levels of LH, and an increase in LH and FSH in response to GnRH stimulation, with the response of LH being greater than that of FSH. A significant increase in LH and FSH in response to GnRH excludes the diagnosis of premature thelarche. An increase in FSH only to GnRH administration may occur in both premature thelarche and the very early stages of idiopathic precocious puberty and is, thus, not helpful in distinguishing between the two entities.

Children who are hypothyroid and present with precocious puberty usually have a delayed bone age compared to their chronologic age. Thyroid function tests will confirm the diagnosis and serve as a baseline from which the effects of therapy can be judged.

A GnRH stimulation test differentiates CPP from PPP. Children with PPP may have an advanced bone age, but they fail to manifest a significant increase in gonadotropins (especially LH) following GnRH stimulation.

A rectal-abdominal examination and pelvic ultrasonography will identify ovarian tumors and ovarian cysts. Serum hCG concentrations are elevated in the presence of germ cell tumors. Adrenal tumors are diagnosed with the use of adrenal sonograms and/or other imaging studies. Exogenous sources of sex steroids can only be detected by a thorough medical history and a careful review of the child's environment. McCune–Albright syndrome is diagnosed by physical examination with findings of facial asymmetry, skeletal deformities, and irregularly bordered *café-au-lait* spots. A radiographic skeletal survey or technetium bone scan will confirm the presence of dysplastic bone lesions.

Children with CPP have an advanced bone age and demonstrate an increase in gonadotropin levels in response to GnRH, with a preferential rise in LH over FSH. Children with CPP have symmetrically increased ovarian volume for age and pubertal uterine size as determined with pelvic ultrasonography. CNS disease is confirmed with the use of neurologic and ophthalmologic examinations, skull x-ray, EEG, and MRI studies of the brain. The diagnosis of idiopathic CPP is made by the exclusion of all demonstrable specific causes of precocious puberty.

Treatment

The treatment of precocious puberty depends upon the specific etiology. Incomplete forms of precocious puberty are usually self-limiting and do not require treatment. The hypothyroid child is managed with thyroid replacement therapy. If exogenous sources of estrogen or androgen are identified, they should be eliminated from the child's environment. Ovarian and adrenal tumors causing precocious puberty should be removed surgically. Testolactone, a first-generation aromatase inhibitor, has been successfully used in the treatment of children with McCune–Albright syndrome. Testolactone is started with a total daily oral dose of 20 mg/kg body weight in four divided doses. Over a 3-week interval, the total daily dose is increased to 40 mg/kg body weight. As a result, estrogen concentrations in the peripheral circulation are reduced, ovarian volume measured by ultrasound is reduced, and the frequency of menses diminishes, with little effect on the regression of breast development or pubic hair growth. The newer aromatase inhibitors, anastrazole and letrazole, may also have some promise. The estrogen receptor blocker, tamoxifen, has also been used to treat girls with McCune-Albright syndrome. Secondary CPP may ensue in these girls requiring the addition of a GnRH agonist.

Long-acting GnRH agonists have become the treatment of choice for CPP. GnRH agonists produce an initial rise in pituitary secretion of gonadotropins, followed relatively quickly by downregulation of pituitary GnRH receptors which causes estrogen levels to decline to the prepubertal range. Ovarian volume and uterine size as determined by ultrasound regress, breast development is halted or regresses, menstruation ceases, and the rates of linear growth and skeletal maturation decrease. Children with CPP treated with GnRH agonists will usually achieve a greater height than predicted as the result of their therapy. Full recovery of the reproductive axis can take up to 12–18 months when the GnRH agonists are discontinued. Limited long-term data from Japan and Italy suggest normal fertility rates (~80%) in women previously treated as children with GnRH agonists.

The ultimate decision to use GnRH agonists is dependent on the rate of height growth, bone age change, and estimated adult height. Some authorities prefer a more conservative approach to the use of GnRH agonists if the estimated height prediction is above 150 cm in girls and if the pace of sexual maturation is not causing major psychosocial dysfunction.

Several GnRH analogs are available for the treatment of precocious puberty. Leuprolide (Lupron® Depot Ped) contained in microcapsules, administered as an intramuscular injection at a dose of 60 μg/kg every 3–4 weeks, is by far the most common formulation used. Histrelin acetate (Supprelin®), the newest FDA-approved GnRH agonist product, is an ultralong-acting, slow-release formulation that is surgically implanted in a muscle with a duration of action of 1 year. The implant must be removed and replaced annually. GnRH analogs are recommended for the treatment of CPP, but not PPP. The dose of the chosen GnRH agonist is titrated to maintain an estradiol level of less than 10 pg/mL, as is present in prepubertal girls. Side effects observed with the use of GnRH agonists to treat precocious puberty include sterile abscesses at the injection site. Menopausal symptoms are rarely reported. Therapy should be started as early in the clinical presentation as possible and continued until at least the mean age for pubertal development and/or when an acceptable height has been attained.

Suggested reading

Cameron FJ, Scheimberg I, Stanhope R. Precocious pseudopuberty due to a granulosa cell tumor in a seven-month old female. *Acta Paediatr* 1997; 86: 1016–1018.

Cavallo A, Richards GE, Busey S, Michaels SE. A simplified gonadotrophin-releasing hormone test for precocious puberty. *Clin Endocrinol* 1995; 42: 641–646.

Elders MJ, Scott CR, Frindik JP, Kemp SF. Clinical work-up for precocious puberty. *Lancet* 1997; 350: 457–458.

Eugster EA, Rubin SD, Reiter EO, *et al*. Tamoxifen treatment for precocious puberty in McCune–Albright syndrome: a multicenter trial. *J Pediatr* 2003; 143: 61–67.

Feuillan PP, Jones J, Cutler GB Jr. Long-term testolactone therapy for precocious puberty in girls with the McCune–Albright syndrome. *J Clin Endocrinol Metab* 1993; 77: 647–651.

Herman-Gidens ME, Slora EJ, Wasserman RC. Secondary sexual characteristics and menses in young girls seen in office practice: a study from the Pediatric Research in Office Settings Network. *Pediatrics* 1997; 99: 505–512.

Ibanez L, de Zegher F, Potau N. Anovulation after precocious pubarche: early markers and time course in adolescence. *J Clin Endocrinol Metab* 1999; 84: 2691–2695.

Jensen A-M, Brocks V, Holm K, *et al*. Central precocious puberty in girls. Internal genitalia before, during and after treatment with long-acting gonadotropin-releasing hormone analogs. *J Pediatr* 1998; 132: 105–108.

Jung H, Carmel P, Schwartz M, *et al*. Some hypothalamic hamartomas contain transforming growth factor alpha, a puberty-inducing growth factor, but not luteinizing hormone-releasing neurons. *J Clin Endocrinol Metab* 1999; 84: 4695-4701.

Kaplowitz PB, Oberfield SE. Reexamination of the age limit for defining when puberty is precocious in girls in the United States: implications for evaluation and treatment. *Pediatrics* 1999; 104: 936–941.

Kornreich L, Horev G, Blaser S, *et al*. Central precocious puberty: evaluation by neuroimaging. *Pediatr Radiol* 1995; 25: 7–11.

Neely EK, Bachrach LK, Hintz RL, *et al*. Bone mineral density during treatment of central precocious puberty. *J Pediatr* 1995; 127: 819–822.

Neely EK, Wilson DM, Lee PA, *et al*. Spontaneous serum gonadotropin concentrations in the evaluation of precocious puberty. *J Pediatr* 1995; 127: 47–52.

Rosenfield RL. Selection of children with precocious puberty for treatment with gonadotropin releasing hormone analogs. *J Pediatr* 1994; 124(6): 989–991.

Stewart L, Steinbok P, Daaboul J. Role of surgical resection in the treatment of hypothalamic hamartomas causing precocious puberty. Report of six cases. *J Neurosurg* 1998; 88: 340–345.

Teles MG, Bianco SD, Brito VN, *et al*. A GPR54-activating mutation in a patient with central precocious puberty. *NEJM* 2008; 358: 709–715.

Verrotti A, Chiarelli F, Montanaro AF, Morgee G. Bone mineral content in girls with precocious puberty treated with gonadotropin-releasing hormone analog. *Gynecol Endocrinol* 1995; 9: 277–281.

Chapter 89
Primary Amenorrhea

Briana Rudick and Karine Chung
Department of Medicine and Obstetrics and Gynecology, Keck School of Medicine, University of Southern California, CA, USA

Introduction

Amenorrhea is defined as the absence or the abnormal cessation of menses. The term primary amenorrhea refers to the failure to menstruate by age 15 in the presence of normal secondary sex characteristics or within 5 years after breast development if thelarche occurs before age 10. Other clinical situations which require investigation include failure to initiate breast development or absence of other secondary sex characteristics by age 13.

The causes of primary amenorrhea are numerous and may be physiologic, endocrine or anatomic. Pregnancy is an example of a physiologic cause of both primary and secondary amenorrhea. Endocrine causes include failed maturation of the hypothalamic-pituitary-ovarian (HPO) axis or gonadal failure as seen in Turner's syndrome. Gonadal failure accounts for over 40% of cases of primary amenorrhea. Anatomic causes include obstruction of the lower reproductive tract as in mullerian agenesis or Mayer Rokitansky Kuster Hauser syndrome (MRKH). This accounts for another 15% of primary amenorrhea. Another 10% of primary amenorrhea will be due to constitutional delay. Finally, in rare cases, polycystic ovarian syndrome (PCOS) may present as primary amenorrhea, as metabolic syndrome and obesity are now epidemic in the adolescent population. PCOS is the subject of Chapter 93. This chapter will focus on the endocrine causes of primary amenorrhea.

In order to understand how primary amenorrhea is evaluated, it is necessary to understand the basic embryology of sex development, how the internal and external genitalia form and under what influences. Prior to 6–9 weeks of gestation, the fetus contains bipotential gonads, and both the mullerian and wolffian ducts. The SRY region on the Y-chromosome then acts on the bipotential gonad to differentiate into a testis instead of an ovary (the default). Once formed, the testes secrete two substances. The first is testosterone, which causes further growth of the wolffian ducts and testicular descent. Eventually the wolffian ducts become the seminal vesicles, the vas deferens, and the epididymis. Testosterone is converted into dihydrotestosterone which is responsible for male secondary sex characteristics such as changes in voice, penile growth, and pubic hair growth. The second substance secreted by the testis is mullerian inhibiting substance (MIS), which causes regression of the mullerian ducts.

In women, with the absence of the SRY gene, the germ cells in the bipotential gonad develop into the ovaries and there is no MIS to inhibit the growth of the mullerian ducts. Since there is nothing to support wolffian duct development, they regress. The mullerian ducts eventually become the fallopian tubes, uterus, and the upper third of the vagina. The lower two-thirds of the vagina is formed from the urogenital sinus. The estrogen secreted by the ovaries supports female secondary characterstics such as breast development at puberty.

Keeping this embryology in mind, when encountering a patient with primary amenorrhea, the history should focus around several key questions. Is there a history of abnormal or delayed growth as a child? This might suggest an endocrine cause at the level of the hypothalamus or pituitary. Any history of pelvic pain and is it cyclic? This would suggest lower genital tract outflow obstruction. Any history of breast discharge, headache or visual symptoms suggesting a prolactinoma? It is important to ask about activity and nutritional status since extremes of weight are associated with hypothalamic amenorrhea. Any history of childhood cancers, chemotherapy or pelvic radiation? These treatments are associated with gonadal failure from accelerated oocyte loss. Finally, it is important to take a complete history, focusing on present systemic illnesses, family history and reproductive history, as well as any medications that the patient is currently taking.

Management of Common Problems in Obstetrics and Gynecology,
5th edition. Edited by T.M. Goodwin, M.N. Montoro,
L. Muderspach, R. Paulson and S. Roy. © 2010 Blackwell
Publishing Ltd.

Physical exam should focus on the presence or absence of secondary sex characteristics. Breast development (Tanner staging) reflects estrogen status while pubic hair growth reflects androgen exposure. Bodyweight and height should be noted. A careful skin exam could reveal hirsutism, virilism, neurofibromas, *café-au-lait* spots, acne, acanthosis, myxedema, striae on the abdomen or male-pattern hair distribution. Head and neck exam should rule out the presence of exophthalmos, cleft lip or palate. Abdominal exam should include the presence or absence of palpable abdominal masses, and an inguinal exam. Finally, careful examination of the external genitalia should be performed since it will be abnormal in 15% of women with primary amenorrhea. Ultrasound should then be performed to look for the presence of a uterus.

Based on the presence or absence of a uterus and breast development, there are four distinct phenotypes of individuals with primary amenorrhea (see Table 89.1).
• Group I: absent breast development but uterus present
• Group II: breast development present but uterus absent
• Group III: absence of both breast and uterus
• Group IV: presence of both breast development and uterus

Group I

Individuals with primary amenorrhea who lack breast development but who have a uterus have a defect in estrogen action somewhere along the HPO axis, either at the level of the hypothalamus/pituitary (hypothalamic hypogonadism) or at the level of the ovary (hypergonadotropic hypogonadism). These two etiologies can be differentiated by measuring serum FSH and LH. Serum gonadotropin levels are low in hypothalamic/pituitary causes, while they are elevated in primary gonadal disorders.

The most common chromosomal abnormalities associated with hypergonadotropic hypogonadism are 45,X (Turner's syndrome), 46,X (abnormal X chromosome), mosaicism, pure gonadal dysgenesis (46,XX and 46,XY), and 17α-hydroxylase deficiency with a 46,XX karyotype. Turner's syndrome is the most common cause of gonadal failure, and it occurs in 1/2500 livebirths. The principal features of this syndrome include sexual infantilism, short stature, and streak gonads, but other organ systems are commonly affected and include cardiac, renal, and autoimmune manifestations. These individuals require estrogen replacement to induce breast development and protect the skeletal system from osteoporosis. Progestin should be added for the sole purpose of protecting the endometrium from the unopposed estrogen or alternatively, OCPs may be used. In order to maximize final height, low-dose androgens, steroids or growth hormone can be administered before or during hormone replacement therapy. While greater than 90% of Turner's patients have gonadal failure, 2–5% do have spontaneous menses and thus may conceive spontaneously. Alternatively,

Table 89.1 Classification of disorders with primary amenorrhea according to breast and uterine development

Group I Breast development absent Uterus present	Group II Breast development present Uterus absent	Group III Breast development absent Uterus absent	Group IV Breast development present Uterus present
Gonadal failure • 45,X (Turner's) • 46,X, abnormal X (short or long arm deletion) • mosaicism • 46,XX or 46,XY pure gonadal dysgenesis • 17α-hydroxylase deficiency, 46,XY *Hypothalamic failure* • insufficient GnRH secretion • inadequate GnRH synthesis • congenital anatomic defect in CNS *Pituitary failure* • isolated gonadotropin deficiency • chromophobe adenomas • mumps, encephalitis • newborn kernicterus • prepubertal hypothyroidism	*Androgen insensitivity* • testicular feminization *Congenital absence of uterus* • Mullerian agenesis • MRKH syndrome	*17,20 desmolase deficiency* *Agonadism* *17α-hydroxylase deficiency* *(46,XY)*	*Hypothalamic* *Pituitary* *Ovarian* *Uterine*

Adapted and modified from Mashchak CA, Kletzky OA, Davajan V, *et al.* Clinical and laboratory evaluation of patients with primary amenorrhea. *Obstet Gynecol* 1981; 57: 715. Used with permission from the American College of Obstetricians and Gynecologists.

these patients may undergo *in vitro* fertilization with egg donation to carry a pregnancy, However, recent surveys of egg donation programs have demonstrated a 100-fold increase in maternal mortality in pregnancy from undiagnosed cardiac disease. It is important to counsel these patients about the risks of pregnancy prior to conception, and all patients should have an echocardiogram preconceptually.

Gonadal dysgenesis can be associated with more than one genotype, including 45,XO, 46,XX, and 46,XY. Genetically XY individuals with gonadal failure will have female genitalia because MIS and testosterone will not be produced, so these patients will have a uterus. Gonadal tumors occur in up to 25% of women with a Y chromosome; unlike in androgen insensitivity (see group II), these gonads do not secrete hormones and should be removed at the time of diagnosis.

A few individuals have gonadal failure due to a deficiency of 17α-hydroxylase in the biosynthetic pathway and they are unable to produce sex steroids. The diagnosis is established by the determination of serum progesterone (elevated) and serum 17α-hydroxyprogesterone (decreased) levels and confirmed by an adrenocorticotropic hormone (ACTH) challenge test. Individuals with 17α-hydroxylase deficiency have a life-threatening disease due to the defect in the synthesis of cortisol and require cortisone administration as well as HRT. They also have sodium retention, hypokalemia, and hypertension due to the increase in the synthesis of mineralocorticoid precursors in the aldosterone pathway.

Individuals with primary amenorrhea who lack breast development but have an intact uterus have hypogonadotropic hypogonadism if their serum FSH level is normal or low. These individuals have a hypothalamic-pituitary disorder. Very rarely, an anatomic defect of the hypothalamic-pituitary region is the cause of the disorder. A CT scan or a MRI study of the sella turcica and serum prolactin and thyroid-stimulating hormone (TSH) levels should be performed for all individuals with hypogonadotropic hypogonadism to diagnose an anatomic lesion. Individuals with hypogonadotropic hypogonadism who do not have a CNS lesion should have a qualitative test for olfaction with coffee, tobacco, orange, and cocoa, as some of these patients may present with anosmia (Kallman's syndrome). A karyotype is not necessary for individuals with hypogonadotropic hypogonadism as they have a normal female karyotype, in contrast to hypergonadotropic hypogonadism which is commonly associated with chromosomal abnormalities. For individuals with a hypothalamic-pituitary disorder who desire pregnancy, human menopausal gonadotropins (hMG) or pulsatile GnRH can be used to successfully induce ovulation. Clomiphene citrate is generally not effective in the induction of ovulation in hypoestrogenic individuals, since this medication requires an intact HPO axis. For those who do not currently desire fertility, HRT should be prescribed to promote breast development as well as to derive long-term benefits from HRT.

Group II

Individuals with primary amenorrhea who have normal breast development but lack the presence of a uterus have either the congenital absence of the uterus (mullerian agenesis) or androgen insensitivity syndrome (also called "testicular feminization"). A karyotype will confirm the diagnosis since patients with mullerian agenesis are 46,XX while patients with androgen insensitivity are 46,XY. However, obtaining a testosterone level is just as effective in making the diagnosis; patients with androgen insensitivity will have a normal to high testostosterone level in the male range while patients with mullerian agenesis will have a testosterone level in the female range.

Mullerian agenesis is the second most common cause of primary amenorrhea and occurs once in every 4000–5000 female births. Fifteen percent of individuals with primary amenorrhea have a congenital absence of the uterus. It is a noninherited event due to the failure of development of the mullerian system, and there can be varying degrees of agenesis. These patients have a normally functioning HPO axis, including ovulation, and since estrogen and androgen production is normal, breast development and axillary and pubic hair growth are normal. Absence of the vagina in addition to absence of the uterus is referred to as Mayer Rokitansky Kuster Hauser (MRKH) syndrome.

Women with congenital absence of the uterus have a normal complement of ovarian follicles, normal ovarian steroidogenesis, and are ovulatory. Using a surrogate mother, these women may donate their own eggs and have their own genetic children. HRT is not necessary until the menopause, which occurs at the same average age as in ovulatory women with a uterus. Women with congenital absence of the uterus who have a short or absent vagina can use a series of progressively larger dilators or can undergo vaginoplasty to create a functional vaginal vault.

Women with congenital absence of the uterus with or without a vagina also have an increase in congenital anomalies of the renal system and the skeletal system. Congenital anomalies of the renal system occur in one-third or more of these individuals (absence of the kidney 15%, a double collecting system 40%). Any woman with uterine agenesis should be evaluated with an intravenous pyelogram. Skeletal abnormalities occur in 5–10% of women with congenital absence of the uterus. One of the most common skeletal anomalies is congenital fusion of the cervical vertebrae. The presence of this anomaly will impede successful endotracheal intubation should the individual ever require general anesthesia.

Androgen insensitivity syndrome may be complete or, less commonly, incomplete. The clinical features of the complete form include the absence of or decreased axillary and pubic hair, normal breast development, and a blind vaginal pouch, so the patient is phenotypically female. It is inherited via X-linked recessive mutation of the gene that encodes the intracellular androgen receptor. As a result, the genetic (46,XY) and gonadal (testes) male fetus fails to masculinize *in utero* or at puberty but the MIS secreted by the testes still blocks the development of the uterus and oviducts.

Patients with complete androgen insensitivity appear normal at birth but it is important to look for the presence of inguinal masses denoting undescended testes, since dihydrotestosterone is responsible for complete testicular descent. The incidence of gonadal tumors in patients with androgen insensitivity syndrome varies from 2% to 22% when the testes are left *in situ*. All patients with this syndrome should have their gonads surgically removed after puberty because of the high incidence of malignancy. It is usually recommended that the testes not be removed until the patient has undergone full sexual development since the sexual development obtained with hormone replacement is not as optimal as that achieved with endogenous hormones. Additionally, because most tumors have not been reported to develop until after the patient is older than 20 years, it is felt to be safe to wait until after puberty. Following gonadectomy, the patient should receive continuous unopposed estrogen replacement therapy.

Patients with incomplete androgen insensitivity have some androgen effect. Clinical features at birth may include partial fusion of the labioscrotal folds, clitoromegaly or even a phallus. At puberty there is breast development, although to a lesser degree than seen in the complete form. There is also pubic hair growth and enlargement of the clitoris.

In the past, the accepted way to counsel these patients was to avoid disclosing gonadal and chromosomal sex to the patient. However, many patients appreciate a full understanding of themselves, so educating patients in a sensitive manner is essential. It is important to keep in mind that these patients are almost always female in their gender identity and it becomes the challenge of the physician to educate them in a way that will reinforce this identity.

Group III

The least common group of individuals with primary amenorrhea comprises those who have neither breast nor uterus development. These individuals have a male karyotype (46,XY), elevated serum gonadotropin levels, and serum testosterone levels that are within or below

the normal female range. Individuals with primary amenorrhea who lack both breast and uterine development include those with 17,20-desmolase deficiency, agonadism, and 17α-hydroxylase deficiency. These patients differ from those with gonadal failure who have a 46,XY karyotype in that they lack a uterus while those with gonadal failure have a uterus present. These individuals differ from those with androgen insensitivity syndrome in that they do not have breast development and their serum testosterone levels are in or below the normal female range, and those with androgen insensitivity syndrome have breast development and serum levels of testosterone in the normal male range.

Individuals with a 17,20-desmolase enzyme deficiency cannot convert 17α-hydroxypregnenolone and 17α-hydroxyprogesterone to DHEA and androstenedione respectively, and thus are unable to synthesize all sex steroids. Individuals with 17α-hydroxylase deficiency are unable to convert pregnenolone and progesterone to 17α-hydroxypregnenolone and 17α-hydroxyprogesterone respectively, and this defect also results in the inability to synthesize sex steroids. Those with 17α-hydroxylase deficiency have hypertension.

Agonadism is also known as "vanishing testis syndrome." It is theorized that individuals with agonadism had testicular tissue present for sufficiently long that MIS was present and inhibited the formation of the mullerian system derivatives. Then the testicular tissue vanished. The diagnosis of agonadism is only considered after enzyme deficiencies have been excluded in patients with primary amenorrhea who lack the development of both the breasts and uterus.

When an enzyme deficiency is confirmed, these individuals should have their testes surgically removed. They will then require continuous unopposed estrogen replacement therapy, as will those individuals with agonadism. Patients with 17α-hydroxylase deficiency require cortisol replacement in addition to estrogen replacement.

Group IV

The second largest group of individuals with primary amenorrhea are those who have both spontaneous breast development and the presence of a uterus. The presence of spontaneous breast development and the failure of menarche indicates either a lower genital tract obstruction or a disturbance in the HPO axis occurring some time after the initiation but before the completion of puberty. Examples of anatomic causes include imperforate hymen, transverse vaginal septum, and isolated absence of the vagina or cervix. These lower urogenital tract abnormalities usually present with cyclic pelvic pain. Physical exam can reveal an accumulation of blood behind the obstruction. This build-up can cause retrograde flow of menses, and thus increase the likelihood of pelvic adhesions and endometriosis. In the absence of a lower genital tract obstruction, the endocrine evaluation of individuals with primary amenorrhea who have normal breast and uterine development is very similar to the diagnostic evaluation of women with secondary amenorrhea. This evaluation is presented in Chapter 90.

Suggested reading

ASRM Practice Committee Opinion. Current evaluation of amenorrhea. *Fertil Steril* 2004; 82: 266–272.

Frisch RE, Revelle R. Height and weight at menarche and a hypothesis of menarche. *Arch Dis Child* 1971; 46: 695–701.

Mashchak CA, Kletzky OA, Davajan V, *et al*. Clinical and laboratory evaluation of patients with primary amenorrhea. *Obstet Gynecol* 1981; 57: 715–721.

Mishell DR Jr, Davajan V, Lobo RA (eds). *Infertility, contraception and reproductive endocrinology*, 3rd edn. Cambridge, MA: Blackwell Scientific Publications, 1991.

Warren MP. The effects of exercise on pubertal progression and reproductive function in goals. *J Clin Endocrinol Metab* 1980; 51: 1150–1157.

Ying S-Y. Inhibins, activins and follistatins: gonadal proteins modulating the secretion of follicle-stimulating hormone. *Endocrinol Rev* 1988; 9: 267–293.

Chapter 90
Secondary Amenorrhea

Briana Rudick and Richard J. Paulson

Department of Medicine and Obstetrics and Gynecology, Keck School of Medicine, University of Southern California, CA, USA

Introduction

Secondary amenorrhea is defined as cessation of menses for more than three cycles or 6 months in women who previously had menses. After ruling out pregnancy (the most common cause of secondary amenorrhea), it may be the result of disorders in the central (CNS, hypothalamic-pituitary) axis, ovary or uterus and outflow tract. Amenorrhea associated with hyperprolactinemia is the subject of Chapter 91 whereas polycysytic ovary disease is covered in Chapter 93. This chapter will focus on the diagnosis and management of secondary amenorrhea in the absence of those two conditions.

Etiology

Central nervous system – hypothalamus

Stress is a common cause of menstrual dysfunction, and may lead to amenorrhea if the stress is severe. The exact mechanism of how stress diminishes GnRH release is not clear. It has been observed that the increase in both catechol estrogens and β-endorphins associated with stress appears to inhibit LH (and probably FSH) release, most likely by altering the function of the neurotransmitters responsible for the normal episodic release of GnRH. Amenorrhea results when the low gonadotropin levels fail to stimulate sufficient estradiol production to cause endometrial proliferation.

Strenuous exercise also causes an increase in β-endorphins and catechol estrogens. However, exercise amenorrhea appears to be to limited to runners. Swimming, even when strenuous, is much less likely to cause amenorrhea, suggesting that weightbearing plays a role in limiting

gonadotropin secretion. Menstruation resumes when the stress ceases.

Weight loss can cause amenorrhea in some women. This is presumably by the same "stress" response mechanism as noted above. When the total bodyweight diminishes, amenorrhea persists, even if the weight remains constant. The hypothalamus is responsive to fluctuations of weight as well as the total bodyweight and controls reproductive function. The pituitary and the remainder of the reproductive tract remain normal.

A special case of weight loss is anorexia nervosa. In this condition, both stress and weight loss combine to stop normal hypothalamic GnRH release. Amenorrhea may also occur in bulimia nervosa in which the BMI may remain normal, supporting the idea that weight loss is not the sole cause. If severe weight loss occurs and the patient weighs less than 25% of ideal bodyweight, an abnormal gonadotropin response to GnRH has been observed. This finding suggests that pituitary dysfunction also occurs in persons with anorexia nervosa when the weight loss becomes severe. Because anorexia nervosa is a psychiatric disorder, women with this disease should receive appropriate psychiatric treatment. Individuals with anorexia nervosa, as well as those with dietary weight loss, usually resume ovulatory menstrual cycles when they gain weight and reach a normal BMI.

Anatomic lesions in the brainstem or hypothalamus are an infrequent cause of secondary amenorrhea. Hypothalamic lesions include craniopharyngiomas, granulomatosis disease (tuberculosis and sarcoidosis), and sequelae of encephalitis. When these lesions are present, circulating gonadotropin and estradiol levels remain very low.

Phenothiazine derivatives, antihypertensive agents, and certain other drugs can produce amenorrhea without hyperprolactinemia, although usually prolactin levels are elevated with the use of these agents. Oral and injectable contraceptive steroids inhibit ovulation by acting on the hypothalamus to suppress GnRH as well as acting directly on the pituitary to suppress FSH and LH. In some individuals, this hypothalamic-pituitary suppression persists

Management of Common Problems in Obstetrics and Gynecology, 5th edition. Edited by T.M. Goodwin, M.N. Montoro, L. Muderspach, R. Paulson and S. Roy. © 2010 Blackwell Publishing Ltd.

for several months after the discontinuation of steroid contraceptives, producing the syndrome termed "post-pill amenorrhea." Prolonged gonadotropin suppression is uncommon following discontinuation of the low doses of steroids present in currently used oral contraceptive formulations and does not last more than 6 months. The etiology of amenorrhea persisting more than 6 months after discontinuation of oral contraceptives is unrelated to their use. Amenorrhea after injection of depomedroxyprogesterone acetate (DMPA) may persist for a year or more after the last injection.

Functional hypothalamic amenorrhea

The general term functional hypothalamic amenorrhea (FHA) has been used to characterize secondary amenorrhea in women who do not ingest drugs, do not engage in strenuous exercise, are not undergoing environmental stress, have not lost weight, and do not have pituitary, ovarian or uterine abnormalities.

When sufficient gonadotropins are produced to maintain circulating estradiol levels above 40 pg/mL, the term hypothalamic-pituitary dysfunction has been used to characterize this disorder. When the estradiol levels fall below 40 pg/mL, the term hypothalamic-pituitary failure is used, indicating a more serious disorder. Serum estradiol levels above 40 pg/mL are usually sufficient to stimulate endometrial growth and sloughing of the endometrial tissue usually occurs when progesterone levels fall several days after exogenous progestins are last administered. The presence or absence of the withdrawal bleeding response to progesterone administration has also been used to differentiate between the two diagnostic categories of FHA instead of measurement of estradiol.

Piuitary lesions

Although most pituitary tumors secrete prolactin, some do not. However, they may impede the action of prolactin-inhibitory substance (dopamine) on the lactotrophs and thus result in mild elevations of prolactin. These tumors may cause secondary amenorrhea to occur without hyperprolactinemia. Chromophobe adenomas are the most common nonprolactin-secreting pituitary tumors. In addition, both basophilic (ACTH secreting) and acidophilic (growth hormone (GH) secreting) adenomas may not secrete prolactin.

Pituitary cells can become damaged or necrotic as a result of anoxia, thrombosis or hemorrhage. When pituitary cell destruction results from a hypotensive episode during pregnancy, the disorder is called Sheehan's syndrome. When the disorder is unrelated to pregnancy, it is called Simmond's disease. Diagnosing this cause of secondary amenorrhea is important because pituitary damage (unlike hypothalamic dysfunction) can be associated with decreased secretion of other pituitary hormones. Thus, individuals with pituitary lesions may have secondary hypothyroidism or adrenal insufficiency that seriously impairs their health, in addition to their decreased estrogen levels.

Ovarian factors

The ovaries may fail to secrete sufficient estrogen to produce endometrial growth if the follicles are damaged as a result of infection, interference with blood supply, chemotherapy, radiation or surgical depletion (e.g. bilateral cystectomies). Even without these etiologies, the ovaries may spontaneously stop producing sufficient estrogen to stimulate endometrial growth several years before the age of the physiologic menopause. When this condition occurs before the age of 40, the term premature ovarian failure (POF) is best used to describe the clinical entity. About 1% of women under the age of 40 years develop POF, and the incidence steadily increases from ages 15 to 39.

Many individuals with POF, particularly those with primordial follicles that appear normal, also have an autoimmune disorder such as Hashimoto's thyroiditis. Some individuals with POF who do not have clinical evidence of an autoimmune disorder have antibodies to gonadotropins as well as to several other endocrine organs such as the thyroid and adrenal glands, suggesting that there is frequently an autoimmune etiology for this condition. POF can also occur after gonadal irradiation or systemic chemotherapy. In some instances, the condition may be transient before permanent ovarian failure occurs. Occasionally individuals with POF may ovulate and conceive during this transition period. It is recommended that immunologic screening and tests of endocrine function be performed on all individuals under age 35 who have POF. This entity is more fully discussed in Chapter 95.

Polycystic ovary syndrome (PCOS) is an ovarian condition which is associated with tonically elevated LH levels and impaired follicular maturation. Most women with PCOS have oligo-ovulation, but some may present with amenorrhea. The cardinal features of PCOS are its chronic nature, oligo-ovulation, and hyperandrogenism (either clinical or biochemical). It is also called chronic hyperandrogenic oligo-ovulation. Most women also have polycystic ovarian morphology, which appears as multiple (more than 12) small (< 10 mm) follicles arranged around the periphery of the ovary. PCOS is more fully discussed in Chapter 93.

Uterus and outflow tract

If normal endocrine function is present, menstrual bleeding can be stopped by blocking its outflow. A diagnosis of outflow obstruction should be suspected if there is a temporal relationship between the onset of amenorrhea and a surgical procedure on the uterus, most commonly a uterine curettage. If the curettage is overly vigorous, and especially if it occurs during a hypoestrogenic state (such as postpartum hemorrhage), the denuded endometrium may undergo scarring and form intrauterine adhesions or synechiae (Asherman's syndrome). In milder cases, only the outflow is blocked, typically in the region of the internal cervical os, but in severe cases, the cavity may be entirely obliterated. The diagnosis can be confirmed with a hysterosalpingogram or hysteroscopy. Treatment with hysteroscopy is generally successful but in severe cases, the re-establishment of the cavity may not be successful or the intrauterine adhesions may recur.

Diagnostic evaluation

All women who consult a clinician for the symptom of secondary amenorrhea should have a detailed history and physical examination. After pregnancy has been ruled out, the possibility of intrauterine adhesions (IUA) should be considered. A history of endometrial curettage, especially if related to pregnancy, may suggest that outflow obstruction is responsible for the lack of menses. An attempt may be made to sound the uterus and if there appears to be an obstruction, the diagnosis can be confirmed by an HSG or hysteroscopy.

If Asherman's syndrome is ruled out, the history should determine whether the patient is taking any medications or has recently discontinued oral contraceptives. In addition, information regarding diet, weight loss, stress, and strenuous exercise should be obtained. A history of decreasing breast size or vaginal dryness may suggest estrogen deficiency. In this case, hormonal testing should confirm estradiol levels along with FSH and LH to look for either hypo- or hypergonadotropic hypogonadism.

If the history and physical examination fail to reveal the cause of the amenorrhea, a complete blood count, urinalysis, and serum chemistries should be assessed to rule out systemic disease. A sensitive thyroid-stimulating hormone (TSH) assay should also be performed to determine whether or not an asymptomatic thyroid disorder is present. Serum estradiol, FSH, and prolactin levels should also be measured (Figure 90.1). If prolactin levels are elevated, a diagnostic evaluation for the etiology of the hyperprolactinemia should be undertaken.

The presence of uterine bleeding several days after the administration of injectable progesterone or oral progestins is an indirect means of determining if serum levels of estradiol are sufficient to cause endometrial proliferation. This corresponds to approximately 40 pg/mL. This level of estradiol usually produces sufficient endometrial growth so that after the progesterone levels fall, withdrawal bleeding occurs (progesterone challenge test). With the availability of estradiol assays, there is little need for this procedure except to reassure the patient that menstruation is still possible. However, the progesterone challenge test is liable to false negatives and positives and should not be a substitute for the accurate determination of serum estradiol levels.

Women with PCOS, moderate stress, exercise, weight loss or hypothalamic-pituitary dysfunction will usually have estradiol levels above 40 pg/mL, and withdrawal bleeding after progestin administration usually occurs. Individuals with pituitary tumors, ovarian failure, severe

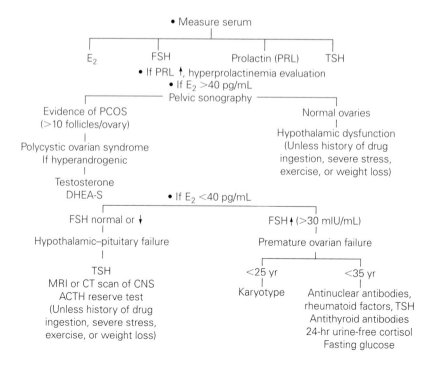

Figure 90.1 Diagnostic evaluation of secondary amenorrhea. Reproduced with permission from Mishell DR Jr. Primary and secondary amenorrhea. In: Stenchever MA, Droegemueller W, Herbst AL, Mishell DR Jr (eds) *Comprehensive gynecology*, 4th edn. St Louis, MO: CV Mosby, 2001: 1099–1124.

dietary weight loss or anorexia nervosa, severe stress or the rare hypothalamic lesions will usually have estradiol levels less than 40 pg/mL, and they will not have withdrawal bleeding after progesterone administration.

The diagnosis of PCOS is suggested by observing the characteristic polycystic ovary morphology by transvaginal ultrasound. This is the observation of 12 or more follicles 2–9 mm in diameter in the periphery of each ovary. When there is sonographic evidence of PCOS, serum testosterone and dehydroepiandrosterone sulfate (DHEAS) levels should be measured to determine if either or both are elevated.

Women with low FSH and estradiol levels who do not have a history of severe weight loss, strenuous exercise or severe stress should have an MRI or a CT scan of the hypothalamic-pituitary region performed to determine whether a lesion is present. If a lesion is seen or the medical history is compatible with possible pituitary destruction, such as the occurrence of hypotension during pregnancy, other pituitary hormones should be measured. These include prolactin, TSH and ACTH. If no lesion is identified, the condition is characterized as hypothalamic amenorrhea (a nonspecific diagnosis). Individuals with this diagnosis may resume normal ovarian function over time without treatment.

If POF is diagnosed because FSH levels are elevated and no cause of ovarian destruction is elicited, the possibility of autoimmune disease should be considered if the woman is younger than age 35. In these individuals, antithyroid antibodies and antiadrenal antibodies should be measured and a 24-hour urine-free cortisol level measured to determine whether Addison's disease is present. In addition, an assay to detect rheumatoid factors should be undertaken. Fasting blood sugar, serum calcium, phosphorus, TSH and thyroxin levels should also be measured to determine if other endocrinopathies are present. To rule out mosaicism, a karyotype should be obtained if POF occurs under the age of 30. Biopsy of the gonads by laparoscopy or laparotomy is not indicated. Individuals with POF are assumed to be hypoestrogenic and need estrogen replacement although residual ovarian function is sometimes present and occasional ovulation can occur.

Management

The appropriate treatment depends upon the diagnosis and whether conception is desired. Women with secondary amenorrhea have low estrogen levels and are anovulatory. Therefore, the goal of therapy is to restore a normal hormonal milieu or to re-establish ovulation if the patient wishes to conceive.

Patients with hypothalamic amenorrhea secondary to a particular behavior pattern may be advised to alter their behavior. Those who are underweight should be advised to gain weight. Those with exercise-induced amenorrhea may be advised to decrease the level of exercise or intensity. If this is not possible, they should be treated with estradiol replacement to prevent osteoporosis.

If women with hypothalamic amenorrhea wish to conceive, ovulation must generally be induced with exogenous FSH. Clomiphene works by opposing estradiol feedback on the hypothalamus and pituitary, and in a hypoestrogenic state, this is not effective. However, some patients may have amenorrhea yet have estradiol levels above 30 pg/mL. In some of these cases, (sometimes called "hypothalamic dysfunction"), clomiphene may be effective in inducing ovulation.

If women with PCOS desire conception, administration of clomiphene citrate is successful in inducing ovulation in the majority of cases. Those who fail clomiphene therapy may be treated with exogenous gonadotropins. If pregnancy is not desired, administration of medroxyprogesterone acetate (10 mg/day for the first 12 days of each month) or low-estrogen oral contraceptives will reduce the increased risk of endometrial cancer associated with unopposed estrogen.

Women with POF are generally quite hypoestrogenic and require estrogen replacement. Younger women may prefer to take combination oral contraceptives, although menopausal doses of estrogen are sufficient. Women with an intact uterus need intermittent progestins to avoid endometrial hyperplasia. If conception is desired, oocyte donation represents the only proven therapy. Attempts at ovulation induction with exogenous steroids or gonadotropins have been shown to be unsuccessful.

Intrauterine adhesions require treatment if the patient wishes to conceive. In these cases, hysteroscopic lysis of adhesions is the treatment of choice. The patient should be treated with estradiol postoperatively to reduce the risk of recurrence. Severe cases may require the placement of a stent to keep the cavity open while the endometrium heals.

Suggested reading

Alper MM, Gartner PR. Premature ovarian failure: its relationship to autoimmune disease. *Obstet Gynecol* 1985; 66: 27.

Berga SL, Mortola JF, Girton L, *et al*. Neuroendocrine aberrations in women with functional hypothalamic amenorrhea. *J Clin Endocrinol Metab* 1989; 68: 301.

Boyer RM, Katz J, Finkelstein JW, *et al*. Anorexia nervosa. Immaturity of 24-hour luteinizing hormone secretory pattern. *NEJM* 1974; 291: 861.

Carr DB, Bullen BA, Skrinar GS, *et al*. Physical conditioning facilitates the exercise-induced secretion of beta-endorphin and beta-lipotropin in women. *NEJM* 1981; 305: 560.

Crowley WF, Filicori M, Spratt KL, *et al*. The physiology of gonadotropin-releasing hormone (GnRH) secretion in men and women. *Recent Prog Horm Res* 1985; 4: 473.

Drinkwater BL, Nilson K, Chestnut CH III, *et al*. Bone mineral content of amenorrheic and eumenorrheic athletes. *NEJM* 1984; 11: 277–281.

Fries H, Nillus SJ, Pettersson E. Epidemiology of secondary amenorrhea: a retrospective evaluation of etiology with special regard to psychogenic factors and weight loss. *Am J Obstet Gynecol* 1974; 118: 473.

Jaroudi KA, Arora M, Sheth KV, *et al*. Human leukocyte antigen typing and associated abnormalities in premature ovarian failure. *Human Reprod* 1994; 9: 2006–2009.

Lloyd T, Myers C, Buchanan JR, Demers LM. Collegiate women athletes with irregular menses during adolescence have decreased bone density. *Obstet Gynecol* 1988; 72: 639.

Mason HD, Sagle M. Reduced frequency of luteinizing hormone pulses in women with weight loss-related amenorrhea and multifollicular ovaries. *Clin Endocrinol* 1988; 280: 611.

McArthur JW, Bullen BA, Beitins I, *et al*. Hypothalamic amenorrhea in runners of normal body composition. *Endocrinol Res Comm* 1980; 7: 13.

Reame NE, Sauder S, Kalch RP, *et al*. Pulsatile gonadotropin secretion during the human menstrual cycle. Evidence for altered frequency of gonadotropin-releasing hormone secretion. *J Clin Endocrinol Metab* 1984; 59: 328.

Rebar RW, Erickson GF, Yen SSC. Idiopathic premature ovarian failure. Clinical and endocrine characteristics. *Fertil Steril* 1981; 37: 35.

Reindollar RH, Novak M, Tho SPT, McDonough PG. Adult-onset amenorrhea. A study of 262 patients. *Am J Obstet Gynecol* 1981; 140: 371.

Russell JB, Mitchell DE, Musey PI, *et al*. The role of β-endorphins and catechol estrogens on the hypothalamic–pituitary axis in female athletes. *Fertil Steril* 1984; 42: 690.

Schenker JG, Margalioth EJ. Intrauterine adhesions: an updated appraisal. *Fertil Steril* 1982; 37: 593–610.

Schlechte JA, Sherman B, Martin R. Bone density in amenorrheic women with and without hyperprolactinemia. *J Clin Endocrinol Metab* 1983; 56: 1120.

Sherman BM, Halmi KA, Zamudio R. LH and FSH response to gonadotropin-releasing hormone in anorexia nervosa: effect of nutritional rehabilitation. *J Clin Endocrinol Metab* 1975; 41: 135.

Snow RC, Hbarhbieri RL, Frisch RE. Estrogen 2-hydroxylase oxidation and menstrual function among elite oarswomen. *J Clin Endocrinol Metab* 1989; 69: 369.

Surrey ES, Cedars MI. The effect of gonadotropin suppression on the induction of ovulation in premature ovarian failure patients. *Fertil Steril* 1989; 52: 36–41.

Vigersky RA, Andersen AE, Thompson RG, *et al*. Hypothalamic dysfunction in secondary amenorrhea associated with simple weight loss. *NEJM* 1977; 297: 1141.

Chapter 91
Galactorrhea and Hyperprolactinemia

Donna Shoupe
Department of Medicine and Obstetrics and Gynecology, Keck School of Medicine, University of Southern California, CA, USA

Introduction

Galactorrhea is defined as nonpuerperal watery or milky breast secretion that contains neither pus nor blood. This secretion may be manifested spontaneously but may be detected after breast and nipple palpation. To detect galactorrhea, the breast examination should include compression of the glands from the periphery of the breasts toward the nipple concentrically. Confirmation of the diagnosis is through observation of microscopic fat globules in the expressed fluid. The incidence of this condition among reproductive-aged women is unknown but has been estimated to occur in 20–25% of women at some time in their life. Galactorrhea with amenorrhea is commonly associated with a pituitary adenoma.

Normal lactation

During pregnancy, the ductal system and lobules of the breast are primed by a multitude of hormones including estrogen, growth hormone, progesterone, insulin, thyroid hormone, glucocorticoids and human placental lactogen. The high levels of estrogen and progesterone that occur during pregnancy, however, block the action of prolactin and prevent milk production. Following delivery, the precipitous fall in these hormones in the presence of elevated prolactin levels results in lactation. Suckling stimulates the release of prolactin and oxytocin as well as thyroid-releasing hormone. The contraceptive effect of lactation is dependent on the intensity and frequency of suckling. Basal levels of prolactin can remain elevated for several months following weaning.

Pathophysiology

Prolactin (PRL), the critical hormone regulating puerperal-related lactation, is often involved in the physiology of galactorrhea. Normally, the anterior pituitary secretes prolactin at a low basal rate as a result of constant suppression by prolactin-inhibiting factor. Dopamine, the main component of prolactin-inhibiting factor, is secreted by the hypothalamus and delivered to the anterior pituitary via the portal system. Excessive secretion of PRL by anterior pituitary cells called lactotrophs results in hyperprolactinemia. A common cause of hyperprolactinemia is an adenoma, often referred to as a prolactinoma. The most common systemic disease resulting in galactorrhea is hypothyroidism. Low levels of thyroid hormone stimulate increased release of thyrotropin-releasing hormone which increases prolactin secretion. Other common causes include excessive breast manipulation, certain medications, and idiopathic (Box 91.1).

Since the predominant control of PRL release from the anterior pituitary is mediated by prolactin-inhibiting factor (PIF), any mechanical compression of the pituitary stalk or destructive process involving the pituitary gland or hypothalamus can interfere with tonic PIF inhibitory action and result in hyperprolactinemia and galactorrhea. Dopamine receptor antagonists, such as phenothiazines, directly inhibit dopamine action. Natural processes such as stress, sleep, nipple stimulation, pregnancy, and exercise also stimulate PRL release. Chronic renal failure may result in galactorrhea due to decreased clearance of prolactin through the kidneys. Some nonpituitary malignancies such as bronchogenic carcinoma or T-cell lymphomas may release prolactin.

Clinical presentation

Two easily recognizable consequences of elevated PRL in women are galactorrhea and menstrual cycle disturbances. Menstrual irregularities associated with hyperprolactinemia include amenorrhea, oligomenorrhea, luteal phase defects, and delayed menarche. Hyperprolactinemia

Management of Common Problems in Obstetrics and Gynecology, 5th edition. Edited by T.M. Goodwin, M.N. Montoro, L. Muderspach, R. Paulson and S. Roy. © 2010 Blackwell Publishing Ltd.

Box 91.1 Causes of hyperprolactinemia

Idiopathic (common cause)
Physiologic
- hypothyroidism
- early morning/sleep
- high-protein meal
- physical exercise
- psychologic stress
- late follicular phase or menstrual cycle or mid-cycle
- suckling/pregnancy
- coitus
- exercise
- breast manipulation
- dehydration
- "witch's milk" in neonates

Hypothalamic-pituitary diseases
- lactotroph hyperplasia
- prolactinoma, micro- or macro-
- Cushing's disease
- pituitary stalk compression or resection
- empty sella syndrome
- infiltrative, destructive or neoplastic diseases
- craniopharyngiomas, sarcoidosis, tuberculosis, schistosomiasis
- encephalitis
- radiation
- acromegaly
- pseudotumor cerebri
- hypothalamic cyst

Drugs
- hormones
  - oral contraceptives (particularly high dose)
  - estrogens
  - medroxyprogesterone acetate
  - danazol
- amphetamines
- anesthetics
  - sumtriptan (Imitrex)
  - opiates
- antidepressants/antianxiety
  - alprazolam
  - buspirone
  - chlordiazepoxide
  - citalopram, fluoxetine, paroxetine, sertraline
  - diazepams
  - MAO inhibitors
  - sulpride
  - tricyclic antidepressants
- antihistamines
  - cyproheptadine
- antihypertensives
  - atenolol
  - methyldopa
  - reserpine
  - verapamil
- antipsychotics
  - butyrophenones
  - chlorpromazine
  - haloperidol
  - perphenazine
  - phenothiazines
  - procholperazine
  - promazine
- gastrointestinal medicines
  - domperidone
  - cimetidine
  - metoclopramide
- glucocorticoids
- thyrotropin-releasing hormone

Herbs
- anise
- blessed thistle
- fennel
- nettle
- red clover

Local nerve stimulation
- breast manipulation
- irritating clothes, ill-fitting brassieres
- herpes zoster
- spinal cord lesion
- chest wall or breast surgery, breast implants
- chest wall lesions or trauma
- atopic dermatitis
- burns

Other causes
- renal failure
- bronchogenic carcinoma
- lymphoma
- multiple sclerosis
- spinal cord surgery or injury
- esophagitis/reflux

Cannabis

may be associated with infertility, decreased libido and vaginal dryness or osteopenia (due to low estrogen levels). Changes in menstrual function are often the result of diminished hypothalamic pulsatile gonadotropin-releasing hormone secretion (GnRH) due to changes in hypothalamic dopamine activity, resulting in abnormal follicle-stimulating hormone/luteinizing hormone (FSH/LH) secretion. A direct inhibitory action of PRL on ovarian folliculogenesis and corpus luteum function is reported.

About one-third of women with hyperprolactinemia have amenorrhea. In women presenting with secondary amenorrhea and galactorrhea, over 75% will have hyperprolactinemia. Due to the many isoforms of PRL and the large variations in the immunoactivity and bio-activity of each isoform, some patients may have large discrepancies between serum measurements of PRL and clinical evidence of hyperprolactinemia.

Headaches or visual field defects in women with elevated PRL suggest the presence of a prolactinoma. Visual field defects, generally bitemporal hemianopia due to compression of the optic chiasm, usually involve a macroadenoma greater than 10 mm in diameter. Tumor extension into the cavernous sinus is rare but may cause compression of cranial nerves. Large macroadenomas may cause partial or complete panhypopituitarism.

Diagnosis

Evaluation of women with hyperprolactinemia or galactorrhea includes a complete history with emphasis on menstrual history, headaches, medications, fertility, and personal and family history of thyroid disease. Physical examination includes expression of a milky secretion from the breast, visual field assessment, and thyroid palpation. The optimum time to measure PRL is in the early to mid-follicular phase of the menstrual cycle, during late morning hours, and not shortly after a breast examination, eating, stress, exercise, sleep or coitus. Normal PRL levels are 20–25 ng/mL but can reach levels as high as 45–69 ng/mL during certain physiologic conditions (see Box 91.1). Strenuous exercise may acutely raise PRL levels to as high as 250 ng/mL. Generally, levels over 200 ng/mL give cause for concern because they are most likely caused by a prolactin-secreting adenoma. The highest risk group is women with amenorrhea and galactorrhea, especially if PRL >200 ng/mL. Laboratory studies include PRL and TSH levels, possibly a β-hCG, and, in patients with amenorrhea, a 17β-estradiol.

Imaging of the pituitary gland is indicated in patients with newly diagnosed hyperprolactinemia with normal TSH. If the PRL is greater than 100 ng/mL, the optimum test is a MRI scan or contrast CT. The presence of a macroadenoma (>10 mm in diameter) requires visual field testing and more frequent monitoring. Patients with low estrogen levels should have a bone mineral density measurement of the femoral neck and lumbar spine.

Treatment

The objectives of therapy for patients with galactorrhea and/or hyperprolactinemia include establishment of normal estrogen levels, elimination of bothersome galactorrhea, establishment of normal menstrual cycles, and in some cases, ovulation induction. Management of patients with pituitary PRL-secreting adenomas includes periodic monitoring, low-dose oral contraceptives, dopamine therapy, surgery or radiation therapy. Factors to consider when selecting the best management plan are listed in Box 91.2 and Box 91.3.

Yearly measurement of prolactin is generally indicated for patients with normal menses and normal or idiopathic elevated serum PRL levels. Patients with oligomenorrhea can be treated with oral contraceptives or cyclic progestin therapy. Microadenomas should be followed up with yearly measurements of serum PRL and follow-up MRI or other imaging of the sella annually for 2 years. Long-term studies have documented that a

---

Box 91.2 Factors to consider regarding treatment of pituitary adnenomas

- Prolactin-producing microadenomas (<10 mm in diameter) are slow growing, rarely progress to a macroadenoma and many spontaneously regress.

- Imaging of the sella and prolactin levels should be done annually for 2 years after diagnosis of a pituitary microadenoma. If no changes occur, follow-up may be limited to annual measurement of the prolactin level.

- A prolactin-producing microadenoma is not a contraindication to treatment with oral contraceptives, progestin or estrogen therapy or pregnancy.

- Dopamine agonist therapy shrinks macroadenomas, often with necrosis of some of the tumor cells. After tumor shrinkage, a low maintenance dose can be used.

- Treatment of pituitary micro- or macroadenomas with dopamine therapy usually results in normalization of menses and ovulation.

- Prolactin levels >1000 ng/mL may indicate a locally invasive tumor. These tumors are often best treated with a dopamine agonist.

- Surgical intervention is usually reserved for those who have persistent suprasellar extension or continued visual impairment after dopamine treatment. Recurrence rates following surgery are high.

small percentage (5–7%) of women with a microadenoma who do not receive any treatment have an increase in the size of the tumor. An increase in tumor size is usually coupled with increases in serum PRL levels. Over time, many patients with untreated microadenomas return to normal prolactin levels. Indications for dopamine treatment or initiation of OCs include hypoestrogenism, decreased libido or osteopenia. The best option for intolerable galactorrhea is dopamine therapy.

Patients with a macroadenoma should be followed yearly with PRL levels and with MRI or other sella imaging at 6 months, 1, 2, 4 and 8 years. Dopamine agonist therapy is the treatment of choice for patients with a macroadenoma. Testing for panhypopituitarism should be carried out prior to treatment. Bromocriptine and cabergoline are dopamine agonists approved by the Food and Drug Administration (FDA). Cabergoline is dosed weekly (0.5–3 mg) or split into two doses per week to lower the side effects. It is often better tolerated than bromocriptine that must be taken 1–3 times per day (2.5–7.5 mg). Side effects include nausea, vomiting, headache, constipation, orthostatic hypotension, and nasal congestion. Treatment is better tolerated if an initial low dose (half tab) is given at night and slowly increased over time. Intravaginal delivery of bromocriptine has fewer gastrointestinal side effects. An injectable long-acting form of bromocriptine (depot bromocriptine 50–75 mg monthly) is effective and well tolerated. Two dopamine agonists also not approved by the FDA are pergolide and quinagolide (CV205-502). The majority of patients treated with cabergoline or bromocriptine will have suppression of galactorrhea, normalization of PRL, and restoration of ovulatory cycles. Part of the management of these patients therefore is contraception or conception counseling. For women attempting pregnancy, bromocriptine may be discontinued following ovulation and restarted with menses if necessary, or alternatively stopped at the time of a missed menses or positive pregnancy test.

Trans-sphenoidal surgery is generally reserved for patients with large macroadenomas with extrasellar extension or for the 10% of patients who fail to respond to dopamine agonist therapy. The long-term cure rate of surgery is around 60% and serious complications can occur. Radiotherapy with or without surgery is associated with long-term hypopituitarism.

Adequate treatment of hypothyroidism normalizes hypothalamic release of thyroid-releasing hormone and should normalize prolactin levels and eliminate galactorrhea. Similarly, within 3–6 months after discontinuation of phenothiazine derivatives, diazepams, opiates, tricyclic antidepressants or other drugs that can cause galactorrhea

---

Box 91.3 Treatment of galactorrhea

- Isolated galactorrhea in an otherwise healthy woman with regular cycles does not require treatment and can be followed with periodic prolactin levels.
- Bothersome galactorrhea can be treated most effectively with a dopamine agonist, even in women with normal prolactin levels.
- Dopamine agonists:
- Bromocriptine 2.5 mg   ½ –1 pill /day up to 7.5–10 mg/day
- Cabergoline   0.5 mg once or twice weekly up to 3 mg/week

---

through hypothalamic suppression, galactorrhea should disappear.

Ovulation induction

Often treatment with dopamine agonist therapy is associated with restoration of ovulatory menstrual cycles. Clomiphene citrate may be used in women with normal estrogen levels and is often preferred. In patients with low estradiol levels, use of a dopamine agonist plus clomiphene citrate is a good option.

Pregnancy

The clinical course of a microadenoma during pregnancy is generally benign and carries a low risk for neurologic complications (<1%). When pregnancy is diagnosed, dopamine agonist therapy should be discontinued and the patient followed for the appearance of headaches or evidence of visual field changes. Dopamine agonists can be added for those in whom headaches or cranial nerve dysfunction develop.

In contrast to the typically benign clinical course seen with microadenomas, visual field changes, diabetes insipidus or neurologic signs can develop in up to 15–40% of pregnant patients with macroadenomas. Visual field testing should be performed monthly in these patients. Bromocriptine is often continued throughout pregnancy. An MRI should be obtained if symptoms develop or if defects in the visual fields are detected. Problems are more likely in patients with larger tumors. Bromocriptine therapy has been successfully used in pregnancies complicated by visual loss. During the postpartum period, breastfeeding does not worsen the clinical course. Some women resume normal menstrual cycles following delivery thought to be due to tumor infarction due to the stimulation, expansion and eventual shrinkage of the tumor during pregnancy.

Suggested reading

Barbieri RL, Ryan KJ. Bromocriptine, endocrine pharmacology, and therapeutic applications. *Fertil Steril* 1983; 39: 727.

Colao A, di Sarno A, Cappabianca P, DiSomma C, Pivonello R, Lombardi G, Withdrawal of long-term caberoline therapy for tumoral and nontumoral hyperprolactinemia. *NEJM* 2003;349: 2023.

Crosignani PG, Mattei AM, Severni V, *et al*. Long-term effects of time, medical treatment and pregnancy in 176 hyperprolactinemic women. *Eur J Obstet Gynecol Reprod Biol* 1992; 44: 175.

Davajan V, Kletzky OA, March CM, *et al*. The significant of galactorrhea in patients with normal menses, oligomenorrhea and secondary amenorrhea. *Am J Obstet Gynecol* 1978; 130: 894.

Donovan LE, Corenblum B. The natural history of the pituitary incidentaloma. *Arch Intern Med* 155; 181: 1995

Jackson RD, Wortsman J, Malarkey WB. Characterization of a large molecular weight prolactin in women with idiopathic hyperprolactinemia and normal menses. *J Clin Endocrinol Metab* 1985; 61: 258–264.

Molitch ME, Elton RL, Blackwell RE, *et al*. Bromocriptine as primary therapy for prolactin-secreting microadenomas; results of a prospective multicenter study. *J Clin Endocrinol Metab* 1985; 60: 698–705.

Passos VQ, Souza JJS, Musolino NRC, Bronstein MD, Long-term follow-up of prolactinomas: normoprolactinemia after bromocriptine withdrawal. *J Clin Endocrinol Metab* 2002; 87: 3578.

Schlechte J, Dolan K, Sherman B, *et al*. The natural history of untreated hyperprolactinemia: a prospective analysis. *J Clin Endocrinol Metab* 1989; 68: 412–418.

Schlechte J, Walker L, Kathol M. A longitudinal analysis of premenopausal bone loss in healthy women and women with hyperprolactinemia. *J Clin Endocrinol Metab* 1992; 75: 698–703.

Shoupe D, Montz FJ, Kletzky OA, diZerega G. Response to TRH stimulation of Concanavalin A –bound and unbound immunoassayable prolactin during human pregnancy. *Am J Obstet Gynecol* 1983; 147: 482.

Vallette-Kasic S, Morange-Ramos I, Selim A, *et al*. Macroprolactinemia revisited: a study on 106 patients. *J Clin Endocrinol Metab* 2002; 87: 581.

Webster J, Piscitelli G, Polli A, *et al*. A comparison of cabergoline and bromocriptine in the treatment of hyperprolactinemia amenorrhea. *NEJM* 1994; 331: 904–909.

Chapter 92
Androgen Excess and Hirsutism

Rebecca Z. Sokol and Donna Shoupe
Department of Medicine and Obstetrics and Gynecology, Keck School of Medicine, University of Southern California, CA, USA

Introduction

Androgen excess includes a vast spectrum of clinical presentations and symptoms. The key to the differential diagnosis and treatment of androgen excess states is to differentiate the patient who presents with hirsutism from the patient who presents with virilization (Box 92.1). A basic understanding of androgen production and actions allows the clinician to make the appropriate diagnosis.

Androgen physiology

Androgens are produced in the ovary and the adrenal gland, and androgen precursors are converted to androgens in the periphery. The ovary produces testosterone, androstenedione, and dehydroepiandrosterone (DHEA). The adrenal gland produces androstenedione, DHEA, and dehydroepiandrosterone sulfate (DHEAS). More than 90% of DHEAS is derived from the adrenal. Regardless of source of origin, androstenedione and DHEA are converted in the periphery to testosterone. Testosterone is further metabolized to dihydrotestosterone (DHT) and its metabolite, 3α-androstanediol glucuronide (3α-diolG), at the receptor sites in the skin and genitalia. Total testosterone production in the woman is 0.35 mg/day, with the majority arising from peripheral conversion.

Most circulating testosterone (85%) is bound to sex hormone-binding globulin (SHBG) and is considered biologically inactive. Biologically active testosterone is mainly albumin associated (10–15%) and "free" (1–2%). Non-SHBG-bound testosterone is elevated in 60–70% of hirsute women. Hypothyroidism, obesity, hyperinsulinemia, and hyperandrogenism are associated with decreased SHBG leading to elevated "free" testosterone. Hyperthyroidism and estrogen increase SHBG and decrease free testosterone levels. In hirsute women there is an excellent correlation between total and non-SHBG-bound testosterone.

Androgens exert their actions when bound to their appropriate receptors. Areas of the body where androgen receptors are present are considered to be androgen sensitive.

Hirsutism and virilization

Hirsutism is increased terminal hair growth usually in areas where it does not normally occur but which contain androgen receptors. Terminal hairs are coarse, long, and pigmented and normally grow in the pubis, scalp, axillae, eyebrows, legs, and arms. Hirsutism may result

---

> **Box 92.1 Differential diagnosis of hirsutism and virilization**
>
> **Ovarian**
> PCOS
> hyperthecosis
> neoplasms
>
> **Adrenal**
> CAH
> neoplasms
> Cushing's syndrome
>
> **Idiopathic**
>
> **Drugs**
> anabolic (testosterone/adrenal) steroids
> danazol
> 19-norsteroid derivative progestogens
>
> **Other endocrine disorders**
> acromegaly
> menopause
> thyroid disease

Management of Common Problems in Obstetrics and Gynecology,
5th edition. Edited by T.M. Goodwin, M.N. Montoro,
L. Muderspach, R. Paulson and S. Roy. © 2010 Blackwell
Publishing Ltd.

from either elevated circulating androgens or increased sensitivity of the pilosebaceous unit to androgens. Androgen stimulation of the hair follicle results in transformation of fine, soft, unpigmented vellus hairs into the coarser terminal hairs. Hirsutism is defined as excessive terminal hair growth over an androgen-sensitive area of the body where hair growth is normally minimal or absent. These areas include the face, chest, areola, lower abdomen, inner thighs, and back. However, what may be considered excessive growth in one culture or family may not be considered excessive in another. The amount of hair is related to the potency of the circulating androgens, quantity of ciculating free androgens, duration of exposure, sensitivity of the hair follicle, and density of the hair follicle.

In general, hirsutism is gradual in onset and often presents as a cosmetic or infertility complaint. Hirsutism is usually associated with normal or minimally elevated levels of serum androgens. However, there are many periods in a woman's life, such as pregnancy, puberty, and after menopause, when hair may appear at an accelerated rate as a result of physiologic changes in circulating sex steroids.

Hirsutism should be differentiated from hypertrichosis, which is a diffuse increase in terminal and vellus hairs that can occur all over the body. Hypertrichosis is a reversible side effect of phenytoin or minoxidil, occurs occasionally with anorexia nervosa, and rarely is a congenital X-linked disorder.

Virilization is the masculinization of a woman. In addition to hirsutism, these women present with temporal hair recession, acne, deepening of the voice, malodorous sweat, clitoral enlargement, atrophy of the breasts, increased muscle mass, loss of female body contours, and amenorrhea. Signs of virilization usually appear over a relatively short period of time and are indicative of serious endocrine disease. Virilization is associated with a marked increase in circulating androgen levels.

History and physical examination

A history is obtained of the age of onset of hair growth, the amount, duration, rate, and distribution. Symptoms of virilization, menstrual history and infertility, drug history, and the co-existence of other medical diseases are also uncovered. The family history of hirsutism or other endocrine disorders aids in the diagnosis of familial or genetic forms of hirsutism.

Physical examination will reveal the severity of the hirsutism, signs of virilization, and other associated endocrine disorders. The Ferriman–Gallwey scoring system assesses the severity of hirsutism and is used to analyze response to treatment. A modified Ferriman–Gallwey, as shown in Figure 92.1, scores the degree of hirsutism from nine androgen-sensitive body sites including chin, upper lip, mid-line hair between the breasts, upper and lower abdomen. A score of 8 or more is considered abnormal. It is important to consider racial and ethnic differences when determining what is truly excessive hair growth. The Ferriman–Gallwey scale was developed in England and a traditionally "normal" score is based on white British women. In research settings, the degree of hirsutism and response to therapy are often determined by shaving a specific

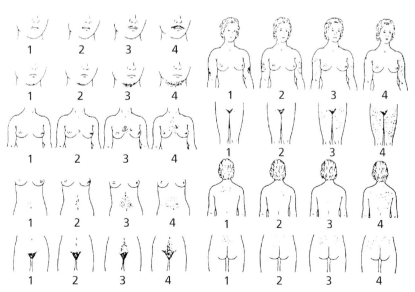

Figure 92.1 Hirsutism scoring from 1 to 4 from nine body sites. Reproduced with permission from Ferriman D, Gallwey JD. Clinical assessment of body hair in women. *J Clin Endocrinol Metab* 1961; 21: 1440-1447. ©The Endocrine Society.

area and either counting the number of hairs or weighing the hair.

Signs of virilization include high scores on the Ferriman–Gallwey system, clitoromegaly, increased muscularity and/or male body habitus, male-pattern balding, and deepening of the voice. Signs suggestive of other endocrine disorders, such as Cushing's syndrome (central obesity, hypertension, striae, easy bruising) and congenital adrenal hyperplasia (CAH) (abnormal blood pressure, short stature) are noted. Signs of metabolic syndrome include abdominal obesity (waist circumference >88 cm (>35 inches)) and an elevated blood pressure.

Laboratory evaluation

Serum testosterone and DHEAS levels are the initial screening tests in the work-up of the hirsute woman. Testosterone levels are primarily derived from the ovary and thus serve as a marker for excess ovarian androgen production. DHEAS levels are a direct reflection of excess androgen production by the adrenal gland. A testosterone level greater than 200 ng/dL is suggestive of an ovarian tumor. Definitive diagnosis is made with imaging studies. A DHEAS level greater than 8 μg/dL suggests an adrenal tumor. Lower yet abnormal values of these hormones may indicate an exogenous or iatrogenic cause, the presence of idiopathic androgen excess, polycystic ovarian syndrome (PCOS), stromal hyperthecosis, CAH or Cushing's syndrome.

Screening for adult-onset CAH is accomplished by measuring 17-hydroxyprogesterone (17-OHP) concentrations. Normal baseline 17-OHP should be less than 200 ng/mL if measured first thing in the morning. Levels between 200 and 800 ng/mL require ACTH testing. Cortisol, 11-deoxycorticol, and 17-OHP are measured in serum before and 30 and 60 minutes after the administration of 250 μg of synthetic ACTH. The blood sample should be obtained during the follicular phase of the cycle. Patients with CAH demonstrate a disproportional increase in 17-OH progesterone compared to cortisol levels. Baseline levels of 17-OHP above 800 ng/mL are diagnostic of a 21-hydroxylase deficiency.

Collection of urine for measurement of 24-hour urinary free cortisol and creatinine is the preliminary screening test for the diagnosis of Cushing's disease. Measurement of fasting glucose and insulin levels is indicated in the work-up of those patients who may be insulin resistant.

Differential diagnosis

Idiopathic hirsutism

Idiopathic hirsutism classically presents as hirsutism in a patient with regular, ovulatory menstrual cycles and normal circulating androgen levels. Idiopathic hirsutism is a diagnosis of exclusion. Patients with idiopathic hirsutism present either with mildly elevated or normal testosterone levels. Many patients with idiopathic hirsutism have elevated levels of 3α-androstanediol-glucuronide (3α-diolG), a marker of peripheral androgen activity. Specifically, 3α-diolG is a marker of 5α-reductase activity in the pilosebaceous unit. This is the enzyme which converts testosterone to the highly androgenic DHT. Although androgens are the main regulators of 5α-reductase activity, another major factor is the genetic expression of this enzyme. If testosterone and DHEAS are normal and 3α-diolG is elevated, a peripheral disorder (i.e. abnormality at the psu unit) is suggested.

Polycystic ovarian syndrome
Polycystic ovarian syndrome (PCOS) generally presents with perimenarchal onset of oligomenorrhea, insulin resistance, mid-line obesity, infertility and mild-to-moderate hyperandrogenism, sometimes with the signs of virilization. Other clinically important physical findings of androgen excess include acne and alopecia. A family history of the syndrome is common (see Chapter 93).

Hyperthecosis
Hyperthecosis is similar to PCOS although the clinical picture is of more severe androgen excess. Women with hyperthecosis often have a longstanding history of progressive, relentless hirsutism, anovulation, and resistance to clomiphene citrate. Their symptoms may include signs of virilization such as temporal balding and clitoral enlargement. Because testosterone levels in this condition often exceed 200 ng/mL, the differential diagnosis must include an androgen-producing tumor and the work-up must include an ovarian ultrasound. On ultrasound, both ovaries are enlarged with extremely dense and excessive stroma, without the subcortical cysts characteristic of PCOS. The diagnosis is confirmed histologically when nests of theca cells are found in the ovarian stroma at some distance from the follicles. Hyperthecosis of the ovaries may be associated with insulin resistance and acanthosis nigricans. Luteinizing hormone (LH) levels are generally lower than see with PCOS. Gonadotropin-releasing hormone (GnRH) agonist therapy with or without oral contraceptives is effective treatment.

Androgen-producing ovarian tumor
Worrisome features associated with hirsutism include rapid onset and progression, severe hirsutism, abdominal or pelvic mass or any virilizing sign including clitoromegaly, temporal balding or deepening voice. Androgen-secreting ovarian tumors are classified as steroid or lipoid cell tumors, sex cord stromal tumors, gonadoblastomas or tumors with functioning stroma. Lipoid cell tumor refers to the morphologic features

associated with steroid-producing cells such as Leydig or luteinized thecoma. The sex cord stromal tumors include the granulosa and Sertoli cell tumors. Gonadoblastomas are composed of germ cell elements and usually contain a Y chromosome. Any ovarian tumor has the potential of androgen secretion including mucinous cystadenomas, Brenner tumors, cystadocarcinomas, and Krukenberg tumors. The mechanism for this is stimulation of functioning ovarian stroma within the tumor that liberated increased amounts of androgens.

Although rare (less than 1% of all solid ovarian tumors), the most common and largest androgen-producing ovarian tumors are the Sertoli–Leydig cell tumors. These are most often diagnosed in women between the ages of 20 and 40, are usually palpable on pelvic examination, and have a low-grade malignant potential. Seventy-five percent of women with lipoid cell tumors are virilized and 10% have Cushing's syndrome. Granulosa-theca cell tumors usually secrete estrogens but infrequently produce androgens. Hilus tumors occur most commonly in postmenopausal women and also have low-grade malignant potential. The general rule of thumb is to begin investigation for an ovarian secreting tumor with any sign of virilization or when total testosterone levels are 150–200 ng/dL or higher or 2.5 or more times the upper range of normal.

Adrenal causes of androgen excess
Congenital adrenal hyperplasia: adult onset

Most women with adult-onset or nonclassic CAH present with androgen excess and irregular bleeding. The characteristic findings of classic CAH, including early growth spurt, shorter adult height, and ambiguous genitalia, are mild or absent. Most women with adult-onset CAH have a partial enzyme deficiency, most commonly an incomplete 21-hydroxylase deficiency. This is not associated with salt wasting. A few have an incomplete 11-hydroxylase deficiency. Both of these defects produce increased serum 17α-hydroxyprogesterone levels, inefficient cortisol production, and inconsistent increases in adrenal androgens such as androstenedione and DHEAS. The 11-hydroxylase deficiency also causes increases in 11-deoxycortisol (substance S) and hypertension in some patients. The administration of intravenous ACTH, which causes marked increases in levels of 17α-hydroxyprogesterone, may confirm both enzyme defects.

A 3β-ol-dehydrogenase defect produces high levels of DHEAS and low or normal levels of androstenedione and testosterone.

Androgen-producing adrenal tumors

Androgen-producing adrenal tumors, either microadenomas or macroadenomas, are rare causes of androgen excess. Adrenal adenomas or carcinomas are usually large enough to be detected on intravenous pyelogram by the time they produce signs or symptoms of androgen excess. Patients usually have extremely high levels of adrenal androgens with serum DHEAS levels over 6–8 μg/mL. Adrenal adenomas rarely produce testosterone or androstenedione but their existence suggests the need for a CT or MRI to exclude an adrenal tumor whenever a testosterone-secreting tumor is suspected but cannot be detected by ovarian imaging.

Cushing's syndrome

Hirsutism, excess lanugo hairs, amenorrhea, osteoporosis. muscle weakness, truncal obesity, hypertension, easy bruisability, ecchymoses, central obesity, thinning of the skin, facial flushing, supraclavicular and dorsal neck fat pads, purple striae, diabetes, alkalosis, and hypokalemia are clinical findings in women with Cushing's syndrome. Excess lanugo hairs of the face and extremities are a result of glucocorticoid excess. A true androgen-related coarse type of hirsutism results from excess adrenal androgen production.

Iatrogenic causes

Drugs associated with hirsutism or other signs of androgen excess include phenytoin (Dilantin), diazoxide, corticosteroids, 19-nortestosterone progestins, anabolic steroids, danazol, DHEA(S), testosterone, androstenedione, and ACTH. Some of these products and other products with androgenic activity are easily available from health food stores.

Obesity

Several factors contribute to the hirsutism associated with obesity. Increased adiposity is associated with decreased synthesis of SHBG and thus higher levels of unbound androgens. Additionally, because of the metabolic activity of adipose cells, obesity is associated with a time- and weight-dependent progression of hirsutism due to androgen stimulation of the pilosebaceous unit. Additionally, adipose cells actively convert androgens into estrogens that can lead to menstrual dysfunction.

Genetic causes

Rare cases of gonadal dysgenesis and incomplete forms of testicular feminization, where a Y chromosome is present, are associated with androgen excess and often primary amenorrhea. This combination requires a karyotype study for the detection of a Y chromosome. If diagnosed, surgical removal of the gonadal tissue is necessary due to the increased risk of neoplasia.

Virilization in pregnancy

The usual source of the excess androgens in pregnancy is thought to be the ovaries in most cases. The most common cause is the luteoma of pregnancy, which usually regresses spontaneously post partum. Conservative management is recommended. Other causes include ingestion of androgens, ovarian tumors associated with functional stroma, and hyper-reactio luteinalis. Half of female infants born to mothers with virilization in pregnancy have ambiguous external genitalia.

Rare causes

Extremely rare causes of androgen excess include acromegaly and porphyria. These diagnoses usually are made prior to the investigation of androgen excess. There is also an association between hirsutism and diethystilbestrol exposure *in utero*.

Treatment

Except for cases of androgen-secreting adrenal or ovarian neoplasms which require surgical intervention or Cushing's syndrome, treatment for hyperandrogenic women is aimed at the primary symptoms reported by the patient: excess facial hair, oligomenorrhea, infertility. It is important to counsel the patient on realistic expectations of therapy and the time course expected. Once a vellus hair follicle has been transformed into a terminal hair by androgen stimulation, pharmacologic treatment will not reverse this process. Suppression of circulating androgens and local suppression of androgen activity around a hair follicle will decrease hair growth, diameter and color and prevent further transformation of remaining vellus hair follicles. In patients with chronic anovulation associated with hirsutism, periodic shedding of the endometrium is necessary to prevent endometrial hyperplasia.

Patients may not notice a decrease in hair growth due to pharmacologic therapy for up to 3 months and they may not see the full benefit of treatment for up to 12 months. Hormonal therapy will inhibit to some extent the growth of existing hairs, but its primary benefit is in preventing the appearance of new terminal hair follicles. Adjunctive use of local methods for removing existing hair follicles substantially increases the overall effectiveness of any treatment plan. It is important to emphasize to the patient that discontinuing medical treatment often allows for an increased androgen activity around the hair follicles and the reappearance or worsening of hirsutism. The use of a scoring system, photographs or detailed charting of the location and thickness of existing hairs are excellent ways to monitor ongoing therapy.

Specific approaches include the following.

Weight loss

Several mechanisms contribute to the fact that the greater the weight and longer the time of excess fat tissue, the greater the hyperandrogenism and hirsutism. The hyperinsulinemia associated with obesity is associated with stimulation of ovarian and adrenal androgen production. Obesity also lowers SHBG levels and thereby increases the levels of unbound, bio-active testosterone. Additionally, obesity is associated with increased production rates of testosterone, dihydrotestosterone, and the peripheral marker of androgen activity, 3α-diolG. The clearance of androgens is increased in skin and adipose tissues in the obese compared to the normal weight woman. In many overweight and obese patients, the increased production rate is balanced by an increased peripheral clearance rate, resulting in normal circulating androgen levels. An elevated serum androgen level is not necessary to initiate treatment because hyperandrogenic symptoms demonstrate that there is increased androgen activity at the target tissues.

Obese and overweight individuals may not initially present with complaints of hirsutism. There appears to be a protective mechanism in the hair follicles of obese women that at least partially blocks the effects of the increased skin turnover of androgens. This protective mechanism diminishes over time. Often, the degree of hirsutism can be correlated to the duration of obesity. Obese individuals with a waist-to-hip ratio greater than 0.85 are most likely to have hyperandrogenism. Acne and alopecia are also results of hyperandrogenism.

Weight loss should be encouraged in the obese as well as the overweight, primarily for the beneficial impact on long-term health. Additionally, weight loss results in decreased insulin and androgen production and increased SHBG levels. Small amounts of weight loss, as little as 7% reduction in bodyweight, often lead to a significant reduction in androgens and to the resumption of ovulatory menses in obese women.

Local measures

Depilation with waxes, creams, electrocoagulation, electrolysis, bleaching, shaving, tweezers, and laser are local techniques used to temporarily or permanently remove or modify unwanted hair. Once a vellus hair has transformed into a terminal hair, pharmacologic treatment can result in slower growth and decreased diameter but will not eradicate the presence of the terminal hair. Thus the addition of local measures to pharmacologic treatment is often the preferred management.

Pharmacologic treatments

Oral contraceptives (OCs) are the first line of treatment for hirsutism and other hyperandrogenic conditions, regardless of whether or not androgens are elevated. OCs suppress ovarian production of testosterone (50%) and adrenal DHEAS production (30%), increase SHBG (thus decreasing free, bio-active testosterone), and inhibit 5α-reductase activity (which decreases target tissue androgen activity). High-dose medroxyprogesterone acetate also inhibits 5α-reductase activity and can be used with less efficacy in patients unable to take OCs. Essentially, all OCs are reported to decrease androgens and improve hirsutism and relatively few comparative trials exist. Generally, OCs with higher estrogen to progestogen ratios and low androgenic activity are preferred. A full clinical response may require up to 6–12 months to appreciate.

For patients with nonclassic, adult-onset CAH, the administration of dexametasone 0.25–0.75 mg/day or prednisone 2.5–7.5 mg/day suppresses androgen levels, slows or prevents the progression of hyperandrogenism, and often results in ovulatory menstrual cycles. Corticosteroids, at low doses, have also been used to treat idiopathic hirsutism. These low doses of dexametasone (0.25–0.37 mg/day or 2.5 mg prednisone) suppress adrenal androgen production without suppressing cortisol secretion. Ovarian testosterone production is also suppressed with this therapy, but not to the extent seen with OC treatment. Prolonged treatment does not appear to produce significant side effects.

Even though androgens, especially DHEAS, may be suppressed by 50% or more following corticosteroid therapy, the clinical response to treatment is often not as dramatic as that seen with other treatment options. This is probably because corticosteroids do not directly suppress the peripheral compartment, an important factor for the treatment of hirsutism. The addition of a peripheral blocker of androgen activity, such as spironolactone, improves the clinical response. Spironolactone may inhibit steroidogenesis; its primary effectiveness lies in its peripheral androgen-blocking ability. Spironolactone is an excellent inhibitor of the androgen receptor in the peripheral compartment. Reports suggest that spironolactone couples with the receptor to create a biologically inactive complex. Additionally, spironolactone also inhibits 5α-reductase activity and increases the clearance of testosterone. Some patients complain of irregular bleeding or spotting after treatment. Use of spironolactone with an OC is often very effective. An OC containing a spironolactone derivative is now available.

Gonadotropin-releasing hormone analogs, given intramuscularly or intranasally, effectively decrease circulating androgens and are an effective treatment for hirsutism. When given alone, GnRH analogs are generally limited to 6 months' treatment because of bone loss associated with estrogen deficiency. The addition of OCs to analog treatment prevents bone loss, extends the treatment phase, and is superior in efficacy to either GnRH analog or OC use alone. After treatment with GnRH analog plus OCs for at least 1 year, many patients report a longer remission than with either treatment alone.

Flutamide is a potent nonsteroidal compound that inhibits the androgen receptor. At high doses, it may decrease androgen synthesis or increase its metabolism. It is necessary to monitor liver enzymes while using this product. Therapeutically, it has an effect similar to that seen with spironolactone treatment.

Finasteride inhibits 5α-reductase activity and is approved for use in men for prostatic hypertrophy or male-pattern baldness. It is effective in treating hirsute women and results are often evident by 6 months. Side effects in women are minimal.

Ketoconazole, technically an antifungal agent, blocks the synthesis of androgens through the suppression of P450-dependent ovarian and adrenal enzymes. Treatment results in a reduction of serum testosterone levels and increases in hydroxyprogesterone levels. Side effects include nausea, hepatic dysfunction, and pruritus. Periodic measurement of liver enzymes is recommended.

Insulin-lowering agents are not approved by the Food and Drug Administration for hirsutism. However, metformin has been tested extensively in women with polycystic ovaries. Treatment often results in lower testosterone and insulin levels, and resumption of ovulation may occur in some patients. Periodic liver testing is recommended and kidney disease is a contraindication.

Surgical management

Laparoscopic ovarian drilling is generally reserved for those who desire ovulation and fail other treatment options. Ovarian electrocautery normalizes ovarian function, decreases androgen production, and restores normal menstrual function in a high percentage of patients for as long as 20 years. Since there is a drop in circulating androgen levels following laparoscopic ovarian drilling, consideration of this procedure for selected women with persistent, untreatable androgen excess may be appropriate.

Suggested reading

Carmina E, Lobo RA. Peripheral androgen blockade versus glandular androgen suppression in the treatment of hirsutism. *Obstet Gynecol* 1991; 78: 849.

Crave J. Fimbel S, LeJeune H, *et al.* Effects of diet and metformin administration on sex hormone-binding globulin, androgens, and insulin in hirsute and obese women. *J Clin Endocrinol Metab* 1995; 80: 2057–2062.

Dunaif A. Insulin resistance and the polycystic ovary syndrome: mechanism and implications for pathogenesis. *Endocrinol Rev* 1997; 18: 774.

Ehrmann DA, Cavaghan MK, Imperial J, *et al.* Effects of metformin on insulin secretion, insulin action, and ovarian steroidogenesis in women with polycystic ovary syndrome. *J Clin Endocrinol Metab* 1997; 82: 524–530.

Ferriman D, Gallwey JD. Clinical assessment of body hair growth in women. *J Clin Endocrinol* 1961; 21: 1440.

Heiner JS, Greendale JA, Kawakami AK, *et al.* Comparison of a gonadotropin-releasing hormone agonist and a low dose oral contraceptive given alone or together in the treatment of hirsutism. *J Clin Endocrinol Metab* 1995; 80: 3412–3418.

Imperato-McGinley J, Gaitier T, Cai LZ, *et al*. The androgen control of sebum production. Studies of subjects with dihydrotestosterone deficiency and complete androgen insensitivity. *J Clin Endocrinol* 1993; 76: 524–528.

Kiddy DS, Hamilton-Fairley D, Bush A, *et al*. Improvement in endocrine and ovarian function during dietary treatment of obese women with polycystic ovary syndrome. *Clin Endocrinol (Oxf)* 1992; 36: 105–111.

Korytkowski MT, Mokan M, Horwitz MJ, *et al*. Metabolic effects of oral contraceptive in women with polycystic ovary syndrome. *J Clin Endocrinol Metab* 1995; 80: 3327–3334.

Kuttenn F, Mowszowicz I, Schaison G, *et al*. Androgen production and skin metabolism in hirsutism. *J Endocrinol* 1977; 75: 83–91.

Lobo RA. Androgen excess. In: Lobo RA, Mishell, DR, Paulson RJ, Shoupe D (eds) *Mishell's textbook of infertility, contraception, and reproductive endocrinology*, 4th edn. Malden, MA: Blackwell Science, 1997: 342–362.

Lobo RA, Paul WL, Goebelsmann V. DHEA as an indication of adrenal androgen production. *Obstet Gynecol* 1981; 57: 69.

Lobo RA, Shoupe D, Serafini P, *et al*. The effects of two doses of spironolactone on serum androgens and anagen hair in hirsute women. *Fertil Steril* 1985; 43: 200–205.

New MI, Lorenzen F, Leiner AJ, *et al*. Genotyping steroid 21-hydroxylase deficiency: hormonal reference data. *J Clin Endocrinol Metab* 1983; 57: 320.

Orth DN. Cushing's syndrome. *NEJM* 1995; 332(12): 791–803.

Taylor AE. Polycystic ovary syndrome. *Endocrinol Metab Clin North Am* 1998; 27(4): 877–902.

Wild RA, Umstot ES, Andersen RN, Givens JR. Adrenal function in hirsutism. II. Effect of an oral contraceptive. *J Clin Endocrinol Metab* 1982; 54: 676.

Chapter 93
Polycystic Ovarian Syndrome

Donna Shoupe
Department of Medicine and Obstetrics and Gynecology, Keck School of Medicine, University of Southern California, CA, USA

Introduction

Polycystic ovarian syndrome (PCOS), also called Stein–Leventhal syndrome, is a heterogeneous endocrine disorder that affects approximately 4–8% of women of reproductive age. PCOS is characterized by anovulation, hyperandrogenism, menstrual irregularities, and insulin resistance. Signs and symptoms of women with this disorder include acne, hirsutism, obesity, infertility, oligomenorrhea or polymenorrhea which usually begin at the time of menarche (Box 93.1). The clinical hyperandrogenemia results from elevated ovarian production of testosterone and androstenedione, adrenal secretion of androstenedione, dehydroepiandrosterone (DHEA) and dehydroepiandrosterone sulfate (DHEAS), increased skin 5α-reductase activity or a combination of these factors. Other common laboratory features of this syndrome include an elevated ratio of (>2) luteinizing hormone/follicle-stimulating hormone (LH/FSH) and decreased sex hormone-binding globulin (SHBG) levels. Testosterone levels are generally elevated but lower than levels seen with ovarian tumors and are typically less than 100–150 ng/dL.

Multiple metabolic sequelae are associated with PCOS and insulin resistance, especially when obesity is present, including increased risk of noninsulin-dependent diabetes mellitus, hyperlipidemia, hypertension, and cardiovascular disease. Other health risks include endometrial hyperplasia or even carcinoma and psychosocial dysfunction. Early recognition and diagnosis of this syndrome, appropriate screening for lipid abnormalities and diabetes, along with close follow-up and treatment are important for both short- and long-term health issues.

Definition and diagnostic criteria

In 1990, the National Institutes of Health defined PCOS as hyperandogenism and chronic anovulation where secondary causes such as hyperprolactinemia, adult-onset congenital adrenal hyperplasia or androgen-secreting neoplasm had been excluded. The presence of insulin resistance or polycystic-appearing ovaries was not included in the diagnostic criteria. Hyperandrogenism is established either by clinical findings such as hirsutism or acne or by elevated androgen levels.

Etiology

Polycystic ovarian syndrome is a heterogeneous syndrome presenting with a wide variety of signs and symptoms (Box 93.2). The exact pathophysiology remains unknown and it is unlikely that any single factor will explain the entire spectrum.

Top-to-bottom theories imply a common central nervous system defect involving neurotransmitters such as dopamine, catecholamines, γ-aminobutyric acid (GABA), and endogenous opioids, and expressed by an imbalance of the LH/FSH ratio, enhanced LH pulsatility, and elevated bio-active LH.

> ### Box 93.1 Criteria for the diagnosis of polycystic ovarian syndrome
>
> - **Clinical evidence of androgen excess:** hirsutism, acne, androgenic alopecia, elevated total or free testosterone
> - **Oligo-ovulation since menarche:** irregular cycles >35 or <24 days
> - **Exclusion of other disorders:** nonclassic adrenal hyperplasia, androgen-secreting tumor, thyroid dysfunction, hyperprolactinemia
>
> Presence of polycystic-appearing ovariesnot necessary for diagnosis

Management of Common Problems in Obstetrics and Gynecology, 5th edition. Edited by T.M. Goodwin, M.N. Montoro, L. Muderspach, R. Paulson and S. Roy. © 2010 Blackwell Publishing Ltd.

Box 93.2 Polycystic ovarian syndrome: important findings in history

- **Menstrual history:** lifetime history of irregular cycles, infertility
- **Onset and progression of hirsutism, acne or alopecia:** use of depilatory creams, dermatologic agents
- **Change in bodyweight**
- **Medication use**: use or abuse of anabolic or androgenic drugs; OCs or other medication, use and response
- **Family history of endocrine disorders**

Box 93.3 Polycystic ovarian syndrome: critical parts of physical examination

Look for:
- excessive hair growth, location, thickness, pattern
- acne, alopecia, acanthosis nigricans
- obesity, fat distribution
- galactorrhea

Exclude:
- pelvic/abdominal masses
- virilization or masculinization (breast size, change)
- thyroid enlargement
- Cushingoid features (muscle weakness, central obesity, hypertension)
- signs of systemic illness

The bottom-to-top theories describe either an ovarian-centered defect in the ovarian FSH receptor or a generalized impaired action of insulin on glucose transport and lipolysis. The insulin resistance of PCOS appears to be a postreceptor signaling aberration, different from the insulin resistance in simple obesity. Evidence strongly supports that insulin stimulates exaggerated production of androgens from ovarian theca cells, excessive growth of skin basal cells (resulting in acanthosis nigricans), abnormal peripheral and hepatic lipid metabolism leading to dyslipidemia, and decreased hepatic SHBG, resulting in higher levels of free androgens. The elevated androgen levels in the ovary inhibit the emergence of a dominant follicle and cause atresia of the follicle. Generalized insulin resistance occurs in up to 75% of all patients with PCOS, strongly suggesting a pathophysiologic role of hyperinsulinemia in the disorder.

Clinical findings

Polycystic ovarian syndrome is associated with prolonged periods of anovulation and extraovarian estrogen production, largely through increased peripheral conversion of androstenedione to estrone coupled with elevated levels of unbound estradiol. Persistent acyclic estrogen in conjunction with an absence of luteal-phase progesterone causes prolonged stimulation to the endometrium and may lead to simple hyperplasia, complex hyperplasia, or endometrial carcinoma. Interestingly, women in the Nurses' Health Study with the most irregular menstrual cycles were reported to have a reduced risk of breast cancer.

Androgen excess in PCOS is associated with hirsutism, acne, excess sebum production, android obesity, and androgenic alopecia (Box 93.3). The hyperandrogenism in PCOS is principally from ovarian overproduction, but the adrenal gland may contribute.

Most PCOS women have lipoprotein abnormalities, with low levels of high-density cholesterol and increased levels of low-density cholesterol and triglycerides. These findings, along with hyperinsulinemia, contribute to a substantial increased risk of cardiovascular disease, hypertension, and diabetes mellitus. Central android obesity is a predictor of cardiovascular disease and menstrual irregularities.

Ovarian morphology

Classically, polycystic ovaries are defined as enlarged ovaries, often 1.5 to 3 times larger than normal, with 10 or more subcapsular follicles located in the periphery of the ovarian cortex which are 2–10 mm in diameter. These multiple follicles are typically arranged peripherally around an enlarged central mass of stromal tissue. Demonstration of stromal hypertrophy on ultrasound is reported in 80% of patients diagnosed with PCOS. The presence of polycystic-appearing ovaries on ultrasound or in surgery does not establish the diagnosis of PCOS, as high levels of circulating androgens from any source may cause the accumulation of small atretic follicles in the cortex. Other conditions that may demonstrate polycystic-appearing ovaries include Cushing's syndrome, congenital adrenal hyperplasia, adrenal tumors, thyroid disorders, bulimia nervosa, obesity, women on oral contraceptives, and normal women. Generally, polycystic-appearing ovaries have an exaggerated response to ovulation induction agents and greater care must be used.

Diagnosis

The major two criteria for the diagnosis of PCOS are hyperandrogenism and chronic anovulation. Hyperandrogenism may arise from either elevated serum androgens or clinical manifestations of hyperandrogenism such as acne or hirsutism. It is important to exclude other androgen disorders such as an ovarian tumor or adrenal hyperplasia. The clinical criteria of the polycystic ovarian syndrome are listed in Box 93.1.

Work-up and laboratory tests

The recommended work-up of women with persistant anovulatory bleeding and hyperandrogenism is shown in Box 93.4. One of the best markers for hyperandrogenism in PCOS is serum total testosterone. It is also recommended that DHEAS, a marker of adrenal androgen production, be measured. Although free testosterone is theoretically the best marker of biologic activity, clinical assays vary considerably and the test is often difficult to interpret. It is not necessary to routinely measure LH and FSH although they may be helpful. A 17-OH progesterone should be measured in those with moderate to severe hirsutism (Ferriman–Gallwey score >8; see Chapter 92).

ADA recommends HbA1C as a screening tool where prediabetes values are 5.7–6.4% and values for overt diabetes are >6.4%. Women with elevated HgA1C or abnormal GTT are good candidates for metformin treatment. Other critieria used to define insulin resistance include BMI >27–30 kg/m^2, a waist/hip ratio >0.85 or the presence of acanthosis nigricans. Screening of obese PCOS women, those over 40 years of age or those with prior gestational diabetes with an oral glucose tolerance test is suggested. Measurement of a lipid profile should be considered in all women with PCOS and repeated every 3–5 years. Close monitoring of PCOS patients for hypertension, especially for those who are obese, with insulin resistance or over 40 years of age, is recommended.

The appearance of polycystic ovaries on ultrasound is a common finding but is not necessary for diagnosis. Ultrasound evidence of polycystic-appearing ovaries is not alone sufficient for the diagnosis of PCOS as these may occur with many other disorders. It is recommended that an endometrial biopsy be performed on patients with long-term anovulation or thickened endometrial echo complex on ultrasound, to rule out malignancy.

Treatment

The aim of treatment is to decrease the long-term and short-term manifestations of PCOS. The objectives are to reduce hyperandrogenism, restore cyclic menses, reduce insulin resistance and other cardiovascular risk factors, protect the endometrium from unopposed estrogen, and restore fertility.

Obesity

Although the insulin resistance directly related to PCOS is not dependent on bodyweight, obesity may further compound the problem. Weight loss is beneficial in reducing hyperinsulinemia, as well as androgens, and may substantially decrease the associated long-term morbidity. Along with weight loss, the treatment

---

Box 93.4 Polycystic ovarian syndrome work-up

Laboratory evaluation and supporting tests
- Total, free testosterone: exclude androgen-secreting tumor, monitor treatment
- DHEAS: exclude neoplasm, monitor treatment, consideration of dexametasone (see Chapter 92)
- Fasting glucose, 2 hour GTT, HbA1C: detect insulin resistance or diabetes, monitor treatment
- Thyroid-stimulating hormone (TSH): exclude thyroid disease
- Prolactin: exclude hyperprolactinemia
- Lipids and lipoprotein profile

In selected clinical situations
- 17-hydroxprogesterone: exclude congenital adrenal hyperplasia (21-hydroxylase deficiency) with moderate to severe hyperandrogenism
- Endometrial biopsy: longstanding irregular bleeding, age >40 or endometrial echo complex >12 mm (even when clinical suspicion low)
- Screen for Cushing's disease: central obesity, muscle weakness, hypertension
- LH and FSH are not routinely necessary although they are diagnostic in certain situations
- Pelvic ultrasound: presence of polycystic-appearing ovaries is not necessary but may support the diagnosis; used to rule out ovarian tumor if testosterone levels >200 ng/dL

---

of choice in patients not seeking immediate fertility is often oral contraceptives (OCs) (Box 93.5). In weight loss clinical trials, metformin has been shown to be as good as or superior to low-calorie diet alone or FDA-approved weight loss medications.

Menstrual irregularities

Treatment is based upon the specific complaint of each patient. Patients with menstrual dysfunction who do not desire fertility may be treated with OCs or cyclic progestins such as oral medroxyprogesterone acetate 10 mg/day for 10 days each month or oral micronized progesterone 300–400 mg/day for 12 nights each month.

Hirsutism

Options in the treatment of hirsutism are shown in Box 93.5 and discussed at length in Chapter 92. Patients with hirsutism, acne or other evidence of hyperandrogenism are often best treated with low-dose OCs. Treatment with OCs serves multiple purposes including decreasing ovarian and adrenal androgen production, increasing SHBG which binds free androgens, and suppressing skin 5α-reductase activity. Occasionally spontaneous

Box 93.5 Polycystic ovarian syndrome: medications for women with hyperandrogenism and irregular bleeding

Low-dose oral contraceptives
First-line agent, substantially reduces androgens, peripheral (skin) action, controls bleeding, decreases risk or endometrial hyperplasia and cancer; OCs with 20 μg and low progestin impact (norgestimate, drosperinone), OCs may be more effective in some patients with moderate-to-severe androgen excess

Cyclic progestins
Medroxyprogesterone acetate 5–10 mg/day, norethinedrone acetate 5–10 mg/day, micronized progesterone 200–400 mg/day for 10–14 days/month; controls bleeding and protects endometrium; will have little or no effect on hyperandrogenism or hirsutism

Glucaphage (metformin) 500 tid or 500–850 mg twice a day
May decrease long-term cardiovascular risks in those with insulin resistance; must follow hepatic function. Metformin decreases androgens and may restore ovulation or improve response to ovulation induction

Spironolactone 50–200 mg/day
Interferes with P450–androgen synthesis, and competitively binds androgen receptors; not given during pregnancy

Dexamethasone 0.25–0.5 mg/day
Decreases DHEAS and androstenedione, may improve response to clomiphene citrate

Depo-medroxyprogesterone acetate 150 mg IM every 3 months
Inhibits 5α-reductase activity, protects the endometrium, generally prevents heavy bleeding

Topical eflornithine
For facial hirsutism

Less commonly used medications
GnRH agonist 3.75 mg/month or 11.25mg every 3 months. Effective, often combined with OCs after 6 months
  Nafarelin acetate 500 μg twice a day nasal spray
  Ketoconazole 400 mg/day. Generally experimental, inhibits P450 steroidogenesis, periodic liver function testing
  Glyburide (Micronase) 1.25–5.0 mg twice a day
  Finasteride 1.5 mg/day. Inhibits 5α-reductase, may feminize fetus (not recommended in fertile women), primarily used to prevent hair loss
  Flutamide 100–500 mg/day. Binds androgen receptor, hepatotoxic effects
  Cyproterone acetate 2–100 mg/day. Binds androgen receptor, used outside USA

ovulation may occur in PCOS patients and another benefit of using OCs is contraceptive protection. Further benefits of OCs include protection from the higher rates of endometrial cancer and ovarian cancer seen in PCOS patients. While all OCs can be used to treat hirsutism or acne, more difficult patients may benefit from OCs with low androgenic progestins including norgestimate, desogestrel or drosperinone. When patients have only a limited response to OCs, addition of spironolactone (or finasteride) should be considered.

One of the effective treatment regimens for hirsutism is a combination of GnRH agonist plus OCs. Hyperandrogenism originating primarily from an adrenal source (DHEA ≥5 μg/mL) is effectively treated with a low-dose corticosteroid such as dexametasone.

A major effort should be made to encourage weight loss. Obesity is associated with multiple alterations that interfere with normal ovulation, including increased peripheral aromatization of androgens to estrogens in adipose tissue, increased insulin levels which stimulate ovarian and adrenal androgen production, and decreased levels of SHBG resulting in elevated levels of free testosterone and estradiol. Therapies that lower circulating insulin levels, such as weight loss and hypoglycemics, may improve menstrual irregularities and decrease androgens by 30–40%. Hypoglycemics improve glucose tolerance and decrease triglycerides, glucose, insulin, and androgens. Lipid-lowering agents may also be considered.

Insulin resistance
Weight loss and exercise are the first-line treatments to reduce the health risks associated with PCOS. Insulin-sensitizing agents, such as metformin, are considered to be beneficial as they improve many of the cardiovascular risk parameters (Box 93.6).

Infertility
In patients wishing to conceive, treatment is aimed towards inducing ovulation. Clomiphene citrate is the first line of therapy. Prior to treatment, pregnancy and possible endometrial pathology should be excluded. If clomiphene citrate fails to produce ovulation, dexametasone or bromocriptine may be added in patients with elevated DHEAS or prolactin levels, respectively. Alternatively, metformin may be added to improve ovulation response. Pretreatment with both metformin 500 mg three times daily and clomiphene citrate induced ovulation in 89% of obese oligomenorrheic women with hyperandrogenemia and polycystic ovaries. Studies report higher fertilization rates and number of embryos produced in women undergoing IVF cycles after treatment with metformin.

Treatment with gonadotropins, either LH and FSH combinations or "pure" FSH, is indicated in clomiphene citrate failures. Care should be taken when using gonadotropins since PCOS patients are at high risk for developing ovarian hyperstimulation syndrome. A low-dose step-up increase is recommended.

Laparoscopic ovarian drilling is generally reserved for those patients who are clomiphene resistant or gonadotropin failures. This surgical attempt to achieve ovulation is

Box 93.6 Metformin

Actions
Inhibits hepatic glucose production
   Increases sensitivity of peripheral tissues to insulin

Benefits
May restore ovulation and menstrual cyclicity
   Pretreatment may increase the effectiveness of clomiphene (60% versus 49%, p = 0.003 in a recent study)
   Generally decreases serum androgen levels and may improve hirsutism
   Lowers fasting serum insulin
   Although poorly studied in women with PCOS, data suggest that it may retard progression to type 2 diabetes in women who have impaired glucose tolerance at baseline

Management
Therapy initiated at low dose (500 mg with dinner) and taken with meals, then progressively increased each week 500 mg with breakfast and 1000 mg with dinner to 1000 mg twice daily
   Cannot be used with renal impairment, hepatic dysfunction, heart failure or alcohol abuse
   Weight loss diet and routine exercise plan are important adjuncts
   Adverse effects include gastrointestinal distress (10–25% of users report nausea or diarrhea), low risk for malabsorption of vitamin B12, rarely lactic acidosis (0.3 per 10,000)
   Category B for pregnancy, no teratogenic effects reported

Candidates
May be considered for all PCOS patients
   Best candidates are those who are overweight or obese, have insulin resistance, low serum high-density lipoprotein and/or high triglycerides

associated with fewer tubo-ovarian adhesions than the traditional wedge resection techniques. Laparoscopic electrocautery is reported to be successful, in that 70–90% of clomiphene citrate-resistant patients ovulated after the procedure and pregnancy rates of 50% are reported. Ovarian electrocautery normalizes ovarian function, including androgen production, which appears to be stable for up to 20 years.

Suggested reading

Azziz Zacur HG. 21-Hydroxylase deficiency in female hyperandrogenemia; screening and diagnosis. *J Clin Endocrinol Metab* 1989; 69: 577–584.

Burghen GA, Givens JR, Kitabchi AE. Correlation of hyperandrogenism in polycystic ovarian disease. *J Clin Endocrinol Metab* 1980; 50: 113–116.

Chang RJ, Nakamura RM, Judd HL, Kaplan SA. Insulin resistance in nonobese patients with polycystic ovarian disease. *J Clin Endocrinol Metab* 1983; 57: 356–359.

Davison RM. New approaches to insulin resistance in polycystic ovarian syndrome. *Curr Opin Obstet Gynecol* 1998; 10: 193–198.

Dunaif A, Scott D, Finegood D, et al. The insulin-sensitizing agent troglitazone improves metabolic and reproductive abnormalities in the polycystic ovary syndrome. *J Clin Endocrinol Metab* 1996; 81: 3299–3306.

Ehrmann DA, Sturis J, Byrne MM. Insulin secretory defects in polycystic ovary syndrome. Relationship to insulin sensitivity and family history of noninsulin dependent diabetes mellitus. *J Clin Invest* 1995; 96: 520–527.

Elkind-Hirsch KE, Anania C, Mack M, Malinak R. Combination gonadotropin-releasing hormone agonist and oral contraceptive therapy improves treatment of hirsute women with ovarian hyperandrogenism. *Fertil Steril* 1995; 63: 970.

Gal M, Eldar-Geva T, Margalioth EJ, et al. Attenuation of ovarian response by low-dose ketoconazole during superovulation in patients with polycystic ovary syndrome. *Fertil Steril* 1999; 72: 26–31.

Gjonnaess J. Late endocrine effects of ovarian electrocautery in women with polycystic ovary syndrome. *Fertil Steril* 1998; 69: 697–701.

Legro RS, Finegood D, Dunaif A. A fasting glucose to insulin ratio is a useful measure of insulin sensitivity in women with polycystic ovary syndrome. *J Clin Endocrinol Metab* 1998; 83: 2694–2698.

Legro RS, Barnhart HX, Schlaff WD, et al. Clomiphene, metformin or both for infertility in the polycystic ovary syndrome. *NEJM* 2007; 356: 551–566.

Li TC, Saravelos H, Chow MS, et al. Factors affecting the outcome of laparoscopic ovarian drilling for polycystic ovarian syndrome in women with anovulatory infertility. *BJOG* 1998; 105: 338–344.

Lobo RA, Carmina E. Polycystic ovary syndrome. In: Lobo RA, Mishell, DR, Paulson RJ, Shoupe D (eds) *Mishell's textbook of infertility, contraception, and reproductive endocrinology*, 4th edn. Malden, MA: Blackwell Science, 1997: 363–383.

Meirow D, Raz I, Yossepowitch O, et al. Dyslipidaemia in polycystic ovarian syndrome: different groups, different etiologies. *Human Reprod* 1996; 11: 1848–1853.

Morin-Papunen LC, Koivunen RM, Ruokonen A, Markainan HK. Metformin therapy improves the menstrual pattern with minimal endocrine and metabolic effects in women with polycystic ovary syndrome. *Fertil Steril* 1998; 69: 691–696.

Nestler JE. Insulin regulation of human ovarian androgens. *Hum Reprod* 1997; 12(suppl 1): 53–62.

Nestler JE. Metformin for the treatment of the polycystic ovary syndrome. *NEJM* 2008; 358: 47–54.

Nestler JE, Jakubowicz DJ, Evans WS, et al. Effects of metformin on spontaneous and clomiphene-induced ovulation in the polycystic ovary syndrome. *NEJM* 1998; 338: 1876–1880.

Polson DW, Wadsworth J, Adams J, Franks S. Polycystic ovaries: a common finding in normal women. *Lancet* 1988; i: 870–872.

Rotterdam ESHR/ASRM-Sponsored PCOS Consensus Workshop Group. *Hum Reprod* 2004; 19: 41–47.

Shoupe D, Kumar DD, Lobo RA. Insulin resistance in polycystic ovary syndrome. *Am J Obstet Gynecol* 1983; 147: 588–592.

Van Montfrans JM, van Hoof MHA, Hompes PGA, Lambalk CB. Treatment of hyperinsulinaemia in polycystic ovarian syndrome? *Hum Reprod* 1998; 13: 5–6.

Chapter 94
Menopause

Lauren Rubal and Donna Shoupe
Department of Medicine and Obstetrics and Gynecology, Keck School of Medicine, University of Southern California, CA, USA

Introduction

Menopause, also known as the climacteric, is a multi-faceted process that includes but is not solely defined by the cessation of menses due to diminished ovarian activity. The decline of ovarian function occurs gradually and the effects of decreased ovarian hormone production manifest as a multitude of symptoms. Virtually all postmenopausal women note some symptoms due to menopause. Treatment options for these women, while plentiful, remain the subject of continued research and debate.

The nomenclature in this area was previously somewhat ambiguous. To correct this issue, the Stages of Reproductive Aging Workshop (STRAW) was convened to establish standard terminology and staging systems for the menopause transition. Menopause is a retrospective diagnosis after 12 months of amenorrhea.

The mean age of menopause in the USA is about 51 years, with the majority of women undergoing menopause between ages 45 and 55 years. Women who experience menopause prior to age 40 have premature ovarian failure, and represent about 1% of the population.

There are certain genetic and environmental influences that affect the timing of menopause. The age at which menopause occurs is strongly genetically predetermined, unlike the age of menarche, which is highly related to body mass. Recent genome association studies demonstrate several single nucleotide polymorphisms that are linked with age at menopause. Other genes potentially related to this include the estrogen receptor gene and the FMR1 premutation. Environmental factors that affect the age of menopause include cigarette smoking, ovarian and pelvic surgery, chemotherapy, and radiation.

Management of Common Problems in Obstetrics and Gynecology, 5th edition. Edited by T.M. Goodwin, M.N. Montoro, L. Muderspach, R. Paulson and S. Roy. © 2010 Blackwell Publishing Ltd.

Endocrinology of menopause

There are dramatic changes in hormone patterns that occur well before the cessation of menses. The initial clinical manifestation of an alteration in the axis is shortening of the menstrual cycle, primarily a shortening of the follicular phase, often beginning as women approach their early 30s. Later in the 40s there are skipped ovulations often leading to a lengthening of the cycle.

As the number of follicles declines, there is a corresponding decrease in serum inhibin B and antimullerian hormone (AMH) levels. The reduction of inhibin B (and its negative feedback on pituitary FSH) leads to a corresponding increase in serum FSH. These higher levels of FSH stimulation often result in higher than normal levels of estradiol in the follicular phase of the cycle. Clinically, these changes may present in women with shorter but heavier menstrual cycles. Aromatase activity increases with age and increased body fat and can also contribute to higher estrogen exposure. In the late menopausal transition, there is increased cycle irregularity and marked variations in serum FSH and estradiol levels. These changes may be compounded by a decreased hypothalamic-pituitary sensitivity to estradiol.

After menopause, ovarian production of estradiol falls dramatically, often reaching its nadir around age 55. The postmenopausal ovarian androgen production falls by about 50% and remains stimulated by high levels of LH. Estrone is now the predominant circulating estrogen and is primarily produced by extraglandular conversion of circulating androstenedione. After menopause, about 85% of androstenedione comes from adrenal secretion and about 15% from the ovaries. The conversion of androstenedione to estrone takes place mainly in adipose tissue; therefore, obese women have higher levels of estrone and are less likely to be as estrogen deficient as their slender counterparts.

Differential diagnosis of menopause

While menopause is the most common diagnosis in women between 40 and 55 years who present with amenorrhea and concomitant flushes and sweats, it is prudent to consider other etiologies if indicated. Pregnancy should always remain in the differential in any woman, even during the menopausal transition, due to the irregular ovulation that may still take place. Hyperthyroidism may mimic symptoms of menopause. Clinical presentation can guide whether TSH, a screening test, is needed.

Rare diagnoses that may be confused with menopausal symptoms include tumors or medications. Carcinoid, pheochromocytoma or other malignancies should be considered if atypical symptoms or physical findings are present. A thorough medication history is always indicated.

Manifestations of estrogen deficiency

Since estrogen plays such a widespread and important role in many tissues in the body, its decline can be manifested in a varied and extensive fashion.

Hot flushes
Hot flushes represent the pathognomonic symptom of menopause. They occur in up to 75% of postmenopausal women. Time of onset varies as they can begin during either the perimenopausal or menopausal years. The majority of women experience spontaneous resolution of hot flushes within a few years after menopause but they can persist for more than 5 years. Typical symptoms of hot flushes include an acute sensation of heat that starts in the face and upper chest and then becomes generalized, perspiration, and palpitations. These sensations last approximately 2–5 minutes, after which time chills or shivering may occur. Flushes can occur during the day and night and can be in groups or appear as single episodes.

A definite pathophysiologic explanation for hot flushes is still unknown, but they are attributed to estrogen withdrawal at the hypothalamus. This deficiency causes thermoregulatory disruption due to inappropriate peripheral vasodilation, leading to heat loss and a decrease in the core body temperature. Readjustment of core temperature to normal occurs with shivering. Sleep disturbance represents an important consequence of hot flushes. In many women these sleep disturbances lead to chronic insomnia and have a significant negative impact on quality of life issues.

Treatment options include reducing room temperatures, wearing layered clothing and avoiding hot foods. The most effective and low-cost treatment for moderate-to-severe hot flushes is hormone therapy. Low-dose conjugated estrogen and 17β-estradiol (oral or transdermal) are both effective, especially if given continuously. A re-evaluation of symptoms may be performed 6 weeks to 3 months after initiation of therapy but can be prolonged up to 1 year after adequate counseling. A yearly discussion on the risks and benefits of hormone therapy, reassessment of symptoms, and review of therapy options is important. When therapy is discontinued, it is best to taper the patient off the medications slowly (discontinue one pill per week or decrease the amount of estrogen in transdermal patches weekly).

Hormone therapy may not be a treatment option due to contraindications, side effects or patient preference. In this case, there are alternative treatments that may be effective. Selective serotonin reuptake inhibitors (SSRIs) and selective norepinephrine reuptake inhibitors (SNRIs) are generally the first alternative treatment option. These medicines are well tested and generally well tolerated but they should be avoided in patients on tamoxifen as adjuvant therapy for breast cancer, since SSRIs decrease its antiestrogenic activity and therefore may affect prognosis. Gabapentin is another agent employed in treatment. The ideal time of administration is at night, since it may cause drowsiness. Clonidine is a less effective option, but may be considered especially in women with hypertension.

Complementary treatments are growing in popularity and include soy, other phytoestrogens, black cohosh, vitamin E, and acupuncture. Many of the studies have mixed outcomes for the treatment of hot flushes. Furthermore, soy and black cohosh may have estrogenic effects on the breast.

Genitourinary atrophy
Vulvar, clitoral, and vaginal atrophy are changes seen after estrogen depletion. The initial alterations in the epithelium manifest as fewer superficial cells, more parabasal cells, with decreased support and elasticity of the tissue. The vaginal pH becomes more basic, thereby providing a more conducive environment for vaginal infections via growth of different types of bacteria. After long-term estrogen deficiency, there is atrophy of the vessels, muscles, and stroma of the vagina. This results in less blood flow to the area and more advanced signs of atrophy, such as a decrease in vaginal length and constriction of the vagina. Atrophic vaginitis can cause itching, burning, discomfort, dyspareunia, and also vaginal bleeding when the epithelium thins.

The trigone of the bladder and urethra are embryologically derived from estrogen-dependent tissue, and estrogen deficiency can lead to their atrophy, producing symptoms of urinary urgency and incontinence, dysuria, and urinary frequency. Another problem that can develop with decreased circulating estrogen levels is decreased synthesis of collagen that forms the connective tissue beneath the vaginal epithelium. These atrophic changes may decrease the support of the posterior urethrovesical angle and urinary stress incontinence can develop. Mild symptoms of vaginal dryness may be managed through the use of vaginal lubricants. However, more symptomatic patients find the most relief with either systemic or vaginal estrogen therapy. The advantages of vaginal estrogen administration are that it often works very quickly and the low systemic levels associated with its use have very low if any impact on coagulation factors, breast tissue, and endometrium. The advantages of systemic estrogen therapy often include ease in use, a lack of the messiness of vaginal products, and its concomitant beneficial effect on hot flushes and osteoporosis.

While estrogen relieves the symptoms of atrophic vaginitis, there are conflicting results in its treatment of urinary incontinence. While a meta-analysis did report subjective improvement in incontinence, the Women's Health Initiative (WHI) demonstrated a worsening of incontinence in older women on both estrogen alone and combination estrogen and progestin.

Osteoporosis

Osteoporosis is defined as a systemic skeletal disease characterized by low bone mass and microarchitectural deterioration of bone tissue, with a consequent increase in bone fragility and susceptibility to fractures. Osteoporosis is a silent disease that is usually asymptomatic until fractures occur. Early diagnosis and treatment are essential to avoid fractures of the skeleton. Postmenopausal osteoporosis initially affects trabecular bone, which is present in the vertebral column and distal radius. Osteoporosis develops more slowly in cortical bone, which is present in the hip and limb bones. Bone mass is increased in black, obese, and athletic women and is decreased in frail, light-skinned, sedentary women. Without antiresorptive treatment, women often lose about 1–1.4% of bone mass each year after menopause. In women undergoing a normal menopause, fractures begin to occur at about age 60 in structures composed mainly of trabecular bone, such as the vertebral spine and distal portion of the radius. By age 60, 25% of white and Asian women have spinal compression fractures. Loss of bone mass in cortical bone occurs at a much slower rate, so osteoporotic fractures of the femur usually do not begin to occur until about age 70 or 75.

Since osteoporosis is asymptomatic, its presence needs to be detected by imaging studies. At least 25% of the bone is lost before osteoporosis is diagnosed by routine x-ray examination. Dual-energy x-ray absorptiometry (DEXA) is the best way to measure bone mineral density in the sites at which fractures are most likely to occur – the spinal column and hip. The National Osteoporosis Foundation has stated that bone mineral density measurements are indicated when clinical decisions will be influenced by the information gained. Indications for measuring bone mineral density in postmenopausal white women include:
• all postmenopausal women under age 65 with at least one risk factor for osteoporosis
• all women 65 or older

• postmenopausal women with fractures
• women taking postmenopausal estrogen for prolonged periods of time
A careful history and physical examination will determine whether risk factors for the development of osteoporosis are present. Factors known to increase the risk of osteoporosis include:
• race: white or Asian
• reduced weight for height
• early spontaneous or surgical menopause
• family history of osteoporosis
• diet: low calcium intake, low vitamin D intake, high caffeine intake, high alcohol intake, and high protein intake
• cigarette smoking
• endocrine disorders, such as diabetes mellitus, hyperthyroidism, and Cushing's disease
• certain medications, such as corticosteroids and GnRH analog
• sedentary lifestyle
Bone mineral density is usually defined by the T score and the Z score. The T score is the difference in the bone density measured in standard deviations compared with a young adult of the same gender (peak bone density), while the Z score is the difference in the standard deviations of bone density compared with an adult of the same age and gender. Definitions of bone loss by bone mineral density are as follows.
• Normal: T score above –1
• Low bone mass (osteopenia): T score between –1 and –2.5
• Osteoporosis: T score below –2.5
• Established osteoporosis: T score below –2.5 and presence of fractures
Indications for pharmacologic treatment include:
• T score less than –2 without risk factors
• T score less than –1.5 with risk factor(s)
• women over age 70 with multiple risk factors without bone mineral density measurement
The clinical utility of measuring biochemical markers of bone turnover has not been definitively established. Adequate calcium and vitamin D intake are critical components of osteoporosis prevention. Postmenopausal women need a daily intake of 1000–1500 mg of calcium, along with 400 IU daily of vitamin D. Supplementation is encouraged if daily intake of calcium is low, lack of sun exposure or measured vitamin D deficiency is determined, or osteopenia or osteoporosis is diagnosed.

US FDA-approved drugs for osteoporosis prevention and/or treatment include the following.
• Estrogen: low doses can be administered orally or parenterally
• Alendronate (Fosamax, a bisphosphonate that induces osteoclast apoptosis): 5 mg/day for prevention, 10 mg/day or 70 mg/week for treatment
• Risedronate (alendronate, bisphosphonate): 5 mg/day, 35 mg/week; 150 mg/monthly for prevention and treatment

• Ibandronate (Boniva, bisphosphonate): 150 mg/month; intravenous calcitonin (peptide hormone that inhibits osteoclasts): nasal spray 200 μg/day, safe but less effective than estrogen
• Raloxifene (Evista, selective estrogen receptor modulator that has a positive effect on estrogen receptors in bone to slow resorption): 60 mg/day for both prevention and treatment
• Teriparatide (Forteo-Parathar, parathyroid hormone) teriparatide daily injection for treatment zoledronic acid (Reclast-bisphonate) 5 mg IV infusion every 2 years (prevention) and yearly (treatment)

Many prospective and retrospective studies have shown that estrogen therapy reduces the amount of postmenopausal bone loss as well as the incidence of vertebral fracture and hip fracture. Women need to take estrogen for more than 5 years to reduce fractures, and when estrogen is stopped the rate of bone loss increases.

Estrogen therapy for osteoporosis should be considered early in menopause, especially if a woman has other concomitant menopausal symptoms or concerns that would also be ameliorated with estrogen. Bisphosphonates are now first line for osteoporosis prevention and treatment. They increase bone mineral density and significantly reduce vertebral and nonvertebral fractures. Their most common significant side effect is gastric irritation and ulceration. Osteonecrosis of the jaw is a rare but serious risk during bisphosphonate therapy. Raloxifene, a selective estrogen receptor modulator (SERM). has agonist effects on bone and antagonist properties on endometrium and breast. It increases bone mineral density and has been proven to decrease vertebral fractures. However, its use carries a rare risk of venous thromboembolism.

Exercise in the premenopausal years increases bone density. However, weight-bearing exercise alone will not prevent postmenopausal bone loss. It has been reported that neither a program of brisk walking nor nonloading back exercise altered the rate of trabecular bone loss postmenopausally. Thus, calcium alone and a moderate exercise program cannot prevent the loss of bone mass in the early postmenopausal woman, but exercise is beneficial for the woman's overall health.

Metabolic effects

With any drug there is a benefit/risk ratio, but the risks of low-dose estrogen replacement therapy are minimal. Orally administered estrogen, especially high dose, causes increases in hepatic proteins, specifically in serum globulins. One of these globulins, angiotensinogen, can be converted to angiotensin and produces an increase in blood pressure, whereas other globulins may produce a hypercoagulable state and possibly thrombosis. Exogenous estrogens may alter lipid levels and other metabolic processes. However, these metabolic changes are related to the dosage and type of estrogen administered, and the dose and type of estrogen given for postmenopausal hormone replacement therapy are much less potent than those used in oral contraceptives. The dosage of estrogen in most of the currently used oral contraceptive formulations is 30–35 μg of ethinyl estradiol, which is the equivalent of about 2.5 mg of conjugated equine estrogens. Therefore, although the usual dosage of 0.3–0.625 mg of conjugated estrogen is 20–40 times greater than the minimum weight of estrogen used in oral contraceptives, it is only about one-fifth as potent in terms of effects on liver globulins and postmenopausal estrogen replacement does not increase blood pressure. However, several studies have shown that it does increase the risk of developing venous thromboembolism. Estrogen appears to have little effect on glucose metabolism, as several recent studies have shown no decrease in glucose tolerance in women treated with doses of estrogen equivalent to 1.25 mg of conjugated equine estrogen. Although some studies have shown a statistically increased risk of gallbladder disease in postmenopausal estrogen users, others have reported no such risk. Estrogens may accelerate the formation of cholelithiasis in susceptible individuals.

Cardiovascular effects

In contrast to the increase in blood pressure that has been reported in some women using oral contraceptives, no such increase has been observed with the use of estrogen replacement therapy. It is safe to prescribe estrogen replacement for postmenopausal women with hypertension, and if blood pressure increases while they are receiving this treatment, it is unlikely that the estrogen is the cause of the blood pressure elevation.

Several studies have reported that the use of oral estrogen postmenopausally is associated with about a 2–3-fold increased risk of venous thromboembolism (VTE). The increased risk is greatest in the first 2 years of use and occurs in women with and without inherited thrombophilic conditions.

The Women's Health Initiative reported that oral estrogen increased the risk of stroke and cardiovascular disease, primarily in women starting oral estrogen after age 65. Hormone therapy's impact on coronary heart disease (CHD) is still under investigation. Multiple observational studies and clinical trials report that when started in the early menopause, estrogen appears to be cardioprotective. The ongoing ELITE and KEEPS trials are large prospective randomized trials that are designed to further clarify the age-dependent manner in which estrogen exerts its effects. The WHI Coronary Artery Calcium Study examined 1064 women, 50–59 years old, who had participated in the estrogen-only arm of the WHI. Evaluation of coronary artery calcium by CT showed significantly less calcification in those who were on estrogen therapy. This can be interpreted as fewer coronary atherosclerotic plaques, a known risk factor for MI. The Kronos Early Estrogen Prevention Study (KEEPS) is a clinical trial designed to specifically address whether estrogen use early in menopause affects CHD markers. Women who are 3 years or less from their last menses and without a known history of CHD will be randomized to oral conjugated estrogens, a transdermal estradiol patch or placebo, along with cyclic micronized progesterone if on any type of estrogen. Carotid intimal medial thickness and coronary calcium will be assessed. These data will hopefully provide answers to the age-related role of estrogen in CHD.

Cognitive function

The role of estrogen in maintenance of cognition and development of dementias such as Alzheimer's disease has not yet been adequately elucidated. Estrogen has been linked to neuroprotection *in vitro*, with improvement in neuron communication, potentiation, plasticity, and regeneration. It has specifically improved markers related to the pathology of Alzheimer's disease, such as a decrease in tau protein hyperphosphorylation, β-amyloid protein formation, and increase in apolipoprotein expression. Multiple neuroimaging studies using functional magnetic resonance imaging (fMRI) and positron emission tomography (PET) demonstrate that estrogen increases neural activity during cognitive tasks in postmenopausal women.

Studies that examine estrogen in relation to cognition in women without overt dementia are divided into women who have just undergone menopause and those who have been menopausal for some time. Observational studies demonstrate that women who have recently experienced natural menopause report mixed results from the use of estrogen on cognitive function. However, women who recently had a surgically induced menopause do show improvement in verbal tasks with use of estrogen. The Cache County cohort was a group of 1889 women with a mean age of 75 years. They had an overall relative risk of dementia of 2.11 compared with men. These women were followed for 3 years to evaluate the relationship between hormone therapy and the risk of Alzheimer's disease. The authors found that women who had previously used estrogen had a decreased incidence of Alzheimer's disease, and this protection was greatest if it had been used for 10 or more years. Interestingly, women who were currently on hormone therapy did not experience any risk reduction for dementia, unless they had been on it for more than 10 years.

The WHI Memory Study (WHIMS) examined a subset of women greater than 65 years old who had no dementia at baseline. These women were randomized to combined estrogen/progestin therapy (*n* = 4932), estrogen alone (*n* = 2947) or placebo and followed for 4–5 years. The rate of dementia, measured by annual Mini-Mental Status Examinations, was significantly higher for those women taking combined therapy, and showed a trend towards increased risk in women taking estrogen only. It appears that estrogen's effect on cognition is similar to its actions on the cardiovascular system – that administration early in menopause has positive effects but initiation in late menopause may cause harm. Clinical trials looking at estrogen as therapy for established Alzheimer's disease generally have not shown any benefit.

Breast cancer

While still controversial, use of hormone therapy in the menopause has been linked to a slight increased risk of breast cancer. This has been shown in both epidemiologic and clinical trials, with the exception of data on unopposed exogenous estrogen use. Indirect evidence suggesting longer exposure to estrogen as a risk factor for breast cancer lies in the increased risk seen with early menarche, late age at menopause, and postmenopausal increased bone and breast density.

A multitude of observational studies have addressed the impact of hormone therapy on breast cancer. Unfortunately, many trials did not discriminate between types of hormone therapy, namely whether estrogen was used with a progestogen. A meta-analysis of 51 studies looking at approximately 50,000 women with and 100,000 women without breast cancer indicated there is a 2.3% increase in risk of breast cancer with each year of postmenopausal hormone use. Other meta-analyses have reported similar increase in relative risk of breast cancer with use of hormone therapy. The risk appears to be higher with combined therapy as opposed to estrogen alone.

The clinical trials in this area have shown similar results for combined estrogen/progestin therapy, but not for estrogen-only treatment. The WHI, as mentioned previously, examined the role of hormone therapy in breast cancer risk. In the combined estrogen/progestin arm, there was a significant increase in risk of breast cancer compared to placebo, with a hazard ratio of 1.2. This was first manifested in the third year of the study in women who had previously been on hormone therapy, and in year 4 in those women who had initiated hormone therapy with the trial alone. The estrogen-only arm of the WHI showed dissimilar results. There was no increase in breast cancer risk with estrogen treatment, and in fact, a trend towards decreased risk was shown, with a hazard ratio of 0.80 and 95% confidence interval of 0.62–1.04. These disparate findings may be due to an effect of progestins on breast tissue or to other factors. The Million Women Study followed more than 1 million women aged 50–64 years and found that current use of both estrogen-only and combined therapies did statistically increase the risk of breast cancer, but that use of combined hormones was associated with a higher risk.

The duration of postmenopausal hormone use may play a role in breast cancer development. There is no appreciable increase in risk if combination hormones are used for less than 4 years. Women who currently have breast cancer or have a history of breast cancer should not use hormone therapy. Although clinical data are somewhat conflicting, a large randomized trial of breast cancer survivors, the HABITS study, reported an increase in breast cancer events in the hormone treatment arm compared with placebo.

Endometrial cancer

Many epidemiologic studies have reported that there is a significantly increased risk of endometrial cancer developing in postmenopausal women who are ingesting estrogen without progestins as compared with nonestrogen users. The risk increases with increasing duration of estrogen use as well as with increasing dosage, and thus the increased risk appears to be causally related to estrogen use. The endometrial cancer that develops in estrogen users is nearly always well differentiated and is usually cured by performing a simple hysterectomy.

The risk of developing endometrial carcinoma for women receiving estrogen replacement can be markedly reduced by giving progestogens. The duration of progestin therapy is more important than the dosage, and one study has shown a greater reduction in endometrial cancer when the progestin is given daily instead of sequentially. The use of progestins lowers the increased risk of developing cancer of the endometrium associated with unopposed estrogen, and therefore progestins should be given to postmenopausal women receiving estrogen if they have a uterus. The addition of a progestin to estrogen therapy acts synergistically with estrogen to cause a slight increase in bone density. The use of synthetic progestins, however, may reverse the beneficial effect of estrogen upon serum lipids. It appears prudent to use the lowest dose of progestin that will prevent the endometrial proliferation produced by estrogen.

Treatment regimens

Estrogen therapy for postmenopausal women should be given in the lowest possible dose that relieves vasomotor symptoms, prevents vaginal-urethral epithelial atrophy, maintains the collagen content of the skin, reduces the rate of bone resorption, and prevents acceleration of atherosclerosis. Estrogen therapy given to postmenopausal women should result in physiologic and not pharmacologic circulating levels of estrogen, so that the risks of hypertension and thromboembolic disease are not further increased. The long-term effects of transdermal estradiol on fracture reduction have not yet been reported, but use of a 0.014–0.05 mg skin patch provides physiologic estrogen replacement and reverses postmenopausal bone loss. The level necessary to prevent bone loss and avoid symptoms of breast tenderness appears to be between 30 and 100 pg/mL. Vaginal administration of estrogen may be used initially to relieve atrophic vaginitis but other routes may offer further systemic benefits and easier long-term use.

A hormonal regimen should be selected that produces the least amount of uterine bleeding. One of the primary reasons why postmenopausal women decide not to use estrogen, or discontinue its use, is the occurrence of uterine bleeding. For this reason combination instead of sequential estrogen-progestin regimens are being increasingly prescribed. Heealthy, nonhypertensive, normal-weight perimenopausal women may consider low-dose oral contraceptives to provide regular scheduled bleeding episodes and contraception. Control of perimenopausal irregular bleeding with hormone replacement therapy options is usually more challenging.

The benefit of including a progestin in the estrogen replacement regimen is protection of the endometrium. Unfortunately, this benefit may be accompanied by an increase of adverse CNS symptoms including changes in mood and sense of well-being. Women who have undergone a hysterectomy are no longer at risk for endometrial cancer and can be treated with estrogen-only options.

A routine pretreatment endometrial biopsy is unnecessary, as it is not cost-effective. Also, routine annual endometrial biopsies are not necessary. If breakthrough, unscheduled bleeding occurs, the lining of the uterine cavity should be sampled if ultrasonography shows the endometrial thickness to be more than 5 mm, or vaginal ultrasonography is not available. Annual mammography should be recommended for all women aged 40 years or older, regardless of whether they are using estrogen therapy, as the incidence of breast cancer steadily increases as a woman ages. Contraindications to estrogen therapy occur infrequently. Contraindications for estrogen therapy in the product labeling include:

• known or suspected pregnancy. Estrogen may cause fetal harm when administered to a pregnant woman
• undiagnosed abnormal genital bleeding
• known or suspected cancer of the breast
• known or suspected estrogen-dependent neoplasia
• liver dysfunction or disease
• hypersensitivity to the ingredients
• active, recent or a history of thromboembolic disorders, both venous and arterial

In women with a history of breast cancer who presents with symptoms due to estrogen deficiency, progestins or clonidine can be given to reduce hot flushes and a vaginal lubricant given to relieve the symptoms of vaginal atrophy. Several studies have reported that women with a positive family history of breast cancer involving either a second-degree or first-degree relative may use estrogen replacement therapy without further increasing their risk of breast cancer.

Estrogen is the treatment of choice for the relief of vasomotor symptoms and symptoms caused by vaginal and urethral mucosal atrophy. In addition, estrogen therapy maintains the integument, improves mood, prevents postmenopausal osteoporosis and possibly Alzheimer's disease, and possibly reduces the morbidity and mortality associated with cardiovascular disease if begun early in menopause. Nearly all postmenopausal women can derive a substantial benefit from the use of estrogen replacement therapy and several studies have shown that estrogen users have decreased overall mortality compared to women of a similar population and age who were not taking estrogen.

Suggested reading

American College of Obstetricians and Gynecologists. *Committee Opinion. Hormone therapy and heart disease.* Washington, DC: American College of Obstetricians and Gynecologists, 2008: 420.

American Society for Reproductive Medicine Practice Committee. Estrogen and progestogen therapy in postmenopausal women. *Fertil Steril* 2008; 90(3): S88.

Anderson GL, Limacher M, Assaf AR, et al. Effects of conjugated equine estrogen in postmenopausal women with hysterectomy: the Women's Health Initiative randomized controlled trial. *JAMA* 2004; 291: 1701.

Cauley JA, Robbins J, Chen Z, Cummings SR. Effects of estrogen plus progestin on risk of fracture and bone mineral density: the Women's Health Initiative randomized trial. *JAMA* 2003; 290: 1729.

Chlebowski RT, Hendrix SL, Langer RD, et al. Influence of estrogen plus progestin on breast cancer and mammography in healthy postmenopausal women: the Women's Health Initiative Randomized Trial. *JAMA* 2003; 289: 3243–3253.

Collins JA, Crosignani PG, Blake JM. Breast cancer risk with postmenopausal hormone treatment. *Hum Reprod Update* 2005; 11: 545–560.

Gold EB, Colvin A, Avis N, et al. Longitudinal analysis of the association between vasomotor symptoms and race/ethnicity across the menopausal transition: study of women's health across the nation. *Am J Public Health* 2006; 96: 1226.

Grady D, Herrington D, Bittner V, et al. Cardiovascular disease outcomes during 6.8 years of hormone therapy: Heart and Estrogen/progestin Replacement Study follow-up (HERS II). *JAMA* 2002; 288: 49.

Grodstein F, Manson JE, Stampfer MJ. Postmenopausal hormone use and secondary prevention of coronary events in the Nurses' Health Study. A prospective, observational study. *Ann Intern Med* 2001; 135: 1.

Hodis HN, Mack WJ, Azen SP, et al. Hormone therapy and the progression of coronary-artery atherosclerosis in postmenopausal women. *NEJM* 2003; 349: 535–545.

Hulley S, Grady D, Bush T, et al. The Heart and Estrogen/progestin Replacement Study (HERS) Research Group. Randomized trial of estrogen plus progestin for secondary prevention of coronary heart disease in postmenopausal women. *JAMA* 1998; 280: 605.

Hulley S, Furberg C, Barrett-Connor E, et al. Noncardiovascular disease outcomes during 6.8 years of hormone therapy. Heart and Estrogen/progestin Replacement Study follow-up (HERS II). *JAMA* 2002; 288: 58.

Loprinzi CL, Sloan J, Stearns V, et al. Newer antidepressants and gabapentin for hot flashes: an individual patient pooled analysis. *J Clin Oncol* 2009; 27: 2831.

Nedrow A, Miller J, Walker M, et al. Complementary and alternative therapies for the management of menopause-related symptoms: a systematic evidence review. *Arch Intern Med* 2006; 166: 1453.

Nelson HD, Vesco KK, Haney E, et al. Nonhormonal therapies for menopausal hot flashes: systematic review and meta-analysis. *JAMA* 2006; 295: 2057.

Rapp SR, Espeland MA, Shumaker SA, Henderson VW. Effect of estrogen plus progestin on global cognitive function in postmenopausal women: the Women's Health Initiative memory study: a randomized controlled trial. *JAMA* 2003; 289: 2651.

Rossouw JE, Anderson GL, Prentice RL, et al. Risks and benefits of estrogen plus progestin in healthy postmenopausal women: principal results from the Women's Health Initiative randomized controlled trial. *JAMA* 2002; 288: 321.

Rossouw JE, Prentice RL, Manson JE, et al. Postmenopausal hormone therapy and risk of cardiovascular disease by age and years since menopause. *JAMA* 2007; 297: 1465.

Salpeter SR, Walsh JM, Greyber E, Salpeter EE. Brief report: coronary heart disease events associated with hormone therapy in younger and older women. A meta-analysis. *J Gen Intern Med* 2006; 21: 363.

Stefanick ML, Anderson GL, Margolis KL, et al. Effects of conjugated equine estrogens on breast cancer and mammography screening in postmenopausal women with hysterectomy. *JAMA* 2006; 295: 1647–1657.

Suckling J, Lethaby A, Kennedy R. Local oestrogen for vaginal atrophy in postmenopausal women. *Cochrane Database Syst Rev* 2006; 4: CD001500.

Utian WH, Archer DF, Bachmann GA, et al. Estrogen and progestogen use in postmenopausal women: July 2008 position statement of the North American Menopause Society. *Menopause* 2008; 15: 584.

Chapter 95
Premature Ovarian Failure

Richard J. Paulson

Department of Medicine and Obstetrics and Gynecology, Keck School of Medicine, University of Southern California, CA, USA

Introduction

Premature ovarian failure (POF) is defined as cessation of ovarian function prior to the age of 40 years. This number roughly corresponds to two standard deviations below the normal age of menopause. The approximate incidence of POF is 1 in 250 at 35 years of age and 1 in 100 at the age of 40 years. POF is associated with elevated levels of follicle-stimulating hormone (FSH) and is also called hypergonadotropic hypogonadism. In most cases, it is associated with amenorrhea, but intermittent ovarian function may occur. A small percentage of affected women may ovulate and even conceive and carry a normal pregnancy.

Diagnosis

As with other medical conditions, the patient should undergo a complete history and physical exam. Common presenting complaints include menstrual irregularity and various symptoms of hypoestrogenism. These include hot flushes and genital atrophy. In the early phase of POF, menstruation may remain regular and the patient may present with infertility. In these cases, the diagnosis is made on the basis of elevated levels of gonadotropins only, as the remainder of the history and physical findings will be normal.

The patient may have a prior history of ovarian surgery, especially if multiple interventions for endometrioma removal were performed. Past history of treatment for malignancies including chemotherapy and/or radiation predispose the patient to POF. There may also be a family history of POF, because up to 10% of cases of POF may be familial.

Physical examination may reveal the stigmata of Turner's syndrome, including short stature, shield chest, wide carrying angle or low posterior hairline. There may be signs of other autoimmune diseases, such as a goiter, suggestive of autoimmune thyroiditis, or increased skin pigmentation, consistent with adrenal insufficiency. There may be signs of hypoestrogenism, such as atrophic vaginitis.

The laboratory evaluation should rule out other causes of oligomenorrhea, and should include serum levels of prolactin, thyroid-stimulating hormone (TSH), and human chorionic gonadotropin (hCG). Elevations of FSH are characteristic of the condition. In the past, a specific value (such as 20 mIU/mL or 40 mIU/mL) was used as a diagnostic criterion. However, FSH levels vary widely among laboratories and thus, no specific value is used. However, the patient with POF should have an FSH level which is above the normal range. Women with residual ovarian function should have FSH levels measured on the third day of menstrual bleeding. This is because follicular development may occur in response to the elevated FSH, and the resulting high estradiol levels produced by the granulosa cells will act to decrease FSH levels, resulting in a false-negative evaluation. It has been observed that women with early follicular phase FSH levels as high as 60 mIU/mL may continue to have normal menstrual cycles, and even continue to ovulate. Normal-appearing oocytes have been retrieved from such cycles and fertilization *in vitro* was achieved. However, none of the embryos implanted. Serum FSH levels are higher than those of luteinizng hormone (LH); this observation may be used to differentiate POF from a mid-cycle gonadotropin surge, in which LH levels are higher than those of FSH.

Etiology

Premature ovarian failure commonly results from accelerated follicular atresia. The classic example of this condition is Turner's syndrome. The lack of a second X chromosome results in a dysregulation of follicular development. Whereas histologic studies of the ovaries of Turner's syndrome fetuses revealed normal numbers of primordial

Management of Common Problems in Obstetrics and Gynecology, 5th edition. Edited by T.M. Goodwin, M.N. Montoro, L. Muderspach, R. Paulson and S. Roy. © 2010 Blackwell Publishing Ltd.

germ cells, it is known that individuals with Turner's syndrome have primary amenorrhea and so-called "streak gonads" which consist primarily of fibrous tissue but no oocytes. Turner's syndrome mosaics have varying degrees of ovarian function, depending on the proportion of ovarian cells, which carry the XO cell line. Partial X chromosome deletions are also associated with POF, suggesting that the genes on the X chromosome are necessary for normal ovarian longevity.

Fragile X syndrome premutation carriers have amenorrhea prior to 40 years of age in 12–28% of cases. In this syndrome, there is a mutation of the FMR1 gene, with affected subjects having more than 200 CGG repeats in the 5′ regions of the FMR1 gene. Individuals with 55–200 CGG repeats are said to have a "premutation." The number of CGG repeats within the premutation range also appears to be associated with the timing of cessation of ovarian function.

Ovarian failure results in the aftermath of treatment with ovarian toxins, such as chemotherapy. The ovaries are also very sensitive to radiation. Ovarian surgery, especially if repetitive, results in diminishment of ovarian tissue, and may lead to ovarian failure later in life. Uterine artery embolization for uterine fibroids involves the injection of microparticles into the uterine arteries; because of the rich anastomotic network in the parametrial vasculature, these particles are frequently carried to the ovaries and may precipitate ovarian failure.

Autoimmunity was first thought to play a role in the etiology of POF when it was noted in association with adrenal insufficiency. POF is also part of the syndromes of polyglandular autoimmune failure, which are associated with autoantibodies to multiple endocrine organs. Therefore, when POF is discovered, the laboratory evaluation should rule out other endocrinopathies, including hypothyroidism (serum TSH), hypoparathyroidism (serum calcium and phosphorus), and diabetes (fasting glucose). Antiadrenal antibodies may also be present.

Rare cases of FSH receptor mutations have been reported, but the majority of POF cases are thought to be idiopathic in nature.

Treatment

Estrogen replacement is necessary for women with POF. Those with an intact uterus must also receive progestins. Younger patients may prefer to use oral contraceptives, but menopausal doses of estrogen replacement are probably adequate. Calcium supplementation, as with women with natural menopause, is advised. When patients reach the age of 50, hormone replacement therapy may be managed as with other menopausal women.

Women who wish to conceive should be informed that whereas spontaneous ovulation may take place in 5–10% of cases, there is no proven effective way of inducing ovulation with medical therapy. Since menopausal estrogen replacement therapy produces only relatively low levels of estrogen, these do not appear to interfere with ovulation. Thus, women who wish to conceive may be treated with low levels of exogenous estrogen (such as a transdermal estradiol patch) with intermittent progestins.

The only effective proven method of achieving pregnancy in women with POF is through oocyte donation. The uterus retains its ability to respond to exogenous estrogen and progesterone and excellent pregnancy rates may be achieved by inducing endometrial receptivity and transferring donated embryos during the synchronous time of the cycle (see Chapter 104).

Women with Turner's syndrome appear to have a defect in their connective tissue, especially in blood vessels, and are at increased risk for aortic dissection during pregnancy. Therefore, pregnancy in these women is relatively contraindicated, even though uterine receptivity is normal. A cardiac evaluation is indicated in all cases. However, even if this evaluation is normal, the risk of aortic dissection is not completely eliminated. Therefore, pregnancy remains highly risky in these individuals. Other POF patients have normal pregnancy outcomes following oocyte donation.

Suggested reading

American College of Obstetricians and Gynecologists. Committee Opinion No. 338. Screening for fragile X syndrome. *Obstet Gynecol* 2006; 107: 1483–1485.

Aiman J, Smentek C. Premature ovarian failure. *Obstet Gynecol* 1985; 66: 9–14.

Allingham-Hawkins DJ, Babul-Hirji R, Chitayat D, *et al.* Fragile X premutation is a significant risk factor for premature ovarian failure: the International Collaborative POF in Fragile X study – preliminary data. *Am J Med Genet* 1999; 83: 322–325.

Bakalov VK, Vanderhoof VH, Bondy CA, *et al.* Adrenal antibodies detect asymptomatic auto-immune adrenal insufficiency in young women with spontaneous premature ovarian failure. *Hum Reprod* 2002; 17: 2096–2100.

Hoek A, Schoemaker J, Drexhage HA. Premature ovarian failure and ovarian autoimmunity. *Endocr Rev* 1997; 18: 107–134.

Ito Y, Fisher CR, Conte FA, *et al.* Molecular basis of aromatase deficiency in an adult female with sexual infantilism and polycystic ovaries. *Proc Natl Acad Sci USA* 1993; 90: 11673–11677.

Krauss CM, Turksoy RN, Atkins L, *et al.* Familial premature ovarian failure due to an interstitial deletion of the long arm of the X chromosome. *NEJM* 1987; 317: 125–131.

Lindheim SR, Sauer MV, Francis MM, Macaso TM, Lobo RA, Paulson RJ. The significance of elevated early follicular-phase follicle stimulating hormone (FSH) levels: observations in unstimulated in vitro fertilization cycles. *J Assist Reprod Genet* 1996; 13: 49–52.

Mallin SR. Congenital adrenal hyperplasia secondary to 17-hydroxylase deficiency. Two sisters with amenorrhea, hypokalemia, hypertension, and cystic ovaries. *Ann Intern Med* 1969; 70: 69–75.

Marozzi A, Vegetti W, Manfredini E, *et al*. Association between idiopathic premature ovarian failure and fragile X premutation. *Hum Reprod* 2000; 15: 197–202.

Nelson LM, Kimzey LM, White BJ, *et al*. Gonadotropin suppression for the treatment of karyotypically normal spontaneous premature ovarian failure: a controlled trial. *Fertil Steril* 1992; 57: 50–55.

Singh RP, Carr DH. The anatomy and histology of XO human embryos and fetuses. *Anat Rec* 1966; 155: 369–383.

Surrey ES, Cedars MI. The effect of gonadotropin suppression on the induction of ovulation in premature ovarian failure patients. *Fertil Steril* 1989; 52: 36–41.

van Kasteren YM, Schoemaker J. Premature ovarian failure: a systematic review on therapeutic interventions to restore ovarian function and achieve pregnancy. *Hum Reprod Update* 1999; 5: 483–492.

van Kasteren YM, Hundscheid RD, Smits AP, *et al*. Familial idiopathic premature ovarian failure: an overrated and underestimated genetic disease? *Hum Reprod* 1999; 14: 2455–2459.

Chapter 96
Human Chorionic Gonadotropin and the Diagnosis of Early Pregnancy

Rene B. Allen, Mario J. Pineda, Frank Z. Stanczyk and Richard J. Paulson

Department of Medicine and Obstetrics and Gynecology, Keck School of Medicine, University of Southern California, CA, USA

Introduction

Although human chorionic gonadotropin (hCG) is known to be secreted by preimplantation embryos, its main utility is in the diagnosis of pregnancy. It can first be detected in serum 8 days following ovulation, approximately at the time of implantation. During this process, hCG is produced by the syncytiotrophoblast cells and is released into the maternal circulation. Serial hCG measurements are now routinely used, along with ultrasonography, to distinguish between normal and abnormal pregnancies and to estimate the prognosis for a livebirth.

Human chorionic gonadotropin production in pregnancy

Human chorionic gonadotropin is a heterodimer glycoprotein hormone, approximately 37 kDa in weight. There are two subunits of human chorionic gonadotropin: α-hCG and β-hCG. The α-subunit is identical to the α-subunits of luteinizing hormone, thyroid-stimulating hormone, and follicle-stimulating hormone. The β-subunit of hCG is unique. β-hCG is composed of 145 amino acids linked by six disulfide bridges. It has two N-linked and four O-linked oligosaccharides.

Multiple hCG-related molecules are present in pregnancy serum and urine samples. These include hCG in various stages of degradation, free α- and β-subunits, individual subunit fragments and hCG with altered glycosylation forms. Compared to normal pregnancies, much greater and variable proportions of hCG-related molecules are detected in Down's syndrome, pre-eclampsia and trophoblastic disease. Additionally, there are temporal differences in the production of hCG variants. Early in pregnancy, a hyperglycosylated form of hCG (HhCG) is detected in serum and urine samples. This HhCG is phenotypically and antigenically similar to the hyperglycosylated hCG produced by gestational trophoblastic disease. Examination of urine pregnancy samples for total hCG and HhCG revealed that 68% of total hCG detected early in pregnancy is HhCG. By the end of the first trimester HhCG comprised less than 3% of total hCG. HhCG is produced by cytotrophoblast cells, which are mostly phenotypically invasive cells, while regular hCG is produced by differentiated syncytiotrophoblasts.

Initial detection of β-hCG is thought to coincide with implantation. Among pregnancies lasting greater than 6 weeks, implantation occurred on days 8, 9 and 10 after ovulation in 84% of women. Risk of early pregnancy loss increased with later implantation; 13%, 26%, 52% and 82% of pregnancies that implanted on day 9, 10, 11 and >11 resulted in early loss, respectively. In another study, hCG was detectable in the serum by day 10 postgonadotropin surge (9 days after ovulation) in 75% of pregnancies and this increased to >95% by day 11 postgonadotropin surge. If hCG was not detected in the serum until day 12, the pregnancy was more likely to result in miscarriage.

Clinical applications of human chorionic gonadotropin measurements

Serial measurements of hCG have been established as a useful tool in distinguishing viable from nonviable pregnancies. In the early 1980s, initial studies described the minimum increase in hCG levels over 48 hours in a normal intrauterine pregnancy to be 66%. More recently (in 2004), utilizing newer assay technologies and a larger cohort of patients, a 99% confidence interval for normal hCG rise was established. This report found the lowest rate of rise to be 53% over 48 hours, with a median rate of rise of 124% over 48 hours. Abnormal gestations are associated with slower doubling times, although a normal rate of rise does not rule out an abnormal gestation.

Management of Common Problems in Obstetrics and Gynecology, 5th edition. Edited by T.M. Goodwin, M.N. Montoro, L. Muderspach, R. Paulson and S. Roy. © 2010 Blackwell Publishing Ltd.

If the circulating hCG level is greater than 1500 mIU/mL and the transvaginal ultrasound notes no gestational sac or pole in the uterus, an ectopic gestation should be suspected. Transvaginal ultrasound studies performed with a 5 MHz probe suggest that a gestational sac should be evident with a serum hCG level of 1500 mIU/mL, approximately 23–29 days from the LMP; a yolk sac should be evident at 5000 mIU/mL, 32–45 days from the LMP; and fetal cardiac motion detected at 13,000–15,000 mIU/mL and 42 days from the LMP with a CRL >5 mm. A note of caution: a 4 mm sac looks similar to 4 mm of fluid. A false-positive sac may represent late follicular-phase endometrium, a pseudosac associated with an ectopic gestation or a venous lake in myometrium.

A useful rule of thumb is that hCG levels are approximately 100 mIU/mL at the time of missed menses (or 14 days after ovulation). Based on a 28-day cycle, production of hCG has been estimated to double within 1.4–1.6 days up to the 35th day from the onset of the LMP and within 2.0–2.7 days from days 35–42. The level of hCG peaks at 8–10 weeks from the LMP at 10,000–80,000 mIU/mL and then drops and remains at approximately 10,000 mIU/mL for the remainder of pregnancy.

Ectopic pregnancies are commonly associated with an abnormal rise of hCG. However, a normal pattern of increase of hCG does not rule out an ectopic gestation. An abnormal pattern of increase of hCG in an asymptomatic patient should be documented by two abnormal values 1 week apart before therapeutic options are discussed with the patient. If the patient is symptomatic or ectopic gestation is suspected for any reason, and the value of hCG is above 1400 mIU/mL, then transvaginal ultrasound should be performed. Transvaginal ultrasound should be able to locate an intrauterine sac with hCG levels between 1500 and 2000 mIU/mL. Laparoscopy is indicated if the patient is symptomatic or the hCG is rising and there is no intrauterine pregnancy by ultrasound. Laparoscopy is also warranted if the hCG plateaus and there are no chorionic villi on endometrial curettage. In settings in which the date of conception is known (i.e. assisted reproductive technologies), failure to detect a gestational sac 24 days post conception or later may also be evidence of an ectopic gestation.

An anembryonic gestation should be suspected if by ultrasound there is no fetal pole with a gestational sac that is greater than 18 mm or if the hCG level is ≥5100 mIU/mL and no fetal pole is seen. Serial hCG and repeat ultrasound should be performed in this clinical presentation. In the event that serial hCG levels plateau or decline, or repeat ultrasound does not reveal a fetal pole with appropriate hCG levels, an anembryonic gestation is presumed.

Reported embryonic loss rates have shown variation depending on the parameters used as a prognostic indicator. Vaginal probe ultrasonography is a useful adjunct in demonstrating early intrauterine embryonic progression and prognosis. Endometrial stripe thickness may be informative in the diagnosis of an abnormal pregnancy. Approximately 97% of subjects who present with a symptomatic early pregnancy in an emergency room setting, with an initial endometrial stripe of 8 mm or less at presentation, were eventually diagnosed with an abnormal pregnancy. Furthermore, when examining anatomic landmarks by endovaginal ultrasound, the subsequent loss of viability in the embryonic period occurred with a frequency of 11.5% among patients with a gestational sac, 8.5% with a yolk sac, 7.2% for an embryo up to 5 mm, 3.3% for an embryo of 6–10 mm, and 0.5% for an embryo larger than 10 mm. The documentation of cardiac motion is also a good prognostic indicator of an early pregnancy. Persistence of cardiac motion beyond 8 weeks of gestation reduces the risk of subsequent embryonic loss to approximately 2–3%.

The half-life of hCG in serum is about 36 hours (range 12–50 h). Examination of 710 patients diagnosed with spontaneous abortion determined that the rate of decline of hCG was dependent upon the initial hCG level: the higher the starting concentration, the more rapid the decline. The rate of decline of hCG ranged from 21% to 35% at 2 days and 60% to 84% at 7 days for initial hCG concentrations of 250 mIU/mL to 5000 mIU/mL. This trend may also be helpful in monitoring the normal regression of hCG, for example following a suction and curettage of a molar gestation or evacuation of an ectopic gestation via salpingostomy.

It has also been previously shown that with IVF pregnancies, both twin and triplet gestations have significantly higher hCG levels than singleton gestations ($p < 0.0001$) and triplet gestations also were significantly higher than twin pregnancies ($p < 0.0001$). Although absolute levels were increased in multiple gestations, there was no effect on rate of rise.

False-positive hCG values

Referred to as "phantom hCG," some patients have a false-positive serum hCG result due to nonspecific heterophilic antibodies in the serum and this often results in inappropriate intervention. These false-positive levels are usually low (<10 mIU/mL) but have been reported at levels higher than 300 mIU/mL. This situation should be suspected when hCG levels plateau at a low concentration and do not respond to further therapeutic attempts, such as methotrexate for a persistent ectopic or molar gestation. Since the heterophilic antibodies are not secreted in the urine, one should measure a urinary hCG level if suspicious. Also, a serial dilution of the patient's serum can be performed, as the false-positive test is not affected by the dilution.

Hyperglycosylated human chorionic gonadotropin

Produced during implantation by the cytotrophoblast cells, the hyperglycosylated form of hCG (HhCG) is formed when a carbohydrate moiety is O-linked to the carboxyterminal end of the hCG molecule and therefore has a higher molecular mass. Detection of this form requires a separate assay in which an antibody is directed against the carbohydrate portion of the hCG protein. HhCG was initially found in molar pregnancies and was termed invasive trophoblast antigen or ITA because the cytotrophoblast cells are invasive in nature. HhCG has been shown to increase more rapidly in early pregnancy and achieves higher concentrations than hCG but also then decreases more rapidly, usually by 6–8 weeks of gestation. Several studies have evaluated using HhCG as a marker for differentiating a viable from a nonviable pregnancy and the ratio of HhCG/hCG has been found to be helpful in predicting pregnancies destined for failure. One study compared both total amount of HhCG and the ratio of HhCG/hCG in urine at the time of implantation and found significantly higher concentrations of HhCG and higher ratios in women who went on to have term pregnancies as compared to those who ultimately miscarried.

Conclusion

Differentiating between early viable intrauterine, nonviable intrauterine, and ectopic pregnancies has long presented a diagnostic dilemma for clinicians. The widespread use of ultrasound in combination with serial hCG levels has led to earlier diagnosis of ectopic gestations and subsequently less morbidity and mortality associated with these. Recent studies have helped to better define the normal rates of rise for hCG. When a viable intrauterine pregnancy has been ruled out, uterine curettage is very helpful in differentiating a nonviable intrauterine gestation from an ectopic pregnancy. When the hCG level is falling, it should fall at a minimum of 21% over 48 hours, and if it falls at a rate less than this, again, a D&C should be performed to accurately make the diagnosis. Recent research has evaluated the use of HhCG in distinguishing viable from nonviable gestations and it may even allow determination of which pregnancies are destined for failure.

Suggested reading

Barnhart K, Katz I, Hummel A, Gracia C. Presumed diagnosis of ectopic pregnancy. *Obstet Gynecol* 2002; 100: 505–510.

Barnhart K, Sammel M, Chung K, Zhou L, Hummel A, Guo W. Decline of serum human chorionic gonadotropin and spontaneous complete abortion: defining the normal curve. *Obstet Gynecol* 2004; 104: 975–981.

Barnhart K, Sammel M, Rinaudo P, Zhou L, Hummel A, Guo W. Symptomatic patients with an early viable intrauterine pregnancy: hCG curves redefined. *Obstet Gynecol* 2004; 104: 50–55.

Boime I, Garcia-Campayo V, Hsueh A. The glycoprotein hormones and their receptors. In: Strauss J, Barbieri R (eds) *Yen and Jaffe's reproductive endocrinology*, 5th edn. Philadelphia, PA: Elsevier Saunders, 2004: 75–92.

Chung K, Sammel M, Coutifaris C, *et al.* Defining the rise of serum HCG in viable pregnancies achieved through use of IVF. *Hum Reprod* 2006; 21: 823–828.

Chung K, Sammel M, Zhou L, Hummel A, Guo W, Barnhart K. Defining the curve when initial levels of human chorionic gonadotropin in patients with spontaneous abortions are low. *Fertil Steril* 2006; 85: 508–510

Cole L. Phantom hCG and phantom choriocarcinoma. *Gynecol Oncol* 1998; 71: 325–329.

Condous G, Kirk E, Lu C, *et al.* Diagnostic accuracy of varying discriminatory zones for the prediction of ectopic pregnancy in women with a pregnancy of unknown location. *Ultrasound Obstet Gynecol* 2005; 26: 770–775.

Condous G, Kirk E, van Calster B, van Huffel S, Timmerman D, Bourne T. Failing pregnancies of unknown location: a prospective evaluation of the human chorionic gonadotrophin ratio. *BJOG* 2006; 113: 521–527.

Garcia A, Aubert J, Sama J, Josimovich J. Expectant management of presumed ectopic pregnancies. *Fertil Steril* 1987; 48: 395–400.

Ho H, O'Connor J, Nakajima S, Tieu J, Overstreet J, Lasley B. Characterization of human chorionic gonadotrophin in normal and abnormal pregnancies. *Early Preg* 1997; 3: 213–214.

Kadar N, Caldwell B, Romero R. A method of screening for ectopic pregnancy and its indications. *Obstet Gynecol* 1981; 58: 162–166.

Kovalevskaya G, Birken S, Kakuma T, *et al.* Differential expression of human chorionic gonadotropin (hCG) glycosylation isoforms in failing and continuing pregnancies: preliminary characterization of the hyperglycosylated hCG epitope. *J Endocrinol* 2002; 172: 497–506.

Lohstroh P, Overstreet J, Stewart D, *et al.* Secretion and excretion of human chorionic gonadotropin during early pregnancy. *Fertil Steril* 2005; 83: 1000–1011.

Pandian R, Lu J, Ossolinska-Plewnia J. Fully automated chemiluminometric assay for hyperglycosylated human chorionic gonadotropin (invasive trophoblast antigen). *Clin Chem* 2003; 49: 808–810.

Rotmensch S, Cole L. False diagnosis and needless therapy of presumed malignant disease in women with false-positive human chorionic gonadotropin concentrations. *Lancet* 2000; 355: 712–715.

Sasaki Y, Ladner D, Cole L. Hyperglycosylated human chorionic gonadotropin and the source of pregnancy failures. *Feril Steril* 2008; 89(6): 1781–1786.

Seeber B, Barnhart K. Suspected ectopic pregnancy. *Obstet Gynecol* 2006; 107: 399–413.

Seeber B, Sammel M, Guo W, Zhou L, Hummel A, Barnhart K. Application of redefined human chorionic gonadotropin curves for the diagnosis of women at risk for ectopic pregnancy. *Fertil Steril* 2006; 86: 454–459.

Chapter 97
Work-up of Infertility

Melanie Landay and Kristin A. Bendikson
Department of Medicine and Obstetrics and Gynecology, Keck School of Medicine, University of Southern California, CA, USA

Introduction

Infertility, or subfertility, is defined as the inability of a couple to conceive after 1 year of regular intercourse without contraception. This definition initially arose following a study of over 5500 English and American women having regular, unprotected intercourse between 1946 and 1956; among the women who conceived, 50% did so within 3 months, 72% within 3 months, and 85% within 1 year. Overall, approximately 10–15% of all couples attempting pregnancy will be defined as having infertility, though this percentage increases significantly with increasing maternal age. Infertility is, therefore, a very common problem. Studies since the 1960s have shown a relatively stable prevalence in the United States of approximately 15%. About 30% of infertile couples in the USA seek therapy and 15% of these undergo some form of artificial reproductive technology.

In evaluating infertility and its treatment, it is useful to utilize the concept of fecundability, defined as the monthly conception rate which, in young fertile couples, is approximately 20%. Because the most fertile couples conceive in the first month of attempting conception, the monthly fecundability rate is probably higher than that in the first month, and then steadily decreases thereafter.

The incidence of subfertility increases steadily with the age of the female partner as a result of ovarian and oocyte aging. This effect of age on pregnancy rates has consistently been observed in all investigations addressing fertility, including population studies and national reports of pregnancy rates after fertility treatment. For example, it was demonstrated in studies of women attempting to conceive by donor sperm insemination. These studies found that the pregnancy rates were constant among women up to age 31 but then steadily declined so that by age 35 only about half as many women became pregnant with a given number of inseminations compared to those under age 31, and by age 40 only about one-third of women inseminated became pregnant in the same number of insemination cycles. Therefore, after 31 years of age, with increasing age, the percentage of women with subfertility steadily increases. Thus two factors influence fecundability rates: the duration of time during which the couple has been attempting to conceive, and the age of the female member of the couple.

Causes of infertility

The exact incidence of the various factors causing infertility varies among different populations. In general, however, the following incidences have been reported.
- Ovulatory disorders: 15–25%
- Endometriosis: 5–10%
- Pelvic adhesions: 10%
- Tubal blockage: 10–15%
- Female factor (alone): 40–50%
- Male factor (alone): 20%
- Combination female + male: 30–40%
- Unexplained: 10–25%

It has not been demonstrated with certainty that other abnormalities, such as antisperm antibodies, luteal-phase deficiency, subclinical genital infection or subclinical endocrine abnormalities such as hypothyroidism or hyperprolactinemia in ovulatory women, are a true cause of infertility. No prospective randomized studies have demonstrated that directed treatment of these latter entities results in greater fecundability than that which occurs without treatment. Therefore, couples with these abnormalities are treated in a manner identical to that of the 10–15% of couples in whom a specific cause is not found and who are considered to have idiopathic or unexplained infertility.

Management of Common Problems in Obstetrics and Gynecology, 5th edition. Edited by T.M. Goodwin, M.N. Montoro, L. Muderspach, R. Paulson and S. Roy. © 2010 Blackwell Publishing Ltd.

Diagnostic evaluation

At the time of the initial consultation for infertility, the clinician should take a complete history and perform a physical examination. In addition, a discussion about the normal reproductive process, normal fecundability, and the optimal time of intercourse should be undertaken. While reviewing the diagnostic evaluation, the clinician should discuss not only the type of tests but also their sequence and relation to the timing in the menstrual cycle as well as the discomfort and costs of the various diagnostic procedures.

The available therapies and the prognosis for treatment of the various causes of infertility can also be included in the dialogue. Methods to increase the fecundability rates of couples with normal diagnostic findings, such as controlled ovarian hyperstimulation and intrauterine insemination (IUI), as well as assisted reproductive technologies (ART), should be discussed.

Each couple should be instructed about the optimal time in the cycle for conception to occur. A study was performed in which fertile couples who stopped contraception in order to conceive recorded the cycle day when they had a single act of sexual intercourse. Hormone analyses were performed to determine the day of ovulation. All the couples who had intercourse after ovulation occurred did not become pregnant. The pregnancy rate was about 30% if intercourse occurred on the day of ovulation as well as 1 and 2 days before ovulation occurred. The pregnancy rate was about 10% if coitus occurred 3, 4 or 5 days before ovulation. No pregnancies occurred when intercourse took place 6 days or more days before ovulation.

Therefore, the optimal time for sexual intercourse is 1 or 2 days prior to or on the day of ovulation. Sperm retain their viability and fertilizing capacity for a longer period than the ovum is capable of being fertilized after ovulation occurs. Therefore it seems reasonable to advise couples to have sperm in the female reproductive tract awaiting the release of the egg, and to err on the early side when timing intercourse.

Ovulation typically takes place 14 days prior to the onset of the next menstrual cycle. Therefore, couples who want to use the "calendar method" for timing intercourse should consider the shortest and the longest menstrual interval of the female partner, and then time intercourse for 14 days prior to the anticipated time of the next menstruation. For example, if the shortest cycle is 24 days and the longest cycle is 32 days, then the couple should have intercourse every other day between cycle days 10 and 18.

Measurement of LH by commercially available urinary LH detection tests is the best way to detect ovulation and thus to determine the optimal time to have intercourse or insemination. Ovulation occurs in most cases 12–24 hours following detection of the LH surge in the urine. Testing should be performed between 10 am and 8 pm, excluding the first morning urine, as the LH surge often begins in the early morning hours and is not detectable in the urine until several hours later.

Initial evaluation

A thorough history should include all obstetric and gynecologic issues, with emphasis on ovulatory history (age of menarche, cycle length, dysmenorrhea), previous gynecologic diseases, abnormal Pap smears and methods of contraception. General medical health (current medical problems, medications, allergies) as well as history of previous surgeries and hospitalizations should be reviewed. Family history should include both medical issues and reproductive history. A thorough review of duration of infertility, coital frequency and previous treatments should occur. A review of systems should take place that includes symptoms of thyroid disease, galactorrhea, hirsutism and dysmenorrhea. A physical exam should include the patient's height and weight, palpation of thyroid, breast exam, evaluation of signs of hyperandrogenism, assessment of vaginal or cervical abnormalities and a pelvic exam to assess uterine size, pelvic or abdominal tenderness, and signs of endometriosis. The initial laboratory tests to consider for the female partner include a complete blood cell count, blood type determination and antibody screen, cervical cytology, and TSH as well as other routine prenatal labs including rubella antibodies, hepatitis B surface antigen, HIV and rapid plasma reagent (RPR).

The four-step infertility evaluation
Step 1: the egg

The first step in attempting to determine a cause for a couple's infertility is to confirm ovulatory status. Although anovulation or oligo-ovulation can be assumed if menstrual cycle length is highly irregular or prolonged, up to 10% of patients with normal cycle length between 21 and 35 days will be anovulatory. Basal body temperature recordings are a simple and inexpensive way to document ovulation, but some women have monophasic temperature patterns and the test is not reliable in defining time of ovulation as the rise in temperature occurs post ovulation. The best way to ascertain that ovulation has in fact occurred is to measure the serum progesterone level in the mid-luteal phase, 7 days prior to the expected menses. Progesterone levels greater than 3 ng/mL are indicative of ovulation, but it has been reported that a progesterone level of at least 10 ng/mL is always found in the luteal phases of cycles during which conception has occurred. Therefore, measurement of a serum progesterone level greater than or equal to 10 ng/mL 7–8 days after a positive urine LH surge is detected is an indication not only that ovulation has occurred, but also that the corpus luteum is producing sufficient progesterone to support implantation.

If the patient has irregular cycles and is thought to be anovulatory, the etiology should be sought. TSH, prolactin, and testosterone should be checked to rule out thyroid disease, hyperprolactinemia and polycystic ovary syndrome. Other underlying causes should also be ruled out: obesity, eating disorders, significant weight loss, and extremes of exercise. 17-hydroxyprogesterone (to rule out congenital adrenal hyperplasia) and DHEAS (to rule out an adrenal tumor) may also be obtained. Menstrual disturbances may also be subtle but have important implications for fertility, including intermenstrual spotting or a shortened luteal phase. In amenorrheic women, serum follicle-stimulating hormone (FSH) should be measured to differentiate between women with premature ovarian failure and those with hypothalamic dysfunction.

Serum follicle-stimulating hormone level should be measured on day 3 of the menstrual cycle to evaluate ovarian reserve, especially in women older than 35. Because FSH levels are not standardized among laboratories, a single value cannot be used for a definitive diagnosis. However, an elevated FSH level (>10 mIU/mL or near the upper range of normal) is an indication of diminished ovarian reserve. This may be reflected in poor egg quality, decreased pregnancy rates and diminished response to ovarian stimulation. A level greater than 20 mIU/mL in most labs provides strong evidence of impending ovulatory failure and is highly predictive of poor response to ovarian stimulation. When oocytes are retrieved in women with elevated FSH levels during treatment with *in vitro* fertilization (IVF), the oocytes are more likely to fail to fertilize and implantation of the embryos is very rare. Women with ovarian failure can achieve normal pregnancy rates with oocyte donation, which is the treatment of choice in this group (see Chapter 95).

Step 2: sperm

After the initial laboratory tests are performed on the female partner, a semen analysis should be performed on the specimen obtained from the male partner. This semen specimen should be obtained after 2–5 days of abstinence, preferably by masturbation at the doctor's office. If this is not possible, specimens may be collected in additive-/spermicide-free condoms with delivery to the office within 1 hour of ejaculation.

Normal values established by the World Health Organization (WHO) for the semen analysis are a volume more than 2 mL and a pH between 7.2 and 7.8. Sperm density should be greater than 20 million per milliliter and sperm motility of 50% or more is considered to be normal. The specimen should contain less than 10 million white blood cells per milliliter of semen. At least 40% of the sperm should have normal morphology by WHO criteria. If the strict morphologic criteria of Kruger are used, 14% is considered "normal" and 5–14% is considered acceptable. Men with 4% or less of normal forms are advised to proceed directly to IVF with intracytoplasmic sperm injection.

Mild cases of oligoasthenospermia may be treated with IUI but more severe forms of male-factor infertility are best treated with IVF. If a patient is found to be azoospermic, referral to a urologist and genetic testing should be considered (see Chapter 99).

Step 3: tubal blockage/pelvic factor

In order to assess tubal patency/structure, hysterosalpingography (HSG) should be performed in the follicular phase of the cycle utilizing water-based contrast media. Tubal evaluation can differentiate between proximal and distal blockage, the former of which may be caused by tubal spasm and not be indicative of disease. If tubal blockage is present, prognosis for fertility following tubal reconstruction depends on location and severity of tubal damage. Hydrosalpinges with significant dilation of the fallopian tube(s) are considered to be largely irreparable and IVF following salpingectomies is recommended. In addition, HSG can suggest the presence of peritubal adhesions when loculation of spill is noted. The HSG also evaluates the characteristics of the tubal mucosa and will show if salpingitis isthmica nodosa is present.

In the past, diagnostic laparoscopy was performed routinely as part of the diagnostic evaluation of all women with infertility. If laparoscopy is performed, indigo carmine can be used to document tubal patency and to identify subtle tubal factors such as fimbrial phimosis that may not be seen on HSG, yet may negatively impact fertility. If proximal blockage is noted on HSG, hysteroscopic cannulation of the fallopian tube under laparoscopic guidance can be performed to document patency or correct proximal blockage. However, since laparoscopy is an invasive procedure requiring general anesthesia and is costly, it should be performed only if there is a substantial likelihood of either improving the prognosis for fertility or changing the course of treatment. In some cases, visualizing peritubal adhesions or endometriosis or further assessing proximal blockage may make a difference in the choice of therapy. However, women with mild-to-moderate endometriosis are likely better served by foregoing surgery and simply proceeding with superovulation and IUI, especially in the setting of advanced reproductive age. If simple therapy with superovulation and IUI fails, IVF is the next course of action. Therefore, in most cases, it is not cost-effective to perform a diagnostic laparoscopy as part of the initial infertility evaluation for women whose initial evaluation (history, physical examination, laboratory tests, pelvic sonography, and HSG) is normal.

Step 4: uterine factor

Though less common, uterine abnormalities can be the cause of infertility and should be evaluated. Developmental anomalies and acquired anomalies such as endometrial polyps, uterine fibroids and intracavitary scarring should be ruled out if suspected. In addition to demonstrating tubal patency, the HSG can demonstrate whether or not there are abnormalities in the uterine cavity, though in the case of a significantly anteverted or retroverted uterus, additional radiographic angles may have to be evaluated in order for the uterine contour to be accurately assessed. Hysteroscopy or hydrosonography can be performed to assess for intracavitary lesions or mullerian anomalies if uncertainties exist after the HSG. Pelvic ultrasound can also be used to assess for submucosal or intramural fibroids, adenomyosis, polyps or uterine anomalies that may affect infertility and pregnancy.

Sonohysterography (also called "hydrosonography" or "saline injection sonography") provides additional contrast and is superior for the identification of lesions in the uterine cavity to pelvic ultrasound without saline injection. Hysteroscopy is the gold standard for the diagnosis and treatment of intracavitary abnormalities, but is generally reserved for cases in which less invasive and expensive testing methods have failed.

Additional diagnostic evaluation

The extent and immediacy of the work-up for infertility should take into account several factors, with emphasis on the least invasive means of diagnosing the most common causes of infertility. Important factors to consider include the duration of infertility and age of female partner. Evaluation, and ultimately treatment, may be tailored to correspond to the wishes of the couple. However, if treatment fails to produce a pregnancy within 3–6 treatment cycles, further diagnostic testing or change of treatment strategy should ensue and a more aggressive course of action is indicated.

Suggested reading

American Society for Reproductive Medicine Practice Committee. Endometriosis and fertility. *Fertil Steril* 2006; 86: S156–160.

Barnea ER, Holford TR, McInnes DRA. Long-term prognosis of infertile couples with normal basic investigations: a life-table analysis. *Obstet Gynecol* 1985; 66: 24–26.

Collins JA, Wrixon W, Janes LB, *et al*. Treatment-independent pregnancy among infertile couples. *NEJM* 1983; 309: 1201.

Deaton JL, Nakajima ST, Gibson M, *et al*. A randomized controlled trial of clomiphene citrate and intrauterine insemination in couples with unexplained infertility of surgically corrected endometriosis. *Fertil Steril* 1990; 54: 1083.

Evans JE, Wells C, Gregory L, *et al*. A comparison of intrauterine insemination, intraperitoneal insemination, and natural intercourse in superovulated women. *Fertil Steril* 1991; 56: 1183.

Fisch P, Collins JA, Casper RF, *et al*. Unexplained infertility. Evaluation of treatment with clomiphene citrate and human chorionic gonadotropin. *Fertil Steril* 1987; 51: 441.

Gunalp S, Onculoglu C, Gurgan T, Kruger TF, Lombard CJ. A study of semen parameters with emphasis on sperm morphology in a fertile population: an attempt to develop clinical thresholds. *Hum Reprod* 2001; 16: 110–114.

Guttmacher AF. Factors affecting normal expectancy of conception. *JAMA* 1956; 161: 855.

Guzick DS, Carson SA, Coutifaris C, *et al*., National Cooperative Reproductive Medicine Network. Efficacy of superovulation and intrauterine insemination in the treatment of infertility. *NEJM* 1999; 340: 177–183.

Guzick DS, Overstreet JW, Factor-Litvak P, *et al*., National Cooperative Reproductive Medicine Network. Sperm morphology, motility, and concentration in fertile and infertile men. *NEJM* 2001; 345: 1388–1393.

Hull MGR. Infertility treatment: relative effectiveness of conventional and assisted conception methods. *Hum Reprod* 1992; 7: 785–796.

Hull MGR, Savage PE, Promham DA, *et al*. The value of a single serum progesterone measurement in the midluteal phase as a criterion of a potentially fertile cycle ("ovulation") derived from treated and untreated conception cycles. *Fertil Steril* 1982; 37: 355–360.

Hull MGR, Glazener CMA, Kelly NJ, *et al*. Population study of causes, treatment, and outcome of infertility. *BMJ* 1985; 291: 1693–1697.

Menken J, Trussell IJ, Larsen U. Age and infertility. *Science* 1986; 23: 1389.

Pearlstone AC, Pang SC, Fournet N, *et al*. Ovulation induction in women age 40 and older: the importance of basal follicle-stimulating hormone level and chronological age. *Fertil Steril* 1992; 58: 674.

Rousseau S, Lord J, Lepage Y, van Campenhout J. The expectancy of pregnancy for "normal" infertile couples. *Fertil Steril* 1983; 40: 768.

Schwartz D, Mayaux MJ. Female fecundity as a function of age: results of artificial insemination in 2193 nulliparous women with azoospermic husbands. *NEJM* 1982; 306: 404.

Toner JP, Philput CB, Joeons GS, Muasher SJ. Basal follicle-stimulating hormone level is a better predictor of *in vitro* fertilization performance than age. *Fertil Steril* 1991; 55: 784–791.

Vermesh M, Kletzky OA, Davajan V, Israel R. Monitoring techniques to predict and detect ovulation. *Fertil Steril* 1987; 47: 259–264.

Wilcox AJ, Weinberg CR, Baird DD. Timing of sexual intercourse in relation to ovulation. Effects on the probability of conception, survival of the pregnancy, and sex of the baby. *NEJM* 1995; 333: 1517–1521.

Chapter 98
Induction of Ovulation

Marsha B. Baker and Kristin A. Bendikson
Department of Medicine and Obstetrics and Gynecology, Keck School of Medicine, University of Southern California, CA, USA

Introduction

Induction of ovulation with clomiphene citrate (Clomid, Serophene) is intended for patients who wish to conceive. There are two distinct approaches to ovulation induction: the first is for treatment of anovulation, whereas the second represents enhanced stimulation of ovulation in the setting of normal ovulation. The first group of patients includes women with oligomenorrhea or with primary or secondary amenorrhea who want to conceive and who do not have ovarian failure. In this group, those anovulatory patients who successfully ovulate on clomiphene, cycle fecundability approaches 15%. The second indication, called "superovulation," is used for ovulatory women experiencing infertility. When clomiphene is used for couples with this indication, cycle fecundability is approximately 5% but increases to 8–10% when combined with intrauterine insemination (IUI).

Mechanism of action

Clomiphene citrate is the pharmacologic agent of choice for ovulation induction in most anovulatory patients and is the first-line therapy for many ovulatory women with infertility. It was approved for clinical use in the United States in 1967, and has since been the most commonly prescribed treatment for infertility. Clomiphene is metabolized by the liver and eliminated in the stool. It is safer, cheaper, and easier to use than gonadotropins for ovulation induction.

Clomiphene is a selective estrogen receptor modulator: it is both an antiestrogen and a weak estrogen. It acts by competing with endogenous estradiol for estrogen-binding sites in the hypothalamus and displaces estradiol from these binding sites. Therefore, it blocks the static negative feedback of estradiol upon the hypothalamus, permitting an increased release of gonadotropin-releasing hormone (GnRH) which stimulates the pituitary to increase follicle-stimulating hormone (FSH) and luteinizing hormone (LH) production and release. This release of gonadotropins causes oocyte recruitment and maturation with an increasing production of estradiol. The estradiol initially produces a negative feedback upon the hypothalamus and pituitary to reduce gonadotropin secretion, limiting the number of growing oocytes. Then, as the endogenous estradiol level increases exponentially, it provides a positive feedback to initiate the LH surge.

Approach to treatment

Prior to treatment, the cause of anovulation should be evaluated and treated appropriately. Anovulatory patients should also be screened for ovarian failure, as well as associated endocrinopathies, including a pituitary tumor, thyroid or adrenal disorders.

Women with either primary or secondary amenorrhea who do not have uterine bleeding after progesterone are likely to be estrogen deficient. These patients should undergo measurement of their serum estradiol (E2) and FSH levels. If the FSH concentration is elevated, a diagnosis of ovarian failure is likely and should be explored. If premature ovarian failure (POF) is confirmed, treatment with ovulatory medications is not effective (see Chapter 95).

The estrogen-deficient amenorrheic woman who has normal or low serum levels of FSH should have an MRI of the central nervous system to rule out a hypothalamic or pituitary tumor. If the MRI is negative and the patient is believed to have hypothalamic amenorrhea, treatment is directed towards gonadotropin therapy, given that clomiphene will rarely work to cause ovulation when a low estrogen environment already exists.

Pretreatment studies should include a pelvic ultrasound to rule out pre-existing uterine abnormalities or adnexal masses. Semen analysis should be performed to verify that the male partner does not have severe oligospermia,

Management of Common Problems in Obstetrics and Gynecology,
5th edition. Edited by T.M. Goodwin, M.N. Montoro,
L. Muderspach, R. Paulson and S. Roy. © 2010 Blackwell
Publishing Ltd.

azoospermia or another gross abnormality. The uterine and tubal factors should be investigated by obtaining a hysterosalpingogram (or hysteroscopy and laparoscopy with chromopertubation).

These pretreatment procedures should insure that multiple causes of infertility are not present. Although multifactorial infertility is not a contraindication to therapy, the chance of a full-term gestation is reduced in such patients and the couple should be afforded a realistic prognosis before undertaking therapy.

Clomiphene is administered, beginning between day 3 and day 5, following a spontaneous or induced menstrual period for 5 days. Ovulation, conception and pregnancy rates are equivalent when treatment is started in this time frame.

Treatment begins with a daily dose of 50 mg for anovulatory patients, while many physicians opt for a higher daily dose of 100 mg for those undergoing "superovulation." During treatment, the patient can be allowed to ovulate spontaneously or monitored by ultrasound for follicle growth with planned ovulation using human chorionic gonadotropin (hCG) injection to mimic the LH surge. Urinary ovulation predictor tests, which detect the preovulatory LH surge, are a reliable method to assist the timing of intercourse and laboratory tests that assess the ovulatory response to clomiphene. If ovulation is going to occur, it will usually do so within 5–10 days, with a mean of 7 days, following the last clomiphene tablet. The ideal day for hCG administration should be based on follicle maturity, best determined by transvaginal ultrasound. The dominant follicle should be at least 18 mm in mean diameter and the endometrial stripe should be at least 7 mm in thickness before hCG is administered.

If the patient is not being monitored and intercourse is planned, ovulation should be documented in each cycle of treatment. Ovulation may be presumed if the serum progesterone level is in excess of 3 ng/mL 2 weeks after the last clomiphene tablet. If the level of progesterone is determined at the time of peak production, it is usually higher than 15 ng/mL. If menstrual bleeding does not occur within 4 weeks after the last clomiphene tablet, it can be assumed that either the patient did not ovulate or that the patient is pregnant. Appropriate evaluation should ensue.

While ovulatory patients will respond to Clomid treatment, not all anovulatory patients will. If the cycle was ovulatory and the patient did not conceive, she may be treated again with the same dose of clomiphene beginning on the same start day used previously. Monthly examinations should be performed, preceding each successive course of therapy. These examinations serve to exclude the presence of pregnancy and functional ovarian cysts that can interfere with the clomiphene treatment. Increasing the dose above 100 mg in the setting of

superovulation is not believed to lead to additional follicular growth.

The majority of anovulatory patients will ovulate in response to 50 mg of Clomid. This number trails downward with each increasing dose (see Table 98.1). If, after an initial clomiphene treatment of 50 mg, the cycle proves to be anovulatory, then the dose should be increased. If there is no bleeding or monitoring shows no follicular growth in response to clomiphene, depending on both hormone levels and endometrial thickness, a higher dose of clomiphene can be administered immediately or progesterone can be administered to induce a withdrawal bleed. Treatment should then begin with clomiphene 100 mg per day for a 5-day period.

If ovulation does not occur at the 100 mg dosage, the dose can be increased, in 50 mg per day increments, up to a maximum of 250 mg per day, for 5 days. Previous reports have suggested that patients may occasionally respond to even higher daily doses of clomiphene or to 250 mg given for 8 days. The regimen outlined includes treatment above the 100 mg per day dosage, which is the maximum recommended in the physician's product brochure.

Given the low incidence of ovulation with doses above 150 mg, it is reasonable to switch to gonadotropin therapy if it is available and ovulation is not achieved with 150 mg. However, approximately 25% of patients who ovulate and conceive with clomiphene citrate will do so only when these higher doses have been employed.

Among patients with unexplained infertility, the use of clomiphene citrate combined with IUI will result in an approximately 25% pregnancy rate within three treatment cycles. In these patients, treatment begins on cycle day 3 in order to maximize follicle recruitment and reduce the chances of dominant follicle selection, which may begin by day 5. The same precautions and monitoring systems are used as in the treatment of anovulatory patients.

Of all patients who conceive during therapy, three-quarters will do so within the first three ovulatory cycles. Therefore, more aggressive treatment with gonadotropins is recommended if pregnancy has not occurred within three cycles, as a dramatic decrease in pregnancy rates is seen with subsequent cycles. However, if gonadotropin

Table 98.1 Ovulation rate by dose of clomiphene citrate

Clomiphene citrate dose	Ovulation rate
50 mg	52%
100 mg	22%
150 mg	12%
200 mg	7%
250 mg	5%

treatment is not available or desired, treatment can be extended beyond the recommended three ovulatory cycles.

Numerous series reports have substantiated the safety and efficacy of exceeding the manufacturer's recommendations for dosing. However, because only 5% of all couples that conceive do so after six ovulatory cycles, the empiric use of other modalities should be considered at that time. The American College of Obstetricians and Gynecologists has recommended that clomiphene treatment be limited to fewer than 12 cycles.

Risks of treatment

It is imperative to inform the patient about the risks inherent in clomiphene treatment. The risk of multiple gestation, almost always twins, is between 5% and 10%. Higher order multiple gestations, such as triplets, are rare. There is no increased risk of congenital anomalies during clomiphene treatment, nor is there an increased risk of spontaneous abortion. However, early studies showed that when clomiphene was administered inadvertently during the first 6 weeks of pregnancy, the incidence of birth defects was 5.1%. Although this frequency is not significantly higher than the 2.4% observed in patients to whom the drug was given prior to conception, there is a concern that the drug may be teratogenic if given during the time of embryogenesis. Therefore, it is important that clomiphene is administered only when a patient has had normal menstrual bleeding and pregnancy has been ruled out. The risk of ectopic pregnancy also appears to be increased, but it is unclear if this is due to the medication or the underlying infertility.

During therapy, the risk of forming a functional ovarian cyst is between 5% and 10%. If a cyst forms, it will regress spontaneously in less than 1 month provided that clomiphene is withheld during that time. Cysts may occur at any dose and during any course of therapy. The use of clomiphene has been associated with borderline ovarian tumors, but not with invasive cancers. One case–control study found that the risk of ovarian tumors was increased in only those treated with 12 or more cycles of clomiphene.

True ovarian hyperstimulation is rare. More common minor side effects observed with clomiphene treatment include hot flushes, abdominal distension and pain, nausea, vomiting, breast discomfort, and visual disturbances.

Approach to treatment failure

While more than 90% of oligomenorrheic patients will ovulate, those patients who fail to ovulate need to be informed of alternatives to clomiphene administration.

Some hyperandrogenic, anovulatory women who do not respond to clomiphene will be found to have elevated serum levels of the adrenal androgen dehydroepiandrosterone sulfate (DHEAS). If the DHEAS level is elevated, treatment with dexametasone can be considered. Several doses of dexametasone for various amounts of time have been proposed for this purpose. Studies indicate that a few more anovulatory patients may be made to ovulate with this combined regimen.

Women with polycystic ovarian syndrome (PCOS) will often be insulin resistant and, at times, they will be resistant to the stimulatory effects of clomiphene. Some of these women ovulate when treated with metformin alone and, in others, treatment with metformin enhances sensitivity to clomiphene citrate. Metformin may be administered 500 mg three times daily or 850 mg twice daily. The clomiphene-resistant PCOS patient may also benefit from laparoscopic ovarian drilling, which may promote spontaneous ovulation or enhance clomiphene responsiveness. However, patients incur risks associated with the surgical procedure, including postoperative adhesion formation, which may further impact fertility potential.

Aromatase inhibitors may also provide another alternative to patients who have failed clomiphene treatment. The inhibition of aromatization by the medications letrozole or anastrozole essentially blocks estrogen production and releases the hypothalamic-pituitary axis from its negative feedback. Follicular growth occurs as a result of gonadotropin stimulation. Although aromatase inhibitors are well tolerated and have a low side-effect profile, their widespread use in the setting of ovulation induction has not yet been FDA approved. Additionally, their use has been controversial due to the possibility of fetal toxicity and malformations brought about by one study, which has since been refuted by additional work.

Ovulation induction with gonadotropins

Exogenous gonadotropins have been used to induce ovulation in gonadotropin-deficient women and those who do not ovulate with clomiphene citrate or for those women whose prognosis mandates more aggressive treatment. Patients should be advised that the chance of conceiving in any one course of therapy is approximately 20%, a rate similar to the conception rate in spontaneous ovulatory cycles. However, as with clomiphene, if pregnancy is not achieved in the first three cycles, pregnancy rates tend to decrease in subsequent cycles. Of all patients who conceive during therapy, the average number of treatment courses needed to achieve a pregnancy is three. Overall, 70% of all patients treated with gonadotropins will conceive, but among women with PCOS, the percentage is lower.

Gonadotropin preparations

Human menopausal gonadotropin (hMG; Repronex, Menopur) is a gonadotropin preparation extracted from the urine of postmenopausal women. Each ampule contains equal amounts of FSH and LH. hMG was the first gonadotropin preparation available on the market and has been used for ovulation induction as well as to cause superovulation in women undergoing IUI. Gonadotropins are also prescribed to induce the growth of multiple oocytes in women undergoing IVF. The basic gonadotropin preparation (such as Repronex) is associated with a 10% incidence of reactions at the site of injection when administered subcutaneously, and must be given intramuscularly in these individuals. The highly purified preparation (Menopur) may be given subcutaneously. Human menopausal FSH (hFSH; Bravelle) is also a purified urinary product and is produced by removing the LH from the combined FSH/LH urinary extract. Each ampule contains mostly FSH and negligible amounts of LH. Recombinant FSH (rFSH; Gonal-F, Follistim) is also available for subcutaneous administration. A recombinant form of LH, (rLH; Luveris) is produced in a similar manner to that of rFSH, via a Chinese hamster ovary cell line transfected with the gonadotropin gene.

Patient selection

The estrogen-deficient amenorrheic woman should be completely investigated to rule out the presence of a hypothalamic or pituitary tumor. If the investigation is negative, the patient should be considered for ovulation induction with one of these agents. Candidates for gonadotropin therapy are anovulatory women who failed ovulation induction with clomiphene citrate, women with hypothalamic amenorrhea, and ovulatory women with infertility who have failed clomiphene or whose clinical picture indicates more aggressive treatment than clomiphene.

Extensive counseling of the couple prior to therapy is an important consideration. Therapy with these medications is inconvenient, expensive and stressful for both partners, each of whom must provide support for the other. These data, together with a thorough explanation of the risks and sequelae of multiple gestations and of hyperstimulation, will insure that the couple is well informed prior to beginning therapy.

Approach to gonadotropin treatment

Treatment with gonadotropins involves the attempt to mimic as closely as possible the follicular development that occurs in a spontaneous cycle. The earliest index of this development is the rising level of estradiol in serum. The amount of medication required to induce adequate follicular development, as well as the duration of therapy, may vary not only from one patient to another but also from one course of treatment to another in the same patient. Therefore, treatment should only be undertaken in settings where estradiol levels may be measured rapidly on a daily basis and where transvaginal ultrasound monitoring is available.

Several different treatment regimens are used for the administration of gonadotropins. Typically, hCG is used to cause ovum release, but spontaneous ovulation may eventually occur and can be detected with urine LH kits or monitoring of estradiol levels and ultrasound measurement of follicular size. Clomiphene citrate can be used in conjunction with gonadotropins, which may decrease the amount of total gonadotropins necessary for treatment. In this setting, clomiphene citrate is administered for 5 days to induce partial follicular development and gonadotropin administration can begin at the same time or be delayed until the Clomid is finished.

With gonadotropin treatment, patients are started on injections on day 2 or day 3 of their menses. At that time, patients typically have ultrasound evaluation of the ovaries and hormone testing. hMG or rFSH (with or without rLH) is administered in the evening. Treatment is usually initiated with a determined dose and this amount is continued daily for 2–4 days. At that point, the patient again undergoes ultrasound evaluation of follicular number and development as well as estradiol measurement so that adjustments may be made to gonadotropin dose if necessary.

In the setting of PCOS, a prolonged course of low-dose gonadotropins can be used to minimize ovarian hyperstimulation and limit follicular growth. Typically, a very low dose of gonadotropins is initiated and then after 1 week of treatment, if the serum estradiol concentration remains unchanged, the dose of hMG or rFSH is increased accordingly. A stepwise increase every 3 or 4 days is continued until the dose is found which will cause a consistent increase of the serum estradiol level above baseline levels. This is thought to be the "threshold dose" and it is generally maintained. However, follicle sensitivity to stimulation can change with increased growth, and continued monitoring is necessary to achieve appropriate dose adjustment.

Whenever a follicle reaches 14 mm, the patient should be monitored no less frequently than every 2 days. Ultrasound monitoring provides immediate feedback, the assurance that there are not too many mature follicles, and verification that at least one follicle has matured (i.e. has reached a preovulatory size). When one or more follicles reach 17–18 mm in mean diameter, ovulation can be triggered with 10,000 IU of hCG. All other gonadotropin preparations are stopped at that time. Release of the oocyte occurs about 37–40 hours later. Therefore, follicle aspiration for IVF is scheduled for about 36 hours later. In the setting of superovulation plus IUI, the couple is instructed to return to the clinic 36 hours later for the insemination.

Risks of gonadotropin treatment

With appropriate protocol and monitoring techniques, almost all patients treated may expect to ovulate with gonadotropin therapy. Pregnancy rates of 15–20% per cycle with a very low rate of high-order multiple gestations and other complications may be expected. Approximately one-fifth of gonadotropin conceptions may result in multiple gestations, most often twins. Although the rate of spontaneous abortion and ectopic pregnancy may be increased, no increase in the incidence of congenital anomalies has been reported.

Ovarian hyperstimulation syndrome (OHSS), while rare, is a serious risk of gonadotropin therapy. Often occurring several days after stimulation, it is characterized by ovarian enlargement, ascites, hemoconcentration, hypovolemia, and electrolyte imbalances. The primary pathophysiologic cause is a shift of intravascular fluid into the peritoneal cavity ("third space"), thought to be due to the secretion of vascular endothelial growth factor (VEGF) from the hyperstimulated ovaries. A full discussion of this entity is beyond the scope of this chapter. Although most cases are mild, severe cases require hospitalization and intensive monitoring.

Suggested reading

American College of Obstetricians and Gynecologists. Management of infertility caused by ovulatory dysfunction. ACOG Practice Bulletin No. 34. Washington, DC: American College of Obstetricians and Gynecologists, 2002.

Biljan M, Hemmings R, Brassard N, *et al.* The outcome of 150 babies following the treatment with letrozole or letrozole and gonadotropins. *Fertil Steril* 2005; 84: S95.

Farquar C, Vandekerckhove P, Lilford R. Laparoscopic "drilling" by diathermy or laser for ovulation induction in anovulatory polycystic ovary syndrome. *Cochrane Database Syst Rev* 2001; 4: CD001122.

Forman, R, Gill, S, Moretti, M, *et al.* Fetal safety of letrozole and clomiphene citrate for ovulation induction. *J Obstet Gynaecol Can* 2007; 29: 668.

Fluker MR, Urman B, MacKinnon M, *et al.* Exogenous gonadotropin therapy in World Health Organization Groups I and II ovulatory disorders. *Obstet Gynecol* 1994; 83: 189–196.

Hammond MG, Halme JK, Talbert LM. Factors affecting the pregnancy rate in clomiphene citrate induction of ovulation. *Obstet Gynecol* 1983; 67: 196–202.

Kallen B, Olausson PO, Nygren KG. Neonatal outcome in pregnancies from ovarian stimulation. *Obstet Gynecol* 2002; 100: 414.

Kerin JF, Liu JH, Phillipou G, *et al.* Evidence for a hypothalamic site of action of clomiphene citrate in women. *J Clin Endocrinol Metab* 1985; 61: 265–268.

Lobo RA, Paul W, March CM, *et al.* Clomiphene and dexamethasone in women unresponsive to clomiphene alone. *Obstet Gynecol* 1982; 60: 497–501.

March CM. Improved pregnancy rate with monitoring of gonadotropin therapy by three modalities. *Am J Obstet Gynecol* 1987; 156: 1473–1479.

Marrs RP, Vargyas JM, March CM. Correlation of ultrasonic and endocrinologic measurements in human menopausal gonadotropin therapy. *Am J Obstet Gynecol* 1983; 145: 417.

McFul PB, Traub AI, Thompson W. Treatment of clomiphene citrate resistant polycystic ovarian syndrome with pure follicle-stimulating hormone or human menopausal gonadotropin. *Fertil Steril* 1990; 53: 792.

Morris RS, Paulson RJ, Sauer MV, Lobo RA. Predictive value of serum oestradiol concentrations and oocyte number in severe ovarian hyperstimulation syndrome. *Hum Reprod* 1995; 10: 811–814.

Rossing MA, Daling JR, Weiss NS, *et al.* Ovarian tumors in a cohort of infertile women. *NEJM* 1994; 331: 771.

Tulandi, T, Martin, J, Al-Fadhli, R, *et al.* Congenital malformations among 911 newborns conceived after infertility treatment with letrozole or clomiphene citrate. *Fertil Steril* 2006; 85: 1761.

Vandernmolen DT, Ratts VS, Evans WS, *et al.* Metformin increases the ovulatory rate and pregnancy rate from clomiphene citrate in patients with polycystic ovary syndrome who are resistant to clomiphene citrate alone. *Fertil Steril* 2001; 75: 310.

Wu CH, Winkel CA. The effect of therapy initiation day on clomiphene therapy. *Fertil Steril* 1989; 52: 564–568.

Chapter 99
Male Factor Infertility

Rebecca Z. Sokol

Department of Medicine and Obstetrics and Gynecology, Keck School of Medicine, University of Southern California, CA, USA

Introduction

Approximately 15% of couples experience some difficulties when trying to conceive. Because up to 50% of these couples will have a degree of male factor infertility, the evaluation of the man and woman should proceed in parallel. An understanding of the male reproductive physiology, sperm physiology, and the diagnosis of the infertile man will allow the obstetrician/gynecologist to provide better care for the female patient and assist in the formulation of a treatment plan for the couple.

Achievement of pregnancy requires the production of spermatozoa with normal fertility potential that travel to the upper female genital tract and fertilize an ovum. Spermatogenesis takes place in the seminiferous tubules of the testes. The orderly process during which spermatogonia differentiate into mature spermatozoa covers a 72-day period. During emission and ejaculation, secretions from the seminal vesicles and prostate are secreted into the urethra. These secretions make up most of the seminal plasma. Following ejaculation, spermatozoa undergo capacitation and the acrosome reaction prior to achieving the ability to fertilize an ovum. Control and co-ordination of testicular function occurs via feedback signals, both positive and negative, exerted by the hormones secreted at each level of the hypothalamic (gonadotropin-releasing hormone (GnRH)), pituitary (luteinizing hormone (LH), follicle-stimulating hormone (FSH)), and testicular (testosterone, inhibin) axis. Any disruption of the delicately co-ordinated interaction between the components of the hypothalamic-pituitary-testicular (HPT) axis, the orderly process of spermatogenesis, the processes of the acrosome reaction, and the steps of fertilization may lead to male infertility.

Management of Common Problems in Obstetrics and Gynecology, 5th edition. Edited by T.M. Goodwin, M.N. Montoro, L. Muderspach, R. Paulson and S. Roy. © 2010 Blackwell Publishing Ltd.

Clinical evaluation

The evaluation of the infertile man includes a history, physical examination, and semen analysis. Baseline reproductive hormone testing (LH, FSH, testosterone, estradiol, prolactin) is performed when indicated by the history and physical examination. The history uncovers any underlying medical or endocrine disease. Failure of the testicles to be descended at birth, delayed puberty, congenital abnormalities of the urinary tract or CNS, history of gynecomastia, and changes in libido and potency are symptoms that suggest an underlying endocrinologic abnormality. A history of genitourinary surgery, testicular trauma, infections or change in semen volume suggests an anatomic defect such as obstruction or ejaculatory duct cyst. Drugs and medications, alcohol, chemical exposures, and other environmental hazards can adversely affect infertility.

A complete physical examination is performed in order to uncover any underlying medical conditions as well as hypogonadism. The latter may present with eunuchoid proportions, female body habitus, gynecomastia or abnormal genitalia. The contents of the scrotal sac are palpated for the presence of the vas deferens, epididymes and varicocele. Testicular volume is measured with an orchidometer or calipers. Small testes are associated with diminished sperm production.

Semen analysis

The semen analysis is traditionally the most important tool in the investigation of male infertility. A normal semen specimen has an adequate number of spermatozoa, the majority of which are motile and morphologically normal. The semen analysis is a means by which the physician can assess the production of spermatogenesis by an individual. However, there is a marked variability in sperm density, motility, and morphology among multiple semen samples from an individual man. A number of studies since the 1960s have documented this variability. Therefore interpretation of a semen analysis must occur in the context of this marked variability for a given individual. The collection of 3–6 samples over 2–3 months increases the reliability of the mean values calculated for the semen parameters recorded for those samples. Standardization of abstinence times also improves the reliability of the interpretation of the results.

The semen sample is assessed for color, volume, pH, motility, sperm concentration, and morphology. The semen analysis procedure is outlined in detail in the World Health Organization Laboratory Manual. Over the past decade, the approach to morphology assessment has become more rigorous. Normal sperm are defined based on specific size and shape criteria, with a standard of 14% determined to be predictive of success in *in vitro* fertilization (IVF).

Although the semen analysis results are helpful in predicting pregnancy success, an abnormal semen analysis does not preclude pregnancy and a normal analysis does not guarantee pregnancy. Because the semen analysis does not definitively predict fertility potential, a number of sperm function tests have been developed. However, none of these tests can definitively predict pregnancy success. Currently, the most common practice utilizes the WHO standards presented in Table 99.1. These results are based on a standardized abstinence time of 2–7 days.

Hormone assessment

The endocrine status of the reproductive hormonal axis (hypothalamus, pituitary, testes) is assessed by measurement of serum LH, FSH, and testosterone. A single sample of 10 mL of whole blood collected in the morning to minimize diurnal variation is usually adequate. However, because of the pulsatile nature of hormone secretion in man, single random serum levels may not accurately reflect the mean concentration of LH, FSH and testosterone over a prolonged period of time. Therefore, if an abnormal result is obtained, the patient should be re-evaluated with a collection of multiple

Table 99.1 Recommended standards for semen analysis

Parameter	Recommended normal value
Volume	2.0 mL or more
pH	7.2–7.8
Sperm density	$>20 \times 10^6$/mL
Total sperm count	$>40 \times 10^6$
Sperm motility	>50% with progressive motility
Vital staining	>50% live (exclude dye)
Sperm morphology	>14% or more
White cell count	$<10^6$/mL

Source: Aitken RJ, Comhaire FH, Eliasson R, *et al. WHO laboratory manual for the examination of human semen and semen cervical mucus interaction*. Cambridge: Cambridge University Press, 1999.

samples (three samples collected through an indwelling cannula at 20 min intervals; by pooling three samples, a more integrated measure of basal hormone secretion is obtained). Estradiol measurements are indicated when a patient presents with gynecomastia, a testicular mass or a history consistent with exogenous estrogen exposure. Prolactin measurement is included in the evaluation of a patient who presents with impotence and/or evidence for a CNS tumor, as well as in men with a relevant drug history.

Diagnosis and treatment

Based on the information obtained from the history, physical examination, semen analysis, and hormone measurements, patients can be placed into five major diagnostic categories: irreversible germ cell failure, hypogonadotropic hypogonadism, androgen synthesis or action disorders, idiopathic infertility, and anatomic defects. The selection of the treatment regimen is based on the diagnosis.

Irreversible germ cell failure

Men with irreversible infertility can be subdivided into two major groups: men with spermatogenic failure who present with elevated serum FSH levels, normal LH and testosterone levels, and small testes, and men who present with classic hypergonadotropic hypogonadism identified by elevated gonadotropins, low testosterone, and severe oligospermia or azoospermia. Klinefelter's syndrome (47,XXY), occurring in approximately 0.2% of adults, is the most common cause of hypergonadotropic hypogonadism. At present, there is no therapy available for the treatment of infertility in these two groups of men. Artificial insemination with donor semen (AID) or adoption are the recommended options. The combination of intratesticular sperm aspiration with intracytoplasmic sperm injection (ICSI) may result in a pregnancy when the male partner has testicular failure, even if the patient has Klinefelter's syndrome. Those men who present with both an abnormality of spermatogenesis and hypogonadism should be treated with androgens to maintain secondary sexual characteristics. However, testosterone replacement acts as a male contraceptive by inhibiting gonadotropins and further suppressing spermatogenesis. Thus, if the patient has any sperm in the ejaculate, and he may want to attempt ICSI, he should not be treated with testosterone until the procedure has been done.

Hypogonadotropic hypogonadism

Men with hypogonadotropic hypogonadism are deficient in LH and FSH secretion. As a result, they are also deficient in testosterone and spermatogenesis. Spermatogenesis can be initiated and pregnancies achieved in many of these hypogonadotropic hypogonadal men when they are treated with exogenous gonadotropins or GnRH. Selection of the type of hormonal therapy as well as the ultimate success of therapy depend on the severity of the defect.

A small number of infertility patients carry the diagnosis of hypogonadotropic hypogonadism. The etiology is either congenital or acquired. The former, Kallmann's syndrome or idiopathic hypogonadotropic hypogonadism, is an abnormality of the secretion of gonadotropin-releasing hormone (GnRH). Acquired causes include tumor, infection, infiltrative diseases, and autoimmune hypophysitis. In general, prolactin-secreting pituitary tumors in men are large at the time of discovery and often present with impotence. Therapy must be primarily directed at reduction of tumor mass. The hyperprolactinemia itself may be treated with dopamine agonists, with usual improvement in the gonadotropin secretion, and testicular hormonal and spermatogenic function. If the tumor is not producing prolactin, the patient may require surgery.

Induction of spermatogenesis is initiated with injections of human chorionic gonadotropin (hCG) in divided doses of 1000–1500 IU two to three times per week. The hCG will stimulate the testes to produce testosterone. In many cases, hCG therapy alone will stimulate spermatogenesis. If sperm are not present in the ejaculate after 6–9 moonths of therapy, recombinant FSH should be added to the regimen in divided doses of 75 IU two to three times per week. Patients not interested in fertility should be treated with testosterone replacement as previously outlined.

Defective androgen synthesis or response

The pathophysiology underlying these disorders is either a deficiency of the enzyme 5α-reductase or an abnormality of the androgen receptor. These patients will often present with ambiguous genitalia at birth.

5α-Reductase deficiency presents with a mild elevation in testosterone, decreased to absent levels of dihydrotestosterone (DHT) and normal LH and FSH levels. Because of the failure to convert testosterone to DHT, DHT-sensitive organs do not develop normally. Patients present with a spectrum of ambiguous genitalia, abnormal prostate development and virilization at puberty. These men usually have sperm production adequate to initiate a pregnancy, but because of their genitourinary anatomic defects, intrauterine insemination may be necessary.

Androgen resistance is associated with elevated testosterone and estradiol levels, borderline elevation of LH and normal FSH. This is due to insensitivity of the androgen receptor to testosterone. The androgen receptor defect results in a deficient cellular response to testosterone, with a secondary increase in serum LH. Because the testes are continually stimulated by an elevation of

serum LH levels, the secretion rate of testosterone may be increased. Androgen receptors in the pituitary gland are also insensitive to the feedback inhibition of testosterone, and LH continues to be secreted in excess. Because testosterone is normally converted to estradiol by aromatization, serum estradiol levels are usually elevated. The altered testosterone/estradiol ratio often produces gynecomastia. The clinical presentation of the patient depends on the severity of the impairment in receptor function.

Idiopathic infertility

There is no proven treatment for idiopathic oligospermia. These patients present with normal gonadotropins and normal testosterone in the face of low sperm counts. Idiopathic oligospermia is not a specific entity but is the result of a variety of abnormalities, each causing a reduction in sperm concentration. A number of causes for a decline in sperm quality have been suggested. These include genetic and environmental. Some men with severe oligospermia will have Y chromosome microdeletions. Others may have been exposed to chemicals toxic to the reproductive tract such as heavy metals, organophosphates, and other pesticides. Others may be taking drugs documented to impact sperm function, i.e. sulfazalazine, β-blockers and calcium channel blockers.

Because of the heterogeneity of this group of men, treating all patients with the same drug will not uniformly result in an improvement in fertility. Medications which have been suggested to be of value in the treatment of idopathic oligospermia can be divided into androgens, gonadotropins, antiestrogens, and miscellaneous drugs. The few placebo-controlled studies published that evaluate the efficacy of these drugs in the treatment of male infertility conclude that these medications do not increase pregnancy rates.

Anatomic defects

Anatomic defects include varicoceles, obstruction (vasectomy, inadvertent ligation or transection of the vasa during herniorrhaphy or pelvic surgery, epididymal obstruction secondary to infection), congenital absence of the vas deferens, ejaculatory duct cysts, and retrograde ejaculation. Congenital absence of the vas is often associated with a mutation of the CFTR gene, the defect responsible for cystic fibrosis.

A varicocele is a dilation of the scrotal portion of the pampiniform plexus/internal spermatic venous system that drains the testicle. The pathophysiology of varicocele-induced infertility remains undefined and the data regarding improvement in pregnancy rates following varicocelectomy controversial. The clinical studies that report improved semen parameters and pregnancy rates after varicocele ligation were uncontrolled. Prospective controlled studies report no improvement in pregnancy rates. One cross-over study does suggest improvement in pregnancy rates.

Obstructive azoospermia is associated with azoospermia, normal-sized testes, and normal hormones. Unless the etiology is a vasectomy or the physical exam is consistent with absence of the vas deferens bilaterally, a testicular biopsy is performed to confirm the results. If normal spermatogenesis is noted, microsurgical repair of the obstruction is the treatment of choice. An alternative approach is transepididymal or testicular aspiration of spermatozoa. Sperm collected in this manner can only be used in an IVF/ICSI setting. Vasectomy reversal is usually successful. Investigators who participated in a large multicenter study reported that post first-time reversal, 86% of the men had sperm present in their ejaculate. Fifty-two percent of the couples established a pregnancy. There was an inverse correlation of patency rate and pregnancy rate with obstruction interval.

Retrograde ejaculation, the consequence of neuropathic disruption of the vasa deferentia and bladder neck, occurs most commonly in diabetic men and men post transurethral and open prostatectomy. The diagnosis is confirmed by identification of large numbers of sperm in a postejaculate urine specimen. Spermatozoa can be harvested from alkalinized urine and used for intrauterine insemination.

Conclusion

The endocrine evaluation of the male partner is an essential part of the work-up of the infertile couple. A careful history, physical examination, and laboratory assessment, guided by an understanding of the physiology of the hypothalamic-pituitary-testicular axis, will allow the clinician to ascertain a diagnosis and appropriate treatment plan.

Suggested reading

Alukal JP, Lamb DJ, Niederberger CS, Maklouf AA. Spermatogenesis in the adult. In: Infertility in the Male. Lipshultz LI, Howards SS, Niederberger CS (eds). 2009; 74.

Attia AM, Al-Inany HG, Proctor ML. Gonadotropins for idiopathic male factor subfertility. Cochrane Database Syst Rev 2006; (1):CD005071.

AUA and ASRM. *Practice Committee Report on Male Infertility*, Vols 1–4. American Urological Association, 2001.

Belker AM, Thomas AJ Jr., Fuchs EF, *et al.* Results of 1,469 microsurgical vasectomy reversals by the vasovasostomy study group. *J Urol* 1991; 145: 505.

Hauser R, Sokol RZ. Science linking environmental contaminant exposures to fertility and reproductive health impacts in the adult male. Fertility and Sterility, 2008, 89(2 supple), e59.

Hughes IA. Minireview: Sex differentiation. Endocrinology 2001;142:3281.

Melmed S. Update in pituitary disease. J Clin Endocrinol Metab 2008;93:231.

Nagler HM, Grotas AB. Varicocele. In Infertility in the Male. Lipshultz LI, Howards SS, Niederberger CS (eds). 2009; 331.

Nachtigall LB, Boepple PA, Pralong FP, Crowley WF Jr. Adult-onset idiopathic hypogonadotropic hypogonadism – a treatable form of male infertility. Engl J Med 1997;336:410.

Vernaeve V, Staessen C, Verheyen G, Van Steirteghem A, Devroey P, Tournaye H. Can biological or clinical parameters predict testicular sperm recovery in 47,XXY Klinefelter's syndrome patients? Hum Reprod 2004;19:1135.

Whitten SJ, Nangia AK, Kolettis PN. Select patients with hypogonadotropic hypogonadism may respond to treatment with clomiphene citrate. Fertil Steril 2006;86:1664–8.

Chapter 100
Uterovaginal Anomalies: Diagnosis and Management

Donna Shoupe

Department of Medicine and Obstetrics and Gynecology, Keck School of Medicine, University of Southern California, CA, USA

Introduction

Structural defects of the uterus and vagina are associated with a host of gynecologic and obstetric clinical problems. The defects are caused by either a genetic error or exposure to a teratogen during embryonic development. The incidence of congenital uterine anomalies is not precisely known but reports suggest that defects occur in 2–4% of all women and in 10–15% of women with recurrent pregnancy losses. Advances in imaging techniques and development of less invasive surgical procedures have advanced the clinician's ability to detect these abnormalities and provide more management options.

The three common developmental defects of the mullerian system are lateral fusion defects, vertical fusion defects, and agenesis. Lateral fusion defects are the most common mullerian developmental defects and septum is the most common fusion defect. Lateral fusion defects occur from failure of formation, fusion or absorption or abnormal migration of one or both of the mullerian ducts. An example of an asymmetric lateral fusion defect is the unicornuate uterus. The bicornuate or arcuate uterus results from a partial fusion defect whereas uterine didelphys occurs when the two mullerian ducts massively fail to fuse.

Vertical fusion defects result from either a failure of fusion between the caudal end of the mullerian duct and the urogenital sinus or a failure of proper vaginal canalization. Vertical fusion defects include cervical agenesis, cervical dysgenesis and vaginal septums and are often responsible for outflow obstruction problems.

Agenesis of the mullerian ducts may result in complete absence of the uterus and vagina known as Mayer Rokitansky Kuster Hauser syndrome, hemiuteri or uterine horns, uterus without a cervix or variable uterine development.

Management of Common Problems in Obstetrics and Gynecology, 5th edition. Edited by T.M. Goodwin, M.N. Montoro, L. Muderspach, R. Paulson and S. Roy. © 2010 Blackwell Publishing Ltd.

Clinical presentation

Uterine abnormalities

It is estimated that as many as 50–75% of congenital uterine abnormalities remain undiagnosed. In one study, 679 women with normal reproductive histories underwent a hysterosalpingogram. In this "normal" population, 3.2% were diagnosed with congenital anomalies, which included septate uterus (90%), bicornuate uterus (5%), and didelphys uterus (5%). It is important to consider the diagnosis of mullerian anomalies in all patients presenting with a history of recurrent miscarriage, premature delivery, abnormal fetal presentation or late abortion or for women presenting with primary amenorrhea, severe dysmenorrhea, dyspareunia or infertility. The clinician should be alerted to the possibility of a uterine anomaly in the clinical settings listed in Box 100.1.

Congenital uterine abnormalities are commonly associated with second-trimester loss because of limited intrauterine space and an associated incompetent cervix. An intrauterine septum may have poor blood supply to the septum, resulting in poor implantation, poor placental growth, and early or mid-trimester pregnancy loss. Premature labor and abnormal fetal presentation are also common problems associated with intrauterine anomalies that limit intrauterine space. Two-thirds of pregnancies in women with a uterine duplication are expected to reach term.

A noncommunicating rudimentary horn with functional endometrium may present as recurrent abdominal pain or hematometra. Many patients with mullerian system anomalies have cervical incompetence. Vaginal septums may present as dyspareunia or obstruct a normal vaginal delivery. Some patients with severe outflow obstruction present with hematocolpos.

Vaginal abnormalities

Abnormalities of the vagina can range from abnormalities of the hymen, transverse or longitudinal vaginal septum, hemivagina or vaginal agenesis. The imperforate hymen may be diagnosed at birth due to bulging mucocolpos

Box 100.1 Conditions associated with uterovaginal anomalies

Obstetric problems
- high presenting part
- abnormal presentation, breech
- retained placenta
- premature birth
- dystocia
- stillbirth
- intrauterine growth retardation
- rupture

Gynecologic problems
- recurrent first-trimester loss
- second-trimester loss
- incompetent cervix
- dyspareunia, penetration problems
- difficult tampon insertion
- ectopic pregnancy
- primary amenorrhea
- cyclic abdominal, pelvic pain, endometriosis
- pelvic or vaginal mass
- foul or bloody discharge

Gynecologic examination findings
- broad uterus or fundal notch noted on examination
- presence of vaginal mass, septum
- cervical anomalies, two cervices
- two separate cornua on bimanual exam
- pelvic or vaginal mass
- blind pouch, shortened vagina

Ultrasound findings
- two-lobed contour of uterus with asymmetric shape of fundus
- hematocolpos, hematometra
- endometrial echo separated by longitudinal septum or wall
- off-center amniotic sac

Hysterosalpingogram findings
- oblong-shaped cavity instead of a normal triangular shape
- V-shaped endometrial cavity
- duplicated cavity
- septum
- prominent horns

or during adolescence when cyclic abdominal or pelvic pain, urinary problems or pain with defecation occur. Incomplete hymenal fenestration may cause partial obstruction, retention of blood or malodorous discharge or interfere with coitus or insertion of tampons.

Longitudinal septum may be associated with uterine anomalies and the patient may note dyspareunia or difficulty with inserting tampons. Transverse vaginal septa most often occur in the upper or middle vagina but 15–20% occur in the lower vagina. They may have a small perforation. The vagina is shortened and may be associated with a mucocolpos, hematocolpos or pyohematocolpos. There are a few reports of women with transverse vaginal septa having obstructed labor necessitating either cesarean section or incision during labor. Vaginal agenesis, also known as Mayer Rokitansky Kuster Hauser (MRKH) syndrome, occurs in women with normal female karyotype and a variable uterine remnant development. The patients often present with primary amenorrhea but have otherwise normal pubertal development.

Associated problems

Obstetric problems

Obstetric problems include miscarriage, intrauterine growth retardation, prematurity, postpartum bleeding, incompetent cervix, abnormal fetal presentation, and cesarean delivery. Increased risk of pregnancy-associated hypertension may be due to co-existing congenital renal anomalies. Pregnancy diagnosed in a rudimentary or obstructed uterine horn is dangerous as it can result in rupture.

Urinary tract abnormalities

The close embryologic development between the urinary and reproductive systems often means that abnormal development in one is commonly associated with abnormal development in the other system. The incidence of combined anomalies varies, but a diagnosis of unilateral absence or underdevelopment in one system is a strong signal to investigate the other. Up to 75% of patients with unicornuate uteri have unilateral renal agenesis. Analogously, 20% of patients with unilateral renal agenesis will have major reproductive tract anomalies. Women with significant uterine or upper vaginal anomalies should have either an intravenous pyelogram or ultrasound scanning of the kidneys.

Endometriosis

Retrograde menstruation appears to play a significant role in the development of endometriosis. The presence of patent tubes, a functioning endometrium, and an outflow obstruction is associated with a high incidence (up to 77%) of endometriosis.

Infertility

The presense of a bicornuate or unicornuate uterus or uterine didelphys does not appear to prevent implantation and may result in favorable pregnancy outcomes.

Multiple studies report good pregnancy rates and term delivery rates in women with bicornuate or unicornuate uteri or uterine didelphys undergoing infertility treatment although pregnancy rates with *in vitro* fertilization (IVF) may be diminished due to mechanical difficulties associated with embryo transfer.

Other

Other associated problems include anomalies of the digestive tract, chiefly imperforate anus, cardiovascular system, eyes, ears, and musculoskeletal system, and increased risk of collagen vascular diseases. Vertebral abnormalities are common in true mullerian aplasia (MRKH syndrome).

Evaluation

Most uterine anomalies can be accurately defined with currently available imaging techniques including hysterosalpingography, ultrasonography, and MRI. Transvaginal ultrasound or hydrosonography is sensitive enough to distinguish the appearance of the endometrium during the proliferative and secretory phases of the menstrual cycle and can clearly assess the contours, cavity size and shape, structural changes, and overall size of the uterus. Transvaginal ultrasound can often distinguish between a bicornuate and septate or subseptate uterus, whereas on hysterosalpingography they often look similar. Transvaginal ultrasound can usually differentiate a small uterine horn from an ovarian mass. Ultrasound is useful in locating hematometra or hematocolpos and presence of ovaries, and for evaluating the presence of kidneys.

Hysterosalpingography and hysteroscopy are also useful techniques for the evaluation of uterine anomalies. On hysterosalpingography, the endometrial cavity of a unicornuate uterus appears as an oblong-shaped contour, instead of a normal triangular shape, and only one fallopian tube arises from the cavity. A uterine didelphys yields a duplicated endocervical canal and two oblong-shaped endometrial cavities. Incomplete fusion of the mullerian ducts results in a bicornuate, V-shaped endometrial cavity.

Magnetic resonance imaging is considered by many as the gold standard for diagnosing uterine anomalies. Accurate measurement of the uterine fundus diameter can distinguish a normal, bicornuate, didelphys or septate uterus. Uterine contours, presence of endometrial tissue in a uterine horn or diameter and length of a septum can be assessed.

Classification system and treatment options

The American Society for Reproductive Medicine (formerly the American Fertility Society) developed a classification system for Müllerian system anomalies associated with fetal wastage. In this system, each group represents a structural change that has similar clinical problems, treatment, and prognosis. This classification system (Fig. 100.1) consists of seven major uterine anatomic types as well as the associated vaginal changes. The vaginal and labial conditions described next are not included in this classification system, but are included here as uterovaginal anomalies.

Labial fusion

Labial fusion is most often a result of exogenous androgen exposure. The most common etiology is congenital adrenal hyperplasia that is associated with clitoral enlargement and labial fusion and is most often due to a 21-hydroxylase deficiency. An elevated blood level of 17-hydroxyprogesterone necessitates cortisol replacement therapy. This condition is often diagnosed at birth or in early infancy. Labial fusion may also result from defects in the anterior abdominal wall or from a local infectious process.

If there is a small opening in the labial fusion plane, a vaginogram prior to surgical separation informs the surgeon about the depth of the fusion present and the dimensions of the upper vagina, and may confirm the presence of a cervix.

Imperforate hymen

The hymen is formed as a result of the fusion of the urogenital sinus and mullerian ducts. With the onset of menstruation and the inability of the menstrual blood to pass through an imperforate hymen, the vagina becomes distended with blood. Imperforate hymen is most often diagnosed at puberty when either primary amenorrhea occurs or when hematocolpos or hematometrium causes pain or urinary retention. Occasionally, a mucocolpos or hydrocolpos causes pain and is diagnosed during infancy or childhood.

The diagnosis is made by inspection of a bulging membrane at the introitus. Treatment consists of a cruciate incision in the hymen. A thick hymen may need a triangular section removed and placement of hemostatic sutures. A thick, fibrous but not imperforate hymen can be easily incised to produce a normal-caliber vagina.

Vaginal septum: transverse or longitudinal

If the area between the junction of the mullerian tubercles and sinovaginal bulb is not properly canalized, a transverse vaginal septum may remain. The septum may be complete or partial and lie in the upper third or lower two-thirds of the vagina. Septa located in the upper third of the vagina are usually the thickest and most difficult to correct surgically. Transverse vaginal septa are extremely rare, occurring in only 1:75,000 women.

With complete septa, hematocolpos or hematometrium may become symptomatic, similar to the imperforate

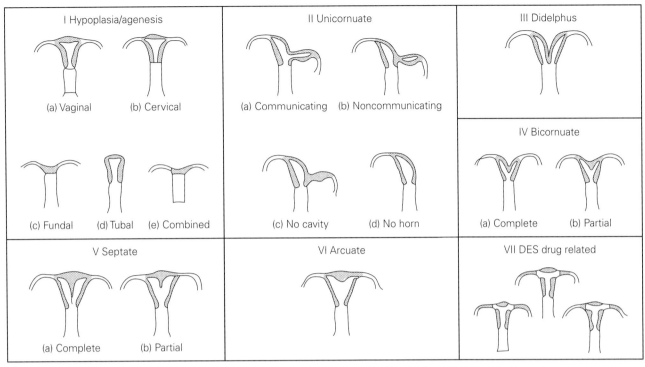

Figure 100.1 Classification of mullerian anomalies developed by the American Fertility Society. DES, diethylstilbestrol.

hymen as described above. With an incomplete septum, cyclic cramping and bleeding, a foul-smelling vaginal discharge, dystocia or sexual problems may be the presenting complaint.

Generally, the septa are thin, less than 1 cm thick, composed of fibromuscular tissue covered with squamous epithelium. If an opening is present, a manual dilation may be possible or a simple incision with suturing of the edges of the septum to the vagina on either side. If a vaginogram reveals a thick septum, either an anastomosis between the lower and upper vagina or a split-thickness skin graft, similar to the McIndoe procedure mentioned below, may be necessary. An intravascular pyelogram (IVP) should be used to exclude renal or ureteral anomalies.

A longitudinal vaginal septum may result from failure of fusion of the lower ends of mullerian ducts that form the vagina. This lesion may present with patients complaining of acyclic or cyclic pelvic pain as a result of a collection of blood in the pouch formed due to the vaginal septum. The septum may be complete or partial and may be associated with a double uterus, vaginal obstruction, ipsilateral renal agenesis and vascular abnormalities.

Surgical treatment of a longitudinal vaginal septum usually involves removal of the septum and suturing together the two edges of normal vaginal tissue over the defect. Care should be taken to avoid injury to the bladder or rectum. Surgery may not be necessary in asymptomatic women.

Vaginal mullerian cysts

Vaginal wall cysts are rare but may present with vaginal bulging, pelvic pressure, dyspareunia or protruding cystic mass. Pelvic MRI may be helpful in revealing nonseptated homogeneous vaginal cysts that are differentiated from a urethral diverticulum. The differential diagnosis also includes Bartholin's duct cyst, epidermal inclusion cyst, Gartner's duct cyst, endometrioid cyst and unclassified cyst. Mullerian cysts are lined by columnar endocervical-like or cuboidal epithelium. Simple removal or marsupialization is indicated with care to avoid the bladder or rectum.

Class I: hypoplasia/agenesis
Vaginal agenesis (with normal uterus)
The vagina is formed after fusion of the mullerian ducts and the urogenital sinus. Further growth results in the formation of a solid mid-line cord of cells called the vaginal plate. Canalization of the vaginal plate occurs as the central cells degenerate. A vestibular dimple may mark the site where the urogenital sinus pushed in from the perineal surface. This dimple marks the location of a potential space filled with loose areolar connective tissue, located between the bladder and rectum. Congenital absence of the vagina is often unrecognized until medical attention is sought for primary amenorrhea, dyspareunia or cyclic cramping.

The work-up includes documentation of the presence of a uterus and ovaries with examination, ultrasound or

MRI, and evaluation of the urinary collection system. Treatment is directed at the creation of a functional (>12 cm) vagina. The first choice of treatment is progressive vaginal dilators that generally take several months in well-motivated patients. A bicycle seat can be used to maintain dilator pressure for 15–20-minute sessions for a total of 2 hours a day. Surgical correction is usually the McIndoe procedure that utilizes a stent over which a split-thickness skin graft is sewn and placed in the dissected space between the rectum and bladder. The success rate is 80%. The Williams procedure utilizes labial skin that is used to create a vaginal pouch. A normal vaginal axis is reported to develop eventually.

Pediatric surgeons may opt to use the sigmoid to form a neovagina. The disadvantage to this procedure is that it is associated with a chronic foul-smelling vaginal discharge. Two other more recently introduced techniques can be done by laparoscopy. The Vecchietti procedure creates a neovagina by using an acrylic "olive" placed into an invagination of the vaginal canal. The "olive" is placed under traction by connecting it to a device resting on the abdomen. The Davydov procedure utilizes peritoneum to create a neovagina.

Absence of the lower vagina is treated by surgical intervention. The hematocolpos is identified, dissection is done to reach the area, and then it is opened and drained. The edges may be marsupialized. The vaginal mucosa is identified, mobilized, brought down to the hymenal ring and then sutured.

Cervical agenesis

Congenital absence of the cervix with functioning endometrial tissue is extremely rare. Primary amenorrhea and cyclic abdominal pain are the usual presentation. Creation of a functional cervix is difficult due to a lack of cervical mucus production. Infection, stenosis, and reoperation are common.

Tubal agenesis

The diagnosis of congenital tubal anomalies is generally made after problems of infertility. Isolated tubal agenesis is extremely rare. Microscopic tubal unification may be possible in cases of segmental tubal agenesis.

Combined uterovaginal agenesis

The most severe vaginal anomaly results from an unexplained inhibition in growth of the mullerian ducts at a very early stage. Vaginal agenesis associated with absence of the uterus is called Mayer Rokitansky Kuster Hauser syndrome and occurs in 1 in 5000 female births. The ovaries are derived from a different embryonic source and are normal. The fallopian tubes are either rudimentary or fairly well developed, and are usually connected near the mid-line to a small bulb of fibrous or muscular tissue located between the bladder peritoneum and the rectosigmoid. Occasionally (8%), this bulb of tissue contains a small amount of endometrial tissue and occult menstruation may occur. While complete vaginal agenesis is usual, about 25% of patients have a short vaginal pouch.

The work-up includes documentation of the absence of a uterus. MRI is very useful for demonstrating ovaries, mullerian and vaginal remnants, and renal agenesis. Renal abnormalities are present in 25–40% of these patients. Additionally, skeletal changes, including congenital fusion or absence of vertebrae, are reported to occur in up to 12% of patients. Treatment is usually directed at the creation of a functional vagina as described above. If a rudimentary uterine anlage is symptomatic, it should be removed.

Differential diagnosis primarily includes testicular feminization. Palpation of a partially descended testis, presence of scant pubic hair or failure to identify ovaries are indications for karyotype testing. Androgen insensitivity syndrome (testicular feminization) has a 46, XY karyotype. There is a high incidence of seminomas and therefore the testes need to be removed after puberty.

Class II: unicornuate
Communicating rudimentary horn

Occasionally, one mullerian duct may be very rudimentary or may fail to develop at all. Many of these anomalies are asymptomatic, although incidences between 10% and 70% of fetal loss in unicornuate uteri are reported. Cervical incompetence may account for much of the increased risk of fetal loss. Congenital alteration of uterine vascularization may compromise uteroplacental blood flow, and may account for early pregnancy loss and greater risk of intrauterine growth retardation. Other obstetric problems include malpresentation and delivery difficulties. There is a frequent occurrence of congenital malformations of the urinary tract, especially absence of the ipsilateral kidney. An imaging study of the urinary tract is indicated in all patients with a unicornuate uterus.

Recurrent first-trimester loss or a single second-trimester loss is an indication for (hydro)sonography, office hysteroscopy or a hysterosalpingogram. Placement of a cervical cerclage should be considered after reproductive loss. Removal of a communicating horn is necessary if it is associated with retrograde flow, an ectopic pregnancy, cyclic pain or mass formation.

Noncommunicating rudimentary horn

In 90% of rudimentary horns, there is no communication with the uterine cavity. The presence of any endometrial tissue in a noncommunicating horn may lead to the problems listed above and is generally an indication for removal of the horn. A pregnancy in a noncommunicating horn is thought to be due to transperitoneal migration of the ova and/or sperm. Rarely a livebirth occurs.

Unicornuate: no cavity in rudimentary horn

These patients are generally asymptomatic but when a unicornuate uterus is associated with increased pregnancy losses, the patient can be managed as for communicating unicornuate uterus (see above).

Unicornuate: single cavity, no horn

A half uterus, arising from only one mullerian duct and its single attached fallopian tube, may be normally formed and may function normally. Early pregnancy loss can be managed in the same way as for communicating unicornuate uterus (see above), often with placement of a cervical cerclage. A 30–50% incidence of unilateral renal malformation can be anticipated.

Class III: didelphys

Complete duplication of the uterus, vagina, and cervix is often diagnosed at the time of the first pelvic examination. Often the two vaginal cavities are asymmetric and vaginal function may be normal in only one vagina. Some patients present with dyspareunia or complaining that a tampon does not obstruct menstrual bleeding.

Overall, reproductive function is normal or modestly compromised. There is a chance that pregnancies may exist in both uteri or remain in one uterus after removal of the pregnancy in the other uterus. Normal vaginal deliveries of simultaneous pregnancies in both uterine cavities have been reported. Didelphic uteri are reported to be associated with a higher rate of incompetent cervix and an increased risk of premature labor. A mean length of gestation of around 35 weeks is reported with a 27% incidence of breech presentation.

The diagnosis is made by inspection of a double cervix and vagina and palpation of a double uterus. A metroplasty is rarely indicated or beneficial. Removal of a longitudinal vaginal septum, in cases of dyspareunia or to improve reproduction efficacy, is indicated.

Class IV: bicornuate

There is generally no conception difficulty in women with a bicornuate uterus, but dystocia, premature birth, and retained placenta are common. Increased rates of early fetal loss are generally thought to be related to inadequate formation and functioning of the cervix. Incompetent cervix is reported to be as high as 38% in women with bicornuate uteri. Implantation problems resulting in early pregnancy loss are less well documented as studies reporting higher incidences generally have included both bicornuate and septate uteri in their series.

The diagnosis can often be made on bimanual examination with detection of two completely separate cornua.

The use of transvaginal ultrasound can assist in differentiating bicornuate from septated uterus, whereas a hysterosalpingogram usually cannot. Placement of a cervical cerclage should be the primary consideration in cases of repetitive fetal loss. The value of a Strassman unification procedure is questionable but the procedure has been advocated by some for cases of repeated reproductive failure.

Class V: septate

The most outstanding feature of the septate uterus is the high incidence of first-trimester fetal wastage, probably related to inadequate blood supply in the septum resulting in placental implantation site malnourishment. Most data suggest that the more complete the septum, the higher the frequency of fetal loss. However, other studies suggest that the more complete the septum, the better the blood supply and the better the chance for a full-term pregnancy. Septate uteri are associated with abnormal fetal presentation, especially breech presentation, and also incomplete expulsion of the placenta leading to postpartum hemorrhage.

A hysterosalpingogram can rarely distinguish a septate from a bicornuate uterus, while a transvaginal ultrasound or MRI can. Treatment by hysteroscopic resection is indicated in cases of repetitive pregnancy losses. Asymptomatic septa do not require treatment.

Class VI: arcuate

The arcuate uterus contains a concave indentation in the uterine fundus with a depth of less than 1.5 cm. The arcuate uterus behaves benignly and may simply be a variant of normal.

Class VII: diethystilbestrol drug related

The changes associated with diethystilbestrol exposure *in utero* include anomalies in all parts of the genital tract. At least 50% of these women have vaginal adenosis, and 20–50% have structural abnormalities of the cervix. A hypoplastic or T-shaped uterus is characteristic but other abnormalities include filling defects, endometrial cavity adhesions or hypoplastic uterus. The cervical changes may include hoods, collars or hypoplasia. Vaginal anomalies include adenosis, transverse septa and ridges. Reproductive performance is reduced in these women as they have increased risk of spontaneous abortion, ectopic pregnancies, premature labor, and perinatal mortality.

Overall, patients with diethylstilbestrol exposure have a good chance for at least one viable pregnancy. After demonstration of a reproductive problem, a hysterosalpingogram is indicated. This population is also at risk of incompetent cervix and a cervical cerclage may be indicated.

Table 100.1 Treatments available in each class of abnormality

Class	Treatments available
IA	Vaginal dilators, vaginal anastomosis, McIndoe procedure
IB	Surgery unwarranted in most cases
IC	Removal of uterine remnant in cases with functional endometrium
ID	Tubal unification in cases of segmental tubal agenesis
IE	Dilator therapy, McIndoe procedure
II	Cervical cerclage, removal of horn when functional endometrium causes clinical problem
III	Cervical cerclage, value of metroplasty unclear, removal of vaginal septum
IV	Cervical cerclage, value of metroplasty unclear
V	Hysteroscopic resection, metroplasty
VI	No treatment needed
VII	Cervical cerclage

Conclusion

The fallopian tubes, uterus, and upper four-fifths of the vagina are created by fusion of the mullerian ducts occurring during the 10th–17th weeks of pregnancy. A disturbance of duct migration, fusion, growth or canalization may result in anatomic changes and functional impairment. The most common site of anomalies is the vagina, while cervical and uterine anomalies are equally common. Anomalies of the cervix and uterus are frequently accompanied by changes in the urinary tract.

Most congenital uterine anomalies can be accurately defined with imaging techniques including ultrasound (hydro)sonography, MRI, and hysterosalpingography. It is important that, prior to intervention, comprehensive examinations be carried out to establish which complaints are due to uterovaginal pathology and which may have other etiologies. Investigation for the cause of reproductive loss should include incompetent cervix, infections, endocrine disorders, chronic illness and karyotypic anomalies. Treatment options for the disorders covered in this chapter are listed in Table 100.1. Advanced operative laparoscopy, microsurgical techniques, and advanced reproductive technologies are now available to minimize operative morbidity and increase successful reproductive outcome.

Suggested reading

American Fertility Society. The American Fertility Society classifications of adnexal adhesion, distal tubal occlusion, tubal occlusion secondary to tubal ligation, tubal pregnancies, Müllerian anomalies and intrauterine adhesions. *Fertil Steril* 1988; 49: 944.

Coskun A, Okur N, Ozdemir O, Kiran G, Arykan DC. Uterine didelphys with an obstructed unilateral vagina by a transverse vaginal septum associated with ipsilateral renal agenesis, duplication of inferior vena cava, high-riding aortic bifurcation, and intestinal malrotation: a case report. *Fertil Steril* 2008; 90(5): 2006.

Damewood MD, Rock JA. Uterine reconstructive surgery. In: Hunt RB (ed) *Text and atlas of female infertility surgery*, 3rd edn. St Louis, MO: Mosby, 1999: 268–286.

DeCherney AH, Russell JB, Braebe RA, Polan ML. Resectoscopic management of Müllerian fusion defects. *Fertil Steril* 1986; 45: 726.

Fedele L, Dorta M, Brioschi D, *et al*. Magnetic resonance imaging in Mayer–Rokitansky–Kustner–Hauser syndrome. *Obstet Gynecol* 1990; 76: 593.

Golan A, Langer R, Bukovsky I, Caspi E. Congenital anomalies of the Müllerian system. *Fertil Steril* 1989; 51: 747.

Green LK, Harris RE. Uterine anomalies. *Obstet Gynecol* 1976; 47: 427.

Grimbizis GF, Camus M, Tarlatzis BC, Bontis JN, Devroey P. Clinical implications of uterine malformations and hysteroscopic treatment results. *Hum Reprod Update* 2001; 7(2): 161–174.

Heinonen PK. Primary infertility and uterine anomalies. *Fertil Steril* 1983; 40: 311.

Heinonen PK, Saarikoski S, Pystynen P. Reproductive performance of women with uterine anomalies. *Acta Obstet Gynecol Scand* 1982; 61: 157.

Hwang JH, Oh MJ, Lee NW, Hur JY, Lee KW, Lee JK. Multiple vaginal Müllerian cysts: a case report and review of the literature. *Arch Gynecol Obstet* 2009; 280(1): 137–139.

Jayaprakasan K, Campbell B, Hopkisson J, Johnson I, Raine-Fenning N. A prospective, comparative analysis of anti-Müllerian hormone, inhibin-B, and three dimensional ultrasound determinants of ovarian reserve in the prediction of poor response to controlled ovarian stimulation. *Fertil Steril* 2008; Nov 29 (Epub ahead of print).

Leung JWT, Hricak H. Role of magnetic resonsance imaging in the evaluation of gynecologic disease. In: Callen PW (ed) *Ultrasonography in obstetrics and gynecology*, 4th edn. Philadelphia, PA: WB Saunders, 2000: 940.

Mazouni C, Girard G, Deter R, *et al*. Diagnosis of Müllerian anomalies in adults: evaluation of practice. *Fertil Steril* 2008; 89; 219.

Oppelt P, van Have M, Palusen M, *et al*. Female genital malformations and their associated abnormalities. *Fertil Steril* 2007; 87; 335.

Rock JA. Surgery for anomalies of the Müllerian ducts. In: Thompson, JD, Rock, JA (eds) *Telinde's operative gynecology*, 7th edn. Philadelphia, PA: JB Lippincott, 1992: 603–660.

Rossier MC, Bays V, Vial Y, Achtari C. Congenital uterine anomalies: diagnosis, prognosis and management in 2008. *Rev Med Suisse* 2008; 4(176): 2253–2260.

Simon C, Martinez L, Pardo F, *et al*. Müllerian defects in women with normal reproductive outcome. *Fertil Steril* 1992; 56: 1192.

Taylor E, Gomel V. The uterus and fertility. *Fertil Steril* 2008; 89(1): 1–16.

Vercelini P, Daguati R, Somigliana E, *et al*. Asymmetric lateral distribution of obstructed hemivagina and renal agenesis in women with uterus didelphys: institutional case series and a systematic lierature review. *Fertil Steril* 2007; 87: 719.

Chapter 101
Tubal Factor in Infertility

Kristin A. Bendikson
Department of Medicine and Obstetrics and Gynecology, Keck School of Medicine, University of Southern California, CA, USA

Introduction

Historically, treatment of tubal factor infertility was limited to surgical restoration of normal pelvic architecture and the opening of obstructed fallopian tubes. Due to the high pregnancy rates achieved with *in vitro* fertilization (IVF), the role of surgical repair for tubal pathology has decreased. IVF bypasses tubal disease by direct retrieval of oocytes and uterine replacement of embryos. Surgical treatment of tubal disease is progressively less successful with worsening tubal pathology, whereas success rates with IVF are unaffected by the extent of tubal damage, except in cases of hydrosalpinges. In addition to lower pregnancy rates, surgical treatment is associated with an average of a 1.6 year delay to conception. Ectopic pregnancies are also more common after surgical treatment (5–20%) in comparison to IVF (1%). The biggest disadvantage to IVF is the significant cost to the patient.

Although the success of surgical repair for extensive tubal damage may be limited, there is a role for tubal repair in the case of minimal-to-moderate tubal damage. Tubal surgery can be justified with moderate-to-severe tubal disease when this is the only viable treatment option available to the patient. The prognosis for fertility after tubal reconstruction depends on the severity of the pre-existing disease. The probability of an intrauterine pregnancy following tuboplasty can range from 3% to 77%, depending on the degree of tubal damage.

The modern microsurgical approach to pelvic reconstruction has nearly doubled pregnancy rates when compared with conventional macrosurgical techniques. Magnification permits pinpoint application of energy sources so that minimal tissue is damaged. Presently, pregnancy rates for laparoscopy appear comparable to rates following laparotomy. However, operative laparoscopy is associated with a faster recovery, lower incidence of postoperative ileus, decreased postoperative pain, and a shorter hospital stay. Additionally, in the closed laparoscopic environment, drying of tissues is minimized and bleeding is reduced secondary to tamponade from the pneumoperitoneum, leading to decreased postoperative adhesion formation.

Prior to surgery, a thorough evaluation including history, physical examination, pelvic ultrasound, semen analysis, assessment of ovulation, and hysterosalpingogram should be performed as well as a review of any prior operative reports. The patient should be counseled extensively about the possible surgical findings and treatment options, as well as the risks of ectopic pregnancy and surgical treatment failure. Surgical treatment for tubal factor infertility can be categorized as adhesiolysis, fimbrioplasty, neosalpingostomy, removal of hydrosalpinx, proximal tubal cannulation, uterotubal junction implantation and tubal reanastomosis.

Adhesiolysis

For those patients with periadnexal adhesions, pregnancy rates can be substantially reduced as pelvic adhesions may impair oocyte pick-up between the ovary and fimbria. Adhesiolysis involves removing peritubal and adnexal adhesions. Tulandi *et al.* calculated cumulative pregnancy rates among infertile patients with adnexal adhesions. After adhesiolysis, these rates were 32% and 45% at 12 and 24 months respectively, but only 11% and 16% in the same time periods in patients who did not undergo adhesiolysis. Although the adhesiolysis was performed by laparotomy in these patients, similar results can be expected via laparoscopy.

Microsurgical techniques minimize the risk of postoperative adhesion formation. Other recommended ways to reduce postoperative adhesion formation include tissue irrigation, delicate handling of tissue, minimal suturing, minimal blood loss, and the use of prophylactic antibiotics. Intraoperatively, physical barriers have been utilized in order to minimize adhesion formation. Both oxidized regenerated cellulose and hyaluronic acid sheets have

Management of Common Problems in Obstetrics and Gynecology, 5th edition. Edited by T.M. Goodwin, M.N. Montoro, L. Muderspach, R. Paulson and S. Roy. © 2010 Blackwell Publishing Ltd.

been shown to be effective in decreasing postoperative adhesion formation.

Fimbrioplasty

Fimbrioplasty refers to repair of the fimbria at the distal end of the fallopian tube. Fimbrial phimosis, damage or loss of the fimbria, can lead to partial obstruction of the fallopian tube. Often, adhesive bands are found surrounding and occluding the distal end of the tube. Surgical procedures can release agglutinized fimbria, lyze adhesive bands or broaden a phimotic fimbrial opening. Repair can be accomplished by either direct release of occlusive bands or by gently opening a forcep after it has been inserted into the end of the tube to release minor agglutination and stretch the opening. Pregnancy rates for patients undergoing fimbrioplasty are excellent. Donnez *et al.* reported a 60% intrauterine pregnancy rate with a 2% ectopic rate after fimbrioplasty. A similar study found a 51% pregnancy rate and 37% livebirth rate after laparoscopic fimbrioplasty in infertile women.

Neosalpingostomy

Neosalpingostomy is the surgical construction of a new distal ostia. This procedure can be carried out via either laparoscopy or laparotomy. The surgical technique may use either laser or suture. With the laser technique, a defocused laser beam of low-power density ($10–50 \, W/cm^2$) is applied to the serosal surface to "flower" the distal end. With suturing, the edges of the newly formed ostia are everted and then sewn back on to the adjacent serosa. Overall, the pregnancy rates after a neosalpingostomy are variable, but are generally below 30% and ectopic pregnancies account for up to 5–15% of pregnancies. However, efficacy of the procedure depends heavily on the condition of the entire tube at the time of surgery, including tubal wall thickness, presence of mucosal folds and ampullary dilation. This accounts for the wide variation in reported postoperative pregnancy rates, as high as 80% when tubal morphology is normal with the exception of the fimbrial end or as low as zero in cases of diffuse and severe tubal disease. Therefore, in cases of severe disease, IVF is more likely to be successful than surgical repair.

Removal of hydrosalpinx

Multiple studies have confirmed that the presence of a hydrosalpinx has detrimental effects on pregnancy rates in IVF cycles. Several mechanisms may account for this negative effect, including a direct toxic effect on the endometrium and embryos via micro-organisms, debris, toxins and cytokines present in hydrosalpinx fluid. In addition, hydrosalpinges may mechanically flush the embryo from the uterus. A meta-analysis published in 1998 demonstrated that the presence of a hydrosalpinx decreased pregnancy rates by one-half, in both fresh and frozen IVF cycles. As with other morphologic aspects of the tubes, the worse the hydrosalpinx, the more likely it is to have a detrimental effect on pregnancy rates, especially when the diameter of the hydroxalpinx is greater than 1.5 cm. Several studies have demonstrated an improvement in IVF outcomes in patients who underwent surgical salpingectomy to remove a hydrosalpinx in comparison to those patients in whom the hydrosalpinx was not removed. Although salpingectomy is preferred prior to IVF, neosalpingostomy can be performed to eliminate the accumulated hydrosalpinx, and has been shown in one small study to have encouraging results. When IVF is not available, neosalpingostomy may be the only option. Prior to IVF, proximal tubal cauterization or clipping can be considered in cases when a salpingectomy cannot be performed secondary to extensive pelvic adhesions.

Proximal tubal cannulation

Proximal tubal cannulation is a method of opening the fallopian tube lumen in cases of minimal proximal blockage. It involves the insertion of a cathether, with a progressively increasing diameter, into the proximal ostia and interstitial fallopian tube in order to break up any adhesions. This procedure is carried out via the hysteroscope but is best performed with concomitant laparoscopy. Selective cannulation is successful in opening blocked tubes in 60–80% of patients, with a pregnancy rate of approximately 24% and a relatively low ectopic pregnancy rate of about 3%. Because of the risk of perforation, this technique can only be used in cases with minimal proximal intraluminal blockage.

Uterotubal implantation

Uterotubal implantation is the reimplantation of a tubal segment into the uterine cornu performed in cases of severe cornual occlusion. The diseased cornual portion of the tube is resected, then the new end of the tube is reattached to the uterus. This procedure requires laparotomy and microsurgical anastomosis. Term pregnancy rates range from 14% to 55%.

Tubal reanastomosis

Although most commonly used for sterilization reversal, tubal reanastomosis can be performed in order to remove abnormal tissue. Tubal reanastomosis has been successfully performed in cases of pathologic mid-tubal blockage, tubal occlusion from an ectopic pregnancy and salpingitis isthmica nodosa ("tubo-cornual reanastomosis"). In all scenarios, the goal is to unite two healthy segments of tube in order to re-establish functional tubal patency. Conception rates correlate with tubal morphology, the final length of the tube after anastomosis, and the type of sterilization previously performed. With tubal reanastomosis, pregnancy rates following tubal ligation are the most successful, with pregnancy rates after reversal operations ranging from 50% to 84%. Success of the reanastomosis is most commonly achieved after sterilization with clips (84%), followed by rings (75%), then the Pomeroy procedure (50%) and is least likely after electrocautery (41%). Magnification, microcautery, atraumatic technique and accurate approximation of tubal segments are critical to the success of this procedure. Pregnancy rates resulting from microsurgical sterilization reversal or laparoscopic tubal anastomosis are equivalent. Sterilization reversals can be considered if there is at least 4 cm of residual tube remaining.

Conclusion

Surgical correction of abnormalities can be successful in cases of minor tubal damage, and remains an important tool in the treatment of infertility. However, when severe morphologic abnormalities exist, prognosis after surgery is poor and IVF is the preferred fertility treatment. Patients need to be carefully selected for appropriate management, which may include surgical exploration to assess the extent of tubal damage. It is important to individualize and patients need to be thoroughly counseled on the risks, benefits and success rates of surgical repair in comparison to the option of IVF.

Suggested reading

Audibert F, Hedon B, Arnal F, *et al*. Therapeutic strategies in tubal infertility with distal pathology. *Hum Reprod* 1991; 6: 1439–1442.

Audibert AJ, Pouly JL, von Theobald P. Laparoscopic fimbrioplasty: an evaluation of 35 cases. *Hum Reprod* 1998; 13: 1496.

Bateman BG, Nubley JWC, Kitenin JD. Surgical management of distal tubal obstruction – are we making progress? *Fertil Steril* 1987; 48: 523.

Blazar AS, Hogan JW, Seifer DB, *et al*. The impact of hydrosalpinx on successful pregnancy in tubal factor infertility treated by *in vitro* fertilization. *Fertil Steril* 1997; 67: 517–520.

Boer-Meisel M, Tevelde ER, Habbema JDF, Kardaun JPF. Predicting the pregnancy outcome in patients treated for hydrosalpinx: a prospective study. *Fertil Steril* 1986; 45: 23.

Camus E, Poncelet C, Goffinet F, *et al*. Pregnancy rates after *in-vitro* fertilization in cases of tubal infertility with and without hydrosalpinx: a meta-analysis of published comparative studies. *Hum Reprod* 1999; 14: 1243.

Diamond MP. Reduction of adhesions after uterine myomectomy by Seprafilm membrane (HAL-F): a blinded, prospective, randomized, multicenter clinical study. Seprafilm Adhesion Study Group. *Fertil Steril* 1996; 66: 904.

Diugi AM, Reddy S, Salen WA, *et al*. Pregnancy rates after operative endoscopic treatment of total (neosalpingostomy) or near total (salpingostomy) distal tubal occlusion. *Fertil Steril* 1990; 54: 390.

Donnez J, Casanas-Roux F. Prognostic factors of fimbrial microsurgery. *Fertil Steril* 1986; 46: 200.

Donnez J, Nisolle M, Casanas-Roux F. CO2 laser laparoscopy in infertile women with adnexal adhesions and women with tubal occlusion. *J Gynecol Surg* 1989; 5: 47–53.

Dubuisson JB, de Joliniere JB, Aubriot FX, *et al*. Terminal tuboplasties by laparoscopy: 65 consecutive cases. *Fertil Steril* 1990; 54: 401–403.

Eyraud B, Erny R, Vergnet F. Distal tubal surgery using laparoscopy. *J Gynecol Obstet Biol Reprod* 1993; 22: 9–14.

Farquhar C, Vandekerckhove P, Watson A, *et al*. Barrier agents for preventing adhesions after surgery for subfertility. *Cochrane Databse Syst Rev* 2000; 2: CD000475.

Fayez JA. An assessment of the role of operative laparoscopy in tuboplasty. *Fertil Steril* 1983; 39: 476–479.

Freeman MR, Whitworth CM, Hill GA. Permanent impairment of embryo development by hydrosalpinges. *Hum Reprod* 1998; 13: 983–986.

Gomel V. Laparoscopic tubal surgery in infertility. *Obstet Gynecol* 1975; 46: 47–48.

Gomel V. Salpingo-ovariolysis by laparoscopy in infertility. *Fertil Steril* 1983; 40: 607–611.

Jauer MV, Zeffer KB, Bustillo M, Buster JE. Sterilization reversals performed by fellows in training; what success rates can we resonably expect? *Microsurgery* 1987; 8: 125.

Mecke H, Lehmann-Willenbrock E, Lesoine B, *et al*. Pelviscopic treatment of female sterility. *Geburtwhilfe Fraueheilkd* 1993; 53: 693–699.

Mettler L, Giesel H, Semm K. Treatment of female infertility due to tubal obstruction by operative laparoscopy. *Fertil Steril* 1979; 32: 384–388.

Musich JR, Behrman SJ. Surgical management of tubal obstruction at the uterotubal junction. *Fertil Steril* 1983; 40: 423.

Nackley AC, Muasher SJ. The significance of hydrosalpinx in *in vitro* fertilization. *Fertil Steril* 1998; 69: 373–384.

Reich H. Laparoscopic treatment of extensive pelvic adhesions, including hydroxalpinx. *J Reprod Med* 1987; 32: 736–742.

Thurmond AS. Pregnancies after selective salpingography and tubal recanalization. *Radiology* 1994; 190: 11.

Zeyneloglu HB, Arici A, Olive DL. Adverse effects of hydrosalpinx on pregnancy rates after in vitro fertilization-embryo transfer. *Fertil Steril* 1998; 70: 492–499.

Chapter 102
Unexplained infertility

Lauren Rubal and Richard J. Paulson
Department of Medicine and Obstetrics and Gynecology, Keck School of Medicine, University of Southern California, CA, USA

Introduction

Infertility in a couple is defined as the inability to conceive after 1 year of sexual intercourse without the use of any contraceptive method. This group can be further subdivided into those who will eventually be able to conceive without intervention and those who cannot conceive without therapy. Couples in the former category have decreased fecundability, since their probability of achieving a pregnancy within one menstrual cycle is lower than the fertile population.

Specific causes of decreased fecundability can be identified in most couples who are unable to conceive after 1 year of unprotected intercourse. The diagnostic infertility assessment determines the putative cause of infertility in the majority of cases. However, in the remaining 10–30% of couples, the etiology of infertility cannot be specifically attributed to a specific cause. Couples with unexplained infertility have a normal work-up. Specifically, this assessment is composed of documentation of ovulation, tubal patency, a normal uterine cavity, a normal semen analysis, and adequate ovarian reserve.

Unexplained infertility may constitute a group at the lowest limit of normal in terms of fertility status or those with abnormalities in aspects of conception that we currently do not have the ability to diagnose. Conception as a whole is composed of many intricate processes, and thus there are multiple areas in which abnormalities may occur. In order for pregnancy to take place, the ovary must release a mature egg that then must be transported to the fallopian tube, where it must be fertilized by a sperm. The resulting embryo must then be transferred to the uterus, where it must implant into the endometrium. A flaw at any one or more of these points may be manifested as unexplained infertility.

Management of Common Problems in Obstetrics and Gynecology, 5th edition. Edited by T.M. Goodwin, M.N. Montoro, L. Muderspach, R. Paulson and S. Roy. © 2010 Blackwell Publishing Ltd.

Cycle fecundability is decreased in couples with unexplained infertility. The duration of infertility and the age of the female partner further affect cycle fecundability. In young couples first attempting conception, it is about 20%. Among couples with unexplained infertility, fecundability decreases with each passing year. After 3 years of unsuccessful attempts at conception, young couples have an approximately 3% fecundability, which drops to about 2% after 5 years. Fecundability among older couples is even lower.

Potential etiologies

Female partner's age

There is a well-documented decrease in female fertility that is age dependent and occurs many years prior to menopause. Eventually, this decline manifests as diminished ovarian reserve. This is reflected in both reduced oocyte quantity as well as oocyte quality. Decreased oocyte quantity results in a diminished response to ovarian stimulation, whereas decreased oocyte quality is reflected by a decrease in embryo implantation. This process occurs even in the absence of a rise in serum FSH levels.

A decline in fertility begins in many women in their early 30s, and becomes more pronounced as they grow older. A recent study examined a cohort of 1654 women undergoing donor insemination for male or situational infertility. The cumulative delivery after 12 cycles of natural, clomiphene or gonadotropin ovarian stimulation varied by age group. Specifically, it was 87% for the group aged 20–29, 77% for ages 30–34, 76% for ages 35–37, 66% for ages 38–39 and 52% for ages 40–45. This difference in age was the only variable that significantly affected the cumulative delivery rate. Prior observational trials in several countries corroborate the finding that fertility decreases with advancing age.

An associated finding is that success with assisted reproductive technologies (ART) decreases with increasing age. Also, the incidence of spontaneous miscarriage increases as the woman becomes older. This is thought to be due to oocyte abnormalities, such as anomalous meiotic spindles, and microtubule matrix changes, which lead to an increase in aneuploidy. These defects contribute to the increased miscarriage rate in older women of over 50% by the the age of 43.

Male partner

Semen analysis parameters have been determined by the World Health Organization (WHO) to evaluate sperm concentration, motility, and normal morphology. However, the normal values are based on limited data. Furthermore, there is sizeable overlap between normal and abnormal ranges in men both fertile and infertile. It is also recognized that the same man may produce semen that varies markedly in these parameters, depending on the sample. Therefore, subtle abnormalities in sperm may result in an intermittent ability to fertilize oocytes and the couple may present with infertility that will appear to be unexplained.

Many tests have been developed over the years to better assess sperm function. The sperm penetration assay, also known as the zona-free hamster oocyte penetration test, is one such evaluation. Normally, the zona pellucida protects the oocyte against multiple sperm entry or sperm from different species. In the hamster oocytes to be tested, the zona pellucida is removed by enzymes, and sperm from the infertile male are introduced. Simultaneously, sperm from a proven fertile male are incubated with another zona-free hamster oocyte. Comparative results are then generated. While this test initially appeared very promising for being able to quantify sperm function, it eventually proved not to be clinically useful, primarily because of variability between samples and overlap between normal and abnormal males. The hemi-zona binding assay evaluated the ability of sperm to bind to the human zona pellucida. Unfortunately, this test was also shown to have limited predictive value.

At the present time, sperm are evaluated with a standard semen analysis including semen volume, sperm concentration, evaluation of the percentage of motile sperm, and a morphologic assessment according to "strict" criteria. This has proven to be as good a predictor of fertilization *in vitro* as any other test. If the percentage of normal forms is less than 5%, intracytoplasmic injection (ICSI) in conjunction with IVF is recommended.

Cervical factor

The cervix is the entry point of sperm into the uterine cavity. Anatomic abnormalities in the cervical area (such as cervical stenosis) may interfere with sperm transport and result in infertility. It has also been hypothesized that abnormal cervical mucus production can impede sperm transport.

It was for this reason that the postcoital test was developed. The test analyzed the volume, consistency, ferning, spinnbarkeit, cellularity, and pH of the cervical mucus. It also assessed the sperm count and motility. Normally, the test was performed a few days before expected ovulation. After intercourse, the woman was examined and a sample of cervical mucus was obtained.

However, the clinical utility of this test was found to be limited. There was no standardized range of normal values, and results from clinical trials demonstrated conflicting results on the utility of the test. Most importantly, a randomized trial showed no difference in pregnancy rates whether the postcoital test was included in the infertility work-up or not. Eventually, the test was abandoned. This does not mean that the cervix may not play a role in unexplained infertility. The utility of intrauterine insemination (IUI) may be inferred as indirect evidence that the cervix may indeed play a role in some cases of unexplained infertility.

Subtle ovulatory dysfunction

Subtle ovulatory dysfunction has also been postulated as an etiology of unexplained infertility. A history of regular menstrual cycles provides an indication that ovulation is most likely taking place. Nevertheless, current diagnostic tests for ovulation (for example, basal body temperature shift and mid-luteal phase serum progesterone) provide only indirect evidence of ovulation and cannot confirm the actual release of the oocyte.

In the absence of an ideal method, the measurement of mid-luteal progesterone levels in plasma is probably the most cost-effective compromise to indicate that ovulation has occurred using hormonal methods. Because progesterone is released in a pulsatile manner, more than one assay may be needed to determine serum levels accurately. The value of 3 ng/mL correlates with a finding of secretory endometrium and has been used for presumptive indication of ovulation. Hull *et al.* found that a value of 10 ng/mL more closely correlates with subsequent conception, suggesting that lower levels, while indicative of ovulation, may be associated with subtle ovulatory inadequacy. The utility of superovulation may thus be inferred as indirect evidence that subtle ovulatory dysfunction may be a part of the etiology of unexplained infertility.

Luteal-phase defect

Luteal-phase defect (LPD) is defined as an abnormality in the endometrium during the postovulatory (luteal) phase of the menstrual cycle. This has been hypothesized to lead to diminished endometrial receptivity and consequent lack of embryo implantation. The diagnosis of LPD has traditionally been confirmed by obtaining a biopsy of the endometrium in the late luteal phase. The biopsy was histologically evaluated to ascertain the day of the cycle to which it corresponded. The date of the biopsy was then established by counting the number of days from the biopsy to the first day of the next menstrual cycle and subtracting this number from 28. The two dates were then compared. If a discrepancy of more than 2 days was found in two separate cycles, a diagnosis of LPD was made.

There is no question that there is such a thing as poor endometrial receptivity, and thus LPD was postulated as a cause of unexplained infertility. However, studies have noted LPD in up to 51% of normal fertile women if a single biopsy was 2 or more days out of phase and a 27% incidence if sequential biopsies were analyzed. By comparison, the incidence of LPD in infertile couples was reported to be less than 5%, similar to a fertile population. Furthermore, the clinical association between LPD and infertility is tenuous at best. Treatment of LPD has not been shown to improve pregnancy outcome. Therefore, it is not necessary to test for LPD during the infertility evaluation. However, empiric progesterone supplementation during treatment with superovulation continues to be utilized, due to a demonstration of the utility of progesterone supplementation during *in vitro* fertilization.

Infections

Clinical infection of the female reproductive tract is associated with inflammatory cells, a purulent cervical discharge, and a hostile environment that can lead to miscarriage and prevent implantation. Therefore, it is tempting to speculate that subclinical infections may play a subtle role in inhibiting conception. It has been previously suggested that *Mycoplasma hominis* and *Ureaplasma urealyticum* in the male and female genital tract could interfere with sperm function and normal sperm transport. An early clinical trial showed improvement in pregnancy rates with antibiotic treatment to eradicate these organisms. However, subsequent randomized controlled trials reported no such difference in pregnancy rates between the treated and placebo groups. At this time, obtaining screening cultures to assess for these organisms is not recommended and empiric treatment with antibiotics is not recommended.

Immunologic factors

The presence of antisperm antibodies in the male or female partner has been suggested to interfere with sperm motility and oocyte fertilization. Clarke and his group described a test with the ability to detect IgA, IgM, and IgG antibodies bound to sperm membranes. This immunobead test can detect the presence of antisperm antibodies in the serum or cervical mucus or directly in the ejaculate. Antisperm antibodies are especially prevalent in men who have experienced testicular infection, injury or surgical procedures (for example, vasectomy reversal). Nevertheless, detection of antibodies as an isolated factor among couples with unexplained infertility has not been shown to alter the prognosis for fertility.

Smarr *et al.* performed a retrospective analysis comparing women with high titers of antisperm antibody who received corticosteroid therapy to those who received no treatment. The study group did not experience any increase in the pregnancy rate. Corticosteroid treatment of infertile men with positive antisperm antibody titers has also not resulted in increased pregnancy rates.

While there possibly is an association between different antibody titers and infertility, the tests employed are variable and the results have been inconsistent. Thus, there is no standardized way to interpret the results of these tests and they are not typically ordered in a work-up for unexplained infertility. However, it has been observed that men with prior proven fertility who subsequently underwent vasectomy and vasectomy reversal may fail to fertilize oocytes during IVF, apparently as a result of autoantibodies. Therefore, these types of antisperm antibodies may indeed play a role in preventing fertilization. And therefore, couples with unexplained infertility after vasectomy reversal in the male partner may benefit from an earlier application of IVF with ICSI.

Implantation failure due to poor endometrial function

An embryo cannot implant on an endometrium that is not receptive to it. The concepts of postcoital contraception and the intrauterine device are based on this principle. In response, inhibition of implantation by poor endometrial function has been suggested as a possible cause of unexplained infertility. Furthermore, uterine trauma, such as that caused by irradiation or uterine surgery, may lead to an endometrium that is persistently thin or one that does not proliferate in response to estrogen. In these instances, the endometrium may never develop adequate receptivity to allow embryo implantation.

Among the many postulated markers of endometrial receptivity are the adhesion molecules, the cathedrins and integrins. To assess uterine receptivity in women with unexplained infertility, Lessey *et al.* evaluated the levels of β-3 integrin subunits in endometrial biopsies obtained during the window of implantation (days 20–24 of the menstrual cycle). All endometrial biopsies from parous controls showed positive immunostaining for β-3 integrin. In contrast, biopsies from women with unexplained infertility revealed significantly reduced β-3 expression. The authors concluded that abnormal endometrial integrin expression was a frequent finding in their population of women with unexplained infertility and suggested that defective uterine receptivity may be an unrecognized cause of infertility in this population.

However, since endometrial development is dependent on adequate stimulation with estrogen and progesterone, it may be that subtle endometrial dysfunction is secondary to subtle ovulatory dysfunction or inadequate stimulation of the endometrium. It has not been demonstrated that specific testing for integrins provides independent information about the endometrium which would point treatment in a direction different from standard superovulation plus IUI. Therefore, as long as the uterine cavity is normal, and as long as the endometrium demonstrates appropriate proliferation (as evidenced by endometrial thickness of ≥7 mm), additional endometrial function testing is not indicated.

Current treatment options

Because couples with unexplained infertility are subfertile (rather than sterile), a substantial proportion of them will conceive without therapy. Thus, the decision to initiate treatment depends on two factors: the duration of infertility and the woman's age. The duration of infertility is negatively correlated with the fecundability rate. A study by Hull showed that cumulative rates of spontaneous conception in couples with unexplained infertility were inversely related to the woman's age and the length of infertility. As a result, the choice between empiric treatment and expectant management must be based on the female partner's age, duration of infertility, and the couple's wishes, based on the best estimates of prognosis given observation or treatment. Since no specific cause is found in patients with unexplained infertility, treatment is therefore considered empiric. All the described therapies increase the number and proximity of oocytes and sperm.

Expectant management

It is important to review the natural history of couples with unexplained infertility before considering therapy. The spontaneous cumulative pregnancy rate (that is, without therapy) in couples with unexplained infertility who were followed for 2–7 years has been reported to range from 30% to 60%. Snick *et al.* followed a cohort of infertile couples in The Netherlands who were not treated for infertility. They found that these subjects still had a cumulative livebirth rate of 52.5% at 36 months. In fact, couples with unexplained infertility had the highest cumulative livebirth rate (60.6%) out of all types of subfertility. Another study examining the natural history of unexplained infertility found that greater than 30% of couples become pregnant after 36 months.

Intrauterine insemination

Introduction of semen into the uterine cavity has been used for more than 100 years as a treatment for infertility. Intrauterine insemination (IUI) has also been employed for the empiric treatment of couples with unexplained infertility. The premise behind IUI is to increase the number of motile sperm in the uterine cavity at the time of ovulation. There are different methods of preparing the semen specimen: the swim-up technique, the density gradient centrifugation method, and the simple wash with centrifugation. The first two techniques differentially

separate the motile sperm by either ability to swim up to the culture media overlying a semen sample or by having the highest density after centrifugation, respectively. The last procedure removes prostaglandins from the semen and concentrates the sperm into a small volume in preparation for placement inside the uterus.

There have not been many randomized trials examining the effect of IUI alone versus timed intercourse in couples with unexplained infertility. One trial in 73 couples with unexplained infertility showed no statistically significant difference in pregnancy rate between the two. Another study examined the difference between IUI and intracervical insemination (ICI, used as a correlate of natural intercourse) in infertile couples with a predominant diagnosis of unexplained infertility. This trial found a statistically significant increase in pregnancy rate with IUI of 4.9% compared with 2.0% of ICI cycles. However, this effect is small. A review of the literature shows that the common odds ratio of IUI as compared with timed intercourse is 2.0, with a 95% confidence interval (CI) of 0.7–6.1; this finding is not statistically significant. Therefore, IUI is commonly combined with superovulation instead of being the sole treatment for unexplained infertility.

Clomiphene citrate with or without IUI

Empiric treatment with clomiphene citrate (CC) is based on the rationale that increasing the number of oocytes available for fertilization in a given cycle may increase the probability of at least one released oocyte producing a viable conception. An alternative mechanism involves correction of subtle abnormalities of ovulation, including LPD and luteinized unruptured follicle. The empiric use of CC has been studied in many comparative trials. Several randomized controlled trials demonstrate that CC use alone does not significantly increase the pregnancy rate over placebo. A recent Cochrane review of use of CC alone for unexplained infertility also stated that there is no evidence that it is more effective than no treatment or placebo.

Several studies have addressed issues related to the combination of CC and IUI, and have shown increased fecundability in such cycles. In a prospective, randomized, cross-over study of couples with unexplained infertility, Deaton *et al.* demonstrated increased cycle fecundability rates with CC/IUI (9.7%) compared with spontaneous cycles with timed intercourse (3.3%); the odds ratio (OR) was 2.8 (95% CI 1.1–7.0). A meta-analysis performed by Guzick *et al.* to examine the effectiveness of various described treatments for unexplained infertility also confirmed that CC/IUI was a cost-effective and beneficial treatment. Even though alternative treatments have higher fecundity rates, CC/IUI is the most cost-effective, and can be attempted for several cycles prior to initiating treatment with either hMG/IUI or IVF.

At our institution, we start CC at a dose of 100 mg beginning on day 3 of the cycle, and continue treatment for 5 days. Patients must be counseled that there is a small but increased risk of multiple pregnancies (approximately 8%) and ovarian hyperstimulation syndrome (OHSS, rare) with the use of CC. Treatment should be initiated before the dominant follicle is recruited, and ideally at least two mature follicles will be present. Plosker *et al.* showed that the pregnancy rate per cycle was significantly greater only when two or more mature follicles were stimulated per cycle, supporting the concept of increased pregnancy rates only with increased follicular recruitment.

Human menopausal gonadotropins with or without IUI

Superovulation with hMG with or without IUI has also been utilized as empiric treatment for unexplained infertility. Gonadotropins appear to increase the baseline fecundability even when used alone, and there is a marked increase when they are combined with IUI. This has been supported by several clinical trials. A Cochrane review of ovarian stimulation protocols combined with IUI in subfertile women indicated that pregnancy rates with gonadotropins were significantly increased compared with CC (OR 1.8, 95% CI 1.2–27). Studies suggest that there is a reduction in fecundability after three cycles of hMG/IUI. Some experts advise that couples should be encouraged to proceed with IVF rather than continue with hMG/IUI after three cycles. The risks of multiple gestation and OHSS are significant with the use of gonadotropins, and the patient must be aware of these possibilities. Even though high-order multiple gestations (triplets or more) are relatively uncommon, the potential need for selective fetal reduction must be discussed with the patient before therapy is initiated.

Assisted reproductive technologies

Couples with unexplained infertility who fail to respond to superovulation with IUI are generally advised to undergo assisted reproductive technologies (ART). Numerous studies have evaluated the benefits of *in vitro* fertilization-embryo transfer (IVF-ET), gamete intrafallopian tube transfer (GIFT), and zygote intrafallopian tube transfer (ZIFT) in couples who fail to conceive with superovulation and IUI. Essentially, all studies have demonstrated a favorable outcome, with pregnancy and fecundability rates similar to couples with tubal disease undergoing IVF, despite a higher incidence of fertilization failure noted in couples with unexplained infertility. In the 2007 Society for Assisted Reproductive Technology national IVF data, the percentage of any type of ART cycle resulting in pregnancy for couples with unexplained infertility was as follows: 46.1% for women <35 years, 39.0% for 35–37 year olds, 33.0% for 38–40 year olds, and 21.3%

for 41–42 year olds. It must be noted, however, that a recent Cochrane analysis of the 10 randomized, controlled trials examining the success of IVF compared with other treatments for unexplained infertility found it difficult to draw conclusions about IVF due to heterogeneity of the studies, lack of power, and inadequate follow-up. The risks of multiple gestations and OHSS are very real risks that must also be addressed.

These cautions notwithstanding, IVF remains an effective treatment of unexplained infertility, especially with couples who have failed the more conservative therapies.

Conclusion

The diagnosis of unexplained infertility is defined as the presence of infertility for at least 1 year despite documented ovulation, tubal patency, and normal semen analysis. All other diagnostic tests advocated for evaluation of infertile couples have unproven value for this condition. Therefore, treatment is empiric by definition. The treatment of unexplained infertility with IUI alone is not indicated. Instead, treatment with hMG or CC combined with IUI should be recommended. Assisted reproductive technologies have the highest fecundability rates per cycle, albeit with the addition of considerable expense.

Based on currently available data, a treatment plan for unexplained infertility can be developed. Individualization of this plan should encompass the desires of the couple, taking into account their financial and emotional status, the woman's age, and the duration of the infertility. The treatment plan information presented to the couple should take into account all these factors. The couple need to be made aware of their prognosis and expected long-term plan.

On the basis of these considerations, the current treatment in our clinic for improving fecundability in couples with a female partner younger than 35 with unexplained infertility involves expectant management or 3–6 months of CC/IUI. The next step in the treatment is hMG/IUI for 3 months. If unsuccessful, one of the assisted reproductive fertilization techniques is advised. Women over the age of 35 are offered more aggressive therapy at an earlier time in their treatment regimen and are usually treated with 3 months of superovulation/IUI, followed by ART.

Suggested reading

Athaullah N, Proctor M, Johnson N. Oral versus injectable ovulation induction agents for unexplained subfertility. *Cochrane Database Syst Rev* 2002; 3: CD003052.

Bhattacharya S, Hamilton MP, Shaaban M, *et al.* Conventional in-vitro fertilization versus intracytoplasmic sperm injection for the treatment of non-male-factor infertility: a randomized controlled trial. *Lancet* 2001; 357: 2075.

Cantineau AE, Cohlen BJ, Heineman MJ. Ovarian stimulation protocols (anti-oestrogens, gonadotrophins with and without

GnRH agonists/antagonists) for intrauterine insemination (IUI) in women with subfertility. *Cochrane Database Syst Rev* 2007; 2: CD005356.

Collins JA, Milner RA, Rowe TC. The effects of treatment on pregnancy among couples with unexplained infertility. *Int J Fertil* 1991; 36: 140.

Collins JA, Burrows EA, Wilan AR. The prognosis for live birth among untreated infertile couples. *Fertil Steril* 1995; 64: 22.

Crosignani PG, Walters DE, Soliani A. The ESHRE multicenter trial on the treatment of unexplained infertility: a preliminary report. *Hum Reprod* 1991; 6: 953.

Davis OK, Berkeley AS, Naus GJ, *et al*. The incidence of luteal phase defect in normal, fertile women, determined by serial endometrial biopsies. *Fertil Steril* 1989; 51: 582.

Deaton JL, Gibson M, Blackmer KM, *et al*. A randomized, controlled trial of clomiphene citrate and intrauterine insemination in couples with unexplained infertility or surgically corrected endometriosis. *Fertil Steril* 1990; 54: 1083.

Foong SC, Fleetham JA, O'Keane JA, Scott SG, Tough SC, Greene CA. A prospective randomized trial of conventional in vitro fertilization versus intracytoplasmic sperm injection in unexplained infertility. *J Assist Reprod Genet* 2006; 23: 137.

Glazener CMA, Coulson C, Lambert PA, *et al*. Clomiphene treatment for women with unexplained infertility: placebo-controlled study of hormone responses and conception rates. *Gynecol Endocrinol* 1990; 4: 75.

Guzick DS, Sullivan MW, Adamson GD, *et al*. Efficacy of treatment for unexplained infertility. *Fertil Steril* 1998; 70: 207.

Guzick DS, Carson SA, Coutifaris C, *et al*. Efficacy of superovulation and intrauterine insemination in the treatment of infertility. *NEJM* 1999; 340: 177.

Hughes E, Collins J, Vandekerckhove P. Clomiphene citrate for unexplained subfertility in women. *Cochrane Database Syst Rev* 2000; 2: CD000057.

Jaroudi K, Al-Hassan S, Al-Sufayan H, Al-Mayman H, Qeba M, Coskun S. Intracytoplasmic sperm injection and conventional in vitro fertilization are complementary techniques in management of unexplained infertility. *J Assist Reprod Genet* 2003; 20: 377.

Kirby CA, Flaherty SP, Godfrey BM, Warnes GM, Matthews CD. A prospective trial of intrauterine insemination of motile spermatozoa versus timed intercourse. *Fertil Steril* 1995; 56: 102.

Lessey BA, Castelbaum AJ, Sawin SW, Sun J. Integrins as markers of uterine receptivity in women with primary unexplained infertility. *Fertil Steril* 1995; 63: 535.

Pandian Z, Bhattacharya S, Vale L, Templeton A. In vitro fertilization for unexplained subfertility. *Cochrane Database System Rev* 2005; 2: CD003357.

Peterson M, Hatasaka H, Jones KP, *et al*. Ovulation induction with gonadotropin intrauterine insemination compared with in vitro fertilization and no therapy: a prospective, nonrandomized, cohort study and meta-analysis. *Fertil Steril* 1993; 62: 3.

Plosker SM, Jacobson W, Amato P. Predicting and optimizing success in an intrauterine insemination program. *Hum Reprod* 1994; 9: 11.

Smarr SC, Hammond MG. Effect of therapy on infertile couples with antisperm antibodies. *Am J Obstet Gynecol* 1988; 158: 969.

Snick HK, Snick TS, Evers JL, Collins JA. The spontaneous pregnancy prognosis in untreated subfertile couples: the Walcheren primary care study. *Hum Reprod* 1997; 12: 1582.

Stolwijk AM, Wetzels AM, Braat DD. Cumulative probability of achieving an ongoing pregnancy after in-vitro fertilization and intracytoplasmic sperm injection according to a woman's age, subfertility diagnosis and primary or secondary subfertility. *Hum Reprod* 2000; 15: 203.

Verhulst SM, Cohlen BJ, Hughes E, Heineman MJ, te Velde E. Intrauterine insemination for unexplained subfertility. *Cochrane Database System Rev* 2006; 4: CD001838.

Chapter 103
Human *In Vitro* Fertilization and Related Assisted Reproductive Techniques

Richard J. Paulson

Department of Medicine and Obstetrics and Gynecology, Keck School of Medicine, University of Southern California, CA, USA

Introduction

The extracorporeal fertilization of mammalian oocytes was first reported over three decades ago by the British team of Steptoe and Edwards. They were the first to report a pregnancy after *in vitro* fertilization (IVF) of a human egg and also the first to achieve the birth of an *in vitro* fertilized baby. Since then, hundreds of thousands of pregnancies have been achieved worldwide by IVF and its modifications, collectively known as assisted reproductive techniques (ARTs). As experience has accumulated, success rates have increased and the indications for the ARTs have expanded. According to the 2006 CDC report, 138,198 ART cycles took place in the United States during that year, resulting in 41,343 live births, and 54,656 infants, representing slightly more than 1% of all US births.

Patient selection

In vitro fertilization essentially performs the function of the fallopian tube in that it brings together the oocyte and sperm, allows for fertilization and then delivers the resulting embryo to the uterine cavity. Therefore, the initial experience with IVF involved women with tubal disease that could not be surgically corrected. With its efficacy established, IVF was progressively made available to patients with other infertility diagnoses. IVF is utilized when conventional therapy fails or when there is little hope that other therapy will be successful. Current indications for IVF include:
- absent or blocked fallopian tubes
- failed tuboplasty
- endometriosis
- male factor infertility
- unexplained infertility

In counseling patients with open fallopian tubes and without a severe male factor, alternative treatment options, including observation, must be considered, as some groups of IVF candidates have substantial treatment-independent pregnancy rates. The difficulty in deciding how soon to proceed to IVF arises in women of advanced reproductive age, in whom further expectant management may risk the occurrence of ovarian failure. In general, women with nontubal factor infertility are offered between three and six cycles of superovulation and intrauterine insemination (IUI) prior to proceeding to IVF. Among younger women, waiting for a total of 2 years of unprotected intercourse and/or conventional treatment is a reasonable guideline which may be used in counseling potential candidates.

One of the principal determinants of IVF success is the age of the female partner. Women over the age of 40 years experience a substantially reduced likelihood of pregnancy (Figure 103.1). This decrease in success

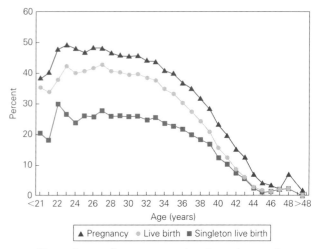

*For consistency, all percentages are based on cycles started.

Figure 103.1 Percentage of ART cycles using fresh nondonor eggs or embryos that resulted in pregnancies, livebirths and singleton livebirths, by age of woman. Reproduced from Center for Disease Control and Prevention: www.cdc.gov.

Management of Common Problems in Obstetrics and Gynecology, 5th edition. Edited by T.M. Goodwin, M.N. Montoro, L. Muderspach, R. Paulson and S. Roy. © 2010 Blackwell Publishing Ltd.

parallels that observed with other forms of fertility treatment. In IVF, the diminished success is due both to a decreased response to gonadotropin stimulation, resulting in a decreased number of embryos available for transfer, as well as decreased per embryo implantation rates. Additionally, pregnancies in older women are associated with increased miscarriage rates.

In addition to the advanced chronologic age of the female partner, elevated follicle-stimulating hormone (FSH) levels in the early follicular phase are associated with poor prognosis for pregnancies with IVF. A single FSH measurement may not be sufficient, as serum FSH levels are known to fluctuate from cycle to cycle. In one study addressing this issue, patients with one prior elevated (>20 mIU/mL) FSH level but normal subsequent levels were observed to achieve a 5.6% pregnancy rate. Patients with two or more previous elevated FSH levels did not achieve any pregnancies.

Recent data suggest that in addition to elevated early follicular phase FSH levels, elevated estradiol (E2) levels are also associated with a poor pregnancy outcome with IVF. One report identified a level of 75 pg/mL as being discriminatory between cycles with good and those with poor prognosis. We consider it reasonable to obtain day 3 serum measurements of E2 and FSH in all women over the age of 35 who are contemplating IVF, and to cancel cycles in those with FSH levels greater than 20 mIU/mL and/or E2 levels greater than 100 pg/mL. If levels are elevated upon repeated measurements, other forms of therapy (e.g. oocyte donation) should be considered. Younger patients who exhibit a poor ovarian response to exogenous gonadotropins should also be tested.

The follicular phase: superovulation

The human ovary normally produces only one dominant follicle and, thus, one mature oocyte. However, if additional stimulation with FSH is provided, the ovary will respond by producing multiple follicles. ART cycles generally utilize some form of ovarian hyperstimulation in order to increase the number of oocytes and subsequently embryos available for transfer, as each embryo has a chance of implanting and thus, pregnancy rates correlate best with the number of embryos replaced.

The most commonly utilized stimulation regimen consists of gonadotropin-releasing hormone agonist (GnRH-a) which suppresses endogenous gonadotropin production (thus maximizing cycle control) and subsequent ovarian stimulation with exogenous gonadotropins. The GnRH-a is initially given for about 2 weeks until pituitary downregulation is achieved. It is then continued during the stimulation phase in order to prevent a premature luteinizing hormone (LH) surge. The dose of FSH is usually started at 225–300 IU/day given intramuscularly.

Patients with polycystic ovarian disease and those who have previously demonstrated an exaggerated response may be given a lower initial dose (75–150 IU/day). The dose is subsequently adjusted according to follicular growth and serum levels of E2.

Monitoring of the ovarian response to stimulation is achieved by transvaginal ultrasonographic measurement of the size of the developing follicles and the measurement of serum E2 levels. Ovulation is triggered with human chorionic gonadotropin (hCG) 10,000 IU intramuscularly when follicle maturity is obtained. Maturity criteria are based on both follicle size and serum E2 levels.

Follicle aspiration

Transvaginal ultrasound-guided follicle aspiration is the most commonly used method of oocyte retrieval. It is performed 34–36 hours after hCG administration with analgesia achieved by conscious sedation. Under direct ultrasonographic visualization, the aspirating needle is introduced sequentially into each follicle and the follicular fluid aspirated (Figure 103.2). The reported incidence of

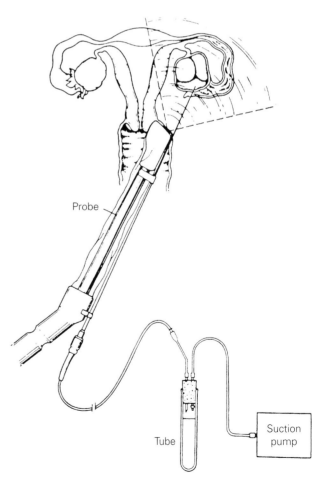

Figure 103.2 Transvaginal ultrasound-guided follicle aspiration. The ultrasound probe is covered with a sterile plastic sheath.

complications of transvaginal follicle aspiration is low; only one series found a substantial risk of infection and the reported 3% incidence of infection dropped to 0% with the use of prophylactic antibiotics. The removal of hydrosalpinges prior to IVF (see below) reduces the risk of infection associated with this procedure.

Oocytes are separated from the follicular fluid in the laboratory under a dissecting microscope. The size of the oocytes (approximately 70–100 μm diameter) allows their visualization and mechanical transport with a pipette to a wash dish, and subsequently a holding test tube containing culture medium. When all the oocytes have been identified and isolated, they are transferred to the incubator where they are kept until insemination approximately 6 hours later.

Fertilization *in vitro*

To achieve fertilization, recovered oocytes are combined with spermatozoa in a small volume of culture medium. In cases of mild male factor, the probability of fertilization may be enhanced by the use of high concentrations of sperm for insemination. However, prior failed fertilization or the presence of a severe male factor requires the use of micromanipulation and intracytoplasmic sperm injection (ICSI). Successful fertilization can be achieved with sperm obtained from the epididymis or directly from the testis. Fertilization rates are approximately 70%, with lower rates associated with testicular sperm and higher rates obtained with ejaculated sperm. In the absence of male factor, ICSI offers no advantage in terms of outcome, and therefore ICSI should be reserved for male factor cases.

Embryo transfer

After fertilization, embryos are maintained in culture for a variable period of time. Pregnancy can be attained after the replacement of embryos back in the reproductive tract at any stage of development. Embryos can be replaced either via the cervix into the uterine cavity or may be placed into the fallopian tubes and then be transported to the uterus by the peristaltic action of the oviducts as normally occurs *in vivo*. Tubal embryo transfer (ET) is generally performed relatively early after fertilization (24–48 hours after follicle aspiration) to allow adequate time for transport to the uterus.

The transcervical route of embryo placement can easily be negotiated in most patients and is, under most circumstances, the least traumatic to the patient. The uterine environment is best suited for more advanced stages of embryo development and embryos are generally transferred 48 or more hours after follicle aspiration, with the most common time being after 72 hours. Embryos

may also be kept in culture for an additional 2–3 days, when they reach the blastocyst stage and implantation is imminent. The advantage of this approach is the greater opportunity to select the best embryos and indeed, it results in the highest per embryo implantation rates. The disadvantage is the lack of development of many of the embryos to the blastocyst stage. Overall per cycle pregnancy rates are similar with 72 hour and blastocyst stage transfers.

Transfer of more than one embryo increases the chances for pregnancy, but also increases the risk of multiple gestations. Embryos that are in excess of the number to be transferred during the (fresh) cycle can be cryopreserved and transferred at a later date. Thus, the incremental benefit of transferring an additional embryo during the fresh cycle must be balanced against the risk of multiple gestations and the potential benefit of pregnancy during the subsequent frozen-thawed ET. Since women over age 40 have decreased per embryo implantation rates compared to younger women, unless donated oocytes are used, it is reasonable to replace a higher number of embryos at one time in this group.

The luteal phase and endometrial receptivity

There is little doubt that endometrial receptivity plays a major role in the success or failure of embryo implantation after IVF. In an effort to optimize endometrial receptivity, it is common practice to supplement the luteal phase with progesterone. Progesterone administration is generally initiated at the time of ET and continued until the end of the first trimester or until a negative pregnancy test is obtained. Progesterone is given by injections or vaginal suppositories.

The presence of a hydrosalpinx is associated with poor IVF outcome: the livebirth rate is about one-half that of women without hydrosalpinges. Furthermore, randomized trials have demonstrated that salpingectomy prior to IVF in women with hydrosalpinges improves pregnancy rates and, therefore, should be recommended. It is thought that the fluid from hydrosalpinges interferes with embryo implantation either by mechanical means or by interfering with endometrial receptivity on a biochemical basis. Therefore, laparoscopic salpingectomy is considered the treatment of choice prior to IVF.

The effect of leiomyomas on IVF is dependent on their location: submucosal myomas decrease the chance of success, whereas subserosal myomas do not appear to have any effect. The effect of intramural myomas is unclear, and probably depends on their size and proximity to the cavity. However, as yet, no study has demonstrated that myomectomy in the setting of intramural myomas improves IVF outcome.

Other assisted reproductive techniques

After it became apparent that IVF could be successfully applied to unexplained infertility as well as other conditions in which the fallopian tubes were open, other investigators attempted to modify the original IVF concept in an effort either to simplify the process and/or to increase its success in this group of patients.

Gamete intrafallopian transfer
The gamete intrafallopian transfer (GIFT) procedure uses IVF methodology for follicle stimulation and oocyte retrieval. Thereafter, oocytes and spermatozoa are replaced directly in the fallopian tube, generally by laparoscopy. Pregnancy is dependent upon fallopian tube function for early embryonic development and ET to the uterus. Since fertilization cannot be verified by direct visualization, GIFT is generally not recommended for male factor, except when donor sperm is used. In the early years of IVF, follicle aspirations were performed almost exclusively with laparoscopic visualization. Thus, the option of placing the gametes in the fallopian tubes rather than requiring the patient to return for the ET represented a significant simplification of IVF. The markedly shortened time of the gametes in the laboratory environment (several minutes rather than 48 h) also meant that less could go wrong. With today's ultrasound-guided follicle aspirations which require neither general anesthesia nor an operating room environment, and improved laboratory techniques, the putative advantages of GIFT must be weighed against the additional cost incurred as a result of the added laparoscopy.

Zygote intrafallopian transfer
Zygote intrafallopian transfer (ZIFT) utilizes standard IVF technology for all phases up to the first 24 hours after oocyte retrieval. By this point of embryonic life, fertilization is apparent by the visible presence of the male and female pronuclei within the zygote. The embryo is replaced at this state of development into the fallopian tube. Pregnancy is dependent upon further embryo development and ET to the uterus. Proponents of these techniques acknowledge the advantage of the verification of fertilization *in vitro*, and point to the more "natural" quality of early embryonic development taking place within the tube rather than in the uterine cavity, as occurs with standard IVF. Most centers offering ZIFT replace the embryos by laparoscopy, although success with transcervical cannulation has been reported.

Tubal embryo transfer
Tubal embryo transfer (TET) is differentiated from ZIFT in that embryos are replaced after cleavage has taken place, 48 or 72 hours after follicle aspiration. Similar arguments as for ZIFT are used by proponents to advocate the additional laparoscopy or mini-laparotomy which is used for the delivery of the embryos into the female reproductive tract rather than transcervical transfer into the uterine cavity.

As experience with *in vitro* culture and transcervical ET has increased, the utilization of these alternative ARTs has decreased. Most programs offer IVF as the primary ART and reserve tubal procedures for patients who have failed IVF or have a mechanical block to transcervical ET.

Natural cycle IVF
From time to time, ART programs re-evaluate the feasibility of IVF without the use of exogenous stimulation to induce growth of multiple follicles. The purely natural cycle is commonly augmented with a mid-cycle dose of hCG to trigger ovulation and allow for optimal timing of follicle aspiration. One series that analyzed implantation rates per embryo implanted and the rate of ongoing pregnancy in spontaneously ovulating women under age 40 years reported a higher implantation rate per embryo transferred for unstimulated as compared with stimulated cycles (13% versus 9%) but the pregnancy rate was one-half that achieved in stimulated cycles (14% versus 28%) because more embryos were transferred. Therefore, the benefit of multiple embryo transfers outweighed the benefit of the more natural uterine environment.

Currently, many IVF centers are using single embryo transfer in stimulated cycles for good prognosis patients to reduce the risk of multiple gestation, and natural cycle IVF is rarely performed. Instead, "gentle" stimulation is being used to take advantage of the additional control and margin for error afforded by the use of fertility medications.

In vitro maturation
In vitro maturation (IVM) of immature oocytes obtained in the absence of ovarian stimulation has some promise among the ARTs. A major advantage is the avoidance of injectable gonadotropins and their associated high costs. However, success rates are still substantially lower than those after standard stimulation. IVM may be applied in conjunction with reproductive tissue cryopreservation, especially in cancer patients (see Chapter 105).

Outcome and pregnancy success after *in vitro* fertilization

Because of the transfer of multiple embryos, monthly pregnancy rates achieved after ART treatment now exceed the monthly fecundability of natural conception cycles in the general population. Furthermore, cumulative pregnancy rates are substantially higher, as life-table analysis has shown that the per cycle pregnancy rate stays relatively constant for up to six cycles of IVF, although some studies have found a slight decline after 3–4 cycles.

Registry data from the United States for 2006 showed that 426 clinics reported 138,198 ART procedures with 41,343 deliveries of 54,656 infants. For fresh nondonor eggs, 99,199 cycles were started, 87,799 egg retrievals were performed, 80,313 embryo transfers were made, and 34,719 pregnancies resulted in 28,404 livebirths. Per cycle pregnancy rates vary with the age of the female partner and are depicted in Figure 103.1. Livebirth rates exceed 40% in young women, but drop precipitously after age 40.

The outcomes of pregnancies conceived via ART have been generally good and no specific anomalies are associated with the use of fertilization *in vitro*. The principal problem is the high incidence of multiple gestation, leading to preterm birth, and low birthweight. Low birthweight among singletons born after ART is thought to be primarily due to the "vanishing twin" phenomenon, in which more than one embryo implants but only one implantation goes on to form a fetus. Outcomes in these pregnancies are thought to have greater similarity to twin gestations in terms of gestational age at delivery and other obstetric complications.

Embryo and oocyte cryopreservation

Advanced stimulation regimens and retrieval techniques now result in large numbers of oocytes being retrieved from a single procedure of follicle aspiration. Since only a limited number of embryos can be transferred in any given cycle, there exists a need for long-term storage. Embryo cryopreservation was first achieved in the mouse and has been widely utilized in the animal husbandry industry. The first successful human pregnancy following cryopreservation was reported in 1983. Today, most programs utilize cryopreservation for embryos that are not transferred. In 2006, 15.9% of procedures consisted of the patient's own frozen embryos.

About 10–20% of embryos do not survive the thawing process. In 2006, the rates of livebirth per transfer for frozen and fresh embryos were 27.7% and 34%, respectively. The lower pregnancy rate with frozen embryos is thought to be due to subtle damage suffered by the embryo during the freezing and thawing process; however, fetal abnormalities do not appear to be increased.

There is no scientific basis for a maximum duration of storage. The couple has the option of transferring the cryopreserved embryos at a later date, donating them to other couples ("embryo adoption") or research, or disposing of them.

Recent advances in oocyte cryopreservation have now made it a viable alternative to embryo cryopreservation. Nevertheless, at the present time, there is much greater experience with embryo cryopreservation and oocyte cryopreservation is reserved for women wishing to preserve their fertility (see Chapter 105).

Future considerations

Human IVF and related ARTs are now clearly a major part of the armamentarium of the infertility specialist. In the past three decades, continued refinements in technology have enhanced the probability of success with these technologies and made them widely available. Whereas ICSI has made fertilization possible with virtually any spermatozoa, oocyte donation has made pregnancy possible in virtually any woman with an intact uterus (see oocyte donation, Chapter 104). The future application of ART may well be in fertility preservation, especially for those who are rendered sterile by cancer therapy (see Chapter 105). There is no question that the detailed study of the reproductive process made possible by ART has been helpful in understanding reproduction and thus, the optimization of related techniques, such as contraception.

Suggested reading

American Society for Reproductive Medicine Practice Committee in collaboration with Society for Reproductive Endocrinology and Infertility. Progesterone supplementation during the luteal phase and in early pregnancy in the treatment of infertility: an educational bulletin. *Fertil Steril* 2008; 89: 789.

Daya S, Gunby J, Hughes EG, *et al.* Follicle-stimulating hormone versus human menopausal gonadotropin for *in vitro* fertilization cycles: a meta-analysis. *Fertil Steril* 1995; 64: 347–354.

Edelstein MC, Brzyski RG, Jones GS, *et al.* Equivalency of human menopausal gonadotropin and follicle-stimulating hormone stimulation after gonadotropin-releasing hormone agonist suppression. *Fertil Steril* 1990; 53: 103–106.

Evers JL, Larsen JF, Gnany GG, Sieck UV. Complications and problems in transvaginal sector scan-guided follicle aspiration. *Fertil Steril* 1988; 49: 278–282.

Guzick DS, Wilkes C, Jones HW Jr. Cumulative pregnancy rates for *in vitro* fertilization. *Fertil Steril* 1986; 46: 663–667.

Howe RS, Wheeler C, Mastroianni L Jr, *et al.* Pelvic infection after transvaginal ultrasound-guided ovum retrieval. *Fertil Steril* 1988; 49: 726–728.

Hull MGR. Infertility treatment: relative effectiveness of conventional and assisted conception methods. *Hum Reprod* 1992; 7: 785–786.

Hull MGR. Effectiveness of infertility treatments: choice and comparative analysis. *Int J Gynecol Obstet* 1994; 47: 99–108.

Kovacs GT, Rogers P, Leeton JF, *et al. In-vitro* fertilization and embryo transfer: prospects of pregnancy by life-table analysis. *Med J Aust* 1986; 144: 682–683.

Licciardi FL, Liu H-C, Rosenwaks Z. Day 3 estradiol serum concentrations as prognosticators of ovarian stimulation response and pregnancy outcome in patients undergoing *in vitro* fertilization. *Fertil Steril* 1995; 64: 991–994.

Martin JS, Nisker JA, Tummon IS, *et al.* Future *in vitro* fertilization pregnancy potential of women with variably elevated day 3 follicle-stimulating hormone levels. *Fertil Steril* 1996; 65: 1238–1240.

Nagy Z, Liu J, Janssenwillen C, *et al.* Using ejaculated, fresh, and frozen-thawed epididymal and testicular spermatozoa gives rise to comparable results after intracytoplasmic sperm injection. *Fertil Steril* 1995; 63: 808–815.

Pados G, Devroey P. Luteal phase support. *Assist Reprod Rev* 1992; 2: 148–153.

Palermo G, Joris H, Devroey P, van Steirteghem AC. Pregnancies after intracytoplasmic injection of a single spermatozoon into an oocyte. *Lancet* 1992; 340: 17–18.

Paulson RJ, Sauer MV, Francis MM, *et al. In vitro* fertilization in unstimulated cycles: a clinical trial using hCG for timing of follicle aspiration. *Obstet Gynecol* 1990; 76: 788–791.

Paulson RJ, Sauer MV, Lobo RA. Embryo implantation after human *in vitro* fertilization: importance of endometrial receptivity. *Fertil Steril* 1990; 53: 870–874.

Paulson RJ, Sauer MV, Francis MM, *et al.* A prospective controlled evaluation of TEST-yolk buffer in the preparation of sperm for human *in vitro* fertilization in suspected cases of male infertility. *Fertil Steril* 1992; 58: 551–555.

Paulson RJ, Sauer MV, Francis MM, *et al. In vitro* fertilization in unstimulated cycles: the University of Southern California experience. *Fertil Steril* 1992; 57: 290–293.

Sauer MV, Paulson RJ, Lobo RA. Reversing the natural decline in human fertility: an extended clinical trial of oocyte donation to women of advanced reproductive age. *JAMA* 1992; 268: 1275–1279.

Silber SJ, van Steirteghem AC, Liu J, *et al.* High fertilization and pregnancy rates after intracytoplasmic sperm injection with spermatozoa obtained from testicular biopsy. *Hum Reprod* 1995; 10: 148–152.

Toner JP, Philput CB, Jones GS, Muasher SJ. Basal follicle-stimulating hormone level is a better predictor of *in vitro* fertilization performance than age. *Fertil Steril* 1991; 55: 784–791.

Chapter 104
Oocyte Donation and Third Party Parenting

Richard J. Paulson

Department of Medicine and Obstetrics and Gynecology, Keck School of Medicine, University of Southern California, CA, USA

Introduction

Oocyte donation is now an integral part of infertility care. When *in vitro* fertilization (IVF) was first introduced, it became clear that oocytes could be transferred from a donor to a recipient in a manner analogous to that of sperm donation, which had been already been in practice for many years. The first successful pregnancy after oocyte donation was reported in 1983. Initially intended as a treatment for infertile women with premature ovarian failure or those who had genetic disease that they did not wish to pass along to the next generation, oocyte donation gradually became increasingly used to circumvent the age-related decline in human fertility. During 2006, 16,976 cycles of oocyte donation were performed in the United States, representing 12% of all assisted reproductive cycles.

Historical background

Oocyte donation is fundamentally different from other assisted reproductive technologies in that it has a precedent in the animal world. Embryo donation, resulting from artificial insemination of the donor and subsequent recovery of the fertilized embryo from the uterus of the donor, has been practiced by veterinarians for many years. This method was initially attempted as a way of accomplishing oocyte donation in humans. The donor monitored her ovulation in a spontaneous ovulatory cycle, then was inseminated with the sperm of the infertile woman's husband at the time of ovulation. Approximately 5 days later, the uterus was lavaged and if a conceptus was retrieved, it was transferred to the uterus of the recipient. This method resulted in the first livebirth after oocyte donation in the United States in 1983, shortly after the world's first birth achieved in Australia in 1982. However, uterine lavage proved to be very inefficient and attempts at ovarian stimulation of donors were unsuccessful in increasing the number of embryos retrieved. Furthermore, concerns about infectious disease transmission and potential retained pregnancy in the donor caused the abandonment of this process.

At its inception, IVF utilized laparoscopy for oocyte retrieval. Whereas laparoscopy was less traumatic than laparotomy, it nevertheless required general anesthesia and an operating room environment, and was prohibitively complex for utilization on oocyte donors. Therefore, early attempts at oocyte donation via IVF typically used excess oocytes donated by infertile women themselves undergoing IVF. When embryo cryopreservation became a reality, IVF patients now had the option of preserving their own embryos for future use and "excess oocytes" were no longer available. The development of the transvaginal ultrasound-guided method for follicle aspiration dramatically changed IVF and made oocyte donation a reality. Oocytes could now be retrieved under conscious sedation in an office setting and donors could now be recruited explicitly for the purpose of donating all their oocytes to a potential recipient.

All recipients at the beginning were women with premature ovarian failure or those with genetic diseases who did not wish to pass them along to their offspring. As experience grew, it became apparent that the pregnancy rate after oocyte donation was not influenced by the age of the recipient. Thus, it became clear that oocyte donation could be used to circumvent the age-related decline in fertility. Oocyte donation then became the treatment of choice for women in their mid-40s and for those who failed standard IVF.

Oocyte donors

Oocyte donors may be anonymous or known and in many instances may be female relatives of the infertile patient. Since pregnancy rates are related to the age of the oocyte provider, the ideal age for oocyte donors is

Management of Common Problems in Obstetrics and Gynecology, 5th edition. Edited by T.M. Goodwin, M.N. Montoro, L. Muderspach, R. Paulson and S. Roy. © 2010 Blackwell Publishing Ltd.

between 21 and 35. Older donors may be utilized but pregnancy rates are lower.

Donors are screened for infectious diseases according to FDA regulations with a questionnaire and serum testing. Their reproductive potential is assessed with a day 3 follicle-stimulating hormone measurement and an antral follicle count by ultrasound. They need to be carefully counseled regarding the psychologic and emotional ramifications of donating their gametes, and should receive informed consent information regarding the physical risks of the procedure. Fortunately, there are very few risks associated with controlled ovarian hyperstimulation and follicle aspiration (see Chapter 103), and these are thought to be even less among young healthy oocyte donors.

The oocyte donation cycle

Oocyte donation is achieved with what is essentially a cycle of IVF, which is divided into two portions: the donor undergoes controlled ovarian hyperstimulation and follicle aspiration, and the recipient undergoes embryo transfer. Ovarian hyperstimulation in oocyte donors utilizes standard regimens and medications. Because the donors are generally good responders, lower doses of gonadotropins are utilized. There is a risk of ovarian hyperstimulation syndrome (OHSS) associated with the good response to stimulation and careful monitoring of donors is required. Fortunately, since the donors do not became pregnant after the procedure, cases of OHSS tend to be mild and self-limited.

Follicle aspiration is performed under conscious sedation (with intravenous narcotics and benzodiazepines) or under heavy sedation with intravenous propofol in a manner that is identical to that of standard IVF. The donors are monitored during the postoperative period and then during the luteal phase for symptoms of OHSS. Donors are commonly seen at the time of their next menstrual period to ensure that their ovaries have returned to normal size.

The recipient endometrium is prepared with a regimen of estrogen and progesterone, which renders the endometrium receptive to embryo implantation. Estrogen may be administeed by the oral, transdermal or intramuscular route and is commonly given in increasing doses for about 2 weeks prior to oocyte retrieval. Estrogen stimulation needs to be adequate to induce endometrial proliferation, which is associated with an ultrasound measurement of endometrial thickness of more than 7 mm. At our institution, the recipients receive 2 mg daily for 4 days in divided doses, then 4 mg daily for 5 days, and then 6 mg daily for 5 days. If the recipient has ovarian function, leuprolide acetate is used to prevent ovulation during the recipient cycle.

The recipient endometrium is synchronized to the embryo by starting progesterone in the recipient on the day of egg retrieval in the donor. Estrogen is maintained at a dose of 2 mg twice daily and progesterone is added in a dose of 200 mg vaginally three times daily. Estrogen and progesterone are continued through the end of the trimester.

Because donor oocytes produce high-quality embryos, typically only one or two embryos are transferred during any one cycle. Up to three embryos may be transferred in exceptional circumstances. The pregnancy rate with oocyte donation is high and is independent of the age of the recipient. In 2006, the national average livebirth rate for oocyte donation was in excess of 50% per cycle.

Specific problems

There are specific issues associated with oocyte donation, which is unique in making pregnancy possible in women who would not naturally become pregnancy by any other means. These include poor response to uterine stimulation, advanced maternal age, and specific health issues associated with ovarian failure.

Women whose uterine lining responds poorly to exogenous steroids may have a decreased probability of success with oocyte donation. Several strategies have been adopted to increase the endometrial thickness in these women, including prolonged estrogen stimulation and vaginal administration of estrogen. Vaginally administered estradiol tablets are well absorbed, and lead to very high serum estradiol levels. Furthermore, endometrial tissue levels appear to be particularly high with vaginally administered steroids (both estrogen and progesterone). It has been shown that in a group of women who could not achieve adequate endometrial thickness with oral estradiol, vaginal estradiol resulted in adequate endometrial thickness and good pregnancy outcome.

Since virtually any woman with a functional uterus may be able to conceive, it is now possible to initiate pregnancy in women beyond the natural age of menopause. But whereas the uterus responds appropriately and achieves normal endometrial receptivity, obstetric complications are dependent on the age of the recipient, and are substantially higher in the older gravida. One study showed a 35% incidence of pre-eclampsia in women over 50 conceiving with donor oocytes. This rate increased to 60% among a small subgroup of women aged 55 or older. Since pre-eclampsia may become severe and may require early delivery, there may be an increased risk of prematurity among these women. Most programs in the US limit oocyte donation to women under the age of 50. Our program extends this age limit up to age 54, as long as the recipient has no underlying medical problems and undergoes a thorough medical screening.

A special class of recipients are those with Turner's syndrome. In this genetic anomaly (45,XO), there is not only primary amenorrhea with streak gonads, but also an associated phenotype of a web neck, shield chest, and other physical stigmata. There appears to be an associated defect in the wall of blood vessels in these individuals, which may lead to aortic aneurysm. Turner's syndrome patients are at particular risk for dissecting aortic aneurysms during pregnancy. Hence, whereas these patients may become pregnant easily with oocyte donation, they must be evaluated for cardiovascular status before this treatment is attempted. However, there is increasing concern that cardiovascular evaluation may not be sufficiently sensitive to exclude the possibility of aortic dissection during pregnancy. Many programs in the US now consider Turner's syndrome to be a contraindication to oocyte donation.

Gestational surrogacy

Oocyte donation was designed to induce pregnancy in a woman whose own oocytes were either absent or nonfunctional or carried an undesired genetic mutation. However, it can easily be applied to gestational surrogacy, in which the intended mother either does not have a uterus or has a medical condition which makes pregnancy dangerous. The method of initiating pregnancy in the gestational surrogate is identical to that of oocyte donation. Since surrogates almost always have ovarian function, their cycles are controlled with the use of exogenous leuprolide acetate. Oocytes are retrieved following controlled ovarian hyperstimulation in the intended mother (or an oocyte donor, if desired). Oocytes are fertilized *in vitro*, and the resulting embryos are transferred to the uterus of the gestational surrogate. As with standard oocyte donation, progesterone is initiated on the day of follicle retrieval. Embryo implantation rates and clinical pregnancy rates are similar to those achieved by women undergoing IVF with their own oocytes. Therefore, increased numbers of embryos may be transferred in older women.

Gestational surrogacy must be managed carefully, primarily due to the legal, psychologic, and ethical issues associated with one woman carrying a pregnancy for another. Laws regulating surrogacy vary widely from state to state. It is important to have psychologic support and follow-up for the surrogate. Nevertheless, gestational surrogacy provides the last best opportunity for a couple's own genetic child in cases where the intended mother has had a hysterectomy or for whom pregnancy would be medically risky.

Future directions

The technique of oocyte donation has made pregnancy possible in virtually any woman with a functional uterus. Since oocytes may now be cryopreserved, it is possible for women to cryopreserve their own oocytes when they are young and then effectively act as their own oocyte donor in the future. Until such time as the age-related decline in fertility may be reversed by direct methods, this type of "fertility preservation" may be the best strategy for women to have their own genetic offspring at later stages of the reproductive lifespan.

Oocyte cryopreservation may also be applied to oocyte donation from anonymous donors. Thus, oocyte banks may become a reality. Advantages of such banks would include the immediate availability of oocytes, the ability to quarantine reproductive tissue prior to transfer, decrease utilization of the cryopreservation of excess embryos, and increase efficiency of the utilization of donor oocytes. At this point, however, oocyte cryopreservation is still a relatively new technology, and fresh oocyte donation continues to have the advantage of greater experience and greater oocyte viability.

Oocytes may, in the future, be obtained from unstimulated ovaries with subsequent *in vitro* maturation (IVM) of the immature oocytes. This method has theoretical appeal in that it avoids the utilization of multiple injections and controlled ovarian hyperstimulation in the donors. However, at present, IVM is quite inefficient when compared with standard methods.

Conclusion

Oocyte donation is now an integral part of the armamentarium of the infertility specialist. It is the most successful of the assisted reproductive technologies with pregnancy rates exceeding 50% per initiated cycle in the United States. With this technology, it is possible to initiate a pregnancy in virtually any woman with a functional uterus. However, health considerations may limit the applicability of pregnancy initiation with this technology.

Suggested reading

Buster JE, Bustillo M, Thorneycroft I, *et al*. Non-surgical transfer of in vivo fertilised donated ova to five infertile women: report of two pregnancies. *Lancet* 1983; 2: 223–224.

Cha KY, Koo JJ, Ko JJ, *et al*. Pregnancy after in vitro fertilization of human follicular oocytes collected from nonstimulated cycles, their culture in vitro and their transfer in a donor oocyte program. *Fertil Steril* 1991; 55: 109–113.

Lutjen P, Trounson A, Leeton J, *et al*. The establishment and maintenance of pregnancy using in vitro fertilization in a patient with primary ovarian failure. *Nature* 1984; 307: 174–175.

Paulson RJ, Boostanfar R, Saadat P, *et al.* Pregnancy in the sixth decade of life: obstetric outcomes in women of advanced reproductive age. *JAMA* 2002; 288: 2320–2323.

Sauer MV, Paulson RJ. Human oocyte and preembryo donation: an evolving method for the treatment of infertility. *Am J Obstet Gynecol* 1990; 163: 1421–1424.

Sauer MV, Paulson RJ, Lobo RA. A preliminary report on oocyte donation extending reproductive potential to women over 40. *NEJM* 1990; 323: 1157–1160.

Sauer MV, Paulson RJ, Lobo RA. Reversing the natural decline in human fertility: an extended clinical trial of oocyte donation to women of advanced reproductive age. *JAMA* 1992; 268: 1275–1279.

Trounson A, Leeton J, Besanko M, *et al.* Pregnancy established in an infertile patient after transfer of a donated embryo fertilised in vitro. *BMJ* 1983; 286: 835–838.

Younis JS, Simon A, Laufer N. Endometrial preparation: lessons from oocyte donation. *Fertil Steril* 1996; 66: 873–884.

Chapter 105
Fertility Preservation and Oocyte Cryopreservation

Karine Chung and Richard J. Paulson

Department of Medicine and Obstetrics and Gynecology, Keck School of Medicine, University of Southern California, CA, USA

Introduction

As the trend to delay childbearing continues among women in the United States and other developed countries, the demand for effective methods of fertility preservation has grown considerably. Perhaps the most pressing need for such technology applies to women facing imminent loss of ovarian function due to impending cancer therapy or other causes of premature ovarian failure. Though many of the techniques to preserve future fertility are still considered experimental, several options show great promise and will be discussed in this chapter.

Age-related decrease in female fertility

The progressive loss of oocytes that occurs from fetal life until menopause is one of the defining features of the age-related decline in female fertility. The oocyte pool peaks while the female fetus is *in utero*, reaching approximately 6–7 million oocytes at 20 weeks' gestation. Subsequently, progressive atresia occurs so that the number of remaining oocytes is approximately 1–2 million at birth and 200,000 at the onset of puberty. During the reproductive years, there is continued atresia, which occurs at an accelerated rate after the age of 37 in normal women. The average age of menopause is 51, at which time there are approximately 1000 oocytes remaining.

As the number of oocytes declines over time, their quality also declines and eventually reaches a critical threshold below which pregnancy is no longer possible. The decrease in quality primarily refers to an increased prevalence of aneuploid oocytes with age, largely due to dysfunctions of the meiotic spindle. Errors in meiotic segregation result in higher rates of chromosomally abnormal embryos, translating into higher rates of spontaneous

abortion and lower chances of pregnancy. It is estimated that the prevalence of aneuploid oocytes approaches 100% after the age of 45. For women who are approaching advanced reproductive age but are not ready to become pregnant or are not in the position to have a child, options to preserve fertility including embryo and oocyte cryopreservation may be considered.

Cancer therapy-induced decrease in female fertility

The need for fertility preservation options is particularly pertinent for women facing imminent loss of ovarian function due to cancer therapy. Over 600,000 women are diagnosed with cancer each year in the United States. Thousands of these women are in their reproductive years and many of them have not yet started or completed their families. Steady advances in cancer treatment have greatly improved survival rates. Unfortunately, the most successful treatment strategies, which include chemotherapy and radiation, often cause infertility and premature menopause, thus rendering many female cancer survivors incapable of having future children.

Ovarian follicles are remarkably vulnerable to agents that cause DNA damage, including ionizing radiation and chemotherapy. These treatments result in a dramatic reduction in follicular and oocyte reserve due to apoptosis, and eventually lead to ovarian atrophy. With respect to radiation, the degree of oocyte depletion depends on the field of treatment, total dose, and fractionation schedule. Ovarian damage resulting from cytotoxic chemotherapy depends on the dose administered and the agent used, with alkylating agents such as cyclophosphamide and ifosfamide posing the greatest risk of infertility. For both forms of cancer therapy, patients who are younger at the time of treatment are less likely to suffer infertility and have later onset of premature menopause than patients who are older at the time of treatment. Overall, the incidence of impaired fertility is not well characterized due to variable definitions, but is reported to range between 15% and 90%. Thus, the potential for infertility is significant and

Management of Common Problems in Obstetrics and Gynecology, 5th edition. Edited by T.M. Goodwin, M.N. Montoro, L. Muderspach, R. Paulson and S. Roy. © 2010 Blackwell Publishing Ltd.

is a known source of stress for female cancer survivors. Therefore, discussion about options for fertility preservation is critical. The algorithm presented in Figure 105.1 should aid the clinician in counseling patients about their options, which are described in further detail below.

Options for fertility preservation

Embryo cryopreservation

Embryo freezing is the most proven method of fertility preservation and is not considered experimental. Since by definition an embryo is a fertilized egg, this process requires sperm. It is an excellent option for women who have a male partner or are interested in using donor sperm. It involves ovarian stimulation with daily injectable gonadotropins, which typically starts at the beginning of a menstrual period and continues for approximately 10–14 days to mature the eggs. Alternative approaches to stimulation include use of tamoxifen or aromatase inhibitors, which can be employed if exposure to high estrogen levels is a concern (as in breast cancer patients). The eggs are removed by a transvaginal ultrasound-guided needle (a procedure which is done under conscious sedation) and are then combined with the sperm in the laboratory. The resulting embryos can be stored indefinitely until the patient is ready to use them. The entire process takes 2–6 weeks to complete, and therefore requires that the patient can safely delay cancer therapy for this amount of time. Pregnancy rates from frozen-thawed embryos depend on the age of the woman at the time of the egg retrieval, ranging from approximately 20% at age 40 to 40% at age 35 per embryo transfer.

While embryo freezing is the standard method of fertility preservation and has been successful in routine use for about two decades, it is only applicable in post-pubertal female patients and those who have a current male partner or are willing to consider sperm donation.

Oocyte cryopreservation

For women who do not have a male partner and are not interested in using donor sperm, oocyte cryopreservation is the preferred option. For many years, sperm freezing prior to chemotherapy has provided a reliable method of fertility preservation in male patients with cancer. Because of the complex biologic properties of the human egg, the science of egg freezing has proven more challenging. Though the first pregnancies from oocyte cryopreservation were reported about two decades ago, overall success with respect to oocyte survival, fertilization rates, and pregnancy rates remained low for many years, discouraging routine application of the technology. Much of the difficulty was related to the high water content of the human oocyte. Thus, recent advances have realized that the principal aims of successful cryopreservation are to avoid formation of ice crystals which can damage intracellular organelles, to limit toxicity of electrolytes and other solutes to the intracellular proteins of the oocyte during the transition from liquid to solid phase, and to prevent sudden drops in extracellular osmotic pressure that could lead to cell swelling and "osmotic shock" during rewarming.

Conventional oocyte freezing protocols are derived from "slow-freeze" techniques which have been used to effectively cryopreserve embryos. The slow-freeze method involves the use of low initial concentrations

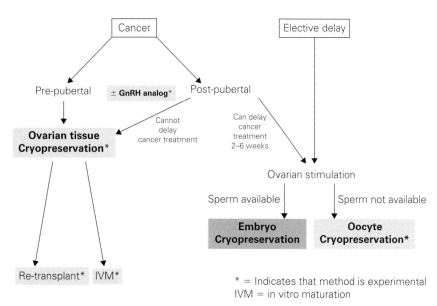

Figure 105.1 Algorithm of fertility preservation options.

of cryoprotectants, which are associated with lower toxicity while the oocyte is still at temperatures at which it is metabolically active. As the temperature decreases gradually and the oocyte's metabolic rate declines, there is an increasing concentration of cryoprotectants to prevent intracellular ice crystal formation. Approximately 2 hours later when the concentration of cryoprotectants is high enough to support solidification of the oocyte without intracellular ice ("glass-like"), rapid exposure to much lower temperatures is possible.

Adjustments to solute concentrations and optimization of cryoprotectants have resulted in dramatic improvements in oocyte survival and pregnancy rates after slow-freezing. In a feasibility pilot study conducted at our institution, we achieved a 64% survival rate and a 63% pregnancy rate in subjects with tubal factor infertility. We used a sodium-depleted culture medium and a modified slow-freeze protocol which had been previously described by others reporting similar results. A recent meta-analysis summarized results from 41 manuscripts that reported outcomes of slow-freezing and estimated fertilization rates of 61% (1346/2217), clinical pregnancy rates of 27% (95/351), and livebirth rates of 21.6% (76/351).

Vitrification is an alternative approach to oocyte freezing which is based upon the concept that metabolically active cells can be cooled so rapidly that ice does not have time to form. During vitrification, permeating cryoprotectants are added at high concentrations. A very short time is allowed for equilibration and an extremely rapid rate of cooling is used. Successful use of vitrification procedures has been reported in animal models and the number of human livebirths resulting from vitrification of oocytes continues to increase. Since the first birth from vitrified human oocytes was reported in 1999, several case series showing promising results have been published. A recent meta-analysis including five reports on vitrification estimated fertilization rates of 74% (637/859), clinical pregnancy rates of 45.5% (61/134), and livebirth rates of 36.6% (49/134). These rates are comparable to those achieved using frozen and thawed embryos.

While these preliminary results are very encouraging, the number of livebirths to date by either method of oocyte cryopreservation remains insufficient to be certain of the safety of these techniques. However, of the approximately 500 livebirths reported from frozen and thawed oocytes, there have been no reports of increased congenital anomalies, aneuploidies or other adverse outcomes. A recent follow-up study of children born from egg freezing showed no abnormalities in karyotype, birthweight, organ formation, intellectual or developmental deficits. Additionally, there have been more than 150,000 livebirths resulting from embryo freezing and over 50,000 livebirths resulting from sperm freezing and studies have shown no increase in adverse outcomes.

While both methods of oocyte cryopreservation have recently yielded promising results, they are considered experimental by the American Society for Reproductive Medicine (ASRM) and should only be performed under research protocols approved by Institutional Review Boards. Similar to embryo cryopreservation, the process of egg freezing involves a 10–14-day interval of ovarian stimulation starting from the beginning of a menstrual period, and is therefore only suitable for women who are post pubertal and able to safely delay cancer treatment for 2–6 weeks.

Ovarian tissue cryopreservation

For patients whose cancer therapy cannot be delayed and prepubertal females, ovarian tissue containing immature eggs can be removed by laparoscopy and preserved for future use. Retransplantation of the tissue to the pelvis has resulted in livebirths in humans, but this strategy is limited by the short-term viability of the transplanted tissue and by concerns of potential reintroduction of malignant cells into a patient who is in remission.

The alternative approach involves isolation of immature follicles from the ovarian tissue followed by the use of *in vitro* maturation (IVM). Because immature eggs cannot be fertilized, techniques to mature the eggs in the laboratory have been developed and refined over the past several decades, leading to consistent improvements in egg survival and fertilization. Recent reports of pregnancies and healthy liveborn babies resulting from this technology in women without cancer and successful freezing of eggs matured in the laboratory in women with cancer indicate that this strategy holds promise for fertility preservation in female cancer patients. This is an option for those patients who cannot or do not wish to delay their cancer treatment. Similar to egg freezing, ovarian tissue freezing is considered investigational and should be performed responsibly under ethics board-approved research protocols. Accordingly, the recent committee opinion from the ASRM states that "although currently investigational, ovarian tissue cryopreservation and oocyte cryopreservation hold promise for future female fertility preservation, particularly following aggressive chemotherapy and/or radiotherapy treatment protocols."

Gonadotropin-releasing hormone (GnRH) analogs

Use of GnRH analogs is an investigational approach to fertility preservation which can be used in postpubertal women who cannot safely delay their cancer therapy. Though the biologic mechanism is not clear, it has been theorized that use of the GnRH agonist prior to and during chemotherapy mimics the protective effect of the prepubertal state, thereby reducing the degree of follicular depletion induced by chemotherapy. The advantage of this approach is that it is relatively noninvasive and does not require a delay in the initiation of cancer therapy. Unfortunately, the majority of studies show little if any benefit. Further investigation is ongoing, but the current recommendation is that GnRH agonists should not be used as the sole method of fertility preservation. However, they may be used in conjunction with the other methods described above as they are unlikely to cause harm.

Pregnancy after cancer: is it safe?

Thus far, research on the safety of pregnancy after cancer is reassuring. Further research is necessary to confirm these findings. In the mothers, research to date suggests that pregnancy after cancer does not trigger recurrence, even after breast cancer. Among the children, the risk of birth defects in those born to cancer survivors is reported to be similar to that of the general public: approximately 2–3%. Children born to cancer survivors do not appear to be at increased risk for getting cancer themselves (except in true inheritable cancer syndromes).

Conclusion

In the face of progressive loss of oocytes due to advancing reproductive age, cancer treatment or other causes, various methods of fertility preservation are now available and offer a reasonable chance of future pregnancy. While embryo cryopreservation is the traditional method, oocyte and ovarian tissue cryopreservation techniques show great promise. However, these methods are still considered experimental and should be offered only in a research setting with IRB oversight.

Suggested reading

American Society for Reproductive Medicine Practice Committee and the Practice Committee of the Society for Assisted Reproductive Technology. Ovarian tissue and oocyte cryopreservation: Practice Committee Opinion. *Fertil Steril* 2006; 86(suppl 4): S142–147.

Blumenfeld Z. How to preserve fertility in young women exposed to chemotherapy? The role of GnRH agonist cotreatment in addition to cryopreservation of embrya, oocytes or ovaries. *Oncologist* 2007; 12: 1044–1054.

Boldt J, Cline D, McLaughlin D. Human oocyte cropreservation as an adjunct to IVF-embryo transfer cycles. *Hum Reprod* 2003; 18: 1250–1255.

Chen C. Pregnancy after human oocyte cryopreservation. *Lancet* 1986; 1: 884–886.

Chen C. Pregnancies after human oocyte cryopreservation. *Ann NY Acad Sci* 1988; 541: 541–549.

Donnez J, Dolmans MM, Demylle D, *et al*. Livebirth after orthotopic transplantation of cryopreserved ovarian tissue. *Lancet* 2004; 364: 1405–1410.

Faddy MJ, Gosden RG, Gougeon A, Richardson SJ, Nelson JF. Accelerated disappearance of ovarian follicles in mid-life: implications for forecasting menopause. *Hum Reprod* 1992; 7: 1342–1346.

Jain JK, Paulson RJ. Oocyte cryopreservation. *Fertil Steril* 2006; 86: 1037–1046.

Jain JK, Francis MM, Bayrak A, Quinn P, Paulson RJ. Pregnancy outcome after cryopreservation of all oocytes from a single ovulatory cohort: a prospective clinical trial. *Fertil Steril* 2005; 84: S350–351.

Kuleshova L, Gianaroli L, Magli C, Ferraretti A, Trounson A. Birth following vitrification of a small number of human oocytes: case report. *Hum Reprod* 1999; 14: 3077–3079.

Kuwayama M, Vajita G, Kato O, Leibo SP. Highly efficient vitrification method for cryopreservation of human oocytes. *Reprod Biomed Online* 2005; 11: 300–308.

Lansac J, Royere D. Follow-up studies of children born after frozen sperm donation. *Hum Reprod Update* 2001; 7: 33–37.

Lobo R. Potential options for preservation of fertility in women. *NEJM* 2005; 353: 64–73.

Lucena E, Bernal DP, Lucena C, Rojas A, Moran A, Lucena A. Successful ongoing pregnancies after vitrification of oocytes. *Fertil Steril* 2006; 85: 108–111.

Meirow D, Nugent D. The effects of radiotherapy and chemotherapy on female reproduction. *Hum Reprod Update* 2001; 7: 535–543.

Meirow D, Levron J, Eldar-Geva T, *et al*. Pregnancy after transplantation of cryopreserved ovarian tissue in a patient with ovarian failure after chemotherapy. *NEJM* 2005; 353: 318–321.

Oktay K, Cil AP, Bang H. Efficiency of oocyte cryopreservation: a meta-analysis. *Fertil Steril* 2006; 86: 70–80.

Pellestor F, Andreo B, Arnal F, Humeau C, Demaille J. Maternal aging and chromosomal abnormalities: new data drawn from in vitro unfertilized human oocytes. *Hum Genet* 2003; 112: 195.

Rao GD, Chian RC, Son WS, Gilbert L, Tan SL. Fertility preservation in women undergoing cancer treatment. *Lancet* 2004; 363: 1829.

Thornton MH, Francis MM, Paulson RJ. Immature oocyte retrieval: lessons from unstimulated IVF cycles. *Fertil Steril* 1998; 70: 647–650.

Volarcik K, Sheean L, Goldfarb J, Woods L, Abdul-Karim FW, Hunt P. The meiotic competence of in-vitro matured human oocytes is influenced by donor age: evidence that folliculogenesis is compromised in the reproductively aged ovary. *Hum Reprod* 1998; 13: 154.

Wallace WHB, Thomson AB, Kelsey TW. The radiosensitivity of the human oocyte. *Hum Reprod* 2003; 18: 117–121.

Wennerholm WB. Cryopreservation of embryos and oocytes: obstetric outcome and health in children. *Hum Reprod* 2000; 15: S18–25.

Winslow KL, Yang D, Blohm PL, Brown SE, Jossim P, Nguyen K. Oocyte cryopreservation: a three year follow-up of sixteen births. *Fertil Steril* 2001; 76: S120–S121.

Chapter 106
Recurrent Pregnancy Loss

Melanie Landay and Richard J. Paulson
Department of Medicine and Obstetrics and Gynecology, Keck School of Medicine, University of Southern California, CA, USA

Introduction

The probability that a pregnancy will end as a miscarriage is highly dependent on the age of the mother, but approximately 15% of all clinically recognized pregnancies end in spontaneous abortion. Recurrent pregnancy loss (RPL) is traditionally defined as three or more consecutive, involuntary losses of pregnancy prior to 20 weeks' gestation or fetal weight less than 500 g. Between 0.4% and 1% of women have three consecutive miscarriages, a higher percentage than would be expected solely by chance (0.15 [mult] 0.15 [mult] 0.15 = 0.3%), suggesting that there is a specific cause for RPL in some women.

The products of conception of women who have three or more abortions are more likely to be chromosomally normal (80–90%) than those of women with a single spontaneous abortion. Women with recurrent abortions also have a tendency to abort later in gestation, with two-thirds of such abortions occurring beyond 12 weeks' gestation, indicating that maternal or environmental factors are a more likely cause of repeated pregnancy loss. If a woman has had no livebirths and three spontaneous abortions, without treatment she has about a 50% chance of having a viable gestation in her next pregnancy, and if she has had one livebirth, this chance is increased to about 70%. Couples with recurrent losses require careful, sympathetic management by the practitioner, because an abortion is an emotionally traumatic experience that can result in as much grief as intrauterine fetal death in late pregnancy or a neonatal death. With RPL, this emotional trauma is magnified, and the practitioner needs to express sympathy and understanding as counseling is performed and a diagnostic regimen is outlined.

An extensive evaluation is not generally recommended after a single first-trimester loss, as this is a relatively common event. However, because the etiology of a mid to late second-trimester loss is more likely to be uterine in origin and thus more likely to be amenable to diagnosis, a diagnostic evaluation should be performed after a woman has had only one second-trimester spontaneous abortion. There is no need to wait for a woman to have three first-trimester abortions, with their accompanying emotional trauma, before beginning a diagnostic evaluation. Work-up should be initiated after two losses because the risk of recurrence is similar to the risk of recurrence after three (25% vs 33%).

Etiology

The etiology of recurrent pregnancy loss can be categorized into: genetic, anatomic (uterine), endocrinologic, immunologic, inherited and acquired thrombophilias, and infectious, and they will be discussed in this order.

Genetic chromosomal abnormalities

Between 40% and 60% of first-trimester losses have chromosomal anomalies, whereas such anomalies are found in only 5–10% of second-trimester losses. Chromosomal anomalies have been identified and reported in 2.5–8% of couples with RPL compared with an incidence of approximately 0.7% in the general population.

Chromosomal abnormalities occur in the female parent about twice as frequently as in the male. About 60% of all chromosomal abnormalities are balanced reciprocal translocations, and 40% are Robertsonian translocations. Sex chromosome mosaicism, chromosome inversions, deletions, duplications and other structural abnormalities can also be present. Therefore, when couples have had two or more spontaneous abortions, karyotypes should be obtained from both partners. If a balanced translocation is found in one parent, about two-thirds of their subsequent pregnancies will abort. If abortion does not occur in a subsequent pregnancy, fetal cytogenetic studies are indicated, because there is about a 3–5% incidence of an unbalanced fetal karyotype in these gestations. Therefore, if an abnormal karyotype is found in one of

Management of Common Problems in Obstetrics and Gynecology, 5th edition. Edited by T.M. Goodwin, M.N. Montoro, L. Muderspach, R. Paulson and S. Roy. © 2010 Blackwell Publishing Ltd.

the members of the couple with RPL, genetic counseling is indicated.

Anatomic factors

Uterine abnormalities, either congenital or acquired, may not provide the optimal environment for nourishment and survival of the embryo and may cause miscarriage of a genetically normal embryo. Congenital uterine abnormalities can be divided into those brought about by abnormal uterine fusion, those produced by maternal diethylstilbestrol (DES) ingestion, and those caused by abnormal cervical function. The latter condition, the incompetent cervix, can also be acquired after mechanical cervical dilation. Other acquired anomalies are intrauterine synechiae and submucous myomas.

Anomalies of uterine development

The prevalence of congenital uterine malformations in the general population is, 3–4%. In comparison, 5–10% of patients with recurrent early loss and up to 25% of women with a late first- or second-trimester loss or preterm delivery will be found to have a uterine anomaly. The septate uterus is the anomaly most commonly associated with poor pregnancy outcome and RPL, with the first-trimester miscarriage rate reported to be 23–67%. The mechanism by which a uterine septum causes miscarriage is not completely understood, but is thought to be secondary to poor vascularization of the septum, leading to poor implantation and placentation. In contrast, unicornuate, bicornuate and didelphys uteri are more commonly associated with second-trimester loss or preterm delivery, possibly secondary to impaired uterine distension or cervical insufficiency.

Minor surgical procedures are most commonly used to treat uterine anomalies associated with pregnancy loss. Hysteroscopic metroplasty, a process by which a uterine septum is incised and thereby removed, is the procedure of choice for this condition. Cervical cerclage can be used to treat patients with uterine anomalies causing recurrent loss by cervical insufficiency. Uterine reunification procedures (for bicornuate and didelphys uteri) and metroplasty by laparotomy are now only rarely performed.

Uterine anomalies after diethylstilbestrol

Comparative studies have shown that women exposed to DES during their fetal life have a significantly greater incidence of spontaneous abortion than controls. Kaufman *et al.* reported that the percentage of first or all pregnancies in women exposed to DES that ended in spontaneous abortion was higher if their hysterograms revealed abnormalities in the shape of the uterine cavity or intrauterine defects. Haney *et al.* reported that the endometrial cavity of women exposed to DES *in utero* had a significantly smaller surface area than normal, which could perhaps

contribute to the increased spontaneous abortion rate in women exposed to DES *in utero*. No therapy, including routine cervical cerclage, has been shown to be beneficial in lowering the abortion rate in women exposed to DES who have abnormalities of the uterine cavity and recurrent losses. The length of gestation tends to increase with subsequent pregnancies, and therefore most of the women who had fetal DES exposure ultimately have a viable pregnancy.

Cervical insufficiency

The diagnosis of cervical insufficiency is best made by a history of second-trimester pregnancy loss accompanied by spontaneous rupture of the fetal membranes without preceding uterine contractions. Cervical insufficiency has been found to be associated with uterine anomalies, including both mullerian anomalies as well as those produced by fetal DES exposure, though the majority of cases occur as a result of cervical trauma including loop electrosurgical excision procedure (LEEP), obstetric laceration and cervical dilation.

Cervical insufficiency is treated with the placement of a concentric Mersilene suture at the level of the internal os (cerclage), using the technique described by either Shirodkar or McDonald. Because these techniques yield a similar rate of success, with a significant increase in the rate of fetal survival, the McDonald procedure is preferable, since this procedure is technically easier and is associated with less morbidity than the Shirodkar technique. It is recommended that the suture be placed electively between 10 and 14 weeks of gestation after major embryogenesis has been completed and the incidence of spontaneous abortion caused by genetic abnormality has decreased. An ultrasound examination should be performed before cerclage to document a normal gestation. Occasionally, if there is a markedly shortened cervix or previous placement of the McDonald cerclage has failed to maintain a pregnancy, a transabdominal cervical cerclage may be performed. If the suture is placed externally, it is usually removed at 38 weeks' gestation, and vaginal delivery allowed. However, because of cervical scarring, cesarean section is required in about 15% of pregnancies.

Outcomes from a randomized, intention-to-treat study of 1292 women with obstetric histories thought to put them at risk for preterm delivery revealed that placement of a preventive cerclage imparts significant benefit in preventing preterm delivery before 33 weeks only in the subgroup of women with three or more second-trimester losses. However, although elective cerclage is recommended only in this subset of patients, many other women with only one or two second-trimester losses thought to be secondary to cervical insufficiency will elect to have a cerclage placed by their care provider so as to minimize the risk of another loss.

Uterine adhesions

Adhesions in the uterine cavity can cause partial or complete obliteration of the endometrial cavity, leading to menstrual abnormalities and amenorrhea, as well as infertility and miscarriage. The latter is thought to be the result of insufficient endometrium to support adequate fetal growth. The major cause of adhesions is curettage of the endometrial cavity in association with a pregnancy or in the early puerperium.

The recommended treatment for intrauterine adhesions is lysis of the adhesions during hysteroscopy. To prevent adhesion reformation, a stent such as a size 8 pediatric Foley catheter can be placed in the cavity immediately postoperatively. The catheter should then be removed after 7–10 days. Alternatively or concurrently, high-dose estrogen (such as oral micronized estradiol 2 mg 2–3 times daily) can be administered for 30 days, with medroxyprogesterone acetate 10 mg per day added for the last 10 days in order to provoke a withdrawal bleed.

Uterine leiomyomas

Submucous uterine leiomyomas have been implicated as a cause of miscarriage. A prospective study of 29 women with submucous fibroids, 14 with primary infertility and 15 with previous poor obstetric outcome, showed that the miscarriage rate prior to 12 weeks' gestational age decreased from 61.6% to 26.3% following hysteroscopic myomectomy. The relationship of intramural and subserosal fibroids to miscarriage is not yet clearly defined; however, available data on intramural and subserosal myomas not distorting the cavity seem to indicate little or no affect on reproductive outcomes in cases of fibroids less than 5–7 cm diameter.

Leiomyomas are most commonly diagnosed by ultrasound. The intracavitary component of each myoma is best determined by either hysteroscopy or saline hydrosonography. A hysterosalpingogram may also be helpful as it provides additional information about the patency of the fallopian tubes. The surgical approach (hysteroscopic vs transabdominal) is based on the imaging studies.

Endocrinologic factors
Diabetes mellitus

Although women with good glucose control have no increased risk of pregnancy loss, diabetic women with elevated blood glucose and glycosylated hemoglobin (Hgb A1C) levels in the first trimester are at increased risk for both early and late spontaneous miscarriage. The risk of pregnancy loss appears to correlate positively with increasing levels of hemoglobin A1C. A study of 116 pregnancies in 79 insulin-dependent diabetic women showed that compared to women who carried pregnancies beyond 20 weeks, women who had spontaneous miscarriages had statistically significantly higher Hgb

A1C levels. At 8–9 weeks' gestation, levels <12% were associated with successful outcomes, whereas levels >12% were associated with increased risk of miscarriage.

Thyroid disease

Although older studies indicate that hypothyroidism may be a cause of abortion, a study by Montoro *et al*. reported that no abortions occurred in 11 pregnancies of nine markedly hypothyroid women. In more recent studies of large numbers of women with RPL, only a few women in one of the studies were found to have abnormal thyroid function. There is no definitive evidence that hypothyroidism is a cause of abortion in humans. In women who have had recurrent losses, some studies have shown an increased incidence of antithyroid antibodies compared with controls, though the published data are largely conflicting on this issue.

Luteal insufficiency

Luteal phase insufficiency is classically defined as a lag of more than 2 days in histologic development of the endometrium compared with the cycle day. Inadequate luteal phase has also been defined as a mid-luteal progesterone of <10 ng/mL. Progesterone concentrations in both normal and abnormal early pregnancy reflect function of the corpus luteum and the developing trophoblast, and these levels fluctuate widely and overlap significantly. Therefore, measurement of serum progesterone in early pregnancy to identify those at risk for miscarriage is largely futile. Diagnosis of poor luteal function in a nonconception cycle is also fraught with difficulty, as concentrations vary widely given the pulsatile secretion of progesterone from the corpus luteum. Ascertainment of a short luteal phase (<13 d) is the most reliable criterion for diagnosis. The true association of luteal phase insufficiency to recurrent pregnancy loss is unknown, and the prevalence in RPL patients has been difficult to identify given the varying methods of diagnosis.

Several investigators have treated women with RPL and evidence or presumption of luteal insufficiency with progesterone beginning 3 days after ovulation and continuing throughout the first trimester. However, no randomized placebo studies have been reported to verify the effectiveness of progesterone in preventing miscarriage in women with luteal insufficiency. There is also no evidence of benefit to initiating progesterone therapy after the expected menstrual period is missed. In spite of the lack of data, however, empiric progesterone therapy is commonly used in women with unexplained pregnancy loss.

Immunologic factors

Both alloimmune and autoimmune factors have been proposed as causes for RPL. Antithyroid and antinuclear antibodies have been proposed to have association with pregnancy loss, but results have been inconclusive as to whether they are or are not present more often or at higher levels in patients with RPL. In addition, no logical or effective treatment is available for these conditions. Alloimmune factors may cause pregnancy loss by a mechanism similar to graft rejection. However, because the exact mechanisms that allow a mother to immunologically tolerate her fetus are not well understood, and because the specific alloimmune mechanisms are not yet well defined, it is difficult to study the roles that various immunologic factors might play in cases of recurrent pregnancy loss. Antiphospholipid syndrome (APS) is the only autoimmune condition that has been well studied and characterized with respect to pregnancy loss.

Antiphospholipid syndrome

Antiphospholipid syndrome is characterized by adverse pregnancy outcomes or arterial and/or venous thrombosis, in addition to the presence of antibodies to phospholipids. The defining criteria of APS (Sopporo Criteria) were initially proposed in 1999 by an international committee and were updated in 2006 as shown in Box 106.1.

Although *in vitro* these immunoglobulins have anticoagulant activity by interfering with activation of the prothrombin–activator complex and thus prolonging the partial thromboplastin time, *in vivo* the presence

---

Box 106.1 Sopporo Criteria for APS

Clinical criteria
History of thromboembolic event (arterial, venous, small vessel)
  Pregnancy morbidity:
- three or more losses <10 weeks of gestational age (wga) unexplained by parental chromosomal, anatomic or hormonal causes
- unexplained fetal death ≥10 wga of morphologically normal fetus
- premature birth <34 wga associated with eclampsia, pre-eclampsia or placental insufficiency

Laboratory criteria
Presence of antiphospholipid antibodies on two or more occasions at least 12 weeks apart as demonstrated by:
- anticardiolipin (aCL) IgG or IgM in moderate or high titer (>40 units GPL or MPL or >99th percentile for the testing laboratory, ELISA)
- antibodies to β2-glycoprotein I (β2-GP I) of IgG or IgM isotype at a titer >99th percentile for the testing laboratory (ELISA)
Presence of lupus anticoagulant (LA) (aPTT, dRVVT, KCT)
  Antiphospholipid syndrome can and should be diagnosed if at least one clinical and one laboratory criteria are met

---

of these antibodies is associated with thrombosis. For example, lupus anticoagulants are antibodies directed against plasma proteins (i.e. β2-glycoprotein I, annexin V, prothrombin) bound to anionic phospholipids; this blocks *in vitro* assembly of prothrombinase complex and causes prolongation of clotting assays. The presence of lupus anticoagulant activity is usually documented by performing an activated partial thromboplastin time (aPTT). If the test is prolonged, an equal amount of normal plasma is added to the patient's plasma and the aPTT is repeated. If it is still prolonged, the presence of lupus anticoagulant is likely and can be confirmed by correcting the aPTT with addition of phospholipid. The antiphospholipid antibodies associated with lupus anticoagulant activity bind several phospholipids, including cardiolipin. The majority of patients with lupus anticoagulant activity, but not all, also have anticardiolipin antibodies. The presence of the anticardiolipin antibody, as well as other antiphospholipid antibodies, can be determined by specific solid-phase or enzyme-linked immunoassays.

Deleze *et al.* reported that about 80% of women with systemic lupus erythematosus and recurrent fetal loss had antiphospholipid antibodies, whereas they were present in only 15% of women with SLE without fetal loss. These antibodies are found also in women with other immunologic disease, with subclinical autoimmune disease, and with recurrent pregnancy loss, thrombosis or thrombocytopenia. Anticardiolipin antibody has been reported to occur in 13–40% of such individuals. The presence of lupus anticoagulant activity, anticardiolipin antibody and anti-β2-glycoprotein I should be determined in individuals with recurrent losses, since a causal relationship has been shown to exist, but there is little evidence that other antiphospholipid antibodies are a cause of RPL.

Although specific treatment of patients with recurrent pregnancy loss and APS is still occasionally debated, most practitioners agree that if diagnostic criteria are truly met, treatment with ASA 81 mg daily as well as prophylactic Lovenox or heparin should be administered throughout pregnancy. Aspirin is usually started prior to conception given its low-risk profile. The appropriate time for starting Lovenox/heparin is still not known definitively, however, and usually ranges from the time of the first normal rise of β-hCG to the time an intrauterine pregnancy is documented by ultrasound.

Inherited thrombophilic factors

The inherited thrombophilias that have been proposed as causes for RPL include factor V Leiden (activated protein C resistance), prothrombin gene mutation (G20210A), proteins C and S deficiency, antithrombin III deficiency, and methylenetetrahydrofolate reductase polymorphisms/hyperhomocysteinemia. The two most common are factor V Leiden and the prothrombin gene mutation; their prevalence in Western populations is 8% and 2–3% respectively.

Evidence regarding the association of thrombophilias and RPL has been conflicting. Several studies have been performed to evaluate this issue and although not completely consistent, frequent associations have been shown between pregnancy loss and factor V Leiden (FVL) and the prothrombin gene mutation; however, most often, FVL has stronger association with late fetal loss, not early recurrent loss. In addition, several studies have shown that multiple thrombophilic defects in either partner significantly increase the risk of miscarriage and are also strongly associated with IUGR.

Despite the controversy surrounding thrombophilias and recurrent pregnancy loss, if detected, most clinicians recommend treatment with ASA and prophylactic Lovenox/heparin during pregnancy.

Infectious causes

Toxoplasma, Ureaplasma urealyticum (*T. mycoplasma*), *Chlamydia*, cytomegalovirus, and herpes simplex have all been associated with abortion. Intrauterine infection is thought to potentially prevent implantation or interfere with organogenesis. Infection may be primarily intrauterine or may result from transplacental transmission from the mother. However, a causal relation between these organisms and recurrent pregnancy loss has not been well documented. Moreover, no properly performed clinical trial has demonstrated improved outcome after therapy.

Diagnostic evaluation

After a thorough history and physical examination are performed, a complete blood count, serum thyroid-stimulating hormone, 2-hour glucose tolerance test, and assays to detect lupus anticoagulant, anticardiolipin antibody and anti-β2-glycoprotein I antibody should be obtained. In our practice, analysis for FVL and the prothrombin gene mutation is performed if the patient is Caucasian (as this is the population in which the mutations are most prevalent) or has a personal history of a DVT/PE. A saline sonohysterogram or hysterosalpingogram should also be performed to rule out congenital uterine anomalies, submucous leiomyomas, and intrauterine adhesions. Finally, a karyotype of the mother and father should be performed.

If any of the diagnostic tests discussed above reveals an abnormality that can be corrected with appropriate surgical or medical therapy, such therapy should be initiated. If no diagnosis can be obtained, as occurs in approximately 50% of all cases of RPL, the couple should be counseled regarding the risk of miscarriage in a subsequent pregnancy. After conception, measurement of human chorionic gonadotropin (hCG) levels twice weekly will allow early prognosis of the outcome of the pregnancy. In normal gestations, the levels of hCG double about every 2 days, and the rate of increase in a particular patient can be compared with the expected normal rate of increase. In most individuals with an early abortion, levels of hCG will rise at a slower rate than normal, plateau, and then decline. If hCG levels are increasing normally, an ultrasound examination should be performed at 6 weeks of gestation, at which time a gestational sac should be found. Fetal heart activity in a normal pregnancy may be detected at 6 weeks of gestation with a highly sensitive ultrasound probe, and 7 weeks in all cases. Serial ultrasound examinations every 1–2 weeks provide reassurance of normal development to both the mother and clinician and thus are of benefit.

Some individuals recommend that low-dose ASA and/or progesterone supplementation be given to all women with unexplained RPL. Although neither of these modalities has been scientifically demonstrated to improve pregnancy outcomes, their low cost and minimal risks make them reasonable choices to offer patients who have no other treatment options.

Several studies have demonstrated that extensive counseling and emotional support throughout early gestation results in significantly greater livebirth rates than when only routine care is given. Thus, intensive emotional support during early pregnancy appears to be very beneficial for improving the prognosis of couples with recurrent pregnancy loss whose etiology remains undetermined. Therefore such support should be given.

Suggested reading

Acien P. Incidence of müllerian defects in fertile and infertile women. *Hum Reprod* 1997; 12: 1372–1376.

American Society for Reproductive Medicine Practice Committee in collaboration with Society of Reproductive Surgeons. Myomas and reproductive function. *Fertil Steril* 2008; 90(5 suppl): S125–130.

Kutteh WH, Yetman DL, Carr AC, Beck LA, Scott RT Jr. Increased prevalence of antithyroid antibodies identified in women with recurrent pregnancy loss but not in women undergoing assisted reproduction. *Fertil Steril* 1999; 71: 843–848.

March CM, Israel R. Hysteroscopic management of recurrent abortion caused by septate uterus. *Am J Obstet Gynecol* 1987; 156: 834–842.

Miyakis S, Lockshin MD, Atsumi T, *et al.* International consensus statement on an update of the classification criteria for definite antiphospholipid syndrome (APS). *J Thromb Haemost* 2006; 4: 295–306.

Rai R, Backos M, Rushworth F, Regan L. Polycystic ovaries and recurrent miscarriage – a reappraisal. *Hum Reprod* 2000; 15: 612–615.

Sugiura-Ogasawara M, Aoki K, Fujii T, *et al*. Subsequent pregnancy outcomes in recurrent miscarriage patients with a paternal or maternal carrier of a structural chromosome rearrangement. *J Hum Genet* 2008; 53: 622–628.

Surrey ES, Lietz AK, Schoolcraft WB. Impact of intramural leiomyomata in patients with a normal endometrial cavity on in vitro fertilization-embryo transfer cycle outcome. *Fertil Steril* 2001; 75: 405–410.

Wilson R, Ling H, MacLean MA, *et al*. Thyroid antibody titer and avidity in patients with recurrent miscarriage. *Fertil Steril* 1999; 71: 558–561.

Chapter 107
Combination Oral Contraceptives, Contraceptive Patch and Vaginal Ring: Indications, Contraindications, Formulations, Monitoring

Daniel R. Mishell Jr

Department of Medicine and Obstetrics and Gynecology, Keck School of Medicine, University of Southern California, CA, USA

Combination oral contraceptives (COCs), the intrauterine device (IUD), progestin-releasing implants, and long-acting steroid injections are the most effective methods of reversible contraception currently available for use by women in the USA. COCs, the contraceptive patch and vaginal ring all contain ethinyl estradiol which increases hepatic synthesis of globulins, enhancing coagulation of blood. Progestins do not have this effect. All estrogen-containing thrombophilic contraceptives can be prescribed for the majority of women in the reproductive age group because they are young and healthy; however, there are certain absolute contraindications for their use:

- current or past history of thrombophlebitis or thromboembolic disorders
- cerebrovascular or coronary artery disease
- known or suspected carcinoma of the breast, endometrium or other estrogen-dependent neoplasia
- undiagnosed abnormal genital bleeding
- cholestatic jaundice of pregnancy or jaundice with prior COC use
- hepatic adenomas or carcinomas
- known or suspected pregnancy

In addition, uncontrolled hypertension, diabetes mellitus with vascular disease, as well as smoking in women over 35 years of age are absolute contraindications to COCs, patch and ring because use of high-dose COCs in women with these disorders increases the risk of stroke and myocardial infarction. Women who are pregnant should not take COCs because of the theoretical but unproven masculinizing effect of the 19 nortestosterone progestins on the external genitalia of the female fetus. The concern that ingestion of COCs during pregnancy is teratogenic has not been proven to be valid.

Women with functional heart disease should not use COCs, since the fluid retention produced by these agents could lead to congestive heart failure. However, there is no evidence that asymptomatic mitral valve prolapse is a contraindication. Women with active liver disease should not use these agents, since steroids are metabolized in this organ. However, women who have had liver disease (e.g. viral hepatitis) in the past but whose liver function tests have returned to normal can receive these agents.

Relative contraindications to COC use include heavy cigarette smoking under the age of 35, the presence of migraine headaches, and undiagnosed causes of amenorrhea. The presence of aura with migraine headaches/classic migraine is an absolute contraindication to these agents; however, common migraine without aura is not a contraindication. Migraine headaches can worsen in frequency and/or severity with use of these agents. If these events occur or peripheral neurologic symptoms accompany the migraine headache, the agents should be discontinued.

These agents can be given to women with hypothalamic amenorrhea but if amenorrhea is due to a prolactin-secreting pituitary macroadenoma, the estrogen component could stimulate growth of the tumor. COC use has not been shown to adversely affect the natural history of women with prolactin-secreting microadenomas. Therefore the presence of these small benign tumors is not a contraindication to COC use if the woman does not wish to become pregnant and is at risk for development of osteoporosis because of low estrogen levels. The cause of the symptom of amenorrhea should be determined before starting COC use. COCs can also be taken by women with amenorrhea due to premature ovarian failure.

Anyone who develops galactorrhea while taking these agents should discontinue them and after 2 weeks, a serum prolactin level should be measured. If the prolactin level is elevated, a further diagnostic evaluation is indicated.

Management of Common Problems in Obstetrics and Gynecology, 5th edition. Edited by T.M. Goodwin, M.N. Montoro, L. Muderspach, R. Paulson and S. Roy. © 2010 Blackwell Publishing Ltd.

Women with a history of gestational diabetes can also take low-dose OC formulations because they do not affect glucose tolerance or accelerate the development of diabetes mellitus. Insulin-dependent diabetes without vascular disease, although previously a relative contraindication to COC use, is no longer considered to be so. Use of low-dose COCs in women with insulin dependency does not accelerate the disease process and these women are at high risk for pregnancy complications.

Medical conditions that were previously believed to be contraindications to COC use but are no longer contraindications include the presence of varicose veins, hypertension controlled with medication, and women with a current or past history of venous thromboembolism who are anticoagulated. In the latter condition, bleeding from a ruptured corpus luteum cyst can cause severe intraperitoneal hemorrhage and the slight thrombophilic changes produced by COCs will be overcome by the anticoagulant therapy. Obesity is an independent risk factor for venous thromboembolism (VTE). Therefore extreme obesity (BMI >40) is a relative contraindication to estrogen-containing contraceptives, as is a family history of idiopathic VTE. Evidence is conflicting regarding the presence of obesity and steroid contraceptive effectiveness but the majority of studies report that steroid contraceptive effectiveness is not decreased in obese women. If a woman has a known thrombophilic mutation she should not take a steroid contraceptive with estrogen, but it is not cost-effective to screen for thrombophilic mutation before use of these agents unless there is a family history or individual history of VTE. The World Health Organization has established medical eligibility criteria for use of estrogen plus progestin, progestin-only agents and the nonhormonal contraceptive. Its recommendations are summarized in Table 107.1.

Initiating oral contraceptive therapy

In deciding whether the pubertal, sexually active girl should use steroid contraception, the clinician should be more concerned about compliance than possible physiologic harm. Provided the postmenarchal girl has demonstrated maturity of the hypothalamic-pituitary-ovarian axis by having at least three regular, presumably ovulatory cycles, it is safe to prescribe hormonal contraceptives without being concerned about causing permanent alterations of hypothalamic-pituitary function. One need not be concerned about accelerating epiphyseal closure in postmenarchal females. Their endogenous estrogens have already initiated the process a few years before menarche, and the contraceptive steroids will not hasten it. These agents can also be prescribed for women with oligomenorrhea, especially those with polycystic

Table 107.1 Medical eligibility criteria for contraception adapted from WHO guidelines (Category 1: No contraindications, Category 2: Benefits outweigh risks, Category 3: Risks outweigh benefits, Category 4: Contraindicated)

	E + P	P	Cu IUD
Venous cardiovascular disease			
Hx of DVT +/or PE	4	2	1
Family Hx of VTE	2	1	1
Thrombophilia	4	2	1
Varicose veins	1	1	1
Superficial VT	2	1	1
Obesity: BMI >30	2	1	1
Arterial CV disease			
Ischemic heart disease	4	3	1
Stroke history	4	2	1
Hypertension			
Uncontrolled	4	2	1
Controlled	3	2	1
Smoking			
Age <35	2	1	1
Age >35 (<15/day)	3	1	1
Age >35 (>15/day)	4	1	1
Hyperlipidemia	2	2	1
Headache			
No migraine	1	1	1
Migraine w/out aura (age <35)	2	2	1
Migraine w/out aura (age >35)	3	2	1
Migraine with aura	4	2	1
Valvular heart disease			
Uncomplicated	2	1	1
Complicated (AF)	4	1	2
Diabetes			
Hx of gestational diabetes	1	1	1
Noninsulin dependent	2	2	1
Insulin dependent	2	2	1
Vascular disease or duration >20 years	4	2	1
Epilepsy			
No drugs	1	1	1
Anticonvulsants	3	3	1
Depression	1	1	1
Thyroid disease	1	1	1
Breast diseases			
Benign	1	1	1
Family Hx of Ca	1	1	1
Personal Hx of breast Ca	4	4	1
Anemias			
Thalassemia	1	1	2
Sickle cell disease	2	1	2
Fe deficiency	1	1	2
Systemic lupus erythematosus			
No vascular disease	2	1	1
Vascular disease	4	2	1
Antibiotics			
Rifampicin	3	3	1
Broad spectrum	2	2	1
Antiretroviral	1	1	2
Antifungals	1-2-3	1-2	1
HIV/AIDS			
HIV	1	1	2
Aids no antiretroviral	1	1	3
Aids with antiretroviral	2	2	2

E + P, ; P, ; Cu IUD, copper intrauterine device. (E + P = estrogen plus progestin, P = progestin only)

ovarian syndrome and dysfunctional bleeding due to anovulation. COCs will inhibit testosterone secretion and, by increasing levels of sex hormone-binding globulins, will increase the binding of biologically active testosterone, thus reducing the manifestations of hyperandrogenism. In both these conditions, COCs, the patch and ring will produce regular uterine bleeding without excessive blood loss. The progestin component of these agents will reduce the incidence of endometrial hyperplasia due to the effect of unopposed estrogen in these anovulatory women.

Following pregnancy

Ovulation occurs sooner after a spontaneous or induced abortion, usually between 2 and 4 weeks, than after a term delivery, when ovulation is usually delayed beyond 6 weeks but may occur as early as 4 weeks in a woman who is not breastfeeding.

Thus after spontaneous or induced abortion of a fetus of less than 12 weeks' gestation, steroid contraception should be started immediately to prevent conception occurring with the first ovulation. For women who deliver after 28 weeks and are not nursing, use of these agents should be initiated 2–3 weeks after delivery. If the termination of pregnancy occurs between 12 and 28 weeks, estrogen-containing contraceptive should be started 1 week after the end of the pregnancy. The reason for the delay in the latter instances is that the normally increased risk of thromboembolism occurring post partum may be further enhanced by the hypercoagulable state associated with estrogen-containing contraceptives. Because the first ovulation is delayed for at least 4 weeks after a term delivery, there is no need to expose the woman to this increased risk.

It is probably best for women who are nursing not to use estrogen-containing contraceptives, as their use, even with the low estrogen dose formulations, has been shown to diminish the amount of milk produced, as estrogen inhibits prolactin's action on the breast. Women who are breastfeeding every 4 hours, including at night, will not ovulate until 6 months after delivery if they do not menstruate and thus do not need contraception before that time. Once any supplemental feeding is introduced after 4 weeks post partum, ovulation can resume promptly. Since only a small percentage of full breastfeeding women will ovulate within 6 months post partum as long as they continue full nursing and remain amenorrheic, there is no need for additional contraceptive use. Progestin-only methods of contraception, in contrast to the estrogen-containing products, do not diminish the amount of breast milk and are effective in this group of women. However, a small portion of these synthetic steroids have been detected in breast milk. The long-term effects (if any) of these progestins on the infant are not known, but none has been detected to date.

All women

At the initial visit, after a history and physical examination have determined that there are no medical contraindications for COCs, patch and ring, the woman should be informed about their benefits and risks. For medicolegal reasons, it is best either to use a written informed consent signed by the woman or note on the woman's medical record that the benefits and risks have been explained to her and that she has been told to read the patient package insert.

Type of formulation

In determining which formulation to use, it is best to prescribe initially a COC formulation with less than 50 μg of ethinyl estradiol, since these agents are associated with less cardiovascular risk, as well as fewer estrogenic side effects, than 50 μg estrogen-containing formulations. It would also appear reasonable to use oral formulations with the lowest dosage of a particular progestin because fewer progestogenic metabolic and clinical adverse effects would be associated with their use. The patch and ring are currently made with only a single amount and type of estrogen and progestin. The development of multiphasic formulations has allowed the total dose of progestin to be reduced compared with some monophasic formulations without increasing the incidence of breakthrough bleeding. However, several monophasic formulations have a lower total dose of progestin per cycle than the multiphasic formulations. In addition, the most recently developed progestins derived from levonorgestrel: desogestrel, norgestimate, and gestodene have less androgenic activity than the older progestins norethindrone and its acetates and levonorgestrel. The progestin drosperinone has antiandrogenic as well as antimineralocorticoid properties and formulations with this agent are approved to treat acne and premenstrual dysphoric disorder in women desiring contraception. Some other formulations are also approved to treat acne.

The Food and Drug Administration (FDA) has stated that the product prescribed should be one that contains the least amount of estrogen and progestin that is compatible with a low failure rate and the needs of the individual woman. Because few randomized studies have been performed comparing the different marketed formulations, until large-scale comparative studies are performed, the clinician must decide which formulation to use based on which have the least adverse effects among women in his or her practice. If estrogenic or progestogenic side effects occur with one oral formulation, a different agent with less estrogenic or progestogenic activity can be given. Oral formulations with 20 μg of estrogen and the same amount of progestin as those with 30 μg appear to cause more unscheduled bleeding. If unscheduled bleeding persists beyond a few months after initiation, a formulation with a higher amount of estrogen can be used.

The contraceptive formulations containing progestins without estrogen have a lower incidence of adverse metabolic effects than the combination formulations. Because the factors that predispose to thromboembolism are increased only by the estrogen component, the incidence of thromboembolism in women ingesting these compounds is not increased. Furthermore, blood pressure is not affected, nausea and breast tenderness are eliminated, and milk production and quality are unchanged. Despite these advantages, these agents have the disadvantages of a high frequency of unscheduled bleeding and other abnormal bleeding patterns, including amenorrhea, and a lower rate of effectiveness. The use failure rate of these preparations is higher than with the combined formulations, and a relatively high percentage of the pregnancies that do occur are ectopic. Because nursing mothers have reduced fertility and are amenorrheic, the major disadvantages of these preparations are minimized in these women. Furthermore, because milk production and quality are unaffected, in contrast to the change produced by estrogen-containing contraceptives, the formulations with only a progestin may be prescribed to nursing mothers.

Follow-up

If the woman has no contraindications to steroid contraceptive use, no routine laboratory tests are needed prior to initiation. However, cervical cytology should be obtained or repeated annually as in all women of reproductive age. At the end of 3 months, the woman should be seen again. At this time a nondirected history should be obtained and the blood pressure measured. After this visit the woman should be seen annually, at which time a nondirected history should again be taken, blood pressure and bodyweight measured, and a physical examination (including breast, abdominal, and pelvic examination with cervical cytology) performed. It is important to perform annual cervical cytologic examinations on users of steroid contraceptives, since they are a relatively high-risk group for development of cervical neoplasia. The routine use of other laboratory tests is not indicated unless the woman has a family history of diabetes or vascular disease. If the woman has a family history of vascular disease, such as myocardial infarction occurring in family members under the age of 50, it would be advisable to obtain a lipid panel before COC use is started, since hypertriglyceridemia may be present and COC use will further raise triglycerides. As the low-dose formulations do not greatly alter the lipid profile, except for triglycerides, it is not necessary to measure lipids, other than routine serum lipid screening every 5 years. Low-dose COCs can be used in women with dyslipidemia, other than hypertriglyceridemia, as they

have a beneficial effect upon the lipid profile, raising high-density lipoprotein (HDL) cholesterol and lowering low-density lipoprotein (LDL). If the woman has a family history of diabetes or evidence of diabetes during pregnancy, a 2-hour postprandial blood glucose test should be performed before steroid contraceptives are started and, if elevated, a glucose tolerance test performed. If the woman has a past history of liver disease, a liver panel should be obtained to make certain that liver function is normal before these agents are started.

Drug interactions

Although synthetic sex steroids can retard the biotransformation of certain drugs (e.g. phenazone and meperidine) as a result of substrate competition, such interference is not important clinically. COC use has not been shown to inhibit the action of other drugs. However, some drugs can clinically interfere with the action of COCs by inducing liver enzymes that convert the steroids to more polar and less biologically active metabolites. Certain drugs have been shown to accelerate the biotransformation of steroids in the human. These include barbiturates, sulfonamides, cyclophosphamide, and rifampin. There is a relatively high incidence of COC failure in women taking rifampin, and these two agents should not be given concurrently. The clinical data concerning COC failure in users of other antibiotics (e.g. penicillin, ampicillin, and sulfonamides), analgesics, and barbiturates are less clear. A few anecdotal studies have appeared in the literature, but there is no reliable evidence for a higher pregnancy rate in women using COCs and these drugs, such as occurs with rifampin. Women with epilepsy requiring medication possibly should be treated with formulations containing 50 μg of estrogen, since a higher incidence of abnormal bleeding has been reported in these women with the use of lower dose estrogen formulations. The first-generation, but not second-generation, antiepileptic medication increases the metabolism of the estrogenic, not progestogenic, portion of the formulation and does not affect the failure rate of COCs.

Noncontraceptive health benefits

In addition to being a very effective method of contraception, COCs provide many other health benefits. Some occur because the COCs contain a potent, orally active progestin as well as an orally active estrogen and there is no time when the estrogenic target tissues are stimulated by estrogens without a progestin (unopposed estrogen).

Both natural progesterone and the synthetic progestins inhibit the proliferative effect of estrogen, the so-called antiestrogenic effect. Estrogens increase the synthesis of both estrogen and progesterone receptors, while progesterone decreases their synthesis. Thus one mechanism by which progestins exert their antiestrogenic effects is by decreasing the synthesis of estrogen receptors. Another way is by stimulating the activity of the enzyme estradiol-17β-dehydrogenase, within the endometrial cell. This enzyme converts the more potent estradiol to the less potent estrone, reducing estrogenic action within the cell.

Benefits from antiestrogenic action of progestins

As a result of the antiestrogenic action of the progestins in COCs, the height of the endometrium is less than in an ovulatory cycle, and there is less proliferation of the glandular epithelium. These changes produce several substantial benefits for the COC user. One is a reduction in the amount of blood loss at the time of endometrial shedding. In an ovulatory cycle the mean blood loss during menstruation is about 35 mL, compared with 20 mL for women taking COCs. This decreased blood loss makes the development of iron deficiency anemia less likely. COC users are about half as likely to develop iron deficiency anemia as controls.

Because the COCs produce regular withdrawal bleeding, users are significantly less likely to develop heavy bleeding episodes, irregular menstruation or intermenstrual bleeding. Because these disorders are frequently treated by curettage and/or hysterectomy, COC users require these procedures less frequently.

Because progestins inhibit the proliferative effect of estrogens on the endometrium, women who use COCs have been found to be significantly less likely to develop adenocarcinoma of the endometrium. After 1 year of COC use, the chance of developing this cancer is reduced by 50%. Further reduction in risk of this cancer is directly related to the duration of use of COCs. The reduced risk persists for at least 15 years after stopping COC use.

Several studies have shown that COCs reduce the incidence of benign breast disease, and two prospective studies have indicated that this reduction is directly related to the amount of progestin in the compounds. Current users of COCs have an 85% reduction in the incidence of fibroadenomas and 50% reduction in chronic cystic changes and nonbiopsied breast lumps, as compared with controls using IUDs or diaphragms. The risk of developing these three problems decreases with increased duration of COC use and persists for about 1 year following discontinuation of COCs, after which no further reduction in risk occurs.

Benefits from inhibition of ovulation

Other noncontraceptive medical benefits of COCs result from their main action – inhibition of ovulation. Some disorders, such as dysmenorrhea and premenstrual syndrome, occur much more frequently in ovulatory than anovulatory cycles. COC users have 63% less dysmenorrhea and 29% less premenstrual syndrome than controls.

Another serious adverse effect of ovulatory menstrual cycles is the development of functional ovarian cysts – specifically, follicular and luteal cysts – that may require surgical excision because of pain, rupture or hemorrhage. When ovulation is inhibited, functional cysts do not usually develop. Users of COCs have a significant reduction in the development of ovarian cysts. The magnitude of the reduction in risk appears to be greater with combination formulations containing 30–35 μg of estrogen than 20 μg and greater with fixed-dose than multiphasic formulations.

Another disorder linked to incessant ovulation is epithelial ovarian cancer. The development of this type of ovarian cancer is significantly reduced in COC users with a duration-dependent decrease in risk. After 1 year of use the risk is reduced by 50% and after 10 years use it is reduced by 80%. Protection against development of this lethal malignancy persists for at least 15 years after COCs are discontinued. COCs reduce the risk of developing ovarian cancer in women with the BRCA mutations as well as in women without these mutations.

Other benefits

Combination OCs with nonandrogenic progestins decrease the severity of acne. Several formulations are approved for the treatment of acne because randomized controlled trials found that the COC users had a greater improvement in the severity of acne than the control group. Several studies have shown that the risk of developing rheumatoid arthritis in COC users was only about half that in controls. Another benefit is protection against salpingitis, often referred to as pelvic inflammatory disease (PID). The risk of developing PID among COC users in most studies is reduced by 50%. It has been estimated that 14–20% of women with cervical gonorrhea will develop PID. In a Swedish study all cases of suspected PID were confirmed by laparoscopic visualization 1 day after hospital admission. Of women who used contraception other than the IUD and COCs, 15% developed PID; only about half as many, 8.8% of those who used COCs, developed PID. The results of this study indicate that COCs reduce the clinical development of PID in women infected with gonorrhea.

Although the incidence of the cervical infection *Chlamydia trachomatis* is increased in COC users compared with controls, the incidence of chlamydial PID in COC users is only half that of control subjects. This protection may be related to the decreased duration of uterine bleeding, which results in a smaller number of organisms which ascend to the upper genital tract, and allows the body's defenses to eliminate them more easily. One sequela of PID is ectopic pregnancy, an entity that has tripled in incidence in the past 15 years. COCs reduce the risk of ectopic pregnancy by more than 90% in current users and may reduce the incidence in former users by decreasing their chance of developing PID.

Because of these many noncontraceptive benefits as well as the fact that there is no evidence that use of low-dose COCs in nonsmoking normotensive women is associated with an increased incidence of serious arterial cardiovascular disease, particularly myocardial infarction and stroke, an FDA advisory committee recommended that COCs can be used by nonsmoking women without vascular disease beyond the age of 40. Of course, older women, as all women who take oral contraceptives, should take the lowest possible dose formulation that is effective.

Several recent studies have shown that use of COCs by perimenopausal women increases the amount of bone mineral density. COCs appear to prevent postmenopausal osteoporosis fractures. Another advantage of COC use is about a 20% reduction in the development of colon and rectal cancer.

Analysis of COC users in the large British General Practitioners Study from 1968 to 1992 reported they had less chance of developing all cancer than controls not using COCs. The risk of breast cancer was not increased in COC users and the risk of ovarian cancer and endometrial cancer was reduced about 50% compared with controls. Breast cancer risk with COC current and past users is not increased compared with nonusers in women aged 35–65. COC use in women with a family history of breast cancer is not increased compared with nonuse and a similar relation of no increase of breast cancer with COC use occurs in women with a BRCA mutation. Oral contraceptives can be prescribed until the woman becomes postmenopausal, as determined by an elevated FSH level (>20 mIU/mL) on a serum sample obtained on the day before starting the next cycle of contraceptives or until she reaches age 55. At this time treatment should be switched to estrogen-progestin hormone replacement because of the lower potency of the latter steroids upon liver globulin synthesis compared to COCs.

Suggested reading

Beral V, Hermon C, Kay C, *et al*. Mortality associated with oral contraceptive use: 25 year follow up of cohort of 46000 women from Royal College of General Practitioners' Oral Contraception Study. *BMJ* 1999; 318: 96.

Burkman R, Schlesselman J, Zieman M. Safety concerns and health benefits associated with oral contraception. *Am J Obstet Gynecol* 2004; 190: S5.

Collaborative Group on Hormonal Factors in Breast Cancer. Breast cancer and hormonal contraceptives: collaborative reanalysis of individual data on 53,297 women with breast cancer and 100,239 women without breast cancer from 54 epidemiological studies. *Lancet* 1996; 347: 1713.

Croft P, Hannaford PC. Risk factors for acute myocardial infarction in women. *BMJ* 1989; 298: 165.

ESHRE Capri Workshop Group. Noncontraceptive health benefits of combined oral contraception. *Hum Reprod Update* 2005; 11: 513–525.

Gerstman BB, Piper JM, Tomita DK, *et al*. Oral contraceptive estrogen dose and the risk of deep venous thromboembolic disease. *Am J Epidemiol* 1991; 133: 32.

Hankinson SE, Colditz GA, Hunter DJ, *et al*. A quantitative assessment of oral contraceptive use and risk of ovarian cancer. *Obstet Gynecol* 1992; 80:708.

Hannaford PC, Kay CR. Oral contraceptives and diabetes mellitus. *BMJ* 1989; 299: 315.

Hannaford PC, Selvaraj S, Elliot AM, Angus V, Iversen L, Lee AJ. Cancer risk among users of oral contraceptives: cohort data from Royal College of General Practitioner's oral contraception study. BMJ 2007; 335: 651.

Holt VL, Cushing-Haugen KL, Daling JR. Body weight and risk of oral contraceptive failure. *Obstet Gynecol* 2002; 99: 820–827.

Marchbanks PA, McDonald JA, Wilson HG, *et al*. Oral contraceptives and the risk of breast cancer. *NEJM* 2002; 346: 2025.

Poulter NR, for the World Health Organization Collaborative Study of Cardiovascular Disease and Steroid Hormone Contraception. Venous thromboembolic disease and combined oral contraceptives: results of international multicentre case-control study. *Lancet* 1995; 346: 1571.

Roumen FJME, Apter D, Mulders TMT, *et al*. Efficacy, tolerability and acceptability of a novel contraceptive vaginal ring releasing etonogestrel and ethinyl oestradiol. *Hum Reprod* 2001; 16: 469.

Schwartz SM, Petitti DB, Siscovick DS, *et al*. Stroke and use of low-dose oral contraceptives in young women: a pooled analysis of two US studies. *Stroke* 1998; 29: 2277.

Sidney S, Siscovick DS, Petitti DB, *et al*. Myocardial infarction and use of low-dose oral contraceptives: a pooled analysis of two US studies. *Circulation* 1998; 98: 1.

Chapter 108
Noncontraceptive Effects of Combination Oral Contraceptives

Daniel R. Mishell Jr

Department of Medicine and Obstetrics and Gynecology, Keck School of Medicine, University of Southern California, CA, USA

Introduction

Combination oral contraceptives (COCs) have been marketed since 1960 and millions of women have used these products during the past 50 years. Much information has accumulated regarding the various actions of these steroids in addition to their primary effect of inhibition of ovulation. These effects can be arbitrarily divided into three categories: neoplastic, reproductive, and metabolic.

Neoplastic effects

Numerous epidemiologic trials have been performed studying the relation of COC use to the most common genital neoplasms, breast, cervix, endometrium, and ovary, as well as several extragenital tumors, namely, hepatic, pituitary and malignant melanoma as well as colon and rectal cancer. Most of the studies thus far published have only determined mean risk in women under age 60 who previously used and did not use COCs. However, a recent paper from the Royal College of General Practitioners large cohort study of COC use reported lifetime risk of all cancers among COC users and age-matched nonusers from 1968 to 2004.

Breast cancer
Because estrogen stimulates the growth of breast tissue there have been concerns that the high dose of exogenous estrogen in COCs can either initiate or promote breast cancer in humans. In 1996 a large international collaborative group reanalyzed the entire worldwide epidemiologic data which had investigated the relation between risk of breast cancer diagnosis and use of COCs. The analysis indicated that while women took

COCs they had a slightly increased risk of having breast cancer diagnosed (relative risk (RR) 1.24, confidence interval (CI) 1.15–1.30). The magnitude of risk of having breast cancer diagnosed declined steadily after stopping COCs, so there was no longer a significantly increased risk 10 or more years after stopping their use (RR 1.01, CI 0.96–1.05). It is of interest that the cancers diagnosed in women taking COCs were less advanced clinically than those that occurred in the nonusers. The risk of having breast cancer which had spread beyond the breast compared to a localized tumor was significantly reduced (RR 0.88, CI 0.81–0.95) in COC users compared with nonusers. Furthermore, by age 50 the cumulative risk of breast cancer diagnosis was the same in COC users and never users. A large case control study by the Centers for Disease Control analyzed the relative risk of breast cancer diagnosis in current and former COC users aged 35–64. The relative risk in this study was 1.0 for current users of COCs and 0.9 for former users. In the Royal College of General Practitioners (RCGP) study of 744,000 women-years of COC users and 339,000 women-years of never users, the relative risk of breast cancer diagnosis was 0.98.

Overall, the large body of data regarding COC use and lifetime risk of developing breast cancer risk is very reassuring. COCs do not initiate breast cancer and women with a family history of breast cancer or those with the BRCA mutation do not have an increased risk of diagnosis of breast cancer with COC use.

Cervical cancer
The majority of well-controlled studies indicate that there is no significant change in risk of cervical intraepithelial neoplasia or epithelial cervical cancer with COC use. In one RCGP study, the risk of diagnosis of inverse cervical cancer with COC use was 1.33, an insignificant increased risk (CI 0.93 – 1.94).

Three case–control studies have reported that the risk of adenocarcinoma of the cervix was significantly increased about twofold among COC users compared with nonusers. Thus COCs probably increase the risk

Management of Common Problems in Obstetrics and Gynecology, 5th edition. Edited by T.M. Goodwin, M.N. Montoro, L. Muderspach, R. Paulson and S. Roy. © 2010 Blackwell Publishing Ltd.

of development of this uncommon tumor and women taking COCs should have annual cervical cytologic screening.

Endometrial cancer

Twelve case–control studies and three cohort studies have examined the relation between COCs and endometrial cancer, and all but two of these studies have found that the use of these agents has a protective effect against endometrial cancer, the third most common cancer among US women. In the RCGP study, the relative risk of diagnosis of uterine cancer was 0.58 (CI 0.42 – 0.79). This protection persists after discontinuation of COC use. Women who use COCs for at least 1 year have an age-adjusted RR of 0.5 for diagnosis of endometrial cancer between ages 40 and 55 as compared with nonusers. This protective effect is related to duration of use, increasing from a 20% reduction in risk with 1 year of use to a 40% reduction with 2 years of use, to about a 60% reduction with 4 years of use. The protective effect of COCs upon endometrial cancer occurs with use of combination formulations with both high and low doses of progestin.

Ovarian cancer

There have been 22 case–control and two cohort studies evaluating the use of COCs with subsequent development of ovarian cancer, and all but two of these found a reduction in risk, specifically of the most common type – epithelial ovarian cancers. The summary relative risk of ovarian cancer among ever users of COCs was 0.6, a 40% reduction. In the RCGP study the risk of ovarian cancer with COC use compared with nonusers was 0.58. Several studies have shown that the risk of developing ovarian cancer in women with BRCA 1 and 2 mutations was reduced by 50% with use of COCs. COCs reduce the risk of the four main histologic types of epithelial ovarian cancer (serous, mucinous, endometrioid, and clear cell), and the risk of invasive ovarian cancers as well as those with low malignant potential is reduced. The magnitude of the decrease in risk is directly related to the duration of COC use, increasing from about a 40% reduction with 4 years of use to a 53% reduction with 8 years of use, and a 60% reduction with 12 years of use. Beyond 1 year there is about an 11% reduction in ovarian cancer risk for each of the first 5 years of COC use. The protective effect continues for at least 20 years after COC use ends. There is a similar level of protection with low-dose monophasic formulations as well as higher dose agents. Insufficient data on ovarian cancer risk with use of phasic formulations or formulations with 20 μg of estrogen are currently available. As with endometrial cancer, the protective effect occurs only in women of low parity (≤4), who are at greatest risk for this type of cancer. COCs also reduce the risk of developing benign ovarian tumors including cystoadenomas, cystic teratoma and endometriomas.

Liver adenoma and cancer

The development of a benign hepatocellular adenoma is a rare occurrence in long-term users of COCs, and the increased risk of this tumor was associated with prolonged use of high-dose formulations, particularly those containing mestranol. There does not appear to be a relation between development of this tumor and use of ethinyl estradiol-containing formulations. Data from a large multicenter epidemiologic study co-ordinated by the World Health Organization found no increased risk of liver cancer associated with COC users in countries with a high prevalence rate of this neoplasm. This study found no change in risk of liver cancer with increasing duration of use or time since first or last use.

Pituitary adenoma

Combination oral contraceptives mask the predominant symptoms produced by prolactinoma: amenorrhea and galactorrhea. When COC use is discontinued, these symptoms may occur, suggesting a causal relation. However, data from three studies indicate that the incidence of prolactin-secreting pituitary adenomas among users of COCs is not higher than that among matched controls.

Malignant melanoma

Several epidemiologic studies have been undertaken to assess the relation of COC use and the development of malignant melonoma. The summary RR from eight case–control studies was 1.0 and for three cohort studies 1.4 – an insignificant increase. A more recent analysis of the two large British cohort studies involving more than 40,000 women which were initiated in 1968 reported that the adjusted RR of incidence of malignant melanoma in COC users was 0.92 and 0.85. The latest data from the RCGP study reported that the risk of melanoma with COC use was 0.92 compared to nonusers. The results of these large studies of long duration indicate that COC use does not increase the risk of malignant melanoma.

Colon and rectal cancer

A recent meta-analysis found that COC use was associated with about a 20% decrease in risk of developing colon and rectal cancer in current users. In the RCGP study, the lifetime risk of developing colorectal cancer with COC use was 0.72, a significant decrease.

Reproductive effects

The magnitude and duration of the delay in the return of fertility is greater for women discontinuing use of COCs with 50 μg of estrogen or more than with those containing lower doses of estrogen. However, use of the low-dose formulations still causes a reduction in conception rates for at least the first six cycles after discontinuation. In women stopping use of COCs in order to conceive, the probability of conception is lowest in the first month after stopping their use and increases steadily thereafter. There is little, if any, effect of duration of COC use upon the length of delay of subsequent conception but the magnitude of the delay to return of conception after COC use is greater among older premenopausal women.

Thus, for 2–3 years after the discontinuation of contraceptives in order to conceive, the rate of return of fertility is lower for users of COCs than for women who have used barrier methods. Eventually the percentage of women who conceive after ceasing to use each of these contraceptive methods becomes the same. Thus, the use of COCs does not cause permanent infertility.

Neither the rate of spontaneous abortion nor the incidence of chromosomal abnormalities in abortuses is increased in women who conceive in the first or subsequent months after ceasing to use COCs.

Several cohort and case–control studies of large numbers of babies born to women who stopped using COCs have been undertaken. These studies indicate that these infants have no greater chance of being born with any type of birth defect than infants born to women in the general population, even if conception occurred in the first month after the COC was discontinued. If these steroids are ingested during the first few months of pregnancy, a review of all prospective epidemiologic studies found there is no increased risk of congenital malformations overall among the offspring of COC users. Furthermore, there is no increased risk of congenital heart defects or limb reduction defects in users of COCs after conception occurs.

Metabolic effects

The synthetic steroids in COC formulations have many metabolic effects in addition to their contraceptive actions. These metabolic effects can produce both the more common, less serious side effects, as well as the rare, potentially serious complications. The magnitude of these effects is directly related to the dosage and potency of the steroids in the formulations. Fortunately, in most instances the more common adverse effects are relatively mild. The most frequent symptoms produced by the estrogen component include nausea (a central nervous system effect), breast tenderness, and fluid retention (which usually does not exceed 3–4 pounds of bodyweight) caused by decreased sodium excretion. Estrogen can also cause melasma, pigmentation of the malar eminences, to develop. Melasma is accentuated by sunlight and usually takes a long time to disappear after COCs are discontinued. The incidence of all these estrogenic side effects is much less with use of lower estrogen dose formulations than that which occurs with high estrogen dose formulations.

Most progestins in COCs, are structurally related to testosterone, and produce certain adverse androgenic effects. These include weight gain, acne, and a symptom perceived by some women as nervousness. Some women gain a considerable amount of weight when they take COCs, and this weight gain is believed to be caused by the anabolic effect of the progestin component. Although estrogens decrease sebum production, progestins increase it and can cause acne to develop or worsen.

Thus women who have acne should be given a formulation with a low progestin/estrogen ratio. Several of these formulations have been shown in randomized controlled trials to reduce acne to a greater extent than placebo. The treatment of acne is now an approved indication for use of these agents.

The final symptom produced by the progestin component is failure of withdrawal bleeding or amenorrhea. Because the progestins decrease the synthesis of estrogen receptors in the endometrium, endometrial growth is decreased, and some women have failure of withdrawal bleeding. This symptom is not important medically, but since bleeding serves as a signal that the woman is not pregnant, for some women it is desirable to have some amount of periodic withdrawal bleeding during the days she is not taking these steroids. The two steroid components can act together to produce irregular bleeding.

Unscheduled (breakthrough) bleeding (which is usually produced by insufficient estrogen, too much progestin or a combination of both), as well as failure of withdrawal bleeding, can be alleviated by increasing the amount of estrogen in the formulation or by switching to a more estrogenic formulation.

Many women taking COCs complain of an increased frequency of headaches. It has not been determined what is the exact relation, if any, between each of the steroids in COCs and the occurrence of headaches.

Protein

The synthetic estrogens used in COCs cause an increase in the hepatic production of several globulins. Progesterone and androgenic progestins do not affect the synthesis of globulins except to decrease sex hormone-binding globulin (SHBG). Synthesis of SHBG is reduced by androgens, including the androgenic progestins. Some of the globulins that are increased by ethinyl estradiol ingestion, such as factors V, VIII, X, and fibrinogen, enhance thrombosis while another globulin, angiotensinogen, may be converted to angiotensin and increase blood pressure in some users. The circulating levels of each of these globulins are directly correlated with the amount of estrogen in the COC formulation. Epidemiologic studies have shown that the incidence of both venous and arterial thrombosis is also directly related to the dose of estrogen.

Although angiotensinogen levels are lower in women who take formulations with 30–35 μg of ethinyl estradiol than in those who take higher estrogen dosage formulations, a slight but significant increase in mean blood pressure still occurs in women who take the lower dosage formulations and about 1 in 200 women will develop clinical hypertension. Thus blood pressure should be monitored in all users of COCs. There is some indirect evidence that the progestin component may also raise blood pressure. However, women who receive progestins without estrogen do not have an increase in blood pressure over time, indicating that the estrogen component is the major cause of elevated blood pressure in a few users of COCs.

Carbohydrate

The effect of COCs on glucose metabolism is mainly related to the dose, potency, and chemical structure of the progestin. Conflicting data exist as to whether the estrogen component affects carbohydrate metabolism. The estrogen may act synergistically with the progestin to impair glucose tolerance. In general, the higher the dose and potency of the progestin, the greater the magnitude of impaired glucose metabolism.

Data from 20 years of experience using mainly high-dose formulations in the large RCGP cohort study indicated that there was no increased risk of diabetes mellitus among current COC users (RR, 0.80) or former COC users (RR, 0.82) even among women who had used COCs for 10 years or more. More than 1 million person-years of follow-up of COC users in the large Nurses Health Study cohort, which was initiated in 1976, were analyzed in 1992. Although type 2 diabetes mellitus developed in more than 2000 women, the risk was not increased among current COC users (RR, 0.71) and only marginally increased in past COC users (RR, 1.11) and occurred only among women who had used high-dose formulations many years previously, not for those who had used lower-dose formulations.

Lipids

The estrogen component of COCs causes an increase in high-density lipoprotein (HDL) cholesterol, a decrease in low-density lipoprotein (LDL) levels, and an increase in total cholesterol and triglyceride levels. The progestin component causes a decrease in HDL and an increase in LDL levels while causing a decrease in both total cholesterol and triglyceride levels.

The older formulations with high doses of progestin had adverse effects upon the lipid profile although they also contained high doses of the synthetic estrogen. These progestin-dominant formulations produced a decrease in HDL cholesterol levels and an increase in LDL cholesterol levels. They also caused an increase in serum triglycerides because the estrogen has a greater effect on triglyceride synthesis than does the progestin. Short-term longitudinal studies of several formulations containing levonorgestrel and norethindrone as well as the newer nonandrogenic progestins found that a significant increase in triglyceride levels still occurred but there was little change in either HDL cholesterol or LDL cholesterol levels, as well as total cholesterol levels, because the effects of each steroid on lipid synthesis were offset by the other.

Other metabolic effects

The estrogen component of oral contraceptives increases the synthesis of several coagulation factors, including fibrinogen, which enhance thrombosis, in a dose-dependent manner. The effect of COCs on parameters that inhibit coagulation, such as protein C, protein S, and antithrombin III, is less clear because of the diversity of techniques used to measure these parameters in different laboratories. Changes in most of these coagulation parameters in COC users are very small, if they occur at all, and there is no evidence that these minor alterations in levels of coagulation parameters measured in the laboratory have any effect upon the clinical risk of developing venous or arterial thrombosis.

Nevertheless, if the woman has an inherited coagulation disorder that increases her risk of developing thrombosis, such as protein C, protein S or antithrombin III deficiency or the more common activated protein C resistance, her risk of developing thrombosis is increased severalfold if she takes estrogen-containing oral contraception. The relative risk of developing deep venous thrombosis (DVT) among women with activated protein C resistance and COC use is increased 30-fold compared with non-COC users without the mutation. The annual incidence of DVT in a woman of reproductive age with this genetic mutation is about 6 per 10,000 women if she does not take COCs and about 30 per 10,000 women if she does. Currently, it is not recommended that screening for any coagulation deficiencies be undertaken before starting COC use as it is not cost-effective unless the woman has a personal or family history of thrombotic events.

Cardiovascular events

Venous thromboembolism

In one large study, among users of COC formulations with less than 50 μg of estrogen, the rate of venous thromboembolism (VTE) per 10,000 women-years was 4.2, with users of 50 μg estrogen formulation the rate was 7.0, and in users of higher than 50 μg estrogen formulations, the rate increased to 10.0 per 10,000 women-years. These data confirm earlier findings which indicate that the risk of VTE is directly related to the dose of estrogen in the formulation. The background rate of VTE in women of reproductive age was previously believed to be about 0.8 per 10,000 women-years but more recent studies indicate that it is about 3 per 10,000 women-years. A large observational study found the incidence of venous thromboembolic events among users of COCs with 20–50 μg ethinyl estradiol was 9 per 10,000 women-years, about three times the background rate of women of reproductive age, but one half the rate of 18 per 10,000 woman years associated with pregnancy.

The increased risk of VTE is similar in women taking the same dose of progestin with 20 μg of estrogen or 30 μg of estrogen. Thus, among users of combined COC preparations containing less than 50 μg of ethinyl estradiol, the risk of VTE is not related to the dose of estrogen.

In 1995 results of four observational studies reported that the risk of VTE among women taking low estrogen dose formulations containing desogestrel or gestodene was increased about 1.5–2.5 times that of women taking formulations with less than 50 μg of estrogen and levonorgestrel. Because these studies were not prospective clinical trials, controversy exists as to whether the increased risk of VTE was causally related to formulations containing these progestins or whether the increased risk was due to certain types of bias. Selection bias, diagnostic bias, and referral bias could have accounted for the differences but a causal relation cannot be disproven. Few data have been published to date regarding the risk of VTE with norgestimate-containing compounds, so it remains uncertain whether or not formulations containing this progestin are associated with an increased risk of VTE compared with use of low estrogen dose levonorgestrel compounds. A large observational study reported that the risk of VTE with a formulation containing drosperinone and 30 μg of ethinyl estradiol was similar to formulations containing levonorgestrel and the same dose of estrogen.

Myocardial infarction

Neither epidemiologic studies of humans nor experimental studies with subhuman primates have observed an acceleration of atherosclerosis with the ingestion of COCs. Epidemiologic studies indicate that there is no increased risk of myocardial infarction (MI) among former users of COCs.

The epidemiologic studies that reported an increased incidence of MI in older users of COCs were published in the late 1970s and thus used as databases women who only took formulations with 50 μg or more of estrogen. In these case–control and cohort studies, a significantly increased incidence of MI was found mainly among older users who had risk factors that caused arterial narrowing, such as pre-existing hypercholesterolemia, hypertension, diabetes mellitus or smoking more than 15 cigarettes a day.

Data accumulated during the first 10 years of the large prospective British study (1968–78), in which the majority of users took formulations with more than 50 μg of estrogen and high doses of progestin, showed that a significantly increased relative risk of death from circulatory disease occurred only among women over 35 years of age who also smoked. A more recent analysis of data obtained during the first 20 years of this study (1968–87) revealed that there was no significant increased relative risk of acute MI among current or former users of COCs who did not smoke any cigarettes. Women who smoked and did not use COCs had a greater risk of MI than nonsmokers whether or not they used COCs. Even though most of the women in this study used high-dose formulations, a significantly increased risk of MI with COC use compared to non-COC use occurred only among cigarette smokers. COC users who were heavy smokers had a greater relative risk than mild smokers. A case–control study analyzed the relation between COC use and the risk of MI among women admitted to a group of New England hospitals between 1985 and 1988. The relative risk of MI among current COC users was not significantly increased (RR 1.1, CI 0.4–3.1). Among women who smoked at least 25 cigarettes a day, current COC use increased the risk of MI threefold. Smoking alone, without use of COCs, increased the risk of MI about ninefold. These data indicate that cigarette smoking is an independent risk factor for MI, but the use of high-dose COCs by cigarette smokers significantly enhances their risk of experiencing a MI, the two factors acting synergistically. Current or prior COC use is not associated with an increased risk of MI in nonsmokers. Both the RCGP and WHO studies reported that the risk of MI in COC users was several-fold greater if they had hypertension than if they did not. Two recent case–control studies in the USA have shown no significantly increased risk of MI in COC users. A WHO report stated that women who do not smoke, who have their blood pressure checked, and do not have hypertension or diabetes are at no increased risk of MI if they use combined COCs regardless of their age.

Stroke

Although epidemiologic data from studies performed in the 1970s indicated that there was possibly a causal relation between ingestion of high-dose COC formulations and stroke, the data were conflicting, with some studies showing a significantly increased risk of thrombotic stroke, others an increased risk of hemorrhagic stroke, and still others no significantly increased risk of either entity. Furthermore, as occurred with MI, the studies that did show a significantly increased risk of stroke in COC users indicated that the increased risk was mainly limited to older women who also smoked and/or were hypertensive.

Data from the epidemiologic studies of COC use and cardiovascular disease performed in the 1960s and 1970s are not relevant to their current use, as the dose of both steroid components in the formulations now being marketed is markedly less, and women with risk factors for stroke with COC use, such as uncontrolled hypertension, and migraine headaches with aura are no longer receiving these agents. Furthermore, it is strongly recommended not to prescribe COCs to women over 35 who also smoke, another risk factor for a stroke.

An analysis of strokes occuring in a large health maintenance organization in California during the years 1991–94 indicated that the COC users had no significant increase of either thromboembolic or hemorrhagic stroke. In this study the relative risk of thromboembolic stroke and hemorrhagic stroke for COC users was 1.18 and 1.13 compared with never users and past users. Another case–control study analyzed these data as well as data from Washington State. The relative risks of ischemic and hemorrhagic stroke in COC users compared to nonusers were 1.4 and 1.3. Neither of these figures was statistically significant.

Conclusion

The results of these epidemiologic studies indicate that use of low estrogen/progestin dose COC formulations by nonsmoking women without risk factors for cardiovascular disease is not associated with an increased incidence of either myocardial infarction or stroke. Smoking is a risk factor for arterial but not venous thrombosis. Combination COCs should not be prescribed to women over the age of 35 who smoke cigarettes or use alternative forms of nicotine.

After analyzing all the published epidemiologic data, it appears that healthy nonsmokers can continue to use COCs until the age of menopause and beyond without having an increased risk of cardiovascular disease provided they are using formulations with less than 50 µg of estrogen and a low dose of progestin. There is no evidence of an increased risk of cardiovascular disease associated with increasing duration of use of COCs or previous use of COCs. Thus women can take COCs for an unlimited time period, no matter how old they are when they start taking them. There is no need for a rest period after a few years of COC use as it does not serve any purpose.

Suggested reading

Collaborative Group on Hormonal Factors in Breast Cancer. Breast cancer and hormonal contraceptives: collaborative reanalysis of individual data on 53,297 women with breast cancer and 100,239 women without breast cancer from 54 epidemiological studies. *Lancet* 1996; 347: 1713.

Dinger JC, Heinemann LAJ, Kühl-Habich D. The safety of a drospirenone-containing oral contraceptive: final results from the European Active Surveillance study on oral contraceptives based on 142,475 women-years of observation. *Contraception* 2007; 75: 344–354.

Gerstman BB, Piper JM, Tomita DK, *et al*. Oral contraceptive estrogen dose and the risk of deep venous thromboembolic disease. *Am J Epidemiol* 1991; 133: 32.

Hankinson SE, Colditz GA, Hunter DJ, *et al*. A quantitative assessment of oral contraceptive use and risk of ovarian cancer. *Obstet Gynecol* 1992; 80: 708.

Hannaford PC, Kay CR. Oral contraceptives and diabetes mellitus. *BMJ* 1989; 299: 315.

Hannaford PC, Selvaraj S, Elliot AM, Angus V, Iversen L, Lee AJ. Cancer risk among users of oral contraceptives: cohort data from Royal College of General Practitioners oral contraception study. *BMJ* 2007; 335: 651.

Heinemann LAJ, Dinger JC. Range of published estimates of venous thromboembolism incidence in young women. *Contraception* 2007; 75: 328.

Heit JA, Kobbervig CE, James AH, Petterson TM, Bailey KR, Melton LJ III. Trends in the incidence of venous thromboembolism during pregnancy or postpartum: a 30-year population-based study. *Ann Intern Med* 2005; 143: 697.

Marchbanks PA, McDonald JA, Wilson HG, *et al*. Oral contraceptives and the risk of breast cancer. *NEJM* 2002; 346: 2025.

Schwartz SM, Petitti DB, Siscovick DS, *et al*. Stroke and use of low-dose oral contraceptives in young women: a pooled analysis of two US studies. *Stroke* 1998; 29: 2277.

Sidney S, Siscovick DS, Petitti DB, *et al*. Myocardial infarction and use of low-dose oral contraceptives: a pooled analysis of two US studies. *Circulation* 1998; 98: 1.

Chapter 109
Injectable and Implantable Contraception

Penina Segall-Gutierrez and Ian Tilley
Department of Medicine and Obstetrics and Gynecology, Keck School of Medicine, University of Southern California, CA, USA

Introduction

There is one method of implantable and one method of injectable contraception available in the United States. Both methods contain only progestins, and are highly effective and safe for use in most women. The method of injectable contraception that is available in the United States is depot medroxyprogesterone acetate (DMPA). DMPA is a long-acting reversible hormonal method of family planning, which is administered as a 150 mg intramuscular (Depo Provera™) or a 104 mg subcutaneous injection (Depo Provera Subcutaneous 104™). The hormone used in this contraceptive method is medroxyprogesterone acetate, which is an acetoxy-progesterone derivative. This is a progestin-only form of contraception.

Although not FDA approved for contraceptive use until 1992, it has been available worldwide for over 40 years.

Approved for use in the United States in 2006, the etonorgestrel implant (Implanon™) contains 68 mg of etonogestrel that is slowly released into the systemic circulation. Insertion into the subdermal tissue of the upper arm is performed through a trocar without a skin incision.

Depot medroxyprogesterone acetate

Mechanism of action and pharmacokinetics

The most important mechanism whereby DMPA protects against unwanted pregnancy is the inhibition of ovulation. The mid-cycle surge of gonadotropins is eliminated. Estrogen levels in the peripheral circulation of DMPA acceptors are within the range usually found in the early follicular phase of a normal menstrual cycle. Additional antifertility effects include the formation of an atrophic endometrium and a thick, viscous cervical mucus, which impedes sperm penetration. Fallopian tube motility may also be decreased.

Based on studies that measured gonadotropin levels in DMPA users, ovulation is suppressed for at least 14 weeks following each intramuscular injection and 15 weeks following subcutaneous injection of DMPA. Following either a single dose or multiple tri-monthly injections of 150 mg DMPA, the levels of medroxyprogesterone acetate (MPA) in the peripheral circulation increase and reach peak concentrations at approximately 8–10 days following the last injection. The serum concentrations of DMPA then gradually decline for the remainder of the 12-week dosing interval. Depending on the sensitivity of the assay, MPA may be found in the serum more than 200 days following a single injection of 150 mg DMPA. Repeat injections of intramuscular DMPA at 12-week intervals do not result in an accumulation of drug as determined by the assay of MPA at frequent intervals. Recovery of the reproductive axis and pregnancy is quite variable from patient to patient. Pregnancy may occur as early as 4 months after the last DMPA injection and as late as 31 months or longer after stopping DMPA in order to conceive. The return of fertility is unrelated to the number of DMPA injections the patient has received.

Candidates for use

Depot medroxyprogesterone acetate is a contraceptive modality which is particularly suited for women who desire a long-acting, coitus-independent, convenient, highly efficacious method of family planning. Women who have medical conditions in which estrogen is contraindicated and who desire very effective contraception may wish to consider the use of DMPA, as it does not increase liver globulin production of angiotensin or clotting factors. For women with sickle cell disease, DMPA is the contraceptive method of first choice as it decreases blood loss and acute sickle cell crises. Another group of

Management of Common Problems in Obstetrics and Gynecology, 5th edition. Edited by T.M. Goodwin, M.N. Montoro, L. Muderspach, R. Paulson and S. Roy. © 2010 Blackwell Publishing Ltd.

women who are especially suited to using DMPA as their contraceptive method are those with seizure disorders as it has been correlated with decreased seizure activity. Additionally, anticonvulsant medications should not interfere with the efficacy of DMPA, as they do with some other methods of hormonal contraception. DMPA is also used to treat endometriosis and may improve other conditions such as dysmenorrhea and anemia. For women who choose not to reveal their contraceptive choice to others, DMPA is ideal as it is not visible or palpable, nor does it require the patient to store the medication. It is also particularly well suited for teens and is associated with significantly fewer repeat teen pregnancies at 1 year than oral contraceptives or nonhormonal methods.

There are some women who should not receive DMPA. Current breast cancer is an absolute contraindication to DMPA. DMPA should be used with caution if there is no acceptable alternative for patients with: past breast cancer with no disease for 5 years; undiagnosed abnormal vaginal bleeding; a current pulmonary embolus or deep vein thrombosis; breastfeeding less than 6 weeks post partum; blood pressure 160/100; vascular disease; history of stroke or ischemic heart disease; migraine headaches with aura; diabetes with retinopathy, neuropathy, nephropathy, other vascular disease or more than 20 years of disease duration; multiple risk factors for coronary artery disease; active viral hepatitis; decompensated cirrhosis; hepatoma or benign hepatic adenoma. Patients must be advised that DMPA does not protect against sexually transmitted infections (STIs). DMPA users who are at risk for STIs should also use barrier methods for STI prevention. It should also not be used for women who wish to become pregnant within a year as only 50% of women who desire fertility after DMPA are pregnant by 6–10 months after the last injection. Women who are unable to return to the clinic every 3 months who desire effective, reversible, long-acting contraception should consider using the implant or an intrauterine device.

Initiating DMPA use

Depot medroxyprogesterone acetate is a long-acting, highly convenient family planning method which is easy to administer. It is an aqueous suspension of microcrystals administered by injection every 12 weeks. While women must currently return to a clinic for reinjection every 11–13 weeks, women could theoretically be taught to give themselves subcutaneous DMPA at home, thus eliminating the need to return to the clinic. The injection site should not be massaged immediately following each injection as this disperses the steroid and shortens its time of effectiveness.

A woman who has been consistently using another method of hormonal contraception may switch over to DMPA at any time. Women undergoing elective

termination of pregnancy may be given DMPA prior to being discharged from the clinic. Postpartum women may also receive DMPA prior to hospital discharge.

For women who are new to using this effective method of contraception, the first injection of DMPA was historically given within the first 5 days after the onset of the last regular menstrual cycle. However, waiting for the next menses may put patients at significant risk for unintended pregnancy either in the interim or because they never return for DMPA injection. If a patient presents outside this 5-day window and has had unprotected intercourse in the preceding 5 days, emergency contraception (EC) should be offered on the day of DMPA injection (see Chapter 113). If unprotected intercourse only occurred more than 5 days prior to presentation, DMPA may be administered without EC. All patients initiating DMPA on the first 5 days of menses should be advised to use a back-up method of contraception for at least 7 days and to take a pregnancy test 2 weeks after injection. There is not an increased risk of pregnancy in those initiating DMPA outside the first 5 days of menses when a back-up method of contraception is used.

The periodic well woman exam is also a time for patient education with respect to current preventive medicine practices. Woman should be advised to have adequate calcium intake and to lead a healthy lifestyle with respect to smoking, diet, and exercise. A provider should also discuss the use of EC if the patient is unable to return on time for her next injection. While a well woman exam is a good time to initiate contraception, an asymptomatic patient requesting DMPA as her method of contraception does not need a pelvic and/or breast exam prior to the first DMPA injection.

Efficacy of DMPA

Jain *et al.* found zero pregnancies among 16,023 women-cycles in which intercourse occurred and DMPA was the only method of contraception used, giving DMPA a Pearl Index of zero. With typical use, 3% of women using the DMPA injection will become pregnant within 1 year. When compared to other progestin-only methods, the failure rate with typical use is higher than the single etonogestrel implant (0.2%) and the levonorgestrel intrauterine system (0.1%) but is significantly lower than oral contraceptive pills (8%).

Pregnancy following DMPA administration is rare. However, information has been collected pertaining to the pregnancy outcome of 241 out of 285 pregnancies that have occurred in DMPA users. The incidence of congenital anomalies, spontaneous abortion, ectopic pregnancy, premature births, stillborn infants, and multifetal gestations was not increased in women who conceived while using DMPA compared to women who conceived when they were not using any method of family planning. *In utero* exposure to DMPA does not appear to be teratogenic or detrimental to pregnancy outcome.

Common problems and side effects

All DMPA users experience a disruption of cycle control. Menstrual irregularities are one of the most common reasons for the discontinuation of this method of family planning. Specific counseling regarding amenorrhea, irregular bleeding, and heavy bleeding prior to DMPA initiation will prepare patients for these common effects and will reduce the termination rates of DMPA for this reason. In the first 3-month treatment interval one-third of the new-start DMPA users experience increased number of days of bleeding and spotting, one-third have a normal number of days of bleeding and spotting, and one-third will experience amenorrhea. There is a positive correlation with the duration of use of DMPA and the percentage of women experiencing amenorrhea. Therefore women who continued to use DMPA are less likely to be anemic. If irregular bleeding is bothersome, adding combined oral contraceptives for 1–2 months (for those patients in whom estrogen is not contraindicated) or ibuprofen 800 mg every 8 hours for 3 days may help.

Data regarding weight gain in DMPA users are conflicting. Pelkman *et al.* found no difference in weight gain, energy intake or energy expenditure among women using DMPA compared with women receiving a placebo. This suggests there is no metabolic explanation for weight gain on DMPA except for increased appetite. However, the average DMPA user gains 5 pounds in the first year, with a decline in rate of weight gain after additional years of use. Overweight and obese women gain more weight than normal-weight women. While contraception is an important part of the well woman exam, this must also include information on the importance of a healthy lifestyle, including diet and exercise. Weight should be monitored if there is concern about overweight and obesity.

The side effects and the percentages of women reporting them while receiving DMPA are as follows: headache (17.1%), abdominal discomfort (13.4%), nervousness (10.8%), dizziness (5.4%), decreased libido (5.4%), asthenia (3.8%), varicose vein pain (3.6%), nausea (3.4%), vaginal discharge (2.8%), breast discomfort (2.7%), peripheral edema (2.1%), backache (2.1%), dysmenorrhea (1.8%), depression (1.7%), acne (1.3%), and hair loss (1.2%). Some women may have symptoms associated with hypoestrogenism, particularly in the perimenopausal period. Perimenopausal patients who wish to continue using DMPA may benefit from estrogen therapy.

DMPA and bone health

Some studies have reported a decrease in bone mineral density in women who have used DMPA for 2 years or longer. In 2004, the FDA issued a black box warning for DMPA: "… it is unknown if use of Depo-Provera Contraceptive Injection during adolescence or early adulthood, a critical period of bone accretion, will reduce peak bone mass and increase the risk for osteoporotic fracture in later life …" DMPA has been used for over 40 years with no reports of increased fracture risk. Similar to lactation, there is a transient loss of bone mineral density (BMD) among women while on DMPA, which recovers after discontinuation. This recovery has also been seen in teenagers. Among postmenopausal patients, BMD was not statistically significantly different among former DMPA users and nonusers. Organizations such as the Society for Adolescent Medicine and the World Health Organization have published positions which do not support the restriction of duration of use suggested by the black box. Additionally, there is no reason to routinely provide bisphosphonates or DEXA screening to DMPA users. Patients at high risk for osteoporosis (i.e. those on chronic steroids) should be treated and screened as appropriate for their respective conditions. All patients should be advised to adopt behaviors associated with bone health, such as weight-bearing exercise, consuming the recommended amount of calcium for their age, and not smoking.

Metabolic impact of DMPA

Data regarding DMPA use and potential diabetogenic or lipogenic effects are conflicting. While some studies have found DMPA to have no effect and even an improvement in carbohydrate metabolism and lipid profiles, others have found potentially negative alterations. Depending on the study, total serum cholesterol has been reported to be unchanged, increased or decreased. LDL cholesterol concentrations were reported as unchanged or increased during DMPA use. Most studies have concluded that HDL cholesterol levels decrease during DMPA use, while triglycerides either decrease or are unchanged. While some studies have found no alterations and even an improvement in carbohydrate metabolism, most suggest a slight increase in both insulin resistance and production and an impaired response to glucose challenge which is unlikely to have any clinical significance in healthy patients. It has been suggested that DMPA use in certain ethnic groups at high risk for diabetes alters progression to diabetes (i.e. Native American women and Latinas). Because patients choose their own contraceptive method, it is difficult to determine if the patients who choose DMPA are at increased risk for developing type 2 diabetes. For example, it may be that women who are not motivated to take a pill every day are also less motivated to exercise on a regular basis. Many studies suggest that lifestyle may play a role in the development of diabetes among DMPA users. Most recently, the increase in development of type 2 diabetes among DMPA users was attributed to an increased risk of diabetes at baseline, high baseline triglyceride level, and weight gain in Latinas with a prior history of gestational diabetes.

Etonorgestrel implant

Like intrauterine devices, an important benefit of contraceptive implants is that a single motivated act can result in the long-term use of a highly effective method of rapidly reversible contraception. Although several implant systems are being used globally, only the single-rod etonogestrel-releasing implant system (Implanon™) is currently available in the United States. It is highly effective for 3 years. Because of insertion and removal problems with multicapsule implants, training sponsored by the manufacturer is required before a practitioner can purchase and insert Implanon.

Implanon is a contraceptive implant system that consists of a single ethylene vinyl acetate capsule that is 4 cm in length and 2 mm in diameter, containing 68 mg of etonogestrel, the active metabolite of desogestrel, that is slowly released into the systemic circulation. Insertion into the subdermal tissue of the upper arm is performed through a trocar without a skin incision. A small incision is required to remove the device. The capsule is not radiopaque, so superficial placement is necessary to ensure that the capsule remains palpable for removal. Etonogestrel is released at rate of 60–70 μg/day immediately after insertion, which steadily decreases over 3 years to a rate of 25–30 μg/day at the end of the third year. This amount is sufficient to prevent pregnancy by systemic action that results in ovulation suppression, increased viscosity of the cervical mucus, and progestational endometrial changes to variable degrees. Contraceptive effectiveness is high, with no pregnancies occurring in clinical trials with correct implant insertion. As with all progestin-only contraceptive methods, the incidence of unscheduled bleeding is also high.

Conclusion

Depot medroxyprogesterone acetate and the etonorgestrel implant are reversible contraceptive methods which are highly efficacious, easy to administer, highly acceptable to patients, do not contain estrogen, and minimize patient responsibility. They may be used safely and without restriction by most patients. While not easily visible, the etonorgestrel implant must be palpated by clinician and patient after insertion to confirm placement, while DMPA injection sites are generally neither visible nor palpable. The time of contraceptive administration is also an optimal time for preventive health maintenance counseling. DMPA and the etonorgestrel implant are important additions to the contraceptive choices for women.

Suggested reading

Croxatto HB, Urbancsek J, Massai R, Coelingh Bennink H, van Beek A. A multicentre efficacy and safety study of the single contraceptive implant Implanon *Hum Reprod* 1999; 14: 976–981.

Jain J, Jakimuik A, Bode F, *et al*. Contraceptive efficacy and safety of DMPA-SC. *Contraception* 2004; 70: 269–275.

Kahn H, Curtis K, Marchbanks P. Effects of injectable or implantable progestin-only contraceptives on insulin-glucose metabolism and diabetes risk. *Diabetes Care* 2003; 26(1): 216–225.

Kaunitz A, Miller P, Rice V, *et al*. Bone mineral density in women aged 25–35 receiving depot medroxyprogesterone acetate: recovery following discontinuation. *Contraception* 2006: 74: 90–99.

Le J, Tsourounis C. Implanon: a critical review *Ann Pharmacother* 2001; 35: 329–336.

Mäkäräinen L, van Beek A, Tuomivaara L, Asplund B, Coelingh Bennink H. Ovarian function during the use of a single contraceptive implant: Implanon compared with Norplant. *Fertil Steril* 1998; 69: 714–721.

Nelson A, Katz T. Initiation and continuation rates seen in 2-year experience with same day injections of DMPA. *Contraception* 2007; 75: 84–87.

Pelkman C, Chow M, Heinbach R, *et al*. Short-term effects of a progestational contraceptive drug on food intake, resting energy expenditure, and body weight in young women. *Am J Clin Nutr* 2001; 73: 19–26.

Stewart F, Harper C, Ellertson C, *et al*. Clinical breast and pelvic examination requirement for hormonal contraception: current practice vs evidence. *JAMA* 2001; 285: 2232–2239.

Wenzl R, van Beek A, Schnabel P, Huber J. Pharmacokinetics of etonogestrel released from the contraceptive implant Implanon. *Contraception* 1998; 58: 283–288.

Xiang a, Kawakuro M, Kios S, *et al*. Long-acting injectable contraception and risk of type II diabetes in Latina women with prior gestational diabetes mellitus. *Diabetes Care* 2006; 29: 613–617.

Chapter 110
Intrauterine Devices

Daniel R. Mishell Jr
Department of Medicine and Obstetrics and Gynecology, Keck School of Medicine, University of Southern California, CA, USA

Introduction

The main benefits of intrauterine devices (IUDs) are:
• a high level of effectiveness
• a lack of associated systemic metabolic effects
• the need for only a single act of motivation for long-term use

Despite these advantages, less than 5% of women of reproductive age use the IUD for contraception in the USA, compared with 15–30% in most European countries and Canada. In contrast to other types of contraception, this method does not require frequent motivation to take a pill daily or to use a coitus-related method consistently. These characteristics, as well as the necessity for a visit to a healthcare facility to discontinue the method, account for the fact that IUDs have the highest continuation rate of all currently available reversible methods of contraception.

Unlike other contraceptives, such as the barrier methods, which rely on frequent use by the individual to be effective and therefore have higher typical-failure rates than perfect-failure rates, the IUD has similar rates of failure for typical or perfect use. First-year failure rates are less than 1% with the copper T 380 A IUD and the levonorgestrel-releasing intrauterine system (LNG-IUS). Pregnancy rates are related to the skill of the clinician who inserts the device. With experience, correct high-fundal insertion occurs more frequently, and the incidence of partial or complete expulsion is lower, with resultant lower pregnancy rates. Furthermore, the annual incidence of accidental pregnancy decreases steadily after the first year of IUD use. The cumulative pregnancy rate after 12 years' use of the copper T 380 A IUD is only 1.7% and after 5 years use of the LNG-IUS is about 1.1%. The incidence of all major adverse events with IUDs, including pregnancy

and expulsion or removal for bleeding and/or pain, steadily decreases with increasing age. Thus, the IUD is especially suited for older parous women who wish to prevent further pregnancies but it can also be used by young nulliparous women.

Types of intrauterine devices

In the past 35 years, many types of IUDs have been designed and used clinically. The devices developed and initially used in the 1960s consisted of polyethylene impregnated with barium sulfate to make them radiographic. In the 1970s, to diminish the frequency of the side effects of increased uterine bleeding and pain, smaller plastic devices covered with copper were developed and widely utilized. In the 1980s, devices bearing a larger amount of copper, including sleeves on the horizontal arm (such as in the Cu T 380A and the Cu T 220C), were developed; the multiload Cu 250 and Cu 375 were also introduced during this period. These devices have a longer duration of high effectiveness, and thus need to be reinserted at less frequent intervals than devices carrying a smaller amount of copper. The copper T 380 A IUD is the only copper-bearing IUD currently marketed in the USA, while the multiload Cu 375 is widely used in Europe.

Because of the constant dissolution of copper, even though the amount lost daily is less than that ingested in the normal diet, all copper IUDs must be replaced periodically. The Cu T 380 A is currently approved for use in the USA for 10 years, although it maintains its high level of effectiveness for at least 12 years according to a WHO study. At the scheduled time of removal, the device can be removed and another inserted during the same office visit.

Adding a reservoir of levonorgestrel to the vertical arm also increases the effectiveness of the T-shaped devices. The currently marketed LNG-IUS realeses 20 µg of levonorgestrel into the endometrial cavity each day. This amount is sufficient to prevent pregnancy by keeping the cervical mucus thick and viscid, preventing sperm

Management of Common Problems in Obstetrics and Gynecology,
5th edition. Edited by T.M. Goodwin, M.N. Montoro,
L. Muderspach, R. Paulson and S. Roy. © 2010 Blackwell
Publishing Ltd.

transport into the endometrial cavity and oviducts. Serum levonorgestrel levels are lower than occur with levonorgestrel implants or oral contraceptives. Because of the progestational effect upon the endometrium, the amount of uterine bleeding is reduced to about 5 mL per cycle and this device has been used to treat heavy menstrual bleeding. The LNG-IUS needs to be replaced after 5 years of use, as the reservoir of levonorgestrel becomes depleted after this time. The surface area of plastic in this small device is insufficient to produce a sufficiently large leukocytic response to yield a high level of contraceptive effectiveness without levonorgestrel. This device is extremely effective, with a 5-year cumulative pregnancy rate of 1.1 per 100 women.

Mechanism of action

The main mechanism of contraceptive action of copper-bearing IUDs in humans involves a spermicidal effect. The presence of the foreign body in the uterine cavity generates a local sterile inflammatory reaction. In addition to causing phagocytosis of spermatozoa, tissue breakdown products of these leukocytes are toxic to all cells, including spermatozoa and the blastocyst. The amount of inflammatory reaction, and thus contraceptive effectiveness, is directly related to the size of the intrauterine foreign body. Copper markedly increases the extent of the inflammatory reaction, which explains why this metal has been added to the small frame of T-shaped devices. In addition, copper impedes sperm transport and viability in the cervical mucus. Because of the spermicidal action of IUDs, very few, if any, sperm reach the oviducts, and the ovum usually does not become fertilized.

The LNG-IUS prevents sperm transport through the thickened cervical mucus, so the ovum is not fertilized. The LNG-IUS, like the copper device, has a very low ectopic pregnancy rate, providing additional evidence that fertilization does not usually occur with both these devices.

Upon removal of the IUD, the inflammatory reaction rapidly disappears. Resumption of fertility following all types of IUD removal is prompt and occurs at the same rate as resumption of fertility following discontinuation of the barrier methods of contraception. The incidence of term deliveries, spontaneous abortion, and ectopic pregnancies in conceptions occurring after IUD removal is the same as in women who do not use any contraception.

Time of insertion

Although it is widely believed that the optimal time for insertion of an IUD is during the menses, data indicate that the IUD can be safely inserted on any day of the cycle as long as the woman is not pregnant. Because IUD insertion introduces bacteria into the endometrial cavity, it is preferable to insert it after the menses cease, to avoid providing a good environment for bacterial growth. IUDs can be safely inserted at the time of the routine postpartum visit after a term delivery when the uterus is involuted, whether or not the woman is nursing her infant. IUDs may also be inserted immediately after completion of a spontaneous or induced abortion.

Adverse effects

Incidence
In the first year of use with both types of IUD, there is less than a 1% pregnancy rate, a 10% expulsion rate, and a 15% rate of removal for medical reasons (mainly bleeding and/or pain). The incidence of each of these events diminishes steadily in subsequent years.

A WHO study of the Cu T 380A found that termination rates for adverse effects continued to decline annually following the first year after insertion for the following 12 years. In this study, the cumulative percentage discontinuation rates for reasons of pregnancy, bleeding and pain and expulsion at the end of 12 years were 1.7%, 35.3% and 12.5%. A large study of the LNG-IUS reported that cumulative termination rates for pregnancy, bleeding and pain and expulsion were 0.5%, 13.8% and 5.8% per 100 women respectively after 5 years.

Uterine bleeding
The majority of women discontinuing this method of contraception do so for medical reasons. Nearly all medical reasons accounting for removal of copper-bearing IUDs involve one or more types of abnormal bleeding, either heavy and/or prolonged menses or intermenstrual bleeding. The amount of blood lost in each menstrual cycle is significantly greater in women using copper-bearing IUDs than in nonusers. In a normal menstrual cycle, the mean amount of menstrual blood loss (MBL) is approximately 35 mL. The copper T 380 A IUD is associated with a 55% increase in MBL. In contrast, with the levonorgestrel-releasing IUD, the amount of blood loss is significantly reduced, declining to approximately 5 mL per cycle after 6 months of use.

In a study of women using the copper T 380, no significant change arose in mean measurements of several hematologic parameters, including hemoglobin, hematocrit, and erythrocyte count, when they were taken 3, 6, and 12 months after IUD insertion when compared with mean values before insertion. No significant change in mean serum ferritin levels was found at 3, 6 and 12 months after IUD insertion.

Excessive bleeding in the first few months following IUD insertion should be treated with reassurance and supplemental oral iron, as well as systemic administration of a prostaglandin synthetase inhibitor during menses. The bleeding usually diminishes with time, as the uterus adjusts to the presence of the foreign body. Irregular and frequent bleeding usually occurs in the first few months after insertion of the LNG-IUS. After this time bleeding is usually scant and about 20% of users are amenorrheic 1 year after insertion of the device.

Mefenamic acid taken in a dosage of 500 mg three times per day during the days of menstruation has been shown to reduce MBL significantly in copper-bearing IUD users. If excessive bleeding persists despite this treatment, the device should be removed. After a 1-month interval, another type of device may be inserted if the woman still wishes to use an IUD for contraception. Consideration should be given to inserting a LNG-IUS, as these devices cause less blood loss than the copper-bearing IUD in a normal cycle. All studies in which MBL has been quantitatively measured found that there is a significant reduction of MBL, about 60%, with use of the levonorgestrel IUD. This reduction is seen as early as 3 months after insertion and persists for the duration of use of the device. The reduction of MBL results in an improvement of blood hemoglobin levels. Thus the levonorgestrel-releasing IUD is useful in the prevention and treatment of iron deficiency anemia and the depletion of iron stores by heavy MBL and treatment of heavy bleeding is now an approved indication for use of this device.

Perforation

Although it occurs only rarely, one potentially serious complication associated with IUD use is perforation of the uterine fundus. Perforation always occurs at the time of insertion. Sometimes only the distal portion of the IUD penetrates the uterine muscle at insertion, and uterine contractions over the next few months then force the IUD into the peritoneal cavity. If an IUD is correctly inserted entirely within the endometrial cavity, it will not wander through the uterine muscle into the peritoneal cavity. Perforation of the uterus is best prevented by straightening the uterine axis with a tenaculum and then probing the cavity with a uterine sound before IUD insertion.

Perforation rates for the copper T 380 A are only about 1 per 3000 insertions. As the perforations occurring at the time of insertion are nearly always asymptomatic, the clinician should always suspect that perforation has occurred if the user cannot feel the appendage but did not observe that the device was expelled. One should not assume that an unnoticed expulsion has occurred when the appendage is not visualized. Sometimes the IUD remains in its correct position in the uterine cavity, but the appendage withdraws into the cavity as the position of the IUD changes. In this situation, after pelvic examination has been performed and the possibility

of pregnancy excluded, the uterine cavity should be probed. If the device cannot be felt with a uterine sound or biopsy instrument, a pelvic sonogram or x-ray should be obtained. If the device is not visualized with pelvic ultrasonography, an x-ray visualizing the entire abdominal cavity should be performed. This procedure is necessary because an IUD that has been pushed through the uterus may be located anywhere in the peritoneal cavity, including the subdiaphragmatic area.

Any type of IUD found to be outside the uterus, even if asymptomatic, should be removed from the peritoneal cavity because complications such as severe adhesions and bowel obstruction have been reported with intraperitoneal IUDs. Consequently, intraperitoneal IUDs should be extracted shortly after the diagnosis of perforation is made. Unless severe adhesions have developed, most intraperitoneal IUDs can be removed by means of laparoscopy.

Complications related to pregnancy

Congenital anomalies

When pregnancy occurs with an IUD in place, implantation takes place away from the device itself, so the device is always extra-amniotic. Although published data remain scarce, so far no evidence suggests an increased incidence of congenital anomalies in infants born with a plastic, copper-bearing or LNG-IUS IUD *in utero*.

Spontaneous abortion

In all reports of series of pregnancies with any type of IUD *in situ*, the incidence of fetal death was not significantly increased. On the other hand, a significant increase in spontaneous abortion has been consistently observed. If a woman conceives while wearing an IUD that is not subsequently removed, the incidence of spontaneous abortion is approximately 55%, about three times greater than would occur in pregnancies without an IUD.

After conception, incidence of spontaneous abortion is significantly reduced if the IUD is spontaneously expelled or if the appendage is visible and the IUD is removed by traction. In one study of women who conceived with copper T devices in place, the incidence of spontaneous abortion was only 20% if the device was removed or spontaneously expelled. This figure is similar to the normal incidence of spontaneous abortion and significantly less than the 54% incidence of abortion reported in the same study among women retaining the devices *in utero*. Thus, if a woman conceives with an IUD in place and wishes to continue the pregnancy, the IUD should be removed if the appendage is visible. Several reports indicate that intrauterine IUDs in the lower uterine cavity without a visible appendage can be removed with sonographic guidance during early gestation and that this procedure will not adversely affect the outcome of the pregnancy.

Septic abortion

There is no evidence that IUDs with monofilament tail strings increase the risk of sepsis during pregnancy. No significant difference was found in the incidence of septic abortion among women who conceived with an IUD in place and those who conceived while using other methods. Approximately 2% of all spontaneous abortions are septic, however, and the continued presence of an IUD is associated with a 50% risk of having a spontaneous abortion. Thus, the overall incidence of septic abortion may be increased with any IUD in place because the incidence of spontaneous abortion is increased, not because the presence of the IUD increases the risk of sepsis by itself.

Ectopic pregnancy

Because copper-bearing IUDs principally act by preventing fertilization through a cytotoxic effect upon spermatozoa, the incidence of both ectopic pregnancy and intrauterine pregnancy is decreased with their use. The risk of the pregnancy being ectopic is increased about threefold, from 1.4% to 6%, if a woman becomes pregnant with a copper IUD in place rather than using no contraception method. However, because the copper T 380 A IUD so effectively prevents all pregnancies, the estimated ectopic pregnancy rate is only 0.2–0.4 per 1000 women-years. This rate is one-tenth the rate in women using no contraception: 3 per 1000 women-years. If a woman uses a copper T 380 A IUD, her risk of having an ectopic pregnancy is reduced by 90% compared with use of no contraception. In the WHO study of the copper T 380 A IUD, the cumulative ectopic pregnancy rate at the end of 7 years was only 0.1 per 100 women. These data confirm that the copper T 380 A greatly reduces the risk of having either intrauterine or ectopic gestations.

The LNG-IUS has a very low rate of both intrauterine and ectopic pregnancies. The 5-year ectopic pregnancy rate with this device is 0.1, similar to the copper 380 A IUD. The increased risk of ectopic pregnancy for a woman who conceives with an IUD *in situ* is temporary and does not persist after removal of the device. If a woman becomes pregnant with either IUD in place, her risk of ectopic pregnancy is increased compared with the overall population of pregnant women. Consequently, appropriate diagnostic studies should take place early in gestation to establish the diagnosis before tubal rupture occurs.

Prematurity

When pregnancy occurs during presence of copper T devices, the rate of prematurity among livebirths is four times greater when the copper T is left in place than when it is removed. If a pregnant woman has an IUD in place and the device cannot be removed, but she wishes to continue her gestation, she should be warned of the increased risk of prematurity, spontaneous abortion, and ectopic pregnancy. She should also be informed of the possible increased risk of septic abortion and advised to report promptly the first signs of pelvic pain or fever. No evidence exists that pregnancies with IUDs *in utero* are associated with an increased incidence of other obstetric complications. In addition, prior use of an IUD has not been shown to result in a greater incidence of complications in pregnancies occurring after its removal.

Infection in the nonpregnant intrauterine device user

In 1966, a study was performed in which aerobic and anaerobic cultures were made of homogenates of endometrial tissue obtained transfundally from uteri removed by vaginal hysterectomy at various intervals after insertion of a plastic IUD. During the first 24 hours after IUD insertion, the normally sterile endometrial cavity was consistently infected with bacteria. Nevertheless, in 80% of uteri removed during the following 24 hours, the women's natural defenses had destroyed these bacteria and the endometrial cavities were sterile. When transfundal cultures were obtained more than 30 days after IUD insertion, the endometrial cavity, the IUD, and the portion of the thread within the cavity were always sterile. These findings indicate that development of PID more than 1 month after insertion of an IUD with a monofilament tail string is due to infection with a sexually transmitted pathogen and is unrelated to the presence of the device.

A large multicenter study co-ordinated by the WHO confirmed these findings. Of 22,908 women who had IUDs inserted, the PID rate was highest in the first 3 weeks after insertion, but remained lower and constant (0.5 per 1000 women-years) during the 8 years thereafter. An IUD should not be inserted into a woman who may have been recently infected with gonococci or *Chlamydia*. Insertion of the device will transport these pathogens from the cervix into the upper genital tract, where the large number of organisms present may overcome the host defense and cause salpingitis. If infectious endocervicitis is suspected, tests to detect pathogens should be obtained and the IUD insertion delayed until the results reveal no pathogenic organisms are present. Administering systemic antibiotics routinely with every IUD insertion is not cost-effective, but the insertion procedure should be as aseptic as possible.

A randomized trial comparing use of azithromycin taken just before IUD insertion with a placebo control reported no significant difference in the subsequent rate of pelvic inflammation. The rate was 0.1% in both study arms. In a study of the copper T 380 A IUD, the rate of removal because of infection during the first year of use was only 0.3%. One comparative study showed that the rate of discontinuation of IUD use was less with use of the LNG-IUS than a copper-bearing device.

These data provide additional evidence that, aside from the insertion process, the presence of an IUD with monofilament tail strings does not increase PID incidence after the insertion process. Additional support for this statement is provided by results of an epidemiologic study investigating the incidence of tubal infertility among former IUD users. In the study, nulliparous women with a single sexual partner who had previously used an IUD had no increased risk of tubal infertility. Another study found that nulliparous women who used an IUD did not have an increased risk of tubal infertility compared to women who had not used an IUD.

Symptomatic PID can usually be successfully treated with antibiotics until the woman becomes symptom free, without removing the IUD. For women with clinical evidence of a tubo-ovarian abscess, the IUD should be removed only after a therapeutic serum level of appropriate parenteral antibiotics has been reached, preferably after a clinical response develops. An alternative method of contraception should be utilized in women who develop PID with an IUD in place.

Evidence exists that IUD users may have an increased risk for colonizing actinomycosis organisms in the upper genital tract, especially after a long duration of use. The relationship of actinomycosis to PID remains unclear, as many women without IUDs have actinomycosis in their vagina and are asymptomatic. If actinomycosis organisms are identified during the routine examination of cervical cytology and the woman is asymptomatic, she may be treated with appropriate antimicrobial therapy, followed without therapy, or have the device removed. The IUD should not be removed from an asymptomatic woman who is colonized with actinomycosis but has no evidence of pelvic infection. If pelvic infection is present the woman should be treated with antibiotics and the IUD removed.

Contraindications

It is logical and consistent with good medical practice that IUDs should not be inserted into women with the following conditions, which are listed as contraindications to IUD insertion in the USA.
• Pregnancy or suspicion of pregnancy
• Acute pelvic inflammatory disease
• Postpartum endometritis or infected abortion in the past 3 months
• Known or suspected uterine or cervical malignancy
• Genital bleeding of unknown etiology
• Untreated acute cervicitis
• A previously inserted IUD that has not been removed

Few data indicate that the complications of Wilson's disease, allergy to copper, and genital actinomycosis are true contraindications for insertion of copper-bearing IUDs. Because of the infrequency of these conditions, it is unlikely that data will ever become available to prove or disprove this relationship.

The remaining contraindications for IUD use listed in the product labeling are:
• abnormalities of the uterus resulting in distortion of the uterine cavity
• a history of pelvic inflammatory disease
• vaginitis, including bacterial vaginosis, until infection is controlled
• multiple sexual partners for the patient or her partner
• conditions associated with increased susceptibility to infections with micro-organisms

These contraindications remain questionable because of the lack of clinical studies of IUD use in women with these conditions.

It is unclear why the IUD is stated to be contraindicated in women who have multiple sexual partners or whose partners have multiple sexual partners. Such women should be counseled to have their partners use condoms to protect against sexually transmitted diseases and to use the IUD to effectively prevent pregnancy if they so desire.

Conditions previously believed to preclude IUD use, but are no longer considered to be contraindications, include: diabetes mellitus, valvular heart disease (including mitral valve prolapse), past history of ectopic pregnancy (except LNG-IUS), nulliparity, treated cervical dysplasia, irregular menses due to anovulation, breastfeeding, corticosteroid use, age less than 25.

Overall safety

Several long-term studies have indicated that the IUD is not associated with an increased incidence of endometrial or cervical carcinoma. In fact, studies have shown a reduced risk of developing these neoplasms with IUD use. The IUD is a particularly useful method of contraception for women who have completed their families, and have contraindications to (or do not wish to use) other effective methods of reversible contraception. IUD users in the USA state they have a higher level of satisfaction with their method of contraception than women using any of the other methods of reversible contraception. Both IUDs are as effective as tubal sterilization and are rapidly and easily completely reversible. Insertion of an

IUD, unlike female interval tubal sterilization, does not require anesthesia.

Suggested reading

Alvarez *et al*. New insights on the mode of action of intrauterine contraceptive devices in women. *Fertil Steril* 1988; 49: 768.

Andersson K, Odlind V, Rybo G. Levonorgestrel-releasing and copper-releasing (Nova T) IUDs during five years of use: a randomized comparative trial. *Contraception* 1994; 49: 56–72.

Andersson *et al*. Levonorgestrel-releasing and copper-releasing (Nova T) IUDs during five years of use: a randomized comparative trial. *Contraception* 1994; 49: 56.

Chi I-C, Potts M, Wilkens LR, *et al*. Performance of the copper T-380A intrauterine device in breast feeding women. *Contraception* 1989; 39: 603.

Curtis *et al*. Neoplasia with use of intrauterine devices. *Contraception* 2007; 75(S6): S60.

Daling JR, Weiss NS, Metch BJ, *et al*. Primary tubal infertility in relation to the use of an intrauterine device. *NEJM* 1985; 312: 937–941.

Eroglu *et al*. Comparison of efficacy and complications of IUD insertion in immediate postplacental/early postpartum period with interval period: 1 year follow-up. *Contraception* 2006: 74: 376.

Farley TM, Rosenberg MJ, Rowe PJ, *et al*. Intrauterine devices and pelvic inflammatory disease: an international perspective. *Lancet* 1992; 339: 785.

Farley *et al*. Intrauterine devices and pelvic inflammatory disease: an international perspective. *Lancet* 1992: 339; 785.

Grimes DA, Mishell DR. Intrauterine contraception as an alternative to interval tubal sterilization. *Contraception* 2008; 77: 6.

Inki P *et al*. Long-term use of the levonorgestrel-releasing intrauterine system. *Contraception* 2007; 75: S166.

Luukkainen T, Lahteenmaki P, Tolvonen J. Levonorgestrel-releasing intrauterine device. *Ann Med* 1990; 22: 85–90.

Milson I, Anderson K, Jonasson K, *et al*. The influence of the Gyne-T 380A IUD on menstrual blood loss and iron status. *Contraception* 1995; 52: 175.

Mishell DR Jr, Roy S. Copper intrauterine contraceptive device event rates following insertion 4–8 weeks postpartum. *Am J Obstet Gynecol* 1982; 143: 29.

Mishell *et al*. (The intrauterine device: a bacteriologic study of the endometrial cavity.) *Am J Obstet Gynecol* 1966; 96: 119.

Nelson AL. Contraindications to IUD and IUS use. *Contraception* 2007; 75(S6): S76.

Sivin I. Dose- and age-dependent ectopic pregnancy risks with intrauterine contraception. *Obstet Gynecol* 1991; 78: 291–298.

Sivin I. Utility and drawbacks of continuous use of a copper T IUD for 20 years. *Contraception* 2007; 75: S70.

Tatum *et al*. Management and outcome of pregnancies associated with the Copper T intrauterine contraceptive device. *Am J Obstet Gynecol* 1976; 126: 869.

United Nations Development Programme/United Nations Population Fund/World Health Organization/World Bank. Special programme of research, development and research training in human reproduction. Long-term reversible contraception. Twelve years of experience with the TCU380A and TCU220C. *Contraception* 1997; 56: 341–352.

Walsh T, Grimes D, Frezieres R, *et al*. Randomized controlled trial of prophylactic antibiotics before insertion of intrauterine devices. *Lancet* 1998; 351: 1005.

World Health Organization. Special programme of research, development and research training in human reproduction. Task force on the safety and efficacy of fertility regulating methods. The TCU380A, Multiload 250 and Nova T IUDs at 3, 5 and 7 years of use. Results from three randomized multicentre trials. *Contraception* 1990; 42: 141–158.

Chapter 111
Barrier Methods of Contraception

De Shawn L. Taylor

Department of Medicine and Obstetrics and Gynecology, Keck School of Medicine, University of Southern California, CA, USA

Introduction

Certain barrier methods have the advantages of decreasing the risk of sexually transmitted infections and the absence of adverse metabolic alterations, and some barrier methods can be obtained without a prescription. In addition, barrier methods of contraception can be used concomitantly with other contraceptive modalities to provide additional protection against pregnancy. Women using a barrier contraceptive should be informed about the use of emergency contraception in case of failure of the barrier contraceptive method (broken condom, failure to use, etc.).

Male condom

The male condom is a thin sheath made of latex, natural animal membrane or synthetic material that fits over the erect penis and prevents semen from entering the vagina and cervix during ejaculation. Most of the currently available male condoms in the US are made of natural rubber latex. Latex condoms provide dual protection against unintended pregnancy and many sexually transmitted infections. Latex condoms are not compatible with oil-based lubricants or medications and cannot be used by persons with latex sensitivity or allergy. A small proportion of male condoms are manufactured from the intestinal cecum of lambs ("natural skin," "natural membrane" or "lambskin" condoms). Any type of lubricant can be used with natural membrane condoms, but they are not recommended for prevention of sexually transmitted infections because they contain small pores that may allow the passage of viruses, including hepatitis B virus, herpes simplex virus, and HIV. Nonlatex condoms made of polyurethane film or synthetic elastomers are generally nonallergenic, compatible with both oil-based and water-based lubricants, and have a longer shelf-life. Synthetic condoms are associated with higher rates of clinical breakage and slippage than latex condoms, which may affect their efficacy against sexually transmitted infections and pregnancy. Condoms prelubricated with the spermicide nonoxynol-9 are no more effective than other lubricated condoms, have a higher cost and shorter shelf-life.

With correct and consistent use, male condoms have an annual 2% failure rate. The typical-use annual failure rate is about 15%. Most failures with this method of contraception occur in the first year of use because the condoms are used incorrectly or not at all. A new condom should be used at every coital exposure. The condom should be applied before any genital contact. The rolled-up condom is placed on the tip of the erect penis. The small pouch at the tip of the condom accommodates ejaculated semen and is grasped while the condom is unrolled over the entire length of the penis. Immediately after ejaculation, the condom should be grasped at the base of the penis and the penis withdrawn from the vagina while still erect to avoid leakage of semen. If the condom breaks or falls off during intercourse but before ejaculation, it should be replaced with a new condom. New condoms should also be used for prolonged intercourse and for different types of intercourse within a single session. The condom should be observed for visible damage after it is removed. There is a risk of pregnancy and infection if the condom breaks, falls off, leaks, is damaged or is not used at all.

The advantages of male condoms include easy accessibility without a prescription, medical examination or special fitting; easily reversible when pregnancy is desired and have no systemic effects; protect against sexual transmitted infections; are inexpensive, easy to use, and easily and discretely carried by men and women. Disadvantages include lower efficacy with typical use than some other nonbarrier methods; disruption of foreplay to put the condom on; reduced sensitivity during intercourse and difficulty for some males to maintain an erection while

Management of Common Problems in Obstetrics and Gynecology, 5th edition. Edited by T.M. Goodwin, M.N. Montoro, L. Muderspach, R. Paulson and S. Roy. © 2010 Blackwell Publishing Ltd.

wearing the condom; partner co-operation is required, and some individuals are sensitive or allergic to latex.

Female condom

In 1994 the female condom was approved for marketing in the US. The female condom is a soft, loose-fitting polyurethane sheath with two flexible polyurethane rings designed for vaginal use only. One ring lies within the closed end of the sheath and is used to insert and retain the sheath in the vaginal vault. The second ring forms the external open edge of the device and remains outside the vagina, covering the external female genitalia after insertion. The female condom is nonallergenic. There is a silicone-based lubricant on the inside of the condom but additional water- or oil-based lubricants may be used.

The female condom prevents pre-ejaculatory fluid and semen from entering the vagina and is used for a single act of coitus. It can be placed in the vagina up to 8 hours before initiating sexual activity and can remain in the vagina for several hours following ejaculation. Theoretically the female condom offers a greater degree of protection from sexually transmitted diseases, especially those transmitted via skin lesions or shedding, than the male condom, due to the external ring forming a physical barrier over the labia. Laboratory data suggest that the female condom provides an impermeable barrier to HIV, cytomegalovirus and other sexually transmitted infections. No clinical studies have specifically evaluated the ability of the female condom to prevent HIV transmission.

Failure rates for the female condom are extrapolated from results of a 6-month trial with the assumption that the probability of pregnancy in the second 6 months of use would be the same. The annual failure rate of the female condom with correct and consistent use is 5%. The annual typical-use failure rate of this method is 21%. The female condom should not be used with a male condom as friction between the two condoms may cause breakage.

To insert the female condom, the inner ring at the closed end is squeezed with the thumb and middle finger and inserted into the vaginal opening. The index finger is then placed inside the condom and used to push the inner ring as far up as it will go without allowing the condom to twist. The outer ring remains outside the vagina and extends about an inch beyond the labia. The condom should be removed before the woman stands up to avoid spillage of semen. The outer ring is twisted to seal the condom and the condom is then pulled out of the vagina.

The female condom is also available without a prescription and offers similar advantages and disadvantages to the male condom. Additional advantages specific to the female condom include insertion in advance of sexual activity, allowing more sexual spontaneity; additional protection for the external genitalia against sexually transmitted infection; the female condom does not have to be removed immediately after ejaculation, providing greater intimacy after intercourse; and it offers an option for women who want protection from sexually transmitted infections and whose partners cannot or will not use the male condom. Disadvantages specific to the female condom include difficulty inserting and removing the condom; discomfort of the inner ring of the device; dislike of the visible external ring on the external genitalia and a higher failure rate than the male condom and other barrier methods. The female condom is more expensive than male condoms; however, when female condoms are made available with male condoms, the self-reported proportion of protected sex acts generally increases.

Diaphragm

The diaphragm is a reusable contraceptive device consisting of a soft dome-shaped cup made of latex rubber or silicone with a flexible rim. Before coitus, the dome of the diaphragm is partially filled with a spermicide and the diaphragm is inserted deep into the vagina and positioned to fit over the cervix. When properly fitted, the anterior rim of the diaphragm is located just behind the symphysis pubis and the posterior rim is situated deep into the posterior fornix so that the cervix is completely covered and ideally behind the center of the membrane. Both a barrier effect and spermicidal action provide contraception. Fewer women are choosing the diaphragm for contraception since the introduction of the IUD and the combined oral contraceptive pill in the 1960s. However, older women in monogamous relationships are more likely to choose this method and use it successfully.

There are three major classes of diaphragms: arcing, flat, and coil spring. The flat spring diaphragm requires a plastic introducer. The arcing spring diaphragm is most commonly used. The annual failure rate of the diaphragm is 6% (4–8%) with correct and consistent use and 16% (13–17%) with typical use.

Diaphragms are manufactured in sizes from 50 to 105 mm in diameter, in 5 mm increments. The largest diaphragm that fits without discomfort should be prescribed. Fitting rings are used to help the clinician determine the correct size for an individual woman's anatomy and to teach the woman how to insert and remove the device. The determination of the correct size of a diaphragm for a specific woman should be repeated at each annual visit, if the woman experiences a weight change in excess of 10 lb (4.5 kg), 2 weeks following an abortion or 6 weeks following a full-term pregnancy, and if the woman has symptoms of vaginal pain, bladder or urethral discomfort, difficulty voiding or urinary tract infection. An increase in urinary tract infections (UTIs) in diaphragm users occurs and is most likely due to mechanical obstruction of the outflow of urine by the diaphragm. UTIs have also been associated with the use of the spermicide nonoxynol-9, which is believed to induce changes in the vaginal flora. A history of toxic shock syndrome is a contraindication to this method of contraception. Most cases of toxic shock syndrome associated with diaphragm use involved leaving the diaphragm in the vagina for more than 24 hours, but the syndrome does not occur any more frequently in diaphragm users than the general population.

The diaphragm should be observed prior to each use to detect any puncture marks or cracks. The device should be inserted into the vagina within 2 hours of sexual intercourse, but may be placed 2–6 hours before intercourse. If the first sexual exposure occurs more than 2 hours after inserting the diaphragm, another applicator of spermicide must be inserted into the vagina. An additional placement of spermicide is recommended for each coital exposure which occurs before the diaphragm is removed. The diaphragm should not be repositioned or removed in order to add additional spermicide. The position of the diaphragm should be checked after intercourse. If the device has moved out of the proper position, it should be pushed back into position and spermicide should be reapplied into the vagina. The diaphragm should remain in place for at least 6 hours after intercourse to maximize effectiveness and should be removed by 24 hours after initial placement.

Advantages of the diaphragm include no hormonal side effects; it is reusable; and does not interrupt sexual intimacy if inserted in advance. Disadvantages include skill to insert; must be inserted before each act of coitus; diaphragm needs to be cleaned after use and cared for; both the diaphragm and spermicide must be physically present within a few hours of coitus, which may be inconvenient; and the use of a diaphragm increases the frequency of urinary tract infection.

Cervical cap

Two types of cervical caps are currently available in the US: the FemCap and the Lea Shield. Both require a prescription to obtain and should be inserted at least 15 minutes prior to sexual intercourse. The FemCap is a reusable sailor hat-shaped silicone device with a removal strap approved for marketing in the US in 2003. When correctly applied, the cap fits over the cervix and provides a barrier to the passage of semen. A portion of the dome of the cap is filled with spermicide and the cap provides continuous contraceptive protection for 48 hours. The device is available in sizes 22 mm, 26 mm, and 30 mm. The cap's position is maintained as the rim forms a seal with the surface of the cervix.

To insert the cap, fold the rim and compress the cap dome so that suction between the rim of the cap and the cervix is created when it is released. After inserting the cap, feel along the entire circumference with one finger to make sure there are no gaps between the cap rim and the cervix. To remove the cap, push the tip of the finger against the dome to break suction. Hook the index finger between the dome and removal strap and gently pull the cap down and out of the vagina. Wait at least 6 hours after the last act of intercourse before removing the cap. Additional spermicide is not required for repeated acts of coitus.

The Lea Shield is a reusable silicone rubber device shaped like an elliptical bowl with an anterior loop that assists in removal. It is thicker at the posterior end, which fits into the posterior fornix of the vagina, helping to hold it in place and decrease rotation. The device was approved for marketing in the US in 2002. It blocks the cervix, but does not require suction. The device contains a one-way valve which allows passage of cervical secretions and air. There is only one size, so fitting is not required. The bowl of the contraceptive is filled with spermicide prior to insertion. Additional spermicide application is not required for repeated acts of coitus. The device should stay in place for 8 hours after the last act of intercourse. The cervical cap can be worn for up to 48 hours. If continuous use exceeds the 48-hour interval, an unpleasant odor, infection, and even cervical ulceration may appear.

Both types of cervical cap are more effective in nulliparous than parous women. In nulliparous women, annual failure rates are 9% with correct and consistent use and 20% with typical use. In parous women, the correct-use annual failure rate is 26% and the typical-use failure rate is 40%.

Advantages of the cervical cap include insertion before sexual intimacy; it is reusable; instantly reversible when pregnancy is desired; and has no hormonal side effects. Disadvantages include decreased efficacy compared to some other barrier methods, and the planning required before sexual intimacy.

Contraceptive vaginal sponge

The Today Sponge is a small disposable polyurethane foam sponge containing 1 g of nonoxynol-9 and an attached loop for ease of removal. The sponge was approved for use in the US from 1983 to 1994 and production resumed in 2005. The device does not require fitting or a prescription. The sponge blocks the passage of semen to the cervix, traps sperm, and releases spermicide. The sponge is moistened with tap water prior to use and inserted deep into the vagina. The device is effective for 24 hours no matter how many times intercourse occurs. After intercourse, the sponge must be left in place for at least 6 hours before it is removed. Failure rates vary significantly between parous and nulliparous women. Correct-use failure rates are 9% and 20% for nulliparous and parous women respectively. The typical-use failure rate for nulliparous women is 20% and 40% for parous women.

Spermicides

Spermicides are available as foams, gels, films, tablets, suppositories or creams. Spermicide immobilizes or kills sperm on contact and prevents passage of sperm to the cervical canal. All spermicidal agents contain a surfactant, usually nonoxynol-9. Spermicides are placed in the vagina prior to each coital episode. They are not highly effective when used without a barrier method. The annual failure rate of spermicides alone with correct and consistent use is 18% and 29% with typical use. Effectiveness is reduced if the woman does not wait long enough for the spermicide to disperse before having intercourse, if intercourse is delayed for more than 1 hour after administration or if a repeat dose is not applied before each additional act of intercourse.

Spermicidal agents should be inserted at each coital exposure as near to the time of coitus as possible and no longer than 1 hour prior to coitus. The spermicide is placed as close to the cervix as feasible and should not be cleared from the vagina for at least 8 hours following intercourse. Spermicides do not prevent sexually transmitted infections. These agents should not be used by women at high risk for HIV or those who are infected with HIV or have AIDS.

Barrier methods of contraception and sexually transmitted diseases

A major advantage of male and female condoms is their efficacy in protecting against sexually transmitted infections. The consistent use of male condoms decreases risk of transmission of HIV, gonorrhea, chlamydia, trichomoniasis, and hepatitis. The female condom may offer greater protection against sexually transmitted infections that appear on the skin as the external labia are also covered by the condom. Observational studies suggest that covering the cervix with a barrier like the diaphragm could play a key role in preventing the transmission of HIV and some STIs. When protection against sexually transmitted infection is a concern, women using any method of contraception (except the female condom) should also ask their male partner to use a condom.

Suggested reading

Centers for Disease Control and Prevention. Nonoxynol-9 spermicide contraception use – United States, 1999. *MMWR* 2002; 51: 389–392.

Farr G, Gabelnick H, Sturgen K, Dorflinger L. Contraceptive efficacy and acceptability of the female condom. *Am J Public Health* 1994; 84: 1960–1964.

FHI. Female barrier methods. *Network* 2000; 20. Available at: www.fhi.org/en/fp/fppubs/network/v20-2/index.html.

Gallo MF, Grimes DA, Lopez LM, Schulz KF. Non-latex versus latex male condoms for contraception. *Cochrane Database Syst Rev* 2006; 1: CD003550.

National Institute of Allergy and Infectious Diseases. Workshop summary: scientific evidence on condom effectiveness for sexually transmitted diseases (STI) prevention. 2001. Available at: www3.niaid.nih.gov/research/topics/STI/PDF/condom report.pdf.

Trussel J, Strickler J, Vaughan B. Contraceptive efficacy of the diaphragm, the sponge, and the cervical cap. *Fam Plan Perspect* 1993; 25: 200–205.

Chapter 112
Fertility Awareness Family Planning Methods

Ian B. Tilley and Ronna Jurow

Department of Medicine and Obstetrics and Gynecology, Keck School of Medicine, University of Southern California, CA, USA

Introduction

Concealed ovulation is a unique human characteristic that limits a couple's ability to identify the day of the menstrual cycle when ovulation occurs [1]. Because conception requires coitus during the 5 days before or on the day of ovulation, the identification of this 6-day fertile period can allow couples to time coitus to either achieve or avoid pregnancy [2]. For couples wanting to avoid pregnancy, methods of identifying this fertile period have been developed so they can abstain from unprotected coitus on these days [3-5]. These are fertility awareness-based methods of family planning, a name that accurately conveys their conceptual foundation. Other names commonly used for these methods include periodic abstinence, the rhythm method, and natural family planning.

Knowledge of reproductive physiology allows awareness of detectable aspects of the menstrual cycle that can improve the ability to predict the day of ovulation and estimate the fertile period. The most important knowledge includes the understanding of the length and variability of the typical menstrual cycle, the awareness of the time of ovulation during the menstrual cycle, the understanding of cervical mucus changes during the menstrual cycle, the recognition that changes in body temperature are associated with the rise in progesterone levels after ovulation, and the understanding of the effect of coital timing relative to ovulation on the probability of conception. Through fertility awareness-based methods of family planning, couples can use their understanding of these phenomena to prevent pregnancy by limiting unprotected coitus to predicted nonfertile days.

Fertility awareness-based methods of family planning can be categorized as either calendar-based methods, for which effectiveness depends on the regularity of a woman's menstrual cycle, or physiology-based methods, for which effectiveness depends on a couple's ability to recognize physiological fertility signs. These methods are generally estimated to have a 25% failure rate during the first year of typical use, which reflects the difficulty of avoiding unprotected coitus during the relatively long fertile period of each menstrual cycle [6]. This high failure rate is similar to that of coitus interruptus, but much higher than those of condoms, hormonal contraceptives or intrauterine devices. Fertility awareness-based methods are most appropriate for couples who are either unwilling or unable to use these other more effective contraceptive methods because of ethical concerns, medical concerns or poverty [7,8].

Couples using fertility awareness-based family planning methods should also be counseled on the use of immediately active contraceptive methods, such spermicides, coitus interruptus and barrier contraceptives, during fertile days, and the availability of emergency contraceptives for recognized contraceptive method failure.

Calendar-based methods

Calendar-based methods of family planning depend upon the regularity of a woman's menstrual cycle because they predict the timing of the fertile period based on the assumption that the upcoming menstrual cycle will be similar to past menstrual cycles. If a woman is not experiencing regular menstrual cycles, then calendar-based methods should be delayed until regular monthly menses resume. Calendar-based methods of family planning include the calendar rhythm method, which uses arithmetic calculations to predict the fertile period, and the Standard Days method, which eliminates the need for these calculations by limiting use of the method to women with regular 26 to 32 day menstrual cycles.

Management of Common Problems in Obstetrics and Gynecology,
5th edition. Edited by T.M. Goodwin, M.N. Montoro,
L. Muderspach, R. Paulson and S. Roy. © 2010 Blackwell
Publishing Ltd.

The biologic rationale for the calendar rhythm method is based on the following assumptions.

• Sperm are not capable of fertilizing an ovum more than 72 hours after coitus.

• An ovum is not capable of being fertilized more than 24 hours after ovulation.

• Ovulation occurs from 12 to 16 days before the onset of the next menses.

A woman using the calendar rhythm method records the length of her menstrual cycles for 6–12 months, noting the length of her longest and shortest menstrual cycles. She then calculates the beginning of her next fertile period by subtracting 18 days from the length of her shortest menstrual cycle. These 18 days account for early ovulation at 16 days before the onset of menses plus 2 days for the time that the sperm are assumed to be potent after coitus. She calculates the end of her fertile period by subtracting 11 days from the length of her longest menstrual cycle [3]. These 11 days account for late ovulation at 12 days before the onset of menses minus 1 day for the time that the ovum is assumed to be fertilizable after ovulation. For example, if the menstrual cycle length varies from 26 to 32 days, the fertile period begins on day 8 and ends on day 21, which is 14 total days. During the upcoming menstrual cycle, the couple should avoid unprotected coitus on these days. The calculations are updated monthly, always using data from the six most recent cycles. The first-year failure rate of this method with perfect use is estimated to be 9% [6].

The Standard Days method is designed to be a simpler alternative to the calendar rhythm method, which is achieved by limiting its use to women with regular menstrual cycles ranging from 26 to 32 days in length. Eligible women using this method simply avoid unprotected coitus from days 8 through 19 of the cycle to avoid pregnancy. Unprotected coitus is allowed on all other days of the menstrual cycle. An additional benefit of this standardized calendar-based approach is that a mnemonic device, CycleBeads, can be used to facilitate compliance. A string of CycleBeads consists of 32 beads for each of the 32 possible days of the menstrual cycle. A single red bead represents the first day of the menstrual cycle. The following six brown beads represent the nonfertile period. Beads 8 through 19 are white, indicating the fertile period where unprotected coitus risks pregnancy. The remaining 13 brown beads represent the remainder of the nonfertile period. A moveable rubber ring, which is advanced to the red bead with the start of every menstrual cycle, marks the current day of the menstrual cycle. When the Standard Days method with the use of CycleBeads was prospectively studied in a cohort of 478 women of reproductive age in Bolivia, Peru and the Philippines, the first-year failure rate with imperfect use was 12%, and with perfect use, it was 5% [9]. Women who have two or more menstrual cycles outside the 26 to

32 day range within the previous 12 months should use the calendar rhythm method or a physiology-based method rather than the Standard Days method.

In general, calendar-based methods are not recommended for women with menstrual cycles shorter than 26 days or with cycle-to-cycle variation greater than 7 days. They are not recommended for women with irregular menstrual cycles, such as adolescent women with recent menarche, premenopausal or perimenopausal women with unpredictable bleeding patterns, and postpartum women. After parturition, women should delay using calendar-based methods alone until at least three postpartum menstrual cycles have been completed, and after abortion women should delay until at least one postabortion menstrual cycle has been completed [10].

Physiology-based methods

Physiology-based methods of family planning depend on the ability of the couple to recognize physiological fertility signs because these signs can suggest a woman's fertility status. They are based on two detectable physiological processes that are influenced by the otherwise occult processes of ovulation. First, there are changes in the quantity and viscosity of cervical mucus near the time of ovulation associated with changing estrogen and progesterone levels, and second, there is a rise in body temperature after ovulation associated with increasing progesterone levels. Physiology-based methods include the cervical mucus method, the TwoDay method, the temperature method, and the symptothermal method. Both the cervical mucus method and the TwoDay method are based on mucus changes alone. The temperature method is based on body temperature changes alone. The symptothermal method incorporates changes in both cervical mucus and body temperature to predict the fertile period.

The cervical mucus method, also known as the ovulation method or the Billings method of natural family planning, is based upon recognition of changes in the quantity and viscosity of cervical mucus during the menstrual cycle. The beginning of the fertile period is marked by the onset of mucus secretion. The day of peak cervical mucus discharge roughly coincides with the day of ovulation. When sampled at this time, the slippery cervical mucus resembles raw chicken egg white. Nonfertile type mucus is sticky. The last day of the fertile period is designated to be the third day after the time of peak cervical mucus discharge. The rules of the cervical mucus method are as follows.

• No unprotected coitus during menstrual bleeding.

• No unprotected coitus during the fertile period itself.

• Between menses and the fertile period, no unprotected coitus on consecutive days.

A woman using this method checks her cervical secretions every day. If there are no secretions after completing menses, then she may safely engage in unprotected coitus. After engaging in unprotected coitus, she then abstains from unprotected coitus or mucus sampling on the following day to avoid confusing cervicalsecretions with other postcoital discharge. Once secretions are noticed, the fertile period has begun. She samples her secretions throughout the fertile period to identify the day of peak cervical discharge. She may resume unprotected coitus on the fourth day after the day of peak secretions.

When the cervical mucus method was prospectively studied in a cohort of 725 women of reproductive age in New Zealand, India, Ireland, the Philippines, and El Salvador, the 1-year failure rate was 20% for imperfect use and 4% for perfect use, despite the participants' completion of three teaching cycles prior to enrollment. This study also found that these women were required to abstain from coitus for 58% of each menstrual cycle, and that most pregnancies were the result of the couple's inability to abstain from unprotected coitus during the times required by this method [11-13].

The TwoDay method is a simpler alternative to the cervical mucus method because it eliminates the requirement that a woman learns to recognize changes in her cervical mucus. Instead, women using this method identify their fertile period simply by noticing the presence of cervical secretions. Women using the TwoDay method determine their fertility status by applying an algorithm in which they ask themselves the following questions: (1) Did I notice secretions today? and (2) Did I notice secretions yesterday? If the answer to either is "yes, " then she considers herself fertile and avoids unprotected coitus that day. Alternatively, if the answers to both are "no, " then she considers herself nonfertile that day. This method allows unprotected coitus on nonfertile days, which includes the day following coitus provided that no secretions are present. When this method was prospectively studied in a cohort of 450 women of reproductive age in Guatemala, Peru and the Philippines, the failure rate with imperfect use was 14%, and with perfect use, it was 4% [14].

Unlike calendar-based methods, both the cervical mucus method and the TwoDay method may be used by breastfeeding women because the return of cervical mucus secretions may signal impending ovulation and the return of fertility. This would allow breastfeeding women to recognize the end of lactational infertility before reaching the end of lactational amenorrhea. Neither method is recommended for women with reproductive tract infections causing vaginal discharge or for women with irregular menstrual cycles.

The temperature method is based upon the rise in basal body temperature caused by elevated progesterone levels after ovulation. This method requires a woman to measure her temperature at the same time every morning before rising from bed [15]. She should measure her temperature with a fertility thermometer accurate to 0.1° F and record it on a temperature graph. The beginning of the fertile period is defined as the start of menses. The end of the fertile period occurs with the thermal shift, which is defined as a rise in the basal body temperature of 0.4° to 1.0° F (0.2° to 0.5° C) that persists for 3 consecutive days. To determine the preovulatory basal body temperature, a line is drawn on the temperature graph that is 0.1° F above the six measurements preceding the perceived rise. If the next three measurements are 0.4° F above this line, ovulation has occurred and the nonfertile period has begun [3]. The fertile period includes the days from menses through ovulation detection, so unprotected coitus is prohibited by this method for the entire preovulatory period in ovulatory menstrual cycles and for the entire menstrual cycle in anovulatory menstrual cycles. Because of the long period of abstinence that the exclusive use of this method requires, the temperature method is not commonly used alone. This method is not recommended for women with febrile illnesses, for women taking medications that affect body temperature or for women with irregular menstrual cycles.

The symptothermal method integrates calendar-based and physiology-based methods. It combines elements of the cervical mucus method, the calendar rhythm method and the temperature method. The calendar method is used at the beginning of the cycle to allow coitus during menses. The cervical mucus method is used during the middle of the cycle to allow coitus until fertile type secretions are detected. The temperature method is used to allow coitus after ovulation. The perfect use first-year failure rate is 2% [6]. However, this method is

Table 112.1 Duration of defined fertile period and first-year efficacy for each method

Method	Length of defined fertile period	% of women with unintended pregnancy in first year of use	
	No. of days (% of cycle)	Typical use	Perfect use
Calendar-based		25	
Calendar rhythm*	14 (44–54%)		9
Standard Days	12 (38–46%)		5
Physiology-based		25	
Cervical mucus	17 (58%)		3
TwoDay	13 (43%)		4
Symptothermal	17 (58%)		2

*For women with 26 to 32 day menstrual cycle lengths.
Adapted from Hatcher et al. [6].

more complex and more difficult to learn than methods that rely on only a single parameter to identify the fertile period because the recommendations of each of these methods must be followed. Also, it requires many days of abstinence when used alone. Relying on such prolonged abstinence and intermittent use of immediately active contraceptive methods during fertile periods are the inherent weaknesses of this and all fertility awareness-based methods of family planning. While highly motivated couples may be able to achieve perfect use pregnancy rates, for most couples fertility awareness-based methods are more likely to result in a 25% typical use first year failure rate [1,6,16,17].

References

1. Diamond J. The third chimpanzee: the evolution and future of the human animal. New York: HarperCollins, 1992.
2. Wilcox A, Weinberg C, Baird D. Timing of sexual intercourse in relation to ovulation: effects on the probability of conception, survival of the pregnancy and sex of the baby. *NEJM* 1995; 333: 1517–1521.
3. Klaus H. Natural family planning: a review. *Obstet Gynecol Surv* 1982; 37: 128–150.
4. Brown J, Blackwell L, Billings J, *et al*. Natural family planning. *Am J Obstet Gynecol* 1987; 157: 1082–1089.
5. Sinai I, Arévalo M. It's all in the timing: coital frequency and fertility awareness-based methods of family planning. *J Biosoc Sci* 2005; 38: 763–777.
6. Trussell J. The essentials of contraception: efficacy, safety, and personal considerations. In: Hatcher R, Trussell J, Stewart F, *et al*. (eds) *Contraceptive technology*, 19th edn. New York: Ardent Media, 2009. Available from: www.contraceptivetechnology.org/ table.html
7. Pope Paul VI. Humanae vitae: encyclical of Pope Paul VI on the regulation of birth, 1968. Available from: www.vatican.va/holy_father/paul_vi/encyclicals/documents/hf_p-vi_enc_25071968_humanae-vitae_en.html.
8. World Health Organization, Department of Reproductive Health and Research. *Medical eligibility criteria for contraceptive use*, 4th edn. Available from whqlibdoc.who.int/publications/2009/9789241563888_eng.pdf
9. Arévalo M, Jennings V, Sinai I. Efficacy of a new method of family planning: the Standard Days method. *Contraception* 2001; 65: 333–338.
10. Arévalo M, Jennings V, Sinai I. Application of simple fertility awareness-based methods of family planning to breastfeeding women. *Fertil Steril* 2003; 80: 1241–1248.
11. World Health Organization. A prospective multicentre trial of the ovulation method of natural family planning. I. The teaching phase. *Fertil Steril* 1981; 36: 152–158.
12. World Health Organization. A prospective multicentre trial of the ovulation method of natural family planning. II. The effectiveness phase. *Fertil Steril* 1981; 36: 591–598.
13. World Health Organization. A prospective multicentre trial of the ovulation method of natural family planning. III. Characteristics of the menstrual cycle and of the fertile phase. *Fertil Steril* 1983; 40: 773–778.
14. Arévalo M, Jennings V, Nikula M, Sinai I. Efficacy of the new TwoDay method of family planning. *Fertil Steril* 2004; 82: 885–892.
15. Frank E, White R. An updated basal body temperature method. *Contraception* 1996; 54: 319–321.
16. Small M. *What's love got to do with it? The evolution of human mating*. New York: Anchor Books, 1995.
17. Eldridge N. *Why we do it: rethinking sex and the selfish gene*. New York: Norton, 2004.

Chapter 113
Emergency Contraception

Penina Segall-Gutierrez and Ian Tilley
Department of Medicine and Obstetrics and Gynecology, Keck School of Medicine, University of Southern California, CA, USA

Introduction

Emergency contraception (EC) has also been referred to as postcoital contraception or the "morning-after" contraception. Emergency contraception is the initiation of a reversible family planning method after coitus has taken place. Some couples, for a variety of reasons, are unable to anticipate the need for adequate contraception until after coitus has occurred. This may be the result of the failure of a contraceptive method (a condom breaks), the misuse or mistiming of a method, sexual assault or both partners neglect to practice contraception. Pregnancy may result from a single sexual encounter if the coital experience was either unprotected or inadequately protected. The risk of pregnancy from one coital exposure at any time during the menstrual cycle, irrespective of the regularity of the woman's cycles and at any age in the reproductive years, has been estimated at 3%. The risk of pregnancy from one coital exposure at mid-cycle has been estimated to be 9% [1]. Thus, there is a need for reversible pregnancy prevention that can be administered after coitus has occurred.

Combination oral contraceptives

The first documentation in the literature of high-dose estrogens used as EC was in a victim of sexual assault in the 1960s. In 1974, a combined estrogen and progestin regimen was later termed the "Yuzpe" method, after the Canadian physician who described it. And a dedicated product, Preven, was introduced in 1998. However, the World Health Organization published a world-wide multicenter randomized control trial showing that progestin-only EC was more effective than the Yuzpe method (85%

versus 57% of pregnancies prevented), with fewer side effects [2]. The rates of nausea and vomiting were 50% versus 23% and 19% versus 6% respectively for Yuzpe and progestin-only, respectively. While still considered a safe method, Preven was withdrawn from the market and the use of combined oral contraceptives is now considered an acceptable method of EC only if progestin-only methods are unavailable. An emergency contraceptive regimen of combined oral contraceptive pills taken initially within 72 hours of unprotected or inadequately protected intercourse which provides a total of 500–600 µg of levonorgestrel and 100–120 µg of ethinylestradiol in each of two doses taken 12 hours apart. It should be administered with an antiemetic, such as meclizine, if possible.

Progestin-only pills

Plan B, consisting of two tablets each containing 750 µg of levonorgestrel, was approved by the FDA in 1999 to be taken as one pill every 12 hours up to 72 hours after unprotected coitus. The efficacy of the regimen is inversely related to the interval between unprotected coitus and the initiation of emergency contraception, but has been shown to be effective up to 120 hours after unprotected intercourse [3]. The sooner this regimen of EC is started after a single act of unprotected sex, the more effective it is. Additionally, both tablets of levonorgestrel can be administered simultaneously with no difference in the side effect profile [4]. This is preferable to the one tablet every 12 hours regimen, because if the second dose is missed, efficacy is decreased.

The risk of pregnancy following a single act of unprotected sex is dependent not only on how soon after coitus the dose is taken, but also on the probability of clinical pregnancy resulting from the single act of intercourse. The overall proportion of pregnancies prevented in the 1998 WHO trial was 85% [2]. A combination of progestin-only pills equivalent to 1.5 mg of levonorgestrel may be used and a generic version Next Choice is currently available. Levonorgestrel EC can safely be used

Management of Common Problems in Obstetrics and Gynecology, 5th edition. Edited by T.M. Goodwin, M.N. Montoro, L. Muderspach, R. Paulson and S. Roy. © 2010 Blackwell Publishing Ltd.

in women of all ages, and is currently available in the United States to women 17 years and older without a prescription. The pharmacokinetics of EC are the same in women <18 years as in adults; they can also correctly and safely self-administer EC without medical supervision, and do not demonstrate an increase in sexual risk taking when provided access to EC [5].

The American College of Obstetricians and Gynecologists recommends offering EC to victims of sexual assault. While effective in preventing pregnancy, levongestrel EC provides no protection against sexually transmitted infections, and so prophylaxis against sexually transmitted infections should be offered [6]. The ACOG also recommends discussing EC in advance of need along with routine methods of birth control at the periodic assessment of patients for every age range starting at age 13, except those 65 and older [7]. Patients must understand the indications for EC use relative to their chosen contraceptive method (Box 113.1) [8]. Providing a prescription for EC in advance of need is not associated with abandonment of user-dependent contraceptive methods and does not increase risk of sexually transmitted infections

While women with advanced provision take EC sooner and more often, some women who theoretically have increased access to EC still fail to use EC with every act of unprotected intercourse and thus advance provision of EC has failed to reduce rates of unintended pregnancy over routinely offering information about EC [9]. EC is not readily available in all pharmacies and advanced provision allows patients to access to Plan B in a more timely fashion.

Levonorgestrel EC is not an abortifacent and does not appear interfere with endometrial receptivity to implantation or with sperm transport or function [10,11].

The primary mechanism by which emergency contraception is thought to work is by delay of ovulation [12]. While pregnancy is a relative contraindication to EC administration, this is because it will not be effective in preventing pregnancy. However, administration of EC during pregnancy is not associated with any maternal or fetal risk [13].

It is important to take a history from a patient seeking EC but a pregnancy test or physical exam is not required prior to administration. Patients can and should start or restart an ongoing method of contraception after EC use, as levonorgestrel EC is not as effective as other methods of contraception. Depot medroxyprogesterone acetate can be given on the day of EC administration. The vaginal ring, the patch, and oral contraceptive pills should be started the next day. The methods requiring alternative methods of contraception until the next normal menses include the contraceptive implant, the levonorgestrel intrauterine system, and the fertility awareness method. There are no absolute contraindications to levonorgestrel EC.

Copper intrauterine device

The most effective method of EC is the insertion of a copper intrauterine device (IUD) after unprotected coitus and prior to the time of implantation. Given that human ovulation is concealed and that implantation occurs as soon as 5 days after ovulation, the typical recommendation for EC is that the copper IUD is inserted within 5 days after unprotected coitus. However, when the time of ovulation can be estimated, the copper IUD can be inserted beyond 5 days after unprotected coitus, provided that the insertion does not occur more than 5 days after ovulation [14]. When the timing of copper IUD insertion follows these guidelines, very few pregnancies will occur. In a meta-analysis of 20 published papers examining more than 8400 insertions of copper IUDs for EC, the failure rate was only 0.1% [15]. In comparison, the failure rates for levonorgestrel or the Yuzpe regimen are between five and 40 times higher, depending on the time interval before hormonal EC treatment [16]. The copper IUD may be removed at the next menses or it may be retained for up to the recommended lifespan of the IUD.

Box 113.1 Indications for use of emergency contraception

- IUD removed, expelled or misplaced for ≤7 days after last act of coitus
- Presents > 14 days late for DMPA injection
- Starting a new cycle of vaginal ring, transdermal patch or combined oral contraceptives ≥2 days late
- Missed ≥2 consecutive combined oral contraceptive pills
- Progestin-only pill administration ≥3 hours late
- Error in use of a male or female condom or in coitus interruptus resulting in possible ejaculate entering vagina or external genitalia
- Diaphragm or cervical cap placed incorrectly, removed prematurely, dislodged or torn
- Intercourse during fertile days in a couple practicing natural family planning
- Not using highly effective contraceptive method while exposed to possible cytotoxic or teratogenic agent
- No contraceptive used at time of intercourse
- Sexual assault

Adapted from reference [8].

Because the copper IUD is approved by the FDA for use for up to 10 years (and clinical data indicate that its high effectiveness lasts at least 12 years), an important benefit of copper IUD insertion as compared with hormonal EC is that copper IUD insertion provides continued contraception. The importance of this benefit was demonstrated in studies of hormonal EC where women who participated in additional acts of unprotected coitus later in the same cycle became pregnant [17].

The contraindications for the use of the copper IUD for EC are the same as those for the initiation of the copper IUD at any other time. Absolute contraindications include pregnancy, active gynecologic infection including pelvic tuberculosis, unexplained vaginal bleeding, cancer of the cervix or uterus, malignant gestational trophoblastic disease or severe distortion of the uterine cavity. Relative contraindications include increased STI risk, AIDS, ovarian cancer, benign gestational trophoblastic disease, and being between 48 hours and 4 weeks post partum. When the copper IUD is used for EC after rape, the benefits of its high efficacy must be balanced against the risk of sexually transmitted infection from the sexual assault [14]. Cost also limits the use of the copper IUD for EC. Whereas hormonal EC is cost-effective as an emergency contraceptive alone, the copper IUD is not [18]. However, when women choose to continue with the copper IUD after its insertion as an emergency contraceptive, the savings exceed the costs when use continues for as few as 4 months [19]. High continuation rates are a benefit of IUD use generally, and in a study of copper IUD use for EC, approximately 80% of the trial participants elected to continue IUD use after completion of the study [20].

The immediate and long-term contraceptive superiority of the copper IUD for EC over hormonal EC in the appropriate patient is clear.

Conclusion

The availability and use of emergency contraception have the potential to reduce the number of unplanned and unintended pregnancies in the USA as well as to reduce the number of pregnancy terminations. The three primary methods of emergency contraception (in order of least to most effective) are combination oral contraceptives, progestin-only (levonorgestrel) pills, and the copper intrauterine device. In addition to being most efficacious at preventing pregnancy from the index act of unprotected intercourse, the copper IUD is the only method of EC that also provides contraceptive benefit for up to 10 years. All three methods have been shown to be effective and safe in most patients. There are no absolute contraindications to progestin-only emergency contraception. The primary mechanism of action is via delay

or inhibition of ovulation and use of levonorgestrel EC will not disrupt an established pregnancy.

References

1. Wilcox A, Dunson DB, Weinberg CR, Trussell J, Baird D. Likelihood of conception with a single act of intercourse: providing benchmark rates for assessment of post-coital contraceptives. *Contraception* 2001; 63: 211–215.

2. Von Hertzen H, Piaggio G, van Look PF. Emergency contraception with levonorgestrel or the Yuzpe regimen. Task Force on Postovulatory Methods of Fertility Regulation. *Lancet* 1998; 352(9126): 428–433.

3. Ngai S, Fan S, Li S, *et al.* A randomized trial to compare 24h versus 12h double dose regimen of levonorgestrel for emergency contraception. *Hum Reprod* 2005; 20(1): 307–311.

4. Von Hertzen H, Piaggio G, Ding J, *et al.* Low dose mifepristone and two regimens of levonorgestrel for emergency contraception: a WHO multicentre randomized trial. *Lancet* 2002; 360: 1803–1810.

5. Harper C, Weiss D, Speidel J, Raine-Bennett T. Over the counter access to emergency contraception in teens. *Contraception* 2008; 77(4): 230–233.

6. American College of Obstetricians and Gynecologists. *Sexual assault.* Washington, DC: American College of Obstetricians and Gynecologists, 1997.

7. American College of Obstetrics and Gynecologists. *Primary and preventive care: periodic assessment.* Washington, DC: American College of Obstetricians and Gynecologists, 2003.

8. World Health Organization. *Selected practice recommendations for contraceptive use.* Geneva: World Health Organization, 2002.

9. Polis C, Schaffer K, Blanchard K, *et al.* Advance provision of emergency contraception for pregnancy prevention (full review). *Cochrane Database Syst Rev* 2007; 2: CD005497.

10. Lalitkumar, P Lalitkumar S, Meng C, *et al.* Mifepristone, but not levonorgestrel, inhibits human blastocyst attachment to an in vitro endometrial three-dimensional cell culture model. *Hum Reprod* 2007; 22(11): 3031–3037.

11. Do Nascimento J, Seppla M, Peridagao A. In vivo assessment of the human sperm acrosome reaction and the expression of glycodelin-A in human endometrium after levonorgestrel-emergency contraceptive pill administration. *Hum Reprod* 2007; 22(8): 2190–2195.

12. Novikova N, Weisberg E, Stanczyk F, *et al.* Effectiveness of levonorgestrel emergency contraception given before or after ovulation – a pilot study. *Contraception* 2007; 75: 112–118.

13. De Santis M, Cavaliere A, Straface G, *et al.* Failure of emergency contraceptive levonorgestrel and the risk of adverse effects in pregnancy and on fetal development: an observational cohort. *Fertil Steril* 2005; 84(2): 296–299.

14. World Health Organization, Department of Reproductive Health and Research. *Medical eligibility criteria for contraceptive use,* 3rd edn. Geneva: World Health Organization, 2004.

15. Trussell J, Ellertson C. Efficacy of emergency contraception. *Fertil Control Rev* 1995; 4: 8–11.

16. Piaggio G, von Hertzen H, Grimes D, van Look P. Timing of emergency contraception with levonorgestrel or the Yuzpe regimen. Task Force on Postovulatory Methods of Fertility Regulation. *Lancet* 1998; 352: 721.

17. Ellertson C, Webb A, Blanchard K, *et al.* Modifying the Yuzpe regimen of emergency contraception: a multicenter randomized controlled trial. *Obstet Gynecol* 2003; 101: 1160–1166.

18. Trussell J, Koenig J, Ellertson C, Stewart F. Preventing unintended pregnancy: the cost-effectiveness of three methods of emergency contraception. *Am J Public Health* 1997; 87: 932–937.

19. Trussell J, Leveque J, Koening J, *et al.* The economic value of contraception: a comparison of 15 methods. *Am J Public Health* 1995; 85: 494–503.

20. D'Souza R, Masters T, Bounds W, Guillebaud J. Randomized controlled trial assessing the acceptability of GyneFix versus Gyne-T380S for emergency contraception. *J Fam Plan Reprod Health Care* 2003; 23: 23–29.

Chapter 114
Medical Abortifacients

De Shawn L. Taylor and Ronna Jurow
Department of Medicine and Obstetrics and Gynecology, Keck School of Medicine, University of Southern California, CA, USA

Introduction

Medical abortion involves the use of medications to induce an abortion and should be considered a medically acceptable alternative to surgical abortion in selected, carefully counseled, and informed women. Eighty-eight percent of all abortions in the United States occur during the first trimester. Medical abortion up to 63 days' gestation accounts for 6% of the cases. Second-trimester abortion comprises 12% of all abortions in the United States and less than 2% of abortions 13 weeks' gestational age or greater are medically induced. Dilation and evacuation (D&E) is the most commonly performed method of second-trimester pregnancy termination. Medical methods of abortion continue to evolve. Mifepristone-misoprostol regimens have become the standard for first-trimester medical abortion while misoprostol-only regimens have become the standard in the second trimester.

Medications used for medical abortion

Mifepristone (RU-486) is an antiprogestin that acts to disrupt pregnancy by progesterone receptor blockade. This agent acts on a pregnant uterus by causing necrosis of the decidua with separation of the trophoblast from the decidua, softening the cervix, and increasing uterine contractility and prostaglandin sensitivity. Mifepristone is administered in combination with a prostaglandin, usually misoprostol.

Misoprostol is a prostaglandin E1 analog in pill form that is inexpensive and stable at room temperature. While not approved by the United States Food and Drug Administration for gynecologic care, misoprostol has been well studied for its use as an abortifacient. Misoprostol causes uterine contractions and softens the cervix at any gestational age. Routes of administration vary. Oral and sublingual misoprostol are absorbed rapidly, resulting in higher peak serum levels and higher incidence of gastrointestinal side effects of nausea, vomiting, and diarrhea than the other routes of administration. Vaginal administration results in greater uterine contractility. Recent studies of buccal administration show a pharmacokinetic profile similar to vaginal administration.

Methotrexate is a folic acid antagonist that is cytotoxic to the trophoblast. Methotrexate has been used in combination with misoprostol to induce abortion in pregnancies up to 56 days' gestational age. It is used less often today due to the greater availability of mifepristone.

First-trimester medical abortion

The mifepristone-misoprostol regimen was FDA approved in 2000 for medical abortion up to 49 days' gestational age. This regimen consists of mifepristone 600 mg orally followed 48 hours later by an oral dose of misoprostol 400 µg. The overall complete abortion rate is 92% and is higher with earlier gestations, approximately 96–98% up to 42 days, 91–95% from 43 to 49 days, and less than 85% beyond 49 days. A follow-up examination is performed approximately 14 days after mifepristone administration. If clinical history and physical exam do not confirm expulsion, a transvaginal ultrasound is performed. Uterine aspiration is typically performed if a persistent gestational sac is seen.

Although not FDA approved, evidence has shown that decreasing the mifepristone dose to 200 mg and administering misoprostol 800 µg intravaginally improves complete abortion rates to 95–98% up to 63 days' gestation, reduces the cost of medical abortion, decreases time to expulsion, and decreases gastrointestinal side effects. Women undergoing medical abortion with these regimens should be offered an antiemetic, as well as sufficient analgesia. These are to be taken before, during or after misoprostol administration or as needed.

Management of Common Problems in Obstetrics and Gynecology, 5th edition. Edited by T.M. Goodwin, M.N. Montoro, L. Muderspach, R. Paulson and S. Roy. © 2010 Blackwell Publishing Ltd.

Investigations have shown that the woman can safely and effectively self-administer the misoprostol in her home 6–72 hours after the mifepristone with similar efficacy. A second dose of vaginal misoprostol may be administered if a gestational sac with or without gestational cardiac activity is present at the follow-up visit approximately 14 days after initiation of treatment. More than half of women with ultrasound evidence of a persistent gestational sac will expel the pregnancy after a second dose of misoprostol. One-third of women with persistent gestational cardiac activity will expel the pregnancy with a second dose, making the second dose of misoprostol a reasonable option.

The methotrexate-misoprostol regimen most commonly utilizes intramuscular administration of methotrexate at the same dose used to treat ectopic pregnancy (50 mg/m^2). Overall complete abortion rates are similar to the FDA mifepristone-misoprostol regimen, with 92–96% up to 49 days' gestation and 82% between 50 and 56 days' gestation. However, 15–20% of women may wait up to 4 weeks for complete abortion to occur. Oral regimens have been shown to be as effective as intramuscular regimens. Misoprotsol 800 μg is administered 3–7 days after methotrexate by the woman at home. If a gestational sac persists on transvaginal ultrasound approximately 1 week after methotrexate administration, the dose is repeated. If the ultrasound also shows gestational cardiac activity the woman returns in 1 week for follow-up; otherwise, follow-up occurs at 4 weeks after administration of the second dose of methotrexate. If gestational cardiac activity persists 2 weeks after initiating treatment or expulsion has not occurred by 4 weeks after initiation of treatment, uterine aspiration is performed.

Misoprostol-only regimens have included varying dosages and routes of administration of misoprostol. Misoprostol 800 μg moistened with water and administered vaginally has complete abortion rates of 90% in pregnancies up to 56 days of gestation. This regimen involves three doses of vaginal misoprostol at 0, 24 hours, and 8 days if abortion has not occurred. The most recent randomized trial compared the regimen of 200 mg of mifepristone and 800 μg of vaginal misoprostol to 800 μg of vaginal misoprostol alone with administration of vaginal misoprostol every 24 hours up to three doses. The complete abortion rate for the vaginal misoprostol group was 88% and the mifepristone-misoprostol success rate was 96%.

Confirmation of completed abortion, by ultrasound examination, falling hCG levels or history and physical exam, is necessary with any regimen. While ultrasound offers an efficient means for confirming completion of medical abortion, the need for the equipment and trained clinicians may limit access for women in settings where one or both are not available. Alternatively, patient history and physical examination demonstrating

uterine involution in conjunction with serial hCG assays is able to confirm completed abortion without ultrasound. Follow-up should occur approximately 10–14 days after misoprostol administration as follow-up too soon after initiation of medical abortion will often demonstrate retained tissue, which usually disappears without intervention within a few days. The only reason to perform vaginal sonography is to determine whether the gestational sac is present. After expulsion, the uterus will normally contain sonographically hyperechoic tissue consisting of blood, clots, and decidua. Rarely does this finding indicate a need for intervention in the absence of excessive bleeding. A failed medical abortion is defined as the presence of gestational cardiac activity on vaginal sonography 2 weeks after the initiation of treatment. Patients have the option of a repeat dose of misoprostol and additional observation or uterine aspiration for management of treatment failure. Contraception can be initiated on the day of misoprostol administration for the combined hormonal contraceptive pill and patch. The contraceptive vaginal ring, injectable preparations, implants or intrauterine devices may be initiated at the follow-up visit.

Second-trimester medical abortion

Dilation and evacuation is the method of second-trimester abortion most commonly used in the United States. The safety gap between medical and surgical regimens has narrowed such that providers should become increasingly comfortable offering patients either modern methods of medical induction or D&E for second-trimester abortion. However, the safety profile of D&E is derived from the surgeon's knowledge, experience, and skills. There has been a steady decline in the number of individuals adequately trained to perform D&E.

The use of prostaglandin (PG) analogs is the most important recent advance in medical abortion procedures in the second trimester. Misoprostol, a PGE1 analog, is the most commonly used PG analog used for induction abortion currently. Misoprostol induces labor more effectively with fewer side effects than PGF2-α and PGE2 and is more effective than second-trimester induction regimens using single-agent oxytocin or oxytocin in combination with other classes of PG. Misoprostol is inexpensive, thermostable, and offers various routes of administration. Single-agent misoprostol has become the most common method of second-trimester abortion in the world.

In regimens using misoprostol alone, median induction abortion intervals are 12–16 hours. The abortion time interval is decreased with more frequent dosing. Randomized clinical trials show a significantly shorter induction time with 400 μg vaginal misoprostol administration at 3-hour intervals than 6-hour intervals without a significant increase in side effects. Approximately 90% of patients who abort with this method will do so within 24 hours. Of those patients who have not aborted by 24 hours of misoprostol treatment, 50% will abort within the second 24 hours of treatment. Thus, it is important to evaluate the patient on an individual basis after 24 hours of treatment in order to decide if an alternative plan of management should be undertaken. Investigations have demonstrated that there may be an advantage in placing the first dose of misoprostol vaginally (which may lead to more effective cervical priming), but there is no advantage in the vaginal administration of subsequent doses. After expulsion of the fetus, an oxytocin infusion of 30 units in 1 liter of 5% dextrose lactated Ringer's solution should be administered for 2 hours. Providers should observe nonbleeding patients for at least 4 hours for spontaneous placental expulsion after fetal delivery. It is important to carefully examine the placenta for completeness. An ultrasound examination of the uterus and curettage should be performed if the placenta is incomplete or if there is continued uterine bleeding despite administration of uterotonic agents.

Recent advances in second-trimester medical abortion involve the use of mifepristone preceding PG use. Mifepristone use permits greater efficacy of PG at lower doses which may minimize side effects. Inductions using mifepristone followed by PG require half the induction time of PG alone and approximately 95% of patients deliver within 24 hours. The Royal College of Obstetricians and Gynaecologists recommends mifepristone 200 mg orally on day 1 and misoprostol 800 µg vaginally 36–48 hours later followed by 400 µg misoprostol orally at 3-hour intervals for a total of four doses. If undelivered 3 hours after the fourth dose, mifepristone 200 mg should be repeated and the induction should be resumed the next day or the patient should undergo surgical abortion.

Many providers induce fetal demise with digoxin prior to second-trimester abortion to avoid violating the US Partial Birth Abortion Act of 2003. Digoxin has a favorable safety profile, requires less skill than fetal intracardiac KCL administration, and does not cause maternal side effects. Intrafetal digoxin administration fails to induce fetal demise in up to 5% of cases and intra-amniotic administration has a failure rate of up to 20%.

Patient selection, counseling, and symptom management

Patient counseling must first include pregnancy options counseling to be sure that the woman is certain of the decision to terminate the pregnancy. Most women seeking abortion will be eligible for both medical and surgical methods. The general advantages and disadvantages of each approach should be discussed during counseling. The advantages of medical abortion include avoidance of an invasive procedure and anesthesia and privacy. Additional advantages of second-trimester medical abortion are that surgeons skilled in D&E are not required and it provides an intact fetus for morphologic examination in cases where this type of evaluation is warranted. The disadvantages of medical abortion in the first trimester include the requirement of two or more visits to ensure completion of the abortion, it may take days to weeks to complete, and bleeding is moderate to heavy for a short time. The disadvantages of medical abortion in the second trimester include hospital admission for induction, labor pain, and participation in the delivery of the fetus and placenta. Patients must be counseled regarding the possibility of surgical intervention for failed or incomplete abortion or hemorrhage.

The increasing cesarean section rate means more women will present for second-trimester pregnancy termination with a history of a prior uterine incision. The absolute risk of uterine rupture during second-trimester medical induction is not known. In most series the risk of uterine rupture with scarred uteri is <1%; therefore, medical abortion is not contraindicated. The impact of PG dose and dosing intervals remains unclear. There is little evidence to guide practice in women with uterine scarring due to myomectomy or surgical correction of uterine anomalies.

Contraindications to first-trimester medical abortion include confirmed or suspected ectopic pregnancy, presence of an intrauterine device, current long-term systemic corticosteroid use or chronic adrenal failure, and uncontrolled seizure disorder. Contraindications to medical abortion in the first and second trimester include severe anemia, known coagulopathy or anticoagulant therapy or allergy to either of the medications being used. Asthma is not a contraindication because misoprostol is a weak bronchodilator.

There is no evidence to date of a teratogenic effect of mifepristone. Methotrexate is an antimetabolite that can cause fetal anomalies. Misoprostol use in early pregnancy has been associated with defects in the frontal or temporal bones and limb abnormalities. This is possibly due to mild uterine contractions resulting in decreased blood flow during fetal development. This underscores the importance of patient follow-up for the diagnosis and surgical management of continuing pregnancies.

Some degree of uterine cramping and bleeding must occur during the process of medical abortion. For women undergoing first-trimester medical abortion, it must be emphasized that bleeding may be much heavier than menses and that cramping may be severe. Patients aborting at home should also be counseled on how to identify excessive bleeding and when to call the health-care provider. Other potential side effects include nausea, vomiting, diarrhea, fever or chills, headache, dizziness, and fatigue. Pain management generally includes narcotic medications. Patients aborting at home should receive appropriate counseling regarding pain and analgesia use.

Endometritis is a rare but potentially serious complication of medical abortion. No data exist to support the universal use of prophylactic antibiotics with medical terminations. Five cases of death secondary to infection have been reported in women using mifepristone 200 mg followed by vaginal misoprostol 800 μg for first-trimester medical abortion. In three of these cases, *Clostridium sordellii* was isolated. The cause of these infections and the relationship between the deaths and the abortion procedure are still under investigation. In the second trimester it is important to differentiate fever due to prostaglandin from that due to endometritis. In general, endometritis is associated with a slower onset of fever and more marked uterine and cervical motion tenderness. Leukocytosis may be increased as a result of infection or may be drug induced; thus, leukocytosis and differential white cell counts may not help to distinguish between the two conditions. The threshold for implementing antibiotic coverage should remain low.

Suggested reading

American College of Obstetricians and Gynecologists. *Practice bulletin. Medical management of abortion. Clinical management guidelines for obstetrician-gynecologists.* Washington, DC: American College of Obstetricians and Gynecologists, 2005: 67.

Ashok PW, Templeton A, Wagaarachchi PT, Flett GMM. Midtrimester medical termination of pregnancy: a review of 1002 consecutive cases. *Contraception* 2004; 69: 51–58.

Creinin MD. Medical abortion regimens: historical context and overview. *Am J Obstet Gynecol* 2000; 183: S3–S9.

Hammond C. Recent advances in second-trimester abortion: an evidence-based review. *Am J Obstet Gynecol* 2009; 200: 347–356.

Reeves MF, Kudva K, Creinin MD. Medical abortion outcomes after a second dose of misoprostol for persistent gestational sac. *Contraception* 2008; 78: 332–335.

Chapter 115
Complications of Surgical Abortions

De Shawn L. Taylor and Ronna Jurow

Department of Medicine and Obstetrics and Gynecology, Keck School of Medicine, University of Southern California, CA, USA

Introduction

Approximately one-half of all pregnancies in the United States are unintended. One of every two women between the ages of 15–44 will experience an unintended pregnancy. Over 40% of all unintended pregnancies end in abortion, making this one of the most common surgical procedures in this country. Nine out of 10 abortions occur before the end of the first trimester.

Multiple advances in technology over the last two decades have significantly improved the safety and ease of surgical abortion. Transvaginal ultrasonography has replaced assessments of uterine size with objective methods to accurately establish gestational age. Effective techniques have evolved for preoperative cervical preparation. Present-day procedures utilize medical abortifacients alone or in addition to osmotic dilators, to soften and dilate the cervix. Finally, the development of the manual vacuum aspirator, a portable nonelectric uterine evacuation device, for use in early pregnancy termination has not only improved the safety of the procedure, but also expanded accessibility in outpatient settings.

As a result of these developments, complications due to surgical abortion are uncommon. Although the complication rate increases slightly with advancing gestational age, the risk of serious morbidity or mortality is far lower than that associated with carrying a pregnancy to term. Overall mortality from first-trimester abortion in the United States is 1 per 100,000 procedures. The National Abortion Federation states that the overall complication rate in first-trimester terminations is 9 per 1000 procedures. The risk of second-trimester complications rate is more elusive: Stubblefield noted nine perforations per 10,000 procedures with a range of 0.9–21 per 10,000 procedures. The number varies widely; however, it has been well established that complication rates are higher in facilities where physicians are training than in facilities where only experienced practitioners perform the procedures.

The complications of first- and second-trimester pregnancy termination consist of those that occur at the time of the procedure: inability to dilate the cervix, hemorrhage, uterine perforation and failure to obtain gestational tissue in early gestations; and those that take place in the following days to weeks: retained products of conception and infection.

Inability to dilate the cervix

Difficulty with cervical dilation is most likely to occur among nulliparous women and women who have undergone cesarean section or other surgery affecting the cervix. In these circumstances prostaglandin use leaves few recalcitrant cases. However, direct ultrasound observation of dilator placement may be used to facilitate dilation and avoid creation of a false tract or perforation. The most common prostaglandin used today is misoprostol (Cytotec), an E1 prostaglandin analog that is inexpensive, stable at room temperature and well tolerated. Although not FDA approved as an abortifacient, misoprostol has been safely used for more than a decade. In our experience, in the first trimester 400 μg of buccal misoprostol used at least 90 minutes prior to the procedure leaves the cervix sufficiently softened so that dilation is often no longer necessary.

In second-trimester gestations, osmostic dilators, natural or synthetic, such as *Laminaria japonicum*, Dilapan or Lamicel may be used prior to prostaglandin use. These materials are compressed tents that slowly expand with the absorption of fluid, dilating the cervix for up to 24 hours prior to the procedure. If more dilation is needed in later terminations, a new set of the osmotic dilators can be placed the morning of the procedure. Misoprostol is often added in later terminations for additional cervical softening and dilation, prior to dilation and evacuation (D&E).

Management of Common Problems in Obstetrics and Gynecology, 5th edition. Edited by T.M. Goodwin, M.N. Montoro, L. Muderspach, R. Paulson and S. Roy. © 2010 Blackwell Publishing Ltd.

Uterine hemorrhage

Hemorrhage is defined as greater than 500 mL of blood loss. It is an infrequent event during or after pregnancy termination, particularly during a first-trimester procedure (<1%) in which blood loss is routinely less than 15 mL. In second-trimester procedures, specifically those 18 weeks' gestation and greater, the use of contractile agents such as 20–30 units of oxytocin diluted in a liter of saline or lactated Ringer's solution started prior or during the procedure, and 0.2 mg ergonovine maleate (Methergine), given intramuscularly or intracervically after completion of the procedure, significantly reduces the risk of substantial blood loss (1–2%). The inclusion of four units of vasopressin in the paracervical anesthesia decreases blood loss by half during both first- and second-trimester procedures.

The most likely cause of minor bleeding is trauma to the external os, usually due to the tenaculum. This diagnosis is made by simple observation and treated with pressure, with or without the application of procoagulants such as silver nitrate or Monsel's solution. Suture placement is rarely necessary. If the anatomy allows, the instrument holding the cervix can be a curved Allis clamp or ring forceps instead of a tenaculum.

The most common cause of hemorrhage in the second trimester is uterine atony, for which a careful bimanual exam is diagnostic. In this case, vigorous bimanual massage and the above-mentioned uterotonics are extremely helpful first-line therapies. Other treatments include 800–1000 µg of rectal misoprostol or 250 µg of carboprost tromethamine (Hemabate), a 15-methyl F2-α prostaglandin, given intramuscularly at 15-minute intervals for up to eight doses.

If bleeding continues, other causes such as uterine perforation, abnormal placental attachment, i.e. placenta accreta, incomplete evacuation, and cervical laceration must be considered. Uterine perforation just above the internal cervical os may cause hemorrhage into the broad ligament. Diagnosis of broad ligament hematomas can be elusive, as the bleeding is often into the peritoneal cavity instead of into the vagina. The possibility of bowel damage exists as well. If these problems are suspected, definitive diagnosis will necessitate laparoscopy or most commonly exploratory laparotomy.

Cervical laceration at the utero-cervical junction, where the cervical branch of the uterine artery is located, is significantly more likely to occur during second-trimester than first-trimester procedures. This laceration is usually caused by a stretch injury at the time of dilation or in later procedures, removal of sharp calcified fetal parts that have not been adequately crushed prior to removal. Laparoscopy or laparotomy may be required in the presence of ongoing brisk bleeding or signs of hemodynamic instability. These are surgical emergencies and if suspected, expeditious movement is required. Uterine artery embolization can be performed, but only if a team with expertise and experience can be rapidly mobilized. Failure to recognize these emergencies can result in significant morbidity and possibly death. Cervical lacerations are preventable preoperatively with adequate cervical preparation using misoprostol in combination with osmotic dilators, and intraoperatively with sufficient decompression of bony fetal parts prior to removal.

Uterine perforation

Uterine perforation is most likely to occur in the second trimester and during first- and second-trimester procedures performed by less experienced abortion providers or physicians in training. Presence of severely anteverted or retroverted uteri, prior cesarean section with subsequent weakness of the anterior uterine wall, multiple abortions or vaginal deliveries, and uterine surgery within the preceding 6 months are all risk factors for perforations. In our population, the combination of one or more cesarean sections and history of multiple pregnancy terminations increased the risk for uterine perforation, particularly, if the surgery had taken place during the prior 6 months. Perforation should be suspected if uterine bleeding is brisk and bright red or when intrauterine instruments pass farther than expected or lack a discernible endpoint. The most common location for perforation is the uterocervical junction, the weakest area in the uterine muscle or the anterior uterine fundus in the scar from a previous cesarean section. Less commonly, perforations can occur in the relatively avascular anterior mid-line uterine fundus or the cervical canal itself, described earlier as in creation of a false tract.

There is a wide range of possible outcomes from uterine perforations. Perforations in the first trimester are usually small and self-contained. If a mid-line perforation occurs while using a uterine sound or metal dilator, expectant management can occur, but if perforation is caused during suction with the cannula, the woman needs further evaluation, i.e. laparoscopy or laparotomy. The patient should be closely observed postoperatively with careful assessments of bleeding, abdominal pain and tenderness, as well as serial hemoglobin levels, orthostatics and observation of vital signs over a 2–4-hour period. If clinically stable, she may be discharged safely with explicit warning signs for emergency referral and a timely follow-up appointment.

Although the risk for uterine perforation is greater during a second-trimester D&E procedure, the risk of mortality is approximately 1 in 100,000. The patient may present either during or immediately following the procedure with moderate to brisk uterine bleeding. If uterine atony, cervical laceration and retained products have been ruled out as potential etiologies or if a uterine defect is palpated on bimanual examination, the patient must undergo laparoscopy or laparotomy in order to include evaluation of all intra-abdominal structures. Due to its central location and size, the small bowel is the abdominal organ most likely to be damaged by uterine perforation.

Although this chain of events may occur quite rapidly in a hospital setting, a bleeding perforation in the outpatient setting requires immediate patient stabilization, including fluid support with two large-bore intravenous lines, packing of the uterus with vasopressin or saline-soaked gauze, and rapid transport to the nearest hospital equipped to manage abortion complications.

It is important to note that a significant uterine perforation may at first present in a benign manner. A concealed perforation that is actively bleeding into the broad ligament or pelvic cul-de-sac may not become manifest until the postoperative period with the gradual worsening of abdominal pain, presence of an enlarging pelvic mass or clinical hemostatic changes. These perforations require laparoscopic evaluation or laparotomy, depending on the size and location of the perforation, the acuity of the bleed and the need to assess the abdominal viscera.

Adequate cervical preparation, using misoprostol alone or in combination with osmotic dilators at least 1.5 hours prior to mechanical dilation, will minimize the risk of uterine perforation. Ultrasound observation beginning at the time of dilation throughout the period of uterine evacuation is also advisable, particularly during second-trimester procedures or when a less experienced clinician performs the procedure.

Failure to obtain fetal tissue

A failed surgical abortion occurs in 10% of cases performed at a gestational age less than 6 weeks. The products of conception are scant and the gestational sac may be easily missed. There is also an increased risk of failed abortion in women with mullerian abnormalities, e.g. didelphic, bicornuate or septate uteri due to instrumentation of the wrong horn or wrong side of the septum. Intrauterine leiomyomata can interfere with complete uterine evacuation by distorting the endometrial cavity. In these cases, an ultrasound-guided procedure is recommended. Tissue examination must visualize the gestational sac in addition to chorionic villi as it is possible to essentially perform a chorionic villus sampling and identify chorionic villi while leaving the pregnancy intact. A very small gestational sac in pieces may be difficult to identify when using the electric vacuum aspirator. Use of the manual vacuum aspirator for early gestations allows tissue to be obtained intact for easier identification. Ultrasound evaluation immediately after the procedure will confirm that the uterus has been evacuated. If doubt exists, histologic diagnosis is definitive.

If the gestational sac is not removed and there is no possibility that an ectopic gestation is present, it is usually considered appropriate to wait 2 weeks to repeat the procedure. If aspiration has been attempted through the end of a falsely created tract or in cases of undiagnosed or occult mid-fundal perforation, there will be failure to obtain tissue. If a gestational sac is not evacuated with a second attempt under ultrasound guidance, the likelihood of an interstitial or cornual ectopic pregnancy that falsely appears intrauterine is a rare possibility.

Retained products of conception

The continued presence of retained chorionic villi or fetal tissue is usually diagnosed in the first or second week following uterine evacuation. Prolonged vaginal bleeding, sharp or cramping low abdominal pain, and, rarely, fever and infection are all symptoms of incomplete abortion. On bimanual examination, the uterus may be enlarged, softened or tender. Ultrasound evaluation usually records an abnormally widened or heterogeneous endometrial echogenic complex or a single intracavitary area of focal hyperechoic shadowing. Although small amounts of decidua, blood, and clots remain after abortion, the presence of the aforementioned findings in combination with continued bleeding or cramping is sufficient for a diagnosis of retained products of conception.

If there are no signs of infection, uterine reaspiration is only one of three treatment options. The patient may also choose medical management using a single dose of 400–800 µg of vaginally, orally or buccally administered misoprostol to facilitate expulsion of remaining uterine contents. This may be repeated in 24–48 hours if there is no bleeding following the first dose. The patient should be advised regarding pain management and appropriate analgesia supplied either directly or with a written prescription. Conservative, expectant management for 1–2 weeks is also a treatment option, based on the comfort level of both patient and provider.

Uterine infection

Postabortal uterine infection is most likely to occur when the products of conception are incompletely evacuated from the uterus, but it may also occur without retained tissue. Patients with underlying cervical infections by organisms such as *C. trachomatis* and *N. gonorrhoeae* are at increased risk for this complication. Fever, chills, uterine cramping, foul-smelling or purulent cervical discharge and pelvic pain are symptoms suggesting a postabortal infection. The sequelae of untreated postabortal infection can be life-threatening, so empiric antibiotic therapy is recommended when patients present with the aforementioned symptoms.

Immediate antibiotic prophylaxis following an abortion procedure has been shown to decrease the rate of postabortal infection by 50%. The most commonly used regimen is doxycycline 100 mg by mouth twice daily for 3–7 days. Screening for sexually transmitted infections in all patients is not cost-effective and generally is not recommended. Screening and empiric treatment among those with suspicious clinical exam findings and history is recommended to lessen the possibility of infection. The woman can be treated if cervicitis is suspected and the surgical procedure should not be delayed. If pelvic inflammatory disease is suspected at the time of the procedure, the woman should be treated and the termination should be delayed until treatment is complete.

If a patient develops signs of a postabortal infection, typically within the first 48–96 hours, antibiotic therapy to cover atypical and anaerobic organisms should be instituted as soon as possible, usually in the outpatient setting. The possibility of uterine perforation or occult bowel damage should be considered if there is poor response to antibiotic therapy. Although blood and urine cultures are rarely informative, cultures from the cervical fluid often grow mixed microbial or sexually transmitted pathogens. Aspiration of an infected uterus is not recommended unless the woman continues to bleed and ultrasound findings are consistent with retained products of conception. Many broad-spectrum antibiotic therapies are available for outpatient therapy in an otherwise stable patient. One common regimen includes ceftriaxone 250 mg intramuscularly in a single dose plus doxycycline 100 mg orally twice a day for 14 days with or without metronidazole 500 mg orally twice a day for the same time period. Infected patients require careful and close observation.

If a patient demonstrates signs of sepsis such as tachycardia, high fever or hemodynamic instability or if she exhibits generalized abdominal tenderness with guarding or rebound tenderness, suggestive of peritonitis, immediate hospital admission is required with aerobic and anaerobic blood cultures and aggressive broad-spectrum intravenous antibiotic therapy. Septic abortions are life-threatening. Parental antibiotics are given 2 hours prior to any attempt to reaspirate the uterus. The woman also requires careful assessment for uterine perforation or other intra-abdominal damage that might have led to the sepsis. Sepsis may present atypically with severe nausea and vomiting associated with a marked leukocytosis but no fever or abdominal pain. If these findings occur, and the patient has been closely monitored and there is no response to parental antibiotics and supportive measures, exploratory laparotomy should be considered. There remains the question as to whether the sepsis occurred as a result of bowel or other organ damage from an undiagnosed uterine perforation.

Ongoing pregnancy

With the advent of ultrasonography for establishing both number of pregnancies and gestational age, continued pregnancy following abortion has become a rare event except among cases of uterine aspiration under 6 weeks' gestational age. While tissue examination by an experienced clinician or pathologist is often sufficient to establish completion of the procedure, undetected continuation of a very early pregnancy is still possible, and occasionally occurs. Therefore, a follow-up quantitative B-hCG or assay or high-sensitivity urine hCG assay 14 days following the procedure is advisable in questionable cases.

Repeated undesired pregnancy

Without initiation of a medically appropriate form of birth control which she is willing to use on a regular basis, a woman seeking abortion services is at high risk for repeated undesired pregnancy. To prevent this complication, adequate time should be dedicated to contraception counseling both before and after pregnancy termination. As ovulation can occur in the first postabortal menstrual cycle, it is prudent to strongly recommend contraceptive initiation on the same day as the abortion procedure. Appropriate options include combined hormonal contraceptive pills, vaginal rings, and patches, subcutaneous implants, and injectable depot medroxyprogesterone acetate. Additionally, a levonorgesterol-containing intrauterine system or copper-containing intrauterine device may easily be placed in most women upon completion of the termination or during the immediate postabortal period with only a slight increase in the rate of expulsion. The etonorgestrel implant may also be inserted safely immediately post-abortion. Since the woman is instructed to avoid sexual intercourse for approximately 2 weeks after the abortion procedure, initiation of vaginal rings and barrier methods should occur after pelvic rest is complete. In addition to contraception, a woman should be given a prescription for emergency contraception.

Conclusion

Pregnancy termination is an extremely safe procedure in the first trimester. The risk of complications increases with increasing gestational age yet remains acceptably low throughout the previable period. The risk of mortality is 1 in 100,000. With rare exceptions, this procedure can safely be undertaken in the outpatient setting by a variety of providers, with hospital-based back-up for serious complications.

Suggested reading

Bartlett LA, Berg CJ, Shulman HB, *et al*. Risk factors for legal induced abortion-related mortality in the United States. *Obstet Gynecol* 2004; 103(4): 729–737.

Edwards J, Creinin MD. Surgical abortions for gestations of less than 6 weeks. *Curr Probl Obstet Gynecol Fertil* 1997; 20: 11–19.

Goldberg AB, Dean G, Kang MS, Youssof S, Darney PD. Manual versus electric vacuum aspiration for early first-trimester abortion: a controlled study of complication rates. *Obstet Gynecol* 2004; 103: 101–107.

Guttmacher Institute. Facts on induced abortion in the United States. Updated May, 2006. Available from: www.guttmacher .org/pubs/fb_induced_abortion.html.

Society of Family Planning. Cervical preparation for second-trimester surgical abortion prior to 20 weeks of gestation. *Contraception* 2007; 76: 487–495.

Stubblefield PG, Carr-Ellis S, Borgatta L. Methods for induced abortion. *Obstet Gynecol* 2004; 104: 174–185.

Chapter 116
Tubal Sterilization

Jessica Jocson and Robert Israel

Department of Medicine and Obstetrics and Gynecology, Keck School of Medicine, University of Southern California, CA, USA

Introduction

Sterilization is the permanent method of contraception. As it plays such a prominent role in fertility termination, sterilization must be an integral part of any contraceptive counseling discussion.

According to the Sexuality Information and Education Council for the United States (SIECUS) report in 2002, sterilization was the most commonly used method of contraception worldwide. In 1980, 99 million couples used some form of permanent sterilization, and this number grew to 223 million by 1995. Additionally, the number of couples using female sterilization grew by 42 million, whereas the number of vasectomies increased by only 1 million from 1990 to 1995. About 700,000 sterilization operations are performed annually in the US, and roughly half are performed in the immediate postpartum period. Not surprisingly, most of the women relying on sterilization are older, age 35–44, and this number continues to increase with age. In women 40–44 years of age using contraception, 51% rely on sterilization. As more women are marrying and starting families at older ages, and physicians are prescribing the newer oral contraceptives and intrauterine devices with more frequency, the number of young women choosing sterilization has declined.

Presterilization counseling

Patients should be informed completely about both male and female sterilization options, as well as the risks and benefits of alternative, long-acting, reversible contraceptives. Although some sterilization techniques have greater potential for reversibility than others, any sterilization operation should be viewed as a final contraceptive method by an individual, concluding his or her reproductive potential. Counseling should include factors that lead to sterilization regret, for example marital instability, death of children, etc. The decision to undergo sterilization must be based *solely* on the desire to have no more children. Utilizing any other factors, for example, to improve a relationship or an economic situation, increases the risk of poststerilization regret. Young age at time of sterilization (age 20–24) is the strongest predictor of sterilization regret. Overall, the incidence of postoperative regret is 6% and 0.2% request a reversal procedure.

Preoperative counseling should also include an explanation of the factors and risks of sterilization failure, including the higher probability of ectopic pregnancy if a gestation occurs, compared to the lower ectopic risk of women who conceive without prior tubal sterilization surgery. According to the US Collaborative Review on Sterilization (CREST) study, the risk of sterilization failure is 1.9%, or 18.5 per 1000 sterilizations. Patients should be reminded that sterilization operations offer no protection against sexually transmitted diseases (STDs), including HIV infection. Potential operative and postoperative complications and the need for their correction should be addressed, such as anesthesia risks, damage to major organs or blood vessels, and infection.

The counseling process should begin in a relaxed environment, well in advance of the operation, so that the patients have ample time to make a well-informed decision. Obtaining consent concurrent with labor or an abortion procedure should be avoided. The stress associated with these events could lead to a higher incidence of poststerilization regret. Physicians should be familiar with federal/state laws and/or insurance requirements that dictate a specific interval between obtaining consent and performing the surgery. Additionally, federal/state regulations may require the use of special consent forms.

Sterilization techniques

Postpartum tubal ligation

According to the CREST study, postpartum partial salpingectomy, performed in the first 48 hours after delivery

Management of Common Problems in Obstetrics and Gynecology, 5th edition. Edited by T.M. Goodwin, M.N. Montoro, L. Muderspach, R. Paulson and S. Roy. © 2010 Blackwell Publishing Ltd.

prior to uterine involution, has the lowest rate of tubal sterilization failure. The Pomeroy, modified Irving, and Uchida tubal ligations performed through small infraumbilical incisions remain the procedures of choice in the immediate postpartum period. The surgery can be performed on the delivery table, often utilizing the same anesthesia. They are simple and rapid with an "acceptable" failure rate well below 1:1000 for the Irving and Uchida methods. Additionally, they do not prolong the postpartum hospital stay. The Pomeroy method, midsegment tubal excision after placement of plain catgut sutures, is the most commonly used technique with a failure rate reported to be about 0.6% at 1 year and a cumulative 10-year pregnancy risk of 7.5%. Although the modified Irving method, where the proximal stump is buried in the myometrium and the distal stump is tied off but not buried in the broad ligament, requires more time than the Pomeroy and has less chance of reversibility, it may be more successful. Only one pregnancy has been documented in the literature. Tubal clips, such as the Filshie, may offer higher chances of reversibility but tubal clips have demonstrated the highest rates of sterilization failure.

Interval sterilization

Interval sterilization refers to any sterilization procedure performed in the nonpuerperal state 6 weeks after delivery or later. The surgical route selected, either a minilaparotomy approach or laparoscopic tubal sterilization, is based on individual patient characteristics, such as patient weight, previous abdominal surgeries or any co-morbid health conditions. In addition, the choice of laparotomy versus laparoscopy depends on the surgeon's skill and comfort with either procedure. As laparoscopic surgical techniques have advanced and improved over time, the laparoscope has become a popular and important tool in female sterilization.

Technique

There are wide variations in preoperative preparation, the majority of which are not crucial to the success of the operation. Unless there are significant medical problems (diabetes, hypertension, pulmonary conditions, etc.) or excessive obesity (200 lb (90 kg) or over), or both, there is no reason why laparoscopic tubal sterilization cannot be performed as an outpatient, same-day procedure. The operation should take place in an operating room equipped and staffed for general anesthesia, and for exploratory laparotomy, if it proves necessary. Although a cross-match is unnecessary, blood bank accessibility is prudent.

Laparoscopic sterilization can be performed under local anesthesia, but most laparoscopists favor a short-acting general endotracheal anesthesia. It is unnecessary to shave either the abdomen or perineum, but the bladder must be emptied with either in-and-out catheterization just prior to the procedure or an indwelling catheter left in place during the surgery. At laparoscopy, it is often helpful to elevate and rotate the uterus via a transvaginal intrauterine manipulator.

The creation of satisfactory pneumoperitoneum is the keystone to any successful laparoscopic procedure. A Veress needle entry or open laparoscopic technique may be performed. Open laparoscopy allows for direct visual entry into the peritoneal cavity and may prevent complications, such as bowel or major vessel injury. However, in a patient with no prior abdominal surgeries, open laparoscopy for tubal sterilization is certainly elective. Once the laparoscope is in place, a brief diagnostic overview of the abdomen and pelvis should be performed to confirm normal anatomy. Laparoscopic sterilization can be performed through a single-incision technique utilizing the operating laparoscope. However, this may limit pelvic manipulation, such as the important identification of tubal fimbria confirming that the actual tube has been secured. Thus, an accessory instrument inserted at a second puncture site is most often employed.

Various instruments and methods of tubal occlusion are available. Whatever tubal occlusion technique is utilized, tissue destruction should be confined to the mid-isthmus. In this way, if sterilization reversal is subsequently requested, enough proximal and distal tubal segments will remain for end-to-end anastomosis.

Bipolar fulguration, usually with transection, remains the most widely used technique. Before transection, fulguration must be complete and must include a portion of the adjacent mesosalpinx to avoid bleeding at the transection site. After transection, each cut tubal stump (especially both proximal ends) should be recoagulated briefly to prevent tubal fistulae or recanalization. Utilizing bipolar equipment for fulguration eliminates the electrical hazards associated with unipolar coagulation. Bipolar conduction reduces electrical "scatter" within the abdominal cavity, thus minimizing surrounding thermal injury.

The Falope ring, in which a Silastic band is used to occlude the tube, a spring-loaded clip (Hulka), and the Filshie clip provide alternatives to electrocoagulation. Postoperative abdominal discomfort is experienced for 24–48 hours in 20–25% of the patients undergoing occlusive ring or spring-loaded clip tubal sterilization. However, the clips destroy less tube than laparoscopic fulguration and may offer better potential for reversibility. The Filshie clip consists of an upper and lower jaw joined at one end by a hinge so the clip can be closed over the tube, thus forming a permanent occlusion. The clip has a rigid titanium body and a medical-grade, cross-linked silicone rubber lining. Attached to the open end of the upper jaw is a small "no-touch" handle that is used to load the clip into the applicator and then is removed from the clip. Over time, the occluded tissue becomes necrotic and the silicone lining expands, keeping the tubal lumen occluded while a reperitonealization process occurs to subsequently cover each stump.

An emerging technique of microlaparoscopy is evolving with studies under way. Microlaparoscopy can be performed under local anesthesia with conscious sedation. Currently, the sterilization technique employed closely mimics the Pomeroy method and utilizes three puncture sites: a 2 mm infraumbilical camera port, a 5 mm suprapubic port through which an endoloop of plain catgut is introduced, and a 14 gauge IV catheter port, 4 cm from the suprapubic port, through which a semirigid hysteroscopic grasper is placed for assistance. At this point, studies have not shown any difference from the more standard methods of laparoscopic sterilization regarding outcomes, complications, and failure rates. However, there appears to be a significant reduction in operating time from 44 minutes to 30 minutes.

Failures (poststerilization pregnancies)

The widely held belief that most tubal sterilization failures occur in the first postoperative year was challenged in 1996 by the first long-term follow-up from the Collaborative Review of Sterilization (CREST) project of the Centers for Disease Control and Prevention. The CREST study was large (over 10,000 women), had a 10-year follow-up, and reported sterilization failures by life-table analysis. The CREST report showed that failures continue to occur well beyond the first year, so that by 5 years more than 1% of women had a sterilization failure, and by 10 years, the overall figure rose to 1.8%. The spring-loaded Hulka clip still led the failure rates/procedure after 10 years (3.7%) followed by bipolar coagulation, silicone band application, and, lastly, unipolar coagulation. Younger age at time of sterilization also increased the risk for failure. From the CREST data, the efficacy of the copper intrauterine device is better than the spring-loaded clip. At this point, if a clip is selected for sterilization, it should be the Filshie.

Any pregnancies occurring after tubal sterilization must be carefully evaluated to rule out ectopic gestation. The CREST study reported that 32% of pregnancies following all types of tubal sterilization procedures will be ectopic. Women conceiving after bipolar laparoscopic fulguration are at the highest risk, as up to 50% of the gestations may be ectopic.

Transuterine approach

To improve safety and simplicity in female sterilization, avoiding penetration of the abdominal cavity would be a necessity. A transuterine approach to the fallopian tubes may be the ultimate solution. The emergence of hysteroscopic techniques represents a new area of development in female sterilization and has the advantage of direct visualization of each tubal orifice.

Essure® (Conceptus Inc., Mountain View, CA, USA) was approved for use in the US in 2002. It is a microinsert containing microcoils that is hysteroscopically inserted into each tubal ostium. The microcoils, when correctly placed, stimulate a tissue response resulting in permanent sterilization within 3 months of insertion. The hysteroscopic procedure can be performed in an outpatient setting under conscious sedation assisted by a paracervical block, thus avoiding general anesthesia. After Essure sterilization, the patient remains on contraception until a hysterosalpingogram demonstrates proximal tubal occlusion.

To date, a few comparative studies comparing laparoscopic tubal sterilization to Essure have found overall higher satisfaction rates among women who underwent the Essure procedure: 94% at 90 days postoperatively, compared to 80% of those who had undergone laparoscopic sterilization, although this difference was not statistically significant. Ninety days postoperatively, 100% of the women who had undergone Essure were significantly more satisfied with the speed of their recovery compared to 80% satisfaction in those sterilized laparoscopically. Additionally, hospital stay was significantly longer with laparoscopy, 396.1 minutes, compared to 188.7 minutes with Essure (p < 0.005), and moderate-to-severe postoperative pain was significantly higher for laparoscopy (63%) than hysteroscopy (32%). Surprisingly, operative time was longer for the Essure procedure, 13.2 minutes, compared to 9.7 minutes for laparoscopy, but was only marginally significant (p = 0.045), and may be attributable to the relatively new hysteroscopic technique. The authors noted that the operating time began with the introduction of the hysteroscope or laparoscope to instrument removal; thus, the length of time for actual abdominal placement of the laparoscope, which might be significantly longer in obese women or those with previous abdominal surgery, was not taken into account. At hysterosalpingography 3 months after Essure, 94–96% of patients had bilaterally occluded tubes.

Case reports have documented a few cases of post-Essure pregnancy. In one case, a woman underwent uncomplicated, bilateral Essure placement, but failed to return for her 3-month postoperative hysterosalpingogram. Two years later she presented with an intrauterine gestation at 16 weeks that concluded with an uncomplicated vaginal delivery. At postpartum tubal ligation, the Essure implants were embedded in the myometrium above the ostia.

The overall failure rate of Essure is low, 2.6 per 1000 procedures. With patient or physican follow-up noncompliance at fault for nearly half of the reported pregnancies, the failure risk should be reduced by better postprocedure verification of tubal occlusion. Obviously, future, long-term trials are needed.

Another hysteroscopic approach, Adiana® (Cytyc LP, Marlborough, MA, USA), is currently being investigated in an FDA study in the United States, Australia, and Mexico. It combines controlled thermal damage to the interstitial endosalpinx with insertion of a biocompatible matrix into the tubal lumen. This activates fibroblasts in contact with the matrix to cause infiltration and subsequent luminal occlusion. One pregnancy has been reported amongst a total of 2445 women-months of device wearing. Long-term studies are ongoing.

Chemical sterilization

The ultimate goal in transuterine sterilization would be to eliminate instrumentation, like hysteroscopy, altogether. By means of a syringe, catheter or specialized delivery system, a chemosterilant that acts on the mucosa of the fallopian tube could be instilled via the uterine cavity. Two groups of chemical agents have been investigated. One consists of nonspecific tissue adhesives or sclerosing agents that produce oviductal obstruction through scar formation. Some agents that have been studied include methylcyanoacrylate (MCA), gelatin-resorcibal formaldehyde, phenol mucilage, and phenol atabrine. However, most of these agents have been abandoned secondary to poor tubal occlusion rates after insertion.

The other chemosterilant group consists of highly specific chemical agents capable of inducing morphologic changes in the interstitial tubal epithelium. Quinacrine is the most tested compound in this group. As no animal studies in the US have fully elucidated the safety profile of quinacrine, most of the long-term human studies utilizing quinacrine have been conducted in international settings.

The typical protocol for quinacrine administration involves monthly intrauterine insertions for 3 months using 252 mg quinacrine pellets, impregnated with 55.5 mg ibuprofen, that are placed high in the endometrial cavity via an IUD inserter. International studies have consistently demonstrated the safety and effectiveness of quinacrine. For example, in Indonesia, 10,000 women who underwent quinacrine pellet insertion were followed for 10 years. The pregnancy rate was 4.3 per 100 at 10 years, with the majority of the pregnancies occurring within the first 4 years after insertion. No long-term side effects were noted. The perceived problems with quinacrine include the need for multiple applications and reliably confirming tubal occlusion. Hysterosalpingography may recanalize the tubes by forcing open the scarred proximal tube.

The possibility of a nonsurgical sterilization technique with a chemical agent of very low toxicity, which can be employed by paramedical personnel without sophisticated delivery equipment, opens exciting perspectives in the area of female sterilization. However, more long-term studies, preferably perfomed in the US, evaluating safety and outcomes are needed before use of quinacrine sterilization in the US can begin.

Conclusion

Female sterilization has become an accepted, integral part of family planning. Laparoscopic sterilization techniques have simplified surgery and introduced new operative approaches to the fallopian tubes. The future is represented by transuterine sterilization that promises to avoid anesthesia, complicated instrumentation, and penetration of the peritoneal cavity. When evaluated against the comparable standard criteria for contraception (acceptability, safety, effectiveness, and cost), surgical sterilization, even as it is performed today, appears to be one of the best family planning methods available.

What we call the beginning is often the end and to make an end is to make a beginning. The end is where we start from. (T.S. Eliot, 1943)

Suggested reading

Abbott J. Transcervical sterilization. *Curr Opin Obstet Gynecol* 2007; 19: 325–330.

Benagiano G. Non-surgical female sterilization with quinacrine: an update. *Contraception* 2001; 63(5): 239–245.

Duffy S, Marsh F, Rogerson L, *et al*. Female sterilisation: a cohort controlled comparative study of ESSURE versus laparoscopic sterilisation. *BJOG* 2005; 112(11): 1522–1528.

Engender Health. Sterilization most widely used contraceptive method in world. In: *SIECUS Report Vol 31 (2)*. New York: SIECUS, 2002: 19–21.

Hastings-Tolsma M, Nodine P, Teal SB, Embry J. Pregnancy outcome after transcervical hysteroscopic sterilization. *Obstet Gynecol* 2007; 110: 504–506.

Levey B, Levie MD, Childers MA. A summary of reported pregnancies following hysteroscopic sterilization. *J Minim Invasive Gynecol* 2007; 14(3): 271–274.

Mazdisnian F, Palmieri A, Hakakha B, Hakakha M, Cambridge C, Lauria B. Office microlaparoscopy for female sterilization under local anesthesia. A cost and clinical analysis. *J Reprod Med* 2002; 47(2): 97–100.

Nardin JM, Kulier R, Boulvain M, Peterson HB. Techniques for the interruption of tubal patency for female sterilisation. *Cochrane Database Syst Rev* 2002; 4: CD003034.

Peterson HB, *et al*. Update on female sterilization: failure rates, counseling issues, and post-sterilization regret. The Contraception Report 1996; vol VII (3): 1–15.

Peterson HB, Xia Z, Hughes JM, *et al*. The risk of pregnancy after tubal sterilization: findings from the US Collaborative Review of Sterilization. *Am J Obstet Gynecol* 1996; 174: 1161–1170.

Ryder RM, Vaughan MC. Laparoscopic tubal sterilization. Methods, effectiveness, and sequelae. *Obstet Gynecol Clin North Am* 1999; 26(1): 83–97.

Siegle JC, Cartmell LW Sr, Rayburn WF. Microlaparoscopic technique for partial salpingectomy using bipolar electrocoagulation. *J Reprod Med* 2001; 46(7): 632–636.

Suhadi A, Anwar M, Soejoenoes A. 10-year follow-up of women who elected quinacrine sterilization (QS) in Wonosobo, Central Java, Indonesia. *Int J Gynaecol Obstet* 2003; 83(suppl 2): 137–139.

Vancaillie T. Initial Sydney experience in hysteroscopic sterilization using the Adiana complete permanent birth control device. *J Minim Invas Gynecol* 2006; 13(suppl): S10.

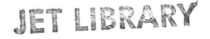

Index

Note: Page numbers in *italics* refer to figures and those in **bold** refer to tables and boxes.